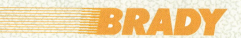

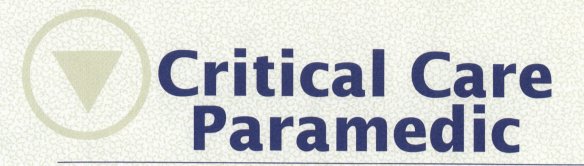

Critical Care
Paramedic

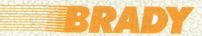

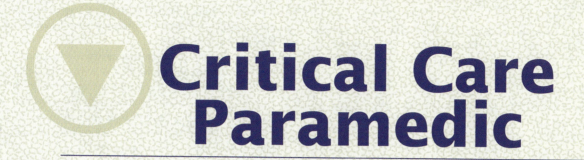

Critical Care Paramedic

BRYAN E. BLEDSOE, DO, FACEP, EMT-P

Adjunct Associate Professor of Emergency Medicine
The George Washington University Medical Center
Washington, D.C.
and
Emergency Physician
Midlothian, Texas

RANDALL W. BENNER, MED, MICP, NREMT-P

Director, Emergency Medical Technology Program
Instructor, Department of Health Professions
Youngstown State University
Youngstown, Ohio

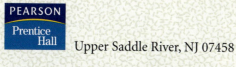

Upper Saddle River, NJ 07458

Library of Congress Cataloging-in-Publication Data

Critical care paramedic / [edited by] Bryan Bledsoe, Randall W. Benner.
    p. ; cm.
    Includes bibliographical references and index.
    ISBN 0–13–119271–X (alk. paper)
    1. Emergency medicine. 2. Emergency medical technicians. 3. Critical care medicine.
    [DNLM: 1. Critical Care—methods. 2. Allied Health Personnel. 3. Emergency
    Medicine—methods. WX 218 C93637 2006] I. Bledsoe, Bryan E., (Date) II. Benner,
    Randall W.
    RC86. 7. C7446 2006
    616.01′5—dc22
                                                                    2005020885

Publisher: Julie Levin Alexander
Publisher's Assistant: Regina Bruno
Executive Editor: Marlene McHugh Pratt
Senior Managing Editor for Development: Lois Berlowitz
Editorial Assistant: Matthew Sirinides
Project Development: Triple SSS Press Media Development, Inc.
Art Program Coordinator: Jeanne Molenaar
Managing Photography Editor: Michal Heron
Director of Marketing: Karen Allman
Executive Marketing Manager: Katrin Beacom
Marketing Coordinator: Michael Sirinides
Director of Production and Manufacturing: Bruce Johnson
Managing Editor for Production: Patrick Walsh
Production Liaison: Faye Gemmellaro
Production Editor: Emily Bush, Carlisle Publishing Services
Manufacturing Manager: Ilene Sanford
Manufacturing Buyer: Pat Brown
Senior Design Coordinator: Christopher Weigand
Cover Design: Michael Ginsberg
Cover Image: Mark Ide
Interior Photographers: Michael Gallitelli, Michal Heron, Craig Jackson/In
    The Dark Photography, Richard Logan, Scott Metcalfe
Interior Illustrations: Rolin Graphics
Interior Design: Jill Little
Composition: Carlisle Publishing Services
Printing and Binding: Courier/Kendallville
Cover Printer: Phoenix Color

Pearson Education, Ltd.
Pearson Education Singapore, Pte. Ltd.
Pearson Education Canada, Ltd.
Pearson Education—Japan
Pearson Education Australia Pty., Limited
Pearson Education North Asia Ltd.
Pearson Educación de Mexico, S.A. de C.V.
Pearson Education Malaysia, Pte. Ltd.
Pearson Education, Upper Saddle River, New Jersey

Notices

It is the intent of the authors and publishers that this text-book be used as part of a formal critical care paramedic education program taught by a qualified instructor and supervised by a licensed physician. The transport of critically ill patients presented here represent accepted practices in the United States. They are not offered as a standard of care. Critical care paramedic emergency care is to be performed only under the authority and guidance of a licensed physician. It is the reader's responsibility to know and follow local care protocols as provided by medical advisors directing the system to which he or she belongs. Also, it is the reader's responsibility to stay informed of emergency care procedure changes.

Notice on Drugs and Drug Dosages

Every effort has been made to ensure that the drug dosages presented in this textbook are in accordance with nationally accepted standards. When applicable, the dosages and routes are taken from the American Heart Association's *Advanced Cardiac Life Support Guidelines.* The American Medical Association's publication *Drug Evaluations,* the *Physicians' Desk Reference,* and the *Prentice Hall Health Professional's Drug Guide* are followed with regard to drug dosages not covered by the American Heart Association's guidelines. It is the responsibility of the reader to be familiar with the drugs used in his or her system, as well as the dosages specified by the medical director. The drugs presented in this book should only be administered by direct order, whether verbally or through accepted standing orders, of a licensed physician.

Notice on Gender Usage

The English language has historically given preference to the male gender. Among many words, the pronouns "he" and "his" are commonly used to describe both genders. Society evolves faster than language, and the male pronouns still predominate in our speech. The authors have made great effort to treat the two genders equally, recognizing that a significant percentage of paramedics and patients are female. However, in some instances, male pronouns may be used to describe both male and female paramedics and patients solely for the purpose of brevity. This is not intended to offend any readers of the female gender.

Notice on Photographs

Please note that many of the photographs contained in this book are taken of actual emergency situations. As such, it is possible that they may not accurately depict current, appropriate, or advisable practices of emergency medical care. They have been included for the sole purpose of giving general insight into real-life emergency settings.

Notice on Case Studies

The names used and situations depicted in the case studies throughout this textbook are fictitious.

10 9 8 7 6 5 4 3 2 1
ISBN 0-13-119271-X

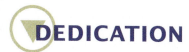DEDICATION

This text is respectfully dedicated to all EMS personnel who have made the ultimate sacrifice. Their memory and good deeds will forever be in our thoughts and prayers.

B.E.B.

I would like to dedicate this work in memory of Kelly Conti, flight nurse, colleague, and friend from University MedEvac in Cleveland, Ohio. In a moment one night in January 2002, Kelly gave her life on a mission to save another. Kelly's faith and skill in the delivery of critical care transport medicine reside in all who have known her.

R.W.B.

Detailed Contents

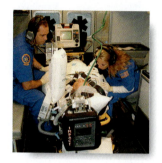
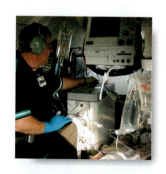

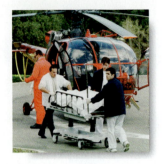

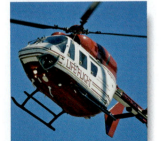

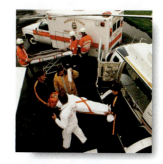

Chapter 6 **Patient Assessment and Preparation for Transport 103**

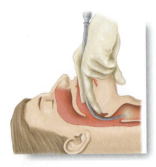

Chapter 7   Airway Management and Ventilation 124

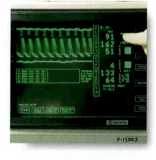

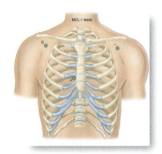

Chapter 10   ECG Monitoring and Critical Care 246

Chapter 11   Critical Care Pharmacology 272

Chapter 12   Interpretation of Lab and Basic Diagnostic Tests 325

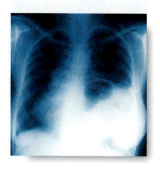

Chapter 13   Introduction to Trauma 355

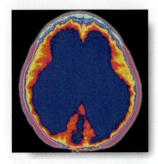

Chapter 16 · Abdominal and Genitourinary Trauma 420

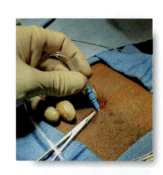

Chapter 17 · Face/Ear/Ocular/Neck Trauma 450

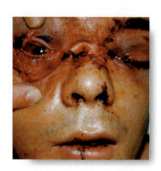

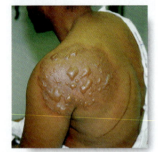

Chapter 18   Burns and Electrical Injuries   485

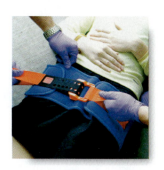

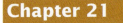

Chapter 21 **Pulmonary Emergencies 578**

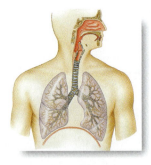

Chapter 22   Cardiovascular Emergencies 620

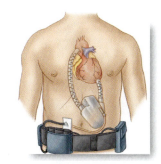

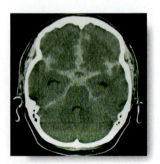

Chapter 23   Neurologic Emergencies   677

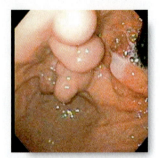

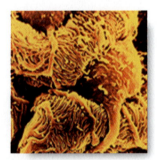

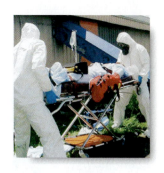

Chapter 26   Infectious Disease Emergencies   771

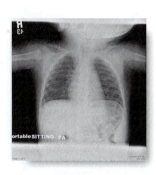

Chapter 27   Pediatric Medical Emergencies   810

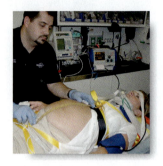

Chapter 28   High-Risk Obstetrical/Gynecological Emergencies 840

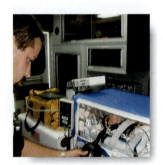

Chapter 29   Neonatal Emergencies 873

Chapter 30 Environmental Emergencies 895

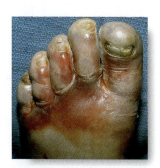

Chapter 31 Diving Emergencies 916

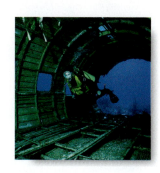

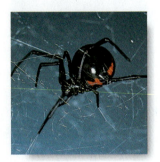

Chapter 32   Toxicological Emergencies 935

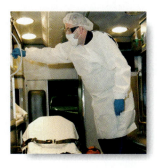
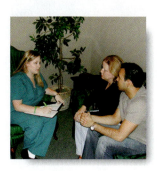

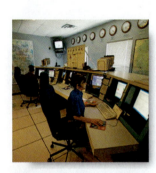

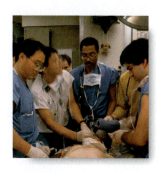

Chapter 37 The Critical Care Paramedic in the Hospital Environment 1050

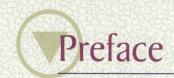

Preface

Welcome to *Critical Care Paramedic*, the first textbook published exclusively for the critical care paramedic. Critical care transport medicine has become an important and integral part of the modern health care system. Today, critical care paramedics, in association with their colleagues in medicine, nursing, and allied health professions, safely and efficiently transport critically ill and injured patients. Whether the transport is by ground ambulance, helicopter, fixed-wing aircraft, or even boat, critical care paramedics ensure that the patient receives the same degree and continued high quality of care during transport.

In this textbook, the authors and the contributors did not repeat material presented in standard paramedic education texts. Instead, this textbook concentrates on the unique knowledge base required of critical care paramedics. To be a good critical care paramedic, you must first be a good EMT and a good paramedic. Even at the critical care transport level, the vast majority of care and skills applied are at the basic life support level. However, when advanced skills are needed, the critical care paramedic must be ready to apply these. It goes without saying that a paramedic must have significant street experience before undertaking the critical care curriculum. As mentioned, we are assuming that the student reading this text is an experienced and competent paramedic.

The text follows the full scope of critical care paramedic education. The initial chapters review the history of critical care transport and critical care medicine. These are followed by basic chapters that address flight operations, flight physiology, and flight safety. The text then moves to basic clinical areas including patient assessment, advanced airway management, advanced shock management, hemodynamic monitoring, advanced 12-lead ECG interpretation, advanced pharmacology, and an introduction to common diagnostic tests and procedures. Next, we explore trauma care from the critical care paramedic perspective including trauma systems; neurotrauma; thoracic trauma; abdominal trauma; head, facial, and neck trauma; burns; orthopedic injuries; and trauma in special populations (pediatric, obstetrical, and geriatric). We address in detail cardiac medical emergencies, neurologic medical emergencies, gastrointestinal and abdominal medical emergencies, renal and genitourinary medical emergencies, infectious diseases, pediatric and neonatal medical emergencies, and obstetrical emergencies. In addition, we present advanced information on environmental emergencies, diving emergencies, toxicological emergencies, and terrorism-related emergencies. Finally, the text ends with an interesting discussion of organ donation, quality improvement and management in critical care, critical care communications, and the role of the critical care paramedic in the hospital setting.

This text is modeled on Brady's award-winning paramedic textbook series *Paramedic Care: Principles & Practice.* Using a similar design, students will easily transition from the paramedic series to this book. In addition, students will find the same features in this book as in the paramedic series including comprehensive objectives, a list of key terms, case studies, a margin glossary, highlighted key ideas, an end-of-chapter review, and a whole lot more! The art program is almost entirely new for this text and meets the needs of the critical care paramedic. Students and instructors will also find the supporting materials for this text that you have come to expect from Brady.

Thank you for choosing Brady's *Critical Care Paramedic* for your critical care paramedic education. It is important to remember that this text is designed to augment classroom instruction, supervised skills practice, and clinical rotations. We close with our best wishes as you embark on what will be a challenging, yet interesting, aspect of your EMS career.

Bryan E. Bledsoe, DO, FACEP

Randall W. Benner, M.Ed., MICP, NREMT-P

Acknowledgments

CHAPTER CONTRIBUTORS

We wish to acknowledge the remarkable talents and efforts of the following people who contributed to *Critical Care Paramedic*. Individually, they worked with extraordinary commitment on this new program. Together, they form a team of highly dedicated professionals who have upheld the highest standards of EMS and Critical Care Paramedic instruction.

Chapter 1 Introduction to Critical Care Transport
Bryan E. Bledsoe, DO, FACEP, EMT-P, Adjunct Associate Professor of Emergency Medicine, The George Washington University Medical Center, Washington, D.C., and Emergency Physician, Midlothian, Texas

Chapter 2 Critical Care Ground Transport
David G. Patterson, BBA, MA, EMT-P, Division General Manager, Rural/Metro Ambulance, Aurora, Colorado
Philip M. DaVisio, BS, PA-C, NREMT-P, EMS Director and Emergency Department Staff, Dameron Hospital, Stockton, California, and Valley Emergency Physicians, Oakland, California

Chapter 3 Critical Care Aerial Transport
Robert M. Brooks, BSN, MBA, CHE, EMT-P, Office of Business Relations and Development, STAT MedEvac, Pittsburgh, Pennsylvania, and Assistant Faculty, Youngstown State University, Youngstown, Ohio
Randall W. Benner, M.Ed., MICP, NREMT-P, Program Director, Emergency Medical Technology, Instructor, Department of Health Professions, Youngstown State University, Youngstown, Ohio

Chapter 4 Altitude Physiology
Larry D. Johnson, NREMT-P, CCT, FP-C, EMS Consultant, Las Vegas, Nevada
Bryan Bledsoe, DO, FACEP, EMT-P, Adjunct Associate Professor of Emergency Medicine, The George Washington University Medical Center, Washington, D.C., and Emergency Physician, Midlothian, Texas

Chapter 5 Flight Safety and Survival
Randall W. Benner, M.Ed., MICP, NREMT-P, Program Director, Emergency Medical Technology, Instructor, Department of Health Professions, Youngstown State University, Youngstown, Ohio

Chapter 6 Patient Assessment and Preparation for Transport
Scott A. Phillips, BS, NREMT-P, CCEMT-P, St. Anthonys Prehospital Services, Flight for Life Colorado, Denver, Colorado,
Randall W. Benner, M.Ed., MICP, NREMT-P, Program Director, Emergency Medical Technology, Instructor, Department of Health Professions, Youngstown State University, Youngstown, Ohio

Chapter 7 Airway Management and Ventilation

Bryan E. Bledsoe, DO, FACEP, EMT-P, Adjunct Associate Professor of Emergency Medicine, The George Washington University Medical Center, Washington, D.C., and Emergency Physician, Midlothian, Texas

William E. Gandy, JD, LP, Paramedic and EMS Educator, Albany, Texas

Chapter 8 The Shock Patient: Assessment and Management

Lee Richardson, NREMT-P, CCEMT-P, FP-C, I/C, Executive Director, TechPro Services Inc., Abilene, Texas

Bryan E. Bledsoe, DO, FACEP, EMT-P, Adjunct Associate Professor of Emergency Medicine, The George Washington University Medical Center, Washington, D.C., and Emergency Physician, Midlothian, Texas

Chapter 9 Cardiac and Hemodynamic Monitoring

Bryan E. Bledsoe, DO, FACEP, EMT-P, Adjunct Associate Professor of Emergency Medicine, The George Washington University Medical Center, Washington, D.C., and Emergency Physician, Midlothian, Texas

Timothy P. Duncan, RN, CCRN, CEN, CFRN, EMT-P, Flight Nurse, St. Vincent Mercy Medical Center Life Flight, Toledo, Ohio

Chapter 10 ECG Monitoring and Critical Care

Bob Page, AAS, NREMT-P, CCEMT-P, I/C, Director of Emergency Care Education, St. John's Health System, Springfield, Missouri

Chapter 11 Critical Care Pharmacology

Timothy P. Duncan, RN, CCRN, CEN, CFRN, EMT-P, Flight Nurse, St. Vincent Mercy Medical Center Life Flight, Toledo, Ohio

Randall W. Benner, M.Ed., MICP, NREMT-P, Program Director, Emergency Medical Technology, Instructor, Department of Health Professions, Youngstown State University, Youngstown, Ohio

Chapter 12 Interpretation of Lab and Basic Diagnostic Tests

Bryan E. Bledsoe, DO, FACEP, EMT-P, Adjunct Associate Professor of Emergency Medicine, The George Washington University Medical Center, Washington, D.C., and Emergency Physician Midlothian, Texas

Chapter 13 Introduction to Trauma

Allan Bulkley, NREMT-P, FP-C, RN, Flight Paramedic, Mercy Flight Central, Canandaigua, New York

Chapter 14 Neurologic Trauma

Donald J. Perreault, Jr., RN, BSN, CCRN, EMT, Boston Medical Center, Menino Pavilion Adult Emergency Department, Boston, Massachusetts

Chapter 15 Thoracic Trauma: Assessment and Management

Lee Richardson, NREMT-P, CCEMT-P, FP-C, I/C, Executive Director, TechPro Services Inc., Abilene, Texas

Chapter 16 Abdominal and Genitourinary Trauma

Scott R. Snyder, BS, NREMT-P, CCEMT-P, Folsom, California

Chapter 17 Face/Ear/Ocular/Neck Trauma

Scott R. Snyder, BS, NREMT-P, CCEMT-P, Folsom, California

INSTRUCTOR REVIEWERS

The reviewers of *Critical Care Paramedic* provided many excellent suggestions and ideas for improving the text. The quality of the reviews has been outstanding, and the reviews have been a major aid in the preparation and revision of the manuscript. The assistance provided by these EMS experts is deeply appreciated.

Rosemary Adam, RN, PS
Emergency Nurse Educator, EMS Nurse
The University of Iowa Hospitals' EMS
    Learning Resources Center
Iowa City, Iowa

Roy L. Alson, MD, Ph.D., FACEP, FAAEM
Associate Professor of Emergency Medicine
Wake Forest University School of Medicine
Winston-Salem, North Carolina

Nikki Atkinson, EMTP
Spring, Texas

Jane Bedford, RN, CCEMT-P
Nature Coast EMS
Chief Training, Public Information, and
    Infection Control Officer
Inverness, Florida

Robert P. Breese, MICP, FP-C
Public Safety Training Center
Monroe Community College
Rochester, New York

Allan Bulkley, NREMT-P, FP-C, RN
Flight Paramedic
Mercy Flight Central
Canandaigua, New York

Lyle Butler, RN, CEN, BS, EMT-PS
Trauma Outreach Coordinator
Creighton University Medical Center
Omaha, Nebraska

Christopher W. Connors, MD, EMT-P
Resident Physician
Brigham and Women's Hospital
Department of Anesthesiology, Perioperative,
    and Pain Medicine
Boston, Massachusetts

Seth D. Guthartz, BA, WEMT-P 1/C
Prehospital Program Manager
Brain Trauma Foundation
New York, New York

Michael Harnois, AA, EMT-P, CPTC, CTBS
Transplant Coordinator
University of Virginia
Charlottesville, Virginia

Laura A. Iacono, RN, MSN, CCRN, CNRN
Quality Improvement Director
Brain Trauma Foundation
New York, New York

Donald A. Locasto, MD
Assistant Professor, Department of Emergency
    Medicine
Director, Division of EMS
University of Cincinnati
Cincinnati, Ohio

Brad Madsen, B.Sc., CCP
Assistant Chief
Clive Fire Department
Clive, Iowa

Steve Maffin, AAS, EMT-P
Firefighter/Paramedic/Flight Paramedic
Medflight of Ohio
Columbus, Ohio

David Marshman, BS, NREMT-P, CPTC
Senior Transplant Coordinator
LifeNet
Lynchburg, Virginia

Alan P. McCartney, CSP, CHCM, CHSP,
    EMT-P
Senior Industrial Hygiene Specialist,
    Information and Electronic Warfare
    Systems, and Paramedic
BAE Systems
Adjunct Professor
Middlesex Community College
Lowell, Massachusetts

David L. McDonald, AHS
Program Faculty
Greenville Technical College
Greenville, South Carolina

Louis N. Molino, Sr., CETFF, NREMT-B, FSI, EMSI
Fire Protection and EMS Instructor and Consultant
Industrial Fire World/Fire and Safety Specialist
College Station, Texas

Greg Mullen, BS, MS
Education Coordinator
National EMS Academy, South Louisiana Community College
Lafayette, Louisiana

Kenneth Navarro, LP
Continuing Education Coordinator
University of Texas Southwestern Medical Center at Dallas
Emergency Medicine Education
Dallas, Texas

Robert G. Nixon, MBA, EMT-P
President/Owner
LifeCare Medical Training
Auburn, Massachusetts

James Richardson, MBA, EMT-P
Field Coordinator
Health One EMS
Englewood, California

Katharine P. Rickey, NREMT-Paramedic, EMS Educator/Consultant
Barnstead, New Hampshire

Lee Ridge, EMT-P, FP-C
University of Iowa Hospitals and Clinics
EMS Learning Resources Center
Iowa City, Iowa

Gina Riggs, AD EMT-P
EMS Coordinator
Kiamichi Technology Center
Poteau, Oklahoma

Rick Rohrbach, RN, CEN, MICP
Flight Nurse
New Jersey Aeromedical Program-Southstar
Voorhees, New Jersey

Philip E. F. Roman, MPH, EMT-P
Mercer University School of Medicine
Macon, Georgia

Michael D. Smith, EMT-P, AAS
Flight Paramedic
Grant Medical Center's LifeLink
Columbus, Ohio

S. Christopher Suprun, Jr., NREMT-P, CCEMT-P
EMS Training Coordinator
Carrollton Fire Department
Carrollton, Texas and Adjunct Instructor in Emergency Medicine
The George Washington University
Washington, D.C.

Scott R. Snyder, BS, NREMT-P, CCEMT-P
Folsom, California

Steven W. Tarbert, EMT-P
North Central EMS
Milan, Ohio

Larry Torrey, RN, EMT-P
Department of Emergency Medicine
New England Medical Center
Boston, Massachusetts

Russell Van Bibber, CCEMT-P
Communications Supervisor
Hopkins County EMS
Sulphur Springs, Texas

Jason C. West, NR/CCEMT-P, FP-C, AAS Degree in Paramedicine
Flight Paramedic
Omaha, Nebraska

PHOTO ACKNOWLEDGMENTS

All photographs not credited adjacent to the photograph were photographed on assignment for Brady Prentice Hall Pearson Education.

ORGANIZATIONS

We wish to thank the following individuals and organizations for their assistance in creating the photo program for this text and for providing technical support during the photo shoots:

Kathy Altergott, BSN, MBA, CRA
Medical Imaging Administrative Director
Banner Good Samaritan Medical Center
Phoenix, Arizona

Children's Medical Center Dallas
Dallas, Texas

Gloria Dow
President-Elect
International Association of Flight Paramedics
Mobile Life Support Services
Newburgh, New York

Martha Holcumb
CareFlite Air
CareFlite Ground Services
Grand Prairie, Texas

James Jackson, Operations Manager
Tim Devine, EMT-P, Manager for Clinical
    Operations
Thomas J. Pelio, CCEMT-P, PNCCT
North Shore–Long Island Jewish Health
    System
Center for Emergency Medical Services
Syosset, New York

Rebecca Marcus, CCEMT
Central Islip–Hauppauge Volunteer
    Ambulance
Central Islip, New York

Rickey Reed, EMT-P
Southwest Helicopters
Terrell, Texas

Sladjana Repic
Franklin Lakes, New Jersey

Suffolk County Police Department
Special Patrol Bureau
Suffolk County, New York

About the Authors

BRYAN E. BLEDSOE, DO, FACEP, EMT-P

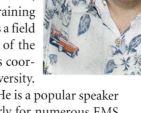

Dr. Bryan Bledsoe is an emergency physician with a special interest in prehospital care. He received his B.S. degree from the University of Texas at Arlington and his medical degree from the University of North Texas Health Sciences Center/Texas College of Osteopathic Medicine. He completed his internship at Texas Tech University and residency training at Scott and White Memorial Hospital/Texas A&M College of Medicine. Dr. Bledsoe is board certified in emergency medicine and is an Adjunct Associate Professor of Emergency Medicine at The George Washington University Medical Center in Washington, D.C.

Prior to attending medical school, Dr. Bledsoe worked as an EMT, a paramedic, and a paramedic instructor. He completed EMT training in 1974 and paramedic training in 1976 and worked for 6 years as a field paramedic in Fort Worth, Texas. In 1979, he joined the faculty of the University of North Texas Health Sciences Center and served as coordinator of EMT and paramedic education programs at the university. Dr. Bledsoe is active in emergency medicine and EMS research. He is a popular speaker at state, national, and international seminars and writes regularly for numerous EMS journals.

Dr. Bledsoe has authored several EMS books published by Brady including *Paramedic Care: Principles & Practice, Essentials of Paramedic Care, Intermediate Emergency Care: Principles & Practice, Anatomy & Physiology for Emergency Care, Prehospital Emergency Pharmacology,* and *Pocket Reference for EMTs and Paramedics.* He is married to Emma Bledsoe. They have two children, Bryan and Andrea, and a grandson, Andrew, and live on a ranch south of Dallas, Texas. He enjoys saltwater fishing and warm latitudes.

RANDALL W. BENNER, M.ED., MICP, NREMT-P

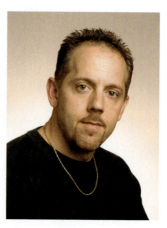

Randall Benner, Instructor in the Department of Health Professions at Youngstown State University, has 20 years of combined experience in the delivery of prehospital medicine, critical care transport medicine, and emergency education. He currently serves as Director of the Emergency Medical Technology Program at Youngstown State University, where he is responsible for all levels of prehospital EMS and critical care paramedic educational programs.

Mr. Benner has contributed to numerous EMS journal publications, books, and instructor resource materials, and he has coauthored several of his own works. He presents regularly both locally and nationally and serves on several EMS committees. Active as an emergency care provider, Mr. Benner is also completing his Ph.D. in education at Kent State University in Kent, Ohio.

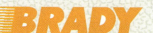

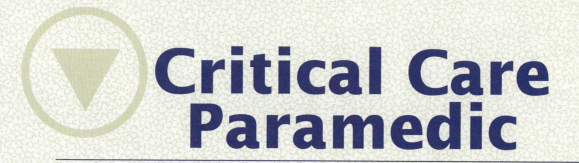

Critical Care
Paramedic

Introduction to Critical Care Transport

Bryan E. Bledsoe, DO, FACEP

Objectives

Upon completion of this chapter, the student should be able to:

1. Define and give examples of behavior that characterizes the health care professional. (p. 3)
2. Provide a brief overview of the history of critical care transport. (p. 4)
3. Define the role of the critical care paramedic. (p. 8)
4. List the duties of the critical care paramedic in preparation for handling critical care transport patients. (p. 8)
5. List the duties of the critical care paramedic during a critical care transport. (p. 9)
6. List the duties of the critical care paramedic after a critical care transport. (p. 11)
7. Define and give examples of professional ethics. (p. 12)
8. List the post-graduation responsibilities of the critical care paramedic. (p. 12)
9. State the benefits and responsibilities of continuing education for the critical care paramedic. (p. 13)
10. List some national organizations for critical care paramedics. (p. 13)
11. Describe the major benefits of subscribing to professional journals. (p. 13)

Key Terms

Case Study

A 54-year-old male walks into the small emergency department (ED) of a rural hospital in a community of 12,000 people. He says to the admission clerk that he thinks he is having a heart attack. The clerk immediately summons a nurse and the patient is taken back to the major medicine treatment area. There he is disrobed, his vital signs taken, and he is placed on the hospital's ECG monitoring system.

The nurse summons a local internist taking emergency department calls for the day. The hospital is too small to have a full-time emergency physician. He comes down from the medical floor where he is doing rounds, he enters the examination room, and sees the patient, who is pale, diaphoretic, and in moderate distress. He introduces himself and performs a brief history. The patient was trying to get his Bush Hog mower off of his tractor so he could attach the bailer. He was having trouble getting the power take-off drive shaft loose and was hitting it with a sledgehammer. While doing so, he developed severe chest pressure and immediately became nauseated and sweaty. He went to his truck and sat in it for a while and drank some water. He failed to feel better, so he decided to drive to the hospital.

The internist orders a standard cardiac workup (12-lead ECG, cardiac enzymes, complete blood count, coagulation panel, portable chest X-ray, standard chemistries) and orders the patient to receive an aspirin orally and a saline lock. The ECG reveals an acute ST-segment elevation myocardial infarction (STEMI). The patient is hypertensive and tachycardic. The internist has an inch of nitroglycerin paste placed on the patient's chest and has 5 milligrams of morphine administered via the saline lock. The chest X-ray and the rest of the lab results are within normal limits. The onset of pain was approximately 45 minutes earlier, making the patient a possible candidate for fibrinolytic therapy.

The internist screens the patient for possible fibrinolytic therapy and, finding no absolute or relative contraindication, orders tissue plasminogen activator (tPA) via a front-loaded protocol. The patient receives additional morphine for pain and promethazine for nausea. The patient continues to have pain and the ST segments remain elevated despite the fibrinolytic therapy. Approximately 2 hours after pain onset, the internist determines the patient needs interventional therapy, which is only available at Saint Francis Hospital 75 miles away.

The rural hospital operates a ground critical care transport (CCT) ambulance and the crew is summoned to the emergency department. The patient is evaluated and prepared for transport by the CCT paramedics while the internist and the nurses arrange the transport. The tPA has been infused and a heparin infusion started. Because the patient continues to have pain and remains hypertensive, a nitroglycerin drip has been started. All of the infusions and monitors have been transferred to the CCT team's equipment and the patient is taken to the ambulance.

The patient has an uneventful trip to Saint Francis Hospital other than requiring additional morphine and an increase in the nitroglycerin drip (managed by the CCT paramedics per standing orders). At Saint Francis, they bypass the ED and take the patient straight to the interventional lab where he is taken in right away. The interventional team and an interventional cardiologist are waiting. They obtain arterial access and get a quick coronary arteriogram. The patient has a 99% lesion of the left anterior descending coronary artery, but is otherwise relatively disease free. Percutaneous transluminal coronary angioplasty (PTCA) is carried out and the vessel opened. Following this, the patient became pain free, the ST segments returned to normal, and the patient was admitted to the coronary care unit for follow-up care. He did well and was discharged 3 days later on various medications. He will follow up with the internist back in his home town.

INTRODUCTION

critical care paramedics
EMT-paramedics who have completed additional formal education in the care and transport of critically ill or injured patients

The critical care paramedic plays an important role in the modern health care system—the safe and efficient movement of critically ill or injured patients between facilities. The best critical care paramedics are excellent technicians who never forget that their patients are human beings with rights and feelings.

In the past 30 years, prehospital emergency care has evolved into a prominent specialty requiring highly sophisticated levels of patient care. **Critical care paramedics** provide highly technological care to patients with complex multisystem problems. (See Figure 1-1 ■.) This advanced level of paramedic care is both an awesome responsibility and an exciting challenge. The critical care paramedic is expected to provide not only competent medical care, but also emotional support for the patient as well as the family members. Experienced paramedics in this specialty assume a high degree of individual responsibility. Within this highly technical setting, it is essential that the critical care paramedic maintain a caring perspective. Caring means that persons, events, projects, and things matter to people. Caring is the moral ideal of the health care profession, whereby the end is protection, enhancement, and preservation of human dignity. Your willingness to accept this role during a critical care transport and an interest in learning how to devise effective treatment plans are the first steps toward becoming a critical care paramedic.

■ Figure 1-1   The modern critical care transport team provides a high level of patient care between hospitals and from the scene to the hospital. *(Eddie Sperling Photography)*

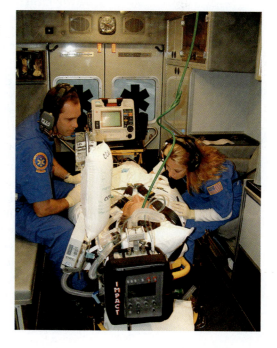

HISTORY OF AMBULANCE TRANSPORT

ambulances *vehicles designed for the safe transport of injured or ill patients.*

As early as the 1790s, during the First Coalition of the Napoleonic Wars, the French began to transport wounded soldiers from the battlefield to hospitals where they could be cared for by surgeons. No medical care was provided to the injured soldier on the battlefield. They were simply carried via horse-drawn carriage to an area where medical care was available. This is the earliest documented emergency medical service.

The Geneva Convention in 1864 resulted in the development of the Geneva Treaty, which established rules related to the care of injured soldiers on the field of battle. **Ambulances** and military hospitals were declared to be neutral and immune from attack. Likewise, persons who worked in ambulances and hospitals were deemed neutral and immune from attack. Neutral medical personnel, including ambulance attendants, wore armbands that displayed their nation's flag and a "red cross."

The first use of an ambulance in the United States occurred during the Civil War around 1865. Famed nurse and founder of the American Red Cross Clara Barton began a battlefield ambulance service. Again, as in the Napoleonic Wars, soldiers were simply ferried from the field of battle to a medical facility where care was provided.

In the latter half of the 19th century, civilian ambulances began to appear at various locations. By 1865, Commercial Hospital (now Cincinnati General) in Cincinnati, Ohio, was operating an ambulance. Bellevue Hospital in New York City established an ambulance service in 1869. Other hospitals gradually developed ambulance services.

In 1899, Michael Reese Hospital in Chicago introduced the first motorized ambulance. The ambulance, built in Chicago, weighed 1,600 pounds and had a top speed of 16 miles per hour. A year later, Saint Vincent's hospital in New York City boasted a motorized ambulance.

Ambulances played a major role in World War I. The U.S. military commissioned an Ambulance Service Corps and sent it to France. Many people in the United States volunteered for this corps. Also, during World War I, selected battlefield casualties were transported by airplane.

Advanced life support was introduced to the prehospital setting in Belfast, Northern Ireland, in the late 1950s. Under the direction of Dr. J. F. Pantridge, physician-staffed mobile intensive care units began providing prehospital advanced medical care to residents of Belfast.

In 1970, advanced life support was first introduced into the United States by Dr. Eugene Nagel. Selected Miami Fire Department personnel received additional education in advanced prehospital care. Nagel is generally credited with creating the first paramedics in the United States. Prior to the development of the Miami program, Saint Vincent's Hospital in New York developed a specialized "mobile coronary care unit." The unit responded to a limited area of Manhattan and included a resident physician.

Today, EMS is a sophisticated part of the health care system. Paramedics are filling more roles both in-hospital and in the prehospital setting. The development of the *EMS Agenda for the Future,* a guidemap for the future EMS, will guide EMS well into the 21st century. (See Figure 1-2 ■.)

HISTORY OF AIR TRANSPORT

Although the first use of aircraft for the transport of patients is lost to history, there are records of hot air balloons being used to transport wounded during the Prussian siege of Paris in 1870. In World War I, selected patients were transported by airplane. The aircraft of this era were small and could usually carry only a single patient. During the retreat of the Serbian Army from Albania in 1915, unmodified French fighter aircraft were used to ferry the injured.

Helicopters were first used for medical transport during the Korean War in the early 1950s. Injured soldiers were provided first aid at the scene and transported rapidly by helicopter to medical facilities such as a Mobile Army Surgical Hospital (MASH) or battalion aid station. More than 20,000 patients were transported by helicopter in Korea. The mortality rate in the Korean War dropped largely because of rapid helicopter transport and the early provision of definitive surgical care in the MASH units near the battlefields. (See Figure 1-3 ■.)

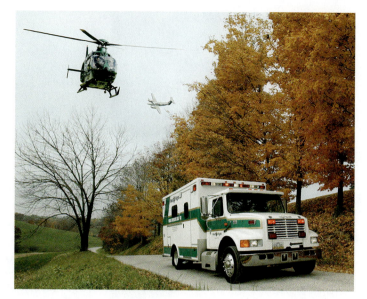

■ **Figure 1-2** Modern critical care transport by specially trained critical care paramedics and other health care providers ensures a high level of patient care during transfer of critically injured or severely ill patients— whether by air or ground. *(MedFlight of Ohio)*

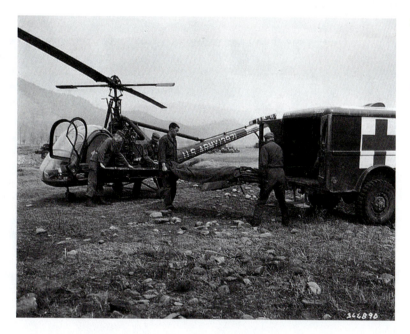

■ **Figure 1-3** Medical helicopters became important lifesaving tools in the Korean War and meant the difference between life or death for many soldiers. *(© Corbis)*

Helicopters played a major role in the Vietnam conflict. Vietnam and Southeast Asia are largely covered by jungles. Military medical personnel followed the Korean model in Vietnam: Wounded soldiers were provided emergency care in the field by corpsmen and medics and then transferred by helicopter to definitive surgical facilities placed a safe distance from the front lines of battle. (See Figure 1-4 ■.) Again, in comparison to previous wars, the mortality rate improved. Nearly 1,000,000 wounded were transferred by helicopter during the course of this prolonged conflict.

During the 1960s, aircraft were used only sporadically for civilian medical transport. It was not until 1969 that the first aircraft used for ambulance work began flying for Samaritan Air Evac in Phoenix, Arizona. The Maryland State Police began providing a combination of police/ambulance helicopter service in 1970. In 1972, Saint Anthony's Hospital in Denver established the first helicopter service dedicated exclusively to patient care. (See Figure 1-5 ■.)

Today, **air transport systems** are a common part of EMS. In fact, some regions of the country are oversaturated. In 1999 Samaritan Air Evac in Arizona was forced to lay off 70 employees because

air transport systems
specialized medical transport of critically ill or injured patients via helicopter or fixed-wing aircraft.

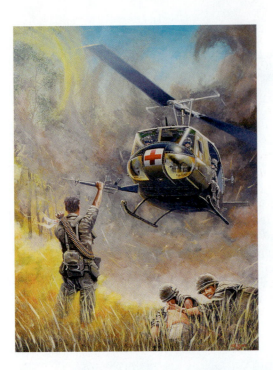

■ **Figure 1-4** The medevac (also called the "Dust Off") helicopter played a major role in decreasing mortality in Vietnam by rapidly moving injured soldiers from the battlefield to definitive care. *(Dust off © 2000, Joe Kline Aviation Art)*

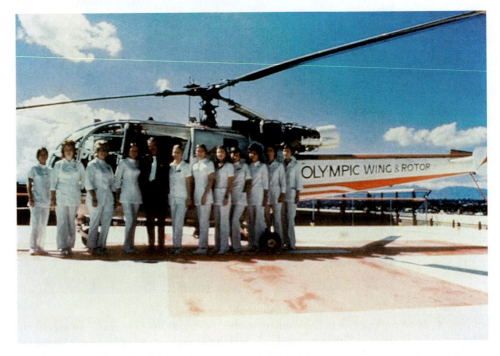

■ **Figure 1-5** The first civilian helicopter in the United States devoted exclusively to patient care was Saint Anthony's Flight for Life in Denver, Colorado. *(Flight for Life Colorado)*

of increased competition in the air medical market. Regardless, air transport remains a major source of patient transport throughout the world. In Australia, most of the state-operated ambulance services also operate a fleet of fixed-wing aircraft and a few helicopters to complement their ground-based fleet.

HISTORY OF CRITICAL CARE MEDICINE

critical care medicine (CCM) *medical specialty dedicated to the care and transport of critically ill or injured patients.*

Critical care medicine (CCM) evolved when physicians and nurses recognized a need to better care for patients who had a life-threatening illness or injury. Initially, such patients were kept on regular nursing floors, yet kept near the nursing station whereby nurses could better monitor the patients.

Later, specialized areas of the hospital were devoted to care of very ill patients. Several events in the history of CCM are noteworthy.

In the mid-19th century, nurse Florence Nightingale wrote about the advantages of establishing a special area of the hospital dedicated exclusively to the care of postsurgical patients.

Intensive care in the United States began early in the 20th century when noted neurosurgeon Dr. W. E. Dandy established a three-bed intensive care unit (ICU) for neurosurgical patients at the Johns Hopkins Hospital in Baltimore, Maryland. The first ICU for premature babies was established in 1927 at Sarah Morris Hospital in Chicago, Illinois.

During World War II, the nursing shortage resulted in the grouping of postoperative patients in recovery rooms to ensure proper care. The resultant benefits resulted in the standardization and development of recovery rooms in all hospitals. The polio epidemic of 1947 and 1948 resulted in the breakthrough in treatment of the respiratory paralysis associated with the disease. A breathing tube was placed into the trachea of polio patients and mechanical ventilation provided. These patients required intensive nursing care and were often grouped together on the same wards. Mechanical ventilation became widely available in the 1950s and commonplace in U.S. and European hospitals. As with recovery room care, the care and monitoring of ventilator patients was more effective when all of the patients were grouped together in the same location. These intensive care units were used for both postoperative and very ill patients. By 1958, approximately 25% of community hospitals with more than 300 beds had an ICU. By the late 1960s, virtually every hospital had at least one ICU bed. By 1997, more than 5,000 ICUs were operational in the United States.

In 1970, 29 physicians with a special interest in the management of critically ill patients met in Los Angeles, California, and formed the Society of Critical Care Medicine (SCCM). In 1973, the American Association of Critical-Care Nurses (AACN) developed achievement examinations for the purpose of recognizing the expertise of registered nurses who were practicing in the specialty of critical care. Two levels of examinations were available: Level I, for entry level, and Level II, for the advanced practitioner. In 1975, AACN established a separate entity, the AACN Certification Corporation, to develop the CCRN Certification Program. The purpose of the program is to use the certification process as a means for developing, maintaining, and promoting high standards of critical care nursing practice. The goals of the program are to establish the body of knowledge necessary for CCRN certification; to test, through written examination, the common body of knowledge needed to function effectively within the critical care setting; to recognize professional competence by granting CCRN status to successful certification candidates; and to assist and promote continued professional development of critical care nurses.

In 1986, the American Board of Medical Specialties recognized the specialty of critical care medicine by approving a certificate of special competence for physicians certified by one of four primary boards (anesthesiology, internal medicine, pediatrics, and surgery).

HISTORY OF PREHOSPITAL CRITICAL CARE

The health care landscape changed drastically in the 1980s. For various reasons, most commonly reductions in federal funding and Medicare reimbursements, small rural and community hospitals in the United States began to close. At the same time, large hospitals became specialized. They found that they could keep costs down and quality high by specializing in a few service areas. Some hospitals began to specialize in such areas as neurosurgical or cardiac care, while others specialized in, say, obstetrics or neonatology. The concept of a "general hospital" became something of the past. In fact, general hospitals could not financially compete with the specialized hospitals and either had to become specialized themselves or face closure.

With this shift from general hospitals to specialized facilities came the need to move more patients between hospitals so that the patient could receive the best possible care in the community. Some of the patients who needed to be moved were in an ICU setting. These patients often were undergoing complicated care such that routine transfer by standard ambulance was unacceptable. Initially, hospitals would send an ICU nurse with the ambulance crew. This required that the ambulance remain out of service while the nurse was returned to the transferring hospital. Also, most ICU nurses, while skilled in critical care, were unprepared for the isolated environment of prehospital medicine. (Nurses later developed a curriculum for flight nursing that was then broadened to encompass air and surface transport with associated specialty certification.) Finally, in the late 1980s and early 1990s the nursing shortage caused several hospitals to close ICU units or reduce ICU beds. As a result of the shortage, nurses were unavailable to accompany ambulance crews.

The advent of medical helicopters, usually staffed by a nurse, allowed the transport of critical patients without a subsequent deterioration in care. But when the weather would not allow helicopter flight, the flight crew would often staff a ground ambulance. Not all critical patients need the speed a helicopter affords—and the associated costs. Thus, ground transport units devoted specifically to critical care transport were developed. The staffing on these typically included a registered nurse.

However, as the demand for ground critical care transport increased, the need arose for personnel other than a nurse to staff the unit. Critical care paramedics (CCPs) evolved somewhat accidentally. One thing that adversely affected aeromedical transport was weather. Often, the weather made it impractical or impossible to move a patient by helicopter. To be able to provide their service, the aeromedical operations would often place their flight crews in ground ambulances to transfer the patient. This resulted in several problems. First, the ground ambulance transports took considerably longer, which tied up the flight crews for an extended period of time. Second, because of the increased time required to complete a ground transfer, it was often necessary to send another flight crew out to transfer a patient. In several instances, the weather cleared and the helicopter was again able to fly only to find that all of the flight crews were tied up in ground transports. In addition, some of the flight crews found ground transport a little less exciting than helicopter transport.

flight paramedics
paramedics with specialized skills and education in the care of critically injured or ill patients transported via helicopter or fixed-wing aircraft.

As the aeromedical programs matured, they began to use their **flight paramedics** for their ground critical care transports. Later, as demand increased, it became obvious that there was a need for paramedics who had critical care training to handle the vast majority of these ground transports. CCP training programs were developed by several ground and aeromedical operations to meet local needs. As the demand for CCPs grew, there was a push to develop and standardize the educational curriculum for CCPs. Educators in Maryland, Iowa, and Texas established the initial educational curriculum for critical care paramedic education. However, no single accrediting body oversaw the process. Today, there are myriad critical care education programs—some more comprehensive than others. However, critical care transport has become a cost-effective way to transport critically ill or injured patients between medical facilities.

Medicare recognizes seven levels of ambulance service. These are detailed in Table 1–1. Reimbursement by Medicare is based on these levels of service and is detailed in Table 1–2.

ROLE OF THE CRITICAL CARE PARAMEDIC

The role of the CCP varies significantly. Critical care paramedics may be assigned to dedicated ground critical care transport vehicles or they may be assigned to standard EMS units and summoned when a critical care transport call is received. Many hospitals operate critical care transport services as a part of their emergency department or ICU. In these cases, critical care paramedics will often work in the emergency department or ICU when not involved in a critical care transport. Critical care paramedics also work as flight paramedics for aeromedical operations. The curriculum for a flight paramedic is very similar to that for a critical care paramedic. Likewise, the curriculum for a flight nurse is very similar to that of a critical care nurse. With most aeromedical operations, a critical care paramedic works with a critical care nurse, although some operations have elected to staff their service exclusively with critical care paramedics. The composition of the team is driven by the specific needs of the patient and the system. (See Table 1–3.) Many long-distance transport services use critical care paramedics to staff their long-haul aircraft for national and international patient transfers. Due to increasing demand, some critical care paramedics have elected to specialize in specific areas of critical care transport such as neonatal or pediatric transport. Such units, by necessity, are only found in the larger cities and usually operated by a children's hospital.

Before becoming a critical care paramedic, it is recommended that a paramedic have 3 to 5 years of experience in a busy ALS system. This is to ensure mastery of ALS and the necessary skills. In critical care transport, paramedics are often called on to use advanced skills much more frequently than they would in the standard prehospital environment. In addition, critical care paramedics will usually acquire skills in procedures that are not commonly used in routine prehospital

Table 1-1	Seven Levels of Ambulance Service as Recognized by Medicare
Type	**Description**
Basic life support (BLS)	Where medically necessary, the provision of BLS services as defined in the *National EMS Education and Practice Blueprint* for the EMT-Basic including the establishment of a peripheral intravenous (IV) line.
Advanced life support 1 (ALS1)	Where medically necessary, the provision of an assessment by an ALS provider and/or the provision of one or more ALS interventions. An ALS provider is defined as a provider trained to the level of the EMT-Intermediate or Paramedic as defined in the *National EMS Education and Practice Blueprint*. An ALS intervention is defined as a procedure beyond the scope of an EMT-Basic as defined in the *National EMS Education and Practice Blueprint*.
Advanced life support 2 (ALS2)	Where medically necessary, the administration of at least three different medications and/or the provision of one or more of the following ALS procedures: • Manual defibrillation/cardioversion • Endotracheal intubation • Central venous line • Cardiac pacing • Chest decompression • Surgical airway • Intraosseous line
Specialty care transport (SCT)	Where medically necessary, in a critically injured or ill patient, a level of interfacility service provided beyond the scope of the paramedic as defined in the *National EMS Education and Practice Blueprint*. This is necessary when a patient's condition requires ongoing care that must be provided by one or more health professionals in an appropriate specialty area (nursing, medicine, respiratory care, cardiovascular care, or a paramedic with additional training).
Paramedic intercept (PI)	These services are defined in 42 CFR 410.40. They are ALS services provided by an entity that does not provide the ambulance transport. Under limited circumstances, these services can receive Medicare payment.
Fixed-wing air ambulance	Fixed-wing air ambulance services are provided when the patient's medical condition is such that transportation by either basic or advanced life support ground ambulance is not appropriate. In addition, fixed-wing air ambulance services may be necessary because the point of pickup is inaccessible by land vehicle, or great distances or other obstacles (for example, heavy traffic) are involved in getting the patient to the nearest hospital with appropriate facilities.
Rotor-wing air ambulance	Rotor-wing air ambulance services are provided when the patient's medical condition is such that transportation by either basic or advanced life support ground ambulance is not appropriate. In addition, rotor-wing air ambulance may be necessary because the point of pickup is inaccessible by land vehicle, or great distances or other obstacles (for example, heavy traffic) are involved in getting the patient to the nearest hospital with appropriate facilities.

care. (See Table 1–4.) While these skills vary from system to system, they must be mastered just like any of the standard paramedic skills.

Certification of the critical care paramedic is currently in a state of flux. The Board for Critical Care Transport Paramedic Certification (BCCTPC), an affiliate of the International Association of Flight Paramedics (IAFP), offers a Certified Flight Paramedic (FP-C) certification. (See Figure 1-6 ■.) Several avenues exist for certification as a critical care paramedic—although these have not been standardized nor universally accepted.

Like all aspects of EMS, critical care paramedics must function under the authority of a licensed physician. Likewise, care must be guided by medical protocols and standing orders that provide guidelines and direction for care of individual patients. Critical care protocols must be customized for the specific operation (adult medicine, pediatrics, neonatal, cardiac). Likewise, the drugs carried should be fairly extensive so that patient care is not interrupted during transport. However, having a more comprehensive formulary places additional responsibilities on the critical care paramedic who must be familiar with all of the various medications available for their use.

Table 1–2	Medicare Reimbursement Based on Levels of Service	
Level of Service	**Relative Value Units (RVUs)**	
BLS (nonemergency)	1.00	
BLS (emergency)	1.60	
ALS1	1.20	
ALS1 (emergency)	1.90	
ALS 2	2.75	
SCT	3.25	
PI	1.75	
Fixed-wing	N/A	
Rotor-wing	N/A	

Table 1–3	Various Critical Care Team Compositions		
Pilot/EMT driver	Physician	Nurse	
Pilot/EMT driver	Physician	Paramedic	
Pilot/EMT driver	Nurse	Nurse	
Pilot/EMT driver	Nurse	Paramedic	
Pilot/EMT driver	Paramedic	Paramedic	
Pilot/EMT driver	Nurse	Paramedic	Respiratory therapist
Pilot/EMT driver	Nurse	Paramedic	IABP perfusionist
Pilot/EMT driver	Paramedic	Neonatal nurse	Respiratory therapist

Table 1–4	Critical Care Paramedic Skills*
Rapid sequence induction/intubation (RSI)	
Central venous line placement	
Arterial line placement	
Pericardiocentesis	
Intraosseous needle placement	
Arterial blood gas interpretation	
Interpretation of common laboratory studies	
Continuous waveform capnography	
Management of complicated pharmacologic infusions	
Mechanical ventilation including PEEP (positive end-expiratory pressure)	
Thoracic needle and tube decompression	
Escharotomy	
Intra-aortic balloon pump	
Management of invasive hemodynamic monitors	
Surgical cricothyrotomy	

* Delegated skills may vary from system to system.

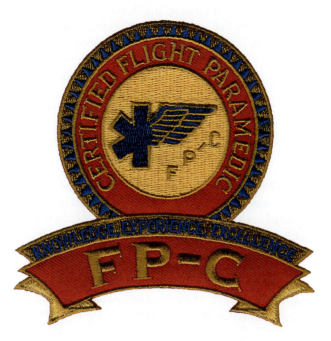

Figure 1-6 Certified Flight Paramedic (FP-C) patch. *(IAFP)*

THE CRITICAL CARE PARAMEDIC IN THE HOSPITAL SETTING

Most paramedics see the hospital only through the emergency department. Critical care paramedics must enter the hospital and continue to perform their assessment and management while the patient remains in their hospital bed. Because of this, it is essential that critical care paramedics understand the culture and environment of the hospital and the intensive care unit. When you enter the hospital, you are out of your "turf."

Your entire EMS educational program, for the most part, has concentrated on treating patients in the field and preparing them for transport to the hospital. With critical care transport, however, you must enter the hospital and adhere to the traditions and requirements of the ICU or emergency department. It is important to remember that you represent the entire prehospital profession each time you enter an ICU or ED to deliver or retrieve a patient. Be careful about what you say or do. Always treat patients, their families, and the hospital staff with the utmost respect and dignity. It is important to remember that small community hospitals may not have the equipment or supplies that you would find in a major teaching hospital. However, they are able to do a good job caring for patients with the equipment they have. Be nonjudgmental when you complete your assessment and care. Ask before looking at the patient's chart. Thank the hospital staff for their assistance and offer to provide them feedback on the patient. Remember the old adage, "You never get a second chance to make a first impression."

PROFESSIONALISM

Professionalism describes the conduct or qualities that characterize a practitioner in a particular field or occupation. Health care professionals promote quality patient care and take pride in their profession; they set high goals. They earn the respect and confidence of team members by performing their duties to the best of their abilities and by exhibiting a high level of respect for their profession.

Attaining professionalism is not easy. It requires an understanding of what distinguishes the professional from the nonprofessional. To develop this skill, keep the following points in mind. Professionals place the patient first; nonprofessionals place their egos first. Professionals practice their

professionalism *the conduct or qualities that characterize the standard of excellence in a particular field or occupation.*

skills to the point of mastery, and then keep practicing them to improve and stay sharp. Nonprofessionals do not believe their skills will fade and see no reason to constantly strive for improvement. Professionals understand the importance of response times; nonprofessionals get to the scene of an emergency when it is convenient. Professionals take refresher courses seriously, because they know they have forgotten a lot and because they are eager for new information. Nonprofessionals believe they do not need training sessions and dislike being required to attend them. Professionals set high standards for themselves, their crew, their agency, and their system. Nonprofessionals aim for the minimum standards and can be counted on to take the path of least resistance. Professionals critically review their performance, always seeking a way to improve. Nonprofessionals look to protect themselves, to hide their inadequacies, and to place blame on others. Professionals check out all equipment prior to the emergency response. Nonprofessionals hope that everything will work, supplies will be in place, batteries will be charged, and oxygen levels will be adequate.

Maintaining professionalism requires effort. But the result of that effort—the admiration and respect of one's peers—is the highest compliment a person can receive. True professionals establish excellence as their goal and never allow themselves to become satisfied with their performance. Professionalism is an attitude, not a matter of pay. It cannot be bought, rented, or faked. Although a young industry, EMS has achieved recognition as a bona fide allied health care profession. Gaining professional stature is the result of many hard-working, caring individuals who refuse to compromise their standards. The critical care paramedic must always strive to maintain that level of performance and commitment known as professionalism.

PROFESSIONAL ETHICS

ethics *self-imposed standards or rules governing conduct by members of a group, profession, or society.*

Ethics are the standards that govern the conduct of members of a particular group. Physicians have long subscribed to a body of ethical standards that were developed primarily for the benefit of the patient. These standards have subsequently been extended to the allied health professions. Ethics are not laws, but standards for honorable behavior designed by the group; conformity by all members is expected. As members of an allied health profession, critical care paramedics must recognize a responsibility not only to their patients, but also to society, to other health professionals, and to themselves.

Whereas legal guidelines obligate the critical care paramedic to certain actions, ethical standards suggest that certain behaviors are right or wrong. The critical care paramedic will encounter many situations that present a moral dilemma. For example, the critical care paramedic must decide between a patient's rights and family members' wishes when called on to resuscitate a terminally ill patient in cardiac arrest. How critical care paramedics act in such cases will depend mostly on their personal values and ethical convictions. Legally, a critical care paramedic must provide for the physical well-being of the patient. Ethically, the critical care paramedic also must care for the emotional welfare of the patient and family members. The best critical care paramedics are excellent technicians who never forget that their patients are human beings with rights and feelings. If you always place the patient's welfare above everything but your own safety, you will probably never commit an unethical act. Treating all patients as you would members of your own family is all that can be expected of you as a critical care paramedic. The best critical care paramedics are aware of not only their legal obligations, but also the ethical and moral responsibilities of the job.

POST-GRADUATE RESPONSIBILITIES

The responsibilities of the critical care paramedic begin with completion of the initial education program. Critical care transport is a high-technology field. It is essential that critical care personnel stay abreast of current developments in EMS and critical care. Because critical care transport is a relatively new aspect of EMS, it may be necessary to develop specialized programs for continuing education.

CONTINUING EDUCATION

There are several methods of keeping up with the rapidly changing field of critical care medicine. First, there are several trade journals directed at EMS and critical care. These often introduce new technologies and procedures in an easy-to-read format. Second, trade shows are an excellent source of information for critical care paramedics. They allow side-by-side comparison of equipment and provide the opportunity to interact with critical care personnel from other operations. Because the critical care paramedic straddles the worlds of EMS and critical care, this provides twice as many opportunities to learn new information. Critical care nursing journals and books are an excellent source of information. Hospitals often have workshops at which representatives of various health care manufacturing companies set up their equipment and provide instruction in its use. They also allow personnel to gain "hands-on" experience with the device being demonstrated.

If you live in a town that has a major hospital or medical school, inquire about the possibility of attending "Grand Rounds." These programs usually begin with a lecture, often by a prominent physician or scientist from the field being discussed. On some occasions, the lecture is followed by presentation of selected patients or lab specimens. In high-technology presentations, attendees are often allowed the opportunity to become familiar with or use the technology being presented.

Many of the advanced skills used by critical care paramedics are only rarely utilized. Because of this, skill degradation becomes a concern. As a rule, the less often a skill is used, the more frequent it should be practiced. With this in mind, critical care operations should track utilization of critical care skills so that refresher training can be provided to personnel who have not had the opportunity to use the skills in their daily work. Periodic rotations through the emergency department, ICU, or operating room allow critical care paramedics the opportunity to review and practice skills and procedures less commonly employed.

Numerous computer-based continuing education programs are available. These include both web-based programs and CD-based programs. This allows for leisurely review of essential material. Also, because of the technology, computer-based programs tend to provide more up-to-date information than that found in books or magazines. Again, programs for both EMS and critical care nursing provide useful continuing education for the critical care paramedic.

PROFESSIONAL ORGANIZATIONS

Because critical care paramedic transport is a relatively new component of EMS, few professional organizations for CCPs exist. The two organizations that are most aligned with critical care paramedic transport are the National Association of Critical Care Paramedics (NACCP) and the International Flight Paramedics Association (IFPA). Traditional organizations can be a valuable source of information through the organization itself and their journals. These include the National Association of EMS Physicians (NAEMSP) and the National Association of Emergency Medical Technicians (NAEMT).

Summary

Congratulations on your decision to further your career by pursuing critical care transport training. This is a challenging, yet rewarding aspect of EMS. As a highly-educated member of the critical care transport prehospital team, you have significant responsibilities. It is important to remember that you represent the entire prehospital profession each time you enter an ICU or emergency department for a patient retrieval or delivery. It is essential that you maintain a professional demeanor and treat the patient, the family, your EMS coworkers, and the hospital staff with the utmost respect and dignity. Your education as a critical care paramedic begins with completion of this program. Because of the technology, and because this is such a new component of EMS, it is essential that you become diligent with regard to ongoing education. You are responsible for keeping yourself current on critical care knowledge.

Review Questions

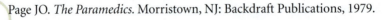

1. Briefly detail the history of ambulance transport in Europe and North America.
2. Discuss the history of air medical transport and detail its role in modern EMS.
3. Detail the history of critical care medicine and the evolution of the critical care paramedic.
4. Describe the role of the critical paramedic in the modern EMS system.

See Answers to Review Questions at the back of this book.

Further Reading

Barkley KT. *The Ambulance: The Story of Emergency Transportation of the Sick and Wounded through the Centuries.* Kiamesha Lake, NY: Load N Go Press, 1978, 1990.

Page JO. *The Paramedics.* Morristown, NJ: Backdraft Publications, 1979.

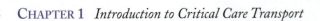

Critical Care Ground Transport

David Patterson, BBA, EMT-P, MA and Phil DaVisio, PA-C, NREMT-P

Objectives

Upon completion of this chapter, the student should be able to:

1. Discuss the history of critical care ground transport. (p. 18)
2. Contrast the benefits and limitations of various ambulance types including ground ambulances, rotor-wing aircraft, and fixed-wing aircraft. (p. 19)
3. Discuss the role of funding as it pertains to critical care transport. (p. 19)
4. Discuss the advantages and disadvantages of various critical care crew configurations. (p. 20)
5. Detail the equipment typically used in modern critical care transport. (p. 21)

Key Terms

ambulance chassis, p. 21
ambulance configuration,
  p. 21

ground transport systems,
  p. 17

specialty care transport
  (SCT), p. 20

Case Study

Today is your first day of employment with a university-based critical care ground service that routinely transports complicated and critical patients across the state. Since you are still in orientation, your primary role is that of an observer and you are excited about the opportunities to see and care for critical patients.

This day, however, is very cloudy and overcast—a typical late fall day in the city where you are based. Approximately 1 hour into your shift, your pager goes off alerting you to an emergency transport from a hospital approximately 100 miles away. You meet up with your crewmates in the dispatch center and review the patient information. You learn the patient is a 36-year-old male who suffered serious burns when he was attempting to burn some leaves. He has been stabilized in a local community hospital and is being transported to the university medical center's burn unit.

In less than 3 minutes you are en route. The EMT driver turns the ambulance onto the interstate highway and you start discussing the case with your coworkers. You talk about airway management, fluid therapy, and pain control—all important concerns in the burn patient.

After an hour and a half the ambulance turns into the community hospital and pulls up to the emergency department entrance. There you are met by a security guard who takes you to the patient. The transport nurse gets a brief history from the emergency nurse and you and your partner don sterile burn gowns and go examine the patient.

The patient has second- and third-degree burns over both arms, his anterior chest, and upper abdomen. There appear to be no circumferential burns. You estimate that approximately 31.5% of the body surface area (BSA) has partial- or full-thickness burns. There is no evidence of airway burns. An IV is running and he is easily arousable. You complete your exam. There is no airway stridor or breathing problems. The patient has received 15 milligrams of IV morphine, 25 milligrams of promethazine, tetanus toxoid, and 1 gram of Ancef. His burns are covered with a sterile burn sheet.

You and the team begin to prepare the patient for transport. However, moving him even slightly causes extreme pain. The team administers 100 mcg of fentanyl IV and the patient's pain is better. Oxygen is started with a venturi mask at 45%.

The transport goes uneventfully although the patient requires additional fentanyl and promethazine. You and the crew calculate fluid replacement therapy using the Parkland formula. Approximately 1 hour later you are pushing the patient into the burn unit and giving a report to the burn unit staff. Finally, you gather your equipment and restock the unit.

After you return to quarters, a standard post-call review is held. No criticism is expressed and all felt the call went well. You questioned whether or not a helicopter would have been a better choice instead of a ground ambulance. You learn that the burn surgeons formerly sent all burn patients by helicopter. However, research had demonstrated that burn patients generally do not require helicopter transport except in cases where there is an airway problem or similar complication. Once the patient is burned, the injury is over and the speed a helicopter offers does not provide the patient any significant benefit. Now, all burn patients in the state are routinely transported by ground.

Just as you are finishing the review, the pager goes off again. This time it is a cardiac patient in the same hospital where you retrieved the burn patient. You grab your kit and head once again for the ambulance.

INTRODUCTION

The purpose of this chapter is to introduce the critical care paramedic (CCP) to the basic configuration of **ground transport systems** for the transport of critically ill or injured patients to an appropriate receiving facility. The use of ambulances themselves however, at this point, should not be something foreign to the practicing paramedic. After all, almost all paramedics' first position is for an EMS system comprised only of ground transport vehicles. (See Figure 2-1 ■.) As such, the focus of the chapter is to prepare CCPs on how best to utilize a ground unit in their practice or how to do so for systems that utilize both aircraft and ground units.

Critical care ground systems play a crucial role in the treatment and transportation of the critically sick and injured. Many differences in equipment and staffing exist between traditional advanced life support units staffed by EMTs and paramedics and the critical care ground ambulances discussed here.

ground transport systems
medical transport of ill or injured patients via ground ambulance.

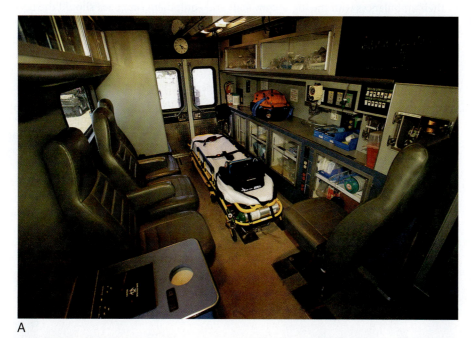

A

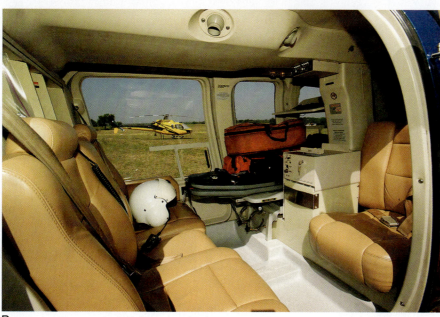

B

■ **Figure 2-1** There is significantly more room for equipment and personnel in ground-based ambulances (A) compared to medical helicopters (B). *(© 2005 Scott Metcalfe LLC, All rights reserved)*

HISTORY

Following the Korean and Vietnam conflicts, in which rotor-wing aircraft were used extensively, the idea made it back to the United States where civilian use of medical helicopters was introduced. (Chapter 3 discusses this in greater detail.) The first helicopter program dedicated exclusively to patient care began in 1972 at Saint Anthony's Hospital in Denver, Colorado. These initial programs were primarily based out of major hospitals in urban areas. The initial purpose of these programs was to respond to emergent scenes and rural hospitals, transporting the critically ill and injured to the facility in which the helicopter program was based.

As critical care programs evolved, many services opted to staff the ground component of their program separately from the air medical service. Other systems utilize the critical care staff for both the air and ground service. This is due in part to the weather limitations of some flight programs, as well as the higher operating costs inherent in air medical transport. In fact, many air medical services that do not have a ground transportation division contract with local EMS services to use one of their ambulances with the flight crew staff and equipment on board should the need arise.

When choosing between air and ground transport, the assumption is often made that a helicopter is faster than ground transport for patient evacuation. But remember that flight times do not reflect patient transfer time, the time needed for aircraft warm-up and shutdown at the origin and destination, nor the time required for other nonflight activities. Another consideration is cost. Critical care ground transport is significantly less expensive than transport by helicopter. Routine critical care transfers by air can cost from $2,000 to $7,000 depending on the distance and operator.

Also, safety is always a concern. Although EMS helicopter operations are relatively safe, the number of medical helicopter accidents in the United States has been steadily increasing. Whether this increase reflects a decline in safety or the fact that there are simply more helicopters in operation is open to conjecture. (See Figure 2-2 ■.)

In the end, many hospitals needed to reexamine their critical care air transport systems, and some were forced to restructure the delivery of these programs. In addition, nonhospital providers began to provide several other options for critical care delivery that utilized ground systems.

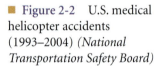 **Figure 2-2** U.S. medical helicopter accidents (1993–2004) *(National Transportation Safety Board)*

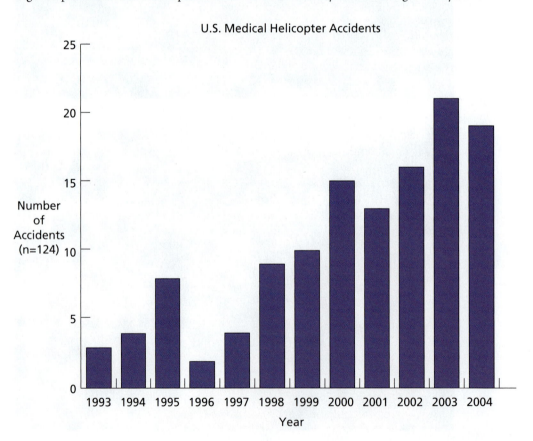

SYSTEM DESIGN

Some advantages of critical care ground transport compared to air transport include:

★ A larger patient compartment

★ Lower transport costs

★ Relative immunity to changing weather conditions

Critical care ground transport is a safe and cost-effective way to move critical patients between facilities.

As mentioned earlier, another advantage is that ground transport is sometimes considered a safer alternative to helicopter or fixed-wing transport, especially when challenging geographical or inclement weather influences exist. Also, other environmental factors can affect both the patient and care providers in air medical operations that might not be experienced in ground transportation. Although more prevalent to fixed-wing operations, some of these factors include oxygen levels, acceleration/deceleration forces, gas volume changes at altitude, cabin pressurization, humidity, noise, and vibration. Table 2–1 illustrates the typical advantages and disadvantages of the various modes of critical care transport.

The most common critical care ground transportation systems continue to be offered by both public and private hospitals. Some of these hospital programs are provided in partnership with external entities, while some of these partners operate their own ground programs. Private, for-profit, nonprofit, and government-based services also exist. And although they all fundamentally provide the same level of service, each has its own idiosyncrasies of billing and reimbursement.

SYSTEM FINANCING

An example of a partnership between a hospital and EMS entity for provision of critical care transports typically finds the hospital contracting with the private EMS service for non–critical care personnel (EMTs and paramedics) and equipment (ambulance), while the hospital provides the critical care personnel and the specialized equipment. The critical care providers who work primarily for the hospital may be assigned internally to the emergency department or critical care units between calls, or even to the air medical portion of the hospital system should it operate a helicopter. In either instance, the hospital decides how and when to utilize the critical care team, and manages the billing for the services as they would any other aspect of the patient's care.

Most of these systems bill third-party payers or patients for services rendered, which provides much of the revenue for operation of the program. These systems are established primarily for the purpose of patient transport within a hospital system. Some systems are supported through government-based tax revenues (such as a hospital district or county-operated facility), while some hospital systems rely on funding from patient revenue received from hospitalization following the transport.

With the advent of the current Medicare fee schedule, critical care transport funding may increase from historical levels. The current fee schedule is designed to recognize this higher level of emergency prehospital and interhospital care, whereas in the past, critical care ambulances were simply recognized as advanced life support units for reimbursement purposes.

Table 2–1	Comparison of Ground, Rotor-Wing, and Fixed-Wing Transport		
Factor	Ground Ambulance	Rotor-Wing Aircraft	Fixed-Wing Aircraft
Departure times	Excellent	Good	Poor to fair
Arrival times	Fair to poor	Excellent	Good
Out-of-hospital time	Poor	Excellent	Fair to excellent
Patient accessibility	Excellent	Good	Good
Weather issues	Excellent	Fair	Fair to good
Cost	Significantly lower	Highest	Higher

Although the specific reimbursements from governmental sources are at the government's discretion, the following discussion offers a brief illustration about the recent Medicare fee schedule change, since reimbursement for a specialty care level of ground transport became available. **Specialty care transport (SCT),** which applies to interfacility critical care transports, is defined by Medicare as "hospital-to-hospital transportation of a critically injured or ill beneficiary by a ground ambulance vehicle, including the provision of medically necessary supplies and services, at a level of service beyond the scope of the EMT-Paramedic. SCT is necessary when a beneficiary's condition requires ongoing care that must be furnished by one or more health professionals in a specialty area, for example, emergency or critical care nursing, emergency medicine, respiratory care, cardiovascular care, or a paramedic with additional training."

Medicare does recognize that the EMT-Paramedic training level is set by each state. So if a paramedic is allowed by his particular state to provide a certain level of critical care service, and the paramedic does not have specialty care certification or qualification, the transport would not qualify for reimbursement under SCT guidelines. If however, a critical care paramedic completes an interfacility transport for a patient that would have previously required the specialty care provided by someone such as a nurse, the transport would be considered a Medicare recognized SCT, and be reimbursed at a higher level.

STAFFING

Staffing configurations on critical care ground transport units range widely from area to area; however, some states have started to take legislative initiative to standardize the teams. In the absence of state regulation in many regions, the local medical communities determine how to best staff critical care ground units.

Medical direction for the critical care paramedic is typically provided through off-line standing orders via medical protocols. On-line medical direction is also utilized, but because of the advanced skill training and education, as well as the rigorous quality assurance programs of critical care transport systems, it is relied on with less frequency than off-line direction. Contributing to this, especially in the case of ground transport units that operate in geographic locations where transport distances to remote locations are great, the use of on-line direction may be inhibited. In the absence of on-line medical direction, the critical care paramedic must rely on standing orders and their clinical expertise to provide appropriate patient care. The critical care practitioner usually possesses a great deal of autonomy for this reason.

Generally, at least one emergency medical technician is assigned to critical care ground transport units for purposes of vehicle operation and assisting with basic patient care. Critical care paramedics, however, are usually educated to a much higher level of care than is found in traditional paramedic programs. The educational underpinnings for these programs, as found in this text, involve a much broader foundation of anatomy, physiology, pathophysiology, symptomatology, and management techniques. Although not an exhaustive description, the critical care paramedic receives knowledge and skills pertaining to advanced airway management techniques (including use of paralytics), chest tube monitoring, thoracic escharotomies, surgical cricothyroidotomy, transvenous pacing, central venous catheter maintenance/interpretation, intra-aortic balloon pumps, blood/blood by-product administration and monitoring, electrolyte interpretation, arterial blood gas measurement, basic radiography interpretation, ventilator management, 12-lead ECGs, pulse oximetry and capnogram interpretation, intracranial pressure monitoring lines, venous cutdowns, infusion pumps, and advanced pharmacologic interventions.

Because paramedics are already accustomed to practicing in a relatively autonomous clinical environment, they typically perform well in critical care after the educational component is complete. Some systems, however, also staff critical care ground units with registered nurses, nurse practitioners, respiratory therapists, physician assistants, or physician residents (physicians in training).

In the end, regardless of staffing configurations on critical care transport units, the local medical community must have a level of comfort with the education, thinking skills, and care provision abilities of the personnel they entrust with the transport of critically ill or injured patients.

EQUIPMENT

Knowledge of the equipment is probably the most comfortable aspect for paramedics entering the critical care transport domain, since they are already acclimated to patient care in a moving ambulance. Nonetheless, the discussion here of **ambulance configuration** is important. Current ambulance design types and **ambulance chassis** include Type I units (see Figure 2-3 ■), which have a truck chassis with a modular-style patient care compartment; a Type II unit, which is the typical van style (see Figure 2-4 ■); and a Type III unit, which is a van chassis with a modular box (see Figure 2-5 ■). Typically, a critical care ground ambulance is a large Type I or Type III unit (see Figures 2-6 ■ and 2-7 ■) due to the additional equipment, staffing, and, in some instances, the need to access the patient from all sides of the cot. The large modular space must usually be mounted on a heavy-duty van chassis or truck chassis.

Generally, a critical care ground ambulance will contain all of the equipment found in a paramedic-level ambulance, such as intubation equipment, medications, and ECG monitoring capability. Some of the specialized equipment commonly found in a critical care unit includes single, triple, or syringe medication pumps (see Figure 2-8 ■); automatic ventilators that allow manipulation of all aspects of ventilatory control (see Figure 2-9 ■); automatic blood pressure monitoring capability (see Figure 2-10 ■); central venous catheters and hemodynamic monitors; arterial catheters and monitors; and intra-aortic balloon pumps (see Figure 2-11 ■).

ambulance configuration *vehicle type, physical layout, electrical, and mechanical design of an ambulance. (Example: USDOT KKK-1822 specifications.)*

ambulance chassis *type of vehicle/cab frame, such as a van or truck, upon which the patient care compartment is mounted.*

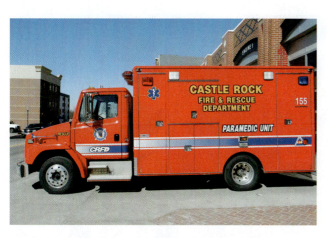

■ **Figure 2-3**   Type I ambulance *(© Jeff Forster)*

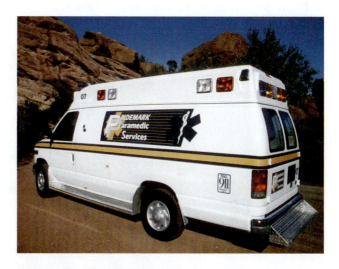

■ **Figure 2-4**   Type II ambulance *(© Jeff Forster)*

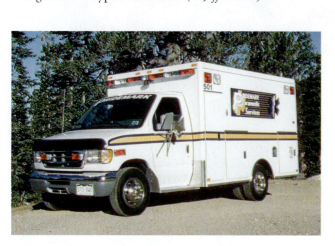

■ **Figure 2-5**   Type III ambulance. *(© Jeff Forster)*

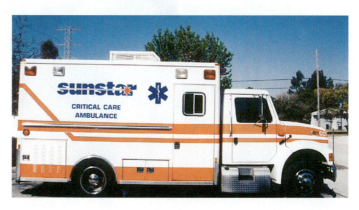

■ **Figure 2-6**   The modern critical care transport vehicle provides virtually all the capabilities of the hospital intensive care unit.

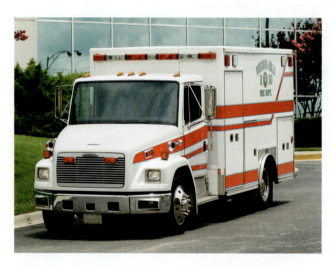

Figure 2-7 Diesel hybrid ambulance. *(© Ken Kerr)*

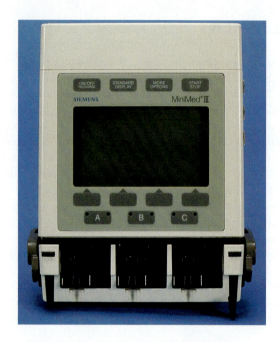

Figure 2-8 Medication infusion pump (multiport).

Figure 2-9 Modern transport ventilator. *(© Craig Jackson/In the Dark Photography)*

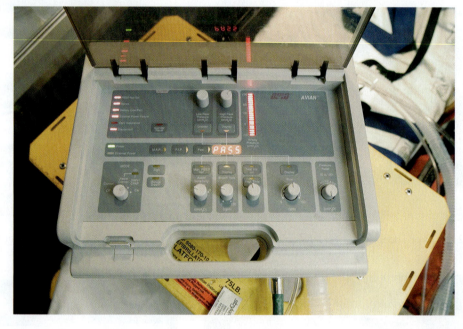

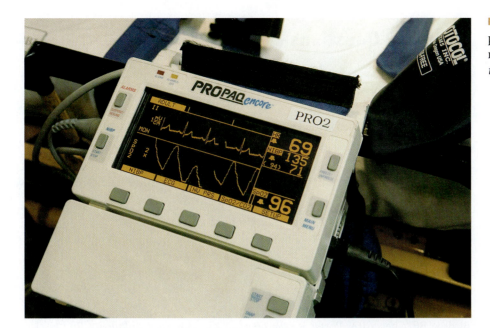

■ **Figure 2-10** Multi-parameter physiologic monitor. *(© Craig Jackson/In the Dark Photography)*

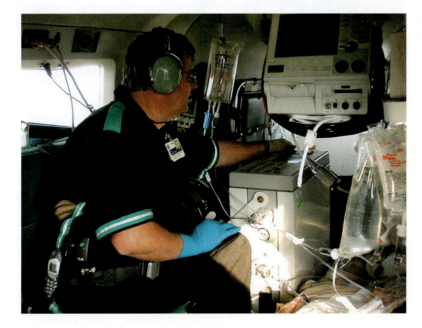

■ **Figure 2-11** Intra-aortic balloon pump in use during transport. *(James Green/Scott and White Hospital, Temple, TX)*

Summary

Critical care ground transport systems share many similarities with their air medical counterparts, although significant differences do exist (as will be discussed in Chapter 3). In some cases, critical patient transportation by ground is advantageous to air transport. Ground system designs, financing, and staffing configurations can, at times, be as diverse as the providers and communities in which they operate. Because many critical care paramedics find themselves employed in services that utilize aircraft as the primary means of transport, issues of staffing, transport protocols, and inclusion criteria for transporting the critical patient are discussed in the next chapter.

Review Questions

1. Describe the historical progression of the paramedic from prehospital care to critical care paramedicine.

2. What is the basic criteria for specialty care transport according to Medicare?

3. List at least three instances when transport of a critical patient may be better served by a ground unit than a helicopter.

4. Why is the critical care paramedic often more reliant on off-line medical direction than on-line medical direction?

See Answers to Review Questions at the back of this book.

Further Reading

Bledsoe BE, Cherry RA, Porter RS. *Paramedic Care: Principles & Practice,* 2nd ed. Upper Saddle River, NJ: Pearson/Prentice Hall, 2005.

Bledsoe BE, Smith MG. "Medical Helicopter Accidents in the United States: A Ten-Year Review." *Journal of Trauma,* Vol. 56 no. 6 (2004): 1325–1329.

Holleran RS. *Air and Surface Patient Transport: Principles and Practice,* 3rd ed. Saint Louis, MO: Mosby, 2003.

Critical Care Aerial Transport

Robert M. Brooks, BSN, MBA, CHE, EMT-P

Objectives

Upon completion of this chapter, the student should be able to:

1. Identify the administrative structure and functions of the administrative team. (p. 27)
2. Discuss the importance of a comprehensive communication center. (p. 29)
3. Discuss the indications and benefits of fixed-wing transport. (p. 29)
4. Describe the indications and benefits of rotor-wing transport. (p. 30)
5. Describe the indications for calling for air medical transport. (p. 40)
6. Indicate general considerations that go into planning and implementing a critical care flight mission. (p. 40)
7. Discuss the advantages and disadvantages of air medical transport. (p. 45)
8. Identify proper packaging of the air medical patient. (p. 46)

Key Terms

communication center, p. 29
fixed-wing transport, p. 29
Instrument Flight Rules (IFR), p. 36
instrument landing system (ILS), p. 38
medical crew configurations, p. 28

medical director, p. 28
microwave landing system (MLS), p. 38
program director, p. 27
rotor-wing transport, p. 30
rotorcraft (helicopter) airframes, p. 31

Visual Flight Rules (VFR), p. 36
wide-area augmentation system with global positioning satellites (WAAS/GPS), p. 38

Case Study

You are working for an air medical service as a flight paramedic. You and your partner have gone about your normal daily duties and have already checked your equipment and your medications to be sure you are prepared for a rapid deployment if summoned. The pilot has given you and your partner your safety brief for the day and you know that the weather is not going to be a factor in any mission today.

Your pagers go off for a scene call. You and your partner package the equipment and head for the aircraft; the pilot prepares the aircraft for departure. The pilot performs his walk-around and removes the cords and checks the covers of the aircraft to ensure they are all properly closed and prepared for flight. You and your partner place your equipment in the aircraft and also do a secondary walk-around to double-check the aircraft for safe departure. The pilot starts the engines and brings the aircraft to idle speed as you and your partner buckle into the aircraft. The pilot brings the rotor speed to "fly" and you depart for the scene.

As you await the coordinates, you start toward the scene using a distance and heading given to you by your communications specialist. As you speed toward the accident scene at approximately 150 miles per hour you start to get the radio ready to make contact with the landing zone coordinator. The dispatch center comes over the radio with your coordinates and ground contact. You enter them into the Global Positioning System (GPS) and radio, and prepare to make contact. As you come over the landing zone (LZ) you see the destructive aftermath caused by an overturned semi-tractor/trailer on an interstate highway. Your LZ is safely marked on the highway about 100 yards from the accident, and your pilot performs a reconnaissance orbit as you and your partner look for any hazards that could obstruct a safe descent into the LZ.

You land safely in the LZ and you and your partner rapidly depart the aircraft "hot" and set up the LZ coordinator to guard the LZ since the aircraft is running. Only now are you able to turn your full attention to the care of the patient. You arrive at the patient's car to find it is crushed underneath the front end of the tractor/trailer. The patient is being extricated with heavy-rescue equipment and the paramedic on scene lets you know that the patient is bleeding profoundly from an open pelvis fracture and that he also suspects a head injury because of repeated questioning and combativeness. After being advised of the patient's current vitals, breath sounds, and findings on the pulse oximeter and cardiac monitor, you reassess the treatment that has been rendered thus far, which includes manual cervical stabilization, administration of oxygen via a nonrebreather mask, and insertion of two large-bore IVs that are infusing NaCl wide open.

You enter the mangled vehicle through a very narrow opening that used to be the driver's side door. You try to talk to the patient, but his mental status is deteriorating rapidly. After reassessing breath sounds, you converse with your partner and determine the best care plan for this severely injured multisystem trauma patient. Because the fire department states that it will be another 10 to 15 minutes before the patient will be extricated, you initiate the steps to perform a rapid-sequence intubation (RSI) procedure, initiate blood administration, and prepare for a right chest wall needle decompression for a suspected tension pneumothorax.

Shortly afterward, the roof of the crushed car has been removed and the patient is ready to be extricated onto the backboard. You and the ground EMS personnel work together to get the patient out of the vehicle and secured onto the backboard in the usual fashion. You package the patient onto your stretcher, ensuring that the endotracheal tube remains properly placed by attaching it to your portable end-tidal CO_2 detector. At this point you are ready to "hot" load the patient. As you recruit three firefighters to assist you to the aircraft with a four-point carry of the cot, your partner departs to the aircraft to act as a safety officer, ensuring that none of the carrying crew gets near the exposed tail rotor. As you load the patient, your partner directs the crew back away from the aircraft the same way they came in. Your partner then enters the aircraft and resumes patient care while you do a walk-around of the aircraft, ensuring that it is once again safe to lift off.

You also now enter the patient compartment of the aircraft and resume patient care while the pilot prepares you for liftoff and advises you that the trauma center is about a 15-minute flight away. Once in the air you continue your care as if in a flying emergency room. You continue your assessments as well as treatment until you arrive in the awaiting trauma room where the patient care will be transferred.

INTRODUCTION

The purpose of this chapter's case study is to highlight that the majority of what the air medical transport crew does to retrieve the patient and get him safely to the hospital has little to do with patient care. Ensuring complete safe operations of the aircraft is a team effort that must be adopted by all of the flight crew. The tasks of performing complete walk-arounds, and setting up LZ safety officers are essential to daily safe operation in the air medical environment. The high-stress environment of air medical transport must be performed by extremely clinically competent and seasoned medical personnel. Once you perform all necessary steps to get to the patient, you must now remember that these severely ill and injured patients still require superior care. The air medical clinician must have substantial knowledge of the treatment of a wide range of patients from neonates to geriatrics, and everything in between, and must be able to perform at the highest of clinical standards to ensure proper prehospital stabilization and transport to tertiary care hospitals.

This chapter will provide basic knowledge about the entire field of aerial transport. The basic setup of air medical programs will be reviewed including administrative and medical crew configuration structures. The criteria that are used to determine if aerial transport is warranted will be reviewed, and the proper packaging of the patient for transport will be explained. Some of the multiple airframes utilized for rotor-wing aerial transport will be discussed.

THE AIR MEDICAL ADMINISTRATIVE TEAM

All air medical organizations have an administrative team that directs the daily operations of the program. Some organizations have very large administrative teams that consist of multiple base site managers, comprehensive outreach teams, and multiple clinical coordinators, while others utilize very basic administrative approaches. There is no right or wrong administrative approach; rather, each organization's administration is tailored to meet the needs and requirements of the mission and size of the organization. Two basic components of this team that are essential are the program director and medical director.

The **program director** is responsible for coordinating all of the daily operations of the flight program, including the direction of the program in terms of strategy and growth. The main responsibilities of the program director include creation of administrative policy, ensuring continuous quality improvement, maintaining the fleet of aircraft through vendors and purchasing or leasing contracts, maintaining the communications center, preparing and planning the operating budget, directing the marketing and growth strategies, and serving as a figurehead for the organization to hospital and nonhospital-based health care organizations. Depending on the size of the

program director *person who coordinates daily operations and directs flight program strategy and growth.*

organization, these duties may be performed directly by the program director or they may be delegated to heads of several departments such as director of operations or director of communications. The position of the program director can be held by any number of flight crew members from flight paramedics to pilots. Whoever holds this position should have a broad understanding of business principles or hold a degree in business.

medical director *physician who creates and implements medical protocols, ensures proper crew training, conducts quality assurance program, and provides on-line medical direction.*

The **medical director** is responsible for creating medical protocols, ensuring proper training of the flight crews, and providing on-line medical direction in the event that a patient case falls outside of the existing written protocols. In many states specific laws and guidelines determine who can perform the duties of the medical director, and in many cases these physicians have backgrounds in emergency or critical care medicine.

The written protocols serve as standing written orders that can be followed by the flight crew without consultation of the physician. As long as the patient fits into the guidelines of the orders in the protocol, he can be treated without a consult. However, very often these comprehensive protocols do not cover the entire spectrum of the critically ill or injured population, and a medical consult is needed. At this point the medical crew will perform a thorough assessment of the patient and report the findings to the medical director, or another physician as directed by the medical director. The care of the patient will be discussed among the physician and the flight crew, and a treatment plan will be formulated that is specific for this patient. As the flight crew initiates the transport and treatment plan, adjustments may be needed that will require subsequent follow-up with the designated physician or medical director via phone or radio.

The initial training of the medical crew and subsequent continuing education are the responsibility of the medical director. These activities are usually performed through an in-house education department that is directed by the medical director. The initial medical crew training is very difficult and tedious. In many instances the medical crew consists of a nurse with critical care or emergency department experience and a paramedic with substantial field training beyond the typical paramedic program requirements. These very competent and experienced clinicians must be molded into medical crew members who can assess and treat any patient in the spectrum of neonate to the elderly, from rare medical illness to multisystem trauma. They are molded over the period of several months to be able to perform advanced emergency procedures, such as RSI, needle thoracotomy, escharotomy, and surgical airway, and to operate and interpret sensitive medical equipment such as a 12-lead ECGs, an end-tidal carbon dioxide ($ETCO_2$) detector, (capnography), intra-aortic balloon pump (IABP), left ventricular assist device (LVAD), and invasive hemodynamic monitors.

This training, as directed by the medical director, prepares the medical flight crew for operation as valuable members of the flight team. However, the training does not stop at the end of this initial training period. Continuing education is essential to the continued competency of the medical flight crew in the form of lecture education days, clinical education days, and clinical competency testing days. The continuing education and competency testing are performed at effective intervals as determined by the medical director.

MEDICAL CREW CONFIGURATION

medical crew configurations *the crew mix for any particular mission, as determined jointly by the program director and the medical director.*

Medical crew configurations are the responsibility of the program director and the medical director. They must determine the appropriate medical crew mix for the mission of the organization. As discussed in Chapter 1, the crew configuration is based on multiple factors—most specifically patient need. Most air medical units are staffed with two medical crew members, and are often staffed with one registered nurse (RN) and one paramedic. This is a marriage of two excellent clinicians, because the RN has had experience with the in-hospital patient population, while the paramedic has had experience with accident scene and prehospital patients. Having these two highly skilled and competent clinicians working together provides a highly effective and efficient medical crew team. A 2000 survey in the *Air Medical Journal* compiled crew configurations for 119 air medical services worldwide, the findings of which are described in Table 3–1.

Table 3–1	Various Air Medical Crew Configuration Worldwide	
Staffing	**Helicopter**	**Fixed-Wing Aircraft**
One attendant	3%	3%
Two attendants	96%	97%
One supplemental staff	1%	0%
RN/paramedic	71%	61%
RN/RN	8%	8%
RN/physician	3%	3%
RN/EMT	1%	5%
RN/other (RRT/PA)	10%	18%
Paramedic/paramedic	5%	0%
Other	2%	5%

Source: From Rau W. *2000 Medical Crew Survey.* Air Medical Journal, Vol. 6, No.5 (September/October 2000): 17–22.

COMMUNICATION CENTER

The heart of every air medical operation is a comprehensive communications center. The **communication center** is responsible for all incoming requests for air medical transports, as well as the gathering of specific required information such as coordinates, ground contact frequencies, destinations, and patient information. Beyond these initial duties, the communications specialists must perform multiple follow-up duties such as following the flight of the aircraft, communicating with the security division of the accepting hospital, and calling back to the requesting agency to get any additional medical or logistical data. The communications center and the communications specialists are very important members of the air medical team and are often not recognized for their importance to the program.

communication center *receives, gathers, disseminates, and coordinates operational and logistical information for each mission.*

FIXED-WING TRANSPORT

Fixed-wing transport is the aeromedical transport of patients in a fixed-wing aircraft (or, more simply stated, a plane). Fixed-wing transport is an efficient and cost-effective mechanism of air transport. Many ambulance services, particularly those in Australia, operate large fixed-wing operations to augment their ground and rotor-wing fleet. (See Figure 3-1 ■.) In the United States, fixed-wing transport is often reserved for use when transport distances are greater than 100 nautical miles or in instances where helicopters cannot fly due to weather conditions that are not prohibitive to the fixed-wing aircraft. (See Figure 3-2 ■.) Many different airframes can be converted to air medical transport planes with commercial devices such as the LifePort. (See Figure 3-3 ■.)

Planning a fixed-wing transport mission within the country of origin is similar to initiating a helicopter transport. However, when international fixed-wing missions become necessary, a substantial amount of extra planning is required. The extra planning includes arranging for safe passage into foreign airspace, ensuring safe and efficient ground transport and refueling, and ensuring crew safety while traveling abroad in sometimes unsafe and unfriendly countries. International fixed-wing missions are often performed to bring critically ill or injured individuals back to their home country from a foreign country where the medical systems may be less advanced, or to a country where the patient's insurance will pay for the medical services.

fixed-wing transport *the transport of a patient by fixed-wing aircraft.*

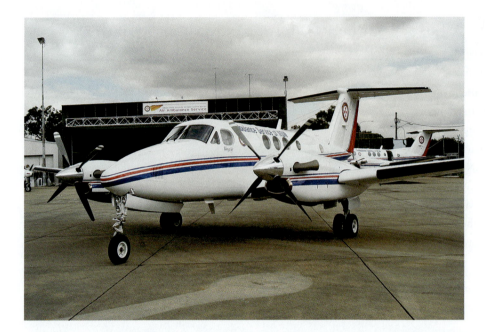

■ **Figure 3-1** Fixed-wing fleet operated as part of the New South Wales, Australia, ambulance service.

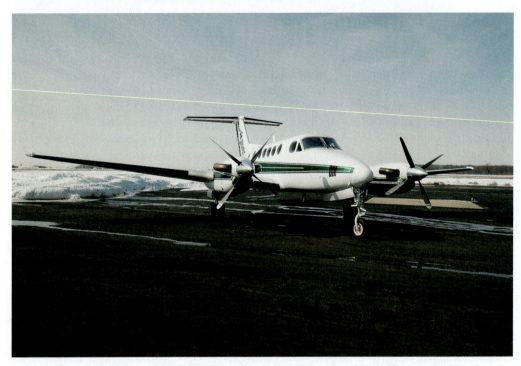

■ **Figure 3-2** Modern fixed-wing air ambulance. *(MedFlight of Ohio)*

ROTOR-WING TRANSPORT

rotor-wing transport *the transport of a patient by rotor-wing (helicopter) transport.*

Aeromedical **rotor-wing transport** of patients occurs when helicopters are used as the mode of transport. Rotor-wing transports make up the majority of the air medical transports in the United States, but are used to a much lesser degree in other countries. Helicopters perform most of the transports within a radius of 100 nautical miles. (See Figure 3-4 ■.) The types of missions that helicopters perform depend on the type of aircraft and the administrative policy of the organization. Some helicopters are equipped to perform search-and-rescue missions utilizing a hoist mechanism that is attached to the side of the aircraft. However, most air medical aircraft are designed just to transport patients from, for instance, an accident scene or between hospitals. Patients who are

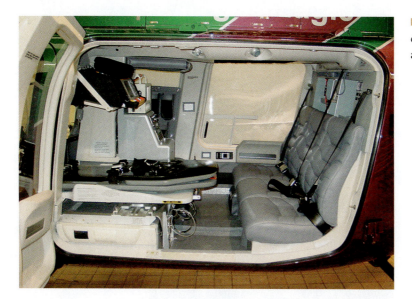

■ **Figure 3-3** LifePort configuration for rotor-wing aircraft. *(LifePort, Inc.)*

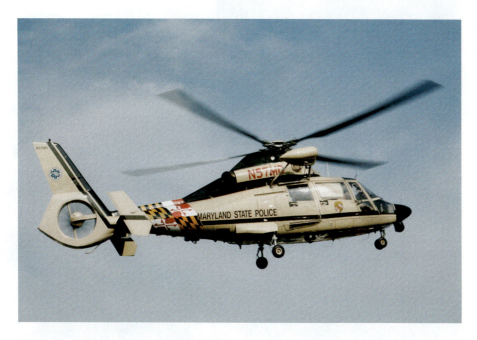

■ **Figure 3-4** Modern medical helicopters usually have responses of 100 nautical miles or less. *(© George Hall/CORBIS)*

moved between hospitals are usually seeking a higher level of care from, say, a cardiac or neurologic specialty unit that is not available where they are currently a patient. These patients are transferred to the care of a specialty physician at the receiving hospital and critical care transport is performed via an air medical helicopter. Patients picked up from a scene run are predominantly trauma victims.

ROTORCRAFT AIRFRAMES

Just as in the fire service, which has a multitude of different types of fire engines to perform different fire-related functions, there are a multitude of **rotorcraft (helicopter) airframes** available to meet the needs of the various administrative and geographical requirements. Some air medical bases may be located in very remote geographical areas that are quite distant from a tertiary care

rotorcraft (helicopter) airframes *aircraft that is kept airborne by air foils rotation, around a vertical axis.*

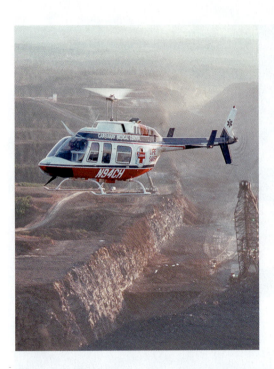

■ **Figure 3-5** Bell 206 L-4. *(Bell Helicopter Textron, Inc.)*

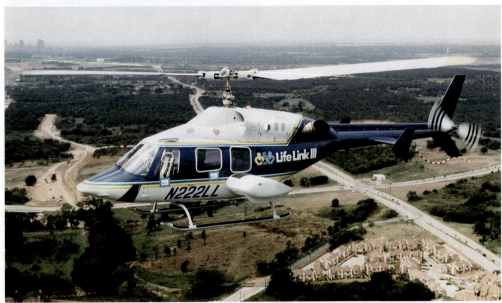

■ **Figure 3-6** Bell 222. *(Bell Helicopter Textron, Inc.)*

hospital. These areas are better served by large helicopter airframes that can cruise at high rates of speed and carry large fuel loads, which allows them to effectively complete the patient mission as rapidly as possible without having to delay for issues such as refueling. Another issue in these remote locations is the fact that if another helicopter is needed for a second patient on scene, the time spent waiting can be detrimental to the patient. Thus it is also important for the helicopter airframe to be able to easily accommodate two patient transports in the event it is required. Large airframes offer the most space for patient care. (See Figures 3-5 ■ and 3-6 ■.)

In other cases the need for such large and expensive helicopter airframes is not justified. In areas that are relatively close to tertiary care centers or in areas that have several other air medical helicopters available for multiple patient missions, smaller less expensive, more efficient helicopter airframes can be utilized. Many of these airframes are also capable of transporting two patients at a time if required, and are also often outfitted with two engines for increased safety in the event of an engine failure. (See Figures 3-7 ■ through 3-17 ■.)

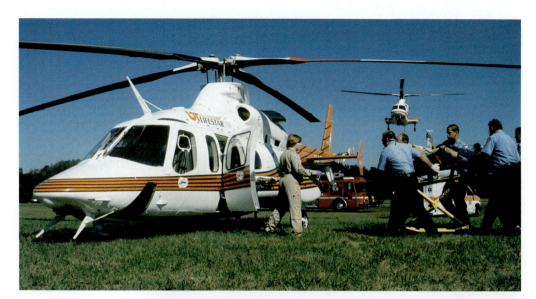

■ **Figure 3-7** Bell 430. (*Bell Helicopter Textron, Inc.*)

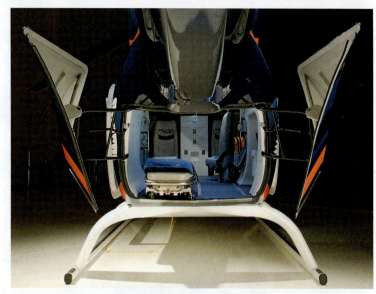

■ **Figure 3-8** Bell 429. (*Bell Helicopter Textron, Inc.*)

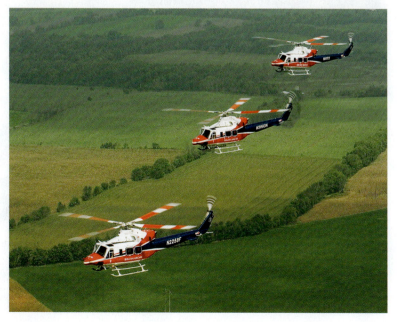

■ **Figure 3-9** Bell 412. (*Bell Helicopter Textron, Inc.*)

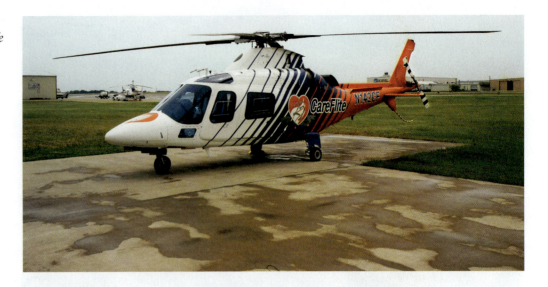

■ **Figure 3-10** Agusta 109 Power. *(© 2005 Scott Metcalfe LLC. All rights reserved)*

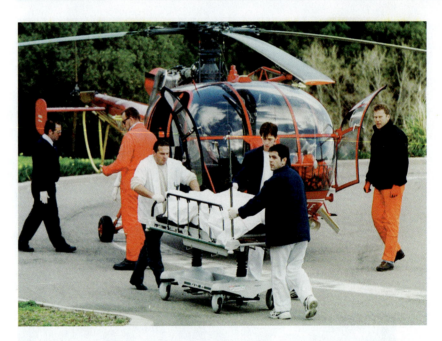

■ **Figure 3-11** Agusta 119 Koala. *(© CORBIS SYGMA)*

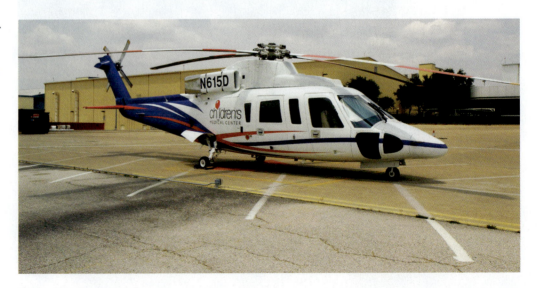

■ **Figure 3-12** Sikorsky S76. *(© 2005 Scott Metcalfe LLC. All rights reserved. Helicopter Courtesy of Children's Medical Center, Dallas)*

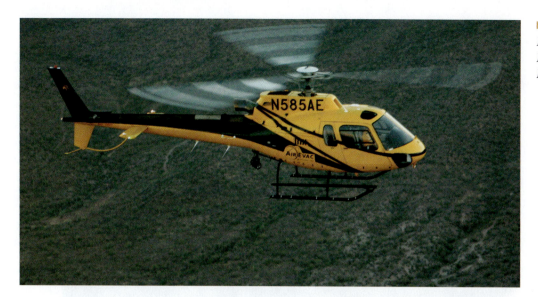

■ **Figure 3-13** AS 350 *(Air Evac Services, Inc., operated by PHI Air Medical Group Phoenix, AZ)*

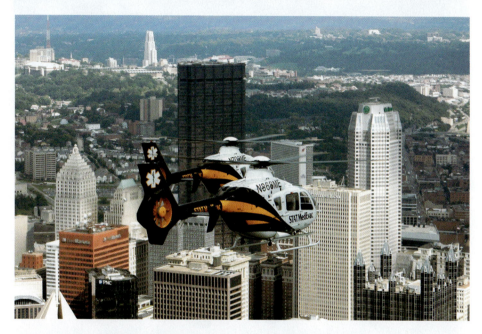

■ **Figure 3-14** Eurocopter EC 135. *(STAT MedEvac, operated by C.J. Systems Aviation Group—West Mifflin, PA)*

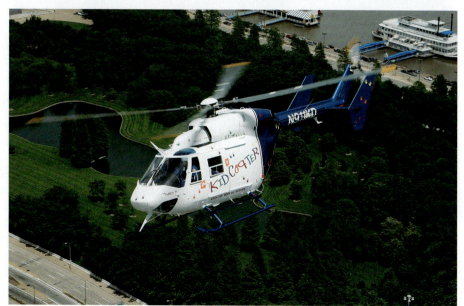

■ **Figure 3-15** Eurocopter BK 117. Aeromed Flight Program *(Aeromed Flight Program, C.J. Systems Aviation Group—Tampa, FL—photo by Gary Chisolm)*

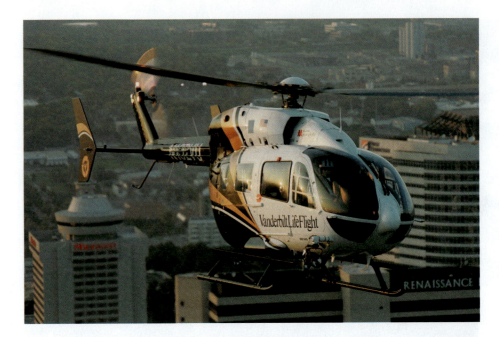

■ **Figure 3-16** Eurocopter EC 145. *(Vanderbilt LifeFlight, operated by Air Methods Corporation— Nashville, TN, photo by Mike Reyno)*

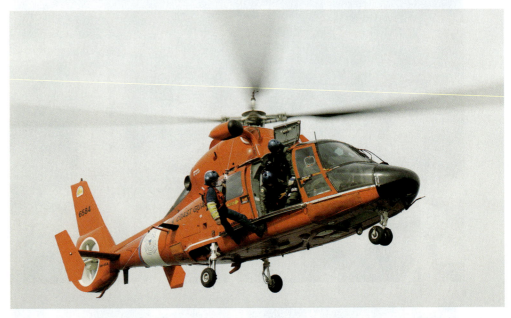

■ **Figure 3-17** Eurocopter AS 365. *(United States Coast Guard, photo by Glenn Grossman)*

Visual Flight Rules (VFR) *FAA regulations mandating minimum visual flight standards for landmark recognition, altitude variables, and weather conditions.*

Instrument Flight Rules (IFR) *FAA Regulations setting minimum standards for use of VFR in conjunction with specialized flight instruments during times of low visibility and/or poor weather.*

VFR VS. IFR

Visual Flight Rules (VFR) and **Instrument Flight Rules (IFR)** are the two modes of flying available to aircraft. All helicopters have the ability to fly VFR, while only specially equipped helicopters can fly IFR. VFR applies when the pilot can clearly see outside the aircraft, uses visual landmarks and cues for the safe operation of the aircraft, and requires the weather to meet minimum standards as outlined and mandated by the Federal Aviation Administration (FAA).

The FAA has several federal aviation regulations (FARs) that specifically define the criteria that must exist for the pilot to operate an aircraft using VFR mode. Although a full listing of the federal aviation regulations can be found on the FAA website, Table 3–2 outlines a few FARs that pertain to weather conditions, visibility, and fuel supplies. The responsibility to understand and maintain IFR or VFR certification rests squarely on the pilot's shoulders; however, it is not a bad idea for the critical care paramedic to have a basic understanding of these. Table 3–3 identifies the weather

Table 3–2	FARs That Pertain to Weather Conditions, Visibility, and Fuel Supplies

Sec. 135.203 VFR: Minimum altitudes.

- Except when necessary for takeoff and landing, no person may operate under VFR
  - (a) An airplane
    - (1) During the day, below 500 feet above the surface or less than 500 feet horizontally from any obstacle; or
    - (2) At night, at an altitude less than 1,000 feet above the highest obstacle within a horizontal distance of 5 miles from the course intended to be flown or, in designated mountainous terrain, less than 2,000 feet above the highest obstacle within a horizontal distance of 5 miles from the course intended to be flown; or
  - (b) A helicopter over a congested area at an altitude less than 300 feet above the surface.

Sec. 135.205 VFR: Visibility requirements.

- (a) No person may operate an airplane under VFR in uncontrolled airspace when the ceiling is less than 1,000 feet unless flight visibility is at least 2 miles.
- (b) No person may operate a helicopter under VFR in Class G airspace at an altitude of 1,200 feet or less above the surface or within the lateral boundaries of the surface areas of Class B, Class C, Class D, or Class E airspace designated for an airport unless the visibility is at least
  - (1) During the day—1/2 mile; or
  - (2) At night—1 mile.

Sec. 135.207: VFR: Helicopter surface reference requirements.

- No person may operate a helicopter under VFR unless that person has visual surface reference or, at night, visual surface light reference, sufficient to safely control the helicopter.

Sec. 135.209: VFR: Fuel supply.

- (a) No person may begin a flight operation in an airplane under VFR unless, considering wind and forecast weather conditions, it has enough fuel to fly to the first point of intended landing and, assuming normal cruising fuel consumption
  - (1) During the day, to fly after that for at least 30 minutes; or
  - (2) At night, to fly after that for at least 45 minutes.
- (b) No person may begin a flight operation in a helicopter under VFR unless, considering wind and forecast weather conditions, it has enough fuel to fly to the first point of intended landing and, assuming normal cruising fuel consumption, to fly after that for at least 20 minutes.

Table 3–3	Weather Guidelines Recommended by the Commission on Accreditation of Medical Transport Systems

Condition	Area	Ceiling (Feet)	Visibility (miles)
Day	Local	500	1
Day	Cross country	1,000	1
Night	Local	800	2
Night	Cross country	1,000	3

guidelines recommended by the Commission on Accreditation of Medical Transport Systems, although they acknowledge that many state regulatory agencies and aeromedical organizations establish their own standards.

Instrument Flight Rules are rules that apply when pilots use their eyesight and also aircraft instrumentation to fly and navigate safely. Generally speaking, a pilot with an IFR rating would utilize instruments to fly IFR when he cannot see the ground or when the weather conditions are less than that imposed by the FAA for VFR. Of course, this is not really that simple, and pilots must go through substantial training to become IFR certified. Furthermore, you can only fly IFR into places where an IFR approach exists (i.e., airports, hospitals). The IFR approach is a way of mapping lateral movements of the aircraft (left or right) in order to ensure that terrain or obstructions are avoided (such as ground elevations and/or mountains, buildings, trees, and wires).

The IFR approaches were initially established for fixed-wing aircraft flying between airports; however, with advancements in technology, IFR approaches now exist for many small outlying community and larger urban/teaching hospitals throughout the country, and can help safely guide IFR helicopters into these facilities. (See Figure 3-18 ■.) To complete our IFR discussion, some of the FARs that pertain to IFR flight that the critical care paramedic should be generally aware of are listed in Table 3–4.

Most aeromedical flight programs may utilize either VFR or IFR at various times during missions, depending on the weather conditions, the certification ratings of the pilot, and the capabilities of the aircraft. Beyond this, additional types of navigational aids might be at the pilot's disposal. These include the **instrument landing system (ILS), microwave landing system (MLS),** and **wide-area augmentation system with global positioning satellites (WAAS/GPS).** What these systems offer primarily beyond IFR navigation is the ability to provide information to the pilot about vertical movement of the aircraft (gaining or losing altitude), via the instruments.

Remember that it is the pilot who will make any needed decisions about the flight plan, navigation concerns, weather, and so on. The information presented here is designed merely to help orient the critical care paramedic to the more common navigational and weather concerns of the pilot; the paramedic is not expected to be responsible for these types of decisions. Simply put, the critical care paramedic does not make weather or navigation decisions, just as the pilot does not make any patient care decisions.

instrument landing system (ILS) *system that provides information to the pilot about vertical movement (that is, gaining or losing of altitude) of the aircraft via the instruments.*

microwave landing system (MLS) *system that provides information to the pilot about vertical movement (that is, gaining or losing of altitude) of the aircraft via the instruments.*

wide-area augmentation system with global positioning satellites (WAAS/GPS) *system that provides information to the pilot about vertical movement (that is, gaining or losing of altitude) of the aircraft via the instruments.*

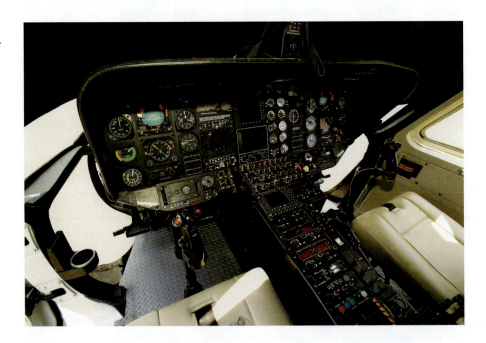

■ **Figure 3-18** Instrument panel. *(© 2005 Scott Metcalfe LLC. All rights reserved. Helicopter Courtesy of Children's Medical Center, Dallas)*

Table 3–4 Selected FARs That Pertain to IFR Flight

Sec. 135.215: IFR: Operating limitations.

- (a) Except as provided in paragraphs (b), (c) and (d) of this section, no person may operate an aircraft under IFR outside of controlled airspace or at any airport that does not have an approved standard instrument approach procedure.

- (b) The Administrator may issue operations specifications to the certificate holder to allow it to operate under IFR over routes outside controlled airspace if

  - (1) The certificate holder shows the Administrator that the flight crew is able to navigate, without visual reference to the ground, over an intended track without deviating more than 5 degrees or 5 miles, whichever is less, from that track; and

  - (2) The Administrator determines that the proposed operations can be conducted safely.

- (c) A person may operate an aircraft under IFR outside of controlled airspace if the certificate holder has been approved for the operations and that operation is necessary to

  - (1) Conduct an instrument approach to an airport for which there is in use a current approved standard or special instrument approach procedure; or

  - (2) Climb into controlled airspace during an approved missed approach procedure; or

  - (3) Make an IFR departure from an airport having an approved instrument approach procedure.

- (d) The Administrator may issue operations specifications to the certificate holder to allow it to depart at an airport that does not have an approved standard instrument approach procedure when the Administrator determines that it is necessary to make an IFR departure from that airport and that the proposed operations can be conducted safely. The approval to operate at that airport does not include an approval to make an IFR approach to that airport.

Sec. 135.217: IFR Takeoff limitations.

- No person may take off an aircraft under IFR from an airport where weather conditions are at or above takeoff minimums but are below authorized IFR landing minimums unless there is an alternate airport within 1 hour's flying time (at normal cruising speed, in still air) of the airport of departure.

Sec. 135.219: IFR Destination airport weather minimums.

- No person may take off an aircraft under IFR or begin an IFR or over-the-top operation unless the latest weather reports or forecasts, or any combination of them, indicate that weather conditions at the estimated time of arrival at the next airport of intended landing will be at or above authorized IFR landing minimums.

Sec. 135.225: IFR Takeoff, approach and landing minimums (partially described).

- (a) Except to the extent permitted by paragraph (b) of this section, no pilot may begin an instrument approach procedure to an airport unless

  - (1) That airport has a weather reporting facility operated by the U.S. National Weather Service, a source approved by U.S. National Weather Service, or a source approved by the Administrator; and

  - (2) The latest weather report issued by that weather reporting facility indicates that weather conditions are at or above the authorized IFR landing minimums for that airport.

- (b) A pilot conducting an eligible on-demand operation may begin an instrument approach procedure to an airport that does not have a weather reporting facility operated by the U.S. National Weather Service, a source approved by the U.S. National Weather Service, or a source approved by the Administrator if

  - (1) The alternate airport has a weather reporting facility operated by the U.S. National Weather Service, a source approved by the U.S. National Weather Service, or a source approved by the Administrator; and

  - (2) The latest weather report issued by the weather reporting facility includes a current local altimeter setting for the destination airport. If no local altimeter setting for the destination airport is available, the pilot may use the current altimeter setting provided by the facility designated on the approach chart for the destination airport.

(continued)

Table 3–4 | **Selected FARs That Pertain to IFR Flight** *(Continued)*

- (c) If a pilot has begun the final approach segment of an instrument approach to an airport under paragraph (b) of this section, and the pilot receives a later weather report indicating that conditions have worsened to below the minimum requirements, then the pilot may continue the approach only if the requirements of Sec. 91.175(l) of this chapter, or both of the following conditions, are met. . . .

- (f) Each pilot making an IFR takeoff or approach and landing at a military or foreign airport shall comply with applicable instrument approach procedures and weather minimums prescribed by the authority having jurisdiction over that airport. In addition, no pilot may, at that airport
  - (1) Take off under IFR when the visibility is less than 1 mile; or
  - (2) Make an instrument approach when the visibility is less than 1/2 mile.

- (i) At airports where straight-in instrument approach procedures are authorized, a pilot may take off an aircraft under IFR when the weather conditions reported by the facility described in paragraph (a)(1) of this section are equal to or better than the lowest straight-in landing minimums, unless otherwise restricted, if
  - (1) The wind direction and velocity at the time of takeoff are such that a straight-in instrument approach can be made to the runway served by the instrument approach;
  - (2) The associated ground facilities upon which the landing minimums are predicated and the related airborne equipment are in normal operation; and
  - (3) The certificate holder has been approved for such operations.

Sec. 135.227: Icing conditions operating limitations.

- (a) No pilot may take off an aircraft that has frost, ice, or snow adhering to any rotor blade, propeller, windshield, wing, stabilizing or control surface, to a powerplant installation, or to an airspeed, altimeter, rate of climb, or flight attitude instrument system, except under the following conditions:
  - (1) Takeoffs may be made with frost adhering to the wings, or stabilizing or control surfaces, if the frost has been polished to make it smooth.
  - (2) Takeoffs may be made with frost under the wing in the area of the fuel tanks if authorized by the Administrator.

- (b) No certificate holder may authorize an airplane to take off and no pilot may take off an airplane any time conditions are such that frost, ice, or snow may reasonably be expected to adhere to the airplane unless the pilot has completed all applicable training as required by Sec. 135.341 and unless one of the following requirements is met:
  - (1) A pretakeoff contamination check, that has been established by the certificate holder and approved by the Administrator for the specific airplane type, has been completed within 5 minutes prior to beginning takeoff. A pretakeoff contamination check is a check to make sure the wings and control surfaces are free of frost, ice, or snow.
  - (2) The certificate holder has an approved alternative procedure and under that procedure the airplane is determined to be free of frost, ice, or snow.
  - (3) The certificate holder has an approved deicing/anti-icing program that complies with Sec. 121.629(c) of this chapter and the takeoff complies with that program.

- (c) Except for an airplane that has ice protection provisions that meet section 34 of Appendix A, or those for transport category airplane type certification, no pilot may fly
  - (1) Under IFR into known or forecast light or moderate icing conditions; or
  - (2) Under VFR into known light or moderate icing conditions; unless the aircraft has functioning deicing or anti-icing equipment protecting each rotor blade, propeller, windshield, wing, stabilizing or control surface, and each airspeed, altimeter, rate of climb, or flight attitude instrument system.

- (d) No pilot may fly a helicopter under IFR into known or forecast icing conditions or under VFR into known icing conditions unless it has been type certificated and appropriately equipped for operations in icing conditions.

INDICATIONS FOR AIR MEDICAL TRANSPORT

The indications for patient transport by helicopter include medical emergencies, trauma emergencies, and search-and-rescue missions. The determination of whether or not the patient needs air medical transport depends on two factors. The first is the clinical status and/or the mechanism of injury, and the second is the transport time by ground vs. the arrival time and transport time of the aircraft. The following list of questions prepared by the National Association of EMS Physicians' Air Medical Task Force will help shape the ultimate decision:

Questions That Can Assist in Determining Appropriate Transport Mode (Air Versus Ground)

1. Does the patient's clinical condition require minimization of time spent out of the hospital environment during the transport?
2. Does the patient require specific or time-sensitive evaluation or treatment that is not available at the referring facility?
3. Is the patient located in an area that is inaccessible to ground transport?
4. What are the current and predicted weather situations along the transport route?
5. Is the weight of the patient (plus the weight of required equipment and transport personnel) within allowable ranges for air transport?
6. For interhospital transports, is there a helipad and/or airport near the referring hospital?
7. Does the patient require critical care life support (e.g., monitoring personnel, specific medications, specific equipment) during transport that is not available with ground transport options?
8. Would use of local ground transport leave the local area without adequate emergency medical services coverage?
9. If local ground transport is not an option, can the needs of the patient (and the system) be met by an available regional critical care ground transport service (i.e., specialized surface transport systems operated by hospitals and/or air medical programs)?

Once the decision to transport a patient by critical care providers is decided, the following guidelines should then be utilized:

General Considerations for Critical Care Transport

1. Patients requiring critical interventions should be provided those interventions in the most expeditious manner possible.
2. Patients who are stable should be transported in a manner that best addresses the needs of the patient and the system.
3. Patients with critical injuries or illnesses resulting in unstable vital signs require transport by the fastest available modality, and with a transport team that has the appropriate level of care capabilities, to a center capable of providing definitive care.
4. Patients with critical injuries or illnesses should be transported by a team that can provide intratransport critical care services.
5. Patients who require high-level care during transport, but do not have time-critical illness or injury, may be candidates for ground critical care transport (i.e., by a specialized ground critical care transport vehicle with level of care exceeding that of local EMS) if such service is available and logistically feasible.

In trauma, the indications for helicopter transport are similar to the indications for trauma center care. These criteria include both mechanism of injury and physiological criteria. However, recent studies have found that mechanism of injury criteria are poor predictors of which patients will benefit from trauma center care and helicopter transport.

Limited research is available that specifically supports when to utilize, or when not to utilize, critical care transport services. It is almost certain though that, with time, critical care transport research will reveal more concrete indicators for making that choice. Until that time, transport of patients with nontraumatic emergencies is limited to logistical considerations, clinical judgment, and medical oversight in determining whether primary air transport is appropriate for such patients.

The National Association of EMS Physicians (NAEMSP) has collaborated with the Air Medical Physician Association (AMPA) and the Association of Air Medical Services (AAMS) to produce the most comprehensive guidelines for guiding decisions for air medical dispatch (for both trauma, interfacilility, and nontrauma). These recommendations are listed here:

★ General trauma and mechanism of injury considerations
   a. Trauma score <12
   b. Unstable vital signs (e.g., hypotension or tachypnea)
   c. Significant trauma in patients <12 years old, >55 years old, or pregnant patients
   d. Multisystem injuries (e.g., long-bone fractures in different extremities; injury to more than two body regions)
   e. Ejection from vehicle
   f. Pedestrian or cyclist struck by motor vehicle
   g. Death in same passenger compartment as patient
   h. Ground provider perception of significant damage to patient's passenger compartment
   i. Penetrating trauma to the abdomen, pelvis, chest, neck, or head
   j. Crush injury to the abdomen, chest, or head
   k. Fall from significant height

★ Neurologic considerations
   a. Glasgow Coma Scale score <10
   b. Deteriorating mental status
   c. Skull fracture
   d. Neurologic presentation suggestive of spinal cord injury

★ Thoracic considerations
   a. Major chest wall injury (e.g., flail chest)
   b. Pneumothorax/hemothorax
   c. Suspected cardiac injury

★ Abdominal/pelvic considerations
   a. Significant abdominal pain after blunt trauma
   b. Presence of a "seat belt" sign or other abdominal wall contusion
   c. Obvious rib fracture below the nipple line
   d. Major pelvic fracture (e.g., unstable pelvic ring disruption, open pelvic fracture, or pelvic fracture with hypotension)

★ Orthopedic/extremity considerations
   a. Partial or total amputation of a limb (exclusive of digits)
   b. Finger/thumb amputation when emergent surgical evaluation (i.e., replantation consideration) is indicated and rapid surface transport is not available
   c. Fracture or dislocation with vascular compromise
   d. Extremity ischemia
   e. Open long-bone fractures
   f. Two or more long-bone fractures

★ Major burns
   a. >20% body surface area
   b. Involvement of face, head, hands, feet, or genitalia
   c. Inhalational injury

d. Electrical or chemical burns

e. Burns with associated injuries

★ Patients with near-drowning injuries

Clinical situations for air transport and interfacility transfers are best summarized as being present when patients have diagnostic and/or therapeutic needs that cannot be met at the referring hospital; and when factors such as time, distance, and/or intratransport level of care requirements render ground transport unfeasible.

The following are the NAEMSP recommendations for dispatching a critical care transport crew for interfacility missions (Thomson, 2003):

Trauma: Injured patients constitute the diagnostic group for which there is best evidence to support outcome improvements from air transport.

★ Depending on local hospital capabilities and regional practices, any diagnostic consideration (suspected, or confirmed as with referring hospital radiography) may be sufficient indication for air transport from a community hospital to a regional trauma center.

★ Additionally, air transport (short or long distance) may be appropriate when initial evaluation at the community hospital reveals injuries (e.g., intra-abdominal hemorrhage on abdominal computed tomography) or potential injuries (e.g., aortic trauma suggested by widened mediastinum on chest X-ray; spinal column injury with potential for spinal cord involvement) requiring further evaluation and management beyond the capabilities of the referring hospital.

Cardiac: Due to regionalization of cardiac care and the time criticality of the disease process, patients with cardiac diagnoses often undergo interfacility air transport. Patients with the following cardiac conditions may be candidates for air transport:

★ Acute coronary syndromes with time-critical need for urgent interventional therapy (e.g., cardiac catheterization, intra-aortic balloon pump placement, emergent cardiac surgery) unavailable at the referring center

★ Cardiogenic shock (especially in presence of, or need for, ventricular assist devices or intra-aortic balloon pumps)

★ Cardiac tamponade with impending hemodynamic compromise

★ Mechanical cardiac disease (e.g., acute cardiac rupture, decompensating valvular heart disease)

Critically ill medical or surgical patients: These patients generally require high level of care during transport, may benefit from minimization of out-of-hospital transport time, and may also have time-critical need for diagnostic or therapeutic intervention at the receiving facility. Ground critical care transport is frequently a viable transfer option for these patients, but air transport may be considered in circumstances such as the following examples:

★ Pretransport cardiac/respiratory arrest

★ Requirement for continuous intravenous vasoactive medications or mechanical ventricular assist to maintain stable cardiac output

★ Risk for airway deterioration (e.g., angioedema, epiglottitis)

★ Acute pulmonary failure and/or requirement for sophisticated pulmonary intensive care during transport

★ Severe poisoning or overdose requiring specialized toxicology services

★ Urgent need for hyperbaric oxygen therapy (e.g., vascular gas embolism, necrotizing infectious process, carbon monoxide toxicity)

★ Requirement for emergent dialysis

★ Gastrointestinal hemorrhages with hemodynamic compromise

★ Surgical emergencies such as fasciitis, aortic dissection or aneurysm, or extremity ischemia

★ Pediatric patients for whom referring facilities cannot provide required evaluation and/or therapy

Obstetric: In gravid patients, air transport's advantage of minimized out-of-hospital time must be balanced against the risks inherent to intratransport delivery. If transport is necessary in a patient in whom delivery is thought to be imminent, then a ground vehicle is usually appropriate, although in some cases the combination of clinical status and logistics (e.g., long driving times) may favor use of an air ambulance. Air transport may be considered if ground transport is logistically not feasible and/or there are circumstances, such as the following:

★ Reasonable expectation that delivery of infant(s) may require obstetric or neonatal care beyond the capabilities of the referring hospital

★ Active premature labor when estimated gestational age is <34 weeks or estimated fetal weight <2,000 grams

★ Severe preeclampsia or eclampsia (pregnancy induced hypertension)

★ Third-trimester hemorrhage

★ Fetal hydrops

★ Maternal medical conditions (e.g., heart disease, drug overdose, metabolic disturbances) exist that may cause premature birth

★ Severe predicted fetal heart disease

★ Acute abdominal emergencies (i.e., likely to require surgery) when estimated gestational age is <34 weeks or estimated fetal weight <2,000 grams

Neurological: In addition to those with need for specialized neurosurgical services, this category is being expanded to include patients requiring transfer to specialized stroke centers. Examples of neurological conditions where air transport may be appropriate include:

★ Central nervous system hemorrhage

★ Spinal cord compression by mass lesion

★ Evolving ischemic stroke (i.e., potential candidate for lytic therapy)

★ Status epilepticus

Neonatal: Regionalization of neonatal intensive care has prompted the development of specialized (air and/or ground) services focusing on transport for this population. Given the fact that, in neonates, rapid transport is often less of a priority than (time-consuming) stabilization at referring institutions, some systems have found that the best means for incorporating air vehicles into neonatal transport is to use them to rapidly get a stabilization/transport team to the patient; the actual patient transport is then performed by a ground vehicle. In some systems, patients are transported (usually with a specialized neonatal team) by air when the ground transport out-of-hospital time exceeds 30 minutes. Examples of instances where air medical dispatch may be appropriate for neonates include:

★ Gestational age <30 weeks, body weight <2,000 grams, or complicated neonatal course (e.g., perinatal cardiac/respiratory arrest, hemodyamic instability, sepsis, meningitis, metabolic derangement, temperature instability)

★ Requirement for supplemental oxygen exceeding 60%, continuous positive airway pressure (CPAP), or mechanical ventilation

★ Extrapulmonary air leak, interstitial emphysema, or pneumothorax

★ Medical emergencies such as seizure activity, congestive heart failure, or disseminated intravascular coagulation

★ Surgical emergencies such as diaphragmatic hernia, necrotizing enterocolitis, abdominal wall defects, intussusception, suspected volvulus, or congenital heart defects

Other: Air medical dispatch may also be appropriate in miscellaneous situations such as the following:

★ Transplant
  ▪ Patient has met criteria for brain death and air transport is necessary for organ salvage
  ▪ Organ and/or organ recipient requires air transport to the transplant center in order to maintain viability of time-critical transplant

★ Search-and-rescue operations are generally outside the purview of air medical transport services, but in some instances helicopter EMS may participate in such operations. Since most search-and-rescue services have limited medical care capabilities, and since most air medical programs have similarly limited search-and-rescue training, cooperative effort is necessary for optimizing patient location, extrication, stabilization, and transport.

★ Patients known to be in cardiac arrest are rarely candidates for air medical transport.
  ▪ NAEMSP's Air Medical Task Force published previously (2000) regarding situations in which resuscitation efforts should be ceased in the field for adult nontraumatic cardiac arrest victims. In such cases air transport should not be considered an alternative to discontinuing (futile) efforts at resuscitation.
  ▪ In situations where patients are in cardiac arrest and do not meet local criteria for cessation of resuscitative efforts, or in jurisdictions in which prehospital providers cannot cease such efforts, air transport is an option only in very rare cases (e.g., pediatric cold-water drowning where helicopter transport to a cardiac bypass center is considered).

ADVANTAGES AND DISADVANTAGES OF AIR MEDICAL TRANSPORT

Air medical transport offers a number of advantages and disadvantages. The advantages include much more rapid transport speed, access to remote locations, access to specialty teams (e.g., neonate, transplant, burn centers), and access to personnel with specialized skills such as surgical airway, thoracotomy, RSI, hemodynamic, and critical care experience. The disadvantages include weather and environmental restrictions on flying. Depending on the size of the aircraft, there may also be limitations on the number of crew members that can care for the patient, or limitations to the physical size of the patient. Again, the NAEMSP Air Medical Task Force has provided guidance as to the benefits and limitations of air medical transport (Thomson, 2003):

★ Comparative considerations for air transport modes
  – Rotor-wing
    ▪ Advantages
      • In general, decreased response time to the patient (up to approximately 100 miles distance depending on logistics such as duration of ground transfer leg)
      • Decreased out-of-hospital transport time
      • Availability of highly trained medical crews and specialized equipment
    ▪ Disadvantages
      • Weather considerations (e.g., icing conditions, weather minimums)
      • Limited availability as compared with ground EMS
  – Fixed-wing
    ▪ Advantages
      • In comparison with rotor wing, decreased response time to patients when transport distances exceed approximately 100 miles

- In comparison with ground transport, decreased out-of-hospital transport time
- Availability of highly trained medical crews and specialized equipment
- In comparison with rotor wing, less susceptibility to weather constraints
  - Disadvantages
    - Requires landing at airport, with two extra transport legs between airports and the patient origin and destination
    - In comparison with ground transport, more subject to weather-related unavailability (e.g., icing, snow)
    - Overall, less desirable as a transport mode for severely ill or injured patients (though extenuating circumstances may modify this relative contraindication to fixed-wing use)

PATIENT PACKAGING FOR TRANSPORT

Preparation for the transport of the air medical patient may vary slightly from the transport of the ground advanced life support or basic life support patient. Usually in the instance of the air medical patient, more equipment is needed to meet the needs of the critically ill or injured patient. This requires setting up and having the equipment in an organized fashion so that it can be accessed when needed. This includes securing hoses, wires, and so on—by coiling up the unneeded length and securing it with tape. This procedure prevents the hoses and wires from being trapped by the stretcher, tangling up, wrapping around crew legs, or from being accidentally cut by sheers. Another important factor is that some of the equipment must be stowed in compartments that are only accessible from the outside of the aircraft. In these cases it is imperative to move the needed equipment into the aircraft before departure, or you may end up delaying transport if you have to land and retrieve the equipment.

Another packaging concern is to protect the aircraft from the need for costly and timely decontamination. This is done by wrapping the patient in a fluid holding material to keep blood and other body fluids from leaking into the aircraft. This foil wrap also protects the patient from environmental elements such as rain, wind, and extreme cold.

Other packaging considerations may need to be considered depending on the specific type of airframe utilized including ear (hearing) protection for the patient, and explaining thoroughly to the patient what to expect. If the airframe has a small patient compartment, the girth or length of the patient may become a factor. In these instances the flight company will provide you with specific information on specialty patient packaging.

SPECIAL CONSIDERATIONS

Aircraft used for medevac purposes are granted special privileges by the FAA regarding flights. One of these privileges is being able to request preferential right-of-way in traffic lanes (over other commercial and industry flight traffic) if they are transporting a patient. They even have the right to request the right-of-way when competing for air traffic lanes with aircraft carrying high-ranking political dignitaries (such as Air Force One). However, 9/11 caused a heightened sensitivity regarding air traffic that the critical care paramedic should be cognizant of. For example, if a high-ranking political figure is within your geographic flight response area, the pilot may have to request a special code or designation from the air traffic control tower prior to lift off. This way, when your aircraft is detected by the radar system, the traffic controller will know you are on a medevac mission. Any unidentified aircraft in the same airspace as the dignitary will likely be met by a military fighter jet.

Another special consideration comes into play when dealing with international flights. It is a requirement for almost all flight programs that each member of the flight crew have a valid passport with him or her at all times. This allows for completion of international missions that are occasionally set up so as to return a citizen to the United States or to bring a foreigner to the United States in order to receive some special medical care. Along these lines, you also need to be cognizant of the various countries and cultures you may encounter. For example, in many Middle Eastern countries a female critical care paramedic cannot care for a Middle Eastern male patient. And for missions that are flown into countries with significant amounts of civil unrest, it is not unheard of for medevac transports to be met at the airport by an armored caravan of vehicles that will transport the team to the patient. Although these are only two examples, the critical care paramedic will learn that there is as much variance to cultures as there are countries and different nationalities. It is the responsibility of the critical care paramedic to stay abreast of significant cultural norms that may be encountered while flying international missions. Fortunately, most international flights are scheduled with a few days of lead time, which will allow the critical care paramedic a chance to research any such concerns.

Summary

This chapter was designed to provide the critical care transport candidate with general information on air medical transport. Every air medical provider operates its organization in a slightly different manner and utilizes slightly different airframes and medical equipment. This chapter covered the basic structure of air medical administration and communications, as well as the basic airframes.

Review Questions

1. What are the main functions of the program director?
2. What are the primary functions of the medical director?
3. What are the advantages of air medical transport?
4. What are the clinical indications for calling for air medical transport?
5. What are the mechanisms of injury indications for calling for air medical transport?
6. What is IFR, and how does it differ from VFR?
7. When is fixed-wing air medical transport utilized?
8. What are the primary functions of the communications center?

See Answers to Review Questions at the back of this book.

Further Reading

Bailey ED, Wydro GC, Cone DC. "Termination of resuscitation in the prehospital setting for adult patients suffering nontraumatic cardiac arrest." *Prehospital Emergency Care,* Vol. 4 (2000): 190–195.

Federal Aviation Administration. http://www.faa.gov/ (last updated March 4, 2005).

Thomas SH. *Aeromedical Transport.* http://www.emedicine.com/emerg/topic717.htm (last updated June 2004).

Thomson DP. *Guidelines for Aeromedical Dispatch.* National Association of EMS Physicians, Air Medical Task Force report. *Prehospital Emergency Care,* Vol. 7, No. 2 (April/June 2003): 265–271.

Altitude Physiology

Larry Johnson, NREMT-P, CCT, FP-C, and Bryan Bledsoe, DO, FACEP

Objectives

Upon completion of this chapter, the student should be able to:

1. Detail the various atmospheric levels and the characteristics of each. (p. 50)
2. Detail the three physiologically important atmospheric zones. (p. 51)
3. Define and describe the significance of the following gas laws:
   ★ Dalton's law (p. 53)
   ★ Boyle's law (p. 53)
   ★ Charles' law (p. 55)
   ★ Gay-Lussac's law (p. 56)
   ★ Henry's law (p. 57)
   ★ Graham's law (p. 57)
   ★ Fick's law (p. 58)
   ★ Avogadro's law (p. 58)
   ★ Ideal gas law (p. 59)
4. Discuss the stressors of altitude and flight including:
   ★ Hypoxia (p. 60)
   ★ Barometric pressure (p. 62)
   ★ Fatigue (p. 63)
   ★ Thermal (p. 63)
   ★ Dehydration (p. 63)
   ★ Noise (p. 64)
   ★ Vibration (p. 64)
   ★ Gravitational forces (p. 64)
   ★ Third spacing (p. 66)
   ★ Spatial disorientation (p. 67)
   ★ Flicker vertigo (p. 67)

5. List the four types of hypoxia. (p. 60)
6. Detail the signs and symptoms of hypoxia. (p. 61)
7. Describe the effective performance time. (p. 62)
8. Describe the time of useful consciousness. (p. 62)
9. Discuss the pathophysiology and treatment of high-altitude pulmonary edema. (p. 68)
10. Describe problems associated with altitude with which the critical care paramedic must be familiar. (p. 68)
11. Discuss the pathophysiology and treatment of high-altitude cerebral edema. (p. 69)
12. Understand the consequences should there be a rapid decompression of the aircraft cabin at altitude. (p. 69)
13. Discuss preventative measures the critical care paramedic can employ in order to reduce the effects of stressors that may occur during flight. (p. 73)

Key Terms

Case Study

You are taking off in a fixed-wing aircraft with a cardiac patient who is being flown across the United States to a cardiac facility in his home state. The patient who was vacationing on the East Coast, suffered a severe myocardial infarction and was initially hospitalized locally. Now, days later, at the request of the patient, his attending physician has arranged transport back to his home state for continuing management and rehabilitation.

You have the patient securely in place on the cot, in a semi-Fowler's position with the head in an aft location to help pool blood in the thorax during the gravitational (G) forces encountered during takeoff. You and your partner belt yourself in beside the patient. You set the patient's chart in your lap so you can continue to review it during takeoff, and you prepare for flight.

As the aircraft taxis toward the runway, the patient turns to you and says, "Back in the war, I used to hate flying . . . ears always hurt, it was loud, cold many times, and noisy. . . . I just never got used to it." You pause from your task of properly securing the infusion pump that is running his IV line and medications and tell him that there have been great strides in aviation technology, so you believe that he will find this flight home much more enjoyable than the missions he was involved with back in his day during the war.

You quickly calculate whether any FiO_2 adjustments will need to be made to his oxygen administration once the aircraft reaches altitude and the cabin is pressurized. Although the cabin is pressurized at 8,000 feet, you recall that the concentration of oxygen decreases as you ascend above sea level, as defined by Boyle's law.

You have just reached altitude with the patient en route to his home state for continued care closer to home. The takeoff was uneventful, and the patient is resting comfortably on the cot. You unbuckle your belt so you can gain better access to the patient as you complete another assessment of him to ensure stability.

Following this, and noting that there are no indications of acute clinical deterioration, you turn your attention to the medical equipment employed in his care. You reevaluate the infusion pump to ensure that the correct flow for the heparin is maintained, the oxygen administration is fine, and the patient's pulse oximetry reading is 97%. The patient does not have a central line nor is he intubated, so there are no concerns about cuff overpressure.

The flight progresses without any remarkable change in the patient's medical condition. You and the patient converse about many topics during the 4-hour flight, and you prepare him for landing as the pilot-in-command starts the final descent. Upon landing, the patient is transferred without incident to a waiting paramedic unit and the aircraft is refueled. You and the other members of the crew grab a quick meal and prepare for the flight home.

INTRODUCTION

Air medical transport must be carried out as safely and expeditiously as possible. The critical care paramedic must have in-depth knowledge of altitude physiology in order to provide optimal patient care. Oftentimes, critical care patients are already compromised by their illness or injury. Thus, the additional stress of air medical transport can often exacerbate an already serious situation. To avoid this, the critical care paramedic must have a thorough understanding of the gas laws and the physiological responses of the human body to changing altitude.

THE ATMOSPHERE

atmosphere (earth) *the gas cloud surrounding earth.*

The atmosphere is essential for survival of life as we know it on the earth.

Weather is primarily located in the troposphere.

The earth's **atmosphere** can be thought of as an ocean of gases that extends from the earth's surface to space. It is composed primarily of nitrogen, oxygen, argon, and trace gases. The atmosphere consists of readily identifiable layers. These layers have unique physical characteristics. The layers of the atmosphere, beginning at the earth's surface, and moving outward are:

★ *Troposphere* (from surface to 5 to 9 miles high)
★ *Stratosphere* (from troposphere to 31 miles high)
★ *Mesosphere* (from stratosphere to 53 miles high)
★ *Thermosphere* (from mesosphere to 372 miles high)

Weather occurs in the troposphere. Beyond this discussion, the critical care paramedic will not find himself involved in using this type of information in critical care decision making. However, in the field of aerospace medicine, the human's physiological response to the environment is of primary concern. Based on research into the physiological responses of the human, the atmosphere can be divided into three zones: the *physiological zone*, the *physiologically deficient zone*, and the *space-equivalent zone*.

PHYSIOLOGICAL ZONE

The **physiologic zone** is the atmospheric zone in which the human body is well adapted. The oxygen level within this zone is sufficient to allow a normal, healthy individual to survive without the aid of special protective equipment. The changes in pressure encountered with rapid ascents or descents within this zone can produce ear or sinus trapped-gas problems. However, these are relatively minor when compared to the physiological impairments encountered at higher altitudes.

PHYSIOLOGICALLY DEFICIENT ZONE

The **physiologically deficient zone** extends from 10,000 feet to 50,000 feet. Here, noticeable physiological deficits begin to occur. The decreased barometric pressure in this zone results in a reduced oxygen deficiency sufficient to cause hypoxia. In addition, problems may arise from trapped and evolved gases. Protective oxygen equipment is necessary in this zone. The critical care paramedic, when participating in fixed-wing aircraft missions, often enters this level (commonly 5,000 to 15,000 feet although jet aircraft may fly as high as 25,000 to 35,000 feet (see Table 4–1).

SPACE-EQUIVALENT ZONE

Physiologically, space is considered to be reached at 50,000 feet, at which point it is called the **space-equivalent zone**. Here, even with the use of 100% supplemental oxygen, there is no protection from hypoxia. The only true protections at these altitudes are pressure suits and sealed cabins. The only additional physiological problems occurring within this zone, which extends from 50,000 feet to 120 miles, are possible radiation effects and the boiling of body fluids (ebullism) in an unprotected individual. Boiling of body fluids will occur when the total barometric pressure is less than the vapor pressure of water, which is reached at an altitude of 63,500 feet (Armstrong's line).

GAS PHYSICS AND PHYSIOLOGY

Since the earth's atmosphere is gaseous, it is important for critical care paramedics to have an understanding of gases and their behaviors. With the exception of plasma, gas is the most disorganized of the four states of matter (solids, liquids, gas, and plasma). Gases share several common properties:

★ Gas molecules are in constant, rapid motion (referred to as *diffusion*).

★ Gas molecules are separated by relatively large distances (on a molecular scale). Because of this, they have much smaller densities than either liquids or solids. In addition, they are compressible and mix readily with one another to form a solution.

★ Gas has neither volume nor shape. Instead, it expands to occupy the available volume and take the shape of the container holding it.

★ Gas molecules collide with the walls of the container holding them, thus producing pressure.

PRESSURE

The pressure of a gas is measured as force *per unit area* and can be represented by the following formula:

$$\text{Pressure (Newtons/meter}^2) = \frac{\text{Force (Newtons)}}{\text{Area (meter}^2)}$$

The greater the unit area, the less the pressure. The less the unit area, the greater the pressure. The pressure unit (N/m^2) is also called a *pascal* (Pa). Although this is the accepted unit for pressure in

physiologic zone *the atmospheric zone in which oxygen levels are sufficient to sustain a normal, healthy individual—up to 10,000 feet above sea level.*

physiologically deficient zone *the atmospheric zone in which barometric pressure is decreased, trapping evolved gases potentially harmful to humans, and causing hypoxia—10,000 to 15,000 feet above sea level.*

space-equivalent zone *the atmospheric zone, sometimes referred to as "space," beginning at 50,000 feet above sea level. Human survival requires the use of pressure suits, self-contained oxygen systems, sealed cabins, and a heat source.*

With the exception of plasma, gas is the most disorganized form of matter.

Table 4-1 | The Earth's Atmosphere

Altitude	Barometric Pressure (mm Hg)	PSI	Temperature (degrees C)
00000	760	14.70	+15.0
01000	733	14.17	+13.0
02000	706	13.67	+11.0
03000	681	13.17	+9.1
04000	656	12.69	+7.1
05000	632	12.23	+5.1
06000	609	11.78	+3.1
07000	586	11.34	+1.1
08000	565	10.92	−0.9
09000	542	10.51	−2.8
10000	523	10.11	−4.8
11000	503	9.72	−6.8
12000	483	9.35	−8.8
13000	465	8.98	−10.8
14000	447	8.63	−12.7
15000	429	8.29	−14.7
16000	412	7.97	−16.7
17000	396	7.65	−18.7
18000	380	7.34	−20.7
19000	364	7.04	−22.6
20000	349	6.75	−24.6
21000	335	6.48	−26.6
22000	321	6.21	−28.6
23000	308	5.95	−30.6
24000	295	5.70	−32.6
25000	282	5.45	−34.5
26000	270	5.22	−36.5
27000	258	4.99	−38.5
28000	247	4.78	−40.5
29000	236	4.57	−42.5
30000	228	4.36	−44.4
32000	206	3.98	−48.4
34000	188	3.63	−52.4
36000	171	3.30	−56.3

the SI system of measurement, it is rarely used because it is so small. Since anything with mass exerts a force as a result of gravitational pull, the gases in the earth's atmosphere produce a force as well. This force is spread over the surface area of the earth and is called **atmospheric pressure.** Since this pressure is usually measured using a barometer, it is sometimes called *barometric pressure.* For example, atmospheric pressure is approximately 101.3 kilopascals (kPa). Thus, a more convenient unit of measurement is the atmosphere (atm). Standard atmospheric pressure at sea level is equal to 1 atm. Here are some equivalencies between pressure units:

$$1 \text{ atm} = 760 \text{ mmHg} = 760 \text{ torr} = 101.325 \text{ kPa} = 29.92 \text{ inches Hg} = 14.7 \text{ lb/in.}^2 = 1.01325 \text{ bar}$$

atmospheric pressure
pressure on the earth and its inhabitants, caused by the weight of atmospheric gases in conjunction with gravity.

GAS MIXTURES

The four principal gases that impact aviation medicine are oxygen, nitrogen, carbon dioxide, and water vapor. The principal function of respiration is to transport oxygen to the tissues and to transport carbon dioxide back to the lungs. This process is accomplished by ventilatory effort that moves gases through the respiratory tract and into the alveoli, allowing the gases within the alveoli and pulmonary capillary bed to exchange. This process can be adversely affected by changes in altitude.

In medicine, pressure is usually measured in mmHg, torr, or atm.

DALTON'S LAW

Because pressure is the constant impact of gas molecules against a surface, the pressure of the gas acting on the surface is the sum of all gas molecules striking the surface at any given instant. Thus, pressure is directly proportional to the concentration of gas molecules. In a mixed gas solution, such as atmospheric air, the pressure is proportional to the pressure caused by each gas alone. This is called the *partial pressure* of that gas. Stated another way, the total pressure of a mixture of gases equals the sum of the pressures that each would exert if it were present by itself and can be represented by the following formula:

$$P_t = P_1 + P_2 + P_3 + \ldots$$

where P_t is the total pressure of a sample that contains a mixture of gases. The P_1, P_2, P_3, and so on, are the partial pressures of the gases in the mixture. This phenomenon is referred to as **Dalton's law,** which states that the total pressure in a container is the sum of the partial pressures of all the gases in the container. Dalton maintained that since there was an enormous amount of space between the gas molecules within the mixture, the gas molecules did not have any influence on the motion of other gas molecules. Thus, the pressure of a gas sample would be the same whether it was the only gas in the container or if it were among other gases. This assumption that molecules act independently of one another works fine as long as there is a lot of space between gas molecules in the mixture and the temperature is not too low. Lowering the temperature and/or compressing the gas will upset that assumption.

Dalton's law *the total pressure in a container is the sum of the partial pressures of all the gases in the container.*

The total pressure of a mixture of gases equals the sum of the pressures that each would exert if it were present by itself.

The partial pressure of a gas can be calculated using the following formula:

$$P_A = X_A \times P$$

where P_A is the pressure of gas A, X_A is the mole fraction of gas A, and P is the total pressure of the mixture. In medicine, we usually use percentage of gas present in the mixture instead of the mole fraction (which is essentially the same thing). For example, the percentage of oxygen in air at sea level is 20.95%, which is usually rounded to 21%. To calculate the partial pressure of oxygen,

$$PO_2 = 0.21 \times 760 \text{ mmHg}$$

Thus,

$$PO_2 = 159.6 \text{ mmHg}$$

The specific composition of the dry atmosphere is presented in Table 4–2. The percentage of each gas present is referred to as the *partial pressure* of that gas.

BOYLE'S LAW

The volume of a gas is directly related to its pressure (assuming the temperature is constant). Thus, as the pressure goes up, the volume goes down. Likewise, as the volume increases, the pressure decreases. **Boyle's law** states that the volume of a gas is inversely proportional to its pressure (assuming temperature remains constant). This means that at 18,000 feet, where the pressure is approximately half that of sea level, a given volume of gas will attempt to expand to twice its initial

The volume of a gas is directly related to its pressure.

Boyle's law *The volume of a gas is inversely proportional to its pressure, assuming temperature remains constant.*

Table 4-2	Composition of the Dry Atmosphere at Sea Level	
Gas	Pressure (mmHg)	Partial Pressure
Nitrogen	593.408	78.08
Oxygen	159.22	20.95
Argon	7.144	0.94
Carbon dioxide	0.288	0.03
Neon	0.013	0.0018
Helium	0.003	0.0005
TOTAL	**760**	**100**

volume in order to achieve equilibrium with the surrounding pressure at that altitude. Or in simple terms, the higher the altitude, the more the gas expands. As an aircraft ascends, the volume of air or gas in a closed space within the patient or equipment can increase, because the external pressure is decreasing. The reverse is true when the aircraft descends. A pressurized aircraft can significantly minimize these effects.

Boyle's law is sometimes used to determine the volume that a gas would have at another pressure and is reflected in the following formula:

$$P_1 V_1 = P_2 V_2$$

where P is the pressure of the gas and V is the volume of the container holding the gas. For example, a sample of gas collected in a 350-cm^3 container exerts a pressure of 103 kPa. What would be the volume of this gas at 150 kPa of pressure (assuming that the temperature remains constant)?

$$P_1 V_1 = P_2 V_2$$

First, list what is given and what is unknown.

$$P_1 = 103 \text{ kPa}$$
$$V_1 = 350 \text{ cm}^3$$
$$P_2 = 150 \text{ kPa}$$
$$V_2 = ?$$

Next, predict what should happen. The pressure is going up by nearly one-third, thus the volume should go down by approximately one-third.

Algebraically adjust the original formula to isolate the unknown, solve, and round to the correct number of significant digits:

$$P_1 V_1 = P_2 V_2$$
$$\frac{P_1 V_1}{P_2} = \frac{P_2 V_2}{P_2}$$
$$V_2 = \frac{P_1 V_1}{P_2}$$

$$P_1 = 103 \text{ kPa}$$
$$V_1 = 350 \text{ cm}^3$$
$$P_2 = 150 \text{ kPa}$$
$$V_2 = ?$$

$$V_2 = \frac{103 \text{ kPa} \times 350 \text{ cm}^3}{150 \text{ kPa}}$$
$$V_2 = 240.333333 \text{ cm}^3$$
$$V_2 = 240 \text{ cm}^3$$

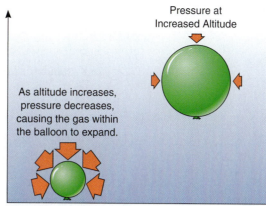

Pressure at
Increased Altitude

As altitude increases,
pressure decreases,
causing the gas within
the balloon to expand.

Pressure at sea level

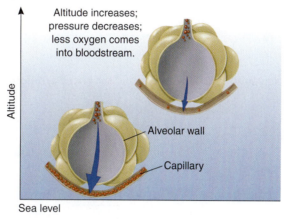

Altitude increases;
pressure decreases;
less oxygen comes
into bloodstream.

Altitude

Alveolar wall

Capillary

Sea level

Oxygen passes through alveolar wall into bloodstream

Check to see that the results match your prediction. The volume did go down by close to one-third. (See Figures 4-1 ■ and 4-2 ■.)

CHARLES' LAW

Charles' law states that the volume of a quantity of gas, held at constant pressure, varies directly with the temperature. Molecular motion (heat) increases with the temperature of the gas. Gases expand as they are heated and contract when they are cooled. In other words, as the temperature of a sample of gas at constant pressure increases, the volume increases. As the temperature goes down, the volume decreases as well. The mathematical expression for Charles' law is as follows:

Charles' law *The volume of a quantity of gas, held at constant pressure, varies directly with the temperature of said gas.*

$$\frac{V_1}{T_1} = \frac{V_2}{T_2}$$

where V is the volume of the gas and T is the temperature (in Kelvins). The following example details Charles' law: A 250 cm³ sample of nitrogen is collected at 44.0 °C. Assuming the pressure remains constant, what would be the volume of the neon at standard temperature? To solve, first change the Celsius temperature to Kelvin:

K = °C + 273

K = 44.0 °C + 273

K = 317

Now list the given quantities and the unknown:

$$T_1 = 317 \text{ K}$$
$$V_1 = 250 \text{ cm}^3$$
$$T_2 = 273 \text{ K (standard temperature in Kelvins)}$$
$$V_2 = ?$$

Now predict the results. The temperature is going down, so the volume must go down as well.

$$\frac{V_1}{T_1} = \frac{V_2}{T_2}$$

Algebraically, adjust the original formula to isolate the unknown, solve, and round to the correct number of significant digits:

$$\frac{T_2 \times V_1}{T_1} = \frac{V_2 \times \cancel{T_2}}{\cancel{T_2}}$$
$$V_2 = \frac{T_2 \times V_1}{T_2}$$

Now substitute, solve, and round to correct significant digits.

$$T_1 = 317 \text{ K}$$
$$V_1 = 250 \text{ cm}^3$$
$$T_2 = 273 \text{ K (standard temperature in Kelvins)}$$
$$V_2 = ?$$
$$V_2 = \frac{T_2 \times V_1}{T_2}$$
$$V_2 = \frac{273 \cancel{\text{ K}} \times 250 \text{ cm}^3}{317 \cancel{\text{ K}}}$$
$$V_2 = 215.2996845 \text{ cm}^3$$
$$V_2 = 220 \text{ cm}^3$$

It is important to point out that the contraction of gas due to temperature change at altitude in no manner compensates for the expansion due to the corresponding decrease in pressure.

GAY-LUSSAC'S LAW

Gay-Lussac's law *the pressure of a fixed amount of gas (fixed number of moles) at a fixed volume, proportional to the temperature.*

Similar to Charles' law is **Gay-Lussac's law,** which states that for a fixed amount of gas (fixed number of moles) at a fixed volume, the pressure is proportional to the temperature. It can be represented by the following formula:

$$\frac{P_1}{T_1} = \frac{P_2}{T_2}$$

Gay-Lussac's law can be used to predict the pressure of a gas at a given temperature. For example, consider a container with a volume of 22.4 L filled with a gas at 1.00 atm at 273 K. What will be the new pressure if the temperature increases to 298 K?

$$\frac{P_1}{T_1} = \frac{P_2}{T_2}$$

Algebraically, adjust the original formula to isolate the unknown, solve, and round to the correct number of significant digits:

$$P_2 = \frac{P_1 \times T_2}{T_1}$$

$$P_2 = \frac{(1.00 \text{ atm}) \times (298 \text{ K})}{(273 \text{ K})}$$

$$P_2 = 1.09 \text{ atm}$$

Thus, Gay-Lussac's law explains why the pressure in a gas cylinder (i.e., oxygen, nitrous oxide) decreases as the temperature decreases.

HENRY'S LAW

Henry's law deals with the solubility of gases above a solution and states that the mass of a gas that will dissolve into a solution is directly proportional to the partial pressure of that gas above the solution. In addition, each gas has a solubility coefficient. Some gases, such as carbon dioxide, are chemically or physically attracted to water molecules. Thus, many more carbon dioxide molecules can be dissolved without generating excess pressure within the solution. Henry's law can be expressed with the following formula:

Henry's law *at equilibrium, the amount of gas dissolved in a given volume of liquid, directly proportional to the partial pressure of that gas in the gas phase.*

$$P = \frac{\text{Concentration of dissolved gasses}}{\text{Solubility coefficient}}$$

The solubility of the respiratory gases (at 1 atm and at body temperature [37°C]) is expressed in the volume of gas dissolved in each volume of water. The solubility coefficients are shown in Table 4–3.

Thus, when a gas is in contact with the surface of a liquid, the amount of the gas that will go into solution is proportional to the partial pressure of that gas. For example, if the partial pressure of a gas is twice as high as that of another gas, then twice as many molecules (on average) will hit the liquid surface in a given time interval, and on average twice as many will be captured and go into solution (see Figure 4-3 ■). For a gas mixture, Henry's law helps to predict the amount of each gas that will go into solution. However, as mentioned before, different gases have different solubilities and this also affects the rate. The constant of proportionality in Henry's law must take this into account. For example, in the gas exchange processes in respiration, the solubility of carbon dioxide is about 22 times that of oxygen when they are in contact with the plasma of the human body.

GRAHAM'S LAW

Graham's law addresses the kinetic energy of gas molecules as the temperature varies. It states that since temperature is proportional to the kinetic energy of the gas molecules, the kinetic energy (KE) of the two gas samples is also the same. When gases are dissolved in liquids, the relative rate of diffusion of a given gas is proportional to its solubility in the liquid and inversely proportional to the

Graham's law *the rate at which gasses diffuse, inversely proportional to the square root of their densities.*

Table 4–3	Solubility Coefficients of Respiratory Gases	
Gas	**Coefficient**
Nitrogen	0.012
Oxygen	0.024
Carbon dioxide	0.57
Carbon monoxide	0.018
Helium	0.008

Figure 4-3 Opening carbonated beverage.

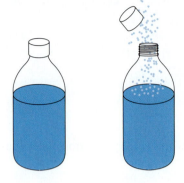

square root of its molecular mass. Since KE = (1/2) mv^2, where m = mass and v = velocity, we can write the following equation:

$$M_1 V_1^2 = M_2 V_2^2$$

You can algebraically manipulate this formula to simplify it:

$$\sqrt{\frac{M_1}{M_2}} = \frac{V_2}{V_1}$$

Thus, Graham's law states that the relative rates of diffusion of gases under the same conditions of temperature and pressure are inversely proportional to the square roots of the densities of those gases. Gases with smaller molecular weights will diffuse more rapidly. This is very important in the transport of the respiratory gases because it impacts the relative diffusion rate of oxygen and carbon dioxide in the plasma of the human body. Carbon dioxide has 22 times the solubility, but is more massive (44 amu compared to 32 amu for oxygen). According to Graham's law, the relative rate of diffusion is given by:

$$\frac{\text{Diffusion rate of CO}_2}{\text{Diffusion rate of O}_2} = 22\sqrt{\frac{32}{44}} = 19$$

FICK'S LAW

Fick's law *the net diffusion rate of a gas across a fluid membrane is proportional to the difference in partial pressure, proportional to the area of the membrane, and inversely proportional to the thickness of the membrane.*

Fick's law states that the net diffusion rate of a gas across a fluid membrane is proportional to the difference in partial pressure, proportional to the area of the membrane, and inversely proportional to the thickness of the membrane. Combined with the diffusion rate determined from Graham's law, this law provides the means for calculating exchange rates of gases across membranes. The total membrane surface area in the lungs (alveoli) may be on the order of 100 square meters and have a thickness of less than a millionth of a meter, so it is a very effective gas exchange interface.

AVOGADRO'S LAW

Avogadro's law *equal volume of all gases under identical conditions of pressure and temperature contain the same number of molecules.*

Avogadro's law states that at the same temperature and pressure, an equal number of molecules of a gas occupies the same volume (1 mol = 22.4 L). Thus, if the amount of gas in a container is increased, the volume increases. If the amount of gas in a container is decreased, the volume decreases. This can be represented by the following formula:

$$n_1 \times V_1 = n_2 \times V_2$$

where n is the number of moles and V is the volume.

IDEAL GAS LAW

Gases behave differently from the other three states of matter (solids, liquids, and plasma). Thus, we must have different methods for treating and understanding how gases behave under certain conditions. As mentioned previously, gases have neither fixed volume nor shape. They are molded entirely by the container in which they are held. The **ideal gas law** is based on relationships described by the classic gas laws:

Boyle's law: $V \propto \dfrac{1}{P}$ (where n and T are constant)

Charles' law: $V \propto T$ (where n and P are constant)

Avogadro's law: $V \propto n$ (where P and T are constant)

ideal gas law *an ideal gas (perfect gas) is one that obeys Boyle's law, Charles' law, and Avogadro's law exactly.*

These three laws can be summarized as:

$$V \propto \frac{nT}{P}$$

We can then add a constant (R) for proportionality; R is the molar gas constant, and $R = 0.0820578$ (L)(atm)(K^{-1})(mol^{-1}):

$$V = R\left(\frac{nT}{P}\right)$$

Thus,

$$PV = nRT$$

Here, P is the pressure in atmospheres, R is the proportionality constant, T is the temperature in Kelvins, and n is the number of moles present. This is known as the *ideal gas equation*. An ideal gas obeys Boyle's law and Charles' law exactly. The ideal gas law assumes several factors about the molecules of gas. The volume of the molecules is considered negligible compared to the volume of the container in which they are held. We also assume that gas molecules move randomly, and collide in completely elastic collisions. Attractive and repulsive forces between the molecules are therefore considered negligible. An ideal gas is modeled on the kinetic theory of gases, which has four basic postulates:

1. Gases consist of small particles (molecules) that are in continuous random motion.
2. The volume of the molecules present is negligible compared to the total volume occupied by the gas.
3. Intermolecular forces are negligible.
4. Pressure is due to the gas molecules colliding with the walls of the container.

It is important to point out that real gases deviate from ideal gas behavior because, at low temperatures, the gas molecules have less kinetic energy (move around less) so they *do* attract each other. Second, at high pressures the gas molecules are forced closer together so that the volume of the gas molecules becomes significant compared to the volume the gas occupies. However, under ordinary conditions, deviations from ideal gas behavior are so slight that they can be neglected. A gas that deviates from ideal gas behavior is referred to as a *nonideal gas*.

We can use the ideal gas equation to determine the volume of 1.0 mol of an ideal gas at 1.0 atm of pressure at 0°C (273.15 K):

$PV = nRT$

$V = nRT/P$

$V = (1.0 \text{ mol})(0.0821 \text{ L atm/mol K})(273 \text{ K})/(1.0 \text{ atm})$

$V = 22.4 \text{ L}$

STRESSORS OF ALTITUDE AND FLIGHT

Altitude places various stresses on the human organism. These stressors can be encountered during flight and are referred to as the *stressors of altitude*. The following stressors are directly related to altitude:

★ Hypoxia
★ Barometric pressure
★ Fatigue
★ Thermal
★ Dehydration

The following are not directly related to altitude per se, but are due to stresses associated with flight and are referred to as *stressors of flight*:

★ Noise
★ Vibration
★ Gravitational forces
★ Third spacing
★ Spatial disorientation
★ Flicker vertigo

HYPOXIA

One of the most frequently encountered hazards in aviation medicine is hypoxia. Records of early balloon and aircraft flights describe tragedies resulting from hypoxia, because even these primitive machines had a higher operational ceiling than the men aboard them. Hypoxia was a serious aviation problem in both World Wars and remains a potential threat even in today's military aviation. Engineering solutions to the problem have been ingenious. Considerable money has been expended on training of aviators and procurement of equipment to prevent hypoxia. Yet, hypoxic incidents continue to occur.

Types of Hypoxia

Hypoxia is an inadequate supply of oxygen for normal cellular function. Hypoxemia is a deficiency of oxygen in the blood. Hypoxia leads to hypoxemia. The amount and pressure of oxygen delivered to the tissues is determined by arterial oxygen saturation, by the total oxygen-carrying capacity, and by the rate of delivery to the tissues. Approximately 97% of oxygen is transported bound to hemoglobin. The remaining 3% is dissolved in the plasma. The four categories of hypoxia are:

The most significant risk factor for ascent to altitude is hypoxia.

1. *Hypoxic hypoxia.* Hypoxic hypoxia is an inadequate PaO_2 caused by reduced oxygen in the atmosphere or inadequate gas exchange at the alveolar–capillary membrane, resulting in inadequate oxygenation of the arterial blood. It is usually caused by a reduced oxygen partial pressure. The reduction of oxygen in the blood as a result of ascent to altitude is called *altitude hypoxia.*

2. *Anemic hypoxia.* Anemic hypoxia results from a reduced oxygen-carrying capacity of the hemoglobin. This is seen in conditions such as anemia, blood loss, carbon monoxide poisoning, or by drugs causing methemoglobinemia. Remember, 97% of oxygen is transported bound to hemoglobin.

3. *Stagnant hypoxia.* Stagnant hypoxia occurs when cardiac output fails to meet the metabolic demands of the tissues, causing shock. This phenomenon, also called *cardiogenic shock,* can lead to venous pooling and cardiac arrest.

4. *Histotoxic hypoxia.* Histotoxic hypoxia results when the tissues are unable to utilize available oxygen. The best example of this is hydrogen cyanide poisoning. With histotoxic hypoxia, there is no oxygen deficiency in the tissues, but rather an inability to use available oxygen. The PO_2 in the tissues may be higher than normal.

Hypoxia is a minimal issue for most helicopter transports (<1,500 feet). The most common type of hypoxia encountered in aviation is hypoxic hypoxia. Other types of hypoxia, such as anemic hypoxia from carbon monoxide poisoning, can affect air crews.

Symptomatology

Many observations have been made on the subjective and objective symptoms of hypoxia:

Objective

★ At 10,000 feet: hyperventilation and impaired performance
★ At 18,000 feet: cyanosis, confusion, poor judgment, and muscular incoordination
★ >20,000 feet: jerking of upper limbs, seizures, and rapid unconsciousness

Subjective

★ At 5,000 feet: blurred vision and/or tunnel vision
★ At 10,000 feet: air hunger, apprehension, fatigue, headache, nausea, dizziness, and hot and cold flashes
★ At 15,000 feet: numbness, tingling, euphoria, and belligerence

A detailed analysis of progressive functional impairment indicates that the effects of hypoxia fall into four stages. Table 4–4 summarizes the stages of hypoxia in relation to the altitude of occurrence, breathing air or breathing 100% oxygen, and the arterial oxygen saturation.

1. *Indifferent stage.* There is no observed impairment. However, night vision decreases by approximately 28%. Some have suggested the need for oxygen use from the ground up during night flights although this may not be practical. During this stage the heart rate and respiratory rates increase slightly. These changes are subtle and the person is unaware of the symptoms, hence the name *indifferent stage.*

2. *Compensatory stage.* During this stage, night vision may be decreased by 50%. Heart rate and respiratory rate increase to compensate for the decreased availability of oxygen.

3. *Disturbance stage.* In this stage, physiological responses are inadequate to compensate for the oxygen deficiency and hypoxia is evident. The person is now aware of the symptoms. These include air hunger, headache, amnesia, decreased level of consciousness, euphoria, and belligerence. Nausea and vomiting may occur—usually in children. At 20,000 feet, the period of useful consciousness is 15 to 20 minutes. In

Table 4–4	Stages of Hypoxia		
	Altitude (feet)		Arterial Oxygen
Stage	Breathing Air	Breathing 100% O_2	Saturation
Indifferent	0–10,000	33,000–39,000	95–90%
Compensatory	10,000–15,000	39,000–42,000	90–80
Disturbance	15,000–20,000	42,000–45,200	80–70
Critical	20,000–23,000	45,200–46,800	70–60

some cases, there are no subjective symptoms noticeable up to the time of unconsciousness. Objective findings include:

Special senses. Peripheral and central vision is impaired and visual acuity is diminished. There is weakness and incoordination of the extraocular muscles and reduced range of accommodation. Touch and pain sense are lost. Hearing is one of the last senses to be affected.

Mental processes. The most striking symptoms of oxygen deprivation at these altitudes are classed as psychological. These are the ones that make the problem of corrective action so difficult. Intellectual impairment occurs early, and the pilot has difficulty recognizing an emergency situation unless he is widely experienced with hypoxia and has been very highly trained. Thinking is slow, memory is faulty, and judgment is poor.

Personality traits. In this state of mental disturbance, there may be a release of basic personality traits and emotions. Euphoria, elation, moroseness, pugnaciousness, and gross overconfidence may be manifest. The behavior may appear very similar to that noted in alcoholic intoxication.

Psychomotor functions. Muscular coordination is reduced and the performance of fine or delicate muscular movements may be impossible. As a result, there is poor handwriting, stammering, and poor coordination in flying. Hyperventilation is noted and cyanosis occurs, most noticeable in the nail beds and lips.

4. *Critical stage.* In this stage of acute hypoxia, there is almost complete mental and physical incapacitation, resulting in rapid loss of consciousness, convulsions, and finally failure of respiration and resulting in death.

The term *effective performance time* is used to describe the amount of time a person is able to perform flight duties in an environment with inadequate oxygen levels. Another term refers to the time from the point of exposure to an oxygen-deficient environment until useful consciousness is lost. This is referred to as **time of useful consciousness.** Table 4–5 reflects the time of useful consciousness at various altitudes for normal flight and sudden cabin depressurization. Of course, the time and response varies from individual to individual.

An important factor in the sequences cited above is the gradual ascent to altitude where the individual can come to equilibrium with the gaseous environment, and physiological compensatory mechanisms have sufficient time to come into play. This phenomenon is more frequently encountered in manual ascents to high altitudes (such as in mountain climbing) than in aviation.

time of useful consciousness *the time from initial exposure to an oxygen-deficient environment until useful consciousness is lost.*

The time of useful consciousness varies by altitude and the speed of decompression.

BAROMETRIC PRESSURE

As stated previously, the critical care paramedic should understand that Boyle's law problems are extremely applicable to critical care flight medicine. When you fly with patients who have had a pneumatic anti-shock garment (PASG) applied, the pressure in the air bladders of the PASG pants may change as you ascend in altitude. (The pants will expand.) Also, the patient's respiratory rate

Table 4–5	Time of Useful Consciousness	
Altitude (Feet)	**Normal**	**Rapid Decompression**
40,000+	15 seconds or less	10 seconds or less
40,000	15–20 seconds	7–10 seconds
35,000	30–60 seconds	15–30 seconds
30,000	1.0–1.5 minutes	30–45 seconds
25,000	3–5 minutes	1.5–2.5 minutes
22,000	10 minutes	5 minutes
15,000	20–30 minutes	

and depth, especially if on a mechanical ventilator, may also vary. Even intravenous flow rates at altitudes can vary (which is why mechanical infusion pumps are commonly used). Due to gas expansion at altitude, patients may experience nausea, vomiting, a need to urinate, and increased pain. Air in the balloons of endotracheal tube (ET) cuffs also may expand and, over time, can cause pressure necrosis to the tissues with which they come in contact. One study measured the tracheal cuff pressures at ground level and at 3,000 feet in 10 intubated patients. With air providing the seal in the cuff, the mean rise in cuff pressure was 23 cm/H_2O, which took the pressures above the critical perfusion pressure of the tracheal mucosa. This could lead to tracheal injury. There are three ways to remedy this problem:

1. Remove pressure from the cuff as needed as you ascend to altitude. Constantly monitor the pilot bulb on the ET tube as an indicator of ET cuff inflation.

2. Use water or saline instead of air in the cuff to minimize this effect (since water is not a gas, expansion at altitude will be minimal). You must remember to remove the water and replace it with air after landing, because water may enhance deterioration of the ETT cuff.

3. An alternative is to use a commercial device to regulate cuff pressure. These include the Posey Cufflator, Rusch Endotest, or a similar cuff pressure monitor.

Generally, these issues are most applicable when flying aboard a fixed-wing aircraft because they reach such high altitudes (although aircraft that cruise at high altitudes pressurize their cabins equivalent to 5,000 to 8,000 feet). Boyle's law can also affect the flight crews that fly with head colds or blocked sinuses. Since the sinuses (and middle ear) essentially become closed containers in such conditions, they well may experience pressure changes. These can be extremely painful. Failure of the middle ear space to ventilate when atmospheric pressure changes are made is referred to as *barotitis media*. This primarily results when changing from low to high pressures as seen on descent from altitude (although it can occur on ascent as well). As a rule, the problem is self-limited and clears without treatment. The efficacy of treatments such as nasal decongestants, oral decongestants, and antihistamines is unclear although these are widely used. Antibiotics and corticosteroids may help in cases of severe barotrauma (pressure-induced trauma).

Monitor ET cuffs constantly at altitude because cuffs containing air can expand and cause pressure-induced tissue necrosis in the trachea.

FATIGUE

Various factors contribute to fatigue in both the patient and air medical crew during flight. These include the person's general health, smoking history, alcohol usage, vibration and noise associated with the aircraft, temperature changes, rotational shifts, diet, hypoxia, gravitational forces, and barometric changes. Thus, it is important to remember that patients requiring medical transport already have a compromised physical condition; therefore, fatigue occurs readily.

In addition, the emotional and physical stress of providing continuous patient care may add to the air medical crew's fatigue. This is especially true for long flights such as international retrievals. The air medical crew should try to minimize fatigue by being well rested, following a good diet, staying wellhydrated, and eliminating unhealthy habits such as smoking.

THERMAL

As one ascends to altitude, the ambient temperature decreases. This change in temperature can dramatically stress the body. Furthermore, hypothermia (and hyperthermia as well) increases the body's oxygen demand. If hypoxia is present, it can be worsened by a change in ambient temperature. High- and low-temperature weather conditions also can create turbulence. Turbulence not only creates its own stress on patients and air medical crews, but also promotes fatigue and heightens motion sickness and disorientation.

DEHYDRATION

The concentration of water vapor in the air is termed *humidity*. The higher the temperature, the greater the number of water molecules the air can hold. As air cools, its ability to hold moisture

The greater the altitude, the lower the temperature and the less humidity the air will hold—hence air becomes drier as you ascend.

decreases. The amount of water vapor in the air at any given time is usually less than that required to saturate the air. The relative humidity is the percent of saturation humidity, generally calculated in relation to saturated vapor density. Stated another way, the relative humidity tells how much water the air is holding compared to how much it could hold at a certain temperature and can be calculated by the following formula:

$$\text{Relative humidity} = \frac{\text{Actual vapor density}}{\text{Saturation vapor density}} \times 100\%$$

The relative humidity can change if the moisture changes or if the temperature changes. The dew point is a much better indicator of moisture in the air. The dew point is the temperature at which the air will be holding all the moisture it could if cooled. Stated another way, the dew point is the temperature at which the relative humidity reaches 100%.

Thus, at higher altitude the air is much drier and the air is cold. Many patients are already dehydrated prior to transport due to age, diet, disease processes, and/or trauma. With the addition of circulatory constriction or dilation caused by altitude changes and the drier atmosphere within the cabin, early fluid replacement should be considered. Oxygen should be humidified to minimize drying of the mucous membranes.

NOISE

Aircraft noise makes reliance on technological monitors more important.

Most aircraft are noisy although modern aircraft have been designed to minimize noise. Regardless, noise is a significant risk for air medical crews. Noise is created by the engines (piston, turboprop, jet), propellers, and rotors of the aircraft. Noise can interfere with the air medical crew's ability to auscultate blood pressures, lung, and abdominal sounds. To compensate for this, blood pressures can be palpated and lung function noted by watching chest excursion and rate, oxygen saturation, and waveform capnography. The condition of the patient's abdomen can be noted by observing abdominal distention and noting increased pain.

Noise also temporarily affects the air medical crew's hearing ability and can contribute to gradual hearing loss, especially at high frequencies. It is recommended that air medical crews wear hearing protection (earplugs) or a headset at all times when around aircraft. Additional headsets should be provided for patients, especially if the patient has a seizure disorder or is preeclamptic or eclamptic.

VIBRATION

Many aircraft vibrate. This is especially true for helicopters whose flight results from multiple forces acting in different directions. Unlike ground vehicles, vibration in aircraft can occur in all three axes. When a person is in direct contact with a vibrating object, such as a helicopter, some of the mechanical injury is transferred to the person. Some of this energy is broken down into heat. This results in an increase in metabolic rate, which causes peripheral vasoconstriction and the redistribution of blood flow. Vibration from the aircraft can cause circulatory constriction and, in some situations, override the body's cooling mechanism, thereby decreasing the ability to sweat. Either hot or cold temperatures can aggravate the effects of vibration.

gravitational forces the forces of attraction between all masses in the universe; more commonly the attraction of the Earth's mass for bodies near its surface.

With hypothermic patients, vibration can worsen the condition. When treating a hypothermic patient, vibration can delay the body's natural cooling ability (through the mechanism described earlier).

GRAVITATIONAL FORCES

Always consider the possible detrimental effect of G-forces on your patients and position them accordingly.

Gravitational forces, commonly called G-forces, are force changes that occur with acceleration. Fortunately, G-forces are not significant with the majority of aircraft used for air medical transport.

Acceleration is the rate of change in velocity and is measured in Gs. Newton's three laws of motion describe the forces of acceleration. Newton's first law describes inertia. It states that a body in motion will remain in motion unless acted on by an outside force. Likewise, a body at rest will remain at rest unless acted on by an outside force. Newton's second law of motion states that the acceleration of an object is dependent on two variables: the net force acting on the object and the mass of the object. The acceleration of an object depends directly on the net force acting on the object, and inversely on the mass of the object. As the net force increases, so will the object's acceleration. However, as the mass of the object increases, its acceleration will decrease. In other words, to overcome inertia, a force (F) is required, the result of which is proportionate to the acceleration (a) applied and the size of its mass (m); that is:

$$F = ma$$

Newton's third law states that for every action (acceleration centripetal force), there is an equal and opposite reaction (inertial centrifugal force).

The critical care paramedic needs to understand where and how accelerative forces—linear, radial or centripetal, and angular—develop in flight.

★ *Linear acceleration.* Linear acceleration is a change in speed without a change in direction. It occurs during takeoffs and changes in forward air speed. This type is also encountered when speed is decreased.

★ *Radial or centripetal acceleration.* Radial acceleration can occur anytime the aircraft changes direction without a change in speed. Crew members may encounter this type of acceleration during banks, turns, loops, or rolls.

★ *Angular acceleration.* Angular acceleration is complex and involves a simultaneous change in both speed and direction. A good example of this is an aircraft that is put into a tight spin.

G-forces and the direction in which the body receives those forces are important physiological factors that affect the body during acceleration. G-forces can affect the body in three axes: G_x, G_y, and G_z. The physiological effects of prolonged acceleration depend on the direction of the accelerative (centripetal) force and on how the inertial force acts on the body. The inertial (centrifugal) force is always equal to, but opposite, to the accelerative force. The inertial force is the most important physiologically. The various G-forces are listed here:

★ Positive G, or $+G_z$, acceleration occurs when the body is accelerated in the head-first (cephalad) direction. The inertial force acts in the opposite direction toward the feet, and the body is forced down into the seat.

★ Negative G, or $-G_z$, acceleration occurs when the body is accelerated in the foot-first (caudad) direction. The inertial force is toward the head, and the body is lifted out of the seat.

★ Forward transverse G, or $+G_x$, acceleration occurs when the accelerative force acts across the body in an anterior to posterior direction. *The G acceleration is experienced during acceleration.*

★ Backward transverse G, or $-G_x$, acceleration occurs when the accelerative force acts across the body in a posterior to anterior direction. The $-G_x$ acceleration is experienced during deceleration.

★ Right- or left-lateral G, or $+/-G_y$, acceleration occurs when the accelerative force impacts across the body from a shoulder-to-shoulder (lateral) direction.

To determine the effects of accelerative forces on the human body, crew members must consider several factors. These factors include intensity, duration, rate of onset, body area and site, and impact direction:

★ *Intensity.* The greater the intensity, the more severe the effects of the accelerative force. However, intensity is not the only factor that determines the effects.

★ *Duration.* The longer the force is applied, the more severe the effects. Crew members can tolerate high G-forces for extremely short periods and low G-forces for longer periods. In general, the longer the force is applied, the more severe the effects. A force of 5 Gs applied for 2 to 3 seconds is usually harmless, but the same force applied for

5 to 6 seconds can cause blackout or unconsciousness. In ejection seats, pilots can tolerate a head-first acceleration of 15 Gs for about 0.2 second without harm, but will become unconscious when the same force is applied for 2 seconds. The body can absorb, without harm, high G-forces applied for extremely short durations.

★ *Rate of onset.* The rate of onset of accelerative or decelerative forces plays a part in the overall effects experienced. When an aircraft decelerates gradually, the decelerative forces are exerted at a rather slow rate. Generally, when the rate of application is higher, such as when an aircraft decelerates suddenly during an accident, the effects are more severe. When an aircraft impacts vertically, the stopping distance is considerably shorter and the rate of application of accelerative forces is many times greater. The rate of application is often slowed down in helicopter crashes by the spreading of the skids and the crumpling of the fuselage, giving the body 3 or 4 extra feet in which to decelerate. Therefore, the distance, as well as the time, is an important factor in acceleration or deceleration. In summary, the shorter the stopping distance, the greater the G-force.

★ *Body area and site.* The size of the body area over which a given force is applied is important. The greater the body area, the less harmful are the effects. The body site to which a force is applied is also important. The accelerative effect of a given force, such as a blow to the head, is much more serious than the same force applied to another part of the body, such as the leg or buttock.

★ *Impact direction.* The direction from which a prolonged accelerative force acts on the body can also impact the physiological effects that occur. The body does not tolerate a force applied to the long axis of the body (G_z) as well as it does a force applied to the G_x axis.

G-forces may be relevant to the patient's position in some aircraft. Their effect on the patient is influenced by weight and distribution, gravitational pull, and centrifugal force, which affect blood pooling. Centrifugal force tends to alter the blood flow in the body in proportion to the amount of force imposed. When positive ($+G_z$) forces are applied to the body, blood tends to pool in the lower portions of the body; the opposite occurs during negative ($-G_z$) applications. Patient positioning in some aircraft may minimize or enhance the effects of G-forces, as follows:

★ *Cardiac.* Consider positioning the patient with head toward the back (aft) position of the aircraft. On ascent, this may enhance the ($-$) G-forces by pooling the blood in the upper part of the body, which may assist in myocardial perfusion.

★ *Fluid overload.* Consider positioning the patient with head toward the front of the aircraft. This may enhance the ($+$) G-forces by pooling the blood in the lower extremities.

★ *Head injury.* Consider positioning the patient head first, with feet toward the back (aft) portion of the aircraft. This may enhance the ($+$) G-forces by pooling blood in the lower extremities. This may help reduce the risk of a transient increase in intracranial pressure (ICP) on liftoff.

★ *Maternal patients.* Among the types of patients transported by air, maternal patients are among the most likely to be affected by gravitational forces. Gravitational forces may enhance labor, pulling the fetus "down," if the patient's head is positioned toward the nose of the aircraft. In addition, acceleration forces may adversely affect uteroplacental perfusion.

THIRD SPACING

third spacing *the loss of fluids from the intravascular space into the tissues, caused by increased intravascular pressures and/or an increased permeability of the cell membranes.*

Third spacing is the loss of fluids from the intravascular space into the tissues and is caused by increased intravascular pressures and/or an increased permeability of the cell membranes. Third spacing can be enhanced by constriction and dilation of the circulatory system. Other physiological stresses, such as temperature, vibration, or G-force changes, can cause or aggravate this phenomenon. Signs and symptoms may include edema, dehydration, increased heart rate, and decreased blood pressure. These occur more frequently with long-distance or high-altitude flights.

SPATIAL DISORIENTATION

Spatial disorientation is a significant factor in aircraft accidents. Regardless of their flight-time experience, all air crew members are subject to spatial disorientation. The human body is structured to perceive changes in movement on land in relation to the surface of the earth. In an aircraft, the human sensory systems (visual, vestibular, and proprioceptive systems) may provide the brain with erroneous orientation information. This information can cause sensory illusions, which may lead to spatial disorientation. **Spatial disorientation** is an individual's inability to determine his or her position, attitude, and motion relative to the surface of the earth or significant fixed objects during hover. When it occurs, pilots fail to see, believe, interpret, or prove the information derived from their flight instruments is accurate. Instead, they rely on the false information that their senses provide.

spatial disorientation an inability to determine position, attitude, and motion relative to the surface of the earth or significant fixed objects.

There are three categories of spatial disorientation:

★ *Type I (unrecognized).* A disoriented crew member does not perceive any indication of spatial disorientation. In other words, he does not think anything is wrong. What he sees, or thinks he sees, is wrongfully corroborated by his other senses. Type I disorientation is the most dangerous type of disorientation. The pilot, unaware of a problem, may fail to recognize or correct the disorientation, usually resulting in a fatal aircraft mishap.

★ *Type II (recognized).* In Type II spatial disorientation, the crew member perceives a problem (resulting from spatial disorientation), but may fail to recognize it as a spatial disorientation problem. For example, the pilot may feel that a control is malfunctioning.

★ *Type III (incapacitating).* In Type III spatial disorientation, the crew member experiences such an overwhelming sensation of movement that she cannot orient herself by using visual cues or the aircraft instruments. Type III spatial disorientation is not fatal if another person, such as the second-in-command pilot, can gain control of the aircraft.

Spatial disorientation cannot be totally eliminated, but it can sometimes be prevented. Air crew members need to remember that misleading sensations from sensory systems are predictable. These sensations can happen to anyone because they are due to the normal functions and limitations of the senses. Training, instrument proficiency, good health, and aircraft design minimize spatial disorientation. Spatial disorientation becomes dangerous when pilots become incapable of properly reading their instruments. All pilots, regardless of experience level, can experience spatial disorientation. For that reason, they should be aware of the potential hazards, understand their significance, and learn to overcome them. To prevent disorientation, air crew members should:

★ Never fly without visual reference points (either the actual horizon or the artificial horizon provided by the instruments).
★ Trust the instruments.
★ Avoid fatigue, smoking, hypoglycemia, hypoxia, and anxiety, which all heighten illusions.
★ Use effective scanning techniques.
★ Never stare at lights.
★ Provide patients with a tactile reference source during flight.

Spatial disorientation can affect all members of an air crew—not just the pilot.

VERTIGO

Vertigo is a disturbance of inner ear equilibrium characterized by a sensation that a person, or objects around the person, are spinning. It is well known that attacks of vertigo can be induced by sudden head movement when pilots are flying. With vertigo, the sense of disequilibrium is due to physiological excess of visual, vestibular, or somatosensory signals that cannot be compensated for by the other systems. In pathological vertigo there is an abnormal sensory signal (from the sensors) or abnormal signal processing (by the central nervous system). Examples of physiological vertigo

vertigo disturbance of the inner ear characterized by a "spinning" sensation.

(due to inappropriate stimulation) include motion sickness, space sickness, height vertigo, visual vertigo, somatosensory vertigo, head extension vertigo, and bending-over vertigo. These physiological vertigo states have significance in aerospace medicine, particularly the type of motion sickness seen in neophyte fliers—air sickness. Vertigo affects passengers as well as crew. Certain medications may help with vertigo, but may be sedating. Focusing the eyes on a fixed object, such as the horizon, will sometimes help alleviate symptoms.

Flicker Vertigo

flicker vertigo *an imbalance in brain cell activity created by light sources that emit a flickering (rather than steady) light.*

Flicker vertigo is a term that describes an imbalance in brain cell activity created by light sources that emit flickering rather than steady light. Light flickering from 4 to 20 times per second can produce dangerous and unpleasant reactions in some people, including nausea, dizziness, migraines, unconsciousness, and even epileptic seizures. Both natural and artificial light sources, especially fluorescent lighting and television screens, may precipitate flicker vertigo. In aviation operations, problematic light sources include wind-milling propellers that cut the sun to give a flashing effect, rotating beacons or strobes in certain lighting and atmospheric conditions, and flashing anticollision strobe lights—especially while the aircraft is in the clouds. Crew members with a history of migraine or a seizure disorder are at risk for flicker vertigo. The effects of flicker vertigo can be minimized by ensuring you have adequate rest, are well hydrated, and avoid looking at flashing lights. Sunglasses and caps can sometimes help.

PROBLEMS RELATED TO ALTITUDE

Air crew members are faced with many hazardous factors when performing flight duties. The purpose of this section is to introduce you to a few of the factors that either occur most often or have the greatest detrimental impact to your and your patient's health and safety. These considerations were not entertained under the stressors of flying, because many of those can be curtailed prior to their emergence. The following problems, however, typically occur suddenly and sometimes without much warning.

HIGH-ALTITUDE PULMONARY EDEMA (HAPE)

high-altitude pulmonary edema (HAPE) *a potentially lethal condition caused by accumulation of fluid in the lungs following rapid ascent to high altitude.*

High-altitude pulmonary edema (HAPE) is an emergency condition in which fluid accumulates in the lungs following ascent to altitude. It is more frequently encountered in mountaineering than aviation. It has been demonstrated that all visitors to high altitudes experience an increase in their pulmonary artery pressure. This finding led to the hypothesis that increased pulmonary artery pressures alone were forcing a transudate (largely water) into the alveolar tissue and air spaces. However, examination of climbers suffering from HAPE demonstrated that the fluid was an exudate, with relatively large proteins, instead of a transudate. This resulted in the hypothesis that major leaks were developing in the pulmonary capillaries. The current theory is that increased intracapillary pressure forces the basement membrane cells apart, thus allowing protein leakage. When the pulmonary artery pressure is reduced, the cells fall together again, sealing off the leak, and accounting for the dramatic recovery associated with descent. Interestingly, pulmonary artery pressures are increased in all persons traveling to high altitude, yet not all people get HAPE.

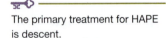

The primary treatment for HAPE is descent.

HAPE is the most common cause of death from high-altitude illness. It usually occurs after the 2 to 4 days at altitude and is associated with rapid ascent to altitudes greater than 8,000 feet. Signs and symptoms include:

★ Crackles or wheezing in at least one lung field
★ Central cyanosis or significant arterial oxygen desaturation relative to altitude
★ Tachycardia
★ Tachypnea
★ Fever (relatively common)
★ Orthopnea

- ★ Pink/frothy sputum (a late finding)
- ★ High-altitude cough

Treatment of HAPE includes administration of high-flow, high-concentration supplemental oxygen, immediate descent, and bilevel positive airway pressure (BiPAP) or positive end-expiratory pressure (PEEP) support. Consider nifedipine and morphine. Hyperbaric therapy is sometimes necessary.

HIGH-ALTITUDE CEREBRAL EDEMA (HACE)

Although originally thought to be separate disorders, **high-altitude cerebral edema (HACE)** is now largely considered to be the end stage of severe acute mountain sickness (AMS). High altitude is generally defined as anywhere higher than 5,280 ft above sea level. At such high elevations, AMS affects almost everyone to some degree. The effects vary for each individual, but the most classic initial symptoms include headache, insomnia, anorexia, nausea, and dizziness. By far, high-altitude headache (HAH) is the most prominent symptom in AMS.

Several hypotheses have been proposed as to the cause of HACE. However, the prevailing theory is that HACE is likely the result of increased cerebral edema, caused by increased cerebral blood flow due to the increased permeability of cerebral endothelium when exposed to hypoxia. Increased cerebral blood flow results in increased intracranial pressure, which is responsible for many of the clinical manifestations of HACE. Hypoxia is the body's primary response to rapid ascent to a high-altitude environment. The lowered barometric pressure of the ambient atmosphere results in diminished alveolar oxygen tension and, as a consequence, arterial partial pressure of oxygen (PaO_2) drops dramatically.

Treatment of HACE must be started immediately because initial symptoms of acute mountain sickness rapidly progress to more serious high-altitude illness. Descent is the most successful treatment for HACE. The goal is to reach the lowest possible altitude as soon as possible. The traditional method of treating altitude sickness is to administer dexamethasone to treat cerebral symptoms. The exact mechanism of action is uncertain, though it does produce profound euphoric effects, which may play a role in the improvement of symptoms. It has been hypothesized that dexamethasone may have the ability to decrease fluid leaks from the micovasculature. Additionally, it acts to relieve nausea, though prochlorperazine (Compazine) or promethazine (Phenergan) can also be used.

Though effective in treatment, dexamethasone is now rarely used prophylactically due to the significant dysphoria and the likelihood of a rebound case of altitude illness occurring with discontinued use of the drug. The diuretic acetazolamide (Diamox) is traditionally used as a preventive measure for all types of altitude sickness. This type of treatment is especially important for those travelers approaching 10,000 feet. Acetazolamide is a sulfonamide carbonic anhydrase inhibitor that enhances the renal excretion of bicarbonate, thus producing a mild acidosis. This serves to reverse the bicarbonate diuresis resulting from the respiratory alkalosis from hyperventilation secondary to hypoxia. Acetazolamide may also work by lowering the cerebral spinal fluid volume and pressure by increasing the minute ventilation oxygen saturation and decreasing periodic breathing at night.

RAPID DECOMPRESSION

Decompression at altitude is one of those factors that can cause significant physiological problems. Decompression is the loss of cabin pressure in a pressurized aircraft. Decompressions are categorized as either "slow" or "rapid." A slow decompression can occur when a leak develops in the seal of the pressurized aircraft cabin. This type of decompression is dangerous because of the possible insidious effect of hypoxia. **Rapid decompressions** are considered more dangerous. They can occur as a result of a perforation of the cockpit or cabin wall or unintentional loss of the canopy or a hatch.

Factors Controlling the Rate and Time of Decompression

The principal factors that govern the total time of decompression of a pressurized aircraft include the volume of the cabin, the size of the opening, the pressure ratio, and the pressure differential.

high-altitude cerebral edema (HACE) *considered to be end-stage, severe, acute mountain sickness (AMS). Classic initial symptoms include headache, insomnia, anorexia, nausea, and dizziness.*

rapid decompressions *at altitude, perforations of the cockpit or cabin wall, or unintentional loss of the canopy or a hatch, causing rapid decrease in pressure. (Also known as "explosive decompressions.")*

Larger cabins will decompress more slowly than smaller ones. The greater the size of the opening, the quicker the egress of the plane's atmosphere and the quicker the subsequent decompression. As discussed in the gas laws section, the pressure within the cabin and the outside ambient pressure affect the rate of decompression. The difference between the internal and external cabin pressures will influence both the rate and severity of the decompression. Thus, the larger the pressure differential between the inside and the outside of the cabin, the more rapid and severe the subsequent decompression.

Physical Characteristics of Rapid Decompression

There are a few physical and observable characteristics that help in the recognition of a rapid decompression. All of the following may indicate a loss of cabin pressurization.

★ *Noise.* When two different air masses make contact, there is a noise that ranges from a "swish" to a loud explosive sound. It is because of this explosive noise that some people use the term *explosive decompression* to describe a rapid decompression.

★ *Fogging.* Air at any temperature and pressure has the capability of holding some water vapor. Sudden changes in temperature or pressure, or both, can change the amount of water vapor the air can hold. In a rapid decompression, temperature and pressure are reduced. This reduction in temperature and pressure reduces the holding capacity of air for water vapor. The water vapor that cannot be held by the air appears as fog. If the environment is cold, the fog can freeze.

★ *Temperature.* Ambient temperatures become colder with increasing altitude. If a decompression occurs, cabin temperature will equalize with outside ambient temperature, resulting in a significant decrease in cabin temperature. Chilling or frostbite is possible depending on the altitude at which the decompression occurs.

★ *Flying debris.* Upon decompression, the rapid rush of air from a pressurized cabin causes the velocity of airflow through the cabin to increase rapidly as the air approaches the hole. The rush of air has such force that items not secured will be extracted through the opening.

Physiological Effects of Rapid Decompression

All patients transported via aircraft are hypoxic. Therefore, they should all be treated as such.

The primary effect of rapid decompression is hypoxia. Other effects can be problems related to gas expansion, decompression sickness, and hypothermia.

★ *Pulmonary.* The lungs are potentially the most vulnerable part of the body during a rapid decompression. Whenever a rapid decompression is faster than the inherent capability of the lungs to decompress, a transient positive pressure will temporarily build up within the lungs. If the escape of air from the lungs is blocked or seriously impeded during a sudden drop in cabin pressure, intrapulmonary pressure can build up high enough to cause tearing and rupture of the pulmonary tissues and pulmonary capillaries. If the expanding gas is free to escape from the lungs through an open airway, the risk of lung damage is nonexistent. Momentary breath-holding, such as swallowing or yawning, will usually not cause excessively high intrapulmonary pressure and overexpansion of lung tissue.

★ *Ears and sinuses.* Decompression of a pressurized cabin is unlikely to cause symptoms in the middle ear and paranasal sinuses. As mentioned previously, it is more likely, however, that individuals will develop pain in the middle ear and paranasal sinuses during the subsequent emergency descent, because they will be exposed to a large and rapid increase of cabin pressure.

★ *Gastrointestinal tract.* During a rapid decompression, one of the potential dangers is the expansion of gases trapped within the gastrointestinal tract. This can cause abdominal distress and/or distention. Abdominal distention, if it does occur, may have several effects. The diaphragm is displaced upward by the expansion of the trapped gas in the stomach. This can impair respiratory movements. In addition, distention of the abdominal organs may also stimulate the abdominal branches of the vagus nerve, resulting in cardiovascular depression and, if severe enough, causing a reduction in blood pressure, unconsciousness, and shock.

★ *Hypoxia.* The effects of hypoxia were addressed in detail earlier in this chapter. Hypoxia is the most significant problem following decompression. The rapid reduction of ambient pressure produces a corresponding drop in the partial pressure of oxygen and reduces the alveolar oxygen tension. A twofold to threefold performance decrement occurs regardless of altitude. The reduced tolerance to hypoxia after decompression is due to a reversal in the direction of oxygen flow in the lung, diminished respiratory activity at the time of decompression, and decreased cardiac activity at the time of decompression. Fortunately, pressurized aircraft have supplemental oxygen delivery systems that deploy in the event of a depressurization.

DECOMPRESSION SICKNESS

Decompression sickness (DCS) describes a condition characterized by a variety of symptoms resulting from exposure to low barometric pressures that cause inert gases (mainly nitrogen), normally dissolved in body fluids and tissues, to come out of physical solution and form bubbles. DCS can occur during exposure to altitude (altitude DCS) or during ascent from depth (mining or diving). In general, decompression sickness does not occur until cabin altitudes of 18,000 feet are reached. The incidence of decompression sickness is small unless the cabin altitude reaches 25,000 to 30,000 feet. As the duration of exposure to the unpressurized environment increases, so does the incidence of decompression sickness. The incidence of decompression sickness following a rapid decompression appears to be only slightly greater than after a slow decompression to the same altitude.

decompression sickness (DCS) *a condition resulting from exposure to low barometric pressure causing inert gases (mainly nitrogen), normally dissolved in body fluids and tissues, to come out of physical solution and form bubbles.*

HYPOTHERMIA

When cabin temperatures drop because of a decompression, it is likely that injuries such as frostbite and hypothermia will occur. Again, the extent and severity will be dependent on the altitude and the type of protective clothing worn during the decompression.

Emergency oxygen systems should deploy in pressurized aircraft in cases of decompression.

TRAPPED GAS EMERGENCIES

During ascent, the free gas normally present in various body cavities expands (per Boyle's law). If the escape of the expanded volume is impeded, pressure within the body cavity increases and pain is experienced. Expansion of trapped gases can cause ear pain, abdominal pain, sinus pain, or toothache.

Most trapped gas problems occur on descent.

Ears

An in-flight ear block can occur on either ascent or descent when air pressure in the middle ear is unable to equalize with ambient air pressure. This normally occurs because the lower orifice of the eustachian tube, which operates as a one-way flutter valve, fails to function adequately. It may also happen if the eustachian tube is swollen from a cold or ear infection. The difference in pressure will cause the eardrum to bulge outward on ascent and inward on descent. This may cause discomfort in the form of pressure or pain (see Figure 4-4).

The symptoms of an in-flight ear block may include:

★ Pressure or pain

★ Muffled sound

★ Dizziness

★ Tinnitus (ringing in the ear)

Descending rapidly from a level of 30,000 to 20,000 feet will often cause no discomfort, whereas a rapid descent from 15,000 to 5,000 feet will cause great distress. This is because the change in

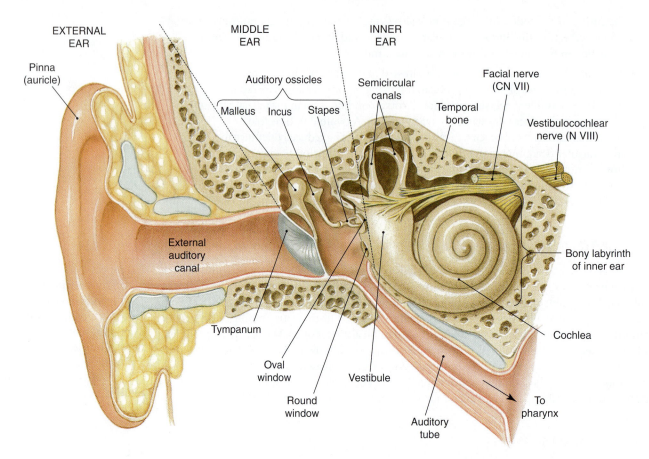

EXTERNAL EAR — MIDDLE EAR — INNER EAR

Pinna (auricle)

Auditory ossicles

Malleus Incus Stapes

Semicircular canals

Temporal bone

Facial nerve (CN VII)

Vestibulocochlear nerve (N VIII)

External auditory canal

Tympanum

Oval window

Round window

Vestibule

Auditory tube

To pharynx

Bony labyrinth of inner ear

Cochlea

■ **Figure 4-4** Inner ear anatomy. *(Fig. 10-19, p. 290, from* Essentials of Anatomy & Physiology, *2nd ed., by Frederic H. Martini, Ph.D. and Edwin F. Bartholomew, M.S. Copyright © 2000 by Frederic H. Martini, Inc. Published by Pearson Education, Inc. Reprinted by permission.)*

barometric pressure is much greater in the latter situation. For this reason, special care is necessary during rapid descents at low altitudes.

Protection against Ear Blocks

Normally, pressure can be equalized during descent by just swallowing, yawning, or tensing the muscles of the throat. Chewing gum during ascent and descent can help, especially with young children who do not know how to clear their ears. These procedures cause contraction of pharyngeal muscles, which opens the orifices of the eustachian tube. If relief is not obtained by this method, a Valsalva maneuver should be performed by closing the mouth, pinching the nose shut, and blowing gently, thus forcing air through the previously closed eustachian tube into the cavity of the middle ear and equalizing the pressure.

Sinuses

The paranasal sinuses present a condition in flight similar to that of the middle ear. The sinuses are air-filled, relatively rigid bony cavities that are lined with mucous membranes. They connect with the nose by means of one or several small openings.

If the openings into the sinuses are normal, air passes into and out of these cavities at any practical rate of ascent or descent, ensuring adequate equalization of pressure. If the openings of the sinuses are obstructed by swelling of the mucous membrane lining (resulting from infection or an allergic condition) or by polyps or redundant tissue, equalization of pressure becomes impossible. Change of altitude produces a pressure differential between the inside and the outside of the cavity and can cause significant pain.

Sinus blocks can occur both during ascent and descent. In about 90% of the cases, however, pain develops during descent. During ascent, the expanding air usually forces its way out past the obstruction. Sinus blocks most often occur in the frontal sinus (70%), followed in frequency by the maxillary sinus. Maxillary sinusitis may produce pain referred to the teeth of the upper jaw and may be mistaken for toothache.

Barodontalgia

Toothache has been reported by individuals during actual or simulated flight. The altitude at which the onset of toothache usually occurs varies from 5,000 to 15,000 feet. Interestingly, a pain in a given tooth in a given individual often may show remarkable constancy in the altitude at which it first becomes manifest. The pain may or may not become more severe as altitude is increased. Pain is invariably relieved on descent—an important feature that helps distinguish **barodontalgia** from pain in the upper jaw due to maxillary barosinusitis.

When first recognized, barodontalgia was thought to be due to expansion of trapped air under restorations such as fillings or crowns. Numerous investigations have experimentally produced air bubbles under dental restorations and exposed the individuals to low barometric pressure. No symptoms were experienced in these cases. It is now thought that gas expansion is responsible for only a very small proportion of these cases.

The specific mechanism of barodontalgia has not been fully identified but it is invariably associated with some degree of preexisting dental pathology—normal teeth are not affected. Imperfect fillings, pulpitis, and carious teeth, which were asymptomatic at ground level, have all been incriminated.

barodontalgia *toothache reported by individuals at actual or simulated altitudes, varying from 5,000 to 15,000 feet. Relieved by descent.*

Gastrointestinal Tract

Discomfort from gas expansion within the digestive tract is frequently experienced with a rapid decrease in atmospheric pressure. Gas is normally present throughout the colon and in parts of the small intestine. As gas expands, it increases the pressure within the colon thus causing pain, Fortunately, the symptom is not serious in most individuals flying at low altitudes. Above 25,000 feet, however, enough distention may occur to produce severe pain.

PREVENTIVE MEASURES

The stressors of flight and the trapping of gases within the body can affect both the air medical crew and the patient. The air medical crew must anticipate the effects of these stressors prior to transport. Appropriate interventions prior to and during air transport should be initiated to minimize the effects on the patient.

Some of these stressors are out of the control of air medical crews or patient. The air medical crew can minimize the effects, however, by following these practices:

1. Be well rested.
2. Avoid smoking at altitude.
3. Remain in the seat, with seat restraints on, to reduce vibration.
4. Avoid gas-producing foods and liquids.
5. Avoid chewing gum on ascent.
6. Avoid flying with a "head cold" or ear infection.
7. In emergencies, consider the time of useful consciousness.

Summary

Flight physiology is a unique, yet important topic for the critical care paramedic. It is one of those topics, like ethics and legalities, that may not directly impact your day-to-day practice, but is instead interwoven into every patient flight. This chapter was intended to provide the critical care student with a basic understanding of the principles associated with this flight medicine. A basic understanding of gas laws and an in-depth knowledge of physiological responses to changing altitude and treatment of altitude-related disease processes are vital to your success in the air medical environment.

Review Questions

1. Of the various gas laws, which one pertains the most to flight medicine?
2. If a patient has medical equipment (such as intubation or central lines) that uses a cuff inflated with air, how should this be managed prior to takeoff?
3. What are the most common stressors to the paramedic with flight missions, how can they affect your practice, and what are the best ways to avoid them?
4. What should the paramedic do if a rapid cabin decompression emergency occurs in flight?
5. Why is patient positioning important when using aircraft for flight?

See Answers to Review Questions at the back of the book.

Further Reading

Department of the Navy. *Virtual Naval Hospital.* http://www.vnh.org/.

Holleran RS. *Air and Surface Patient Transport: Principles and Practice,* 3rd ed. Saint Louis, MO: Mosby, 2003.

Guyton AC, Hall JE. *Textbook of Medical Physiology,* 10th ed. Philadelphia: W. B. Saunders, 2000.

U.S. Department of Transportation. *Air Medical Crew National Standard Curriculum. Advanced Student Manual.* Washington, DC: Author, 1988.

Flight Safety and Survival

Randall W. Benner, M.Ed., MICP, NREMT-P

Objectives

Upon completion of this chapter, the student should be able to:

1. Name and discuss several facets of rotor-wing (and fixed-wing transportation) imperative to the safe completion of each mission. (p. 80)
2. Briefly describe the following helicopter components:
   ★ Airframe (p. 82)
   ★ Fuselage (p. 83)
   ★ Tail boom (p. 83)
   ★ Tail rotor system (p. 83)
   ★ Main rotor system (p. 83)
   ★ Engines (p. 83)
   ★ Transmission (p. 84)
   ★ Landing gear (p. 84)
   ★ Horizontal and vertical stabilizers (p. 84)
3. Briefly describe the following helicopter flight controls:
   ★ Collective pitch control (p. 85)
   ★ Cyclic pitch control (p. 86)
   ★ Throttle control (p. 86)
   ★ Foot pedals (p. 86)
4. Describe the importance of the pilot safety brief. (p. 88)
5. List and describe the common hazards of operating around a helicopter. (p. 89)
6. Explain the importance of perimeter guards at landing zones. (p. 90)

7. Understand the importance of proper rest and nutrition for the flight paramedic. (p. 90)
8. Describe the various types of personal protection equipment, and understand the importance of their use. (p. 91)
9. List and describe the following responsibilities (duties) of each air medical crew member:
   ★ Preflight duties (p. 92)
   ★ In-flight duties (p. 94)
   ★ Post-flight duties (p. 95)
10. Understand and be able to utilize the clock code in relation to describing an object's position relative to the aircraft. (p. 94)
11. Discuss the additional duties of the medical flight crew in instances of in-flight or post-accident emergencies. (p. 97, 98)
12. Describe the "rule of threes" as it pertains to survival situations. (p. 99)
13. Be able to discuss common strategies to provide shelter, fire, and water in a survival situation. (p. 100)

Key Terms

Case Study

You are working for an air medical service as a flight paramedic. Your aeromedical system normally utilizes the twin-engine Eurocopter BK-117 helicopter as the standard aircraft, but since your aircraft is in the hanger for scheduled maintenance, today you will be flying in a Eurocopter EC-135. Your partner, who has previous experience with this airframe, takes a few extra minutes to further familiarize you with this aircraft. He demonstrates how to open and close the rear clamshell doors, how to engage and disengage the cot, where the main oxygen valve is, and how to use the internal radio communication system.

He then walks you around the outside of the aircraft to show where the cowling attachments are, and explains the visual difference between the "fenestrated" tail rotor system on the EC-135 and the open tail rotor system of the BK-117. He points out for safety that the fenestrated tail is no less dangerous than the open tail rotor if someone were to get too close to it. He adds that on the EC-135, the tail boom is shorter than that of the BK-117, and extreme caution must be exercised while loading and unloading the patient while the rotors are running "hot." Following this review of the aircraft, you both complete the additional morning duties of checking all stationary medical equipment aboard the aircraft and the portable medical equipment to be sure all is properly prepared for rapid deployment. Upon reentering the base quarters, your pilot meets with both of you for your daily safety brief, and you learn that the weather is not going to be a factor in any mission today.

About halfway through the shift, your pager alerts you of your first mission of the day—a scene flight. As you and your partner package up the O negative blood and gather your medications, the pilot leaves to prepare the aircraft for departure. The pilot performs his walk-around, removes the rotor tie-down cords, and then checks the cowlings and covers of the aircraft to ensure they are all properly closed and prepared for flight. You and your partner place your equipment in the aircraft and also do a secondary walk-around to double-check the aircraft and helipad for safe departure. The pilot brings the aircraft to its idle speed as you and your partner buckle into your safety harnesses, and, after ensuring that everything is secured for liftoff, the pilot brings the rotor speed to "fly," lifts up on the collective, and the aircraft ascends into the sky.

As you await the coordinates, you start toward the scene using a distance and heading given to you by your communications specialist. As you rapidly fly toward the motor vehicle collision (MVC) scene, you and your partner are both gazing outward into the airspace around your helicopter for any other nearby traffic. You hear your partner say over the headphones, "Small aircraft at 5 o'clock high—moving in the same general direction." The pilot acknowledges back his visual on the aircraft while he makes minor adjustments to the flight direction.

As you near the coordinates for the MVC, the radio starts to crackle in your headset as the on-scene landing zone (LZ) coordinator attempts to make contact with you. As you fly over the LZ, you see a car embedded into a broken utility pole, and about 100 yards away from the car, in a level field, you see the bright orange cones denoting the perimeter of the LZ. Your pilot performs a recon orbit as you and your partner look for any hazards that could obstruct a safe descent into the LZ. The pilot announces his final approach to land, and requests a "sterile cockpit."

You land safely in the LZ at a one-car MVC with entrapment. Once the pilot states it is safe to exit the aircraft, you and your partner unload the cot and portable equipment and make your way to a 10 o'clock position off the nose of the aircraft in a crouched position. You make visual contact with the pilot who gives you the "thumbs up," indicating that it is now safe to exit from under the main rotor system. As you draw near the edge of the LZ, you verbally remind the LZ coordinator to not allow anyone to approach the aircraft since it will be running "hot" the entire time you are on scene. It is only now that you are able to turn your attention to the care of the entrapped patient.

Following extrication by the fire department, and initial management by the on-scene medical personnel, you and your partner assume responsibility for the patient. After completing your necessary care tasks and ensuring that the patient and any loose material are secured to the cot, you determine that you are ready to "hot" load the patient into the aircraft. You notify the pilot via the portable radio of your return, and you recruit three firefighters to assist you to the aircraft with a four-point carry of the cot since the ground is too uneven to push it. Your partner departs ahead of you for the helicopter to act as a safety officer to ensure that none of the carrying crew gets near the tail rotor. The pilot again gives you the "thumbs up" as you near the aircraft, indicating it is safe to enter beneath the rotor disk as you load the patient. After securing the patient in the aircraft, your partner directs the FD personnel to back away from the aircraft in the same way they came in, and he then enters the aircraft and resumes patient care while you do a walk-around of the aircraft, ensuring that is once again safe to lift.

You then enter the back of the aircraft and resume patient care while the pilot prepares you for liftoff. He advises you that the trauma center is about a 15-minute flight away. Once in the air you continue your care in flight, and occasionally look outside the aircraft to quickly scan for any other air traffic. When the pilot draws near the receiving hospital, you ensure that the patient, equipment, and flight crew are all well secured. While the pilot performs his LZ recon orbit at the receiving facility, you and your partner are also watching outside the windows for any potential LZ hazards. A sterile cockpit is maintained during touch down, and after unloading the patient and receiving a "thumbs up" from the pilot, you exit from under the rotor disk and transport the patient safely into the hospital.

INTRODUCTION

As critical care paramedics read this textbook, they will find almost every chapter dedicated to the assessment and management of critical patients. This is done for a good reason because a large part of what the critical care paramedic does is provide ongoing care during transport. This chapter, however, focuses on the safety of the members of the flight crew, who must provide care to these patients in very hazardous environments. The flight crew has a great responsibility for their safety as well as that of the patient, and it is hoped that this chapter will better prepare the critical care paramedic to operate in this environment. Overall, this chapter is intended to provide a brief explanation of helicopter specifics and introduce the paramedic to the safe operations employed in the air medical industry.

Let it first be said, however, that flight medicine is not overtly dangerous. Safe helicopter operations require effective leadership, team member coordination, and assertiveness by everyone involved. The real danger with helicopters arises when the care providers have limited knowledge about aeromedical operations and safety. If a flight crew were to become too lackadaisical in ensuring that safety is the priority of every mission, disaster will inevitably occur. While the axiom of "always err on the side of the patient" refers to the concept of providing the best care even when the patient's condition may not warrant it, it could be said here to "always err on the side of safety," because failure to do so will place the critical care paramedic, his partner, the pilot, and ultimately the patient at risk. The consequence of not keeping a "safety consciousness" about you can easily be a fatal mistake. And not until the flight crew develops a safety consciousness should they assume the responsibility of caring for patients in the aeromedical field.

BECOMING SAFETY CONSCIOUS

Although safety is important in all aspects of EMS operation, it is especially so in the complicated world of flight medicine. In this section we will detail the importance of being safety conscious as it applies to air medical operations.

DEFINING FLIGHT SAFETY

Without a working definition of what flight safety is, it becomes difficult for the critical care paramedic to know if he is meeting safety goals. Flight safety can be defined as those plans that are incorporated into daily flight operations that serve to eliminate risk (when possible) or reduce risk (when unavoidable) so that each mission can be carried out without incident. As mentioned previously, aeromedical transport is not overtly dangerous—but it is not without risk. Because human endeavors entail risk, the procedure taken should be to assess for present risk, prioritize the risk, minimize the known risk by implementation of safety plans, and establish a monitoring or feedback loop designed to assess the effectiveness of the risk reduction program.

FLIGHT SAFETY AWARENESS PROGRAM

Any flight program that enjoys successful operations is one that has a strong commitment to ensuring flight safety. Often times, flight programs include mention of safety in their mission statement—but beyond this they must also be committed by their actions to flight safety. This is often facilitated by a program safety committee, which operates much like other committees within the air medical operation (such as QA/QI), and includes representation by administration, base site managers, aircraft pilots, maintenance personnel, communications, and flight crew members. The committee members' task is to maintain an open forum so that all hazards can be identified and integrated into a risk reduction program. Additionally, they are usually charged with establishing a process that allows for constant review of the safety program to ensure that it is a dynamic process that mirrors the dynamics of the industry itself. As base sites change, helicopter models change, or new areas of service are established, the aeromedical system must ensure that any risks inherent to these changes are eliminated. If the new hazards detected are impossible to avoid (for example, characteristics of the weather or terrain), then attempts to minimize the risk should be taken.

With the expansion of flight programs and the continued evolution of state involvement and regulations within critical care flight medicine, some state and nationwide safety councils are also becoming involved with safety concerns. State programs are commonly comprised of local aeromedical services that meet to exchange program policy information, training guidelines, communication procedures, and criteria about when to (or when not to) fly in adverse weather conditions.

Other sources of information that can be used by program safety committees are the studies and recommendations that come from national organizations. One such organization is the **National Transportation Safety Board (NTSB)**. The NTSB is an independent federal agency charged by Congress to investigate every civil aviation accident in the United States and significant accidents in the other modes of transportation. In the late 1980s, the NTSB released results of an initial investigation into medical flight accidents. From this research, recommendations were made to the **Federal Aviation Administration (FAA)**, whose mission is to provide the safest, most efficient aerospace system in the world; to the **Association of Air Medical Services (AAMS)**, which is an international association that serves providers of air and surface medical transport systems; and to the National Aeronautics and Space Administration (NASA). Recommendations are made from lessons learned through previous aircraft accidents and included the need to improve pilot education in poor weather, the need to prioritize incoming calls, and what type of enhancements need to be made to the interior of medical aircraft to help ensure flight crew safety. The report recognized the need to promote ongoing research into the risks and hazards of flight programs so that lower and lower accident rates can be realized. In the years following this initial research aeromedical accident rates fell, but flight safety is not a subject that can simply be left alone and revisited every few years. The responsibility to have a safe flight program belongs to everyone.

SAFETY CONSCIOUSNESS

Safety consciousness is the last component of a flight safety program, and is the one that becomes internalized by the providers and pilots in the system. This refers simply to the ability of flight crew members to actively look for risks, rather than simply noticing them. To an extent, this is somewhat different from person to person because each individual has an acceptable degree of risk they are willing to

National Transportation Safety Board (NTSB) *federal agency charged with investigating civil aviation accidents and other transportation accidents in the United States.*

Federal Aviation Administration (FAA) *federal Agency whose mission is to regulate, control, and provide for a safe and efficient aerospace system.*

Association of Air Medical Services (AAMS) *an international association, serving the air and surface medical transportation industries.*

assume. This "acceptable risk," however, cannot be greater than what is acceptable to others in the aircraft. If the pilot, for example, feels that the weather conditions they are flying into are not too adverse, he or she may feel that the risk of completing the mission is not too great. But if the medical crew believes that the weather may be too challenging to allow a safe mission and that their personal safety may be at risk, they can become so preoccupied by stress that they cannot focus their attention fully on the task of patient management. Hence, their job performance may suffer. A safety consciousness is not only recognizing and understanding risk, it is decreasing or eliminating risk as well.

To operate with a safety consciousness, the providers must understand their job as well as the external influences that impact it. Critical care paramedics need not be pilots, but they do need to understand the dynamics of how helicopters fly. They need not be meteorologists, but they need to understand how the weather impacts aircraft operations. Critical care paramedics need not be aviation mechanics, but they need to be aware of how they can assist the mechanic in identifying and isolating mechanical problems. And finally, critical care paramedics need not be engineers, but they need to realize how workplace controls and the mounting of medical equipment can impact safe movement around the patient compartment of the aircraft.

The critical care team must take personal responsibility to ensure that every mission meets the highest standards for safe and effective patient care. And this internalization of a safety consciousness is the crux of any safety program. As mentioned previously, a safety consciousness is the ability to look for hazards and fix them, not to simply notice them or try to avoid them (or in the worst case scenario, become complacent and ignore them). Some components of aeromedical critical care transport that the crew needs to perpetually be attentive to (and will be discussed in greater detail later) include:

- ★ Following all program preflight guidelines
- ★ Ensuring that the aircraft is ready to take off
- ★ Noting any irregularities in the takeoff or landing locations
- ★ Preparing all on-board equipment for flight
- ★ Using safety devices (helmets, clothing, restraint systems)
- ★ Properly securing patients within the aircraft
- ★ Utilizing proper communication channels
- ★ Using adequate interior lighting during night missions
- ★ Isolating the pilot and aircraft controls from the patient compartment
- ★ Maintaining good personal physical and mental health

TYPES OF AIRCRAFT

Although many types of rotor-wing and fixed-wing aircraft exist, most aeromedical programs utilize one or two from a core group of available rotor-wing models, such as the Eurocopter BK-117, Sikorsky S76, or Bell 407. (See Figure 5-1 ■.) This is not to say that only one or two types are used exclusively, but that programs only use those aircraft that fit the needs of speed, patient compartment space, distance capabilities (fuel), maintenance/operation costs, weight limitations, and ability to competently navigate the geographical region in which the aircraft is to be operated. What this simply results in is the availability of only a certain number of aircraft that meet all of these needs simultaneously.

Even though the available types of aircraft that meet all of these needs are relatively few, it is likely that the critical care paramedic will only need to become familiar with the one or two models used in his system. At this time, however, it is not our intent to discuss all of the available airframes, but rather to discuss the commonalities between the airframes. (The term **airframe** is used as a general description for what type of aircraft an aeromedical program utilizes.) This provides readers with the widest appreciation of flight safety, and will prepare them for what is likely to be included in the flight safety orientation program present in almost all flight programs for new hires.

Of the available options, an aeromedical program will ultimately select what aircraft to use based on the needs of the service and the capabilities of the aircraft. And the issues of flight safety

airframe *generally refers to the "type" of aircraft, main structure that all other components are attached to.*

can start as early as the decision to use one type of aircraft over another. Although the critical care paramedic will probably not be the one who determines what type of aircraft is purchased, understanding some of the major differences between models will allow early appreciation for potential risk factors. While many of these components were initially introduced in Chapter 3, they are mentioned here again briefly for completeness of discussion, and we now include a basic discussion of their influence on flight safety programs.

SINGLE-ENGINE HELICOPTERS

Single-engine helicopters are primarily used because of their quick start times, lower cost of maintenance, and lower consumption of fuel. Examples of single-engine aircraft include the Eurocopter EC-130, AS 350 A-Star, and the Bell 206 Jet Ranger.

Single-engine designs cost less to purchase and usually need less space for landing. They can be very versatile in situations where flying into confined spaces is commonplace. The concern voiced by those in the industry regarding the use of single-engine aircraft for medical flight programs is that should there be some catastrophic engine failure while in flight, there is no option for anything less than a forced emergency landing. Additionally, the single-engine design typically does not have the payload capability of larger airframes, so this too may serve as a limitation for use in aeromedical operations.

DUAL-ENGINE HELICOPTERS

Dual-engine helicopters are more expensive to operate, have a similar flight range to that of single-engine designs, may remain in flight should one engine suddenly fail, and generally have a greater payload capacity. Examples of dual-engine aircraft used in critical care transport include the Eurocopter EC-135, the BK-117, the AS 355 Dauphin, the Bell 412, and the Sikorsky S76.

Despite the higher purchase price and maintenance costs, dual-engine aircraft are commonly utilized due to their larger payload capabilities, increased patient compartment size, and the fact that if an in-flight engine failure occurs, the second engine can be utilized during the emergency landing.

FIXED-WING AIRCRAFT

Several flight programs in the United States have additional resources available for long-distance patient transports. (Refer to Chapter 3 for criteria for distinguishing among fixed- versus rotor-wing transport.) Fixed-wing aircraft are utilized primarily for transporting a patient long distances within the United States, as well as for completion of the occasional international patient transport mission.

Fixed-wing aircraft also are available in single- or multiple-engine configurations, although multiple-engine configurations are almost exclusively used for air medical transport. Examples of fixed-wing aircraft used in the transport of critical patients include the Beech King Air 200, the Learjet 35A, or the Learjet 55.

Other than the obvious advantage of being able to transport the patient for longer distances at a much greater speed, fixed-wing aircraft also commonly enjoy a quieter and smoother flight. Additionally, there is considerably more room to complete patient management in a fixed-wing aircraft, compared to its rotor-wing counterpart.

Regarding risks or safety hazards, almost all risks present with rotor-wing aircraft transport are shared by fixed-wing aircraft. However, there are a few additional safety hazards unique to fixed-wing transports that the critical care paramedic needs to be cognizant of. As discussed in Chapter 4, safety issues that occur more commonly in fixed-wing aircraft include rapid cabin depressurization at altitude, complications from use of medical equipment at altitude, emergencies involving the regulation of the patient compartment (temperature, humidity, and so on), and inability to land safely elsewhere than an airport should an in-flight emergency necessitate a forced landing.

HELICOPTER SPECIFICS AND OPERATIONS

Part of maintaining a "safety consciousness" is recognizing the hazards surrounding flight medicine and taking the necessary steps to eliminate risks—or at least minimize the risks that cannot be totally eliminated. To be safe, the critical care paramedic must know what components of the aircraft could potentially cause harm. Failure to recognize these, or being unfamiliar with the aircraft in which you are operating, will not allow you to exercise the greatest degree of caution possible (as alluded to in the opening case study). To help the critical care paramedic understand which areas of the aircraft may be potentially harmful, the following discussion identifies the major components of rotor-wing aircrafts.

AIRCRAFT COMPONENTS

★ *Airframe*—the main structure of the aircraft to which all other components are attached. (See Figure 5-2 ■.)

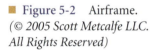
■ **Figure 5-2** Airframe. *(© 2005 Scott Metcalfe LLC. All Rights Reserved)*

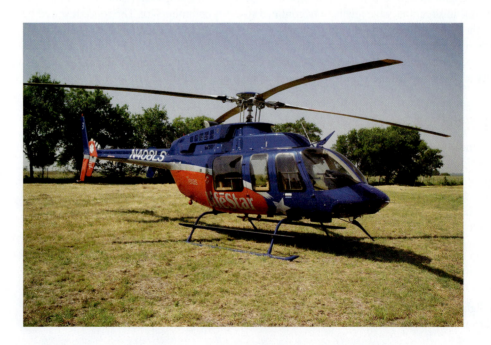

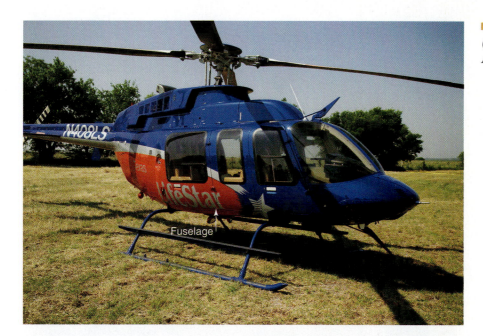

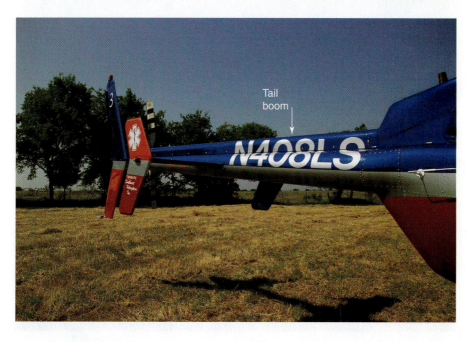

fuselage *external body of the aircraft surrounding the airframe and all of its components.*

tail boom *aft of the airframe, it houses the tail rotor and serves as point of fixation for the stabilizers.*

tail rotor system *vertical rotor blade at the end of the tail boom that compensates for torque induced by the main rotor system.*

main rotor system *horizontal blade above the fuselage that produces lift and thrust for the aircraft as it spins.*

engines *affixed directly to the airframe and supply power to both rotor systems.*

★ **Fuselage**—the external body of the aircraft that surrounds the airframe and all of its components. (See Figure 5-3 ■.)

★ **Tail boom**—the structure that extends aft of the airframe, houses the tail rotor, and provides points of fixation for the horizontal and vertical stabilizers. (See Figure 5-4 ■.)

★ **Tail Rotor System**—the smaller vertical rotor blade that spins at the end of the tail boom. The tail rotor compensates for the torque induced by the turning of the main rotor system. (See Figure 5-5 ■.)

★ **Main Rotor System**—the large horizontal blade located above the fuselage. As it spins, it produces the lift and thrust for the aircraft. (See Figure 5-6 ■.)

★ **Engines**—affixed directly to the airframe (commonly above the patient compartment), and usually hidden behind cowls and coverings of the fuselage. The engines supply power to both rotor systems to accomplish lift.

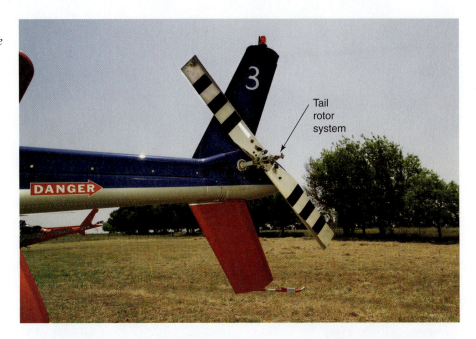

Figure 5-5 Tail rotor system. (© 2005 Scott Metcalfe LLC. All Rights Reserved)

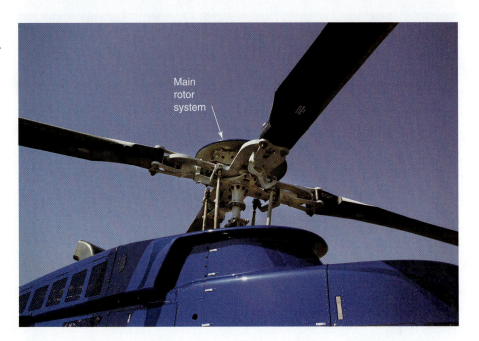

Figure 5-6 Main rotor system. (© Scott Metcalfe LLC. All Rights Reserved)

transmission *converts power from the engines into rotational power that is then transferred to both rotors via drive shafts.*

horizontal and vertical stabilizers *provide stabilization of flight altitude while airborne.*

★ **Transmission**—affixed to the engines and also anchored to the airframe. The transmission converts the power from the engines into rotational power, which is transferred to both the main and tail rotors via drive shafts.

★ *Landing gear*—the portion of the airframe that the helicopter comes to rest on during a normal landing. There are several different forms of landing gear given the different helicopter models and types of surfaces on which they may be landing. They include skids, retractable gear, open wheels, and floats. (See Figure 5-7 ■.)

★ **Horizontal and vertical stabilizers**—these are the structures affixed to the tail boom of the aircraft that provide stabilization of the flight while airborne. The types and physical appearance of stabilizers present on an airframe can vary as much as the different types of aircrafts.

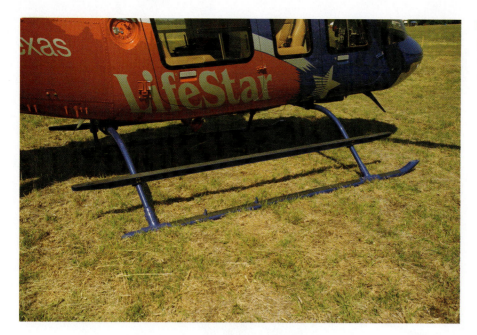

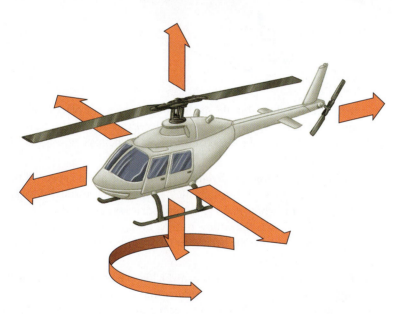

■ **Figure 5-8** Helicopter flight axes.

AIRCRAFT CONTROLS

It was mentioned previously that critical care paramedics need not be pilots, but by understanding some of the controls common to helicopter flying, they can better appreciate the risks and dangers inherent to aeromedical transports. Helicopters are unique in that they can fly in all axes and rotate in flight. (See Figure 5-8 ■.) The following discussion briefly identifies some of these pertinent controls needed for the aircraft to fly.

HELICOPTER CONTROLS

Four essential controls are necessary to achieve flight in a helicopter:

★ **Collective pitch control**—this is commonly a large round lever located to the side of the pilot. When raised upward, it changes the pitch angle of the main rotor blades,

collective pitch control
changes the pitch angle of the main rotor blades to control altitude.

Helicopter Specifics and Operations **85**

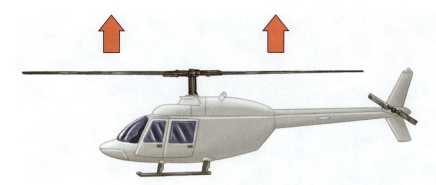

■ **Figure 5-9** Action of collective pitch control.

■ **Figure 5-10** Action of cyclic pitch control.

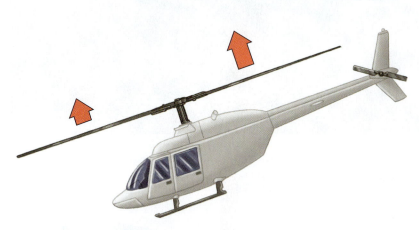

thereby controlling altitude. As the pitch changes, the blades will rotate to a sharper angle. As the pitch becomes sharper, it forces air downward more violently, creating the lift needed to make the aircraft rise. As such, this controls the aircraft's altitude. (See Figure 5-9 ■.)

★ **Cyclic pitch control**—this controls the direction and air speed of the helicopter, and is commonly referred to as the "stick." While flying, a straightforward motion of the stick causes the whole main rotor blade drive system to actually move (tilt) forward slightly. This directs the airflow passing through the main rotor in a downward and aft direction, causing the helicopter to move forward as it simultaneously lifts the aircraft. (See Figure 5-10 ■.)

★ **Throttle control**—the throttle control, like the accelerator pedal in a car, causes the engines to run faster, which translates into the rpm control of the rotor systems. Simply stated, as the engines run faster and cause the rotors to turn quicker, more thrust is provided for flight. (See Figure 5-11 ■.)

★ **Foot pedals**—The foot pedal system allows the pilot to control the pitch angle of the tail rotor. The primary purpose of the tail rotor and its controls is to counteract the torque effect of the main rotor. The foot pedals also allow for the turning of the aircraft. (See Figure 5-12 ■.)

cyclic pitch control
controls the direction and airspeed of the helicopter, and is commonly referred to as the "stick."

throttle control *valve assembly that controls air and fuel flow into an engine, controls desired thrust to the rotor systems.*

foot pedals *allows the pilot to control the pitch angle of the tail rotor.*

■ **Figure 5-11** Action of throttle.

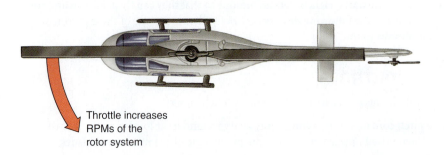

Throttle increases
RPMs of the
rotor system

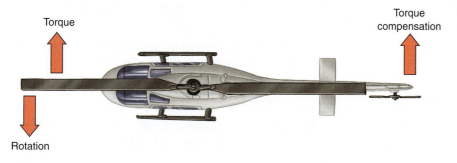

Torque

Rotation

Torque
compensation

■ **Figure 5-12** Effects of foot rotor.

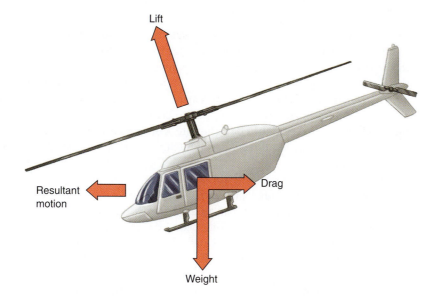

Lift

Resultant
motion

Drag

Weight

■ **Figure 5-13** Helicopter forces.

AIRCRAFT AERODYNAMICS (WEIGHTS AND BALANCES)

All helicopters are designed for certain load limits and balance conditions in order to allow safe flight. (See Figure 5-13 ■) While the pilot is ultimately responsible for making sure that the weight and balance limitations are met prior to takeoff, the critical care paramedic may be called on to help decide what equipment must be off-loaded while on a scene flight, for example, prior to taking off with an obese patient (or multiple patients). In some instances, the pilot will lift off with the aircraft and fly in large circles above the landing site while the critical care paramedics on the ground prepare a patient for transport. These scene orbits will "burn off" fuel, which in turn reduces the aircraft's overall weight. This is done on occasion so that the helicopter is able to accommodate a larger weight load.

Four kinds of "weight" must be considered in the loading of the helicopter, and the pilot needs to account for each type with every mission flown. These include the empty weight, useful load, gross weight, and maximum gross weight. Simplistically speaking, if the weight of the aircraft and its contents exceed the aircraft's flight capabilities, a safe flight cannot be assured. The computation of weights and balances is one of the most important preflight duties the pilot has.

★ **Empty weight**—the weight of the helicopter, including the airframe structure, all fixed equipment, engine fuel, transmission oil, and total quantity of hydraulic fluid. It is the weight of everything but passengers and equipment.

★ **Useful Load (payload)**—the specific weight of the pilot, passengers, and portable medical equipment taken aboard the aircraft for flight.

★ **Gross weight**—the totality of weight given the combination of the aircraft's empty weight, plus the useful payload.

★ **Maximum gross weight**—the maximum weight for which the helicopter is certified for safe flight.

empty weight *weight of the helicopter (includes structure, fixed equipment, fuel/hydraulic liquids) minus passengers and portable equipment.*

useful load (payload) *total weight of pilot, passengers, and portable medical equipment.*

gross weight *total of empty weight plus useful payload.*

maximum gross weight *certified maximum weight for safe flight operations.*

Safety and communications in air medical operations go hand in hand. True safety can never be achieved without adequate communications among all involved.

CREW RESOURCE MANAGEMENT (CRM)

It is important for critical care paramedics to realize that their safety and that of the crew is everyone's responsibility. Documented cases have illlustrated how an error of judgment (or lack of attention) by just one of the crew members has led to a helicopter accident. Consider the following true story:

> An aeromedical flight program received dispatch information from their communications center for a mission. The pilot was first to leave the base quarters when he went out to ready the helicopter for flight, which included removing the rotor blade tie-downs and storing them. One of the tie-downs, however, fell from the pilot's hand without him realizing it, and after completing his preflight check, he started the helicopter's twin engines. Following him, carrying the refrigerated drugs, were the two critical care flight members. They completed their preflight check as they had done hundreds of times before, but this time they were perhaps too lackadaisical, because neither of them noticed the rotor tie-down strap lying there on the helipad.
>
> The medical crew entered the aircraft, which was still warming up; they secured themselves and prepared for liftoff. Upon initial liftoff, the pilot started to rotate the aircraft while hovering just above the landing pad to align themselves with their intended direction of travel. As the tail boom became positioned closer to where the tie-down strap had been dropped on the helipad, the strap was sucked into the rotating tail rotor. This immediately damaged the tail rotor and resulted in the inability of the pilot to safely control the aircraft's flight pattern.
>
> The skilled pilot was able to successfully set the aircraft back down on the helipad with only minor damage from landing "hard," and the crew was undoubtedly taken by surprise. Fortunately this mishap did not result in the loss of the aircraft or human life, but it illustrates how being inattentive (even on your own helipad) can result in a lack of safe practices with disastrous results.

Each air medical crew member has a responsibility to employ and maintain the highest level of safety possible. Ensuring the safety of each mission begins even before the aircraft leaves the ground. Several components constitute **crew resource management** (CRM), which refers to the totality of factors within the aeromedical provider's control that ensure each mission is completed safely.

PILOT SAFETY BRIEF

At the beginning of each pilot shift, and usually before each mission, a **pilot safety brief** is conducted. This is when the pilot discusses with the medical crew such issues as weights and balances of the aircraft, fuel capacity, weather conditions and forecast, and any operational issues existing with the aircraft. The pilot safety brief not only serves the purpose of maintaining a safe working environment, but also facilitates an understanding of normal flight operations and reinforces the constant need for communication between pilot and crew members.

COMFORT OF FLIGHT

It is a general understanding among air medical crew members that every mission will be conducted, or "flown," at the lowest comfort level of any individual team member. What this allows for is the discontinuation (or aborting) of the mission by any one of the flight crew members. This ensures that no one is uncomfortable during the flight or is operating under the impression that a safety margin has been compromised. Failure to do this can easily result in the medical crew being more concerned about the perceived safety issue (for example, inclement weather) than they are for the patient. Not only is the aircraft and crew in jeopardy if, in fact, the weather is suboptimal for

crew resource management (CRM) *operational implementation of pilot safety briefings, flight crew "comfort levels," education, and a safety conscious culture.*

pilot safety brief *a mission specific operational discussion led by the pilot that includes aircraft and weather information, as well as landing zone and other safety issues.*

flight, but the patient is also at risk for omissions or errors in care from the preoccupied critical care flight crew. Several factors can affect this "comfort level":

★ Inclement weather conditions

★ Poor visibility (for example, night flights)

★ Unfamiliar or potentially dangerous landing zones (especially with scene flights)

★ Real or perceived mechanical issues with the aircraft

ANNUAL SAFETY TRAINING

Education and training are the first steps in promoting the safe performance of duties in aeromedical transport programs. Ongoing review of flight communications, flight physiology, helipad and flight safety, survival training, and stress management should be core components of an annual safety training session.

A more in-depth understanding of helicopter operations to include the use of transponder codes, proper arming and use of the emergency locator transmitter (ELT), and aircraft-specific emergency shutdown procedures should be provided.

To promote safe and effective performance by all members in the aeromedical program, a firm commitment to ensuring a foundation of safe practice is required. It is best if this safe practice education has a classroom component (for core knowledge), field experience in the hanger with the aircraft (for flight safety issues), and field experience in the mission environment (for survival techniques). It is through the application of knowledge and experience gained in these annual safety sessions that confidence is built, and the ability to perform safely and effectively is ensured. Ultimately, "safety consciousness" becomes internalized and exuded by all critical care team members.

SAFE OPERATIONS IN HELICOPTER ENVIRONMENTS

Fulfilling your role as a critical care paramedic starts with the performance of day-to-day operations in and out of the helicopter, whether it is sitting still on the base helipad or running hot at the scene of a multiple-car MVC. Critical care paramedics must keep safety foremost, and they can do so by their attentiveness to the following hazardous areas of helicopter operations:

★ *Main rotor system.* The main rotor system of a helicopter generally consists of two to five blades that turn at a range of 290 to 400 rpm (depending on aircraft model), and can result in the tips of the rotor blades moving as fast as 500 mph. It is also important to remember that the rotor blades may flex as low as 4 feet from the ground due to wind gusts while turning at a low rpm. For these reasons extreme caution is mandatory whenever operating under the main rotor system. It is important to remember that all equipment and personal gear must be secured when functioning around the helicopter, because such items can quickly be pulled into either rotor system or projected away from the helicopter at a very high rate of speed.

★ *Tail rotor.* The tail rotor system is much lower to the ground than the main rotor system, therefore increasing the probability for serious injury or death. The tail rotor spins at greater than 2,000 rpm and is virtually invisible to see when at operating speeds.

★ **Rotor wash.** Rotor wash is the airflow produced around the helicopter while the rotor systems are spinning. During warm-up or cooldown, the rotor wash is approximately 25 mph. At closer to operating speed, the rotor wash can be in excess of 50 to 150 mph. This strong rotor wash can project objects at a high rates of speed, potentially causing injury to emergency personnel.

rotor wash *the airflow (wind currents) produced around a helicopter while the rotor systems are spinning.*

★ *Landing zone issues.* Helicopters are often summoned directly to an accident scene. In some instances the LZ is unsecured. In this case extreme caution is needed. All crew members must be observant to obstacles that may be encountered during approach, takeoff, and while operating at the scene. Hazards that may be encountered include utility poles, trees, fences, and wires. All hazards that are encountered must be pointed out to the pilot to ensure a safe approach and departure route.

★ *Approaching/departing the aircraft.* After safely landing at the designated location, the medical crew departs the aircraft at the pilot's discretion. Approaching and departing the aircraft while "hot" (when both rotor systems are functional) should be done in direct visualization of the pilot, by positioning yourself at a ten o'clock or two o'clock position in relation to the nose of the aircraft. In either instance, the crew should await a gesture from the pilot, usually a "thumbs up," indicating that it is safe to depart from under the main rotor system.

perimeter guards *ground personnel who secure the landing zone, normally stationed at least 50 feet from the aircraft, and remain in direct visualization of the pilot.*

★ **Perimeter guards.** Perimeter guards are essential to ensuring safe operation at an incident scene. In most cases, ground EMS/fire personnel can assist in securing the LZ. The perimeter guard should be outside of the main rotor system, usually no less than 50 feet from the aircraft, and remain in direct visualization of the pilot. He or she should also have no direct involvement with patient care, extrication, or rescue so as to remain focused on overall scene safety. As an added degree of safety, any personnel who need to approach the aircraft should only do so under direct supervision of the flight crew. Upon return to the aircraft, the medical crew should once again obtain a "thumbs up" from the pilot and approach from a safe angle. Once under the main rotor system, a tail guard should be utilized. The tail guard will position himself or herself below the tail boom and forward of the horizontal stabilizer. This is to protect any additional personnel from inadvertently walking into the tail rotor system while operating in the aft area of the aircraft.

★ *Air traffic.* Many flight programs operate in areas where air traffic is moderate to heavy at times. It is the responsibility of each crew member to assist the pilot in identifying other aircraft. All visualized air traffic should be relayed to the pilot using the clock code. (The clock code is discussed later in this chapter.)

PERSONAL SAFETY (FITNESS STANDARDS)

Functioning as an air medical crew member can be mentally demanding and physically challenging, and requires a high degree of emotional stability in order to provide the best care possible. This work environment demands constant alertness on the part of the critical care paramedic for both patient management and safety issues. To be the best prepared care provider (beyond your clinical capabilities), consider the following recommendations for emotional/physical fitness as well as personal safety:

★ *Rest.* It is important that all crew members are well rested prior to a shift. Medical crew members should have at least 8 to 10 hours of uninterrupted rest prior to a shift. Most flight programs employ a "downtime" policy allowing crew members to obtain rest during the shifts when call volume permits.

★ *Physical capability.* The first consideration is that some helicopter manufacturer specifications (and flight programs) may limit the physical size of the flight crew. While not an industry standard, one such example of a policy (from a flight program that utilizes the Eurocopter EC-135 airframe) requires that flight crews be 200 pounds or less, and 6 feet, 0 inches or shorter in height in order to function. Beyond meeting these overall guidelines, critical care paramedics must also be able to properly restrain themselves in the aircraft's installed seat belt system and be able to work competently within the space limitations of their particular aircraft. Finally, the critical care flight crew should not have preexisting medical conditions that limit their flexibility or strength or compromise cardiovascular, neurologic, or mental stability.

★ *Nutrition.* It is important that each crew member maintain an adequate nutritional intake while operating as part of the transport team. The stressors of flight combined with the potential for extended periods of time to pass between meals can have a significant impact on individual performance. Crew members should eat several small, high-energy meals through the course of a shift.

PERSONAL PROTECTIVE EQUIPMENT

Helmets

It is generally accepted that the use of protective head gear (helmets) by flight crews is not detrimental beyond the expense of equipping the crew. However, the use of helmets in aeromedical transport is not an industry standard despite its shown benefit in the military for reducing injuries. The use of helmets can not only provide eye and ear protection, it can also contribute to the reduction of head injuries resulting from survivable helicopter accidents. Beyond the popular belief that "no one survives a helicopter crash," one recently published study spanning 10 years found that only 23% of aeromedical crashes resulted in death of all occupants, with another 10% of helicopter accidents having a mixture of fatalities and injuries (the balance of the accidents were either injuries only or no injuries at all). What can be gleaned from this is that the majority of helicopter accidents do *not* result in occupant death, and the use of protective helmets may lower the fatality rate even more. Helmets are typically constructed from a graphite or Spectra® composite shell, and are also used to protect against impact with the airframe or moving objects as the flight paramedic moves about MVC scenes and/or the aircraft.

Fire-Resistant Clothing

The goal of wearing flame-resistant clothing is to help protect the critical care paramedic from burns in a post-accident fire. While the protective clothing typically withstands high temperatures for less than 20 seconds, this may be enough time for the provider to remove himself from the burning wreckage. Flight suits are usually a one-piece uniform made of Nomex® or Kevlar® fibers, and should be worn over cotton, silk, or wool/cotton mix undergarments (that include both briefs and T-shirts). Gloves are also a very valuable piece of protective equipment, and are typically constructed from a Nomex® fiber and leather.

Protective Footwear

This is an important consideration, especially if your flight system responds to scene runs. Leather boots with thick, oil-resistant soles, steel toes, and support extending several inches above the ankles should be used. The boots should be ventilated to avoid moisture from being trapped. And when worn in conjunction with a flight suit, the pant legs should be tucked into the boot prior to lacing.

Hearing Protection

The noise created by aircrafts at times can be extremely loud. And although your exposure to this noise is somewhat episodic (depending on the number of missions you complete), the use of hearing protection devices can only be beneficial to reducing long-range hearing loss. Some hearing protection devices include headphones, ear muffs, and earplugs. Many systems use an integrated communication system of headphones built into the flight helmets, which allows for easy verbal communication among the crew and also offers protection from the external noise.

Eye Protection

Eye protection is necessary due to possible fluid exposure during patient care and is also helpful outside the aircraft while completing "hot" loading or unloading of the patient. Again, in an attempt to provide the best protection possible, some helmets are designed with dual pull-down visors (dark and clear), have built-in hearing protection, and are equipped with headphones and a voice-activated microphone. (See Figure 5-14 ■.)

CREW MEMBER RESPONSIBILITIES

Mentioned repeatedly throughout this chapter is the fact that safety is *everyone's* concern. This is true, however, certain tasks are assigned to specific members of the flight crew, and it is imperative to the safety of all that each member of the crew carry out all assigned tasks efficiently and competently.

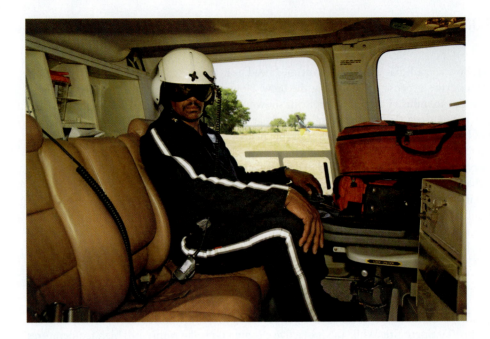

While doing so, communication between each member must be maintained at all times for there to be a good working relationship between the medical flight crew and pilot before, during, and after each mission.

PREFLIGHT PROCEDURES AND SAFETY ISSUES

preflight procedures *tasks completed prior to each mission designed to ensure the highest degree of flight safety for each flight is maintained.*

Preflight procedures refer to those tasks that should be completed prior to each mission that will ensure the highest degree of flight safety is being maintained. At the beginning of each shift (and again prior to entering the aircraft for liftoff), all crew members should approach the aircraft with their eyes glancing downward. What you are looking for is any type of debris on the ground that may be picked up by the tail rotor or be thrown by the rotor wash from the main rotor system. This is especially true when landing/taking off from unknown locations. Because helicopters are versatile enough to be able to land on almost any surface, caution must be exercised to ensure no foreign objects or debris is present. You must actively look for this debris, not just simply notice it. If something is found, the crew should immediately move the debris to a safe location away from the aircraft. Another important thing to remember while looking downward as you approach the aircraft is to remain within view of the pilot and to occasionally look at the pilot to see if she is trying to contact you. As you approach the aircraft, it is impossible for you to hear the pilot if she tries to speak to you (and vice versa); therefore, when you approach always check to see if the pilot is cognizant of your approach.

The critical care paramedic should then complete a "walk-around" of the aircraft prior to liftoff. What you are looking for is anything regarding the aircraft itself that may be a hazard to flight. The critical care paramedic should recite the following to himself at least once while performing the walk-around check: "Cords, covers, and cowlings." *Cords* refers to two things. First, while approaching the aircraft, be sure that all electrical cords plugged into the helicopter have been removed. (These electrical cords provide electricity for the ongoing functioning of internal heaters, batteries chargers, and so on, while the aircraft is sitting silent on the helipad.) Second, it refers to the visual assessment of the rotor blades to ensure that the rotor tie-down straps have been removed and properly stowed.

Covers refers to the visual assessment of the fuselage to ensure that any covers over the windows have also been properly removed and stowed. (Flight programs may use covers on the windows to protect from sun/heat in the summer months, and snow/ice buildup in the winter months while the aircraft sits on the helipad.) This also includes ensuring that the fuel cover is tightly secured. If the fuel cover is loose or open, the vacuum created during flight is great enough to empty the fuel from the aircraft.

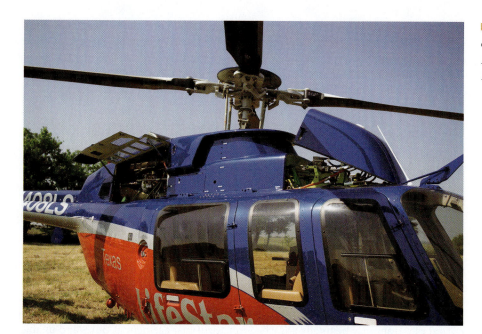

Cowlings refers to the visual assessment of the hinged portions of the fuselage that encase the engine and transmission compartment. These cowlings typically have two or more attachment points where the locking mechanism must be turned a certain direction in order for the cowling to remain closed. The point in this inspection is to ensure that all locking mechanisms are properly engaged so that the cowlings do not open during flight. The locking mechanisms may slowly become disengaged over time from the vibration of the engines. Discuss the location of these cowlings with your flight mechanic so he can point out all the pertinent cowlings and their points of attachment, and show you the visual difference in the locking mechanism appearance between the locked and unlocked position. (See Figure 5-15 ■.)

After ensuring the helipad is free from debris and the aircraft walk-around is complete, the critical care team should now enter the aircraft and secure any portable equipment for flight. Following this, protective equipment should be donned if not done so already (helmets, gloves, eye protection, and so on). Then buckle yourself into your restraint harness. If your flight program employs an internal communication system while in the aircraft, be sure to plug your headset in so you can communicate with others.

The pilot will often have his back to the crew and be unable to see your actions, so just prior to liftoff the pilot may ask the crew if portable equipment has been secured, seat belts fastened, and if everything is ready for liftoff. After confirming that the medical crew is ready, the crew observes a "sterile" cockpit. The *sterile cockpit* is an FAA regulation that necessitates all nonessential communication be ceased during critical phases of flight. Critical phases include lifting off, taxiing, and landing. The sterile cockpit serves numerous purposes. First, it eliminates any distraction of the pilot from nonessential or casual conversation by the crew. Second, it keeps frequencies clear for airport communications or your communications center to relay important information to the pilot that he needs to receive immediately. Third, it allows the pilot to carefully listen to the sounds of the engines during these critical power phases. (Landing, lifting, and taxiing are three instances when the aircraft's engines are run at maximum power, and if some mechanical failure occurs under this heavy strain, it is hoped that the pilot will hear it and take corrective action immediately.) The only time the medical crew can violate the sterile cockpit is when they identify some type of safety concern to themselves or the aircraft. For example, on final approach for a scene landing, if the flight paramedic sees an electrical power line from her side of the aircraft that was not identified by the pilot, she should immediately alert the pilot of the threat through the headset.

In those instances when a patient is being loaded for flight, the crew still has the responsibility of assessing the ground around the aircraft for any debris and doing a complete walk-around for cords, covers, and cowling status. (The pilot most likely will also be taking these precautions, but the built-in redundancy allows for a safer flight.) Furthermore, if the patient is being loaded while the engine is running "hot" (main rotor engaged), the crew should approach the aircraft in a crouched position with their eye protection donned so as to limit any harm from debris that may get picked up and thrown from the rotor wash. In the same vein, ensure that the patient and medical equipment are well secured so that nothing is picked up or blown away. After safely loading the patient, the rest of the liftoff sequence should occur as previously described.

IN-FLIGHT PROCEDURES AND SAFETY ISSUES

in-flight procedures *safety tasks designed to assure the highest degree of safety is maintained during flight operations.*

In-flight safety procedures are those safety tasks that will ensure the highest degree of safety is being maintained while in flight to your destination. First and foremost, the flight crew should always use their seat belts and shoulder harnesses while in flight. Although there are times when the flight crew needs to unbuckle to retrieve a piece of equipment or perform some skill on the patient, this should done only after alerting the pilot that you are going to release your safety belts. Immediately upon completion of the task, resecure your belts for continued safety.

The flight crew should also ensure that they are properly "plugged in" to the internal communication system so they can communicate with other members. Make sure that the mobile equipment is well secured and does not shift or fall while in flight. (Helicopters more than fixed-wing aircraft experience roughness of flight due to air turbulence.) Whenever possible, the flight crew should also be scanning the outside airspace for the presence of any other small aircraft. While the critical care team may be totally absorbed in patient management at times and unable to help the pilot out with this task, if at all possible they should scan the airspace around the helicopter for other aircraft. Another common saying within the profession is that "If your eyes are not looking at the patient, they should be looking outside the aircraft."

If some other air traffic or obstacle is spotted, the flight crew should announce this to the pilot by using the "clock method." (See Figure 5-16 ■.) This method assumes that the nose of the aircraft is pointing toward the 12 o'clock position, thus 3 o'clock is off to the right side of travel, 9 o'clock is off to the left side of travel, and the 6 o'clock position is at the rear of the aircraft. Furthermore,

■ **Figure 5-16** Clock method of describing objects in relation to the aircraft.

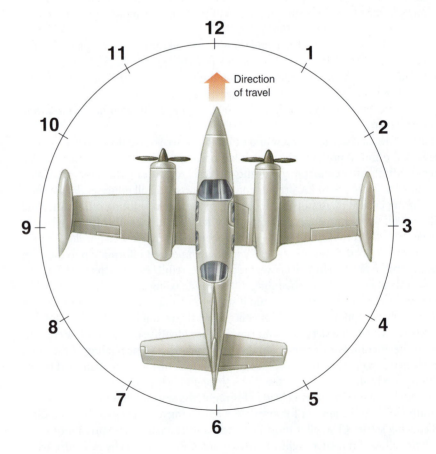

if the object is seen above the aircraft the term *high* is used, and if beneath the aircraft, the term *low* is used. For example, if another helicopter is seen off to the left side and above you, but behind your aircraft, the critical care paramedic might say something like "helicopter at 7 o'clock high." This will alert the pilot that he needs to look above, to the left, and slightly behind his current position to see the other aircraft.

POST-FLIGHT PROCEDURES AND SAFETY ISSUES

Post-flight safety procedures are those that allow for safe landing and exiting of the aircraft once you have arrived at your destination. Perhaps the most critical times when potential safety hazards could appear are during the liftoff and landing procedures in aeromedical transport. During this phase, the flight crew must assume additional roles. First, they again need to ensure that the patient is well secured, the portable equipment is well secured, and the flight crew is secure in their safety harnesses. Additionally, any significantly invasive procedures should be completed prior to descent. As mentioned before, if at all possible, all eyes should be looking outside the aircraft for hazards.

post-flight safety procedures *tasks designed for safe landing and exiting of the aircraft upon arrival.*

The pilot will customarily complete one "fly around," which is one complete reconnaissance orbit above the landing site in order to view it from all sides. The goal is to identify any potential safety hazards prior to starting the final approach to land. During this time, the flight crew (as much as possible) should be assisting the pilot in assessing the landing zone. This is probably nowhere more important than when landing at a scene flight. Although there should be a landing zone co-ordinator on the ground (usually a fire department person), there may be things spotted from the air that were missed by the LZ coordinator. Some of the more common hazards to look for include uneven terrain, radio/electrical towers, trees, wires, vehicles, people, and articles on the ground that may get dislodged by the rotor wash. Once the recon orbit is complete and the pilot announces that you are on "final approach" to land, remember to maintain a sterile cockpit—unless a safety hazard is seen.

How the flight crew exits the aircraft is somewhat dependent on the nature of the flight. If there is no patient on board, and you are landing on the helipad of the requesting hospital, typically the pilot will shut down the aircraft prior to your exiting with your equipment. If however, time is more pressing, or if landing at the scene of an MVC and your assistance is needed immediately, the crew will have to exit the aircraft while it is still running hot. This is a critical point where task delineation by the flight crew is necessary for a smooth and safe transition from the helicopter.

Typically, prior to the final approach, the flight crew has already determined who is going to exit first and open the aircraft doors, and who is going to grab the portable equipment and handle the cot. Since the crew will be unplugged from the internal communications of the aircraft, you will have to rely on eye contact and hand gestures. Be cautious of any foreign material picked up by the wind of the rotor wash, and ensure that all portable equipment is secured well to the cot so it does not become dislodged by the wind as well. Exit from under the rotor disk from the nose of the air-craft so the pilot can see the crew exiting, and remember to stay low. Remember also that during the warm-up and cooldown phases of the helicopter, the main rotor blades can still "flap" due to wind gusts, and come precariously close to the ground.

If the terrain is sloped, exit the aircraft from the downhill side if landing on slightly uneven ground. Failure to do so will cause the person to walk "uphill" and right into the spinning main ro-tor blades. Also keep an eye out for individuals on scene who, believing you need help with your equipment, come rushing up to the aircraft. Generally speaking, they do not have the same famil-iarity as you about working around a helicopter and, hence, could create a safety hazard. Finally, when you are unloading the cot from aircraft with rear-facing clamshell doors, remain cognizant of the exhaust coming from the engines. The temperature of the exhaust gases can exceed 400° C (which is more than 750° F).

IN-FLIGHT EMERGENCIES

An **in-flight emergency** is not one that involves an emergency with the patient, but rather one that influences the flight of the helicopter (or airplane) itself. Because many of these in-flight emergen-cies that lead to an accident occur due to pilot error (64%) or mechanical failure (22%), they are

in-flight emergency *situation affecting flight stability or safety of the aircraft itself.*

caused by something that the medical flight crew cannot necessarily prevent—but must deal with nonetheless.

There are generally two categories of in-flight emergencies. After discussing the source of these emergencies, focus will shift to how critical care paramedics can best prepare themselves and their patient to survive such situations.

Controlled Flight into Terrain (CFIT)

controlled flight into terrain (CFIT) *refers to any aircraft flying into the ground, into water, or in/on some other stationary object without adequate awareness or warning by the pilot.*

Controlled flight into terrain (CFIT) occurs when an airworthy aircraft is inadvertently flown into the ground, water, or some other stationary object without adequate awareness or warning by the pilot to avert such an accident. This most commonly occurs on takeoff and final approach, and can transpire from many situational factors such as pilot fatigue, loss of situational awareness, loss of visual landmarks, or sudden changes in meteorological conditions. A crash secondary to mechanical failure is not considered to be a CFIT since the mechanical failure causing the emergency typically renders the aircraft no longer airworthy.

Mechanical Failure

As mentioned previously, mechanical failure was found to be the second most common cause of accidental air medical crashes. Although even one accident due to mechanical failure is considered one too many, the FAA does keep strict guidelines on the maintenance of rotor-wing and fixed-wing aircraft for just this reason. Listed next are some of the more common in-flight emergencies that have occurred historically and what the critical care paramedic should expect during such an event:

autorotation *a sequence of collective pitch and foot pedal controls that allow a pilot to harness air flowing through the main rotor to control the aircraft's descent and landing.*

★ *Complete engine/turbine failure.* This may occur due to a host of mechanical problems in the engine(s). The end result however is the same—loss of drive to the rotor system. To survive the landing, the pilot may perform what is called an **autorotation** procedure. This procedure is loosely akin to what would be considered gliding an airplane (or coasting to a stop in your car when the motor has stopped running). Through a sequence of collective pitch control and foot pedal controls movements, the pilot may be able to harness the air flowing through the main rotor as a mechanism to control the aircraft's descent and landing.

★ *Single engine/turbine failure.* As mentioned previously, the most common airframe used in flight medicine is a dual-engine design for rotor-wing aircrafts. Should one engine fail, the pilot can usually still control the flight and landing with the second engine. Granted, the landing may be forced (not at the intended destination) and/or harder than desired, but it is usually survivable. The pilot may also be able to use the autorotation procedure in this instance to help control descent and landing.

★ *Tail rotor failure.* Failure of the tail rotor can be caused by equipment malfunction in the driveshaft assembly that transfers power from the engine and transmission to the rear rotor. If this occurs suddenly during lift-off while the pilot is using maximum power (creating maximum torque), the aircraft can start to spin wildly from the torque of the main rotor system. If still only feet from the ground (with no forward momentum), the pilot may opt to cut power to the main rotor and let the aircraft drop back to the surface of the ground (or helipad). If the tail rotor fails while in flight, the pilot may still be able to control the aircraft as the airflow over the rear vertical and horizontal stabilizers helps to keep the aircraft from spinning. From here, the pilot can implement autorotation to descend and land, or attempt a more dangerous maneuver called a *running landing* in which the aircraft is set down while still traveling 10 to 20 knots/hour (allowing airflow over the stabilizers to help stabilize the tail). This latter attempt at landing is generally more dangerous since rotor-wing aircraft are top heavy and have a tendency to roll over.

★ *Fuselage damage.* Fuselage damage can occur should the aircraft impact another object (such as a large bird), while in flight. This typically results in windshield, window, or cowling damage, and the damaged piece could then detach from the aircraft following impact. Generally, the pilot will have to implement the best solution possible for the change in aircraft aerodynamics or controls, and attempt an emergency landing.

★ *Patient compartment environment.* Although a rare occurrence, a problem may occur with the heating/cooling systems of the aircraft, allowing smoke or fumes to accumulate in the patient compartment. Or, a fire may erupt in the cabin that would necessitate the use of the onboard fire extinguisher. Should any of these occur, immediately notify the pilot and take corrective actions as practiced previously. If noxious fumes or excessive heat persist, consider opening the sliding windows on the aircraft doors (with discretion). If the problem is an electrical or lighting one, the problem is usually managed by unplugging all electrical devices and disabling the power inverter. Rely on the battery packs present on all portable patient monitoring devices, and using battery-operated flashlights if lighting becomes an issue. After eliminating the immediate hazard, refocus your attention back to the patient while the pilot plans for an emergency landing.

IN-FLIGHT EMERGENCY PROCEDURES AND SAFETY ISSUES

Each individual involved in the mission should be very familiar with emergency procedures and aware of all exit routes from the aircraft. In fact, the practicing of what should be done given a certain type of emergency should be part of the annual safety training exercise completed by each crew member. Generally, the class should include the use of fire extinguishers, the emergency locator transponder device, and emergency communications including specialized codes.

If an in-flight emergency is called (by the pilot or medical crew), the critical care paramedic should first obey any specific pilot directions, and secondly (or simultaneously if possible) tend to the following tasks if there is a chance that the aircraft is going down or needs to make an emergency landing:

1. Confirm that an emergency does exist (per pilot).
2. Relay as much information as possible to your communications center (your current coordinates and a brief description of emergency).
3. Disable the power inverter and shut off the main oxygen supply.
4. Prepare the patient for an emergency landing:
   —Place patient in supine position.
   —Tighten all straps on the stretcher.
5. Prepare crew for emergency landing:
   —Tighten all safety straps and harnesses.
   —Assume survival position by placing your arms across your chest in an "X" formation with your hands grasping the shoulder harnesses and placing knees together and feet slightly apart.

EMERGENCY EGRESS PROCEDURES AND SAFETY ISSUES

An emergency landing is, at best, a stressful and disorienting event. Flight crews that have practiced what to do and are mentally prepared for such an event will afford themselves and the other occupants of the aircraft the greatest chance of survival in an emergency landing. In the best case scenario, the pilot is able to land the aircraft with minimal or no damage, and after shutting everything down, all occupants aboard the aircraft can safely depart. In the worst case scenario, the aircraft impacts the ground hard, and results in significant if not total destruction of the aircraft.

With this latter scenario comes an increased risk of occupant entrapment, smoke inhalation, fire, and death to the flight crew and/or patient.

Following impact, the first thing that needs to be done is the shutting down of certain aircraft components. This is normally a task for the pilot. However, if the pilot is incapacitated, the critical care paramedic should know how to shut off the engines, the fuel supply, and the main batteries. (All of these reduce the chance for fires following impact.) Generally, the emergency controls that disable these components of the aircraft can be identified by red switches located in the cockpit area. (Again, the flight crew should become familiar with the particulars of their aircraft during annual safety training sessions.)

The critical care paramedic should then attempt a self-extrication. First ensure that any moving components of the aircraft have come to a stop. Following this, grasp a known component within the aircraft as a reference point as you move toward the closest available exit. (Darkness, smoke, and water within the cabin can all disorient the care provider and inhibit an expedient egress.) This is especially true in forced water landings as the aircraft will flip over, and the patient compartment will fill with water. Given the disorientation of being upside down and underwater, the grasping of a known reference point in order to find the exit may be the difference between life and death.

Most emergency landing protocols have the flight crew meeting at a specific location, usually off the 12 o'clock position of the aircraft. Once the crew has assembled at the predetermined point and the threat of fire has passed, they should return to the aircraft wreckage cautiously to assist with any other persons injured or entrapped within the wreckage. Following this, post-accident duties and survival principles become the next order of business.

POST-ACCIDENT DUTIES AND SAFETY ISSUES

post-accident duties
hazard mitigation, rescue operations, and location and/or activation of emergency locator transmitter (ELT) immediately following an unplanned landing (regardless of significance of impact).

Post-accident duties are those that are completed immediately following an unplanned landing (regardless of significance of impact). As just mentioned, the first duty following an accident is meeting with other surviving team members at the designated location. Once the threat of fire or explosion has passed, attempt rescue of anyone else still trapped in the wreckage as soon as possible. Remember to use scene size-up principles as you approach the wreckage; one thing you want to prevent is secondary injuries to yourself or other surviving flight members as you attempt to rescue others. Once the size-up is successfully completed, the crew should then take a moment and assess each other's conditions. Because aircraft crashes often result in injuries, if any flight members are injured, attempt initial stabilization as best possible. Rely on your experience as a street paramedic to guide you with management of these injuries. Any type of salvageable medical supplies should also be secured from the wreckage and brought to a safe location. After tending to the immediate medical needs of those injured, turn your focus to maximizing the survival of everyone until rescue operations can be completed.

emergency locator transmitter (ELT) *device mounted to the aircraft designed to emit a distress radio signal upon impact of the aircraft.*

One requirement of the FAA for all aeromedical services is that each aircraft be equipped with an **emergency locator transmitter (ELT)** These are devices mounted on the aircraft that will automatically emit a distress radio signal upon impact of the aircraft. If the ELT can be found in the wreckage, ensure that it activated. (They are designed to automatically activate if there is an impact exceeding 4 *G*.) If it did not activate, follow the directions on the device to manually activate it. The purpose of the ELT is to emit a radio signal that transmits the call letters of the aircraft, which is then picked up by satellites and relayed to rescue personnel. Although it does not provide a "pinpoint" to the exact location of the crash scene, it will provide a clue to the general location of the downed aircraft. (See Figure 5-17 ■.)

Unless the accident occurs in a populated area, or at a location where a visible road or building can be seen, the crew should remain with the aircraft. It is much easier for the rescue personnel to spot the wreckage from the air than it is to spot individuals attempting to walk to safety. Additionally, based on the remoteness of an accident site, the walk to civilization may be more detrimental to the crew's health than just staying put and preparing to signal the rescuing personnel. Your goal should be to minimize secondary injuries by not placing yourself or your crew in a situation where one's health status is at a great risk by traveling some unknown terrain. Plus, given the distress signal from the ELT, those attempting the rescue are likely to find a remote crash site before a crew member could walk to safety.

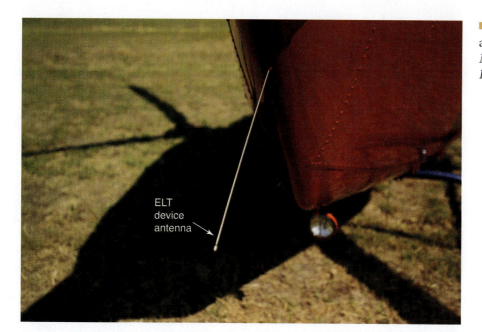

ELT device antenna

SURVIVAL PRINCIPLES AND SAFETY ISSUES

An emergency is the situation most likely to tax the physical and mental stability of the flight crew. The surviving members of the downed aircraft cannot allow fear, isolation, and uncertainty to undermine attempts at survival should the aircraft accident occur in a remote location. Although the majority of flight accidents do occur in more populated areas where rescue personnel can arrive almost instantly, the critical care paramedic cannot rely on always being in that situation. Proper preparation through education, training drills, and survival training will increase the success of those thrust into a survival situation secondary to an aeromedical accident.

The first task is to assess the status of the survival kit housed in the aircraft. Most survival kits include basic medical supplies, some type of high-energy food, tablets for making water potable, waterproof matches, space blanket, signaling device (i.e., flare gun, signaling mirror), and other terrain-specific devices (such as snowshoes or inflatable raft). Also consider how the following components of the aircraft wreckage may aid in survival or in signaling rescue personnel:

★ *Fuselage*—if no threat of fire is present, the fuselage can be used for shelter.

★ *Wings and stabilizers of the aircraft*—wind break, shelter construction, signal panels.

★ *Fuselage cowlings*—wind break, shelter construction, signal panels, collect water, fire pit.

★ *Fuselage doors*—wind break, shelter construction, signal panels.

★ *Upholstered seats*—insulation, cushions for sleeping, fire material.

★ *Intact engine batteries*—illuminate any functional lights, signaling, radio communication.

★ *Tires from the landing gear*—burning will create black signal smoke.

★ *Fuel and engine/transmission oil*—fire starter, signal fire.

Once there is an inventory of usable material, the next task for survival is establishing priorities. One way of doing this is by understanding the "rule of threes" when in outdoor survival situations. The rule states that a person can survive 3 minutes without oxygen, 3 hours in extreme weather without shelter, 3 days without water, and 3 weeks without food. The critical care paramedic can use this as a guide to establish priorities given the estimated likelihood and time frame for rescue personnel to reach the crash site. This would dictate then that, after tending to the immediate medical needs of those injured, the first priority would be creating shelter, the second priority would be creating fire to get heat and allow the boiling of water, and the last priority would be finding food. Unless the rescue is anticipated to take longer than 4 or 5 days, the rationing of foodstuff found in the survival kit will suffice. The following discussion of general **survival techniques** is aimed at preparing the critical care paramedic for survival in an extreme situation.

Shelter

The establishment of a shelter is the first component of any survival situation. Shelters provide protection from the environment and help preserve heat. A proper shelter also serves as a psychological boost for those in the rescue situation. If possible, the fuselage of the aircraft is good shelter that needs little physical preparation. Be cautious however about hypothermia because the heat of the body can conduct rapidly to the aluminum/metal surfaces in cold environments. The use of layered clothing, dry blankets, and upholstered material from the aircraft helps to minimize this effect.

If the fuselage is not a functional option for shelter, one will need to be created using available aircraft structures and suitable items found in nature (branches, rocks, snow, and so on). If building a shelter and construction resources are limited, create the roof of the shelter first, the floor second, the windward wall third, and the remaining walls last. Finally, attempt to build the shelter within site of the aircraft wreckage.

Fire

The establishment of a fire, like shelter, is a strong psychological boost to the mental health of those in a survival situation. Fire is psychologically associated with warmth, stability, and a sense of security. It also, fortunately, provides needed warmth in cold climates, allows for drying of wet clothing, provides light during the nighttime hours, and its smoke can be used as a signal for approaching rescue personnel.

The location of the fire should be carefully considered so that it does not have to be moved. Consider the direction of the prevailing wind, the type of combustible material used, and the physical proximity of the fire pit to the shelter. Preplanning for survival situations will allow the flight crew to understand the best methods and materials to use for fire, and how to employ the fire starter kit available in the aircraft survival pack.

Water

Adequate hydration is imperative to those in the survival situation. An absence of running water made potable by the water purification tablets in the survival pack, or by boiling, should not overly stress the flight crew prematurely. Unless used for medical purposes, remember that intravenous fluids found in the wreckage can be consumed for hydration (and many contain electrolytes and glucose as well). Water can also be trapped from condensation, or be melted from ice and snow if the outside weather conditions permit this. Although third on the list of priorities, a water source should be actively sought, and rationed as needed to ensure the health of those awaiting rescue.

Food

Unless the rescue is not anticipated for a number of days, food is the last priority. The body's ability to use carbohydrates, fats, and protein as energy can allow the body to maintain sufficient energy stores for a number of days. In consuming food found in the survival kit, ration it to all persons present to keep health at a maximum. Do not automatically search for consumable food in the environment (unless absolutely necessary) because a mistake in identifying edible foods in nature can have significant gastrointestinal effects that merely serve to hasten dehydration.

Preparing to Signal Rescuers

Although listed last in this prioritization of duties for survival, it is one task that should be readily prepared and implemented at first notice of rescuer arrival. Ready the flare gun (be cautious however in discharging the flare gun in extremely dry wooded areas), have items near the fire that will easily produce smoke (leaves, upholstery, or tires), and don't forget to attempt communication by the radios on the aircraft (if still operable), or the use of satellite or cellular/digital phones that may be carried by flight personnel.

ENVIRONMENTAL CONSIDERATIONS FOR SURVIVAL

The aforementioned discussions on survival techniques are generic guidelines that would apply to most flight accident instances. Depending on the geographical location of your flight program, there may be additional environmental concerns about which the flight crew should receive education. These would include services that transport patients over large bodies of water, in desert-like conditions, or over large expansions of artic terrain.

When operating over water, the flight crew should consider the donning of personal flotation devices with every mission since an unexpected in-flight emergency may cause a forced landing in water. With agencies that operate in the hot dry climates characteristic to the southwestern United States, additional education on water collection techniques and prevention strategies for heat-related illnesses should be included in annual safety training programs. In extremely cold environments, shelter and heat preservation techniques should be stressed.

The goal of every flight program should be the creation of post-accident strategies that will maximize the survival capability of those involved in an aeromedical accident. These strategies should include the availability of equipment and gear specific to the environment most likely to be encountered in a survival situation.

RESCUE EXTRICATION AND SAFETY ISSUES

Once rescue arrives, naturally those removed first from the scene are those most critically ill or injured. Flight members can assist in the prioritization of the evacuation order, but should leave the actual work of extrication to the adequately prepared rescue personnel. When rescue has arrived, the crew should also realize that their work in maintaining their own health and that of others is completed, and should patiently wait until it is their turn for removal from the accident site.

All individuals involved in the accident, regardless of how minor sustained injuries from the crash may have been, should receive a full medical evaluation once they arrived at a medical facility. In time, debriefing of the crew will occur, the accident will undergo a rigorous investigation by the appropriate authorities, and lessons learned from the accident will be incorporated into future policy decisions.

Summary

The intent of this chapter was to introduce the critical care paramedic to the dynamic environment surrounding aeromedical transport, and to identify risk factors inherent to the system. The critical care paramedic should assume an air of "safety consciousness" regarding every action taken while performing duties in the treatment and transport of critically ill or injured patients. While it is hoped that the flight crew will never find themselves in a situation where an in-flight emergency precipitates a forced emergency landing (or crash), failure to heed basic safety and survival techniques may have a greater detriment on the occupants of the aircraft than did the initial flight emergency.

To this end, the critical care paramedic should remember the following guidelines:

★ *Safety is everyone's responsibility.* Ongoing assessment during every step of a flight mission is essential to the safe completion of every flight mission. Teamwork is the foundation of safety.
★ *Safety is not a "sometimes" thing.* Repetitive review and practice of safety policies and procedures is the best way to avoid complacency.

★ *Safety begins before the flight.* A preflight briefing, clear delineations of duties, effective communication, and thorough walk-around inspection ensure that each mission begins with the highest level of safety possible.

★ *Safety precedes all actions.* Regardless of the myriad of situations in which the flight crew will find themselves, no action should be taken if it even remotely may result in an unsafe situation. Flight is likely the most unforgiving mode of transportation should an error in judgment or action occur.

Review Questions

1. What does it mean to maintain a "safety consciousness"?
2. What is the purpose of the pilot safety brief?
3. List three preflight responsibilities of all flight crew members.
4. What is meant by a "sterile cockpit" and why is it important for a safe flight?
5. What are the most common causes of an in-flight emergency that can result in a forced landing?
6. What is the role of the flight paramedic should the pilot announce that a forced (or crash) landing is inevitable?
7. What is the first thing the flight crew should do following a forced landing, while still in the aircraft?
8. What is meant by the "rule of threes" phrase regarding survival situations?
9. What are the first three priorities that should be tended to by the flight crew in a situation where the aircraft has gone down, and rescue personnel are probably 2 to 3 days off?
10. What are common ways for the flight crew to signal their location to those attempting the rescue operation?

See Answers to Review Questions at the back of this book.

Further Reading

Association of Air Medical Services. http://www.aams.org (last updated November 23, 2004).

Bledsoe BE, Porter RS, Cherry RA. *Paramedic Care: Principles & Practice, Volume 5,* 2nd ed, Upper Saddle River, NJ: Pearson/Prentice Hall, 2005.

Bledsoe BE, Smith MG. "Medical Helicopter Accidents in the United States: A Ten-Year Review." *Journal of Trauma,* Vol. 56, No. 6 (2004): 1325–1329.

Bush C. "Emergency Egress Scenarios." *Journal of Air Medical Transport,* Vol. 10, No. 3 (1991): 35.

Holleran RS. *Flight Nursing: Principles and Practice,* 2nd ed. St. Louis, MO: Mosby, 1996.

Sole ML, Lamborn ML, Hartshorn JC. *Introduction to Critical Care Nursing,* 3rd ed. Philadelphia: W. B. Saunders, 2001.

Wright AE, Campos JA, Gorder T. "The Effect of an In-Flight Emergency Training Program on Crew Confidence." *Air Medical Journal,* Vol. 13, No. 4 (1994): 127.

Patient Assessment and Preparation for Transport

Scott A. Phillips, BS, NREMT-P, CCEMT-P and

Randall W. Benner, M. Ed., MICP, NREMT-P

Objectives

Upon completion of this chapter, the student should be able to:

1. Understand the differences between the prehospital assessment and the critical care provider assessment. (p. 106)
2. Identify steps necessary to obtain comprehensive objective and subjective assessment data through history taking, physical examination techniques, and review of preexisting medical documentation. (p. 107)
3. Explain how to categorize a patient's physiologic status as either a high or low priority. (p. 110)
4. Be able to incorporate all assessment and pertinent diagnostic findings into a working field impression or diagnosis for management. (p. 118)
5. Become familiar with procedures to minimize complications of critical care transports. (p. 120)

Key Terms

Case Study

You and your partner, an RN, are working an overnight shift at a tertiary adult and pediatric referral center. Around 0200 your pager goes off, and you are directed to the helipad for a mission. After completing the aircraft walk-around, climbing in and attaching your safety harnesses, the pilot informs you that you are going to a rural emergency department (ED) about 80 miles northwest of the city. Approximately 8 minutes into your flight, you receive the following information across your pager: "Fifty-four-year-old male, difficulty breathing with a history of asthma, diabetes mellitus, and coronary artery disease. Patient will be returning to University Hospital ED."

While traveling through the night skies, you remember your previous flight transfers from this remote facility. It is a rural hospital with an eight-bed emergency department and a capable staff; it is a health care facility that typically does not call for your service unless the patient is extremely bad. After landing, unloading the equipment on the portable cot, and making your way into the ED, the unit clerk directs you to the patient in room #2. As you arrive at the patient's bedside, you quickly size up the scene and start forming your initial impression of the male patient, while a nurse and ED technician set up an in-line nebulizer mask. You see the ED physician standing at the foot of the bed analyzing blood gas results.

The patient is sitting in a high-Fowler's position, is in moderate distress and appears slightly dusky. The first thing you do is introduce yourself and your partner to him. Following this, you complete your initial examination of the patient. At 54 years of age, you note he appears quite "aged." His skin is dusky in color, and he doesn't make eye contact or acknowledge the presence of you and your partner. As you prepare to place your stethoscope on his chest, you hear the physician giving a brief oral report to your RN partner; "54-year-old male came into the ED about an hour ago. His complaint was primarily difficulty breathing and weakness. Exam revealed wheezing in the bases, tachypnea, and a poor pulse ox. He has received albuterol nebulizers for approximately 50 minutes and IV steroids, but he has steadily deteriorated despite our treatment. I've arranged for transport to your facility for ongoing diagnosis and management for his respiratory distress . . . rule out *status asthmaticus* versus cardiac complication." Your partner continues to converse with the ED staff as he gathers pertinent information while you focus on the patient assessment. After learning of the initial impression of the ED staff, you continue your assessment in order to support that initial diagnosis.

You have already introduced yourself, and when doing so you notice that the patient doesn't even have enough energy to raise his head or to make eye contact; however, he does stick out his hand. Your initial assessment and rapid physical exam proceed in a stepwise fashion as you concurrently ask him the normal history questions while utilizing the SAMPLE and OPQRST mnemonics. Over the noise of the nebulizer mask, you learn that his shortness of breath has progressively gotten worse during the past 6 hours, with no relief from his "home inhalers." The patient stated he felt like he was smothering, so he came into the ED. His history includes coronary artery disease, asthma, and insulin-dependent diabetes mellitus.

Initial assessment findings are as follows: He is a 54-year-old, white male with mild obesity and a diminishing mental status. His airway is patent with a respiratory rate that was initially 40 per minute, but has been decreasing (currently it is 24 per minute), but the tidal volume has likewise been diminishing as the patient becomes increasingly fatigued from the heightened respiratory effort. You also note intercostal muscle retractions, diaphragmatic movement, and jugular venous distention at a 45-degree angle. Peripheral perfusion is intact, but his pulse is tachycardic and irregular. His skin is cool and diaphoretic; the cardiac monitor shows sinus tachycardia with multiple PVCs. The most current 12-lead reading shows left ventricular hypertrophy with a mild left axis deviation.

While auscultating the chest, you listen to heart sounds which reveal an abnormal sound—almost like a late split of S1. Vital signs on the automated BP machine reveal a heart rate of 114, BP 96/62, RR 10, and an SpO_2 reading of 89%. Quickly your partner shares with you the medical charting and you incorporate that into your assessment to this point. You think to yourself:

> ". . . a 54-year-old male with a complaint of shortness of breath for 6+ hours, no relief with home nebulizers . . . came into ED, breathing fast with wheezes in bases . . . after 60 minutes of in-line nebulizers and steroids, the dyspnea is not resolving. . . . Vitals are failing as is his respiratory status . . . this patient is obviously a high priority—but he should have been getting better. . . . "

Your partner then hands you the recent ABGs, which read: pH of 7.32, $PaCO_2$ of 55, PaO_2 of 76, HCO_3 of $^-12$, SpO_2 of 89%. His chest X-ray shows basal bilobular fluid infiltration with a moderately enlarged heart. You turn back to the patient and expose his abdomen (which you note is quite large for his age) and find facial grimacing from pain while palpating the upper right quadrant, and there is a positive hepatojugular reflux. Bowel sounds are present, and in finishing his GI/GU assessment you find that the patient has received nearly a liter of NaCl and hasn't urinated. The patient moves all extremities, and you note +1 pitting edema in lower extremities to which the patient adds ". . . that happens sometimes."

The balance of the rapid physical exam and detailed exam is negative and noncontributory to the patient's clinical presentation. After consulting with your partner, and again with the ED physician, the three of you collectively decide to alter the diagnosis to that of cardiac asthma induced by congestive heart failure (CHF). This is supported by the following rationalization:

> The patient does have a history of asthma; however, the physical examination reveals signs of biventricular failure with cardiac decompensation. Signs and symptoms of right ventricular failure (RVF) include jugular venous distention (JVD) fullness in the RUQ, and peripheral pitting edema. Signs and symptoms of left ventricular failure (LVF) include tachypnea, tachycardia, pulmonary V/Q mismatch with wheezing in lower lobes caused by fluid buildup, dysrhythmias, and poor peripheral perfusion. In concert with the ABGs, chest X-ray, 12-lead findings, and an absence of response to the bronchodilatory treatment, it adds up to acute CHF.

Since this is a high-priority patient, you elect to begin treatment immediately in an attempt to stabilize the patient. You initiate noninvasive ventilatory pressure support with a BiPAP, and slow the IV infusion down to a KVO rate. Your management goals, other than the reversal of hypoxemia and hypercapnia, are to increase myocardial contractility and decrease afterload pharmacologically. The resultant increase in perfusion pressures should in turn stimulate a gentle diuresis by the kidneys in an attempt to eliminate the relative hypervolemia.

After deciding a care plan with your partner and contacting your medical director to confirm the treatment with him, you initiate your interventions. During your reassessment of the patient you start to see an improvement in the patient's hemodynamic stability, so appropriate preparations for transport are begun. The patient's wife and family are allowed to see the patient once again before lifting off. Following this, you and your partner make sure all paperwork is signed, medical records obtained, and the patient is secured to the transport cot. Following this, he is taken to the waiting aircraft for the flight back to your hospital. The flight is uneventful, and you discuss the assessment findings and treatment interventions with the receiving physician.

INTRODUCTION

An accurate and reliable patient assessment is one of the most important skills the paramedic performs in both the prehospital and critical care environments.

An accurate and reliable patient assessment is one of the most important skills the paramedic performs in both the prehospital and critical care environments. Critical care paramedics must be able to efficiently and reliably gather and incorporate information on the patients they are summoned to transport from multiple sources. This includes information gathered from the patient during the physical examination, information from the initial care providers (prehospital or hospital), results of various diagnostic tests already performed, and any medical information shared by the patient's family. Developing a systematic assessment routine for each patient encounter will increase the critical care paramedic's confidence in assessment skills and ensure that emergent or life-threatening conditions are managed immediately.

The patient assessment, identification of the patient's condition, and initiation of critical and noncritical interventions will then provide a framework for preparing the patient for transport. It cannot be stressed enough that each of these tasks must be performed in a structured, rapid, and thorough manner in order to provide optimal patient care and ensure a smooth transport to the destination facility. As such, the intent of this chapter is to reinforce to the paramedic the components of patient assessment and preparation for transport. The chapter also includes how a discussion about assessment, management, and transport considerations change in light of the critical care environment you are now entering.

PATIENT ASSESSMENT

The patient assessment performed by the critical care paramedic continues to be the most frequently utilized skill. It is the one skill that must be thoroughly and efficiently performed on every patient encountered before treatment can be provided.

As with the use of patient assessment skills in the prehospital environment, the patient assessment performed by the critical care paramedic continues to be the most frequently utilized skill. It is the one skill that must be thoroughly and efficiently performed on every patient encountered before treatment can be provided. During your practice in critical care, you will care for patients who fall along a continuum ranging from very stable at one end, to extremely unstable with ongoing deterioration at the other. In all instances, the critical care paramedic must efficiently gather data, methodically complete a physical exam, and synthesize the information into a working diagnosis on which proper patient management will be based. Failure to do so will invariably lead to errors in judgment, and ultimately errors in patient management. In this sense, assessment is the key to proper treatment.

Remember also that assessment is not a one-time-only task. Experienced clinicians know that in order to provide the best care possible, one must constantly reassess the patient's status after each intervention and be prepared to alter the care provided at a moment's notice. If the patient the critical care paramedic is being summoned to treat and transport is unstable and may rapidly decompensate, the importance of assessment cannot be overemphasized.

Unlike the prehospital environment though, where the paramedic is used to formulating his management plan primarily from clinical assessment findings, the critical care environment oftentimes allows the paramedic to utilize a working diagnosis that has been formulated by a tier of medical professionals. This working diagnosis still does not relieve the critical care paramedic of the responsibility of reviewing all pertinent information and performing a physical assessment.

The critical care paramedic needs to be aware that she will be practicing in many types of situations, each of them unique. Although the goal is consistency in your assessment format, you may have to make dynamic changes given the particular situation. This is fine, as long as the critical care paramedic preserves the focus of assessment. Although many of your patient missions will occur between two medical facilities where the exchange of patient information may be more reliable, the critical care team is also requested by EMS providers for prehospital missions where the availability of patient information is limited. Again, in all of these situations, the critical care team must stay abreast of the situation, focus on the patient, and provide the best care possible.

By now, the critical care paramedic should be well acclimated to prehospital medicine and the importance of staying focused on the patient—and not allowing the scene to detract from the mission. Similar to prehospital medicine, critical care paramedics face many of the same distractions during a mission—if not more. The critical care paramedic will be subject to noise, temperature and/or environmental extremes, family and/or patient confusion, differing/conflicting opinions, and distractions from other medical professionals, and will always be affected by the influence of time.

PREARRIVAL INFORMATION AND ITS RELATION TO THE ASSESSMENT

The assessment of the patient in the critical care environment begins long before the provider makes contact with the patient. Many times the critical care paramedic will obtain information that is relayed to him from the initiating care facility. This information comes either before or while in transit to the hospital that initiated the request. This information, listed later, allows the transporting crew the ability to preplan treatment and procedures before coming in contact with the patient. It also gives the critical care paramedic an opportunity to ensure that he has the necessary equipment or personnel to safely make the transport.

After the patient arrives at the initial destination (either by private vehicle or an EMS vehicle), the medical personnel at that facility begin assessing and treating a myriad of medical problems and/or injuries. Upon deciding that transport by a critical care service is warranted, the personnel initially caring for the patient will amass the basic and advanced assessment information they have learned from the patient, which can be shared with the critical care paramedic to use and begin a systematic plan for the patient's transport.

Information gathered that assists the critical care paramedic in developing an initial assessment and management plan may include (but not be limited to) the following:

1. Reason for transport
2. History of the present illness
3. Interventions and/or medications currently in place
4. Responses to interventions and/or medications
5. Expected interventions during transport
6. Current physiologic status of the patient and a review of any diagnostic or advanced imaging finding

Each of these types of information is discussed in the following sections.

REASON FOR TRANSPORT

Chapter 2 (Critical Care Ground Transport) and Chapter 3 (Critical Care Aerial Transport) both provide specific criteria in greater detail that explain what would necessitate transport of a patient from one medical facility to another. They also provide criteria the prehospital providers may consider in determining if a scene transport by the critical care service is warranted. Although the specific reasons for transport missions are varied, the request for critical care transport usually falls into one of the following categories:

1. The patient is still in the prehospital environment due to entrapment or isolation issues (remote locations), and flying them to the medical facility is a viable option due to distance and time issues.

2. If already at one medical facility, the patient may need additional therapies or treatments that are not available there.

3. The patient is being admitted to another facility due to economic or insurance reasons.

4. The patient or his or her family requests the transport.

The first reason that the critical care team may be called to transport a patient is because the patient may benefit from the rapid transport inherent to rotor- or fixed-wing aircraft. But this does come with exceptions. As discussed in Chapter 3, air medical transport offers a number of advantages and disadvantages. The advantages include much more rapid transport speed, access to remote locations, access to specialty teams (e.g., neonate, transplant, burn care), and access to personnel with specialized skills such a surgical airway, thoracostomy, rapid-sequence intubation (RSI), and critical care experience. The disadvantages include weather, altitude effects, vibration, noise, air/motion sickness, and environmental restrictions to flying. Limitations on the number of crew members during transport can also be influenced by the size of the aircraft, fuel load, and landing zone or airstrip limitations. These dynamics also play a role in being able to complete a mission due to the physical size of the patient as well.

The second reason the critical care team may be called is when a facility is unable to provide necessary interventions to benefit the patient. They must transfer that patient to a facility that has the necessary resources and can provide this higher level of care. Regardless of the ability to definitively treat the patient's medical condition, the sending facility has the legal obligation to provide initial medical screening and stabilization. The transporting facility must also ensure that the critical care team assigned to the patient is able to provide the type of current and anticipated care required by this particular patient. Although a full discussion of **EMTALA and COBRA legislation** is well beyond the scope of this chapter, suffice it to say that this legislation requires the transporting personnel to have the appropriate licensure and skills to maintain, initiate, or reinitiate ordered treatment necessary to deal with the known (or potential) problems encountered during transport. It also requires that the sending facility take every step necessary within its power to ensure that the patient is as stable as can be expected prior to transport.

Medical stability requires that the hospital ensure that the patient is not at reasonable risk of deteriorating as a result of, or during or following, the transfer. The hospital is also bound not to transfer patients who are potentially unstable if it has the capability to treat the patient. The critical care paramedic should be relatively assured that if the patient falls into this category for transport, the sending facility has made every effort to ensure the stability of the patient prior to transport.

The third reason for critical care transport missions arises when smaller outlying hospitals or clinics do not have the massive resources of larger health care facilities typical of the larger cities. In such cases, the smaller hospitals often agree to be part of a hospital network system for insurance and/or business purposes. With this arrangement, the insurance carriers and network hospitals have a vested interest in where the patient receives care. It is also preferable for the receiving hospitals and the insurance carrier for the patient transfer to take place within network facilities. Some systems will establish a rotor-wing or ground transport critical care team to perform these interfacility transfers. With this arrangement, an integrated system of initial assessment, stabilization, transfer, and ongoing treatment becomes more seamless and allows the most critically ill individuals to be transported for ongoing diagnosis and treatment in an expedient fashion.

The final reason for transport of the patient by a critical care team arises when a patient or family requests a specific doctor or facility. This request may take the patient across town, the state, the country, or, in some situations, around the world.

In conclusion, once the critical care paramedic has identified the reason for transport he may also develop a bit of insight into the acuity of the patient. He may also have the opportunity to preplan portions of the transport, especially in the case of longer distance transports.

EMTALA and COBRA legislation *federal legislation addressing appropriate licensure and skills of medical personnel involved with patient care and transport, as well as stabilization of patients prior to transport.*

HISTORY OF THE CURRENT ILLNESS

The history of the current illness becomes important for planning interventions and foreseeing potential complications of transport. Unlike the prehospital environment, the critical care paramedic has the ability to review all of the potential information gathered about the current illness. Once the information has been reviewed, the critical care paramedic should be able to reasonably anticipate the level of care necessary for the patient during transport and be prepared to deliver that care.

If, however, the critical care paramedic has just arrived on scene for a medical or trauma patient still being cared for by prehospital providers, the completeness of the medical history may be in question. If this is ever the case, just follow the SAMPLE history and OPQRST mnemonic so that this information can be gained prior to leaving the scene. Since the critical care paramedic typically has a larger array of medications and interventions at her disposal, the need to complete the patient history cannot be overstated so that appropriate interventions can be administered. (See Figure 6-1 ■.)

CURRENT INTERVENTIONS AND MEDICATIONS ADMINISTERED

The interventions in place also tell the critical care team quite a bit about the condition of the patient. Is the patient on multiple medication infusions? Does the patient have invasive lines or tubes in place that may give an indication of the severity of the injury or illness? The incorporation of this important information into your assessment will be more thoroughly discussed later in the chapter.

RESPONSES TO INTERVENTIONS AND MEDICATIONS

How has the patient responded to the interventions and medications currently in place? Once this question is answered, the critical care paramedic will have a better understanding of treatments potentially needed during transport. Generally speaking, the answer to these questions will advise you if first-, second-, or third-line interventions have been attempted and, if so, how the patient responded.

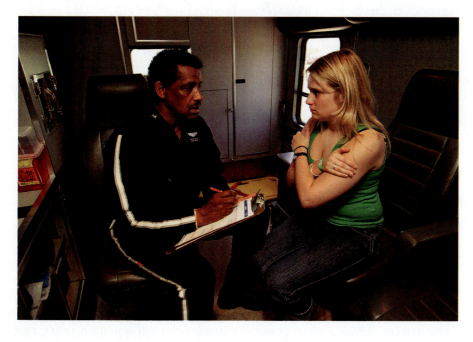

■ Figure 6-1 It is essential for the critical care paramedic to gather as much patient information as possible utilizing multiple sources. (© 2005 Scott Metcalfe LLC. All Rights Reserved)

EXPECTED AND ANTICIPATED INTERVENTIONS DURING TRANSPORT

Anticipating the patient's needs during transport can be one of the most valuable assets of the critical care paramedic. Prearrival information gives the critical care paramedic the ability to preplan and review several of the areas that may prove difficult to take care of once en route. The review of the anticipated needs of the patient may also dictate the mode of transport, which will ensure timely response of the critical care team. Constraints, such as limited space, make the initiation or maintenance of some interventions difficult, if not impossible. For example, the transport of a patient receiving intra-aortic balloon pump (IABP) therapy may require ground transport as opposed to air transport because the local aeromedical system may not have the ability to place the IABP in the aircraft.

CURRENT PHYSIOLOGIC STATUS OF THE PATIENT

The degree of stability the patient demonstrates after you complete your assessment will help the crew anticipate the future needs of the patient. It also provides the crew with a better understanding of the patient's stability for the transport. Many patients may have conditions that preclude transport until further stabilizing measures have been performed. The case of the OB patient in active labor is an excellent example of the need to review the current patient status prior to transport.

But determining the current status of the patient is based on much more than simply their medical diagnosis. The status of the patient also includes the assessment of how the patient is presenting given the diagnosis. Take, for example, two patients experiencing a myocardial infarction. Patient A has a left coronary artery occlusion with a high lateral infarction and stable hemodynamics. Patient B also has a left coronary artery occlusion, but the occlusion is in the left common coronary artery and the patient is suffering infarction to the septal, anterior, and lateral walls of the left ventricle. This latter presentation (known as the "widow maker") will cause the patient to present much more hemodynamically unstable than patient A. The point is that they both have the same diagnosis, but their hemodynamic response to the emergency is drastically different.

What does the current status of the patient include? The current status includes those assessment and diagnostic findings that will tell you how the patient is faring physiologically with his medical or traumatic emergency. Although the type of information provided to you about the status of the patient is a function of what has been performed by the sending facility, the information the critical care medic needs includes the following:

- ★ Current mental status, to include any trends in Glasgow Coma Scale (GCS) scoring
- ★ Respiratory rate and breathing adequacy
  - – Pulse oximetry, end-tidal capnography, peak flow, and so on
  - – Mechanical ventilator compliancy if patient is paralyzed and intubated
- ★ Cardiovascular and peripheral perfusion assessment
  - – Pulse, capillary refill, skin characteristics
  - – ECG rate and rhythm
  - – Hemodynamic pressure findings (if assessed)
- ★ Any laboratory values and blood chemistry studies
- ★ Results of any X-rays or other advanced imaging and diagnostic studies

DIAGNOSTICS

Unlike your prehospital care counterparts, you may have access to various diagnostic studies that have been completed before your arrival. These may include such things as laboratory tests, X-rays, ECGs, pulmonary function testing, echocardiography, ultrasound, and CT and MRI imaging. These tests can provide a tremendous amount of information as to the patient's condition. However, it is not within the scope of this text to provide detailed information about all types of medical imaging. An overview of diagnostic testing is presented in Chapter 12 (Interpretation of Lab and Basic Diagnostic Tests).

ASSESSMENT OF THE BODY SYSTEMS ON ARRIVAL

As with the prehospital environment, the critical care paramedic must complete a physical assessment. The goal is to reconfirm what the sending facility has provided to you, and reassess for any changes in status. The type of patients commonly seen by the critical care paramedic are often critical, and significant changes in the patient's stability can occur rapidly and almost without warning. Without repeated assessments both on scene and while in transit, changes in the patient's status may go unnoticed until significant disturbances present (like lethal cardiac dysrhythmias or unresponsiveness).

The process by which the critical care paramedic provider will complete his or her assessment of the patient closely mirrors the assessment phases used by prehospital providers. With only slight modifications, the critical care paramedic will still complete a scene size-up, an initial assessment of the patient, a history and physical exam, which in this case is actually a rapid physical exam (as time and patient conditions permit), and finally the ongoing assessment phase. These phases are discussed in more detail in the following sections.

SCENE SIZE-UP

Each phase of assessment has a "purpose," or a reason why the steps of that phase are completed. And for the **scene size-up** phase of assessment, the purpose is to *control the scene.* Controlling the scene means employing those techniques that will best ensure your safety and that of your crew and patient immediately upon arrival at the patient's side. In also includes considering additional resources to better enable you to control the ongoing assessment and management of the patient. The steps necessary to "control the scene" during the scene size-up include the following:

★ *BSI precautions.* Body substance isolation (BSI) precautions involve employing the appropriate personal protective equipment (PPE) necessary to ensure a low risk of bloodborne exposure to the critical care crew. The bare minimum would be examination gloves, but access to protective eye, face, and mouth equipment is necessary.

★ *Mechanism of injury (MOI) versus nature of illness (NOI).* MOI and NOI refer to the same thing for the critical care paramedic as it does for other prehospital providers. Often, the NOI is provided by the sending facility's personnel because they are familiar with the patient. If responding to a scene, the on-scene EMS providers should be able to provide the MOI or NOI as appropriate prior to your arrival at the patient's side. In any instance though, the critical care paramedic can use the MOI and NOI as another clue to the patient's status.

★ *Additional resources (not enough or too many).* While completing interfacility missions, additional resources typically include hospital personnel from departments such as pulmonary or respiratory care, OB/GYN, pediatrics, and the like. These individuals are sometimes called on to help with the management of patients with specific emergencies. These providers, however, may know nothing about critical care transport or even flight medicine. Two of your roles here are to help with patient care and to help facilitate the other providers' transition into your world of critical care.

Additionally, when considering additional resources remember that there will be times when too many additional resources (referring to care providers) are at the patient's side. In an emergency, critical patients often require multiple care providers completing tasks simultaneously. Although this may sometimes be necessary, at other times, the critical care paramedic will arrive at an ED or land at the scene of an

With only slight modifications, the critical care paramedic will still complete a scene size-up, an initial assessment of the patient, a history and physical exam, a detailed physical exam (as time and patient conditions permit), and finally the ongoing assessment phase.

scene size-up *assessment of scene safety and the resources needed to control a scene, effect appropriate rescue or extrication, and initiate transport of patients.*

accident only to find that there are just too many people wanting to participate in the patient care. Naturally, all providers have the best intentions in mind and want the optimum care for the patient, but you will find yourself in situations where the critical care team has to actually ask the unnecessary providers surrounding the patient to step back. Too many people can create confusion.

★ *Cervical spine precautions.* For the medical transfer patient, cervical precautions are rarely taken since they haven't the mechanism for a spinal injury. The traumatically injured patient is a different story, however, so as-necessary spinal precautions should be taken immediately by way of manual cervical immobilization with subsequent full spinal immobilization. Since the critical care paramedic is never (or rarely ever) the first person on scene, spinal precautions should have been established already by the initial care providers. This does not mean the critical care paramedic can be lackadaisical about this. Many flight programs may require a patient with a suggestive history to be immobilized even though the EMS providers on scene or the physician in the ED has ruled out the need based on symptomatology or exam (to include X-ray interpretation).

★ *Number of patients.* Although this is another step in the scene size-up, it is rarely one with which critical care paramedics have to concern themselves. When responding to an interfacility transport, you should be provided with reliable information from the sending facility. And rarely, if ever, are you called to transfer two patients simultaneously. On scene flights, however, there may be a chance that two critically injured patients will need transport by the critical care team. In these situations, the pilot of the aircraft needs to be involved in the decision making since some airframes have weight limitations. If you are limited to transporting only one patient, and two are critically injured, you will have to triage them both and transport the most critical first.

Controlling the scene means employing those techniques that will best ensure your safety and that of your crew and patient immediately upon arrival at the patient's side.

The scene size-up is the initial phase of patient assessment completed by the critical care paramedic. Determining the BSI precautions needed, the MOI/NOI, the need for additional resources, the appropriateness of spinal precautions, and the number of patients allows the critical care provider to rapidly determine what is needed in order to take control of the scene. From there, focus the balance of the assessment and treatment on the patient. Even though the completion of this phase of the assessment can be done quicker than it takes to read about it in this chapter, the importance of completing it cannot be overstated. As the old EMS adage goes, "Either control the scene, or the scene will control you."

INITIAL ASSESSMENT

initial assessment
immediate assessment of life threats and transport priority.

The goal for the **initial assessment** is to identify and support any lost vital bodily function. Although you may be assessing other parameters not directly related to vital bodily functions, everything that you do in this phase should be done to determine if a life-threatening injury or illness is present that must be immediately treated. While working in this environment, the critical care provider must assume that all patients encountered are either extremely sick or critically injured, until proven otherwise.

An initial assessment is done to identify and support any lost vital bodily functions.

To a certain extent, reviewing the life threats of the patient can be easily done because individuals who have assessed and initiated care prior to your arrival can share this information with you. And although this will help you in forming your impressions as you do your assessment, it does not alleviate the critical care paramedic from reassessing the airway, breathing, and circulatory functions of the patient. The following subsections outline the steps in completing the initial assessment. The critical care paramedic should keep in mind that the only conditions that are sought and treated during this phase are those that will have a negative impact on the airway, breathing, and circulatory systems of the body.

FORMING A GENERAL IMPRESSION

The first component of the initial assessment is the general impression of the patient. While the emergency care personnel on scene should be able to give a fairly detailed report of the airway, breathing, and circulatory status of the patient, the critical care paramedic should still form his own general impression, while incorporating what was told to him as he does so.

The general impression is the step in the initial assessment in which the critical care paramedic rapidly synthesizes a quick description of the patient. This is often a visual assessment that is completed as you approach the patient. More specifically, this would include the patient's age, gender, ethnicity, confirmation of the MOI/NOI, and a basic interpretation of stability (i.e., responsive or unresponsive). From this general impression as well the critical care paramedic can make an initial determination of "sick versus not sick," which refers to the overall stability with which the patient presents.

MENTAL STATUS ASSESSMENT

Assessment of the mental status is an ongoing process that starts during the initial assessment. Your assessment of mental status is crucial for all patients. Almost any problem (medical or traumatic) can result in an alteration in the mental status. Additionally, the mental status can deteriorate as the patient's physical condition deteriorates. Use this as a clue to the patient's overall stability. To assess your patient's mental status, use the AVPU method and be cognizant to trend changes in the GCS. The critical question the critical care provider should ask herself here is "Does my patient have an acute change in mental status?" If the answer is "no," move on to airway assessment. If the answer is "yes," consider this patient to be a high priority, in probable need of airway and breathing support.

AIRWAY ASSESSMENT

The airway assessment is performed identically to how it is done by other emergency care providers, with the intent being to ensure that the airway is patent. Patients who are exchanging air freely and silently and are able to speak (if conscious) are exhibiting reliable indicators that the airway is patent. Any less than this is suspect, and should be managed immediately. The general progression of initial airway maintenance includes the sequential implementation of:

★ A manual airway technique (tongue occlusion)

★ Oropharyngeal and/or nasopharyngeal suctioning (as needed for fluid)

★ Insertion of a simple mechanical adjunct (OPA or NPA)

★ Placement of an endotracheal tube or CombiTube (or RSI protocol)

★ Consideration for transtracheal airway interventions (needle or surgical cricothyrotomy) if all preceding interventions fail

The critical question to ask is "Does my patient have an adequate airway?" If the answer is "yes," move on to breathing assessment. If the answer is "no," open the airway. At this point, since the critical care paramedic is only trying to establish an open airway during the initial assessment, employ only those techniques needed to ensure airway patency in the obtunded patient. Commonly, this is achieved initially with suctioning, manual techniques, and the use of a simple mechanical airway. Securing the airway as needed will occur after the initial assessment is completed, but for now, support the lost airway function as identified previously.

BREATHING ADEQUACY

Many times assessment and management of the airway and breathing occur simultaneously. But that is not always the case, so the critical care provider should still assess breathing adequacy as a separate component of the initial assessment. Adequate breathing is characterized by an acceptable rate *and* depth of breathing. Assessing the rate is simple; you just count respirations against a measure of time. More important though is assessment of the depth of breathing (or the quality of the tidal volume).

The patient's tidal volume may provide better insight into the patient's breathing adequacy than the rate alone because it will actually indicate whether alveolar ventilation is occurring. This is done by watching the amount of chest wall excursion during breathing, listening for the volume of air exchange, and assessing for breath sounds in the vesicular regions of the lungs. The critical care paramedic needs

The patient's tidal volume may provide better insight into the patient's breathing adequacy than the rate alone because it will actually indicate whether alveolar ventilation is occurring.

to remember that almost all disturbances in breathing adequacy occur because of a change in tidal volume and alveolar ventilation (consider the effects of a flail chest, a pneumothorax, a hemothorax, significant pneumonia, or COPD disorders), and not because of extreme changes in the respiratory rate. With the exceptions of a depressant drug overdose or significant brainstem dysfunction, the respiratory rate rarely slows down. In actuality, the rate has a tendency to increase due to the insult, which taken to an extremely tachypneic rate, will contribute to diminished tidal volumes and drops in alveolar ventilation.

When dealing with breathing assessment, the care provider has another critical question to ask himself. It is simply, "Is my patient breathing adequately or inadequately?" If the answer is "adequately," apply oxygen if you have not done so already and move onto circulatory assessment. If the answer is "inadequately," support lost function by providing mechanical ventilation with oxygen. The options for achieving this include:

★ Mouth-to-barrier ventilation

★ Two-person bag-valve-mask (BVM) ventilation

★ One-person BVM ventilation

★ Utilization of an oxygen-powered ventilatory device

★ Consideration of an automatic transport ventilator

Like airway assessment and management, failure to ensure or provide adequate ventilations will lead to further patient deterioration and hasten cardiac arrest. The focus here though is simple: Support inadequate breathing. Note that you are assessing and treating breathing inadequacy, not the illness or injury underlying the deficit. That will be done momentarily during the rapid physical exam. But for now, ensure that the patient is being oxygenated and ventilated, then move on to the next component of the initial assessment.

CIRCULATORY ASSESSMENT

Once the patient's airway patency and respiratory function have been assessed, the next thing to review is the cardiac and circulatory systems of the patient. This particular step is somewhat more involved at the critical care level than in the prehospital setting for the paramedic. The major goal in reviewing the circulatory and cardiovascular status is to allow the critical care paramedic the opportunity to minimize potential problems during the transport.

Confirmation of central and peripheral pulses must be completed. A comparison of the rate and quality of the two locations will also provide an indirect measure of the hemodynamic status of the patient. Also the temperature, color, and skin condition also give insight into the quality of peripheral perfusion.

The cardiac assessment should also include a review of ECG findings, which may dictate potential therapies en route. If the patient is at risk for a fatal dysrhythmia, it is preferable to apply multifunction cardiac pads (pacing/cardioversion) prior to transport instead of wrestling with the patient in a confined environment to get the pads in place.

The critical care paramedic will also have the opportunity to review IV access, fluids, and medications that are in place to assist the patient's circulatory status. There will be times that the patient is being transported from a hospital with ongoing hemodynamic monitoring. The critical care paramedic should also review these pressures and consider the need for acute management of any noted disturbances.

Finally, like the prehospital realm, if the patient is found to have a life-threatening hemorrhage, direct pressure as well as any needed subsequent interventions should be employed to eliminate the bleeding.

Like the previous steps of the initial assessment, there is also a critical question that the care provider needs to ask himself prior to moving to the next phase of assessment: "Does my patient have a life-threatening circulatory deficit present?" If the answer is "no," initiate steps to move the patient from the hospital bed (or scene location) to the critical care provider's cot, and begin switching any medical equipment over to your portable equipment. If, however, the answer to this critical question is "yes," additional immediate treatment is warranted. Critical cardiovascular findings suggestive of loss in function or acute deterioration include (but may not be limited to):

★ External hemorrhage
★ Lethal prearrest or arrest dysrhythmia
★ Significantly altered perfusion status
★ Any hemodynamic findings suggestive of acute deterioration
★ Significantly altered vital signs (heart rate and/or blood pressure extremes)

If any of the above critical circulatory findings are discovered, immediate treatment should be initiated in order to prevent acute deterioration or cardiac arrest. How to perform these critical interventions is what the balance of this textbook is dedicated to providing, with the focus being the various interventions for the types of emergencies seen in the critical care environment.

DETERMINATION OF PATIENT PRIORITY STATUS

This portion of the assessment is actually a critical thought process leading to a categorizing of the patient's overall condition. Again, in the critical care environment, this is typically done prior to your arrival and the critical care team confirms this determination through its assessment. As needed though, the patient should be regarded as a high priority if any deficits are noted during the initial assessment.

Determining the patient's priority status is actually a critical thought process that leads to a categorizing of the patient's overall condition.

You were probably taught a list of critical findings or conditions that would lead to the determination of "high-priority" status during initial education courses. An easier way to determine high-priority status is the finding of any initial assessment disturbances. Simply put, any patient should be considered a high priority if he has a loss of function in:

★ Airway patency
★ Breathing adequacy
★ Circulatory status
★ Mental status (acute alteration)

Any patient should be considered a high priority if he has a loss of function in airway patency, breathing adequacy, circulatory status, or mental status (acute alteration).

RAPID PHYSICAL EXAM

The **rapid physical exam** is a head-to-toe exam geared toward rapid assessment of key findings in order to provide specific interventions. The overall goal is to assess the patient rapidly from head to toe, looking for those critical injuries or clinical findings that contributed to the loss of function identified earlier in the initial assessment.

rapid physical exam *a head-to-toe assessment designed to identify critical injuries or findings that may contribute to the loss of function or life.*

To illustrate this with an injury example, the critical care paramedic will first identify the patient with inadequate breathing during the initial assessment of the breathing status. In response to this critical finding, the care provider will initiate the critical intervention of positive-pressure ventilation with a BVM and oxygen to support that lost function—while completing the rest of the initial assessment. Then, during the rapid physical exam, the critical care paramedic will attempt to identify the injury (for example, a flail chest) that caused the inadequate breathing to occur, and then provide appropriate critical interventions. Stated more simply, during the initial assessment you support the lost function, then during the rapid physical exam you attempt to find and treat the injury (or illness) that caused the lost function. In reality, this is already done by the initial care providers tending to the patient prior to your arrival. However, do not develop a false sense of security that all findings and interventions will be done every time prior to you arrival. Remember that the patient's status may rapidly deteriorate, or even more simply, a critical finding or illness may yet need to be diagnosed in your patient.

Similar to the rapid trauma physical exam or rapid medical physical exam performed by prehospital providers, the critical care paramedic will perform her rapid physical exam in the following general order (paying attention to only critical injuries or illnesses requiring additional immediate interventions):

★ *Head.* Critical findings: pupil abnormalities, airway disturbance, acute change in mental status, open skull fractures

★ *Neck.* Critical findings: open soft tissue injury, vertebral crepitus, JVD, tracheal deviation

★ *Anterior and lateral thorax.* Abnormal auscultation or percussion findings, palpable instability, soft-tissue trauma, punctures/penetrations

★ *Abdomen.* Open soft-tissue injuries, distention, palpable masses

★ *Pelvis.* Instability to palpation

★ *Extremities.* Large open long-bone fractures, or those with significant pulse, motor, or sensory deficits

★ *Posterior surface.* Open soft-tissue injury to back, flailed posterior ribs, palpable vertebral instability

From here, the critical care paramedic performing the assessment can move onto the next phase of assessment. During this time, the other member(s) of the critical care team should still be preparing the patient for transport by readying the patient for transfer to the team's cot and replacing the hospital/EMS medical equipment with the critical care team's portable equipment (e.g., infusion pumps, mechanical ventilation, ECG, and hemodynamic monitoring).

DETAILED PHYSICAL EXAM

detailed physical exam
methodical assessment designed to identify non-life-threatening conditions, general abnormalities, and adequacy of interventions.

The critical care paramedic should perform a detailed physical exam on every patient that he transports. This will ensure that information is not missed, and will enable the paramedic to review all pertinent information for the patient. The goal of the **detailed physical exam** is twofold: first, to identify any non–life-threatening conditions or general abnormalities and, second, to reassess the adequacy of interventions already being provided. Oftentimes, the critical care provider will have the opportunity to review the patient chart at the same time that he performs the detailed exam. This allows for a thorough patient review and decreases the chance that portions of the assessment will be missed.

Like all other phases of assessment, the detailed exam should be done in a systematic fashion, occurring much in the same order as the rapid physical exam, but, it is done very methodically and attention is given to every aspect of the patient and the interventions she is already receiving.

HEAD AND AIRWAY

The head and airway, by the time the detailed exam is done, have already been evaluated in the initial exam. During the detailed portion of the exam, the critical care paramedic has the opportunity to once again review all of the components of the initial assessment, as well as augment them. For the critical care paramedic who is providing transport by air, the detailed exam provides the ability to check several of the areas that are seldom worried about in the prehospital environment. With conscious patients, there is the opportunity to ask them if they have problems clearing their ears while flying. This may allow the critical care team to foresee any problems that may be encountered related to altitude and prevent or minimize them. This is also the time in the exam when the team may opt to insert an NG or OG tube to minimize the risk of aspiration. Generally speaking, the detailed assessment of the head should include:

★ Pupils (ophthalmoscope as warranted)

★ Mucous membranes and conjunctiva

★ Airway patency (or maintenance)

★ Facial structure integrity (skeletal and skin)

- ★ Ears (otoscope as warranted)
- ★ Nasal cavity

NECK

Assessing the neck is fairly straightforward. Reassess for jugular venous distention and tracheal deviation. These two findings may provide information on the circulatory and respiratory status of the patient. In addition to assessing the neck, this is an ideal time to place a cervical collar on all intubated patients. This will help to minimize patient movement and maintain endotracheal tube placement during transport. Other components of the detailed assessment of the neck include:

- ★ Tracheal location
- ★ Carotid bruits
- ★ Palpable cervical abnormalities
- ★ Crepitus from subcutaneous emphysema
- ★ Cervical X-rays if available

CHEST

Review of the patient's chest provides the critical care paramedic the ability to reassess respiratory status. Assessing breath sounds in all locations is imperative at this point of the assessment. In addition to assessing breath sounds, the critical care paramedic should review any chest X-rays that the sending facility has available. This is especially true in the case of a potential pneumothorax if the patient is being transported by air. Most critical care services have policies in place that dictate that chest tubes are placed if a pneumothorax is present that involves a certain percentage of the chest. The critical care paramedic should also assess the patient who has an existing chest tube or chest drainage system in place. Evaluation of chest tube patency and amount of drainage should be documented in the patient care record. (These specific medical interventions, as well as others, will be discussed in later chapters.) In review, the components of thoracic assessment during the detailed physical exam should include:

- ★ Inspection for soft-tissue trauma (especially in hard to see areas such as the axillary region)
- ★ Assessment for indications of respiratory distress
- ★ Auscultation for tracheal, bronchial, bronchovesicular, and vesicular sounds; auscultation also for normal and abnormal heart tones as needed
- ★ Palpation for instability, crepitus, and chest excursion to the thoracic cage and clavicles
- ★ Percussion for differences in resonance from one hemithorax to the other
- ★ Evaluation of any thoracic intervention (chest tube, needle decompression, drainage system, central line insertion, and so on)
- ★ Review of any chest X-rays for flailed ribs, pneumothoracies, hemothoracies, fractured ribs or clavicles, mediastinal trauma, and endotracheal tube placement

ABDOMEN

Assessment of the abdomen in the critical care environment utilizes the skills of inspection, auscultation, palpation, and perhaps percussion. In the event that the critical care paramedic is going to auscultate for bowel sounds, this should be done prior to manipulation or palpation to ensure accurate findings and assessment. In the event that X-rays have been taken, it is once again helpful to review the findings so that any complications or treatment requirements can be established for the patient prior to transport. The assessment skills to perform while completing the detailed exam to the abdomen are:

★ Visual assessment for trauma and distention

★ Auscultation for bowel sounds, renal bruits, and an absence of air entering the stomach in an intubated patient

★ Proper placement of NG or OG tube

★ Palpation for organomegaly, tenderness, and guarding

★ Evaluation of placement of any abdominal (or intestinal) drainage devices

★ Assessment for Grey Turner's or Cullen's sign

★ Review of abdominal X-rays

PELVIS/GENITOURINARY

Assessment of the pelvis in a critical care situation is similar to that for a prehospital assessment. One difference that should be evaluated in the critical patient is whether or not a Foley catheter has been placed (or needs to be placed). Consider the placement of a Foley catheter prior to transport, especially if the transport will be long enough that the patient may become uncomfortable if he needs to urinate. In the event that a Foley is in place, the critical care paramedic should assess the drainage bag for patency, and the contents for clarity, color, and volume. The presence of a Foley catheter provides an excellent means to determine hydration status and renal function in the critical patient. As will be discussed later in the book, the urine output should be between 30 and 40 cc per hour. If the presence of gross hematuria is noted, the critical care team should assess whether this is due to the patient's condition (or probable condition) or whether the blood is a result of the insertion of the catheter. In review, the detailed physical exam of the pelvis and genitourinary system should include:

★ Visual inspection for musculoskeletal or soft-tissue trauma

★ Gentle palpation for pelvic stability

★ Review of pelvic X-rays, if taken

★ Placement of (or need for) urinary catheter

EXTREMITIES AND THE POSTERIOR SURFACE

When assessing the extremities and posterior surface, the critical care paramedic is once again looking for more than just injuries. Review of any medical devices should be assessed and evaluated (IV lines, PICC lines, immobilization devices, and so on). The number and types of IV catheters should be documented, and their patency ensured. In the event that the critical patient has central lines placed, the location and patency should be assessed, with the determination as to whether they can be utilized for fluid or medication administration en route. The detailed assessment of the extremities includes:

★ Determination of peripheral perfusion, motor, and sensory findings

★ Inspection for musculoskeletal and soft-tissue trauma

★ Palpation for crepitus, deformity, and areas of warmth

★ Evaluation of medical devices already placed

★ Assessment for degree of peripheral perfusion (pulses, skin findings, capillary refill)

★ Review of any available X-ray films (See Figure 6-2 ■.)

REVIEW AND INTEGRATION OF PREVIOUS ASSESSMENTS, DIAGNOSTIC STUDIES, AND CURRENT PATIENT STATUS

Typically during the assessment, the critical care paramedic has the opportunity to review the medical interventions already utilized in patient management. Also during this time, the other team

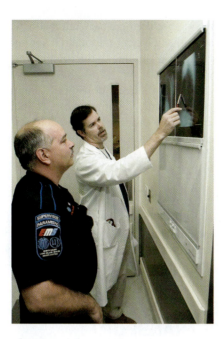

■ **Figure 6-2** If time permits, review all essential diagnostic studies, including X-rays. (© *Craig Jackson/In the Dark Photography*)

member usually reviews the charted information and gathers information orally from the providers initially caring for the patient. At some point in time, however, usually after the assessment is completed, there needs to be an integration of what has happened (to the patient), what interventions are being rendered, how the patient is responding to these interventions, what the patient's current clinical status is, what interventions are warranted now, and finally what interventions may be warranted en route. This is also a good time for the critical care team to share information and review any differences found between previous assessments and the current assessment. As we have all experienced, the condition of the patient or the documented condition of the patient may change drastically depending on the point of view of the assessor.

It is also a good time to review with your partner and the providers already caring for the patient any of the pertinent diagnostic studies, if they have not already been reviewed. Several of the things that should be reviewed are lab results, X-rays, 12-leads, capnograms, hemodynamic waveforms, and any other diagnostic studies that may have been performed prior to the critical care team's arrival. The critical care paramedic does need to be wary of "negative" results. In the event that the patient's clinical condition appears to differ from the diagnostic findings, err on the side of concern for the patient and be more diligent in your assessment and thorough in your management. Consider the case of an elderly patient who was involved in a motor vehicle accident. The patient was short of breath, but the initial X-ray appeared negative for problems. However, based on the patient's continuing clinical presentation, the doctor ordered a CT of the chest, and the CT showed a significant pneumothorax. The moral for the critical care paramedic is to have the ability to recognize the limitations of the diagnostic studies and "see" beyond the technology to assess the patient's complaints effectively and objectively.

> Have the ability to recognize the limitations of the diagnostic studies and "see" beyond the technology to assess the patient's complaints effectively and objectively.

CURRENT INTERVENTIONS FOR PATIENT CARE

During the assessment of the patient, the critical care paramedic has the opportunity to evaluate interventions that have been initiated for patient care. The paramedic should also use the time during assessment to evaluate how well the interventions are working for the patient. It is always preferable to optimize the treatments prior to departure, as opposed to having to play "catch-up" while in transport. It is also a good time to identify the necessary interventions that are not in place. Constantly ask yourself if the patient's condition warrants performing an intervention or applying some piece of equipment prior to initiating transport.

For illustrative purposes, one example of this would be the application of multifunction pacing/cardioversion pads prior to the transport of a cardiac patient. This will not only save precious time

> Constantly ask yourself if the patient's condition warrants performing an intervention or applying some piece of equipment prior to initiating transport.

should pacing or electrical cardioversion become necessary, but it also decreases the risks to the patient and crew. In the transport environment, it can be difficult, if not impossible, to correctly place the pads. It also increases the risk to the patient, due to the need to unstrap the patient from seat belts in order to manipulate him.

Another example of an intervention that is better done prior to transport is airway control. It is always preferable to control the airway prior to initiating transport due to the physical constraints of the transport environment. It is certainly easier to confirm endotracheal tube placement in a quiet, controlled environment as opposed to the loud, and sometimes-chaotic environment encountered in a helicopter or ambulance during transport.

PREPARATION OF THE PATIENT FOR TRANSPORT

Throughout this chapter, you have read multiple times how the patient assessment and patient preparation for transport can occur simultaneously. Naturally the preparation for transport will not supersede the need for immediate treatment of some conditions, but rarely is this ever the case. The following section outlines a few additional items that are part of patient preparation for transport.

DOCUMENTATION, EMTALA/COBRA, AND CRITICAL CARE TRANSPORT

Several important documents need to be gathered prior to the initiation of the transport. These documents are outlined in the EMTALA/COBRA legislation.

Concurrently with the critical care team's assessment of the patient, the other team members can begin the preparation of the patient and necessary documents for transport. (See Figure 6-3 ■.) Several important documents need to be gathered prior to the initiation of the transport. These documents are outlined in the EMTALA/COBRA legislation and typically include the following paperwork:

1. Physician certification that the risks of transport do not outweigh the anticipated benefits
2. Written request for the transfer by the patient, without suggestion or pressure of the facility or physician to induce the request
3. Advanced acceptance, which is documented in the record, by the destination hospital
4. Signed consent to transfer the patient

■ Figure 6-3 Critical care patient being prepared for transport. (© Bob Krist/CORBIS)

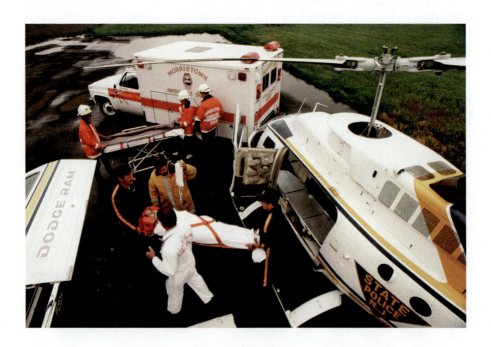

5. Medical orders for the transporting critical care team

6. Copies of the medical records, tests, and X-rays unless delays for these might jeopardize the patient

The majority of this information is usually found on a special consent to transfer form provided by the sending facility. One recommendation with regard to the destination facility is that the transporting team get a contact name and phone number to confirm bed assignment and provide updates on the ETA as necessary.

PATIENT PACKAGING FOR TRANSPORT

The packaging of the patient can also be a concurrent part of the critical care paramedic's assessment of the patient. Proper patient packaging provides the critical care team with the ability to troubleshoot problems before they occur. IV lines should be identified, separated, and straightened prior to transport. This identification provides the critical care paramedic with the ability to readily identify compatible lines for medications that may need to be administered during transport. An acceptable method for identification is to use cloth tape and mark the line at its source, its termination at the catheter, and at any injection ports in between. While this seems like overkill, it will quickly prove invaluable in the event that emergency interventions need to be performed en route.

The packaging of the patient can also be a concurrent part of the critical care paramedic's assessment of the patient.

Along with the IV lines, any medications that are infusing via medication pumps should be switched to the transport team's IV pump. In the event that the facility pump tubing is not compatible with that of the transporting unit, most manufacturers provide an extension or half set to attach to IV tubing in place. This will save time and may also save the patient the cost of having to replace medication containers due to incompatible pump tubing. Consider also the amount of medications or fluids infusing. Is there enough present to complete the mission?

In addition to the IV lines being prepared, any cables or attachments to monitoring equipment should be isolated and bundled to prevent the tangling of cables that can occur during transport. Many transport teams will "pre-bundle" the cables for equipment, especially equipment that is used for multiparameter monitoring. With the equipment and lines all straightened, the patient can be easily moved from the facility's bed to the transport cot. Make sure that all of the tubes and lines have been contained with the patient or have enough length to safely make the move (to include the ventilator tubing if the patient is mechanically ventilated). If the patient is intubated, it is wise to assess breath sounds prior to and immediately following the move to the transport cot. Intubated patients may also benefit from having a cervical collar applied to minimize the chance of dislodging the ET tube during movement.

When the critical care paramedic is comfortable with the assessment, packaging, and stability of the patient and he is ready to transport, a quick review to make sure nothing has been missed is all that is necessary before transport.

DISCUSSION OF PATIENT CONDITION WITH FAMILY

Prior to departure, the transporting crew members should update the immediate family. Oftentimes, the family is experiencing a great deal of anxiety for their loved one. (See Figure 6-4 ■.) The critical care paramedic can help to alleviate some of this apprehension by detailing the events that will occur during transport. One of the questions that the critical care team will need to be able to answer is whether family members are allowed to travel with the patient. Generally, this should be a well-established guideline within the company standard operating procedures. The majority of the time family members are not allowed to accompany the patient during air transport due to space constraints in rotor-wing aircraft, but with fixed-wing aircraft it is more common for a family member to accompany the patient during flight. Ultimately though, this is up to the discretion of the crew and the pilot. In the event that a family member is allowed to accompany the patient, the crew must ensure that the family member will follow all safety requirements. Safety equipment such as seat belts and hearing protection must be readily available for any family member who is accompanying the patient.

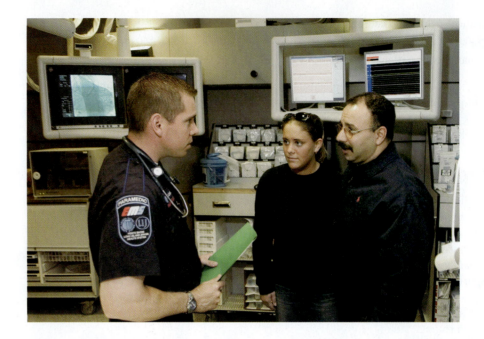

The same also applies to ground transport of patients by critical care paramedics. Similar to the family riding in the EMS vehicle in the prehospital environment, the critical care paramedic needs to brief the family member(s) who may be accompanying the patient and crew in the ambulance regarding expected behavior while traveling. This typically includes the family member agreeing to wear a safety belt, abstaining from smoking while in the ambulance, refraining from distracting the driver of the ambulance with unnecessary conversation, and not attempting to engage the critical care providers caring for the patient in dialogue about the patient's condition. Consider also assisting the person who is accompanying the patient with entering and exiting the ambulance because the step up into the front of the ambulance can be difficult (especially for the elderly).

Family members who are not going to accompany the patient should be given information about how to find the receiving hospital. While personnel at the sending facility can provide this, it is a nice consideration by a transport team member to ensure that this information is available. Oftentimes, the family is not thinking about how to get to the destination. In situations where the transport is occurring by a ground unit, the family should be informed about the dangers of trying to follow the vehicle, especially if there is a possibility that the crew will be utilizing emergency lights and sirens. A valuable technique that has worked in some ground transporting systems is to have the sending facility provide the maps and additional paperwork for the family *after* the transport has started. This allows the transporting unit a chance to get ahead of the family to avoid any confrontations and potentially dangerous situations in the event that the patient's family does try to follow right behind the emergency vehicle.

In addition to the operational aspects of the transport, the family may have medical questions that they would like answered. Similar to questions asked of the paramedic in prehospital situations, the critical care paramedic should attempt to answer them as truthfully and diplomatically as possible.

Summary

Patient assessment and preparation for transport is one of the cornerstones of patient care in the critical care transport environment. Components from the initial assessment to the continued ongoing assessment during transport can set the framework for either a smooth and trouble-free transport, or can serve as the weak links that plague the critical care paramedic with problems throughout the transport. The information presented in this chapter should assist not only in providing optimal patient care, but provide helpful hints to make medical transports as trouble free as possible.

Review Questions

1. Why should the critical care paramedic complete a scene size-up when approaching the patient?
2. What are the six individual steps that comprise the initial assessment?
3. What is the overall goal of the initial assessment?
4. What is the overall goal for the rapid physical exam?
5. Why must the critical care paramedic be attentive to EMTALA/COBRA legislation?
6. Name at least three non–patient care-related things that need preparation prior to departing any scene or hospital with a patient.
7. Why should the critical care paramedic still complete a thorough patient assessment rather than simply adopting the findings of the sending facility?
8. What are the four primary reasons for requesting the transport of a patient by a critical care team?
9. What should the critical care paramedic do if his impression of the patient's primary problem differs from the impression given by the sending facility?
10. Name two situations in which the critical care team may not be able to fly a patient who is hemodynamically unstable.

See Answers to Review Questions at the back of this book.

Further Reading

Bickley LS. *Bates' Guide to Physical Examination and History Taking,* 8th ed. Philadelphia: Lippincott Williams & Wilkins, 2003.

Bledsoe BE, Porter RS, Cherry RA. *Paramedic Care: Principles & Practice, Volume 2,* 2nd ed. Upper Saddle River, NJ: Pearson Prentice Hall, 2005.

Holleran RS. *Flight Nursing: Principles and Practice,* 2nd ed. St. Louis, MO: Mosby, 1996.

Marino PL. *The ICU Book,* 2nd ed. Baltimore, MD: Williams & Williams, 1998.

Martini FH, Bartholomew EF, Bledsoe BE. *Anatomy and Physiology for Emergency Care.* Upper Saddle River, NJ: Pearson Prentice Hall, 2002.

Sole ML, Lamborn ML, Hartshorn JC. *Introduction to Critical Care Nursing,* 3rd ed. Philadelphia: W. B. Saunders, 2001.

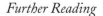

Airway Management and Ventilation

Bryan E. Bledsoe, DO, FACEP, and William E. Gandy, JD, LP

Objectives

Upon completion of this chapter, the student should be able to:

1. Discuss the importance of airway management and ventilation in modern critical care transport. (p. 127)
2. Discuss the advantages and disadvantages of the following specialized laryngoscope blades:
   A. Grandview (p. 129)
   B. Viewmax (p. 129)
3. Detail the use of the gum elastic bougie in advanced airway management. (p. 129)
4. Describe use of the following blind nasotracheal intubation adjunct devices:
   A. Burden nasoscope (p. 131)
   B. Beck airway airflow monitor (BAAM) (p. 132)
5. Describe the application of the BURP maneuver and the advantage it may offer. (p. 133)
6. Detail the indications, contraindications, and techniques for the following intubation procedures:
   A. Digital intubation (p. 133)
   B. Blind nasotracheal intubation (p. 135)
   C. Sky hook technique (p. 135)
   D. Lighted stylet (p. 137)
   E. Retrograde intubation (p. 140)
7. List the four phases of RSI pharmacology. (p. 142)

22. Describe the various phases of the capnogram and the clinical significance of each. (p. 174)
23. Detail the types of mechanical ventilators used in critical care and critical care transport. (p. 176)
24. List and describe common ventilator controls. (p. 177)
25. Set up and select the initial ventilator settings for a simulated patient. (p. 178)
26. Discuss the importance of proper documentation in critical care airway management. (p. 182)
27. Detail the various methods of documenting proper endotracheal tube placement. (p. 182)

Key Terms

Case Study

A 16-year-old male is riding a 250-cc dirt motorbike in a local pasture frequented by dirt bike riders. After making several jumps, he accelerates to approximately 40 miles per hour along the back fence line of the pasture. Before he realizes what is happening, he strikes a telephone pole support cable with his neck. EMTs and paramedics from the local EMS service are called to the scene. They find the patient in moderate distress. He is having difficulty breathing and difficulty speaking. The on-scene EMS providers apply full cervical immobilization given the mechanism of injury and the physical complaints. They make several attempts to visualize the airway without success. The patient, being awake, had an intact gag reflex and could not tolerate the laryngoscope. The patient is becoming more agitated, his screaming becomes more stridorous and his SpO_2 levels are starting to slowly fall—even with 100% supplemental oxygen. Because of the long transport time and deteriorating patient condition, on-scene paramedics request the assistance of the critical care team.

Fortunately, the critical care crew were eating barbecue only 3 miles from the scene. They respond in less than 4 minutes. The lead critical care paramedic quickly reviews the patient's findings with the on-scene EMS providers. It is readily apparent that the patient's airway is closing and immediate intervention is necessary.

First, the patient is moved to the inside of the critical care transport ambulance where the lighting is better and emergency equipment readily available. After deciding that the patient should undergo rapid-sequence intubation (RSI), equipment is prepared and the drugs selected, drawn up, and laid out in the order they will be used. Oxygenation is continued with 100% oxygen with some ventilations being assisted with the bag-valve-mask device. All monitors (pulse oximetry, ECG, waveform capnography, and vital signs) are in place. The lead critical care paramedic administers etomidate as the induction agent, followed by succinylcholine as a neuromuscular blockade. As the succinylcholine takes effect, manual ventilations are provided. The patient's SpO_2 improves and there are no further episodes of desaturation. Once the patient is paralyzed, a critical care provider makes an attempt to visualize the airway while another crew member performs Sellick's maneuver. There is significant soft-tissue swelling and a little bleeding. The intubating critical care provider can not see the glottis. He stops and resumes mechanical ventilation. After 30 seconds, he attempts again, this time with the other paramedic performing the BURP maneuver. Still, the glottic opening is not visible. A laryngeal mask airway (LMA) is opened, but it is feared that the edema will close off the trachea making the LMA ineffective. After identifying the cricothyroid membrane and preparing the site with a povidone-iodine solution, he inserts a transtracheal needle through the patient's cricothyroid membrane. A small amount of blood is noticed after placement. He feeds a guidewire from the retrograde kit into the needle until the tip of the wire is visible in the patient's oropharynx. A 6.5-mm endotracheal tube is advanced along the guidewire and into position in the trachea. The critical care team decide to use a smaller than normal tube because of the massive airway swelling. Once the tube is in place, placement is confirmed by a self-inflating bulb, bilateral breath sounds, the absence of sounds over the epigastrium, improving SpO_2 levels, and finally by waveform capnography. The guidewire is removed, the endotracheal cuff inflated, and mechanical ventilation continued. After reconfirming correct tube placement, the patient is transported to a level 1 trauma facility. During transport, tube placement is reconfirmed every 3 to 4 minutes and the times documented.

As the intubating critical care paramedic is writing his documentation, he includes a detailed summary of the patient's airway management going into extra detail due to the severity of the injury to the patient's airway and the possible complications that might arise.

At the trauma center, the patient was found to have massive blunt trauma to the neck and a fractured hyoid bone. His cervical spine was OK. He required prolonged mechanical ventilation and several surgical procedures. He was later discharged with a paralyzed vocal cord. The injury was a complication of the trauma and not a result of the critical care providers' actions.

INTRODUCTION

Airway management is the most important emergency skill. In the critical care setting, providers are apt to encounter a difficult airway or an airway problem. Likewise, paramedics in the critical care setting often perform mechanical ventilation for longer intervals compared to their non–critical care counterparts. Because of this, critical care paramedics must have excellent airway management skills and master procedures used to manage the difficult airway. (See Figure 7-1 .)

Airway management is the most important prehospital skill.

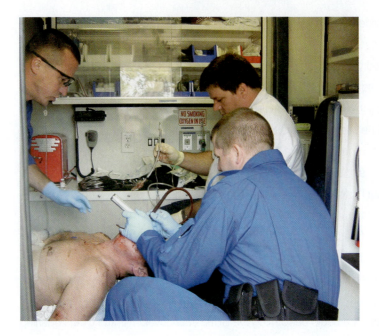

■ **Figure 7-1** Paramedics intubating patient. *(STAR Flight/Austin-Travis County EMS)*

In this chapter, we will assume that you are competent at common airway management skills including:

manual airway maneuvers *manual manipulations of the airway, including head-tilt/chin-lift, jaw-thrust maneuver, and modified jaw-thrust.*

Manual Airway Maneuvers

★ Head-tilt/chin-lift

★ Jaw-thrust maneuver

★ Modified jaw-thrust

basic mechanical airways *nasopharyngeal airway; oropharyngeal airway.*

Basic Mechanical Airways

★ Nasopharyngeal airway (NPA)

★ Oropharyngeal airway (OPA)

Advanced Airway Management

★ Orotracheal intubation

★ Nasotracheal intubation

★ Trauma patient intubation

★ Pediatric intubation

rapid-sequence induction (RSI) *advanced airway technique; includes the use of sedation, anesthesia, neuromuscular blockade, oxygen therapy, and endotracheal intubation.*

Given that assumption, we will instead emphasize advanced airway techniques including **rapid-sequence induction (RSI)** and management of the difficult airway. In addition, we will present information on mechanical ventilation and ongoing respiratory status monitoring.

ADVANCED AIRWAY MANAGEMENT TECHNIQUES

Numerous devices and techniques are available to assist in airway management. (See Figure 7-2 ■.) Normal EMS operations will usually carry a basic airway kit that includes an assortment of laryngoscope blades (Miller and MacIntosh), tubes of various sizes, McGill forceps, stylets, a rescue airway, and equipment for a surgical airway. In the critical care setting, airway problems should be anticipated and additional equipment and supplies should be readily available. In the following sections we will discuss adjuncts, techniques, and alternative airways.

The simplest airway that will do the job should be used.

SPECIALIZED LARYNGOSCOPE BLADES

Two special laryngoscope blades have been developed to assist with visualizing the airway. These attach to a laryngoscope handle. Each has special optics to enhance visualization of the difficult airway. These blades are the *Grandview* and *Viewmax*.

Grandview

The **Grandview™ blade** has an 80% wider blade surface than standard laryngoscope blades, thus helping to keep the tongue out of the way. This also reduces the need to reposition the blade. The blade has a unique design that provides a more anatomically appropriate curve, which improves direct visualization. The adult blade is 165 mm in length to fit the majority of adult patients, creating a universal blade for most cases. The Grandview fits all standard laryngoscope handles with no special connections required. (See Figure 7-3 ■.) A pediatric version (120 mm in length) is available.

Grandview™ blade
laryngoscope blade with an 80% wider blade surface and anatomically appropriate curve for improved visualization.

Viewmax

The **Viewmax™ blade** requires no special training and is used in a similar fashion to a traditional curved blade. (See Figure 7-4 ■.) However, the Viewmax has a viewing tube with a patented lens system that refracts the image approximately 20 degrees from horizontal. This refraction allows visualization of the most anterior larynx through the eyepiece. This should improve success in a patient with an anterior larynx or otherwise difficult airway. The Viewmax fits only fiber-optic laryngoscope handles. A pediatric version is available.

Viewmax™ blade
laryngoscope blade with built-in viewing tube and lens system that refracts images approximately 20 degrees from horizontal useful for intubation of very anterior airways.

INTUBATION ADJUNCTS

Several devices are available to assist with the process of endotracheal intubation. These are particularly useful when the glottic opening is difficult to visualize.

GUM ELASTIC BOUGIE

The **gum elastic bougie** (also called an Eschmann tracheal tube introducer by some manufacturers) is a straight, semirigid stylette-like device with a tip bent at about 30 degrees. (See Figure 7-5 ■.) It is

gum elastic bougie *a straight, semirigid stylette-like device with a tip bent at about 30 degrees to facilitate difficult intubations. (Also called Eschmann tracheal tube.)*

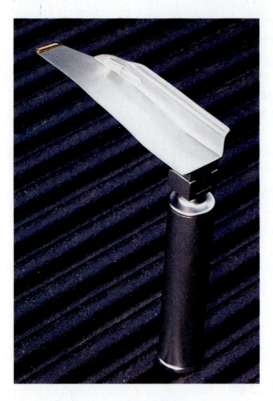

Figure 7-3 Grandview laryngoscope blade. *(Hartwell Medical)*

used to facilitate endotracheal intubations when intubation is (or is anticipated to be) difficult. Patients that often present airway difficulties include those who:

★ Have a short, thick (bull) neck
★ Are pregnant
★ Have laryngeal edema (anaphylaxis, burns)
★ Have other anatomical variations
★ Have supraglottic tumors
★ Are unable to be positioned appropriately (entrapment, confined space)
★ Are Cormack and Lehane Class II or higher view

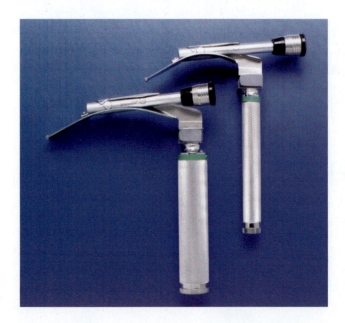

Figure 7-4 Viewmax laryngoscope blade. *(Viewmax™, Rusch Inc., a division of Teleflex Medical)*

The gum elastic bougie comes in several different versions and is 60 to 70 cm long and suitable for use with endotracheal tubes that have an internal diameter of 6.0 mm or greater. The greater length of the 70-cm version makes it easier than the 60-cm version to thread the tube. During laryngoscopy, the bougie is carefully advanced so that the bent tip is in contact with the posterior (underside) of the epiglottis, then into the larynx and through the cords until the tip enters well into the trachea. When the bougie enters the trachea, the operator should be able to feel "bumps" as the tip of the bougie slides over the tracheal rings. The bougie should be advanced until the 25-cm mark is about at the corner of the mouth. When the tip arrives at the carina, usually at about 27 cm, the bougie will be felt to "hold up," and further advancement will not be possible. The combination of "bumps" and "hold up" confirms that the bougie is in the trachea. If the bougie can be advanced further than about 27 cm, it is probably in the esophagus.

While maintaining the laryngoscope in place (this is important—do not remove the laryngoscope) and the bougie in position, an assistant threads an endotracheal tube (ETT) over the end of the bougie, into the larynx. Once the ETT is in place, the bougie is removed. (See Figure 7-6 ■.) The patient can then be ventilated normally. The gum elastic bougie should not be used in children younger than 14 years of age.

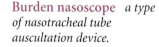

The gum elastic bougie should be in every paramedic airway kit.

NASOTRACHEAL TUBE AUSCULTATION DEVICE

Nasotracheal tube auscultation devices, such as the **Burden nasoscope,** can be used to facilitate blind nasotracheal intubation in patients who are breathing. (See Figure 7-7 ■.) With this device

Burden nasoscope *a type of nasotracheal tube auscultation device.*

■ **Figure 7-6** Gum elastic bougie in place.

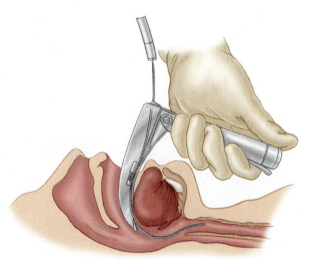

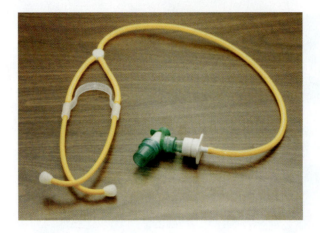

■ **Figure 7-7** The Burden nasoscope, a commercial nasotracheal tube auscultation device. *(Brant Burden, EMT-P)*

you can listen closely to the patient's breathing when blindly inserting a nasotracheal tube. The device functions like a stethoscope with an in-line diaphragm that connects to the endotracheal tube. Most of these are disposable single-use devices. They can only be used in patients who are breathing.

BECK AIRWAY AIRFLOW MONITOR

Beck airway airflow monitor (BAAM) *a device used to facilitate blind nasotracheal intubation in patients who are breathing.*

The **Beck airway airflow monitor (BAAM)** is another device to facilitate blind nasotracheal intubation in patients who are breathing. (See Figure 7-8 ■.) To use, connect the BAAM to a 15-mm endotracheal connector. When the tube is advanced into the posterior pharynx, the patient's breathing will activate the BAAM and a whistling sound will be produced with both inhalation and exhalation. Once in place, the endotracheal tube is then advanced into the larynx and trachea, which will increase the intensity and pitch of the whistling sound. Deviation out of the airflow tract, primarily into the esophagus, will result in immediate loss of the whistling sound. If this occurs, the tube should be withdrawn until the whistle sound is audible, and the tube should be redirected and reinserted.

■ **Figure 7-8** BAAM airflow monitor.

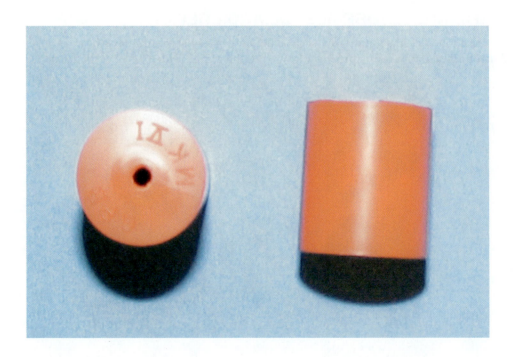

SPECIAL AIRWAY MANAGEMENT TECHNIQUES

BURP MANEUVER

The **BURP maneuver** can enhance visualization of the cords during endotracheal intubation and can often improve a Cormack and Lehane Class III or IV view at least one class better. (Airway classification systems will be discussed later in this chapter.) BURP is an acronym for **B**ackward, **U**pward, and **R**ightward **P**ressure. The laryngoscope operator, with his or her right thumb and index finger, applies pressure to the thyroid cartilage (commonly known as the Adam's apple) in a backward (toward the patient's back) or downward motion, toward the patient's right, and upward toward the patient's jaw. As this pressure is applied, often the glottis will move posteriorly, or down, into view, or at least the tip of the epiglottis will come into view. As soon as the operator sees the glottic opening or a significant part of it, he directs an assistant to place his fingers exactly where the operator's fingers have been and the operator directs the assistant's movements until the optimum view is achieved. Then the gum elastic bougie can be placed into the airway or an ET tube placed directly. (See Figures 7-9 ■ and 7-10 ■.)

DIGITAL INTUBATION

Some situations may require you to perform digital intubation. This technique dates to the eighteenth century, when people performed intubations without the benefit of a laryngoscope. Instead, they used digital (finger), or tactile (touch), intubation. (See Figure 7-11 ■.)

Digital intubation is still useful for a number of situations in the critical care transport setting. It is suggested when a patient is deeply comatose or in cardiac arrest and when proper positioning is difficult. The classic example is an unresponsive trauma patient with a suspected cervical spine injury. Since the digital technique does not require manipulation of the head and neck, it is of great value here. It may also be useful in extrication situations when the confined space prevents proper positioning of the patient. (*Note:* See discussion of the sky hook technique in the next section.)

Because digital intubation does not require visualization, it may be helpful when facial injuries distort the patient's anatomy or when you cannot suction copious amounts of blood, vomitus, or other secretions for a proper view of the airway.

Digital intubation is risky for the paramedic; it may stimulate even a deeply comatose patient to clamp down and bite your finger. Do not use it with conscious patients or with unconscious patients who have a gag reflex.

BURP (Backward, Upward, Rightward Pressure) maneuver *Technique for facilitating visualization of the vocal cords during endotracheal intubation.*

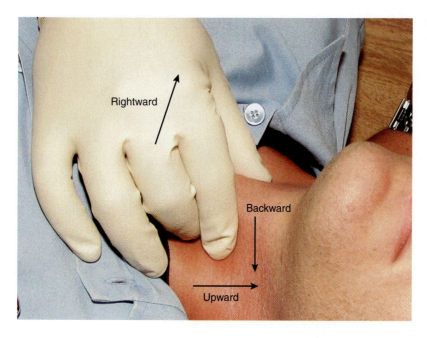

■ Figure 7-9   Initial hand placement for BURP.

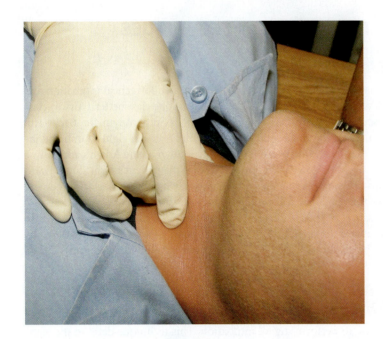

To perform digital intubation:

1. Use blood and body fluid precautions.

2. While maintaining ventilatory support with basic manual and adjunctive airway maneuvers, hyperventilate the patient with 100% oxygen.

3. Prepare and check your equipment. You will need the following items: an appropriately sized ETT, a malleable stylet, water-soluble lubricant, a 5- to 10-mL syringe, a bite block, and umbilical tape or a commercial anchoring device. Insert the stylet into the endotracheal tube and bend the ETT/stylet into a J shape.

4. While another team member stabilizes the patient's head and neck in an in-line (neutral) position, kneel at the patient's left shoulder, facing his head. Place a bite block device between the patient's molars to help protect your fingers.

■ **Figure 7-11** Digital intubation. Insert your middle and index fingers into the patient's mouth.

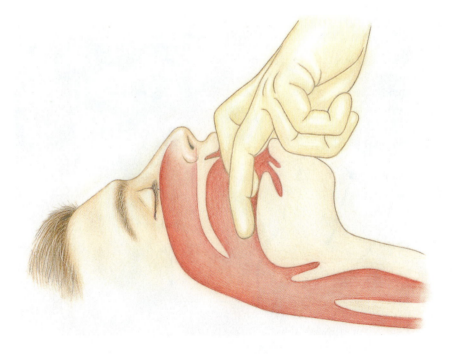

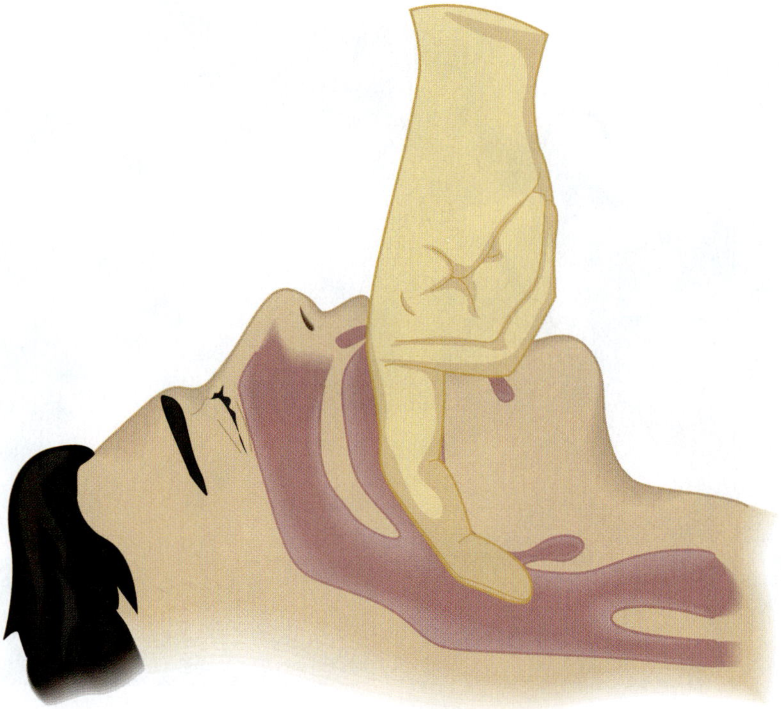

■ Figure 7-12 Digital intubation. Walk your fingers and palpate the patient's epiglottis.

5. Insert your left middle and index fingers into the patient's mouth. (See Figure 7-12 ■.) By alternating fingers, "walk" your hand down the midline while simultaneously tugging gently forward on the tongue. You may also use gauze to hold and extend the tongue more effectively, which may facilitate palpation of the glottis. This lifts the epiglottis up and away from the glottic opening, within reach of your probing fingers.

6. Palpate the arytenoid cartilage posterior to the glottis and the epiglottis anteriorly with your middle finger. (See Figure 7-13 ■.) Press the epiglottis forward, and insert the endotracheal tube into the mouth, anterior to your fingers. (See Figure 7-14 ■.)

7. Advance the tube, pushing it gently with your right hand. Use your left index finger to keep the tip of the ETT against your middle finger. This will direct the tip to the epiglottis.

8. Use your middle and index fingers to direct the tip of the ETT between the epiglottis (in front) and your fingers (behind). Then with your right hand advance the ETT through the cords while simultaneously maneuvering it forward with your left index and middle fingers. This will prevent it from slipping posteriorly into the esophagus.

9. Hold the tube in place with your hand to prevent its displacement. Attach a bag-valve device with an $ETCO_2$ detector to the 15/22-mm connector on the ETT; inflate the distal cuff with 5 to 10 mL of air; check for proper tube placement.

10. Hyperventilate the patient with 100% oxygen. Gently insert an oropharyngeal airway to serve as a bite block. Secure the ETT with umbilical tape. Repeat steps to confirm proper ETT placement and maintain ventilatory support. Continue your airway assessment periodically.

SKY HOOK TECHNIQUE

The **sky hook technique** is another difficult airway management technique in which the laryngoscope is in the hands of an assistant to facilitate visualization of the glottis.

sky hook technique *a two-person technique facilitating visualization of the glottis in a seated or upright patient.*

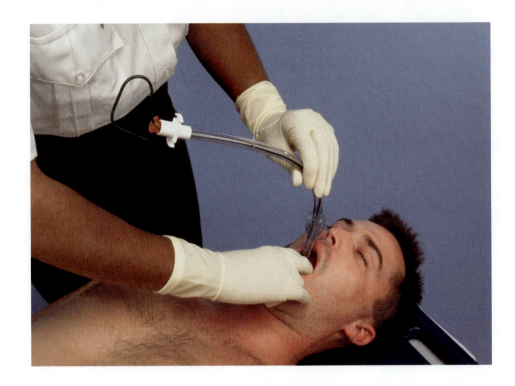

■ **Figure 7-13** Blind orotracheal intubation by digital method.

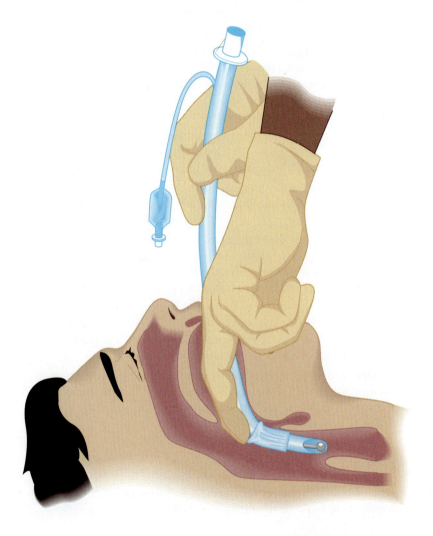

■ **Figure 7-14** Digital intubation—insertion of the ETT.

The "sky hook" may be used with a patient in the sitting position, such as one trapped in a vehicle, or in semi-sitting or supine positions. The technique is as follows:

1. The patient's cervical spine is stabilized in an appropriate fashion.

2. The operator who will place the ET tube stands behind the patient or at the patient's side, so that he can look into the patient's mouth, and holds an appropriately sized ET tube with stylet in place.

3. Another assistant maneuvers in front of the patient or to the patient's front and to the side. This assistant may position himself on the hood of a safely stabilized vehicle with windshield removed to reach a patient sitting in a car.

4. Using a #3 or #4 MacIntosh blade, the assistant in front of the patient opens the patient's mouth and "hooks" the blade behind the tongue and jaw, pulling forward at a 90-degree angle to the patient's vertical axis. This has the same effect as a jaw-thrust/chin-lift maneuver.

5. When the intubating operator looks down into the patient's mouth, he should be able to see the glottis without difficulty. The tube can then be placed.

With the patient in a semi-sitting or supine position, the operator holding the laryngoscope blade straddles the patient and performs the same maneuver as described above, being careful to always pull in a right angle to the patient's vertical axis. The intubating operator will be at the patient's head and can then place the tube from the usual position.

With this technique, flexion or extension of the neck is minimized since there is no temptation to "pry" with the blade as sometimes happens when visualization is attempted with the patient lying supine and the operator at the usual position at the patient's head.

This technique can be very helpful when the operator cannot get into the usual position for intubation, and it can also help with short, bull-necked patients and those with other anatomical features that make direct visualization difficult.

LIGHTED STYLET

Since a bright light in the trachea is visible (transilluminates) through the soft tissue of the anterior neck, an ETT with a lighted stylet can facilitate correct intubation. (See Figure 7-15 ■.) The stylet is a plastic cable with a malleable, retractable wire running through its center and a small, high-intensity bulb at its distal end. An on–off switch and power supply at the stylet's proximal end control the bulb, which begins to blink about 30 seconds after it is turned on. This blinking makes detecting the light's transilluminations easier and also reminds the operator when 30 seconds have passed.

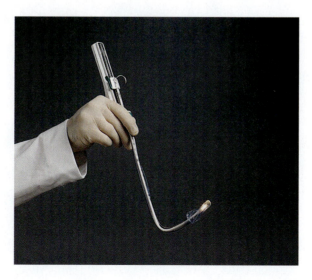

■ Figure 7-15   Lighted stylet for endotracheal intubation.

You can confirm correct ETT placement by observing the stylet's light through the anterior neck's soft tissue; esophageal intubation results in little or no light being visible. Because you can place the ETT safely and correctly without directly visualizing the glottic opening, you can perform endotracheal intubation without manipulating a trauma patient's head and neck. Several studies have shown the transillumination technique to be fast, dependable, and atraumatic.

This technique's biggest limitation is that bright ambient light can make the transillumination difficult to see. Therefore, it works best in a darkened room and with thin patients. When attempting this procedure, reduce ambient light; in direct or bright daylight, shade the patient's neck.

To perform transillumination intubation:

1. While maintaining ventilatory support, hyperventilate the patient with 100% oxygen.

2. Prepare and check your equipment. The endotracheal tube's diameter should be 7.5 to 8.5 mm. You will need to cut the ETT to a length of 25 to 27 cm to accommodate the stylet. Place the stylet in the ETT and lock the ETT in place at its proximal end. Using the sliding mechanism on the handle, adjust the stylet and bend it into a hockey-stick shape just proximal to the distal cuff.

3. With the patient supine and his head in neutral position, kneel along either his right or left side, facing his head.

4. Turn on the stylet light.

5. With your index and middle fingers inserted deeply into the patient's mouth and your thumb under his chin, lift his tongue and jaw forward. (See Figure 7-16 ■.)

6. With the proximal end of the ETT directed toward the patient's feet, insert the tube/stylet into the mouth and advance it gently through the oropharynx into the hypopharynx.

7. Use a "hooking" action with the tube/stylet to lift the epiglottis out of the way. (See Figure 7-17 ■.)

8. When you see a circle of light at the patient's Adam's apple, the stylet is placed correctly. (See Figure 7-18 ■.) A diffuse, dim, hard-to-see, or absent light indicates

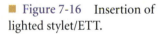

■ Figure 7-16   Insertion of lighted stylet/ETT.

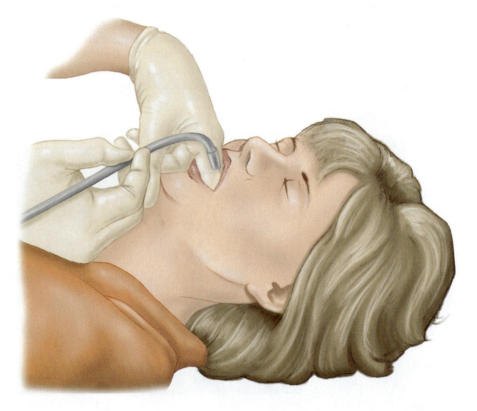

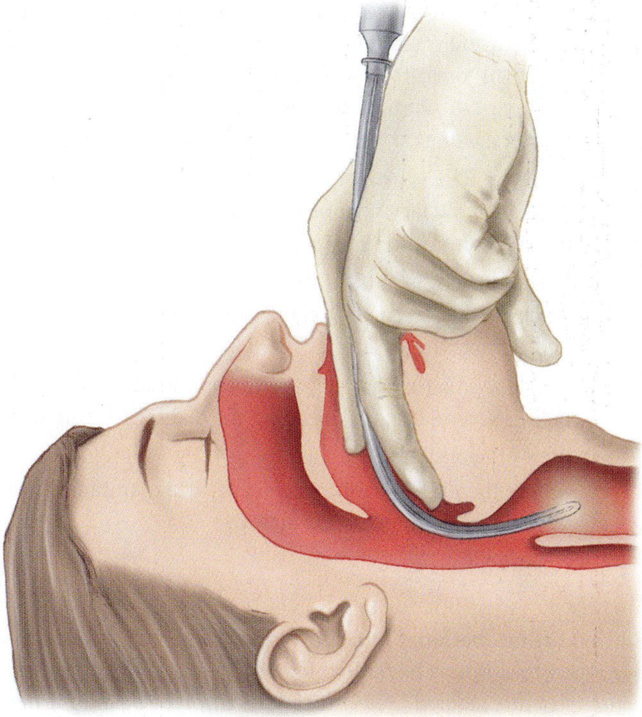

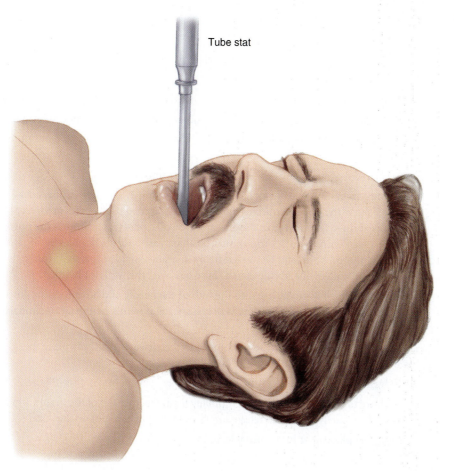

Figure 7-17   Lighted stylet/ETT in position.

Tube stat

Figure 7-18
Transillumination of a lighted stylet.

that the ETT/stylet combination is in the esophagus. A bright light lateral and superior to the Adam's apple indicates that it has moved into the right or left pyriform fossa. To correct either of these placements, withdraw the tube and reattempt intubation after ventilating the patient with 100% oxygen for several minutes, using proper basic manual and adjunct airway maneuvers.

9. After the ETT is properly placed, hold the stylet stationary. Advance the tube off the stylet into the larynx approximately 1 to 2 cm, while simultaneously retracting the internal wire from the stylet using the O-ring at its proximal end.

10. Once the light is in the correct position and you have partially advanced the ETT while partially retracting the stylet wire, hold the tube firmly in place with one hand and remove the stylet.

11. Attach the bag-valve device to the endotracheal tube's 15/22-mm connector and deliver several breaths, inflating the distal ETT cuff and checking for proper placement as usual.

12. Secure the ETT, recheck placement, and maintain ventilatory support. Continue periodic assessment of the airway.

The ambient environment must be darkened to use a lighted stylette.

RETROGRADE INTUBATION

retrograde intubation

intubation technique involving placing a needle into the patient's cricothyroid membrane through which a flexible wire is "snaked" upwards into the oropharynx, facilitating orotracheal intubation.

Retrograde intubation is typically reserved for situations in which routine endotracheal intubation is not possible. It may be performed on any patient who is unconscious as well as on conscious patients who are sedated. The procedure involves placing a needle into the patient's cricothyroid membrane. Once in place, a flexible guidewire is advanced retrograde from the puncture to the oropharynx. Once in the oropharynx, the wire is grasped with forceps and brought further out of the oropharynx so that a special guide stylet can be threaded down over the guidewire. This stylet is then placed into the distal tube opening and the endotracheal tube is then advanced until it is in the proper position.

To perform retrograde endotracheal intubation:

1. While maintaining ventilatory support, hyperventilate the patient with 100% oxygen.

2. Prepare and check your equipment.

3. Position the patient's head and neck so that the anterior neck is readily accessible.

4. Prep the anterior neck with a povidone-iodine or similar antiseptic solution.

5. Select the proper size endotracheal tube. The tube should be 7.5 to 8.5 mm in diameter.

6. With a gloved hand, locate the cricothyroid membrane.

7. Using a large-bore needle attached to a syringe with 1 to 2 cc of saline, advance the needle into the cricothyroid membrane and aspirate until bubbles are freely formed in the syringe (needle tip in the airway). Do NOT penetrate through the posterior wall. (See Figure 7-19 ■.) You should be able to aspirate air bubbles easily, and the needle should be able to be moved freely in a side-to-side motion. If the tip is in the posterior wall, or the needle is in a "false passage," this will not happen.

8. Insert the flexible guidewire into the hub of the needle and advance it up into the oropharynx until it can be seen. If necessary, tag it with a hemostat or similar sterile clamp.

9. Pass the guide stylet over the wire and into the airway (or simply place the endotracheal tube on the stylet). (See Figure 7-20 ■.)

10. Advance the endotracheal tube into the airway over the stylet. (See Figure 7-21 ■.)

11. Remove the stylet and guidewire by pulling them together out of the mouth while holding the tube securely. Be sure to release any clamp that you have put on the distal end.

12. Confirm placement in the usual fashion.

13. Provide mechanical ventilation as needed.

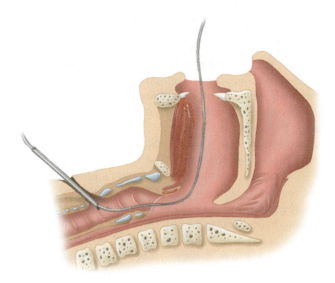

■ **Figure 7-19** Retrograde intubation. (Guidewire in place.)

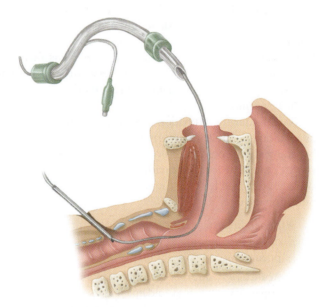

■ **Figure 7-20** Retrograde intubation. (ET tube inserted on proximal guidewire.)

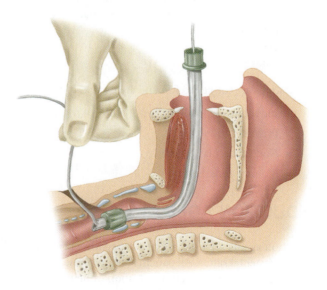

■ **Figure 7-21** Retrograde intubation. (ET tube advanced into trachea.)

RAPID-SEQUENCE INDUCTION/INTUBATION

Your most immediate concern with every patient you treat is to maintain a patent airway and adequate oxygenation and ventilation. Clearly, if a patient is in cardiac or respiratory arrest, or is unconscious or obtunded and not protecting his airway, endotracheal intubation is indicated. Quite commonly, however, you may have an awake patient, perhaps with significantly altered mental status, who is hypoxic even on 100% oxygen because of respiratory distress or a worsening airway disorder. The patient is working his hardest to breathe but does not have adequate gas exchange to support life. An altered mental status indicates that some level of significant hypoxia is putting essential brain functions at risk.

You cannot perform orotracheal intubation on this patient until the patient fatigues enough to have respiratory failure, with resultant unconsciousness and decreased muscle tone. By then, however, the patient will have suffered prolonged hypoxia, possibly accompanied by a myocardial infarction, brain damage, or vomiting with aspiration. If a patient clearly is precipitously failing maximal aggressive medical management, or if the history of his problem clearly indicates that he will not be able to or already cannot protect his airway, then active intervention is appropriate to control the airway and provide adequate ventilation. The safest way to do this is an advanced airway procedure called rapid-sequence induction or rapid-sequence intubation (RSI).

Classic rapid-sequence induction is an anesthetic procedure whereby patients rapidly receive induction of general anesthesia followed by endotracheal intubation. In emergency medicine, we do not administer general anesthesia, but we have borrowed other elements of this technique in order to rapidly obtain an airway in a patient who has altered mental status. While the term *rapid-sequence induction* describes the classic procedure, it has been modified in the emergency medicine setting to *rapid-sequence intubation*. Again, the difference is that the latter does not utilize a general anesthetic agent.

Rapid-sequence intubation involves preoxygenating the patient to the best level possible given his condition, carefully monitoring him, and giving medications to induce (sedate) and temporarily paralyze him. You then proceed with orotracheal intubation in a controlled manner. Patients who are candidates for RSI are either awake, responsive, agitated, or combative, or have a significant gag reflex, clenched teeth, or too much airway muscle tone to allow intubation. Indications for RSI intubation include:

★ Impending respiratory failure due to intrinsic pulmonary disease such as chronic obstructive pulmonary disease (COPD), congestive heart failure (CHF), asthma, or pneumonia

★ Acute airway disorder that threatens airway patency such as facial burns, laryngeal or upper airway trauma, and epiglottitis

★ Altered mental status with significant risk of vomiting and aspiration, as in head trauma (a Glasgow Coma Score of 8 or less), drug or alcohol intoxication, status epilepticus

RSI PHARMACOLOGY

Medications are the key to RSI and are used in four phases:

★ Induction
★ Premedication
★ Neuromuscular blockade
★ Maintenance therapy

INDUCTION AGENTS

induction agents
medications used for sedation, prior to paralysis, during RSI.

Induction agents are used to provide sedation prior to paralysis. The neuromuscular blockers do not affect mental status. All patients (except those already unconscious) must receive sedation with a blocking agent prior to administration of neuromuscular blockade. The prototypical drug used in RSI in the anesthesia setting is thiopental sodium (Pentothal). However, in emergency medicine and EMS, other agents are generally used, as listed next.

Barbiturates and Other Hypnotics

★ *Thiopental sodium (Pentothal).* Thiopental is a short-acting barbiturate. Barbiturates are central nervous system (CNS) depressants and can induce anything ranging from mild sedation to deep coma. Thiopental's onset of action is about 10 to 20 seconds and its duration of effect about 5 to 10 minutes. The typical dose is 2 to 5 mg/kg IV. Thiopental has significant adverse hemodynamic effects and should not be used in patients with hypotension or hypovolemia. Thiopental decreases intracranial pressure, which makes it an attractive induction agent in the setting of head injury.

★ *Methohexital (Brevital).* Methohexital is a barbiturate similar to thiopental. However, it is extremely short acting, which makes it an attractive sedative for brief procedures. It is rarely used in prehospital care. Methohexital's onset of action is less than a minute. The duration of effect is 5 to 7 minutes. A typical dose is 1 to 2 mg/kg IV.

★ *Etomidate (Amidate).* Etomidate is a short-acting, nonbarbiturate hypnotic agent. Because of its excellent safety profile, it is widely used in emergency department and prehosital RSI. In fact, it has been studied in the prehospital setting and found to be safe and effective. Etomidate's onset of action is 10 to 20 seconds and duration of effect is 3 to 5 minutes. The typical dose is 0.2 to 0.3 mg/kg IV over 15 to 30 seconds.

★ *Propofol (Diprivan).* Propofol is an extremly short-acting induction and sedative agent. It is highly lipid soluble and rapidly penetrates the blood–brain barrier. Propofol causes apnea early, making it somewhat unsuitable for RSI. Propofol's onset of action is 10 to 20 seconds. The duration of effect is 10 to 15 minutes. A typical dose is 1 to 3 mg/kg IV. (See Table 7–1.)

Opiates

★ *Fentanyl (Sublimaze).* Fentanyl is a short-acting opiate. Chemically unrelated to morphine, fentanyl is widely used in anesthesia practice as an induction agent. Fentanyl does not seem to cause any significant histamine release. This, combined with its short duration of effect, makes fentanyl an attracive agent for patients with multiple trauma. Since it is metabolized by the liver but not excreted by the kidneys, it is appropriate for use in patients with end-stage renal disease. Fentanyl's onset of action is immediate and duration of effect is 30 to 60 minues. The typical induction dose is 2 to 10 mcg/kg IV.

★ *Morphine.* Morphine can be used as an induction agent. However, it is less effective than fentanyl and its hemodynamic properties make it somewhat unattractive. Morphine is converted into a metabolite that remains active until excreted by the kidneys. Therefore, it is relatively contraindicated for patients with renal failure. If used in patients with renal failure, its dose should be decreased by 75%. Morphine's onset of action is 3 to 5 minutes. The duration of effect is 2 to 7 hours. A typical induction dose is 0.1 to 0.2 mg/kg IV. (See Table 7–2.)

Table 7–1	Barbiturates and Sedatives			
Drug	**Dosage**	**Onset**	**Duration**	**Disadvantages**
Thiopental	1–5 mg/kg	10–20 seconds	10–30 minutes	Hypotension, Bronchospasm, Porphyria
Methohexital	1–2 mg/kg	<1 minute	5–7 minutes	Hypotension
Propofol	2–3 mg/kg	<1 minute	10–15 minutes	Hypotension
Etomidate	0.2–0.3 mg/kg	<1 minute	1 minute	Cortisol suppression, Vomiting

From Stewart, CE. *Advanced Airway Management.* Upper Saddle River, NJ: Pearson Prentice Hall, 2002.

Table 7–2 | Opiates

Drug	Dosage	Onset	Duration	Disadvantages
Morphine	0.1–0.2 mg/kg	2–5 minutes	4–6 hours	Histamine reaction
Fentanyl	2–10 mcg/kg	<1 minute	30–60 minutes	Variable effect on ICP, chest wall rigidity
Alfentanyl	10–20 mcg/kg	<1 minute	~1 hour	?increased ICP

From Stewart, CE. *Advanced Airway Management.* Upper Saddle River, NJ: Pearson Prentice Hall, 2002.

Neuroleptic Agents

★ *Ketamine.* Ketamine is a dissociative drug often used as a general anesthestic in pediatric anesthesia and veterinary medicine. With dissociative drugs, the patient enters deep anesthesia, but appears awake. The patient is amnestic and unresponsive to pain. Ketamine, unlike most of the other induction agents, increases the blood pressure, heart rate, and cardiac output. This inreases myocardial oxygen demand and may increase intracranial pressure. Ketamine's onset of action is less than a minute. The duration of effect is 10 to 20 minutes. A typical induction dose is 1 to 4 mg/kg IV. (See Table 7–3.)

Benzodiazepines

★ *Midazolam (Versed).* Midazolam is a potent benzodiazepine and a popular induction agent for RSI. It is moderately long acting, water soluble and has potent amnestic effects. Midazolam is two to four times more potent than diazepam. The onset of action is typically 1 to 2 minutes. The duration of effect is 30 to 60 minutes. A typical induction dose is 0.1 to 0.3 mg/kg IV. Midazolam can be administered IM when immediate administration is needed prior to establishment of an IV.

★ *Diazepam (Valium).* Diazepam has features similar to midazolam. However, it is not water soluble and is less potent. Hypotension is common with all of the benzodiazepines, but appears a little worse with diazepam. Diazepam's onset of action is approximately 2 to 4 minutes. The duration of effect is 30 to 90 minutes. A typical induction dose is 0.25 to 0.4 mg/kg IV.

★ *Lorazepam (Ativan).* Lorazepam is a long-acting benzodiazepine. It is rarely used for RSI because the onset of action is so long. However, it is useful in the long-term sedation of intubated patients. Lorazepam's onset of action is 1 to 5 minutes. The duration of effect is 1 to 2 hours. The typical induction dose is 50 mcg/kg IV. (See Table 7–4.)

Table 7–3 | Neuroleptic Agents

Drug	Dosage	Onset	Duration	
Ketamine	1–4 mg/kg	<1 minute	10–20 minutes	Increases ICP, increases secretions

From Stewart, CE. *Advanced Airway Management.* Upper Saddle River, NJ: Pearson Prentice Hall, 2002.

Table 7–4 | Benzodiazepines

Drug	Dosage	Onset	Duration	Disadvantages
Midazolam	0.1–0.3 mg/kg	1–2 minutes	30–60 minutes	Slow onset, wildly variable dosage range
Diazepam	0.25–0.4 mg/kg	2–4 minutes	30–90 minutes	Variable dosage range
Lorazepam	0.1–0.4 mg/kg	1–2 minutes	30–90 minutes	Preferred for long-term sedation

From Stewart, CE. *Advanced Airway Management.* Upper Saddle River, NJ: Pearson Prentice Hall, 2002.

PREMEDICATION

It is sometimes necessary to premedicate certain patients prior to the administration of the neuromuscular blocking agent. The principal reason for using **premedications** is to blunt or attenuate some of the adverse side effects associated with the neuromuscular blockers. Common premedications include (See Table 7–5.):

★ *Lidocaine.* Lidocaine (1.0 to 1.5 mg/kg IVP) 2 to 3 minutes before intubation is thought to help control intracranial pressure (ICP) in patients with possible head injuries and for patients with CNS pathology (hypertensive crisis or bleed). Whether lidocaine is effective in this remains controversial. It is also used for dysrhythmia control in patients at risk for ventricular dysrhythmia. Lidocaine is contraindicated if there is known hypersensitivity to the drug.

★ *Atropine.* Atropine (0.5 mg IVP) is used in adults exhibiting bradycardia or at risk for developing bradycardia following succinylcholine administration. The pediatric dosage is 0.01 mg/kg IVP. This should be administered prior to RSI in all pediatric patients less than 3 years of age.

★ *Vecuronium.* A small dose of the nondepolarizing blocker vecuronium (Norcuron) will help minimze fasiculations and possible injury from the depolarizing effects of succinylcholine. The typical premedication dose is 0.10 mg/kg of vecuronium IVP in adults and in children older than 3 years of age. Children less than 3 years of age may require slightly higher doses.

premedications *medications used to blunt or attenuate various adverse side effects of neuromuscular blockers.*

The evidence regarding the effectiveness of lidocaine as a premedication to prevent increased intracranial pressure is poor at best.

NEUROMUSCULAR BLOCKING AGENTS

Establishment and protection of the airway, together with adequate ventilation, has the highest priority in emergency care. On certain occasions patients who are still responsive may have trouble maintaining their airway and may require endotracheal intubation. This situation most commonly occurs in patients with drug overdoses, in patients with status epilepticus, and in trauma patients with closed-head injuries. Often, however, intubation is difficult because of the presence of gag reflexes, clenched teeth, or general combativeness. In these cases endotracheal intubation can be carried out after administration of a neuromuscular blocking agent.

Neuromuscular-blocking agents are drugs that cause muscle relaxation, thus facilitating endotracheal intubation. (See Table 7–6.) All skeletal muscles, including the muscles of respiration, respond to these drugs. Following administration, the patient will become apneic and require mechanical ventilation. Neuromuscular blocking agents have no effect on the patient's level of consciousness or pain sensation. Neuromuscular blocking drugs are classified as depolarizing and nondepolarizing based on their mechanism of action. The most commonly used depolarizing drug is succinylcholine, and vecuronium and pancuronium are the most frequently used nondepolarizing agents.

1. *Succinylcholine (Anectine).* Succinylcholine is a depolarizing neuromuscular blocker commonly used in emergency medicine. It acts in approximately 60 to 90 seconds and lasts approximately 3 to 5 minutes. Succinylcholine causes muscle fasciculations progressing to total paralysis, including paralysis of the diaphragm.

Neuromuscular blockers DO NOT alter mental status.

neuromuscular-blocking agents *medications used to induce muscle relaxation, thus facilitating endotracheal intubation.*

Table 7–5	RSI Premedication Agents		
Agent	**Dose**	**Indication**	**Contraindication Precaution**
Atropine	0.01–0.02 mg/kg (min.–max./0.1–0.4)	Pediatric patients, bradycardia	Cannot give less than 0.1 mg
Lidocaine	1 mg/kg	Head injury	Allergy
Vecuronium	0.10 mg/kg	Minimize fasiculations	Allergy

Table 7–6	Neuromuscular Blocking Agents			
Drug	**Priming Dose**	**Effective Dose**	**Onset**	**Duration**
Succinylcholine	1 mg/kg	1.5 mg/kg IV	15–30 seconds	5–12 minutes
Vecuronium	0.01 mg/kg	0.1–0.2 mg/kg	1–4 minutes	20–60 minutes
Mivacurium		0.15–3 mg/kg	75–120 seconds	10–30 minutes
Rocuronium		0.6–1.0 mg/kg	30–60 seconds	30–60 minutes
Pancuronium	0.01 mg/kg IV	0.1–0.2 mg/kg	120 seconds	45–90 minutes
Cisatracurium		0.15–0.2 mg/kg	90–120 seconds	60 minutes
Curare		0.6 mg/kg	2–6 minutes	45–90 minutes

From Stewart, CE. *Advanced Airway Management.* Upper Saddle River, NJ: Pearson Prentice Hall, 2002.

2. *Pancuronium (Pavulon).* Pancuronium is a long-acting, nondepolarizing neuromuscular blocking agent. It acts in 30 to 45 seconds and lasts 30 to 60 minutes.

3. *Vecuronium (Norcuron).* Vecuronium is a nondepolarizing neuromuscular blocking agent with a rapid onset and short duration of action. It has fewer cardiovascular side effects than succinylcholine and does not cause fasciculations.

4. *Atracurium (Tracrium).* Atracurium is a nondepolarizing neuromuscular blocking agent with a rapid onset and short to intermediate duration of action.

5. *Rocuronium (Zemuron).* Rocuronium is a nondepolarizing neuromuscular blocking agent with a rapid to intermediate onset, depending on dose, and an intermediate duration of action. At equivalent doses, rocuronium has approximately the same clinically effective duration of action as vecuronium.

DEPOLARIZING BLOCKING AGENTS

depolarizing blocking agent *short acting medications that depolarize the synaptic membrane of the muscle, causing total paralysis from 3 to 5 minutes.*

Succinylcholine is the only therapeutic **depolarizing blocking agent.** Although it is similar to nondepolarizing blockers in its therapeutic effect, its mechanism of action differs. Because succinylcholine is absorbed poorly from the gastrointestinal tract, the preferred administration route is IV. Succinylcholine is metabolized in the liver and excreted via the kidneys.

Pharmacodynamics

Succinylcholine has a biphasic effect. In phase I blockade, it acts like acetylcholine and depolarizes the synaptic membrane of the neuromuscular junction (NMJ). However, succinylcholine is not inactivated by cholinesterase, so the depolarization persists, resulting in brief periods of excitation, manifested by muscle fasciculations (uncoordinated contractions of muscle fibers) followed by muscle paralysis and flaccidity. Phase II is normally not seen except in high drug concentrations. Succinylcholine is the drug of choice for short-term muscle relaxation, such as during intubation. The primary adverse drug reactions to succinylcholine are the same as those to nondepolarizing blockers: prolonged apnea and cardiovascular alterations. Patients commonly experience muscle pain from the fasciculations that occur in phase I. Therefore, adequate sedation should have been ensured before administration of succinylcholine. A "defasiculating" dose of another agent, such as vecuronium, can be given prior to succinylcholine to prevent these fasiculations.

NONDEPOLARIZING BLOCKING AGENTS

nondepolarizing blocking agents *medications that block acetylcholine's neurotransmitter action, rendering muscles flaccid without depolarizing the synaptic membrane.*

The **nondepolarizing blocking agents,** also called competitive or stabilizing agents, are derived curare alkaloids and their synthetic analogues. These drugs produce intermediate to prolonged muscle relaxation, such as that required for intubation and ventilation during surgery. Because nondepolarizing blockers are poorly absorbed from the gastrointestinal tract, they are administered parenterally, with the IV route preferred. A variable but large proportion of the nondepolarizing

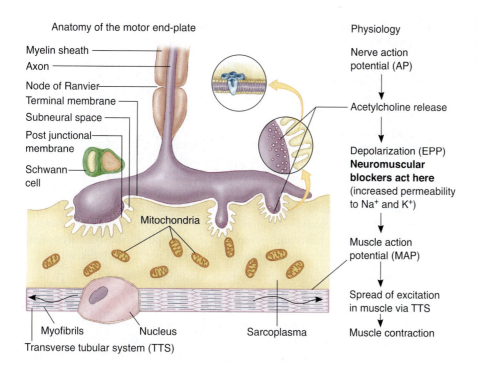

Anatomy of the motor end-plate

- Myelin sheath
- Axon
- Node of Ranvier
- Terminal membrane
- Subneural space
- Post junctional membrane
- Schwann cell
- Mitochondria
- Myofibrils
- Nucleus
- Sarcoplasma
- Transverse tubular system (TTS)

Physiology

Nerve action potential (AP)
↓
Acetylcholine release
↓
Depolarization (EPP)
Neuromuscular blockers act here
(increased permeability to Na⁺ and K⁺)
↓
Muscle action potential (MAP)
↓
Spread of excitation in muscle via TTS
↓
Muscle contraction

■ Figure 7-22
Neuromuscular blockers at the neuromuscular junction.

agents are excreted unchanged in the urine. Some of the newer drugs, such as pancuronium and vecuronium, are metabolized partially in the liver. (See Figure 7-22 ■.)

Pharmacodynamics

The nondepolarizing blockers compete with acetylcholine at the cholinergic sites of the skeletal muscle membrane. This action blocks acetylcholine's neurotransmitter action, preventing the muscle membrane from depolarizing. The effect can be counteracted clinically by anticholinesterase drugs, such as neostigmine or pyridostigmine, which inhibit the action of acetylcholinesterase, the enzyme that destroys acetylcholine.

The initial muscle weakness produced by the drugs quickly changes to flaccid paralysis that affects the muscles in a specific sequence. The first muscles to exhibit flaccid paralysis are those innervated by the motor portions of the cranial nerves and small, rapidly moving muscles in the eyes, face, and neck. Next, the limb, abdomen, and trunk muscles become flaccid. Finally, the intercostal muscles and diaphragm are paralyzed. Recovery from the paralysis usually occurs in the reverse order.

Because these drugs do not cross the blood–brain barrier, no alterations in consciousness or pain perception occur. Thus patients are aware of what is happening to them and may experience extreme anxiety and pain, but they cannot communicate their feelings. It is therefore essential that adequate sedation and pain control be accomplished and maintained both prior to paralysis and during the entire time that the patient is paralyzed. Failure to do this will not only subject the patient to extreme distress, but may render the caregiver vulnerable to damage claims and litigation.

Nondepolarizing blockers are used for intermediate or prolonged muscle relaxation. They facilitate endotracheal intubation and are used during surgery to decrease the amount of anesthetic required and to facilitate surgical procedures through relaxation of the nearby muscles. They are also used to paralyze patients who need ventilatory support but who fight the endotracheal tube and ventilator.

CRITICAL CARE TRANSPORT USE OF NEUROMUSCULAR BLOCKERS

Paralyzing the patient causes complete muscular relaxation and allows you to take control of his precarious clinical condition. In addition to paralyzing the airway muscles, these agents also immobilize the respiratory muscles, so the patient becomes apneic and requires mechanical ventilation.

Esophageal and stomach muscles, and therefore sphincter tone, also relax, posing the risk of vomiting and aspiration.

- ★ *Succinylcholine (Anectine).* As mentioned above, succinylcholine, the agent preferred for neuromuscular blockade in emergency medical care, is a depolarizing drug. It causes fasciculations just before initiating paralysis. These fasciculations may increase the tendency to vomit and may increase intracranial pressure. Conditions that elevate serum potassium preclude the use of succinylcholine, which transiently increases serum potassium, and thus can lead to life-threatening hyperkalemia. Side effects, which are dose related, include bradycardia and other dysrhythmias, as well as hypertension. The typical dose of succinylcholine is 1.5 mg/kg IV bolus in adults, or 2.0 mg/kg IV bolus in children less than 10 years old. The onset of action is 30 to 60 seconds. The duration of effect is 3 to 5 minutes. Contraindications to succinylcholine include penetrating eye injuries, patients with burns greater than 8 hours' duration, patients with paraplegia or quadriplegia, muscular dystrophy, massive crush injuries, and neurologic injuries greater than 1 week out.

- ★ *Vecuronium (Norcuron).* Vecuronium is a nondepolarizing agent; thus, it does not cause fasciculations. It is generally the second-line paralytic when succinylcholine is contraindicated, because it has fewer cardiac and hypotensive side effects than other nondepolarizing agents. In much smaller doses as a premedication, or priming dose, to succinylcholine or to a paralyzing dose of vecuronium, it effectively reduces or prevents fasciculations. It also blunts succinylcholine's bradycardic effect. This priming (or premedication) dose is given 2 minutes before the paralytic agent. The typical dose of vecuronium is 0.15 mg/kg IV bolus (paralyzing), 0.01 mg/kg IV bolus (priming). The onset of action is 2 to 3 minutes. The duration of effect is approximately 45 minutes.

- ★ *Atracurium (Tracrium).* Atracurium is a nondepolarizing paralytic useful for patients with kidney or liver disease because these conditions do not prolong its duration. Some patients experience hypotension from the histamine release that this drug causes. The usual dosage of 0.5 mg/kg IV has a duration of effect of 20 to 30 minutes.

- ★ *Pancuronium (Pavulon).* Pancuronium is a nondepolarizing paralytic that has been used frequently in the past. The advantage of its relatively rapid onset (3 to 5 minutes) is offset by its major disadvantage, a long (60-minute) duration. It also produces tachycardia due to its effects on the heart. Better agents are currently available.

- ★ *Rocuronium (Zemuron).* Rocuronium is a nondepolarizing paralytic with a rapid to intermediate onset (30 to 60 seconds) and intermediate duration of effect (30 to 60 minutes). The RSI dose for adults and children is 0.6 mg/kg. Because of its short onset of action, rocuronium is the agent of choice for patients who cannot be given succinylcholine.

If you cannot intubate a paralyzed patient, he has no definitive airway. You must ventilate him mechanically for the duration of the paralysis (assuming you can mechanically maintain a patent airway). If the airway is lost during the procedure, you must be prepared to insert a rescue airway or initiate a surgical airway (cricothyrotomy). Nothing works as fast as succinylcholine or is of as short a duration; therefore, it is the preferred neuromuscular blocking agent for emergency RSI.

Neuromuscular blocking agents do not affect mental status or pain sensation; therefore, you must use sedating and amnestic drugs to ease the awake, aware patient's anxiety and discomfort and to decrease his gag reflex, thereby increasing patient compliance and enhancing the ease of intubation. If the patient is already obtunded (from a drug overdose or head injury, for example), sedating him is pointless; omit that step. If the patient's injuries are causing significant pain and his clinical condition does not contraindicate their use, give small doses of pain medications as indicated. However, do not withold pain medications for fear of depressing a patient's respiratory drive. You are managing the patient's respirations with mechanical ventilation. It is important to monitor the heart rate. An increase in heart rate in the setting of a euvolemic patient may indicate pain. It is imperative that the critical care paramedic be especially sensitive to the patient's pain sensations.

When hypovolemia is present or when significant trauma is present with hypotension or a strong likelihood for hypotension, avoid induction agents that cause hypotension. Agents that blunt ICP response are good choices for the patient with head injury. If you are able to identify that the patient has an allergy or sensitivity to a particular agent, you should not administer that agent.

Three other agents, atropine, vecuronium, and lidocaine, are appropriate for use as premedication agents in RSI, if indicated. Table 7–5 outlines their use.

Most patients with emergent airway conditions have eaten or drunk something within a few hours before the onset of their emergency conditions. Thus, you should consider every emergency patient to have a full stomach and be at risk of vomiting and aspiration. This is another reason why you should expediently intubate the patient after the onset of paralytic effect and apnea. Remember to always have a working suction device at the patient's side during airway maneuvers. Likewise, application of Sellick's maneuver will help prevent aspiration.

Never begin the RSI sequence before you have all necessary equipment, supplies, and medications prepared and readily available. All medications should be drawn up in syringes and laid out in sequence. Suction must be on and readily available. Always have a plan for maintaining the airway in case you are unable to intubate the patient once he is paralyzed.

MAINTENANCE MEDICATIONS

Patients who are paralyzed via a neuromuscular blockade must remain sedated. In addition, some patients are intubated and mechanically ventilated without neuromuscular blockade. In these cases, sedation must be maintained. The choice of a maintenance medicine is slightly different from an induction medication. With a maintenance medication, choose an agent that is longer acting. Commonly used maintenance sedatives include morphine, diazepam, and lorazepam. With patients who have increased intracranial pressure, barbiturates are usually used—although this is uncommon in the prehospital setting. Some of the short-acting neuromuscular blockers may wear off during transport. If this occurs, additional doses should be administered or the patient switched to a longer-acting agent such as pancuronium.

REVERSAL AGENTS

Rarely, it may be necessary to reverse neuromuscular blockade. Several reversal agents are available, but these are rarely used in the critical care setting. Reversal agents are limited to the nondepolarizing blockers. There is no reversal agent for succinylcholine.

The reversal agents inhibit the enzyme acetylcholinesterase at the neuromuscular junction, thus allowing the levels of the enzyme to gradually rise. Commonly used reversal agents are:

★ Neostigmine (0.05 mg/kg not to exceed 5 mg slow IVP)

★ Pyridostigmine (0.2 mg/kg slow IVP)

★ Edrophonium (0.5 mg/kg slow IVP)

Atropine is used in combination with these agents to attenuate the strong parasympathetic response (bradycardia, heart blocks, bronchoconstriction).

RAPID-SEQUENCE INTUBATION PROCEDURE

To perform rapid-sequence intubation:

1. *Preoxygenate.* Preoxygenate the patient with 100% oxygen using basic manual and adjunctive maneuvers, and using a bag-valve mask (BVM) if indicated.

2. *Prepare.* Prepare your equipment, supplies, and patient. In addition to the usual intubation equipment, be certain you have at least one, and preferably two, secure and working IV lines. Place the patient on a cardiac monitor and pulse oximeter. Draw the appropriate doses of medications into syringes and label them. Have at least one, if not two, secondary devices readily available, such as the CombiTube, the laryngeal mask

airway, or another rescue airway. Always have the equipment to perform a cricothyrotomy available as well as equipment to perform a true surgical airway.

3. *Induce.* If the patient is alert, administer a sedative (induction) agent, such as midazolam or etomidate, prior to administering any neuromuscular blocking agents. Communicate with your patient, tell him what to expect, and reassure him that even though his respirations will be in your hands, you will make certain that he is adequately ventilated. Use patient communication to ascertain when your patient has reached the necessary level of sedation. Never proceed beyond this point until you are absolutely sure that your patient is sedated to the degree that he is unaware of what is happening and that amnesia will occur following the procedure. Don't forget to document this finding. Also be certain that if your patient has sustained an injury, has complained of pain, or is obviously experiencing pain, you have administered adequate analgesia to blunt the pain responses. Sedation does not necessarily blunt pain responses. Be aware that both analgesia and sedation are necessary.

4. *Sellick's maneuver.* Apply Sellick's maneuver (pressure on the cricoid cartilage just below the Adam's apple) and maintain until you confirm proper ETT placement. If, at any time, the patient shows signs of vomiting, release cricoid pressure immediately. Failure to do so may result in esophageal rupture.

5. *Consider premedication.* Per local protocols, consider premedicating the patient with a priming dose of vecuronium. This is especially important in children, where fasiculations from succinylcholine can cause musculoskeletal trauma. The typical premedication dose is 0.10 mg/kg of vecuronium IVP in adults and in children greater than 3 years of age. Children less than 3 years of age may require slightly higher doses. Also, if indicated in local protocols, consider premedicating with lidocaine and atropine.

6. *Paralyze.* Paralyze the patient, administering succinylcholine 1.5 mg/kg IV bolus and continue oxygenation. Alternatively, vecuronium (Norcuron) can be used as a blocking agent. It has a slower onset of action. Rocuronium may be a better choice than vecuronium in patients who cannot be given succinylcholine because of contraindications because it has a more rapid onset than vecuronium and a similar duration of action.

7. *Intubate.* Once adequate relaxation is obtained, insert the ETT through the patient's vocal cords at the onset of apnea and jaw relaxation, using the orotracheal intubation procedure previously explained. Because you have preoxygenated the patient, BVM ventilation is generally not indicated before the first intubation attempt, unless prolonged. Not ventilating the patient at this juncture will help prevent gastric distention and regurgitation. If you are unable to pass the tube after 20 to 30 seconds, stop, hyperventilate the patient with 100% oxygen for 2 minutes, and then try again. Remember that the patient's lower esophageal sphincter tone is decreased, so ventilating during paralysis makes gastric distention and vomiting more likely, even with cricoid pressure. Your goal is to rapidly place the ETT properly in the trachea to minimize these complications, but do not avoid BVM hyperventilation with 100% oxygen in the hypoxic patient.

8. *ET confirmation.* Confirm proper placement of the ETT into the trachea. Inflate the distal cuff, apply a self-inflating bulb syringe, ventilate with a bag-valve device that has an end-tidal CO_2 detector attached, and look for the appropriate color change. Watch for the chest to rise and fall with ventilations. Auscultate with each ventilation for bilateral breath sounds over the chest and no gastric sounds over the stomach. Rememer that if the patient has recently ingested a carbonated beverage, it make take six to eight breaths to eliminate the CO_2 from the carbonation and achieve a reliable reading.

9. *Release Sellick's maneuver.* Release cricoid pressure.

10. *Secure tube.* Insert a bite block device, secure the ETT in place, reconfirm placement, and continue ventilating the patient. Continually assess the patient's condition and

recheck ETT placement, documenting each recheck with times. Be sure, at some point, to set forth the observations that were done to reconfirm tube placement.

11. *Maintain paralysis.* Check with medical direction or follow your local protocol for indications for continuing paralysis with vecuronium during transport. This will depend largely on your patient's medical condition and combativeness after the paralytic and induction agent wear off, as well as on your anticipated transport time to the hospital. Do not forget that sedation and pain management must be maintained.

ALTERNATIVE (RESCUE) AIRWAYS

Every EMS system must have alternative or **rescue airways** available in case endotracheal intubation (including RSI) fails. Many good devices are on the market, each with different advantages and disadvantages. Regardless, one of these should always be available.

ENDOTRACHEAL COMBITUBE (ETC)

The **Esophageal Tracheal CombiTube®**(ETC) is a dual-lumen airway with a ventilation port for each lumen. It is basically two tubes laminated together. One tube is close ended but has holes for air/oxygen to exit. The other tube is open and has no perforations. (See Figure 7-23 ■.)

When inserted, the tubes will either enter the esophagus or the trachea, depending on the patient's anatomy. Either way, the patient can be ventilated. This is due to the structure of the device, which is designed to allow ventilation regardless of whether the device enters the esophagus or the trachea.

There is a large inflatable cuff proximal to the end of the device. (See Figure 7-24 ■.) This cuff is designed to rest in the oropharynx and prevent air from escaping through the mouth and also to decrease the possibility of blood and secretions from above the airway entering the trachea. There is a distal cuff that is roughly the size of the cuff on an ET tube. This cuff, when inflated, will occlude either the esophagus or the trachea surrounding the tubes.

CombiTubes come in two sizes, small adults (37 F) for patient between 4 and 5½ feet tall and standard CombiTube (41F) for adults greater than 5 feet. More recent studies suggest the CombiTube SA for patients between 4 and 6 feet tall and the standard CombiTube for patients greater than 6 feet.

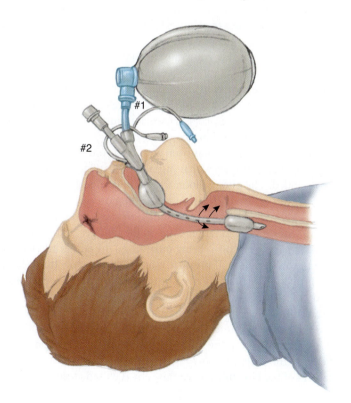

rescue airways *alternative airway management tools and techniques used when endotracheal intubation (including RSI) fails.*

Anytime you perform RSI, you MUST have a rescue airway available.

Esophageal Tracheal CombiTube® (ETC) *a dual-lumen airway device with a ventilation port for each lumen, designed for blind insertion that permits ventilation with BVM via either tube, as required.*

■ **Figure 7-23** ETC airway. First ventilate through the longer blue tube (#1). Ventilation will be successful if the tube has been placed (as is most common) in the esophagus.

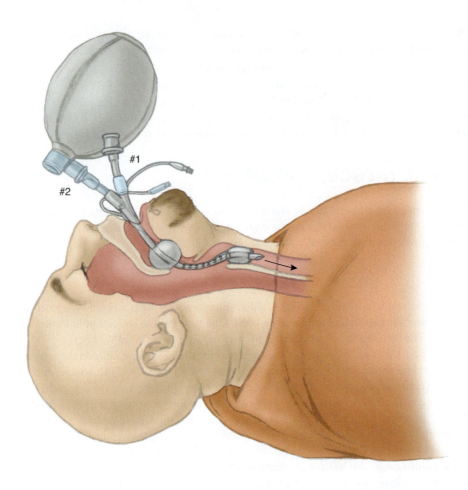

Figure 7-24 ETC airway. If ventilation through tube #1 is not successful, then ventilate through the shorter clear tube (#2). Ventilation will be successful if the tube has been placed in the trachea.

The CombiTube is inserted blindly through the mouth into the posterior oropharynx and then gently advanced until the teeth rest between the two prominent black lines on the device. The proper way to introduce the CombiTube is to perform a jaw thrust, pulling the mandible outward at a 90-degree angle to the patient's vertical axis, and, after placing a bend in the distal portion of the device, gently insert it. The head must be in the neutral position. Do not hyperextend the neck. If resistance is encountered, it may be because the distal end of the device has gone into one of the pyriform fossae. If the patient is in cardiac arrest or paralyzed, muscle tone will be absent, and the operator may need to use a laryngoscope to help thrust the lower jar and make it easier to place the CombiTube. If the laryngoscope is used, it is purely to achieve jaw thrust, not to visualize the airway. The CombiTube is placed blindly.

Once the CombiTube has been advanced so that the patient's teeth lie between the two black lines on the tubes, the large pharyngeal cuff is inflated using either 85 or 100 mL of air in the syringe provided. The pilot balloon for the pharyngeal cuff is blue. It will have printed on it either. "No. 1, 85 mL" or "No. 1, 100 mL," depending on whether it is a 37 F or a 41 F device.

Attach the large syringe to the inflation valve and put either 85 or 100 mL of air into the cuff. This will require substantial pressure on the plunger of the syringe. DO NOT hold onto the device while the pharyngeal cuff is being inflated. As the cuff is inflated, the device will move upward and seat in the proper place. If pressure is applied to it while this is happening, the device may not seat in the proper place and may not form a complete oropharyngeal seal.

After inflating the pharyngeal cuff through the blue valve, inflate the distal cuff using the other valve. Instill 12 or 15 mL of air, depending on the size of the device. The pilot balloon of the distal cuff will have the amount of air to be instilled printed on it.

Attach the BVM to the blue tube and ventilate. If compliance is easily felt, the CombiTube has settled into the esophagus and you are now ventilating the patient through the perforations in the distal end of the blue tube. Since this tube is closed at the end, air or oxygen has no place to go except through the perforations and into the glottis, which is in front of the tube openings. The distal cuff and the pharyngeal cuff preclude gas from going anywhere but into the glottis.

On the other hand, if you encounter poor compliance as you ventilate the blue tube with the BVM, your CombiTube has probably gone into the trachea. Switch the BVM from the blue tube to the other tube and ventilate. Good compliance should be felt, which indicates that the CombiTube is in the trachea. You are now ventilating through the tube which is open ended, and you have, in effect, an endotracheal intubation.

When the CombiTube is in the esophagus, you may place an orogastric tube through the open-ended tube into the stomach and aspirate stomach contents. You may not, however, instill drugs down the tube because it is in the esophagus.

When the CombiTube is in the trachea, you will not be able to place an orogastric tube into the esophagus, but you will be able to instill drugs into the trachea and the bronchial tree through the tube that is open ended.

Now auscultate the epigastrium and the chest to confirm tube placement as with a standard ET tube. If you hear breath sounds over the chest and none over the stomach, continue ventilating through the blue tube. If you hear ventilation sounds over the stomach without breath sounds over the chest, stop ventilating through the longer port and attach the bag-valve device to the shorter port. The distal cuff isolates the distal port, and the larger proximal cuff isolates the proximal port, encouraging air that is insufflated into the hypopharynx to enter the trachea. Inability to ventilate a patient through the CombiTube usually means either that the tube has been placed too deeply and the large cuff is occluding the glottic opening, or there is sufficient foreign matter, such as vomitus, to occlude the openings in the device. In either case, deflate the cuffs, withdraw the tube, clean it as needed, and reinsert.

Advantages of the Esophageal Tracheal CombiTube

★ It provides alternate airway control when conventional intubation techniques are unsuccessful or unavailable.

★ Insertion is rapid and easy.

★ Insertion does not require visualization of the larynx or special equipment.

★ The pharyngeal balloon anchors the airway behind the hard palate.

★ The patient may be ventilated regardless of tube placement (esophageal or tracheal).

★ It significantly diminishes gastric distention and regurgitation.

★ It can be used on trauma patients, since the neck can remain in neutral position during insertion and use.

★ If the tube is placed in the esophagus, gastric contents can be suctioned for decompression through the distal port.

Disadvantages of the Esophageal Tracheal CombiTube

★ Suctioning tracheal secretions is impossible when the airway is in the esophagus.

★ Placing an endotracheal tube can be difficult with the ETC in place.

★ It cannot be used in conscious patients or in those with a gag reflex.

★ The cuffs can cause esophageal, tracheal, and hypopharyngeal ischemia.

★ It does not isolate and completely protect the trachea.

★ It cannot be used in patients with esophageal disease or caustic ingestions.

★ It cannot be used with pediatric patients.

★ Cannot be used in patients shorter than 4 feet or taller than 7 feet.

★ Placement of the CombiTube is not foolproof—errors can be made if assessment skills are not adequate.

PHARYNGOTRACHEAL LUMEN AIRWAY

The **pharyngotracheal lumen (PtL) airway** is a two-tube system. (See Figure 7-25 ■.) The first tube is short, with a large diameter; its proximal end is green. A large cuff encircles the tube's lower third.

pharyngotracheal lumen (PtL) airway *a dual-lumen airway device designed for blind insertion that permits ventilation with BVM via either tube, as required.*

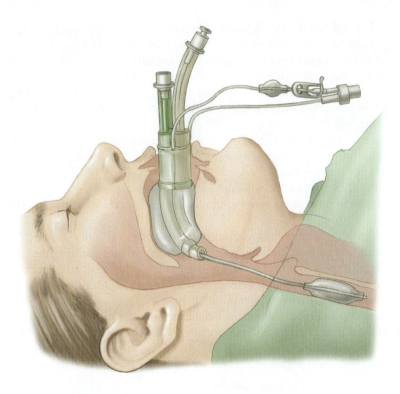

When inflated, the cuff seals the entire oropharynx. Air introduced at this tube's proximal end will enter the hypopharynx. The second tube is long, with a small diameter, and clear. It passes through and extends approximately 10 cm beyond the first tube. This second tube may be inserted blindly into either the trachea or the esophagus. A distal cuff, when inflated, seals off whichever anatomical structure the tube has entered. The second tube, which enters the trachea, is used to ventilate the patient.

Each of the PtL's tubes has a 15/22-mm connector at its proximal end, allowing the attachment of a standard ventilatory device. A semirigid plastic stylet in the clear plastic tube allows redirection of the oropharyngeal cuff while the other cuff remains inflated. An adjustable, cloth neck strap holds the tube in place. When the long, clear tube is in the esophagus, deflating the cuff in the oropharynx allows you to move the device to the left side of the patient's mouth. This may permit endotracheal intubation while continuing esophageal occlusion. However, placement of an endotracheal tube with a PtL already in place is difficult at best.

Advantages of the Pharyngotracheal Lumen Airway

★ It can function in either the tracheal or esophageal position.

★ It has no face mask to seal.

★ It does not require direct visualization of the larynx and, thus, does not require the use of a laryngoscope or additional specialized equipment.

★ It can be used in trauma patients, since the neck can remain in neutral position during insertion and use.

★ It helps protect the trachea from upper airway bleeding and secretions.

Disdvantages of the Pharyngotracheal Lumen Airway

★ It does not isolate and completely protect the trachea from aspiration.

★ The oropharyngeal balloon can migrate out of the mouth anteriorly, partially dislodging the airway.

★ Intubation around the PtL is extremely difficult, even with the oropharyngeal balloon deflated.

★ It cannot be used in conscious patients or those with a gag reflex.

★ It cannot be used in pediatric patients.

★ It can only be passed orally.

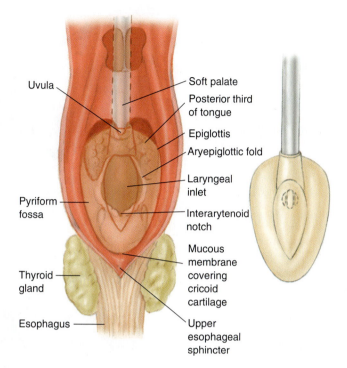

■ Figure 7-26 Laryngeal mask airway in proper anatomical position.

Uvula

Soft palate

Posterior third of tongue

Epiglottis

Aryepiglottic fold

Laryngeal inlet

Pyriform fossa

Interarytenoid notch

Mucous membrane covering cricoid cartilage

Thyroid gland

Esophagus

Upper esophageal sphincter

Laryngeal Mask Airway (LMA)

The **laryngeal mask airway** (LMA) may assist with ventilations in the unconscious patient without laryngeal reflexes when tracheal intubation is unsuccessful. It has an inflatable distal end (similar to a face mask) that is placed in the hypopharynx and then inflated. (See Figure 7-26 ■.) When inflated it surrounds and covers the supraglottic area. A bag-valve device at the proximal end assists respirations (similar to an endotracheal tube). The laryngeal mask airway is available in a reusable and disposable form and comes in various sizes. Its blind insertion requires less skill and training than endotracheal intubation. The LMA's disadvantage is that it does not isolate the trachea; therefore, it does not protect the airway from regurgitation and aspiration. Also, it cannot be used in a patient who has a gag reflex or is semiconscious. You must weigh these disadvantages against the benefits of establishing a patent airway. (See Figures 7-27 ■ and 7-28 ■.)

laryngeal mask airway (LMA) *a noninvasive, single lumen airway device designed to occlude the supraglottic area and facilitate ventilation.*

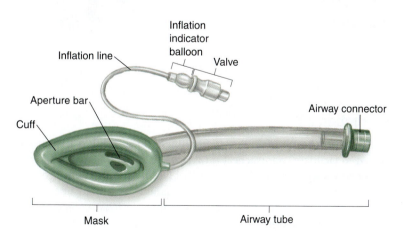

■ Figure 7-27 Laryngeal mask airway.

Inflation indicator balloon

Inflation line

Valve

Aperture bar

Airway connector

Cuff

Mask

Airway tube

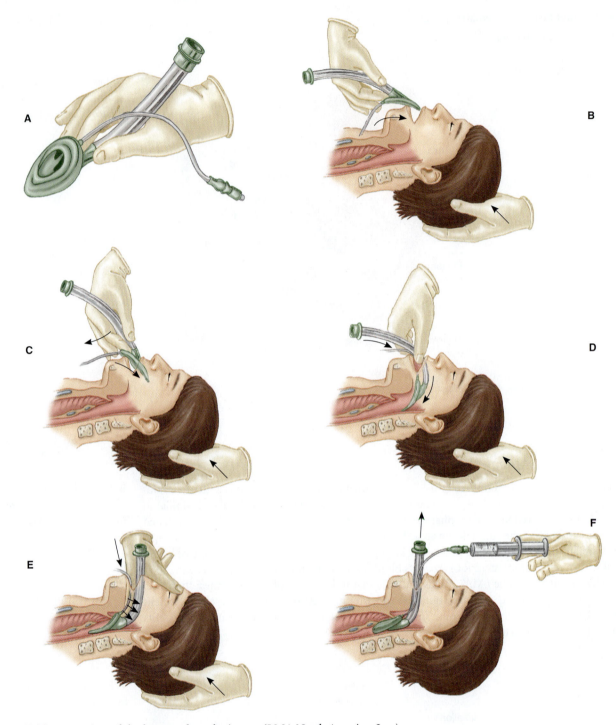

■ **Figure 7-28** Insertion of the laryngeal mask airway. *(LMA North America, Inc.)*

Intubating LMA

intubating laryngeal mask airway (LMA Fastrach®)
a single lumen airway device designed to facilitate endotracheal intubation and ventilation.

The **intubating laryngeal mask airway** (also called the **LMA Fastrach®**) (Figure 7-29 ■) is designed to facilitate endotracheal intubation. It is a rigid, anatomically curved airway tube that is wide enough to accept an 8.0-mm cuffed ETT and is short enough to ensure passage of the ETT cuff beyond the vocal cords. It has a rigid handle to facilitate one-handed insertion, removal, and adjustment of the device's position to enhance oxygenation and alignment with the glottis. (See Figure 7-30 ■.) It requires no visualization of the airway and is relatively easy to insert from any

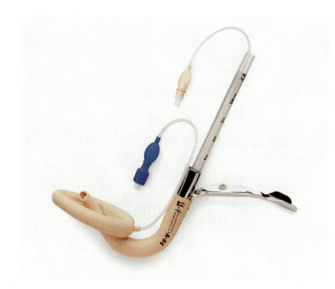

Figure 7-29 Intubating laryngeal mask airway. (*LMA North America, Inc.*)

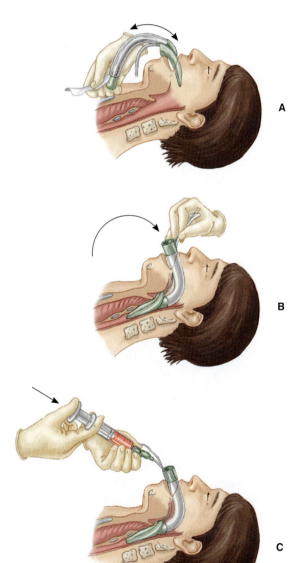

Figure 7-30 Insertion of the intubating laryngeal mask airway (ILMA). (*LMA North America, Inc.*)

A

B

C

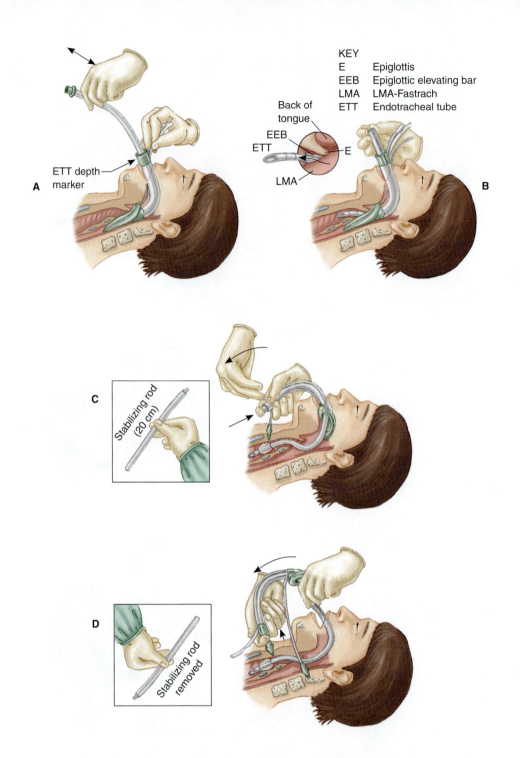

KEY
E   Epiglottis
EEB   Epiglottic elevating bar
LMA   LMA-Fastrach
ETT   Endotracheal tube

ETT depth marker

Back of tongue

EEB

ETT

LMA

E

A

B

Stabilizing rod (20 cm)

C

Stabilizing rod removed

D

position, making it suitable for use in patients who cannot be placed in the supine position for intubation. An epiglottic elevating bar in the mask aperture elevates the epiglottis as the ETT is passed through, and a ramp directs the tube centrally and anteriorly to reduce the risk of arytenoid trauma or esophageal placement. (See Figure 7-31 ■.)

Currently, it is available in three adult sizes in the United States, and it is designed for reuse. No pediatric sizes are available. A disposable model is currently available in Europe and may soon be available in the United States.

An advantage of this device is that its use is similar to that of a standard LMA. After the ET tube is placed, it achieves the advantage over the LMA of having a cuffed ET tube in place. The device may either be left in place with the ET tube remaining inserted through its lumen, or the LMA por-

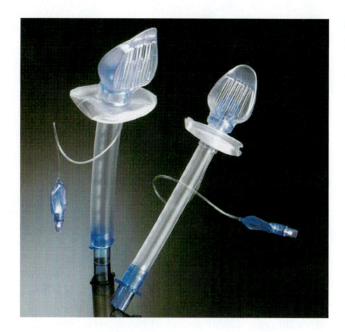

■ Figure 7-32 Cobra
perilaryngeal airway (PLA).
*(Engineered Medical Systems,
Inc., Indianapolis, IN)*

tion may be removed, leaving the ET tube in place. Like the CombiTube, this device requires a minimum of training and practice for use and is inserted blindly, without a laryngoscope.

Cobra Perilaryngeal Airway

The **Cobra perilaryngeal airway (PLA)** is similar to the laryngeal mask in that it is a supraglottic airway (inserted just above the glottis). (See Figure 7-32 ■.) It is a single-use, disposable airway. The "cobra head" of the airway holds both the soft tissue and the epiglottis out of the way. Ventilations are provided through fenestrated (slotted) openings in the distal airway. Like the LMA, it comes in a variety of sizes from pediatric to adult.

Cobra perilaryngeal airway (PLA) *a single lumen airway device designed to occlude the supraglottic area and facilitate ventilation.*

Ambu Laryngeal Mask Airway

The **Ambu laryngeal mask (ALM)** is a supraglottic, single-use, disposable airway. (See Figure 7-33 ■.) It features a special curve that replicates the natural human airway anatomy. This curve is molded directly into the tube so that insertion is easy, without abrading the upper airway. The curve ensures that the patient's head remains in a neutral position when the mask is in use.

Ambu laryngeal mask (ALM) *a supraglottic, single-use, disposable airway designed for insertion when maintaining neutral position is desired.*

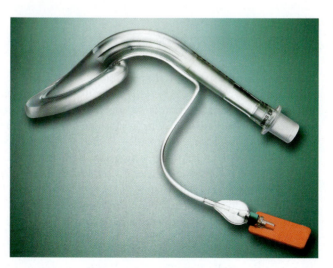

■ Figure 7-33 Ambu
laryngeal mask. *(Ambu Inc.,
Baltimore, MD)*

King LT Airway

The **King LT airway** is a supraglottic airway with a large silicone cuff that disperses pressure over a large surface area. This serves to stabilize the airway at the base of the tongue, thus minimizing risk to the vocal cords and trachea. The King LT allows up to 30 cm/H$_2$O ventilation pressure. It is supplied in three sizes: one for adults less than 61 inches in height, one for adults taller than 61 inches and but less than 71 inches in height, and one for adults taller than 71 inches. The device can be cleaned, sterilized, and reused. (See Figure 7-34 ■.)

SURGICAL AIRWAYS

With proper training and frequent practice, including the use of RSI procedures, you will be able to secure most airways in the field by endotracheal intubation. Occasionally, however, extreme circumstances prohibit successful endotracheal intubation. In these situations, performing a surgical airway technique may be the only way to ensure your patient's survival. Two different techniques, needle cricothyrotomy (also called translaryngeal cannula ventilation) and open cricothyrotomy, both provide access to the airway through the cricothyroid membrane. A needle cricothyrotomy is generally the easier procedure but makes providing adequate ventilation more difficult; an open cricothyrotomy is the more difficult procedure but allows for more effective oxygenation and ventilation.

You should use surgical airway procedures only after you have exhausted your other airway skills and have decided that no other means will establish an airway. Even when performed correctly, these procedures are highly invasive and prone to complications that you must recognize and treat immediately. The major long-term complication, tracheal stenosis, can cause difficulty if the patient requires intubation at some point in the future. You must master the skills for performing surgical airways and continually practice them under the direct supervision of the physician medical director, who should determine that you can perform the technique and that you understand and can treat its possible complications. Extracted animal airways obtained from meat processing plants or biological specimen suppliers can be used for practice.

Indications that warrant a surgical cricothyrotomy include problems that prevent intubating or ventilating a patient by the nasal or oral routes. Massive facial or neck trauma is the most common cause. Some cases involve so much facial or airway distortion that you cannot identify normal landmarks. Other indications of a surgical cricothyrotomy include total upper airway obstruction due to epiglottitis, severe anaphylaxis, burns to the face and respiratory tract, posterior laceration of the tongue, or the inability to open the mouth. You can perform surgical airways with the patient's head and neck in the neutral position. Contraindications to performing surgical airways in the field include inability to identify anatomical landmarks (including trauma and short, fat necks), crush injury to the larynx, tracheal transection, and underlying anatomical abnormalities such as trauma, tumor, or subglottic stenosis.

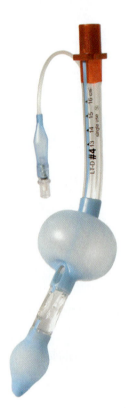

■ **Figure 7-34** King LT airway. *(King Systems Corporation, Indianapolis, IN)*

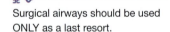

Surgical airways should be used ONLY as a last resort.

NEEDLE CRICOTHYROTOMY

Though it is an invasive surgical procedure that you must master before performing it in the field, a needle cricothyrotomy is technically easier to accomplish than an open cricothyrotomy and has a lower complication rate. It can be rapidly performed, does not manipulate the cervical spine, and provides adequate ventilation when performed properly. It is a temporary airway, used until a larger diameter, definitive airway is provided. It does not interfere with subsequent intubation attempts because it uses a 14-gauge needle, which has a relatively small diameter so that an ETT can pass beside it. However, because the catheter does not fill the tracheal diameter, needle cricothyrotomy cannot protect the patient against aspiration. Needles larger than 14 gauge can be used also, if available.

This procedure requires different oxygenation and ventilation techniques than other airway maneuvers. Transtracheal jet insufflation (ventilation) uses a high-pressure jet ventilator to force oxygen through the small-diameter catheter and provide adequate oxygenation and ventilation. Because very high pressures insufflate large volumes of oxygen, barotrauma, including pneumothorax, is a potential complication. This procedure is not indicated if exhalation is not possible or if adequate high-pressure ventilation equipment is not available. An alternative to transtracheal jet insufflation is to remove the BVM adapter from a #3 ET tube and insert the adapter into the hub of the needle. BVM ventilation with 100% oxygen can then be accomplished through slow but firm pressure on the BVM. A problem with exhalation may be encountered. An additional 14-guage needle may be inserted next to the original one and will afford an additional exhalation port.

NEEDLE CRICOTHYROTOMY COMPLICATIONS

The potential complications of needle cricothyrotomy with jet ventilation include:

★ Barotrauma from overinflation

★ Excessive bleeding due to improper catheter placement

★ Subcutaneous emphysema from improper placement into the subcutaneous tissue, excessive air leak around the catheter, or laryngeal trauma

★ Airway obstruction from compression of the trachea secondary to excessive bleeding or subcutaneous air

★ Hypoventilation from use of improper equipment, incorrect use of the jet ventilator, or misplacement of the catheter

Avoid subcutaneous emphysema by ensuring that the end of the needle is actually in the trachea, not in a tissue plane or "false" passage. Be certain that you can aspirate air into the syringe at all times, and that the needle moves freely. The BVM technique may be safer than jet ventilation since you will be able to experience decreased compliance if the needle is not in the tracheal lumen.

NEEDLE CRICOTHYROTOMY TECHNIQUE

To perform needle cricothyrotomy with jet ventilation:

1. Place the patient supine and hyperextend the head and neck (maintain neutral position if you suspect cervical spine injury). Position yourself at the patient's side. Manage the patient's airway with basic maneuvers and supplemental oxygen, and prepare your equipment.

2. Gently palpate and locate the inferior portion of the thyroid cartilage and the cricoid cartilage and find the cricothyroid membrane between the two cartilages. (See Figures 7-35 ▪ and 7-36 ▪.)

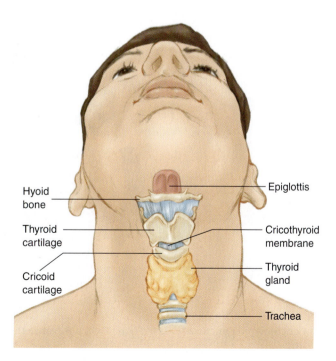

■ Figure 7-35 Anatomical landmarks for cricothyrotomy.

Hyoid bone

Epiglottis

Thyroid cartilage

Cricothyroid membrane

Cricoid cartilage

Thyroid gland

Trachea

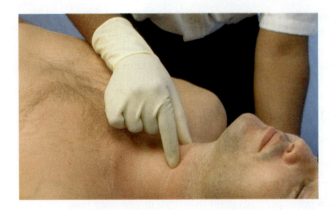

■ Figure 7-36
Locate/palpate the
cricothyroid membrane.

3. Prepare the anterior neck with povidone-iodine swabs. Firmly grasp the laryngeal cartilages and reconfirm the site of the cricothyroid membrane.

4. Attach a large-bore IV needle, with a catheter (adults: 14 or 16 gauge; pediatrics: 18 or 20 gauge), to a 10- or 20-mL syringe. Carefully insert the needle into the cricothyroid membrane at midline, directed 45° caudally (toward the feet). (See Figure 7-37 ■.) Often you will feel a pop as the needle penetrates the membrane.

5. Advance the needle no more than 1 cm, then aspirate with the syringe. If air returns easily, the catheter is in the trachea. If blood returns or you feel resistance to return, reevaluate needle placement. After you confirm proper placement, hold the needle steady and advance the catheter. Then withdraw the needle. (See Figure 7-38 ■.)

6. Reconfirm placement by again withdrawing air from the catheter with the syringe. Secure the catheter in place. (See Figure 7-39 ■.)

7. Check for adequacy of ventilations. Look for chest rise with each ventilation, and listen for bilateral breath sounds in the chest. If spontaneous ventilations are absent or inadequate, begin transtracheal jet ventilation or ventilation with a bag-valve device.

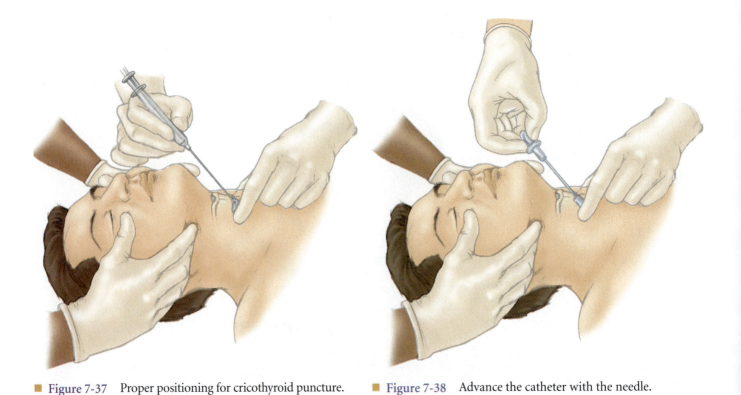

■ Figure 7-37 Proper positioning for cricothyroid puncture.   **■ Figure 7-38** Advance the catheter with the needle.

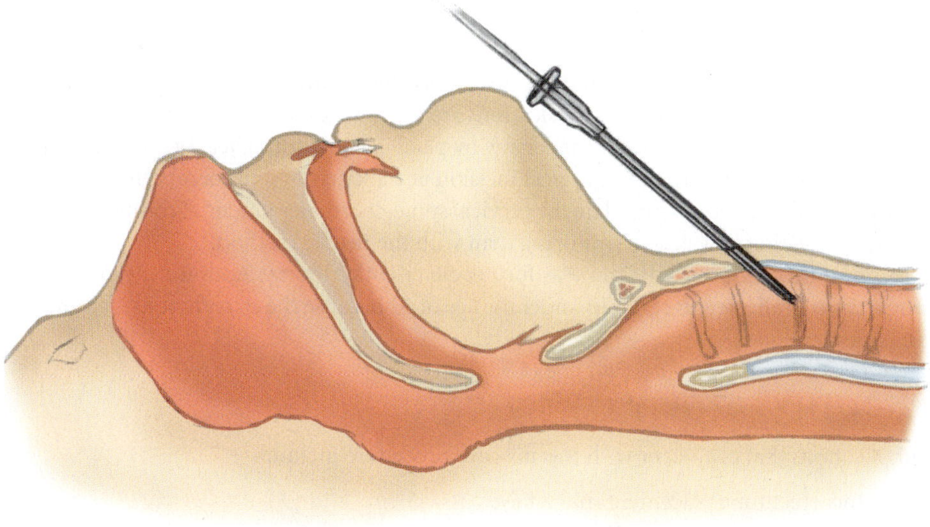

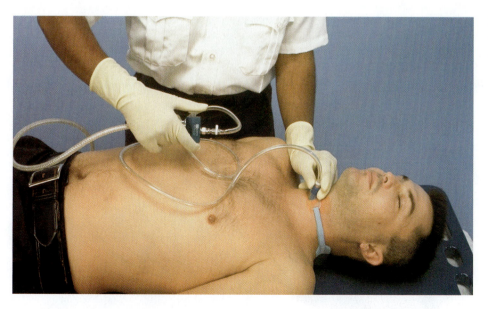

■ Figure 7-39 Cannula properly placed in the trachea.

8. When using jet ventilation, connect one end of the oxygen tubing to the catheter and the other end to the jet ventilator.

9. Open the release valve to introduce an oxygen jet into the trachea. (See Figure 7-40 ■.) Then adjust the pressure to allow adequate lung expansion (usually about 50 psi, compared with about 1 psi through a regulator).

10. Watch the chest carefully, turning off the release valve as soon as the chest rises. Exhalation then occurs passively through the glottis, due to elastic recoil of the lungs and chest wall. Deliver at least 20 breaths per minute to ensure adequate oxygenation and ventilation. The inflation-to-deflation time ratio should be approximately 1:2, as with normal respirations. Keep in mind that you may need to adjust this to the patient's needs, particularly in COPD and asthma patients, who often require a longer expiration time.

11. Continue ventilatory support, assessing for adequacy of ventilations and looking for the development of any potential complications.

■ Figure 7-40 Jet ventilation with needle cricothyrotomy.

OPEN CRICOTHYROTOMY

An open cricothyrotomy is preferred to needle cricothyrotomy when a complete obstruction prevents a glottic route for expiration. Indications are the same as for needle cricothyrotomy. An open cricothyrotomy involves obtaining an airway by placing an endotracheal or tracheostomy tube directly into the trachea through a surgical incision at the cricothyroid membrane. It can be rapidly performed and does not manipulate the cervical spine. Its greater potential complications mandate even more training and skills monitoring than with the needle method.

Contraindications are the same as for needle cricothyrotomy. Additionally, open cricothyrotomy is contraindicated in children under the age of 12 because the cricothyroid membrane is small and underdeveloped.

CRICOTHYROTOMY COMPLICATIONS

Complications that can occur with this invasive procedure include:

- ★ Incorrect tube placement into a false passage
- ★ Cricoid and/or thyroid cartilage damage
- ★ Thyroid gland damage
- ★ Severe bleeding
- ★ Laryngeal nerve damage
- ★ Subcutaneous emphysema
- ★ Vocal cord damage
- ★ Infection

OPEN CRICOTHYROTOMY TECHNIQUE

To perform an open cricothyrotomy (Figure 7-41A through 7-41I ■):

1. Locate the thyroid cartilage and the cricoid cartilage. Find the cricothyroid membrane between the two cartilages.

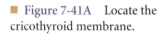 **Figure 7-41A** Locate the cricothyroid membrane.

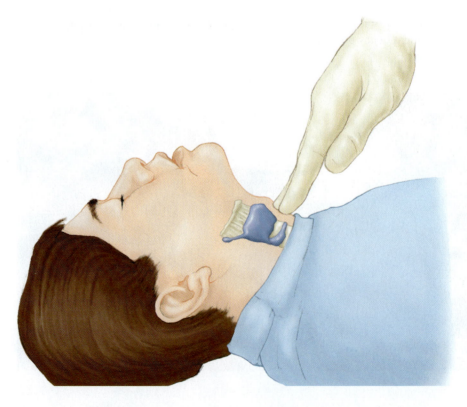

2. Clean the area with iodine-containing solution if time permits, while your partner sets up suction, pulse oximetry, and cardiac monitor.

3. Stabilize the cartilages with one hand, while using a scalpel in the other hand to make a 1- to 2-cm vertical skin incision over the membrane.

4. Find the cricothyroid membrane again and make a 1-cm incision in the horizontal plane through the membrane, avoiding nearby veins and arteries, as well as the recurrent laryngeal nerve.

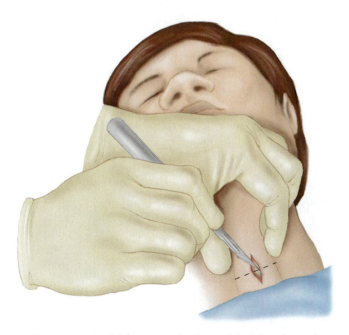

■ **Figure 7-41C** Make a 1 cm horizontal incision through the cricothyroid membrane.

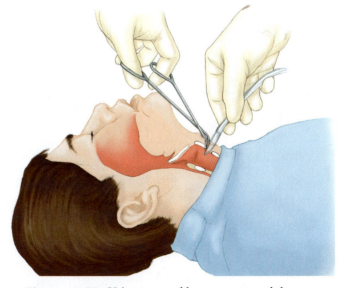

■ **Figure 7-41D** Using a curved hemostat, spread the membrane incision open.

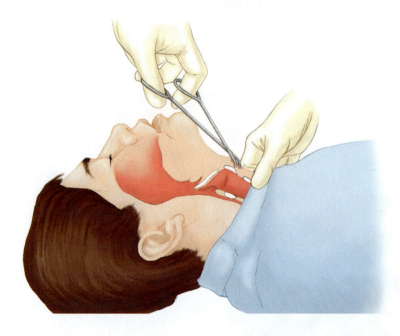

■ **Figure 7-41E** Insert an ETT (6.0 or 7.0) or Shiley tracheostomy tube (6.0 or 8.0).

5. Insert curved hemostats into the membrane incision and spread it open.

6. Insert either a cuffed 6.0- or 7.0-mm endotracheal tube or 6 or 8 Shiley tracheostomy tube, directing the tube into the trachea.

7. Inflate the cuff.

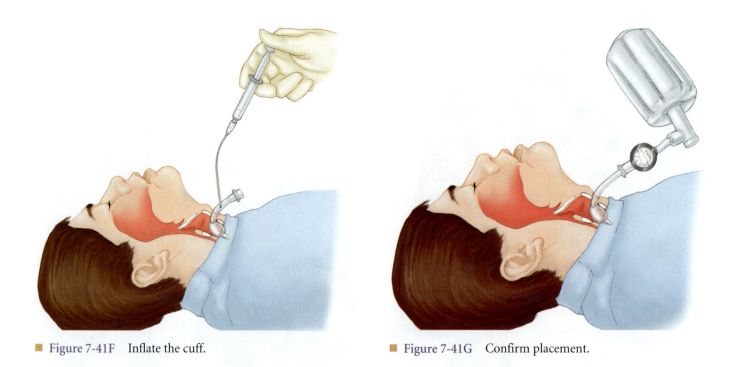

■ **Figure 7-41F**   Inflate the cuff.

■ **Figure 7-41G**   Confirm placement.

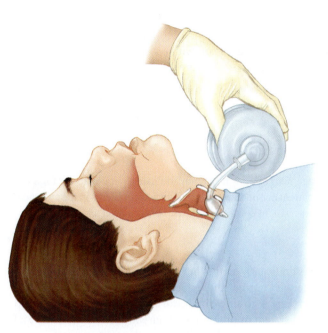

■ Figure 7-41H   Resume ventilation.

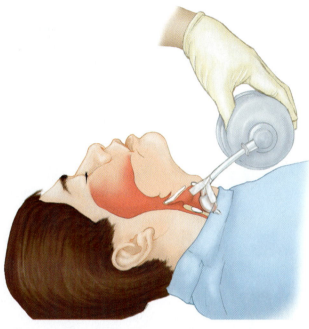

■ Figure 7-41I   Secure the tube, reconfirm placement, and evaluate the patient.

8. Confirm placement with auscultation, end-tidal CO_2 detector, and chest rise.
9. Resume ventilation as appropriate.
10. Secure the tube in place.

We cannot stress enough that you must continuously practice this skill with the medical director's involvement before you are allowed to perform it.

APPROACH TO THE DIFFICULT AIRWAY

As a critical care paramedic, you will be expected to be able to effectively manage patients where establishment of the airway may be difficult. It has been estimated that 1 out of 10 endotracheal intubations can be classified as "difficult." Furthermore, it has been estimated that endotracheal intubation may be impossible in 1 out of 100 patients when conventional techniques are attempted. Terms used in relation to the difficult airway include (modified from the American Society of Anesthesiologists Task Force definitions):

★ **Difficult airway.** A clinical situation in which a conventionally trained paramedic experiences difficulty with mask ventilation, difficulty with endotracheal intubation, or both.
★ *Difficult mask ventilation.* The (1) inability of the unassisted paramedic to maintain an $SpO_2 > 90\%$ using 100% oxygen and positive-pressure mask ventilation in a patient whose SpO_2 was 90% before airway intervention; or (2) inability of the unassisted paramedic to prevent or reverse signs of inadequate ventilation during positive-pressure mask ventilation. (Signs include cyanosis, absence of chest movement, auscultatory signs of severe airway obstruction, gastric entry or gastric distention, and hemodynamic changes associated with hypoxemia or hypercarbia.)

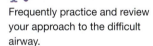

Frequently practice and review your approach to the difficult airway.

difficult airway *a clinical situation in which a conventionally trained paramedic experiences difficulty with mask ventilation and/or endotracheal intubation.*

★ *Difficult laryngoscopy.* Not being able to see any part of the *vocal cords* with conventional laryngoscopy.

★ *Difficult intubation.* Situation where proper insertion with conventional laryngoscopy requires either (1) more than three attempts or (2) more than 10 minutes.

When the issue of difficult airways has been investigated, several factors seem common. These include historical information, anatomical factors and poor technique on the part of the person performing the intubation.

HISTORICAL FACTORS

A history of problems with airway management or anesthesia may indicate a patient at risk for a difficult airway. However, being able to ask a patient about anesthesia and airway problems in the emergency setting is uncommon. However, if time and patient condition allows, obtain a brief airway history.

ANATOMICAL FACTORS

The anatomy of the upper airway varies significantly across the human species. In addition, disease processes and tumors can distort an otherwise normal airway. Several anatomical factors are associated with the difficult airway. However, there is no single indicator that will point specifically to a difficult airway. The most frequently used system of preintubation airway assessment is the **Mallampati classification system.** With this system, the tonsillar pillars and the uvula are assessed. The more concealed the tonsilar pillars and the uvula, the more difficult the intubation. Based on these features, the patient's airway is classified into four grades:

★ *Class 1:* Entire tonsil clearly visible

★ *Class 2:* Upper half of tonsil fossa visible

★ *Class 3:* Soft and hard palate clearly visible

★ *Class 4:* Only hard palate visible

The higher the grade, the more difficult the airway is suspected to be.

While airway classification systems are great, they have little application to emergency medicine. This is especially so in the case of the austere critical care environment. Rarely will a critical care provider have time to assess the Mallampati class prior to intubation attempts. The Mallampati assessment is done with the patient awake and sitting up. The patient opens his mouth and sticks his tongue out. However, knowing the features of this system will allow you to better anticipate the difficult airway.

Recognizing that the Mallampati system is of little use in the unconscious patient, Cormack and Lehane adapted the system to classify the view one sees with a laryngoscope. The revised **Cormack and Lehane classification system** is similar to Mallampati's (Figure 7-42 ■):

Mallampati classification system *four "class" level airway assessment for use in conscious patients, defined by the ability to visualize all, part, or none of the tonsillar pillars and/or the uvula.*

Cormack and Lehane classification system *four "grade" level airway assessment for use in unconscious patients, defined by the ability to visualize all, part, or none of the glottic opening and/or the vocal cords.*

■ Figure 7-42 Airway scoring systems. Mallampati classification system (top); Cormack and Lehane classification system (bottom).

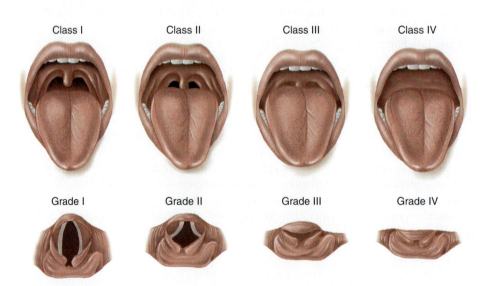

Class I Class II Class III Class IV

Grade I Grade II Grade III Grade IV

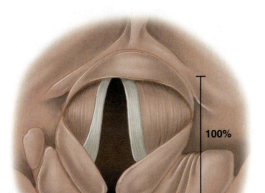

Percentage of glottic opening (POGO) scale.

★ *Grade 1:* Entire glottic opening and vocal cords can be seen.

★ *Grade 2:* Epiglottis and posterior portion of glottic opening can be seen, with a partial view of vocal cords.

★ *Grade 3:* Only epiglottis and (sometimes) posterior cartilages can be seen.

★ *Grade 4:* Neither epiglottis nor glottis can be seen.

Another scoring system used in EMS is the percentage of glottic opening (POGO) system. With the **POGO classification system,** the percentage of glottis that can be visualized is scored. The score ranges from 0 (none of the glottis visualized) to 100 (vocal cords fully visualized). This system also helps predict the difficulty of endotracheal intubation. (See Figure 7-43 ■.)

Knowing the features of these systems will allow you to better anticipate the difficult airway. Other factors associated with a difficult airway include:

★ *Short neck.* People with short necks, as a rule, are more difficult to intubate than those with necks of normal length or long necks. In addition, people with short necks tend to have a restricted range of motion of the neck.

★ *Thick neck.* The thickness of the neck ("bull neck") can cause patients to be difficult to intubate. This can occur with obesity or simply with normal body habitus.

★ *Restricted range of motion in the neck (immobile neck).* Patients who cannot touch the tip of their chin to their chest or who cannot extend their neck have restricted range of motion in the neck. This condition places these patients at increased risk for presenting a difficult airway. In addition, cervical immobilization in trauma can limit the range of motion of the neck, making intubation more difficult.

★ *Dentition.* The teeth can make intubation difficult. Certainly, fractured or dislodged teeth are problematic. However, normal dentition variants can be problematic during intubation. If the maxillary (upper) incisors are long or are protruding, then the patient may have a difficult airway. Likewise, the presence of a prominent "overbite" and the inability of the patient to bring the mandibular (lower) incisors anterior to the maxillary incisors increase the risk.

★ *Small mouth.* Patients with a small oral opening can be more difficult to intubate because there is less room for the laryngoscope and endotracheal tube. If possible, have the patient open his mouth as wide as possible. Patients with oral openings less than 3 cm (about three finger breadths) between the upper and lower incisors when the mouth is fully open are at increased risk for having a difficult airway.

★ *Short mandible.* A short mandible also places patients at risk for having a difficult airway. A short mandible can make visualization of the glottis quite difficult.

★ *Anterior larynx.* The thyromental distance is the distance from the midline of the mandible (mentum) to the thyroid notch. This measurement is performed with the

POGO classification system *airway assessment used by some EMS personnel to rate the percentage of glottic opening (POGO) one can visualize from "0" to "100" percent (all).*

adult patient's neck fully extended. If this thyromental distance is short (less than three finger breadths), the laryngeal axis makes a more acute angle with the pharyngeal axis, and it will be difficult to achieve alignment. In addition, there is less space for the tongue to be displaced during laryngoscopy.

★ *Obesity.* Obesity, especially morbid obesity, increases the risk of encountering a difficult airway. With obesity, a combination of factors is usually involved: short neck, decreased neck range of motion, and a small (relatively) oral opening.

★ *Anatomical distortion.* Distortions of the upper airway anatomy can lead to difficulty in establishing an airway. This can be due to trauma (swelling, bleeding) or medical conditions (tumors, angioedema, tension pneumothorax with tracheal shift).

Figure 7-44 ■ shows an algorithm that will help the critical care paramedic with decision making when a difficult airway is encountered.

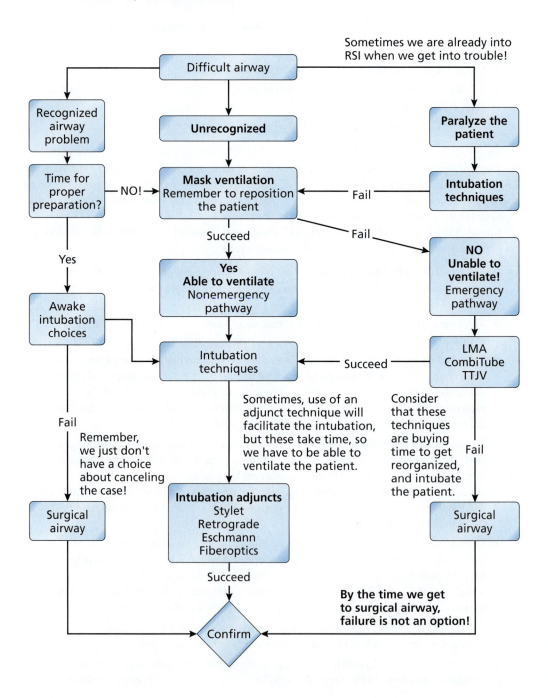

■ **Figure 7-44** Difficult airway algorithm *(From Stewart, CE.* Advanced Airway Management. *Upper Saddle River, NJ: Pearson Prentice Hall, 2002).*

POOR TECHNIQUE

Endotracheal intubation is a fundamental paramedic skill. A poor technique in application of this skill can be disastrous for the patient. Recent studies have indicated that intubation has been associated with periods of hypoxia or hyperventilation. These can be avoided by following established guidelines and the use of monitoring methods such as waveform capnography and pulse oximetry. Patients should be well oxygenated prior to attempting endotracheal intubation. In addition, an alternative or "rescue airway" must always be available and within reach in case endotracheal intubation fails.

NONINVASIVE RESPIRATORY MONITORING

Several available devices will help you measure the effectiveness of oxygenation and ventilation. Those measurements used most commonly in critical care transport are pulse oximetry and waveform capnography.

PULSE OXIMETRY

Pulse oximetry is widely used in prehospital and critical care transport medicine. A pulse oximeter measures hemoglobin oxygen saturation in peripheral tissues. (See Figure 7-45 ■.) It is noninvasive (does not require entering the body), rapidly applied, and easy to operate. Pulse oximetry readings are accurate and continually reflect any changes in peripheral oxygen delivery. In fact, oximetry often detects problems with oxygenation faster than assessments of blood pressure, pulse, and respirations.

To determine peripheral oxygen saturation, you place a sensor probe over a peripheral capillary bed such as a fingertip, toe, or earlobe. In infants, you can wrap the sensor around the heel and secure it with tape. The sensor contains two light-emitting diodes and two sensors. One diode emits near-red light, a wavelength specific for oxygenated hemoglobin; the other emits infrared light, a wavelength specific for deoxygenated hemoglobin. Each hemoglobin state absorbs a certain amount of the emitted light, preventing it from reaching the corresponding sensor. Less light reaching the sensor means more of its type of hemoglobin is in the blood. The oximeter then calculates the ratio of the near-red and infrared light it has received to determine the oxygen saturation percentage (SpO_2).

pulse oximetry *use of an electronic device to measure hemoglobin-oxygen saturation in peripheral tissues.*

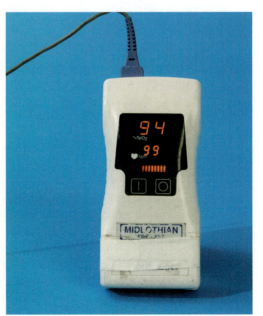

■ **Figure 7-45** Pulse oximeter. *(© Scott Meltcalfe)*

Pulse oximeters display the SpO_2 and the pulse rate as detected by the sensors. They show the SpO_2 either as a number or as a visual display that also shows the pulse's waveform. The relationship between SpO_2 and the partial pressure of oxygen in the blood (PaO_2) is very complex. However, the SpO_2 does correlate with the PaO_2. The greater the PaO_2, the greater the oxygen saturation. Since hemoglobin carries 97% of oxygen in the blood while plasma carries only 3%, pulse oximetry accurately analyzes peripheral oxygen delivery. Pulse oximetry is often called the "fifth vital sign." When available, you should use it in virtually any situation to determine the patient's baseline value, to guide patient care, and to monitor the patient's responses to your interventions.

As a guide, normal SpO_2 varies between 95% and 99%. Readings between 91% and 94% indicate mild hypoxia and warrant further evaluation and supplemental oxygen administration. Readings between 86% and 90% indicate moderate hypoxia. You should generally give these patients 100% supplemental oxygen, exercising caution in those with COPD. Readings of 85% or lower indicate severe hypoxia and warrant immediate intervention, including the administration of 100% oxygen, ventilatory assistance, or both. Your goal is to maintain the SpO_2 in the normal (95% to 99%) range.

False readings with pulse oximetry are infrequent. When they do occur, the oximeter often generates an error signal or a blank screen. Causes of false readings include carbon monoxide poisoning, high-intensity lighting, and certain hemoglobin abnormalities. The absence of a pulse in an extremity also will cause a false reading. In hypovolemia and in severely anemic patients, the pulse oximetry reading may be misleading. While the SpO_2 reading may be normal, the total amount of hemoglobin available to carry oxygen may be so markedly decreased that the patient will remain hypoxic at the cellular level.

Pulse oximetry provides key information about the patient and is an important part of emergency care. However, it is only one more assessment tool and does not replace other physical assessment or monitoring skills. Do not depend solely on pulse oximetry readings to guide care. Always consider and treat the whole patient.

CAPNOGRAPHY

End-tidal carbon dioxide ($ETCO_2$) monitoring is a noninvasive method of measuring the levels of carbon dioxide (CO_2) in the exhaled breath. Recordings or displays of exhaled CO_2 measurements are called **capnography.**

capnography *recordings or displays of exhaled CO_2 measurements.*

Various terms have been applied to capnography, and a review of them may help you to understand the material in this section. These terms include:

★ *Capnometry.* Capnometry is the measurement of expired CO_2. It typically provides a numeric display of the partial pressure of CO_2 (in torr or mmHg) or the percentage of CO_2 present.

★ *Capnography.* Capnography is a graphic recording or display of the capnometry reading over time.

★ *Capnograph.* A capnograph is a device that measures expired CO_2 levels.

capnogram *the visual representation of the expired CO_2 waveform.*

★ *Capnogram.* A **capnogram** is the visual representation of the expired CO_2 waveform.

★ *End-tidal CO_2 ($ETCO_2$).* End-tidal CO_2 is the measurement of the CO_2 concentration at the end of expiration (maximum CO_2).

★ *$PETCO_2$.* $PETCO_2$ is the partial pressure of end-tidal CO_2 in a mixed gas solution.

★ *$PaCO_2$.* The $PaCO_2$ represents the partial pressure of CO_2 in the arterial blood.

CO_2 is a normal end product of metabolism and is transported by the venous system to the right side of the heart. It is then pumped from the right ventricle to the pulmonary artery and eventually enters the pulmonary capillaries. There it diffuses into the alveoli and is removed from the body through exhalation. When circulation is normal, $ETCO_2$ levels change with ventilation and are a reliable estimate of the partial pressure of carbon dioxide in the arterial system ($PaCO_2$). Normal $ETCO_2$ is 1 to 2 mm less than the $PaCO_2$, or approximately 5%. A normal $PETCO_2$ is approximately 38 mmHg (0.05×760 mmHg = 38 mmHg at sea level). When perfusion decreases, as occurs in shock or cardiac arrest, $ETCO_2$ levels reflect pulmonary blood flow and cardiac output, not ventilation.

Decreased $ETCO_2$ levels can be found in shock, cardiac arrest, pulmonary embolism, bronchospasm, and with incomplete airway obstruction (such as mucous plugging). Increased $ETCO_2$ levels are found with hypoventilation, respiratory depression, and hyperthermia.

Capnometry provides a noninvasive measure of $ETCO_2$ levels, thus providing medical personnel with information about the status of systemic metabolism, circulation, and ventilation. The use of capnography has become commonplace in the operating room, in the emergency department in the prehospital setting and in critical care transport.

When first introduced into prehospital care, $ETCO_2$ monitoring was used exclusively to verify proper endotracheal tube placement in the trachea. The presence of adequate CO_2 levels following intubation confirms the tube is in the trachea through the presence of exhaled CO_2. CO_2 is detected by using either a colorimetric or an infrared device. The colorimetric device is a disposable $ETCO_2$ detector that contains pH-sensitive, chemically impregnated paper encased within a plastic chamber. (See Figure 7-46 ■.) It is placed in the airway circuit between the patient and the ventilation device. When the paper is exposed to CO_2, hydrogen ions (H^+) are generated, causing a color change in the paper. The color change is reversible and changes from breath to breath. A color scale on the device estimates the $ETCO_2$ level. Colorimetric devices are not designed to detect hypercarbia (increased CO_2 levels) and have limited usefulness in detecting hypocarbia (decreased CO_2 levels). If gastric contents or acidic drugs (e.g., endotracheal epinephrine) contact the paper in the device, subsequent readings may be unreliable.

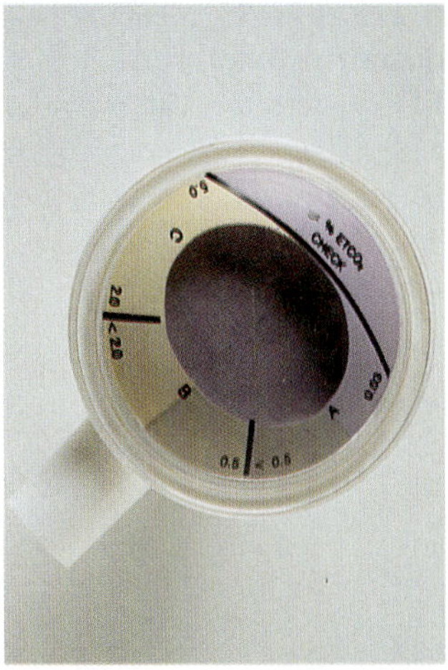

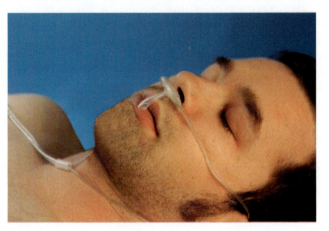

■ **Figure 7-46** Colormetric end-tidal CO_2 detector.

ELECTRONIC DEVICES

Electronic $ETCO_2$ detectors use an infrared technique to detect CO_2 in the exhaled breath. (See Figure 7-47 ■.) A heated element in the sensor generates infrared radiation. The CO_2 molecules absorb infrared light at a very specific wavelength and can thus be measured. Electronic $ETCO_2$ detectors may be either qualitative (i.e., they simply detect the presence of CO_2) or quantitative (i.e., they

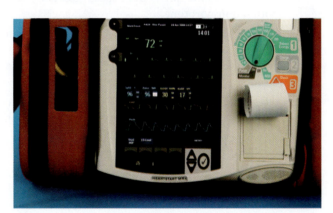

■ **Figure 7-47A** Electronic end-tidal CO_2 detector.

■ **Figure 7-47B** Electronic end-tidal CO_2 detector on a patient. (© *Scott Metcalfe*)

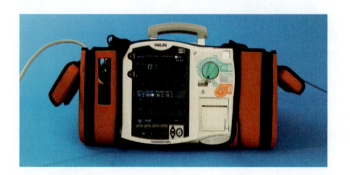

Figure 7-48 Most quantitative electronic $ETCO_2$ detectors can provide a digital waveform (capnogram) that reflects the entire respiratory cycle. (© Scott Metcalfe)

determine how much CO_2 is present). Quantitative devices are now routinely used in critical care transport medicine. Most can provide a digital waveform (capnogram) that reflects the entire respiratory cycle. (See Figure 7-48 ■.)

CAPNOGRAM

The capnogram reflects CO_2 concentrations over time. It is typically divided into four phases (Figure 7-49 ■):

★ *Phase I.* Phase I (AB in Figure 7-49) is the respiratory baseline. It is flat when no CO_2 is present and corresponds to the late phase of inspiration and the early part of expiration (in which dead-space gases without CO_2 are released).

★ *Phase II.* Phase II (BC in Figure 7-49) is the respiratory upstroke. This represents exhalation of a mixture of dead-space gases and alveolar gases from alveoli with the shortest transport time.

★ *Phase III.* Phase III (CD in Figure 7-49) is the respiratory plateau. It reflects the airflow through uniformly ventilated alveoli with a nearly constant CO_2 level. The highest level of the plateau (point D in Figure 7-49) is called the $ETCO_2$ and is recorded as such by the capnometer.

★ *Phase IV.* Phase IV (DE in Figure 7-49) is the inspiratory phase. It is a sudden downstroke and ultimately returns to the baseline during inspiration. The respiratory pause restarts the cycle (EA in Figure 7-49).

CLINICAL APPLICATIONS

Initially, as noted earlier, $ETCO_2$ detection was used only to determine proper endotracheal tube placement. Typically, a qualitative $ETCO_2$ device was applied to the airway circuit following intubation. If $ETCO_2$ levels were detected, then proper tube placement was verified. However, it is difficult to continuously monitor the airway with a quantitative device. Now, continuous waveform capnography is available and allows continuous monitoring of airway placement and ventilation

Figure 7-49 Normal capnogram. AB = *Phase I:* late inspiration, early expiration (no CO_2). BC = *Phase II:* appearance of CO_2 in exhaled gas. CD = *Phase III:* plateau (constant CO_2). D = highest point ($ETCO_2$). DE = *Phase IV:* rapid descent during inspiration. EC = respiratory pause.

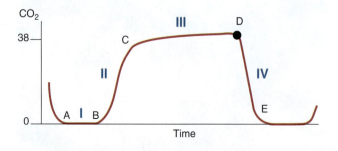

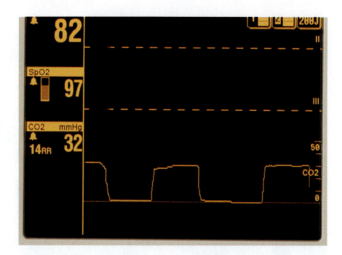

■ **Figure 7-50** Continuous waveform capnography. (*© Scott Metcalfe*)

for intubated patients. Continuous waveform capnography also has utility in monitoring nonintubated patients. By following trends in the capnogram, critical care providers can continuously monitor the patient's condition, detect trends, and document the reponse to medications.

$ETCO_2$ detection is also useful in CPR. During cardiac arrest, CO_2 levels fall abruptly following the onset of cardiac arrest. They begin to rise with the onset of effective CPR and return to near-normal levels with a return of spontaneous circulation. During effective CPR, $ETCO_2$ levels have been found to correlate well with cardiac output, coronary perfusion pressure, and even with the effectiveness of CPR compressions.

Continuous waveform capnography is rapidly becoming a standard of care in EMS. (See Figure 7-50 ■.) Misplaced endotracheal tubes represent a significant area of liability in EMS, and the documentation provided by this technology can provide irrefutable evidence of proper endotracheal tube placement.

VENTILATION

Many of your cases in the field will call for ventilatory support. These situations will range from apneic patients to less obvious instances when patients are experiencing depressed respiratory function. Remember that an unconscious patient's respiratory center may not function adequately. A significant decrease in the patient's rate or depth of breathing will lead to decreased respiratory minute volume, hypercarbia, hypoxia, and a lowered pH. If you do not correct this, respiratory or cardiac arrest may occur.

In the critical care setting, mechanical ventilation is used for multiple reasons including:

★ Apnea

★ Protection of upper airway

★ Relief of airway obstruction

★ Improved pulmonary hygiene (toilet)

★ Refractory cardiogenic pulmonary edema

★ Respiratory failure

★ Anticipated rapid deterioration (It is better to intubate and ventilate early before the patient's condition deteriorates, thus decreasing the chances of complications.)

★ Serious myocardial ischemia (in cases where the added work of breathing can worsen myocardial ischemia)

★ A $PO_2 \leq 50$ mmHg despite the administration of supplemental oxygen

For this discussion, we will assume that you are competent in use of the bag-valve-mask device and similar ventilatory devices. Thus, we will concentrate on the use of transport mechanical ventilators.

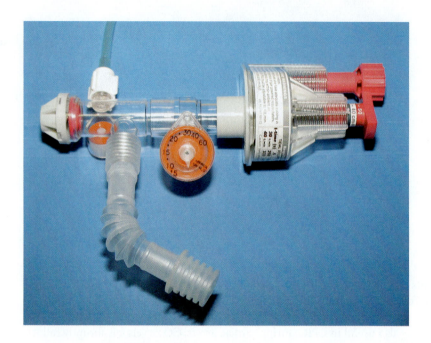

■ Figure 7-51   SureVent. *(Hartwell Medical, Carlsbad, CA)*

AUTOMATIC TRANSPORT VENTILATOR

automatic transport ventilators *compact mechanical ventilators that can be used in out-of-hospital transport.*

Several compact mechanical ventilators, called **automatic transport ventilators** are available for critical care transports. Designed for convenience and ease of use during patient care and transport, these lightweight and durable portable devices offer a number of advantages. They maintain minute volume better than bag-valve devices, and they tolerate temperatures ranging from −30° to 125° F with great dependability. In cardiac arrest, the automatic ventilator allows you to interpose chest compressions between mechanical breaths. It is mechanically simple and adapts to a portable oxygen supply.

The compact ventilator typically comes with two or three controls: one for the ventilatory rate, the other for tidal volume. (See Figure 7-51 ■.) It also has a standard 15/22-mm adapter, so that you can attach it to a variety of airway devices. Some of these automatic units deliver controlled ventilation only. Others function as intermittent mandatory ventilators, reverting to controlled mechanical ventilation in patients who are not breathing. Tidal volume in most is adjustable, while the ventilatory rate may be either fixed or adjustable. The inspired oxygen concentration is usually fixed at 100%, but it may be adjustable.

Many of these ventilators have a pop-off valve that prevents pressure-related injury. When airway pressure exceeds a preset level (typically 60 cm/H_2O), the valve opens, venting some of the tidal volume. This feature can hinder ventilating patients with cardiogenic pulmonary edema, adult respiratory distress syndrome (ARDS), pulmonary contusion, bronchospasm, or other disorders in which high airway pressures must be overcome. Consider using a bag-valve device if this problem occurs. Also, these devices generally have no alarms to warn of possible tube displacement or barotrauma.

As a rule, you should not use mechanical ventilators in children younger than 5 years old, awake patients, or patients with obstructed airways or increased airway resistance, as described earlier. Otherwise, when indicated, the device can prove a valuable tool. In intubated patients, the mechanical ventilator allows you to perform other vital tasks. Its disadvantages are that it can be difficult to secure and proper functioning depends on oxygen tank pressure.

TYPES OF VENTILATORS

There are two types of ventilators: *negative-pressure ventilators* and *positive-pressure ventilators*. Negative-pressure ventilators, such as the iron lung, encircle the patient and generate a negative pressure outside the body. These are rarely used in the critical care setting. The most commonly encountered mechanical ventilators are positive-pressure ventilators. Inspiration occurs when the air is pushed into the airway through positive pressure. Exhalation results when the positive pressure stops.

Positive-Pressure Ventilators

Positive-pressure ventilators can be classified as pressure cycled or volume cycled. With a pressure-cycled ventilator, inspiratory flow is delivered until a predetermined pressure is reached and then it shuts off. With a volume-cycled respirator, inspiratory flow is delivered until a predetermined volume of air has been delivered and then it shuts off. Advantages of pressure-cycled ventilators are that they are relatively inexpensive, compact, mobile, and can operate on compressed oxygen or air. Disadvantages of pressure-cycled ventilators include variances in tidal volumes based on lung compliance, increased intrathoracic pressures that can cause decreased venous blood return to the heart thus decreasing cardiac output, barotrauma, and the requirement for a sealed airway (endotracheal intubation). The primary advantage of volume-cycled ventilators is that they accurately deliver a set tidal volume regardless of lung compliance. Disadvantages of volume-cycled ventilators include increased intrathoracic pressures that can cause decreased venous blood return to the heart thus decreasing cardiac output, barotrauma, and the requirement for a sealed airway (endotracheal intubation).

Control   Control determines how the ventilator determines how much flow to deliver.

- ★ *Volume controlled.* The volume is set and the pressures are variable.
- ★ *Pressure controlled.* The pressures are set and the volume is variable.
- ★ *Dual controlled.* The volume is set and limits are placed on the pressures.

Support   Most ventilators can be set to deliver the tidal volume in a control mode or a support mode.

- ★ *Control mode.* The ventilator delivers the preset tidal volume once it is triggered regardless of patient effort. If the patient is apneic or has limited respiratory drive, the control mode can ensure delivery of appropriate minute ventilation.
- ★ *Support mode.* The ventilator provides inspiratory assistance through the use of an assist pressure. The ventilator detects inspiration by the patient and supplies an assist pressure during inspiration. When the patient enters the exhalation phase, the ventilation is terminated. Use of the support mode requires an adequate respiratory drive. The amount of assist pressure can be selected by the operator.

Cycling   Cycling determines how the ventilator switches from inspiration to expiration.

- ★ *Time cycled.* The ventilator will deliver a certain number of breaths per minute.
- ★ *Flow cycled.* The ventilator switches when preset pressure levels are reached.
- ★ *Volume cycled.* The ventilator is set to cycle to expiration once a set tidal volume has been delivered. If an inspiratory pause is added, then the breath is both volume and time cycled.

Triggering   Triggering is the stimulus that causes the ventilator to cycle to inspiration. Ventilators may be time triggered, pressure triggered, or flow triggered.

- ★ *Time.* The ventilator cycles at a set frequency as determined by the controlled rate.
- ★ *Pressure.* The ventilator senses the patient's inspiratory effort by way of a decrease in the baseline pressure.
- ★ *Flow.* With modern ventilators, a constant flow of gas is delivered around the circuit throughout the respiratory cycle (flow-by). A deflection in this flow-by patient inspiration is monitored by the ventilator and it delivers a breath. This mechanism requires less work by the patient than pressure triggering.
- ★ *Breathing.* Patient-initiated respirations cause the ventilator to cycle from inspiration.
- ★ *Mandatory.* Ventilation is controlled by the set respiratory rate.
- ★ *Assisted.* The ventilator will assist the patient's native respirations.
- ★ *Spontaneous.* No additional assistance is provided on inspiration (used with CPAP or BiPAP).

VENTILATOR MODES

Modes are the parameters by which the ventilator determines when to initiate inspiration.

★ *Assist/control.* With assist/control the ventilator provides the full tidal volume at a minimum preset rate. The patient can also initiate breaths in this mode, thus providing additional full tidal volumes. Assist/control is useful in that it provides near complete resting of ventilatory muscles. In addition, it can be used in patients who are awake, sedated, or paralyzed. However, because patients can trigger ventilations, they can hyperventilate and become alkalotic. They can also "stack" breaths, thus resulting in air trapping and the possibility of barotrauma.

★ *Synchronized intermittent mandatory ventilation (SIMV).* With SIMV, the ventilator delivers a fixed tidal volume at a preset respiratory rate. When a ventilator breath is to occur, the ventilator will wait a predetermined amount of time to see if any patient-initiated breaths trigger the programmed ventilator-delivered breath. With SIMV the patient can take additional breaths but the tidal volume of these extra breaths is dependent on the patient's inspiratory effort. The advantage of SIMV is that it is thought to result in improved blood return to the right ventricle owing to intermittent negative-pressure (spontaneous) breaths. In addition, patients are often more comfortable since they have more control over their ventilatory pattern and minute ventilation. SIMV can result in chronic respiratory fatigue if the respiratory rate is set too low. This, in turn, may cause an increased respiratory rate, a rising pCO_2, and air trapping.

★ *Pressure support.* Pressure support is a mode in which the patient triggers the ventilator at a predetermined pressure during the patient's inspiration. The ventilation is terminated when the patient ceases to inspire. Pressure support is not a volume-cycled mode because the tidal volume and minute ventilation are dependent on the patient. Pressure support is more comfortable since the patient has full control over his ventilatory pattern and minute ventilation. This also avoids asynchrony between the ventilator and the patient. Pressure assist also helps avoid breath stacking and auto-PEEP (especially in patients with COPD). It allows the patient to self-determine his respiratory rate. Pressure support cannot be used in heavily sedated, paralyzed, or comatose patients. As with SIMV, respiratory muscle fatigue can develop if the pressure support is set too low.

★ *Pressure control.* Pressure control limits airway pressures rather than airflow volumes. It is usually used with patients who have ARDS where it can sometimes increase the pO_2 by 0% to 15%. The downside to pressure control is that there is no guaranteed tidal volume and thus there is no guaranteed minute ventilation. Therefore, the critical care team must be very attentive to changes in the patient's respiratory mechanics since unstable reactive airway disease can dramatically affect minute ventilation. With pressure support air trapping can occur as can CO_2 retention. As a rule, patients must be heavily sedated when pressure support is used because it can be quite uncomfortable.

★ *Positive end-expiratory pressure (PEEP).* Mechanical ventilators can be set to provide a fixed positive airway pressure (above atmospheric pressure) at the end of expiration. This is typically used with assist-control ventilation. PEEP opens closed alveolar units thus improving lung compliance and oxygenation up to a point. As more alveoli open, airway pressures tend to decline. PEEP may improve secretion drainage from otherwise closed alveoli. However, it can reduce right ventricular venous return and also lower left ventricular afterload. PEEP, especially at high pressures, can cause barotrauma (pneumothorax, pneumomediastinum) and can be risky and counterproductive in patients with obstructive airway disease. In addition to causing hypotension, PEEP can increase intracranial pressure. Typical PEEP settings range from 2.5 to 10.0 cm/H_2O. PEEP over 20 cm/H_2O is rarely beneficial and usually results in additional pressure-induced lung injury.

★ *Airway pressure release ventilation (APRV).* With APRV, the ventilator supplies a low level of continuous positive airway pressure (CPAP) alternating with a relatively high level of CPAP. This permits rapid exhausting of the gas in the expiratory reserve volume and results in a higher tidal volume. APRV can be coupled with pressure support. APRV reduces the potential for barotrauma and overdistention. In addition, it preserves venous return and allows spontaneous breaths. The disadvantages of APRV are that it requires the use of relatively high CPAP levels. In addition, CPAP reductions can result in hypoxemia. APRV is usually used for postoperative and mildly diseased lungs, and its role in severe respiratory failure is unclear.

MECHANICAL VENTILATION PARAMETERS

There are several controls that are common to most ventilators. They vary according to the patient's problem and needs. Common controls include:

★ *Mode.* The mode of ventilation should be tailored to the needs of the patient. Initially, the critical care paramedic may need to make initial settings quickly, which can be changed later. SIMV and assist/control are good initial setting modes.

★ *Sensitivity.* Sensitivity (when in assist mode) is the amount of inspiratory effort required to initiate an assisted breath. Common settings are -1 to -2 cm/H_2O.

★ *Minute ventilations (V_{min}).* The minute ventilation is a function of tidal volume (V_T) and respiratory rate and is normally 6 to 10 liters per minute (lpm) in an adult. The minute ventilation is represented by the following formula:

$$V_{min} \text{ (mL/min)} = V_T \text{ (mL)} \times \text{Respiratory rate (minute)}$$

★ *Tidal volume (V_T).* The tidal volume is the volume of each delivered breath. Some air in the tidal volume simply fills dead space (V_D) in the lungs while the remaining air ventilates the alveoli (V_A). The tidal volume is represented by the following formula:

$$V_T \text{ (mL)} = V_A + V_D$$

Tidal volume can be estimated at 5 to 15 mL/kg of ideal body weight.

★ *Respiratory rate.* The respiratory rate varies from 8 to 12 per minute normally. The rate must be matched with the tidal volume to ensure an adequate minute volume. Rates up to 20 breaths per minute are sometimes indicated.

★ *Inspiration/expiration (I/E) ratio.* The normal starting I/E ratio is 1:2. If the patient has obstructive airway disease (i.e., COPD), then the ratio should be reduced to 1:4 or 1:5 to avoid air trapping.

★ *Flow rate.* The flow rate can be adjusted so that the inspiratory volume can be delivered in time to allow for adequate exhalation. An inspiratory flow rate of 40 to 80 lpm is most commonly used. Patients with normal lungs can be adequately ventilated with low flow rates. Patients with obstructive lung disease often need higher flow rates.

★ *Oxygen concentration (FiO_2).* The oxygen concentration, or FiO_2, can be adjusted as needed for adequate oxygenation. Initially the FiO_2 is set at 1.0 (100%) and titrated downward based on blood gas values. Once a blood gas value is known, it is possible to predict the needed FiO_2 setting with the alveolar gas equation:

$$PaO_2 = FiO_2 \times (P_B - P_{H_2O}) - PaCO_2/R$$

where

FiO_2 = fractional concentration of inspired oxygen (0.21 if room air)

P_B = barometric pressure (approximately 760 mmHg at sea level)

P_{H_2O} = Water vapor pressure (47 mmHg when air is fully saturated at 37° C)

R = respiratory quotient (the ratio of CO_2 production to O_2 consumption, usually assumed to be 0.8)

★ *Sigh.* Sighing is an important physiological function in that it helps to reexpand collapsed alveoli. Ventilators can be set to provide a sigh (usually 1.5 to 2.0 times the normal tidal volume), usually 10 to 15 times an hour.

★ *Humidification.* Ideally, ventilations should be warmed and humidified (usually 37° C and 100% humidified).

VENTILATOR ALARMS

There are several alarms on mechanical ventilators. These include:

★ *High-pressure alarm.* A high-pessure alarm is activated when the pressure exceeds 10 to 20 cm/H_2O over the patient's peak inspiratory pressure. This can result from either increased airway resistance such as increased secretions, kinking of the tubing, movement of the airway, bronchospasm, or the patient coughing during inspiration. The alarm can also be triggered by decreased respiratory system compliance. Causes include pneumothorax, atelectasis, pneumonia, acute pulmonary edema, and ARDS.

★ *Low-exhaled-volume alarm.* The low-exhaled-volume alarm is usually set to activate when the tidal volume falls by 50 to 100 mL of the set tidal volume. This usually indicates a problem in the breathing circuit such as a disconnected segment or an ET tube cuff leak.

★ *Apnea.* The apnea alarm sounds when the patient stops breathing. Causes are usually physiological and include decreased mental status, overmedication, and fatigue.

★ *Low FiO$_2$.* A low FiO_2 reading results when the oxygen source is disconnected or depleted.

Several ventilators are available for use in critical care transport. (See Figures 7-52 ■ through 7-55 ■.) They vary significantly in cost and sophistication. Longer transports and aeromedical transports (even when a pressurized cabin is used) often require more sophisticated ventilators where additional parameters can be manipulated as needed.

Example. You have just performed an RSI on a victim of a motorcycle accident. His Glasgow Coma Score was 6 prior to RSI. You initially paralyzed the patient with succinylcholine following induction with etomidate. About 5 minutes after intubation, the patient began to twitch and you administered pancuronium for continued paralysis. You have a 1.5-hour transport. How would you set up the ventilator for this patient?

1. Set the mode to SIMV. You do not anticipate the patient initiating breaths.
2. Set the FiO_2 to 1.0. Hypoxemia worsens head injuries so start with 100% oxygen. This can be titrated later.
3. Set the tidal volume. The patient weighs 200 pounds.

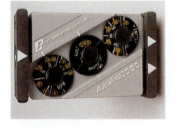

■ **Figure 7-52** Portable mechanical ventilator.

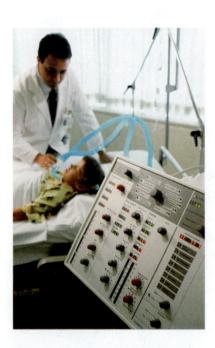

■ **Figure 7-53** Typical multi-function hospital ventilator. *(Allan H. Shoemaker/Getty Images, Inc.-Taxi)*

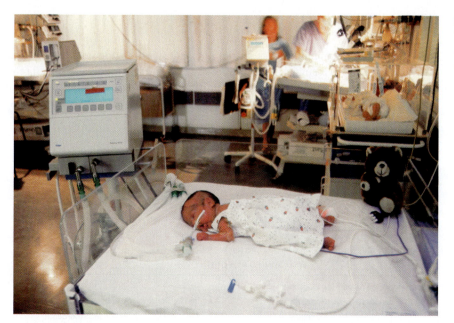

■ **Figure 7-54** Premature baby on a ventilator in an intensive care unit. *(Garry Watson/Photo Researchers, Inc.)*

200 pounds divided by 2.2 pounds/kilogram = 91 kg

91 kg × 10 mL/kg = 910 mL, so set the tidal volume at 900 mL

4. Set the rate. With head injury it is important to avoid hyperventilation. Set the respiratory rate at 12. This will give you a minute volume of 900 mL and a minute volume of 10,800 mL/minute or 10.8 lpm.
5. Set the I:E ratio at 1:2.
6. Set the sigh rate at 10 per hour.
7. If necessary, set the flow rate at 60 lpm.

Monitor the patient with oximetry and capnography and periodically adjust ventilations to keep these parameters within selected tolerances.

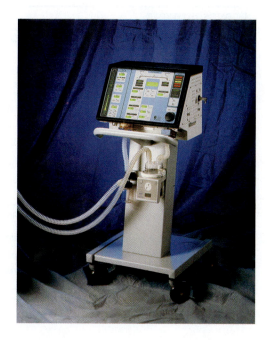

■ **Figure 7-55** Bennett ventilator. *(Mallinckrodt, Inc.)*

DOCUMENTATION

No other part of documentation is more important than the documentation of airway management. A significant percentage of the claims and lawsuits that are filed against prehospital and in-hospital providers involve inadequate patient ventilation. Therefore, it is crucial that the provider learn to document in medically correct and legally sufficient terms exactly what was done in man-

■ **Figure 7-56A** Airway reporting form. *(American Medical Response of El Paso County)*

AMERICAN MEDICAL RESPONSE OF EL PASO COUNTY
AIRWAY REPORTING FORM

Turn in this form attached to a copy of your PCR to CES mailbox immediately

DEMOGRAPHICS

PCR #:_____ Date:_____ Time called:_____ Time arrived:_____

Pt. Age:_____ Gender:_____ Patient Initials:_____ Pt. Weight:_____ Kg

Attending Emp ID#_____ Attending Emp Name:_____

Hosp MR #:_____ Receiving ED Physician:_____

INDICATIONS FOR AIRWAY MANAGEMENT

☐ Apnea or agonal respiration   ☐ Injury or illness involving airway

☐ Airway reflexes compromised   ☐ Anticipated compromise or decompensation

☐ Ventilation Compromised   ☐ Other: (describe)_____

ALL PROCEDURES PERFORMED (select all performed)

☐ BVM   ☐ OETT (no medications)   ☐ NETT   ☐ LMA

☐ OPA   ☐ OETT (awake)   ☐ Digital Intubation   ☐ Cricothyrotomy (surgical)

☐ NPA   ☐ OETT (RSI)   ☐ Combitube   ☐ Cricothyrotomy (needle)

STATE OF AIRWAY PRIOR TO INTERVENTION

☐ Clear   ☐ Blood   ☐ Gag Reflex: ABSENT   ☐ Combative/ Resistive

☐ Emesis   ☐ Teeth/ Foreign objects   ☐ Gag Reflex: PARTIAL   ☐ Burns

☐ Sputum/ Secretions   ☐ Trismus -OR- Biting   ☐ Gag Reflex: PRESENT   ☐ Other:_____

BASIC INTERVENTIONS

Procedure	Size:	Done By:(emp # or agency)	Time
☐ NPA			
☐ OPA			
☐ BVM Vent	--- N/A ---		

INTUBATION INTERVENTIONS

AN ETI ATTEMPT IS DEFINED AS INSERTING THE TUBE INTO THE NOSTRIL OR INSERTING THE BLADE PAST THE TEETH/GUMS AMR PROTOCOL IS A MAXIMUM TOTAL OF THREE ATTEMPTS.

Pulsox pre-attempt: [_____]   Pulsox drop < 90 during attempt? ☐ Yes ☐ No ☐ N/A (unable to get pulsox > 90 pre-attempt)

Cricoid pressure used: ☐ Yes ☐ No   Was Surevent used: ☐ Yes ☐ No

Attempt	Intubation Method: nett, oett,digital,RSI, etc.	Performed By (emp#)	Successful: (yes/no)	Time Performed:
# 1				
# 2				
# 3				
# 4				

PLACEMENT CONFIRMATION STEPS PERFORMED (Check only those actually performed)

YES/NO   YES/NO   YES/NO

☐ ☐ Visualized Through Cords   ☐ ☐ ETCO2 Colormetric Used (color):_____   ☐ ☐ Lung Sounds PRESENT

☐ ☐ Negative EDD (In Trachea)   ☐ ☐ ETCO2 Capnography Used (peak #)_____   ☐ ☐ Gastric Sounds ABSENT

☐ ☐ Positive EDD (In Esophagus)   ☐ Capnography Waveform Present   ☐ ☐ Chest Rise/ Fall

☐ -- Equivocal EDD (unsure placement)

Tube Size: [_____]   Tube Depth: [_____]   How Secured: [_____]

aging the airway. Such documentation can save you from a claim or lawsuit being filed or, in the unfortunate event that one is filed, can help you to win. In this case, proper documentation was crucial, given the massive trauma to the patient's airway prior to intubation attempts. These practitioners may well have seen a claim filed if the patient suffered a disabling injury. The detailed documentation shown could go a long way toward warding off such a claim and demonstrating that correct standard of care was in fact delivered. (See Figure 7-56 ■.)

When possible, use a special airway documentation form (see Figure 7-56).

■ **Figure 7-56B** *continued.*

MEDICATIONS USED: (check mark all meds used)

Medication	Dosage	Given By	Time Given	Medication	Dosage	Given By	Time Given
☐ Etomidate				☐ Fentanyl			
☐ Succinylcholine				☐ Morphine			
☐ Vecuronium				☐ Valium			
☐ Atropine				☐ Neosyn.			
☐ Lidocaine				☐ Viscous			
☐ Topical Spray				☐ Other			

IF FAILED INTUBATION, INDICATE SECONDARY (RESCUE) AIRWAY / VENTILATION TECHNIQUE USED (check all that apply)

Procedure	Done By:	Ventilation Yes/ No	Time	Procedure	Done By:	Ventilation Yes/ No	Time
☐ BVM (rescue)				☐ Cric (surgical)			
☐ Combitube				☐ Cric (needle)			
☐ LMA				☐ Other			

IF COMBITUBE WAS USED:

☐ Ventilation successful with # 1 blue tube (esophageal placement) **Peak ETCO2:** _____ (from the tube used)

☐ Ventilation successful with #2 white tube (tracheal placement)

IF ALL ATTEMPTS AT INTUBATION **FAILED,** INDICATE SUSPECTED REASONS FOR FAILURE (check all that apply)

☐ Unable to visualize glottic opening   ☐ Difficult anatomy: (anterior, overbite, obesity, edema, tumor, etc.)

☐ Unable to pass vocal cords   ☐ Secretions / Blood / Vomit

☐ Complete obstruction; unable to clear   ☐ Unable to locate anatomical landmarks

☐ Inadequate patient or muscular relaxation   ☐ Poor patient access: (extrication, spinal immob., confined space, etc.)

☐ Poor jaw/ neck mobility   ☐ Arrival at hospital prior to completion of procedure

☐ Severe trauma   ☐ Other: _____

ED PHYSICIAN CONFIRMATION OF PROPER ETT / CRICOTHYRIODOTOMY PLACEMENT:

☐ Correct Placement   ☐ Incorrect Placement

Comments:_____

_____

PHYSICIAN SIGNATURE:

MEDICAL DIRECTOR EVALUATION:

☐ Appropriate Intervention   ☐ Confirmation criteria MET

☐ Inappropriate Intervention   ☐ Confirmation criteria NOT met

MEDICAL DIRECTOR COMMENTS:

_____

_____

MEDICAL DIRECTOR SIGNATURE: _____ DATE REVIEWED: _____

TURN IN THIS FORM ATTACHED TO A COPY OF YOUR PCR TO CES MAILBOX IMMEDIATELY

Summary

Airway assessment and maintenance are the most critical steps in managing any patient. If you do not promptly establish a definitive airway and provide proper ventilation, the patient's outcome will be poor. Frequently reassessing the airway is mandatory to ensure that the patient has not decompensated, requiring additional airway procedures. Successful management of all airways requires the critical care paramedic to follow the proper management sequence. And, the critical care paramedic is expected to provide prolonged airway and ventilator management and must be proficient at these. In adddition, the critical care paramedic must be familiar with current monitors including continuous waveform capnography. Without adequate airway and ventilation, any other intervention will be useless.

Review Questions

1. List alternative airway techniques beyond basic airway maneuvers and endotracheal intubation.
2. Discuss the role of rapid-sequence induction (RSI) in modern critical care transport.
3. List the steps in performing RSI.
4. List ways of ensuring proper airway placement in the critical care setting.
5. Discuss the importance of analgesic and hypnotic therapy in RSI.
6. Discuss the importance of documentation in critical care airway management and ventilation.
7. Discuss the physiologic changes that occur due to mechanical ventilation in the critical care setting.

See Answers to Review Questions at the back of this book.

Further Reading

American Society of Anesthesiologists Task Force on Difficult Airway Management. *Practice Guidelines for Management of the Difficult Airway.* Park Ridge, IL: American Society of Anesthesiologists, 2002.

Bledsoe BE, Clayden D. *Prehospital Emergency Pharmacology,* 6th ed. Upper Saddle River, NJ: Pearson Prentice Hall, 2005.

Bledsoe BE, Porter RS, Cherry RA. *Paramedic Care: Principles & Practice,* 2nd ed. Upper Saddle River, NJ: Pearson Prentice Hall, 2005.

Cormack RS, Lehane J. "Difficult Tracheal Intubation in Obstetrics." *Anaesthesia,* Vol. 39 (1984): 1105.

Dennison RD. *Pass CCRN!* 2nd ed. Saint Louis, MO: Mosby, 2000.

Levitan RM, Everett WW, Ochroch EA. "Limitations of Difficult Airway Prediction of Patients in the Emergency Department." *Annals of Emergency Medicine,* Vol. 44, No. 4 (2004): 307–313.

Mallampati SR. "Clinical Signs to Predict Difficult Tracheal Intubation (Hypothesis)." *Canadian Anaesthesia Society Journal* (1983): 310–316.

Mallampati SR *et al.* "A Clinical Sign to Predict Difficult Tracheal Intubations: A Prospective Study." *Canadian Anaesthesia Society Journal,* Vol. 32 (1985): 429–434.

O'Shea JK, Pinchalk ME, Wang HE. "Reliability of Paramedic Ratings of Laryngoscopic Views during Endotracheal Intubation." *Prehospital Emergency Care,* Vol. 9 (2005): 167–171.

Stewart CE. *Advanced Airway Management.* Upper Saddle River, NJ: Pearson Prentice Hall, 2002.

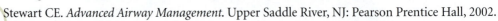

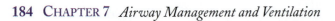

The Shock Patient: Assessment and Management

Lee Richardson, NREMT-P, CCEMT-P, FP-C, and Bryan E. Bledsoe, DO, FACEP

Objectives

Upon completion of this chapter, the student should be able to:

1. Define shock. (p. 188)
2. Describe what happens to the cell during a shock state. (p. 188)
3. Identify vital organs versus nonvital organs. (p. 192)
4. Discuss and describe neurohumoral transmitters involved in shock. (p. 193)
5. Identify the stages of shock. (p. 193)
6. Describe general treatment modalities involved with shock including hemodynamic monitoring. (p. 197)
7. Discuss the four classifications and subclassifications of shock. (p. 200)

Key Terms

anaphylactic shock, p. 201
cardiogenic shock, p. 202
distributive shock, p. 201
dysoxia, p. 189
hypoperfusion, p. 188
hypovolemic shock, p. 201
lactic acid, p. 189

metabolic requirement for oxygen (MRO_2), p. 188
MODS (multiple organ dysfunction syndrome), p. 194
neurogenic shock, p. 202
neurohumoral response, p. 193

obstructive shock, p. 201
oxygen delivery (DO_2), p. 188
oxygen uptake (VO_2), p. 188
septic shock, p. 201
shock, p. 187
sodium/potassium pump, p. 191

Case Study

You and your critical care transport unit have been summoned to a small community hospital about 70 miles from your base. The hospital is really nothing more than an outpatient clinic. Upon arrival you are met by a nurse who takes you to the "first aid room." There you find your patient, a 17-year-old girl, who is resting quietly with an IV of 5% dextrose and water running at a TKO rate. The nurse tells you that the community family practitioner has seen the girl and determined that she has "sepsis" from a ruptured appendix.

You begin the patient assessment while your partner ensures that the paperwork is in order. She is a timid, soft-spoken 17-year-old in mild distress. She said that approximately 72 hours ago she developed right lower quadrant pain. She had some vomiting and diarrhea the first 24 hours after onset. The pain has continued to worsen and has started to radiate to her right shoulder forcing her to seek care at the clinic. Her history is unremarkable. She thinks she may have run a fever but was not sure. A quick review of her lab work reveals that her electrolytes, BUN, and creatinine are relatively normal as is her urinalysis. Her complete blood count revealed a WBC of 12.4. Her hemoglobin is 9.6 grams and her hematocrit is 31%. You question the nurse about the anemia and she said Dr. Roja said it was due to iron-deficiency anemia.

You complete a physical exam before transport. Her HEENT exam is unremarkable except for dry mucous membranes. Her neck is supple and there are no meningeal signs. Her heart has a normal rhythm with a rate of 106 at rest. Heart tones are normal and her lungs are clear to auscultation. You ask her to point to where she hurts and she points and makes a circular motion around her right lower quadrant. You first listen to her abdomen and do not hear any bowel sounds. You begin soft palpation of the abdomen in the left upper quadrant. It is soft and relatively nontender until you move to the right lower quadrant where she has moderate tenderness and a hint of rebound. Her extremities are normal and peripheral pulses are equal. A brief neurologic examination is normal. Her blood pressure is 98/60 mmHg, pulse 110, and respirations 24. Her ECG reveals a sinus tachycardia and her SpO_2 on 2 lpm oxygen via nasal cannula is 100%. She last had 25 milligrams of meperidine and 12.5 milligrams of promethazine about 90 minutes ago IV.

You package her and move her to the vehicle. About 25 minutes into transport she becomes uncomfortable and starts to writhe around on the stretcher. You notice that her heart rate is up to 130. You reassess her vital signs and find her blood pressure to be 88/56, a pulse of 130, and respirations of 30. You decide to try a fluid bolus and remember that D_5W is hanging. You change the D_5W to normal saline and give her a 500-mL fluid bolus. Her heart rate slows to 116 and her blood pressure increases to 90/60. You sit back and think to yourself, "Something is not right here." You repeat your physical exam and find it unchanged. You ask her again to detail her history. She denies chest pain. She says has been able to eat. That rings a bell. Anorexia is a sign of appendicitis and sepsis, not eating. You question her further, "Have you had any injuries in the last week?" She thinks for a minute and says, "No, not that I recall." You ask, "Have you taken any medications—prescription or otherwise—in the last week?" She says, "No." You think and ask about blood in her stool or vomitus and she denies these. You then ask, "When was your last menstrual period?" She says, "What?" You say, "You know, your last menses—period." She thinks and says, "About 2 months ago." You ask about the regularity of her periods. They are usually normal, occurring about the same time each month, and last 2 to 3 days. You ask her, "Is there a chance you could be pregnant?" She says, "I don't think so." You quickly review the chart and do not see a pregnancy test. You go back to the patient and say, "I know this is a hard question—but very important. Please tell me if there is a chance you might be pregnant—have you had sex in the last 2 months." She stares at you for what seems like an eternity and says, "Well, yes—sort of."

Then, the picture becomes clear. This is not a case of "sepsis" from a ruptured appendix—it is a ruptured ectopic pregnancy—the pieces all fit. You give her another fluid bolus to maintain her blood pressure above 90 mmHg and contact the receiving hospital. She arrives in good shape. A stat βHCG is positive. A subsequent ultrasound shows a mass in her right fallopian tube and free blood in the abdomen. She is taken to surgery where a tubal pregnancy is removed via laparoscopy. In the ED her hemoglobin dropped to 7.1 grams and hematocrit was now 19%. Prior to surgery she was typed and crossmatched for a transfusion. Two units of packed red blood cells were administered prior to surgery. She tolerated the surgery well and went home 5 days later.

INTRODUCTION

In 1862, Samuel Gross described shock as a "rude unhinging of the machinery of life," and it was subsequently defined this way for more than 100 years. Today, this description still remains basically unchallenged. Shock states can be some of the most challenging situations the critical care paramedic will face. Shock is often overlooked and unrecognized in the early stages because clinical signs and symptoms are often very subtle and can have many different presentations. Because of this, the critical care paramedic must be very cognizant of trends in the clinical status of the patient.

Shock is never a primary diagnosis but is a physiological adaptation to a potentially life-threatening physical insult. When the body is in **shock** it is attempting to preserve its most vital functions. No matter what the underlying cause of the shock state, the common denominator is the amount of oxygen consumed by the cells. Under normal conditions the body will provide sufficient oxygen to the cells to meet metabolic needs, but when the body is placed under stress it will consume oxygen more rapidly and compensatory mechanisms will initiate to restore oxygen and perfusion to the cells.

Shock can develop from changes in circulating volume, cardiac function, or alterations in peripheral vascular resistance. Shock can cause multiple physiological changes in the cardiovascular, respiratory, nervous, renal, and gastrointestinal systems.

There are various types and categories of shock. However, shock is typically divided into four categories with each category having several causes or subcategories. Shock is further classified into stages: the compensatory stage, the progressive stage, and the irreversible stage. This chapter will provide a brief but thorough review of pathophysiology as it relates to shock states, differentiation of the different categories and stages of shock, and comprehensive management strategies.

shock *a state of inadequate tissue perfusion associated with anaerobic cellular metabolism.*

PREREQUISITES

The objectives for this chapter assume that the student has a thorough knowledge of the following topics and information prior to beginning this chapter:

★ Anatomy and physiology

★ Assessment and management of the different types of shock

★ Basic pharmacological agents used in treating patients in shock states

DEFINING SHOCK

hypoperfusion *lack of adequately oxygenated blood to effectively sustain tissue at the cellular, organ, or system level.*

To maintain homeostasis (the state of normal balance) of the body, you must have adequate perfusion to all organs and organ systems. Shock is often referred to as **hypoperfusion.** Hypoperfusion can be isolated to a particular organ or tissue or it can be systemic. Shock is considered a state in which perfusion is inadequate to meet the demands of the cellular activity. It can have a variety of causes and may result from problems involving the heart, lungs, vessels, blood, nervous system, or a combination of these. When the body is in a state of shock (hypoperfusion) its compensatory mechanisms are activated to compensate and counter its effects. If hypoperfusion is not corrected, it will ultimately lead to death. This is why it is essential that the critical care paramedic be able to recognize the clinical presentation of the different shock states; understand its various etiologies, types, and classifications; and be able to provide appropriate resuscitative management both generalized and cause specific.

PATHOPHYSIOLOGY

Although the pathophysiology of shock is presented in EMT and paramedic education, we will highlight important features of the pathophysiology of shock as they pertain to the critical care paramedic.

THE CELL IN SHOCK

oxygen delivery (DO_2) *the amount of measurable oxygen delivered to the tissues.*

metabolic requirement for oxygen (MRO_2) *the rate at which oxygen is utilized in the conversion of glucose to energy and water, via the glycolysis/tricarboxylic acid (TCA) cycle.*

oxygen uptake (VO_2) *the actual amount of oxygen withdrawn from the circulation at the capillary level.*

Oxygen cannot be stored in the peripheral tissues. Thus, the amount of oxygen delivered to the tissues must meet the oxygen requirements of the tissues. (See Figure 8-1 ■.) The oxygen delivered to the tissues is commonly referred to as the rate of **oxygen delivery (DO_2).** The **metabolic requirement for oxygen (MRO_2)** at the tissue level is the rate at which oxygen is utilized in the conversion of glucose to energy and water through glycolysis and the tricarboxylic acid (TCA) cycle. (See Figures 8-2 ■ and 8-3 ■.) The **oxygen uptake (VO_2)** is the actual amount of oxygen withdrawn from the circulation at the capillary level. Thus:

$$VO_2 \geq MRO_2 = \text{Normal metabolism}$$

When the rate of oxygen uptake fails to meet the metabolic demand for oxygen, shock occurs:

$$VO_2 < MRO_2 = \text{Shock}$$

Normally, 1 molecule of glucose will yield 36 molecules of energy in the form of adenosine triphosphate (ATP) and water as an end product. If oxygen is not present, the glucose will be metabolized

■ **Figure 8-1** Peripheral oxygen demand.

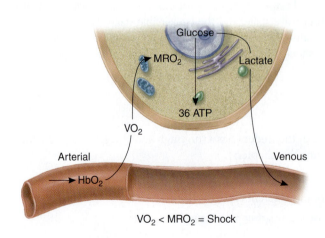

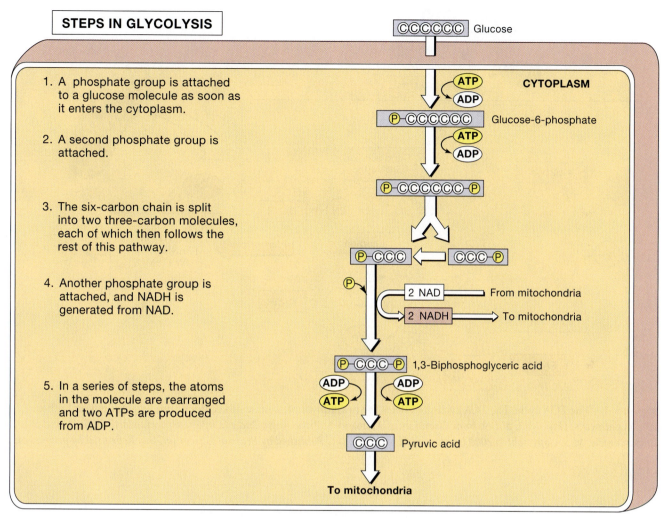

STEPS IN GLYCOLYSIS

1. A phosphate group is attached to a glucose molecule as soon as it enters the cytoplasm.

2. A second phosphate group is attached.

3. The six-carbon chain is split into two three-carbon molecules, each of which then follows the rest of this pathway.

4. Another phosphate group is attached, and NADH is generated from NAD.

5. In a series of steps, the atoms in the molecule are rearranged and two ATPs are produced from ADP.

Glucose

CYTOPLASM

Glucose-6-phosphate

2 NAD — From mitochondria
2 NADH → To mitochondria

1,3-Biphosphoglyceric acid

Pyruvic acid

To mitochondria

■ **Figure 8-2** Glycolysis. Glycolysis breaks down a six-carbon glucose molecule into two three-carbon molecules of pyruvic acid. This process involves a series of enzymatic steps. There is a net gain of two ATPs for each glucose molecule converted to pyruvic acid. *(Fig. 18-2, p. 498 from* Essentials of Anatomy & Physiology, *2nd ed., by Frederic H. Martini, Ph.D. and Edwin F. Bartholomew, M.S. Copyright © 2000 by Frederic H. Martini, Inc. Published by Pearson Education, Inc. Reprinted by permission.)*

through glycolysis only. In this case, 1 molecule of glucose will result in only 2 molecules of ATP and the production of pyruvic acid as an end product. Pyruvic acid is converted to **lactic acid** (a toxic metabolic acid) (See Figure 8-4 ■.) In summary, when the oxygen supply to the tissues falls, the energy yield from glucose then drops dramatically, resulting in a phenomenon known as **dysoxia.** When cellular dysoxia causes a change in organ function, the condition is referred to as shock.

The common denominator of shock is the amount of oxygen consumed by the cells. When the body is under normal conditions, the oxygen uptake (VO_2) is independent of oxygen delivery (DO_2), which means that if the cells need to consume additional oxygen to produce energy, they can extract the necessary amount of oxygen required to produce energy in the form of ATP. Thus, in a normal physiologic state:

$$VO_2 = CO \times 13.4 \times Hb \times (SaO_2 - SvO_2)$$

That is, VO_2 is a function of cardiac output (CO), available hemoglobin (Hb), and the difference in oxygen saturation between arterial (SaO_2), and venous blood (SvO_2). The 1.34 term represents the amount of oxygen transported per gram of hemoglobin (and is multiplied by 10 to preserve units). "Hb" means grams of hemoglobin per 100 mL blood. Normal VO_2 is 100 to 160 mL/minute/m^2.

lactic acid *toxic metabolic by-product of pyruvic acid, as a result of anaerobic metabolism.*

dysoxia *falling energy yield from glucose when oxygen supply to tissue fails or is reduced dramatically.*

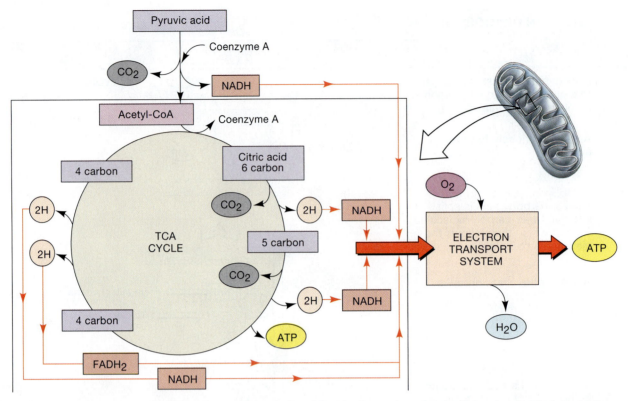

■ **Figure 8-3** The TCA cycle. The TCA cycle completes the breakdown of organic molecules begun by glycolysis and other catabolic pathways. *(Fig. 18-3, p. 499, from* Essentials of Anatomy & Physiology, *2nd ed., by Frederic H. Martini, Ph.D. and Edwin F. Bartholomew, M.S. Copyright © 2000 by Frederic H. Martini, Inc. Published by Pearson Education, Inc. Reprinted by permission.)*

■ **Figure 8-4** Pyruvate degradation.

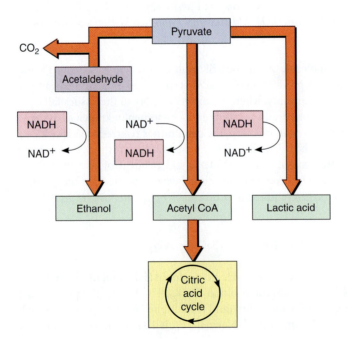

From this equation it is apparent that a problem with cardiac output, available hemoglobin, the ability of the hemoglobin to carry oxygen, or arterial oxygen saturation can result in shock.

Most of the energy produced by the cell drives the **sodium/potassium pump,** which maintains an ionic gradient across the cell wall. Intracellular sodium levels are approximately 10 mEq/L and intracellular potassium levels are 140 mEq/L. Both of these levels are kept at a constant. Extracellular sodium levels are 140 mEq/L and extracellular potassium levels are 4 mEq/L; both of these levels are also kept at a constant. The maintenance of the levels is crucial in maintaining cell size, shape, and function. With anaerobic metabolism the cell is in an energy crisis, causing the sodium/potassium pump to fail and various cells to start to lose their specialized function. With failure of the sodium/potassium pump, extracellular sodium moves into the intracellular space. Sodium is followed by water entering the cells. All of this fluid that enters the cell will cause it to swell and become an irregular shape. (See Figure 8-5 ■.)

A point of no return is reached when the cell lyses. (See Figure 8-6 ■.) Depending on the number of cells involved and the distribution of cells lost, clinically significant organ damage may follow. In early shock this presents as subtle signs and symptoms of organ dysfunction and may be overlooked.

sodium/potassium pump
maintains the ionic gradient across cell walls; driven by energy produced in the cells.

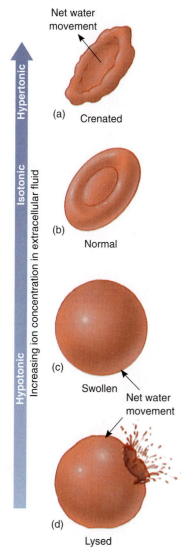

■ **Figure 8-5** The effects of hypertonic, isotonic, and hypotonic solutions on red blood cells.

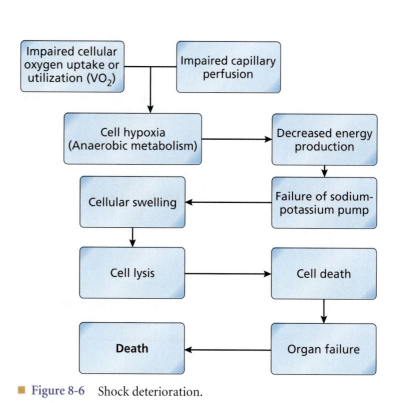

■ **Figure 8-6** Shock deterioration.

Table 8–1 | Consequences of Shock on Organ Systems

Nonvital Organs

Gastrointestinal Tract
- Decreased motility leading to an intestinal obstruction
- Impaired absorption of nutrients
- Inflammation of intestinal and gastric lining

Skeletal Muscle
- Production of lactic acid leading to metabolic acidosis
- Respiratory muscle fatigue leading to failure
- Destruction of muscle to be used as source of energy

Immune System
- Increased risk of infections

Skin
- Ulcer formation
- Prolonged wound healing

Liver
- Gluconeogenesis is eventually impaired so hypoglycemia will follow
- Protein and fat metabolism is altered

Kidneys
- Alters the production of urine
- With prolonged decreased blood flow it can lead to permanent renal damage or failure

Lung
- Carbon dioxide retention
- Atelectasis
- Poor ventilation
- Prolonged shock can lead to development of ARDS

Vital Organs

Heart
- Increase in rate and force
- Possible dysrhythmias
- Risk of infarction

Brain
- Decrease in cerebral function secondary to decreased cerebral perfusion
- Cerebral edema
- Neurotransmitter failure
- Irreversible brain damage

Table 8-2	Effects of Neurohumoral Agents on Shock
Neurotransmitter	**Actions**
Norepinephrine	– Vasoconstriction – Increases cardiac contraction
Epinephrine	– Increases skeletal muscle control – Increases myocardial contraction and heart rate
Angiotensin II	– Vasoconstriction – Promotes ADH secretion
Antidiuretic hormone	– Promotes water reabsorption by the kidneys
Aldosterone	– Promotes sodium and water retention by the kidneys
Cortisol	– Suppresses immune and inflammatory response – Promotes protein catabolism – Increases blood sugar

ORGAN SYSTEMS IN SHOCK

Body organs are composed of billions of specialized cells. The organ dysfunction that is clinically significant in patients in shock represents the impaired function of billions of individual cells. The consequences of shock on organ systems are described in Table 8–1.

NEUROHUMORAL RESPONSES IN SHOCK STATES

Numerous neurohumoral agents work together to produce a stress response while the body is in a shock state. The overall effects of the **neurohumoral response** are to support cardiac output by increasing heart rate and contractility, produce vasoconstriction to distribute the cardiac output to vital organs, retain salt and water to maintain circulating plasma, and assemble metabolic fuels for use. Activation of these responses can only be tolerated for a short period of time (compensation). For example, vasoconstriction will maintain blood flow to the vital organs but it will cause decreased circulation to nonvital organs, which leads to ischemia and the accumulation of lactic acid. If the activation is sustained for long periods, the organ and the organ systems will ultimately be destroyed. Long-term activation (days to weeks) is incompatible with survival.

Neurohumoral agents that are released in shock are listed and described in Table 8–2.

The overall effects of the various neurotransmitters are to support the cardiac output, vasoconstrict to deliver the cardiac output to the vital organs, retain salt and water to maintain plasma volume, and use fuels such as glucose and lipids for the production of ATP. Activation of these neurotransmitters is not without problems. Widespread vasoconstriction will result in tissue ischemia in the underperfused tissues. When hemodynamics and metabolism are altered to support the shock patient, the patient cannot tolerate these compensatory mechanisms for long.

neurohumoral response
stress mechanism that increases cardiac output through increased heart rate contractility, vasoconstriction, fluid retention, and supports other metabolic functions in response to shock states.

STAGES OF SHOCK

Shock is ultimately an event that takes place at the cellular level and progresses in stages ranging from mild to lethal—from compensated, to decompensated, to irreversible. In compensated shock the body is able to compensate for the fall in cardiac output (decreased cardiac output is present in all types and stages of shock). When baroreceptors in the body (i.e., in the aortic arch and carotid arteries) detect a fall in cardiac output, they immediately begin to compensate for the decrease. In this stage the body's compensatory mechanisms are strong enough to overcome the decrease in cardiac output (compensation). The neurotransmitters described earlier are then secreted into the systemic circulation where they precede to their target organs, initiate the desired effects, and cause the appropriate compensatory action to take place. Vasoconstriction will occur in the nonvital organs first (skin, GI tract). Vasoconstriction causes an increase in peripheral vascular resistance, which increases preload, stroke volume, and ultimately cardiac output. Vasoconstriction also causes several clinical signs the critical care paramedic should be familiar with such as pallor, which is most noticeable around skin under the eyes, around the mouth and nose, and in the extremities (especially in the distal region). In critical situations, the critical care paramedic can get a rough indicator of cardiac output by evaluating clinical signs/symptoms such as level of consciousness (cerebral perfusion) and vital sign trends (systemic perfusion). Typically, if the body is in a compensatory state, the blood pressure will remain in normal range, the heart and respiratory rates will increase, and the level of consciousness will be maintained at the patient's normal level. At this stage, with appropriate assessment and treatments, shock can be reversed. If the cause of the shock is not found and treated, the compensatory mechanism will eventually collapse leading to the next stage, which is called the progressive or uncompensated stage of shock.

When shock moves into the uncompensated (progressive) stage, further compensatory mechanisms are engaged. During this stage the effects of anaerobic metabolism and tissue hypoxia are seen. Additional neurotransmitters are secreted into the circulation, which promotes even more vasoconstriction and reabsorption of sodium which acts to conserve water. With further vasoconstriction blood becomes trapped in the capillary beds, which causes a mottled appearance in the skin. Pallor will deteriorate to cyanosis because of the worsening hypoxemia and tissue hypoxia. Additional effects on the cardiovascular system will include a decreased preload and an increase in contractility and heart rate; in the latter stages of progressive shock myocardial contractions will decrease. During the progressive stage of shock, the patient will exhibit decreasing levels of consciousness such as mental status changes, cool/cold or clammy pale skin, diaphoresis, tachycardia, tachypnea, delayed capillary refill, and decreased urine output, and the blood pressure will start a downward trend.

If shock continues uninterrupted, cellular damage will occur. The cell membrane lyses, releasing highly acidic substances from within the cell. At this stage patients typically present unresponsive with decreasing pulse rates, dysrhythmias develop, and the blood pressure is typically not detectable. Respirations are agonal and diaphoresis will cease. With prolonged hypoperfusion, adult respiratory distress syndrome (ARDS) is commonly seen. Decompensation may occur suddenly or it may be delayed from 1 to 3 days. If hypoperfusion persists, the patient may develop **multiple organ dysfunction syndrome (MODS)**. MODS is a progressive impairment of two or more organ systems. It usually results from an uncontrolled inflammatory response after a severe illness or injury. In clinical practice, both sepsis and septic shock are the most common causes of MODS, with MODS being the end stage. The progression from infection to sepsis to septic shock to MODS is known as systemic inflammatory response syndrome (SIRS). Failure of the gut is a major factor in the development of MODS and allows direct invasion of the body by bacteria leading to infection and sepsis. Even if the patient is successfully resuscitated at this phase, his prognosis is quite poor. The mortality from MODS is high (30–80%) and MODS is responsible for 50–80% of ICU deaths. The treatment for MODS remains primarily supportive.

MODS multiple organ dysfunction syndrome *a sequential or concomitant occurrence of a significant derangement of function in two or more organ systems of the body, against a background of a critical illness.*

GENERAL MANAGEMENT

The overall management for a patient in any shock state is to correct the underlying problem. It cannot be emphasized enough that the critical care paramedic must have good assessment skills as well as a comprehensive understanding of pathophysiology related to shock states in order to rapidly identify the specific cause, halt its progression, and begin aggressive treatment. The general management of all shock states is to provide generalized supportive care while trying to identify the cause. Generalized shock management includes ensuring the patient has a patent airway, adequate oxygenation, ventilation, perfusion, and body temperature while identifying and correcting the underlying cause(s). Typically, generalized shock management will include resuscitation based on the patient's hemodynamic status. This could include everything from volume resuscitation (to include blood administration) to administering vasoactive drips (such as dopamine, norepinephrine, and epinephrine) or a combination of these. Also, identifying and correcting any acid-base abnormalities and maintaining a normal body temperature should be addressed.

INITIAL ASSESSMENT AND MANAGEMENT

The initial assessment of the shock patient is no different than with any other critically ill or injured patient. Once you have determined that the scene is safe for you to enter, you should follow a systematic approach, giving particular attention to life-threatening and potentially life-threatening conditions first. A systematic assessment approach, such as the following, will ensure the patient is appropriately evaluated and trusted:

★ Determination of mental status

★ Airway maintenance with cervical spine protection if needed

★ Breathing and ventilation

★ Circulation with bleeding control

Assess Mental Status

Typically, most shock patients initially present awake, alert, and oriented. If this is not the case, the critical care paramedic should consider associated injuries/illnesses that could be causing the altered state of consciousness such as trauma (i.e., head injuries), substance abuse (i.e., ETOH), hypoxia, or pre-existing medical conditions (i.e., diabetes, seizures). Use the AVPU method to assess the patient's LOC:

★ A—**Alert**

★ V—Responds to **V**erbal stimuli

★ P—Responds to **P**ainful stimuli

★ U—**U**nresponsive

While the AVPU system is often used, the Glasgow Coma Scale (GCS) can also be used and is more accurate. Also, always evaluate motor and sensory function.

Airway

The airway should be your first priority and assessed immediately. A compromised airway may be controlled by:

★ Chin lift

★ Jaw thrust

★ Insertion of an oropharyngeal airway (OPA) or nasopharyngeal airway (NPA) in patients with a decreased level of consciousness (LOC)

★ Assessment of the need for endotracheal intubation

If there is a potential cervical spine injury, it is important to protect the integrity of the cervical spine before doing anything that will cause flexion or extension of the neck. In-line manual cervical immobilization is performed during the initial assessment, in general, and during endotracheal intubation, in particular, for those patients in whom cervical spine injury is suspected because of the mechanism of injury or for those with altered mental states from unknown etiology.

Breathing and Ventilation

Adequate ventilation requires adequate functioning of the lungs, chest wall muscles, and diaphragm. Each of these must be evaluated as part of the initial assessment:

★ Verify breath sounds (bilaterally) by auscultation of the chest.

★ Assess adequacy (rate and depth) of respirations.

★ Administer high concentrations (100%) of oxygen via appropriate device (this not only treats hypoxia but helps to wash out CO_2).

★ Assess ventilatory status with capnography.

★ Expose the chest.

★ Inspect the anterior, lateral, and posterior chest for trauma.

Circulation

Assessment of the adequacy of circulation includes evaluation of blood pressure, pulse rate and quality, and skin color/condition/temperature. Intravenous cannulation is performed by inserting two large-bore catheters to begin fluid administration. Additional indicators of decreased circulation include decreased sensation, diminished distal pulses, and decreased capillary refill time.

DETAILED EXAM/HISTORY

As with any critically ill or injured patient, addressing the ABCDEs and managing any life threats found should be the first priority in the care of the shock patient. Once this is complete and proper resuscitative efforts are well established, more detailed exam and patient history can be addressed if time allows. Typically this detailed exam consists of reevaluation of the initial assessment and then a detailed head-to-toe examination of the patient. A complete detailed exam/history is necessary to ensure that all injuries and preexisting diseases are identified and appropriately managed to minimize any potential complications. A detailed examination also provides the critical care paramedic with trends in the patient's condition. A complete neurologic exam should be performed and any diagnostic studies obtained if time allows. (Do not delay treatment or transportation to obtain these.)

PATIENT HISTORY

Every effort should be made to obtain as much information as possible regarding the circumstances surrounding the incident. Initial management as well as definitive care is dictated by things such as preexisting disease processes, mechanism of injury (MOI) in trauma patients, and the duration and severity of the injury. The following information must be obtained:

1. **Mechanism of injury (MOI):**
   —How did the injury occur?
   —What was the patient doing at the time of the injury?
   —Was the patient ejected from the vehicle?
   —How did the patient escape (extrication, self-extrication, or extricated by bystanders)?
   —What type of collision (rollover, head-on, frontal) was it?
   —What was the speed of the vehicle (highway vs. residential)?
   —Is the injury caused by blunt trauma or penetrating trauma or possibly a combination?
   —Were others killed at the incident?
   —Was the patient unconscious at the scene?
   —Was there a motor vehicle crash (MVC), motorcycle crash, or was the patient hit by a car?
   —How badly was the patient's vehicle damaged?
   —Was there a vehicle fire?
   —Is there any associated trauma?
   —Are there injuries that can cause the patient to have an altered mental status or to be unconscious?
   —Are there hidden injuries (i.e., injuries caused by seat belts, steering wheels, windshields)?
   —What was the distance the patient fell or how far was the patient ejected?
   —Was a medical condition the cause of the incident or could it be complicating the condition?

2. **Medical history taking (history of present illness):**

a. **Things to consider**

- Are there any preexisting diseases or associated illnesses (e.g., diabetes, hypertension, cardiac or renal disease, seizure disorders)?
- Medications/alcohol/illegal drugs (These may mask signs or symptoms, possibility of ETOH withdrawal.)
- Allergies
- Tetanus immunization history

b. **An easy to remember mnemonic is "Get an SAMPLE history."**

S—Symptoms

A—Allergies

M—Medications

P—Pertinent past history

L—Last oral intake

E—Events/environment related to the injury

PERFORMING THE DETAILED EXAM

The head-to-toe exam includes:

- ★ Head/face (maxillofacial)
- ★ Neck/cervical spine
- ★ Chest
- ★ Abdomen
- ★ Perineum/genitalia
- ★ Back/spine (including the buttocks); this can be done while placing patient on long board or cot
- ★ Extremities (musculoskeletal)
- ★ Vascular
- ★ Neurological

MANAGEMENT AND FURTHER EVALUATION OF THE SHOCK PATIENT

As discussed earlier the management of the shock patient is essentially the same as any other critically ill or injured patient; that is, use the ABCDE method to address any life threats (i.e., other trauma or abnormalities with the ABCs) first. Once life-threatening and potentially life-threatening injuries have been addressed, specific treatments can be started based on the patient's needs and the etiology of the shock state.

GENERAL TREATMENT CONSIDERATIONS

As with any critically ill or injured patient, airway management and ventilation are the priority. Assessing the airway of a shock patient is of particular concern, and management decisions may prove difficult for the critical care paramedic. A high index of suspicion should be used with shock patients who are thought to have a compromised airway, and aggressive airway management should be started early so as to avoid the need for more invasive techniques such as a tracheostomy, which leads to a higher mortality/morbidity rate due to the inherent complications associated with such a procedure.

In critical patients the airway should be secured with an appropriately sized endotracheal tube (ETT). This may require the use of pharmacologic agents such as amnestics, sedatives, paralytics, and analgesics (rapid-sequence induction). The critical care paramedic must be thoroughly familiar with each agent's pharmacodynamic properties, particularly with paralytic agents such as succinylcholine, so that the patient is not further compromised by the paramedic's actions: *First, do no harm!*

Once the patient's airway has been secured with an ETT, the tube's placement must be not only confirmed initially but monitored throughout transport to ensure tube vigilance. In addition to the standard methods of confirming tube placement that the critical care paramedic learned during initial training, there are several newer methods to confirm the placement of the ETT such as $ETCO_2$ monitoring (capnography), which is rapidly becoming the "gold standard"; the esophageal detector device (EDD); arterial blood gas analysis; and chest X-ray. Once placement is confirmed continuous monitoring with the use of capnography is the preferred method for avoiding the potentially lethal consequences associated with inadvertent and unrecognized tube displacement.

In addition to ETT placement, the patient must be ventilated at an appropriate rate and administered 100% oxygen. The critical care paramedic must be familiar with making adjustments to airway adjuncts such as PEEP valves, CPAP/BIPAP, and the advanced mechanisms/settings on mechanical ventilators such as peek airway pressures and I:E ratios, rates, and volumes so that patient care can be optimized based on the clinical responses of the patient.

FLUID RESUSCITATION

Proper fluid management is critical to the survival of patients with fluid loss. Aggressive fluid replacement is sometimes needed to maintain homeostasis. The initial step to fluid resuscitation is with two large-bore peripheral IVs. In hypovolemia from trauma it is now common practice to not elevate a patient's blood pressure to more than 75% of the patient's preinjury blood pressure. This is referred to as permissive hypotension. Several of the body's compensatory mechanisms operate best at a systolic blood pressure between 70 and 85 mmHg. Increasing the blood pressure to normal levels in patients where the bleeding has not been controlled (i.e., blunt abdominal trauma) can actually worsen bleeding, resulting in a fall in circulating hemoglobin and coagulation factors. If IV access cannot be obtained, consider the placement of a central line early (or interosseous) if peripheral access is difficult to obtain, or when large volumes of fluid are anticipated (such as a severe burn injury). In these cases these lines can be used to facilitate further hemodynamic monitoring if needed. A fluid bolus can be tried to improve the patient's blood pressure. If no signs of pulmonary edema are present, a bolus of 100–200 mL of a crystalloid solution may be instituted.

HEMOGLOBIN-BASED OXYGEN-CARRYING SOLUTIONS (HBOCs)

Hemoglobin-based oxygen-carrying solutions (HBOCs) represent a major development in the field of emergency and critical care. These products differ from other intravenous fluids in that they have the capability to transport oxygen. HBOCs contain long chains of polymerized hemoglobin. This hemoglobin is obtained from either expired donated human blood or bovine (cow) blood. The hemoglobin is removed from the red blood cells and then repeatedly filtered to remove any infectious substances of antigenic proteins. Finally, the individual hemoglobin molecules are joined in a large chain through a chemical process known as *polymerization*. HBOCs are compatible with all blood types and do not require blood typing, testing, or crossmatching.

★ *PolyHeme* is a HBOCs derived from expired donated human blood. PolyHeme contains 50 grams of hemoglobin per unit, which is the same as human blood. PolyHeme must be refrigerated and the shelf life is 1 year.

★ *Hemopure* is a HBOCs derived from bovine (cow) blood. It has been widely used in South Africa. Hemopure does not require refrigeration and has a shelf life of 3 years.

OTHER FLUIDS

★ *Isotonic crystalloids* are the most commonly used intravenous fluids. These have electrolyte concentrations similar to that of blood. The most common solutions are lactated Ringer's and normal saline.

* *Hypertonic saline.* Hypertonic saline solution (1%–3%) had shown some promise in early animal studies in the treatment of shock. However, more recent studies have shown it to be no more effective than standard isotonic crystalloids. The role of hypertonic saline in head injury remains under investigation.

* *Colloids.* Colloids are more commonly used in prehospital care in the Commonwealth countries (i.e., Australia). They are comparable to isotonic crystalloids but appear to be no more or less effective.

* *Blood and blood products.* If blood is required immediately O-negative can be used until patient's blood type is available. Typed and crossmatched packed red blood cells are preferred.

* *Pharmacologic agents.* For shock that is unresponsive to fluid challenges, the critical care paramedic may also have to start pharmacologic agents, such as catecholamine infusions (i.e., epinephrine) or vasoactive drugs (i.e., dopamine) along with fluid administration. However, in hypovolemic shock the instances when these are required are exceedingly rare.

HEMODYNAMIC MONITORING

The initial way to obtain the hemodynamic status of the shock patient is through noninvasive means such as obtaining the blood pressure, cardiac rate, and rhythm. Urine output is measured through a Foley catheter. Normally blood pressure can be obtained with a cuff and stethoscope. If you are unable to detect a blood pressure, you can try the use of a Doppler or insert an invasive monitoring method such as a central venous catheter to monitor CVP (central venous pressure), or an arterial line to measure the arterial blood pressure. Hemodynamic monitoring is discussed in greater detail in Chapter 9. Some common hemodynamic values and trends typically seen in shock states are listed in Tables 8–3 through 8–5.

Table 8–3	Hemodynamic Findings by Shock Type			
Type	CO	SVR	CVP	PAOP
Hypovolemic	Decreased	Increased	Decreased	Decreased
Cardiogenic	Decreased	Increased	Increased	Increased
Obstructive	Decreased	Increased	Increased	Increased
Distributive	Increased	Decreased	Increased	Increased

Key: CO, cardiac output; SVR, systemic vascular resistance; CVP, central venous pressure; PAOP, pulmonary artery occlusion pressure.

ADDITIONAL MANAGEMENT (DIAGNOSTIC TESTS)

Because shock can cause dysfunction of any organ system, certain diagnostic evaluations should be performed on every patient to aid in resuscitation. Any abnormal values should be treated appropriately if they pose a danger to the patient's condition or mortality/morbidity. The following are the standard initial tests that should be performed:

Table 8–4	Normal Arterial Blood Gas Values
pH: 7.35–7.45	
PaO_2: 80–100 mmHg	
Oxygen saturation: 96–98%	
$PaCO_2$: 35–45 mmHg	
HCO_3^-: 21–28 mEq/L	
Base/excess: ±3 mEq/L	

Table 8–5 | Normal Hemodynamic Measurements

Left ventricular pressures:
  Systolic: 100–130 mmHg
  End diastolic: 4–12 mmHg

Left atrial (pulmonary artery wedge) pressures:
  Mean: 4–12 mmHg
  A wave: 4–15 mmHg
  V wave: 4–15 mmHg

Pulmonary artery pressures:
  Systolic/end diastolic: 15–30 mmHg/6–12 mmHg
  Mean: 9–18 mmHg

Right ventricular pressures:
  Systolic/end diastolic: 25–30 mmHg/0–8 mmHg

Right atrial pressures:
  Mean: 0–8 mmHg
  A wave: 2–10 mmHg
  V wave: 2–10 mmHg

Cardiac Output: 4–8 lpm

Stroke volume: 60–130 mL

Central venous pressure: 8–12 dynes/sec

Systemic vascular resistance (SVR): 800–1200 dynes/sec

Normal urine output: 0.5–1.0 mL/ka/hour

★ Complete blood cell count and differential (CBC with diff, which includes hematocrit and hemoglobin levels)

★ Platelet count

★ Complete serum chemistry profile (includes electrolytes)

★ Prothrombin and activated partial thromboplastin times (PT and PTT); the International Normalized Ratio (INR) is often easier to use

★ Serum lactate

★ Urinalysis

★ Serum amylase

★ Arterial blood gases

★ 12-lead ECG

★ Pregnancy test for all females of childbearing age

★ Blood, sputum, and urine gram stains and cultures, which should be done in cases of possible sepsis

★ If blood loss is observed, suspected or anticipated, the patient should be typed and crossmatched for several units of packed red blood cells or fresh frozen plasma

★ Other possible tests: CT scans, ultrasounds, X-rays, or echocardiograms

★ Drug toxicity screening if indicated

These tests should be done prior to transport if possible, but transport must not be delayed to accomplish them.

CLASSIFICATION OF SHOCK

Shock is classified into four categories: hypovolemic, obstructive, distributive, and cardiogenic. We will now look at each type of shock, its causes, and treatments.

HYPOVOLEMIC SHOCK

Hypovolemic shock results from a reduction in circulating intravascular volume. It is most commonly seen with hemorrhage, third-space fluid shifts, or as a result of large amounts of fluid loss such as that seen with patients who are dehydrated. Hypovolemia is the most common cause of shock the critical care paramedic will encounter and it frequently complicates other types of shock.

Hemorrhage may be caused by open wounds, open fractures, GI bleeding, or intrathoracic bleeding resulting in hemothorax. Third-space fluid shifts can occur with massive swelling, sepsis, peritonitis/intestinal obstruction, ascites, and large burn injuries. Dehydration can occur with excessive use of diuretics, GI losses, high fever, or excessive sweating (heat exhaustion). Common signs and symptoms include altered mental status, diaphoresis, tachycardia, tachypnea, pallor/mottling, thirst, collapsed hand and neck veins, increased skin turgor, concentrated urine, oliguria, and hypotension (late sign). Treatment for hypovolemic shock is fluid resuscitation with either crystalloid solutions or colloid solutions or a combination of these. Pharmacologic agents may be used, if needed, once adequate volume has been introduced.

hypovolemic shock *shock caused by reduced intravascular circulating volume, resulting from hemorrhage, third-space fluid shifts, and/or systemic fluid loss (dehydration).*

OBSTRUCTIVE SHOCK

Obstructive shock is a result of impedance of the circulatory flow. Obstructive shock can result from problems such as cardiac tamponade, tension pneumothorax, pericarditis, compression of great vessels (supine hypotension syndrome typically seen in the late stages of pregnancy), pulmonary embolism, or aortic dissection. Common signs and symptoms are the same as hypovolemic and cardiogenic shock (i.e., low cardiac output and end-organ perfusion), the presence or absence of jugular venous distension (JVD) depending on mechanism, muffled heart tones, and pulsus paradoxus. Treatment of obstructive shock is aimed at treating the underlying cause. Treatment may be as simple as repositioning the patient (i.e., pregnant patients) to relieving a tension pneumothorax with pleural decompression or chest tube placement or relieving a pericardial tamponade by performing a pericardiocentesis.

obstructive shock *shock caused by impedance of the circulatory flow, resulting from blockage, compression, embolic, dissecting, and/or tamponade type insults.*

DISTRIBUTIVE SHOCK

Distributive shock is characterized by a decrease in vascular resistance or increased venous capacity from a vasomotor dysfunction. Distributive shock can further be classified into septic shock, anaphylactic shock, and neurogenic shock.

distributive shock *shock caused by decreased vascular resistance, or increased venous capacity, resulting from vasomotor dysfunction.*

Septic Shock

Septic shock is the result of an overwhelming infection. This type of shock is caused by a wide variety of infectious agents. Factors that can predispose the patient to a systemic infection are decreases in the immune system (i.e., HIV, cancer), primary infections, or hospital-acquired sources (nosocomial). The patient's underlying disease or physical condition is of great importance in determining the outcome. In the initial stage the cardiac output is increased because toxins (endotoxins) in the blood cause vasodilation, thus preventing a higher blood pressure. In the last stage, toxins have built up to the point where they cause an increase in cell permeability and dilation of the vasculature and a precipitous fall in blood pressure is seen. Common signs and symptoms include fever, chills, sweating, petechiae, hypotension, and pulmonary edema. A good patient history is paramount to determining the source of the infection. Treatment is generally supportive until the source is found and specific treatments can be started and includes the use of fluids and pressors.

septic shock *shock caused by toxins in the blood, as a result of disease or infection, that can cause potentially lethal systemic vasodilation.*

Anaphylactic Shock

Anaphylactic shock is the result of an exaggerated response to an allergic reaction. The reaction can occur within seconds or can take up to several hours to manifest. The speed and severity of the reaction depend on the degree of sensitivity the patient has to the allergen. The target organs of anaphylaxis usually include the vascular system, lungs, GI tract, and skin. Causes vary greatly; some common ones are anesthetic or analgesic agents, foods, drugs, blood products, diagnostic agents, and venoms. Common signs and symptoms include dyspnea, wheezing, flushing, itching, whelps,

anaphylactic shock *shock caused by exaggerated systemic response to an allergen.*

swollen tongue or face, voice changes, difficulty swallowing, coughing, and possibly petechiae (small skin hemorrhages). Treatment is aimed at stopping and reversing the reaction. This is usually accomplished with the use of epinephrine and some type of antihistamine.

Neurogenic Shock

neurogenic shock *shock caused by damage to the sympathetic nervous system causing reduction in PVR secondary to widespread vasodilation.*

Neurogenic shock results from damage to the sympathetic nervous system. Neurogenic shock occurs when there is a severe reduction in peripheral vascular resistance due to widespread vasodilation. Normally not all the vessels will dilate at the same time; however, when there is an insult to the body that causes neurogenic shock a large number of—sometimes all—the vessels dilate. The most common causes of neurogenic shock are an injury to the spinal cord. Common signs and symptoms are decreased blood pressure with normal or slow heart rate, warm dry skin below the injury, and sometimes normal or even shortened capillary refill time. Patients with spinal injuries should be frequently reevaluated for possible neurogenic shock. Treatment includes fluid administration and possibly vasoconstrictive medications such as dopamine.

CARDIOGENIC SHOCK

cardiogenic shock *shock caused by failure or inability of the heart to maintain a level of cardiac output sufficient to perfuse tissues with oxygenated blood.*

Cardiogenic shock occurs when the heart is unable to maintain a sufficient cardiac output. Damage to either the right or left ventricle can cause a decrease in the amount of blood pumped to the cells to maintain normal activity. The biggest difference between hemorrhagic shock and cardiogenic shock is the presence of pulmonary edema. Damage to the left ventricle will cause a backup of blood in the pulmonary vein, leading to the formation of pulmonary edema in the lungs. Acute myocardial infarction is the most common cause. Other causes include dysrhythmias such as tachycardias and bradycardias, myocardial contusions or rupture, and valvular insufficiency. Common signs and symptoms include chest pains, dyspnea, dysrhythmias, pulmonary edema, diminished lung sounds, white or pink-tinged sputum, and cyanosis. Patients with cardiogenic shock have very high mortality/morbidity rates. Treatment is aimed at restoring cardiac output. Although most of the treatments used for treating cardiogenic shock are pharmacologic in nature, other treatments may include IABP placement, LVAD placement, pacemaker placement, or surgical interventions such as CABG.

Summary

Critical care paramedics should be very familiar with the various types and stages of shock and the standard treatment modalities for each. Careful and vigilant evaluation of the patient clinical trends will guide continued treatment. They should also be familiar with the resources available in the area in which they work. Critical care paramedics must be proficient with the advanced equipment that may be needed to treat and transport their patients and, if needed, should use the services of specialists, such as perfusionists, when the situation dictates.

Review Questions

1. Discuss the role of oxygen uptake and metabolic oxygen requirement in effusion.
2. Contrast the efficiency of glycolysis alone compared with glycolysis and the TCA cycle.
3. Define shock as it applies to critical care transport.
4. List early indicators of shock that can be noted during the compensated change.
5. Discuss the neurohumoral response to shock.
6. Detail the stages of shock.

7. What are the different types of shock that may be seen by the critical care paramedic?

8. Discuss the role of fluid resusciation in the shock patient.

See Answers to Review Questions at the back of this book.

Further Reading

Bledsoe BE, Porter RS, Cherry RA. *Paramedic Care: Principles & Practice,* 2nd ed. Upper Saddle River, NJ: Pearson Prentice Hall, 2005.

Marino PL. *The ICU Book,* 2nd ed. Philadelphia: Lippincott Williams & Wilkins, 1998.

Martini FH, Bartholomew EF, Bledsoe BE. *Anatomy and Physiology for Emergency Care.* Upper Saddle River, NJ: Pearson Prentice Hall, 2002.

Cardiac and Hemodynamic Monitoring

Bryan E. Bledsoe, DO, FACEP, and
Timothy P. Duncan, RN, CCRN, CEN, CFRN, EMT-P

Objectives

Upon completion of this chapter, the student should be able to:

1. Define hemodynamic monitoring. (p. 206)
2. Define the physiological difference between noninvasive vs. invasive pressure monitoring. (p. 209)
3. Identify common sites for arterial line insertion, central line insertion, and pulmonary artery catheter insertion. (p. 211)
4. List four complications of pulmonary artery catheter insertion. (p. 219)
5. Identify the waveforms of RA, RV, PA, and PAWP. (p. 224)
6. Define normal values of CVP, RV, PAP, PAWP, CO/CI, MAP, SVI, SVRI, and PVRI. (p. 230)
7. Identify the hemodynamic parameter that best reflects the pressure in the left ventricle. (p. 231)
8. Identify the hemodynamic parameter that best reflects right ventricular afterload. (p. 231)
9. Identify from which port of a pulmonary artery catheter a mixed venous blood sample is drawn. (p. 235)
10. Discuss how the PA waveform changes when the pulmonary artery catheter floats from the right ventricle into the pulmonary artery. (p. 238)
11. Describe how an intra-aortic balloon pump (IABP) cannula is inserted. (p. 241)
12. Describe how an IABP operates. (p. 241)
13. Identify complications of IABP devices. (p. 242)
14. Describe the use of a ventricular assist device (VAD). (p. 243)

Key Terms

Case Study

One morning, after completing your equipment check and receiving the daily safety brief by your pilot, your crew is alerted to respond to an outlying facility for the interhospital transport of a 55-year-old male patient. After completing the walk-around of the aircraft to ensure there is no material on the pad, and that all cords and cowlings are properly stowed or secured, you and your crew lift off 4 minutes after alert time. While en route to the sending facility, you receive an update from communications that your patient was being cared for at the original facility for persistent dyspnea when he acutely deteriorated. He was moved from the ED to the CCU where he had been the last 3 days. After being seen by consulting physicians, the decision was made to transfer the patient to your destination facility for ongoing diagnosis and care.

Twenty-one minutes from the alert time, you touch down on the designated landing pad for the hospital, and exit the aircraft. You are met by a security officer who escorts you to the hospital's CCU, where you are given an updated report by the nursing staff. They relay to you that the patient's presenting complaints on admission included fatigue, shortness of breath, and a recent 15-pound weight loss. The patient's past medical history includes hypertension, myocardial infarction 2 years prior, congestive heart failure, and morbid obesity (weight: 145 kg). On day 3 of admission, the patient suffered acute dyspnea with hypoxia, requiring intubation. Vasopressor administration with dopamine for hypotension, along with insertion of a pulmonary artery catheter, was initiated. You and your partner move to the patient's bedside, and while you initiate your physical assessment, your partner begins to review the medical equipment and medications being utilized so that a smooth transition to the portable equipment and cot can be ensured. Following your assessment, you determine the following:

- Heart rate: 106/min, sinus tachycardia
- Pulmonary artery pressure: 42/28 mmHg
- Respiratory rate: 16/min
- Pulmonary artery wedge pressure: 14 mmHg
- Blood pressure: 100/54 mmHg
- Temperature: 37.8° C (100.0° F)
- Right atrial pressure: 18 mmHg
- Pulse oximetry: 97%
- Cardiac output: 3.6 L/min
- Lung sounds: Clear but diminished

— Heart tones:	Slightly rapid, regular, distant
— Jugular vein distention:	None at 30°
— Peripheral edema:	3+ lower extremities
— BSA:	3.2 m²
— Electrocardiogram:	ST with nonspecific ST changes
— Chest radiograph:	Right lower lobe infiltrate
— Continuous IV meds:	Dopamine at 4 mcg/kg/min
	Midazolam at 2 mg/hr
	D₅W in 0.9% NaCl at 50 mL/hr

Since the patient was sedated and intubated for acute respiratory failure, you note the ventilator settings so you can preset these values into your transport ventilator:

— Vent mode:	SIMV
— Demand ventilatory rate:	12/min
— Tidal volume:	800 mL
— Flow rate:	45 L/min
— FiO₂	0.4
— PEEP	5 cm/H₂O
— Inspiratory waveform	Sine

You and your partner start the process of moving the patient's medication infusions to your syringe pumps, while asking additional questions about how well the patient has been tolerating the ventilator. After completing the preparation of the equipment, the patient is moved to your cot, and the medical records and appropriate transfer documents obtained. Since the family has already left the hospital and is driving to the second destination, you start to transfer the patient to the helicopter. Your partner notifies your pilot that you are en route back to the aircraft so that he can start up the engines and prepare for return to the tertiary care facility.

INTRODUCTION

It is important to monitor the electrocardiogram and the hemodynamic status of the critical care patient. Subtle changes in a hemodynamic parameter may be the earliest indicator of deterioration in the patient's condition. Critical care paramedics frequently transport and care for patients with various hemodynamic monitors in place. Because of this, it is important to understand the common monitoring devices used in modern critical care. It is also important to interpret what changes in the patient's various physiological parameters may indicate. Commonly monitored **hemodynamic parameters** include, but are not limited to, the following:

hemodynamic parameters *may include ECG, ABP, CVP, CO, PCWP, SV, and DO₂ saturation. These (and others) can assist the practitioner in trending and diagnosis.*

★ Electrocardiogram (ECG)
★ Arterial blood pressure (ABP)
★ Central venous pressure (CVP)
★ Cardiac output (CO or Q)
★ Pulmonary capillary wedge pressure (PCWP)
★ Stroke volume (SV)
★ Oxygen delivery (DO₂)

Close attention to the hemodynamic parameters listed above will help with diagnosis and treatment. Continued monitoring of these parameters will aid in determining patient trends. In other words, is the patient getting better or is he getting worse? They will also aid in determining the effectiveness of administered medications and treatments.

ELECTROCARDIOGRAPHIC MONITORING

Technology has evolved to a point where portable 12-lead ECG monitoring is readily available. Many manufacturers now make high-quality 12-lead machines for the prehospital and critical care transport environments. Most machines have sophisticated electronics, many with ECG diagnostic packages. Some now have a defibrillator/pacer unit. The principles of 12-lead monitoring are similar to those for routine ECG monitoring.

The classic 12-lead ECG is designed to detect the most common types of cardiac problems—usually those involving the left side of the heart and the left anterior descending coronary artery. However, problems that arise in the right ventricle and the posterior wall of the left ventricle may not be readily visible on the standard 12-leads ECGs. Because of this, some clinicians recommend the use of a 15-lead or 18-lead ECG to increase the sensitivity of the test. These supplemental leads specifically look at the right ventricle and the posterior wall of the left ventricle.

To the standard 12 leads (I, II, III, aVR, aVL, aVF, and V1 through V6), the 18-lead ECG adds three right-sided chest leads (V4R, V5R, and V6R) and three posterior leads (V7, V8, and V9). (See Figure 9-1 ■.) The 15-lead ECG is a subset of the 18-lead ECG, using V4R, V8, and V9 as additional leads to the standard 12-lead ECG. Placement of the right chest electrodes mirrors left chest placement. The V4R electrode is placed in the fifth intercostal space at the right midclavicular line. V5R is placed level with V4R at the right anterior axillary line. V6R is placed level with V5R at the right midaxillary line. The V7 to V9 electrodes extend in a horizontal line from V6. V7 is placed lateral to V6 at the posterior axillary line. V8 is placed at the level of V7 at the midscapular line. V9 is placed at the level of V8 at the paravertebral line.

> Always consider the possibility of a right ventricular infarction and be prepared to obtain a 15-lead or right-sided ECG.

12-LEAD ECG MONITORING IN CRITICAL CARE

The following skill sequence details 12-lead ECG monitoring:

1. Explain what you are going to do to the patient. Reassure him that the machine will not shock him.

2. Prepare all of the equipment and ensure the cable is in good repair. Check to make sure there are adequate leads and materials for prepping the skin.

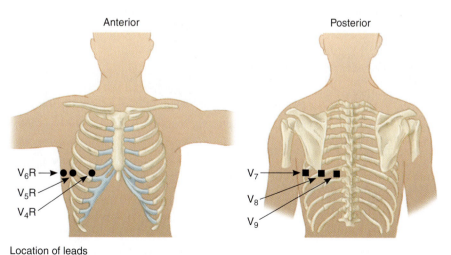

Anterior   Posterior

V₆R
V₅R
V₄R

V₇
V₈
V₉

Location of leads

■ **Figure 9-1** Supplemental lead placements for an 18-lead ECG.

3. Prep the skin. Dirt, oil, sweat, and other materials on the skin can interfere with obtaining a quality tracing. The skin should be cleansed with an appropriate substance. If the patient is diaphoretic, dry the skin with a towel. On very hot days or in situations where the patient is very diaphoretic, tincture of Benzoin can be applied to the skin before attaching the electrode. Occasionally, it may be necessary to slightly abrade the skin to obtain a good interface. Patients with a lot of body hair may need to have the area immediately over the electrode site shaved to ensure a good skin/electrode interface.

4. Place the four limb leads according to the manufacturer's recommendations.

5. Following placement of the limb leads, prepare for placement of the precordial leads. (See Figure 9-2 ■.)

6. First, place lead V1 by attaching the positive electrode to the right of the sternum at the fourth intercostal space.

7. Next, place lead V2 by attaching the positive electrode to the left of the sternum at the fourth intercostal space.

8. Next, place lead V4 by attaching the positive electrode at the midclavicular line at the fifth intercostal space.

9. Next, place lead V3 by attaching the positive electrode in a line midway between lead V2 and lead V4.

10. Next, place lead V5 by attaching the positive electrode at the anterior axillary line at the same level as V4.

11. Finally, place V6 by attaching the positive electrode to the midaxillary line at the same level as V4.

12. Ensure that all leads are attached.

13. Turn on the machine.

14. Ensure that a good tracing is being received from each channel.

15. Record the tracing.

16. Examine the tracing. Do not completely rely on the machine's interpretation of the tracing. If necessary, confirm with medical direction.

17. Provide the tracing to the receiving hospital. If you do not start fibrinolytic therapy in the field, you can reduce the door-to-needle time by providing a quality 12-lead tracing to the emergency staff as soon as the patient arrives.

18. Perform patient pass-off to the hospital personnel.

■ Figure 9-2 Proper placement of the precordial leads.

Angle of Louis

Lead V₁ The electrode is at the fourth intercostal space just to the right of the sternum.
Lead V₂ The electrode is at the fourth intercostal space just to the left of the sternum.
Lead V₃ The electrode is at the line midway between leads V₂ and V₄.
Lead V₄ The electrode is at the midclavicular line in the fifth interspace.
Lead V₅ The electrode is at the anterior axillary line at the same level as lead V₄.
Lead V₆ The electrode is at the midaxillary line at the same level as lead V₄.

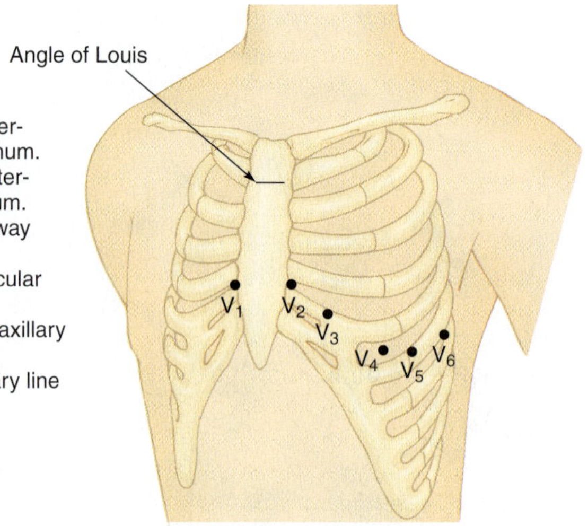

Chest lead placement

19. Restock equipment for next call.
20. Compare your field interpretation with the emergency department and cardiology interpretations.

ARTERIAL BLOOD PRESSURE

The arterial blood pressure is one of the most important physiological measurements utilized in medical practice. Unfortunately, it is also one of the most unreliable. Hypertension, an elevation in arterial blood pressure, is one of the most common medical disorders encountered in our society. Despite this, the standard method of measuring blood pressure with a sphygmomanometer is highly inaccurate.

In the following discussion, the techniques for measuring and monitoring arterial blood pressure in critically ill patients will be discussed. The first section will present indirect/noninvasive techniques while the second section will detail techniques that directly measure arterial pressures with intravascular catheters.

Physiological monitors are essential to monitoring multiple important parameters in the critically ill or injured patient.

INDIRECT (NONINVASIVE) PRESSURE MONITORING

An indirect measurement of arterial blood pressure can be obtained with a sphygmomanometer. The sphygmomanometer contains an inflatable rubber bladder that is covered with cloth. The cloth cuff is wrapped around an arm or leg and the bladder inflated. A manometer containing a column of mercury is attached to the bladder in order to measure the pressure within the bladder. Inflation of the bladder generates pressure that compresses the underlying artery and veins. Bladder inflation continues until blood flow through the artery is completely stopped. The bladder is then slowly deflated, allowing the compressed artery to open and blood flow to resume. The arterial blood pressure can be determined by detecting sounds (Korotkoff's sounds) created when blood flow resumes in the artery (auscultation method) or by detecting the pulsations that occur when blood flow resumes (oscillometric method).

Multiple potential problems are associated with indirect measurement of blood pressure. The most common source of error in indirect blood pressure is use of an incorrectly sized cuff. To be effective, the cuff must be of an appropriate size to produce uniform compression of the underlying artery. Cuffs that are too small will artificially elevate the blood pressure reading. Despite the potential problems, indirect measurement of blood pressure is usually adequate for most medical conditions. However, critical care patients often require a more accurate measure of arterial blood pressure. In these instances, direct blood pressure monitoring may be necessary.

DIRECT (INVASIVE) PRESSURE MONITORING

The direct recording of blood pressure is recommended for critical care patients who require accurate monitoring of arterial pressure. However, direct monitoring of arterial blood pressure is an invasive procedure that requires sophisticated equipment and frequent calibration and maintenance.

For direct arterial monitoring, a catheter is placed into a suitable artery. Most commonly, the radial or femoral artery is used. Other arteries suitable for pressure monitoring in adults include the brachial, axillary, or dorsalis pedis arteries. In neonates, the umbilical or temporal arteries may be used.

Using sterile technique, the arterial catheter is inserted into an artery that is large enough to accommodate the catheter without occluding the artery or significantly impeding flow. The catheter is usually filled with heparinized saline or dextrose solution that serves as a fluid column between the blood and the diaphragm of the pressure transducer. A transducer is a device that changes energy from one form to another. In this case, the transducer changes the mechanical pressure pulse into an electrical signal. The electrical signal from the transducer is often weak and an amplifier is usually required. Finally, the signal is displayed on an oscilloscope or graph. (See Figure 9-3 ■.) Most critical care units utilize an electronic monitor that displays the arterial waveform and also provides a numerical value for the systolic, diastolic, and mean arterial pressure. However, a simple manometer can be attached to the arterial line instead of the pressure transducer. Heparinized fluid (saline or D_5W) is used to fill and flush the system and to prevent blood clotting within the catheter.

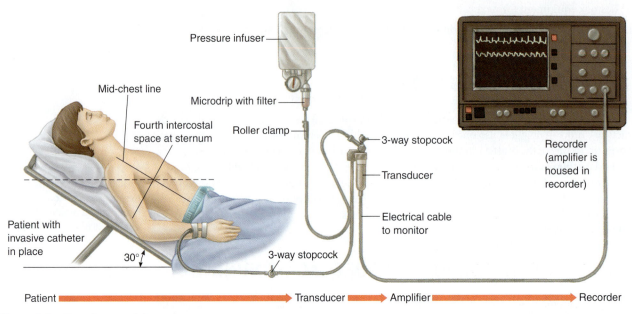

Figure 9-3 Invasive arterial monitor.

The flush solution is placed in a pressure bag that is inflated to 300 mmHg in order to maintain constant pressure through the transducer and flush device.

When setting up an arterial monitoring system, it is necessary to level and zero the pressure transducer. The zero reference point is the intersection of the midaxillary line with the fourth intercostal space. This point, referred to as the *phlebostatic axis,* places the transducer at the level of the patient's right and left atrium when supine. Placing the transducer above or below this point can result in erroneous readings. It is not a valid reference point when the patient is in the lateral recumbent position. In addition to leveling, the transducer must be zeroed in order to negate any effect of atmospheric pressure on the pressure reading. The transducer should be zeroed any time there is a change in the patient's position, the elevation of the head of the bed, or patient transport. Thus, once the patient is situated in the transport vehicle, the pressure transducer should be leveled and zeroed to ensure that any readings obtained are accurate.

The normal arterial waveform has a characteristic configuration. (See Figure 9-4 ■.) There is a rapid upstroke that represents the rapid ejection of blood from the left ventricle into the aorta. This increase in pressure follows the QRS complex on the ECG. Following the rapid upstroke, there is a dicrotic notch that reflects the slight backflow of blood in the aorta that follows closure of the aortic valve. This occurs because the aortic pressure is slightly higher than the left ventricular pressure. This event corresponds with the end of ventricular repolarization as evidenced by the T wave on the ECG tracing. The value measured at the peak of the waveform is the systolic pressure. The lowest point on the waveform is the diastolic pressure. The dicrotic notch indicates the end of ventricular systole (aortic valve closure) and the beginning of ventricular diastole.

Figure 9-4 Arterial pressure waveform. The dicrotic notch indicates aortic valve closure.

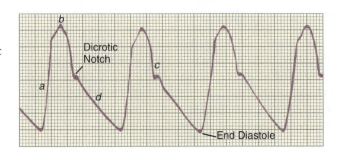

An important parameter that can be determined from arterial pressure monitoring is the **mean arterial pressure (MAP).** Many of the modern pressure monitors automatically measure the MAP. This is accomplished by integrating the area under the pressure waveform and dividing this by the duration of the cardiac cycle. This electronic measurement of the MAP is preferred to the calculated MAP, which can be estimated using the following formula:

$$\text{MAP} = \frac{[(2 \times P_{\text{diastolic}}) + P_{\text{systolic}}]}{3}$$

Or it can be written as:

$$\text{MAP} = P_{\text{diastolic}} + 1/3\,(P_{\text{systolic}} - P_{\text{diastolic}})$$

Diastole counts twice as much as systole because two-thirds of the cardiac cycle is diastole.

The MAP is considered superior to the systolic pressure for arterial pressure monitoring because the MAP is the true driving pressure for peripheral blood flow.

mean arterial pressure (MAP) *true systemic "driving" pressure for peripheral blood flow.*

Invasive blood pressure monitors must be calibrated and checked often to ensure acurate readings.

PLACEMENT OF THE ARTERIAL CATHETER

The following information details placement and use of an arterial catheter:

INDICATIONS

★ Continuous monitoring of intra-arterial pressure in the critical care setting
★ Arterial access for frequent blood gas samples
★ Titration of vasoactive medications during transport

INSERTION OF THE ARTERIAL CATHETER

Arterial pressure readings can be taken from virtually any artery within the cardiovascular system. However, human anatomy does not allow for the placement of a catheter just anywhere.

The most common sites for arterial catheter placement include the radial, brachial, and femoral arteries (and, rarely, the ulnar artery). The waveform will vary somewhat by artery. (See Figure 9-5 ■.) Regardless of the specific site chosen for the arterial line, the successful placement of the catheter is also dependent on many factors beyond that of site selection. These include:

★ The experience of the practitioner placing the catheter
★ A patient history, if any, of peripheral vascular disease
★ The relative hemodynamic status of the patient at the time of catheter placement

These factors may also be the rationale for placement of the catheter at a specific site. For example, if a patient is hemodynamically compromised and requires arterial catheter placement for pressure monitoring and vasopressor administration, a femoral catheter may be placed instead because of the size, location, and ease of insertion into the artery given the poor peripheral perfusion status of the patient overall. However, it is important to remember, femoral arterial catheters are associated with higher infection rates and occlusion problems. Because of this, all sites should be evaluated for their risks and benefits. Conversely, if a patient who requires ventilatory assistance needs arterial line placement for frequent blood gas samples, a radial or brachial catheter may be placed.

As a rule, in most critical care transport systems, critical care paramedics will not be inserting an arterial line. However, you will be responsible for caring for patients with one. So, being familiar with common arterial cannulation sites and knowing the insertion technique can only help to better prepare you to manage them.

Prior to placement of any arterial catheter into a distal artery (i.e., radial, ulnar artery), a simple test must be performed to ensure good collateral arterial blood flow. If the critical care paramedic is

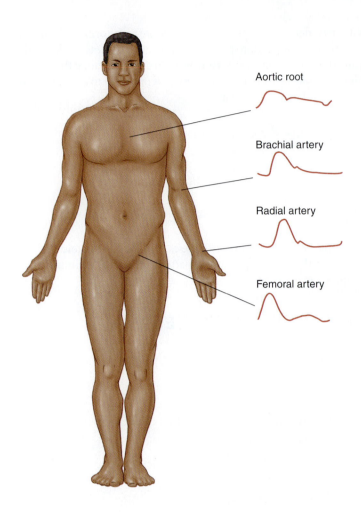

Aortic root

Brachial artery

Radial artery

Femoral artery

assisting in the arterial line placement, he may be asked to first assess the perfusion status of the distal tissues by performing an *Allen's test.* (See Figure 9-6 ■.) By asking the patient to clench his fist (thereby aiding venous flow from the hand), and digitally occluding both the radial and ulnar arteries, the distal perfusion to the hand becomes altered and the palmar region will blanch. From a position where the hand is clenched and both arteries are occluded digitally, the patient is then instructed to open his hand, and the care provider will release pressure from the artery that will NOT be cannulated with the arterial catheter. If the blanching subsides in less than 3 seconds, there is sufficient indication that collateral perfusion is intact and that the artery (still occluded digitally) may be used for catheter placement. (Again, typically the radial artery is preferred since there are some risks inherent to using the ulnar artery.) This maneuver is important, because arterial catheter placement does diminish distal blood flow through the artery being cannulated, and without collateral perfusion, tissue injury may occur. A positive Allen's test is when a blush indicates ulnar patency. A negative Allen's test indicates occlusion of the ulnar artery, and the radial artery should not be punctured. You will sometimes hear of a modified Allen's test. The difference between the true Allen's test and the modified Allen's test is the fact that with the Allen's test the examiner is supposed to occlude both arteries, have the patient clench his fist several times, and release compression on one of the two arteries. This is then repeated on the remaining artery. With a modified Allen's test, only the ulnar artery is compressed and released. If the blanching disappears, the modified Allen's test is positive and the radial artery can be cannulated.

All arterial catheters are placed by using a catheter-over-needle or Seldinger technique under sterile conditions. (See Figure 9-7 ■.) Local administration of 1% Xylocaine (lidocaine) may be used at the insertion site to decrease the discomfort of placement. Any catheter-over-needle intravenous device may be used for distal arterial placement if the patient's body habitus allows. If the femoral artery is being cannulated, or if patient's size is large, specific catheters manufactured for

🔑⟶ ─────────────

Always document an Allen's or
modified Allen's test anytime you
perform a radial artery puncture.

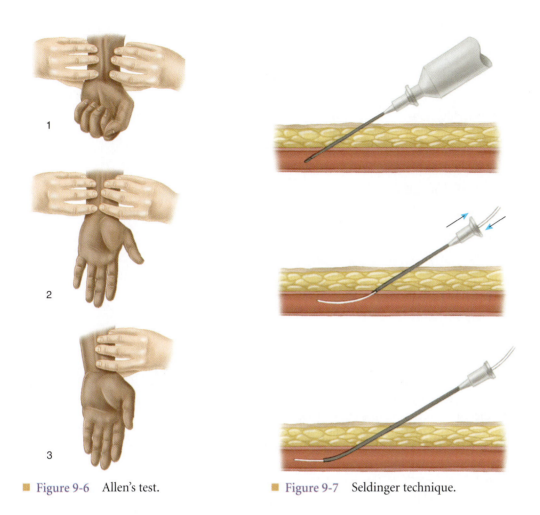

■ Figure 9-6   Allen's test.

■ Figure 9-7   Seldinger technique.

arterial line placement must be utilized, because these contain a guidewire that can be used to successfully cannulate the deeper artery.

COMPLICATIONS

The most common complications associated with arterial catheter placement include pain, bleeding, and vasospasm. Pain associated with arterial catheter placement is described by some patients as "much worse" than intravenous catheter placement, due to the location of the nerve fibers running directly beside arteries. Arteries are also much more vasoactive than veins, and vasospasm can occur, especially with repeated attempts to cannulate the same artery. If vasospasm occurs, the success rate of placement of the catheter drops significantly and repeated attempts further decrease the success rate. If multiple attempts to cannulate a particular artery are unsuccessful, the practitioner should consider a different site for successful placement.

Because blood flow is at a much higher pressure within the arterial system, when compared to the venous system, bleeding is a major concern in the placement of an arterial catheter. If an artery is damaged during cannulation, rapid bleeding can occur either externally or subcutaneously. If this is the case, prolonged direct pressure at the insertion site must be maintained for a minimum of 10 minutes, followed by the application of a pressure dressing. Peripheral perfusion status must then be monitored to assess for distal ischemia.

Waveform distortion can occur with arterial monitoring. Because of this, the arterial line should be periodically flushed and rezeroed to ensure accurate readings. However, if the reading does not improve after flushing, then the system may be overdamped or underdamped. (See

Figure 9-8 (A) Arterial line—normal waveform. (B) Arterial line—flattened waveform. Flattened arterial waveform indicates damping. Damping results from obstruction in arterial line or imbalance of transducer.

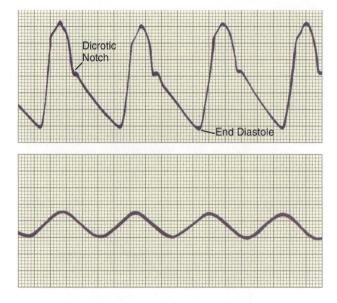

Figure 9-8 ▪.) Damping prevents a system from overshooting after responding to a change, particularly at frequencies close to that of the monitoring system. Overdamping can result from blood clots, air bubbles in the tubing, or a kink in the tubing. It will cause a slurred upstroke, loss of the dichrotic notch, and loss of other fine details in the tracing. Underdamping, on the other hand, causes exaggerations in the peaks and troughs of the waveform. It can cause false elevations in the systolic blood pressure and a false low reading in the diastolic blood pressure. Causes of underdamping include long connecting lines, small tubing, or a catheter that completely occludes the vessel. To correct these, the underlying problem must be addressed.

After successful placement of an arterial catheter, diligent monitoring by the critical care paramedic is mandatory to prevent accidental catheter displacement and kinking of the catheter because either of these will result in inaccurate pressure readings. Bleeding usually results from dislodgement of the arterial catheter or a disconnection of the catheter from the flush system. Rapid blood loss, including exsanguination, can occur if disconnection is not corrected immediately. Ensuring that all connections are tight during arterial placement and constantly assessing the catheter insertion site is, again, paramount. Kinking of the catheter within the artery is also associated with poor distal perfusion and tissue ischemia. To decrease the possibility of catheter kinking, the critical care paramedic may immobilize the extremity after the catheter is successfully placed.

For femoral placement, utilizing a knee immobilizer or a soft restraint around the ankle that is secured to the end of the patient cot will limit hip and knee flexion. If catheter placement is at the radial or ulnar artery, placing an armboard dorsally with the wrist slightly extended keeps the catheter on an even plane and decreases the likelihood of kinking.

Arterial puncture must be used with extreme caution in patients on blood thinners, fibrinolytics, and glycoprotein 2b3a inhibitors because bleeding may be very difficult to control. It is important to continually reassess the patient for bleeding at the puncture site. Also, look for the presence of swelling, redness, or a hematoma because this may indicate bleeding under the skin.

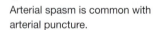

Arterial spasm is common with arterial puncture.

CHECK THE ARTERIAL CATHETER WAVEFORM

Once successfully placed, the arterial catheter is connected to a flush system (discussed later in the chapter) to maintain catheter patency. The systolic peak is indicative of the peripheral systolic blood pressure. The systolic peak begins to fall just after ventricular depolarization (QRS complex) on the ECG is recorded. The normal range for the systolic pressure is 90 to 140 mmHg. The diastolic valley, the low point in the waveform, is indicative of peripheral end diastole, and has a normal range of 60 to 90 mmHg. The dicrotic notch, the third characteristic finding on the arterial wave, occurs on the downslope of the systolic waveform and is indicative of closure of the aortic valve—signifying the beginning of diastole.

The pressure measurement at the dicrotic notch is an indicator of mean arterial pressure, or the average of arterial pressure recorded throughout the entire cardiac cycle. This pressure is important in that it establishes the ability of the circulatory system to maintain a pressure gradient to the various tissues and capillary beds of the body. In short, it is an excellent indicator of end-organ perfusion status. Normal values for MAP are 65 to 100 mmHg. A MAP pressure of less than 60 mmHg is indicative of a hypoperfusion state, and if the MAP drops below 55 mmHg, a significant hypoperfusion state is present. (It is important to note that the presence of a low MAP only identifies a problem. The critical care paramedic must still incorporate other assessment parameters to determine the cause of the lowered MAP and provide corrective therapies.) The MAP is also an important component of other hemodynamic assessments such as cerebral perfusion pressure, renal perfusion pressure, status of fluid resuscitation, and titration of vasopressor medication. If necessary, the MAP can also be calculated manually, without the use of an arterial line. As mentioned earlier, to calculate the MAP:

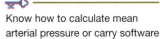

Know how to calculate mean arterial pressure or carry software that can perform the calculation.

$$MAP = \frac{[(2 \times P_{diastolic}) + P_{systolic}]}{3}$$

CENTRAL CIRCULATION MONITORS

Hemodynamic monitoring of the central circulation can provide important information about the hemodynamic status of the critically ill or injured patient. The two most frequently used techniques for monitoring components of the central circulation are the *central venous pressure monitor* and the *pulmonary artery catheter monitor*.

CENTRAL VENOUS PRESSURE MONITOR

The **central venous pressure** (CVP) reflects the pressure of blood within the vena cava or right atrium. Thus, it provides information about intravascular blood volume, right-ventricular end-diastolic pressure, and right ventricular function—in essence, preload.

To perform CVP monitoring, the CVP catheter is inserted into a central vein using standard central venous access techniques. (See Figure 9-9 ■.) The most frequently used access routes are the

central venous pressure (CVP)   *the pressure of blood within the vena cava or right atrium.*

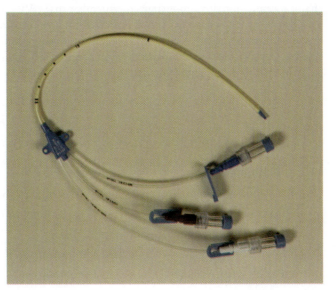

■ **Figure 9-9**   Triple-lumen central venous catheter.

subclavian vein or the internal jugular vein. Alternatively, the CVP catheter can be placed via femoral puncture. When central venous access is impossible or difficult, a special CVP catheter can be introduced through the antecubital vein in the forearm and slowly advanced into the vena cava. Placement of a CVP catheter via the femoral or antecubital route usually requires a catheter that is slightly longer than those inserted via the jugular or subclavian routes.

When properly placed, the tip of the CVP catheter should be in the vena cava, close to the right atrium. The pressure can be measured with a water manometer or an electronic pressure transducer. Most pressure transducers record the pressure in millimeters of mercury (mmHg), while water manometers record the pressure in centimeters of water (cm/H_2O). Mercury is 13.6 times more dense than water. Because of this, pressures measured in cm/H_2O are divided by 1.36 to convert the units to mmHg:

$$CVP \ (mmHg) = CVP \ (cm/H_2O)/1.36$$

To measure with a water manometer, the manometer is placed in line between the IV fluid and the CVP catheter using a three-way stopcock. To measure the CVP, the stopcock is opened to the manometer and the patient. Pressure within the vena cava equilibrates with the column of fluid in the manometer. The point at which the fluid level settles is the CVP. Some variation in the CVP level will be seen with respiration due to changes in intrathoracic pressure. The fluid level will fall with inspiration and rise with expiration.

The water manometer has been replaced by the pressure transducer in the modern critical care unit. The pressure transducer and system components are identical to that used for arterial pressure monitoring. As with the arterial monitor, the CVP transducer must be leveled and calibrated. The zero reference point in the thorax is the intersection of the midaxillary line with the fourth intercostal space. This corresponds to the position of the right and left atrium when the patient is supine. Once it has been established, the patient's chest should be marked to ensure that the pressure transducer remains stable for subsequent pressure readings. Also, the system should be zeroed in order to negate any chance of atmospheric pressure interference.

CVP is measured in centimeters of water (cm/H_2O) or millimeters of mercury (mmHg). Normal CVP, as measured with a water manometer, is approximately 5 to 8 cm/H_2O while normal CVP, as measured by a pressure transducer, ranges from 0 to 6 mmHg. The most important aspect of CVP monitoring is the trend. Isolated measurements mean little. However, continuous monitoring can provide important information about the patient's hemodynamic status.

Central venous pressure provides important information about the patient's state of hydration.

Low CVP readings indicate hypovolemia, which usually requires the administration of fluids. Diuretics, vasodilation from shock, and administration of vasodilating drugs can also lower the CVP. High CVP readings are due to multiple factors including right ventricular failure and mechanical ventilation. It is important to remember that CVP readings will vary somewhat with the various phases of mechanical ventilation. It is important to remember the global situation (i.e., changing intrathoracic pressures from mechanical ventilation) when evaluating CVP waveforms. Overall, the CVP reading should be used in conjunction with other hemodynamic parameters as well as physical assessment information.

PLACEMENT OF A CENTRAL VENOUS CATHETER

The following subsections detail placement and use of a central venous catheter.

Indications

* ★ Patients with hypotension who are not responding to basic clinical management
* ★ Continuing hypovolemia secondary to major fluid shifts or loss
* ★ Patients requiring infusions of inotropic agents
* ★ Requirement for large-volume fluid administration
* ★ For use when peripheral access sites are unavailable

★ Patients in need of total parenteral nutrition (TPN)

★ Patients who need long-term venous access for blood draws or medications (i.e., chemotherapy)

Insertion of the Central Venous Catheter

Central venous catheters are most commonly inserted through the subclavian, internal jugular, or femoral veins. (See Figures 9-10 ■ and 9-11 ■.) In special situations, the catheters can be inserted in the antecubital vein or external jugular vein. Like arterial catheters, central venous catheters are placed by the Seldinger technique under sterile conditions. (See Figure 9-12 ■.) Because of the length of the catheter, a catheter-over-guidewire procedure is used. The most common sites used for insertion include the internal jugular, subclavian, and femoral veins. Always prep the puncture site with the appropriate solution. It is preferable to anesthetize the puncture site with 1% lidocaine. Also, for larger catheters and introducers, consider making a small skin

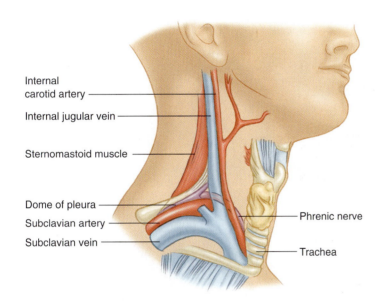

■ Figure 9-10 Neck anatomy.

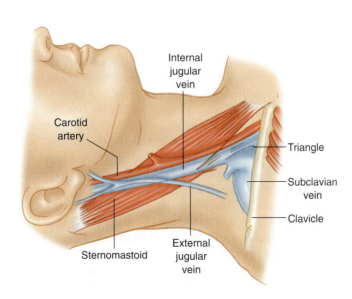

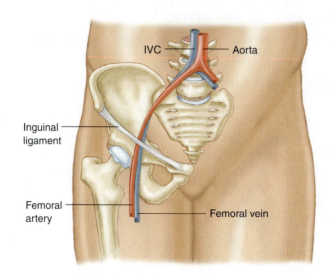

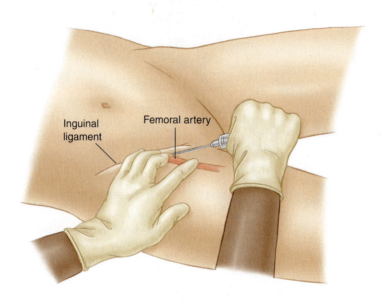

nick with a #11 blade at the puncture site. Once venous access is obtained by venipuncture and placement of venous access is confirmed by aspirating venous blood, a guidewire is passed through the needle and into to the vein. The needle is then removed carefully overtop the guidewire, and, while still grasping the guidewire, the practitioner then threads the central venous catheter over the guidewire and advances it into position. The final step is the removal of the guidewire and attachment of the central line tubing.

CVP catheters are attached to a manometer system or to a central monitor. Critical care paramedics should be familiar with both types of monitors because each may be encountered during interhospital transports. (See Figure 9-13 ■.)

Because multiple types of central venous catheters are available, the choice of which type to place is dependent on what the need is for central venous access (monitoring, fluid resuscitation, medication administration, and so on), and the practitioner's preference when placing the catheter. Critically injured or ill patients with intravascular volume loss may receive a single-lumen, large-bore catheter for rapid volume resuscitation or blood transfusion. Patients requiring central venous access for hemodialysis may have a dual-lumen dialysis catheter, and critically

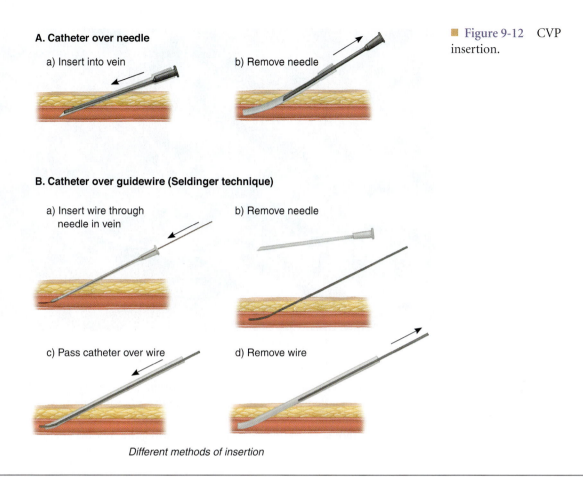

A. Catheter over needle

a) Insert into vein

b) Remove needle

B. Catheter over guidewire (Seldinger technique)

a) Insert wire through needle in vein

b) Remove needle

c) Pass catheter over wire

d) Remove wire

Different methods of insertion

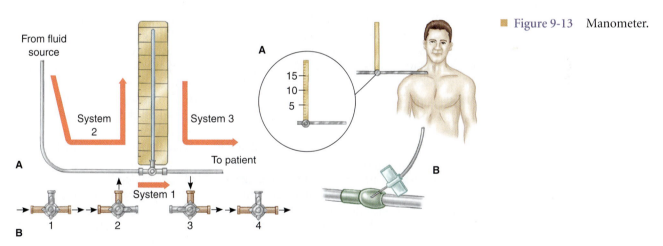

■ Figure 9-13   Manometer.

From fluid source

System 2

System 3

To patient

System 1

A

B

1   2   3   4

A

15
10
5

B

ill patients who require multiple drug interventions may have a multiple-lumen central catheter placed. (See Figure 9-14 ■.)

Complications

Placement of a central venous catheter may have some significant, even life-threatening complications. Bleeding, pnuemothorax, and dysrhythmias are the most serious complications during insertion. Accidental cannulation of an artery is not uncommon. In some cases, direct pressure may not control bleeding (i.e., carotid or subclavian arteries), which is problematic, especially if the patient is receiving anticoagulants or has bleeding dyscrasias. Venous perforation during venipuncture or

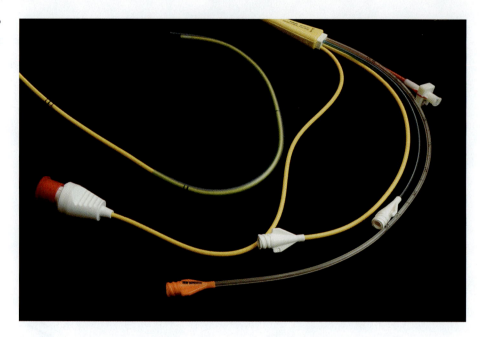

during the advancement of the guidewire may also result in a hemorrhage. Finally, if the needle (or cannula) becomes dislodged from the vessel during the procedure, or at some later time, hemorrhage may result as well.

A pneumothorax can occur with cannulation using the subclavian approach since the apex of the lung and the subclavian vessel lie close to each other. It is for this reason that an upright anterior/posterior chest X-ray (CXR) is essential following successful insertion of a central venous catheter to assess for placement of the catheter and to assess for pneumothorax.

Finally, during the insertion technique, if the catheter is being advanced with the tip passing through the atria, atrial dysrhythmias may occur. As the tip of the catheter is being floated through the right ventricle and into the pulmonary artery for pulmonary artery pressures, ventricular dysrhythmias may occur as well. While this complication is usually self-limiting, with ventricular irritability abating after the guidewire is removed, the patient with hypovolemia or electrolyte imbalance may be at risk for sustained ventricular dysrhythmia even after the guidewire is removed. Cases have been reported in which the guidewire punctured the wall of the heart. Although rare, this is always a possibility.

After successful placement of a central venous catheter, complications include infection, bleeding, accidental dislodgement, and extravasation of fluids. Most central venous catheters are made of synthetic materials that can be irritating to blood vessels if left in for greater than 7 to 10 days. The critical care paramedic should carefully assess the insertion site for signs and symptoms of infection. They include redness, purulent drainage, and pain at the insertion site. A sterile, occlusive dressing over the insertion site will help to minimize environmental exposure and contamination, and routine dressing changes performed under sterile conditions will also aid in limiting contamination risks. If, during transport, a central venous catheter dressing is loosened, a sterile gauze dressing can be placed over the original dressing to reinforce and maintain sterility at the insertion site.

If the central venous catheter becomes dislodged (pulled out) for any reason, manual pressure dressings should be applied to the insertion site for at least 5 minutes to minimize bleeding, followed by placement of an occlusive dressing to decrease the risk of air entering the chest cavity through the original insertion site (although this is not a big concern because the size of the hole from the catheter is so small). If the patient exhibits signs of dyspnea or hypoxia or complains of chest discomfort, place the patient in a left side-lying position and treat appropriately for possible air embolism.

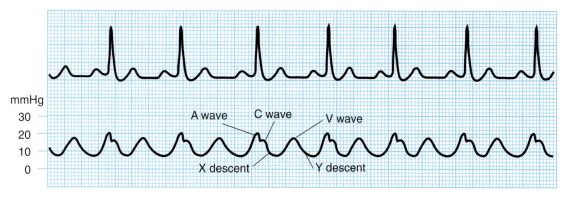

■ **Figure 9-15** Central venous waveform.

Extravasation of certain intravenous fluids that may be administered into the surrounding subcutaneous tissues can lead to tissue necrosis and infection. If extravasation is suspected, first stop all intravenous administration occurring through the central venous catheter. Attempts should be made, as needed, for peripheral intravenous access to continue any specialized medication infusions. If vasopressor agents infiltrate into subcutaneous tissues, the subcutaneous administration of phentolamine (Regitine) in a circular pattern at the site of infiltration should be performed to minimize tissue necrosis caused by the vasoconstrictive properties of the vasopressor.

Central Venous Catheter Waveform

When properly placed in the central circulation, vena cava, or the right atrium, a central venous catheter attached to a transducer will generate a characteristic waveform and provide the corresponding numeric value. (See Figure 9-15 ■.) Because it is a part of the venous system, a low-pressure system, the systolic and diastolic pressures of central venous catheters are essentially indistinguishable. As such, a mean pressure is used to describe the pressure in the venous system. The normal value for CVP can vary between 1 and 6 mmHg. The waveforms and pressure values seen throughout the central venous circulation and the right atrium (RA) are similar because there are no structures (such as valves) that divide these locations into different chambers.

Interpretation of the CVP is an important indicator of venous return to the right side of the heart, and many times will allow the critical care paramedic to validate noninvasive physical assessment findings. For example, an elderly patient presents with a chief complaint of chest pain and dizziness. Vitals signs reveal tachycardia at 112 bpm, and a BP of 84/40. There is evidence of poor peripheral perfusion, and further evaluation reveals a 12-lead electrocardiogram demonstrating evidence of an inferior wall myocardial infarction. During transport to an interventional cardiac catheterization facility, the critical care paramedic can monitor the central venous catheter pressures. If during this monitoring, the CVP is found to be extremely low, then the hypotension may be a result of venodilation and peripheral pooling of blood. If, conversely, the CVP is found to be elevated, then the hypotension may be a result of right ventricular extension of the inferior wall infarction, causing decreased right ventricular contractility and diminished left-sided preload. The CVP provides information when determining a plan of action for the patient. Table 9–1 demonstrates typical causes of high and low CVPs.

Treatment of low CVP starts first with interpreting why it is low, so that the treatment provided is reflective of the problem. Common interventions may include elimination of vasodilator drugs (such as nitroglycerin), and fluid resuscitation to increase right-sided preload. Treatment of high CVP (again, after understanding why it is too high) may include the initiation of vasodilator drugs, the administration of diuretics, or, in the case of right ventricular infarction, fluid resuscitation to increase right ventricular filling pressures to optimize right ventricular function and maintain left-sided preload.

Table 9–1	Common Causes of Abnormal CVP Pressures

Low	High
Venodilation	Vasoconstriction
Hypovolemia	Fluid volume overload
	Right ventricular failure
	Right ventricular infarction
	Chronic left ventricular failure
	Tricuspid insufficiency
	Chronic pulmonary diseases
	Cardiac tamponade
	Positive end-expiratory pressure (PEEP)

PULMONARY ARTERY PRESSURE MONITORING

Placement of a catheter into the pulmonary artery (PA) allows monitoring of several important physiological parameters. With a flow-directed, balloon-tipped pulmonary artery catheter (i.e., Swan-Ganz catheter), it is possible to measure right ventricular function, pulmonary vascular status, and, indirectly, left ventricular function. (See Figure 9-16 ■.) Parameters that can be measured with a pulmonary artery catheter include:

- ★ Cardiac output (CO or Q)
- ★ Right atrial pressure (RAP)
- ★ Right ventricular pressure (RVP)
- ★ Pulmonary artery pressure (PAP)
- ★ Pulmonary artery wedge pressure (PAWP)

Several types of flow-directed balloon-tipped PA catheters are available in different sizes. The basic PA catheter is 110 cm in length and has an outside diameter of 2.3 mm (7 French). There are two internal channels. One channel runs the entire length of the catheter and opens at the very tip of the catheter (the distal port). The other channel is shorter and opens 30 cm from the catheter tip (the proximal port). The tip of the catheter is equipped with a balloon that has a 1.5-mL capacity. The balloon is used to "float" the catheter into position and for measuring pulmonary capillary wedge pressures. Finally, a thermistor is located on the outer surface of the catheter 4 cm from the catheter tip. (See Figure 9-17 ■.) The thermistor senses changes in temperature and is used for determining cardiac output. (See Figure 9-18 ■.) Specialized PA catheters are available depending on the particular needs of the patient. A popular PA catheter

■ **Figure 9-16** Balloon-tipped catheter has multiple lumens (internal tubes) with openings used to measure intracardiac pressures.

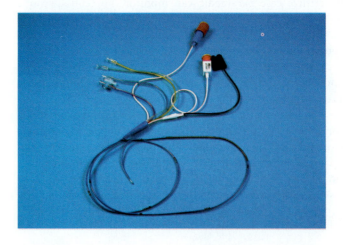

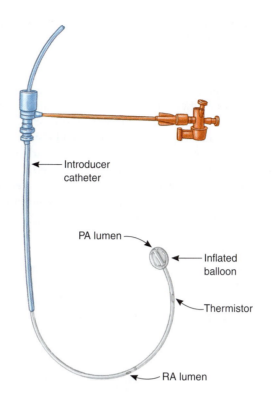

■ **Figure 9-17** Pulmonary artery catheter with thermistor.

Introducer catheter

PA lumen

Inflated balloon

Thermistor

RA lumen

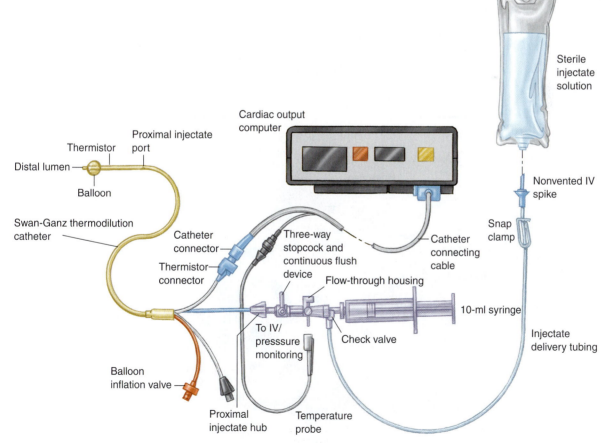

Cardiac output computer

Sterile injectate solution

Thermistor

Proximal injectate port

Distal lumen

Balloon

Swan-Ganz thermodilution catheter

Catheter connector

Thermistor connector

Three-way stopcock and continuous flush device

Flow-through housing

Nonvented IV spike

Snap clamp

Catheter connecting cable

10-ml syringe

Balloon inflation valve

To IV/ presssure monitoring

Check valve

Injectate delivery tubing

Proximal injectate hub

Temperature probe

■ **Figure 9-18** Swan-Ganz setup.

contains an extra channel that opens 14 cm from the catheter tip. This allows for fluid infusion through the catheter or for insertion of a transvenous pacemaker.

Waveform Interpretation

The PA catheter is usually introduced through the internal jugular vein or the subclavian vein. Waveforms and pressures are continuously monitored as the catheter is floated into place. As the catheter is advanced through the heart, pressure readings are obtained. The pressure changes detected are caused by myocardial contraction (systole) and relaxation and filling (diastole). Four distinct waveforms can be seen as the catheter advances through the heart and into the pulmonary artery. The waveforms are classified as *right atrial, right ventricular, pulmonary artery pressure,* and *pulmonary artery wedge pressure.* Many of the pressure waves measured during pulmonary artery catheterization are related to specific parts of the ECG. Figure 9-19 ■ illustrates essential waveforms seen during right heart catheterization.

Right Atrial Pressure

right atrial pressure (RAP)
the pressure in the right atrium, normally less than 8 mmHg.

As the catheter is advanced through the vena cava, it first enters the right atrium. The right atrium is a low-pressure chamber that receives blood passively from the vena cava. The pressure in the right atrium is normally less than 8 mmHg. This is referred to as the mean **right atrial pressure (RAP)** (See Figure 9-20 ■.) Three pressure waves can be seen during RAP monitoring. The first wave, re-

■ **Figure 9-19** Swan-Ganz and the circulatory system.

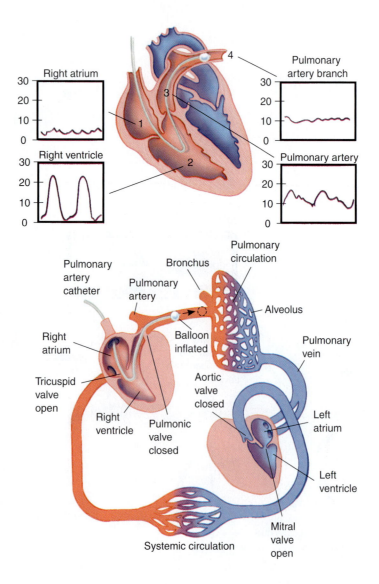

Right Atrial (RA) Pressure

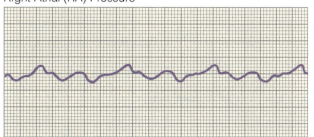

■ **Figure 9-20** Right atrial pressure (RAP).

ferred to as the *a wave,* is caused by atrial contraction and follows the P wave of the electrocardiogram. As the pressure falls from the peak of the *a* wave, a small positive deflection, referred to as the *c wave,* can be seen. The *c* wave results from the building of the tricuspid valve. After full atrial relaxation, the pressure in the atrium starts to rise due to atrial filling from peripheral venous return. Then, right ventricular contraction occurs. The *v wave* results from passive filling of the atrium. The *v* wave reaches a peak just prior to the opening of the tricuspid valve. Following opening of the tricuspid valve, the right atrium empties into the right ventricle, causing pressure in the right atrium to again fall. In addition to the positive *a, c,* and *v* waves, there are two negative waves referred to as descents. The *x descent* follows the peak of the *a* wave and results from atrial relaxation at the beginning of atrial diastole. The *y descent* follows the *v* wave and results from the initial, passive atrial emptying into the right ventricle as the tricuspid valve opens. At the end of the *y* descent, the pressure in the right atrium equals the ventricular diastolic pressure and slowly increases as the ventricle fills. (See Figure 9-21 ■ and Table 9–2.)

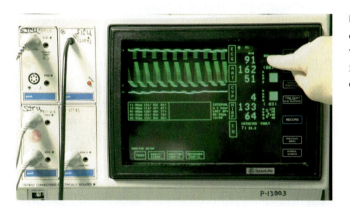

■ **Figure 9-21** Monitor display of ECG pressure waveforms, and digital readouts for continuous client assessment.

Table 9–2	Right Atrial Pressure (RAP)
Abnormal Low Pressures	**Abnormal High Pressures**
Peripheral pooling	Fluid volume overload
Venodilation	Right ventricular failure
Fluid volume deficit/hypovolemia	Chronic left ventricular failure
Transducer placement above the level of the phlebostatic axis	Tricuspid valvular abnormalities (stenosis/regurgitation)
	Transducer placement below the level of the phlebostatic axis
	Physiological increases in intrathoracic pressure (coughing, vomiting, seizure)
	Mechanical increases in intrathoracic pressure (positive pressure ventilation, positive end-expiratory pressure, continuous positive airway pressure)

Figure 9-22 Right ventricular (RV) pressure.

Right Ventricular (RV) Pressure

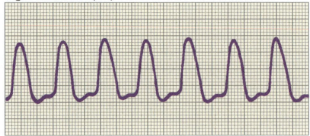

Right Ventricular Pressure (RVP)

right ventricular pressure (RVP) *pressure within the right ventricle; required to open pulmonic valve and release blood into pulmonary arteries.*

From the right atrium, the pulmonary artery catheter is advanced through the tricuspid valve and into the right ventricle. Like the right atrium, the right ventricle is considered a low-pressure chamber. **Right ventricular** end-diastolic **pressure** is normally 0 to 8 mmHg, equal to right atrial pressure when the tricuspid valve opens. Right ventricular systolic pressure is normally 15 to 30 mmHg. This is enough pressure to open the pulmonic valve and move blood into the low-pressure pulmonary vascular system. The diastolic phase of the right ventricular pressure wave consists of an early rapid filling wave, during which approximately 60% of ventricular filling occurs. This is followed by a slow filling period that accounts for 25% of ventricular filling. Next, an atrial systolic wave (*a*) occurs causing the final 15% of ventricular filling. During diastole, right atrial and right ventricular pressures are nearly equal due to the low resistance to flow across the tricuspid valve. Two pressures are usually measured during right ventricular monitoring: the peak systolic right ventricular pressure and the end-diastolic right ventricular pressure (immediately following the *a* wave). See Figure 9-22 ■, which illustrates the normal right ventricular waveform, and Table 9–3.

Pulmonary Artery Pressure (PAP)

pulmonary artery pressure (PAP) *pressure within the pulmonary artery throughout the cardiac cycle.*

Advancing the catheter will cause the tip to exit the right ventricle through the pulmonic valve and enter the PA. The pulmonary vascular system is a relatively low-pressure, low-resistance system in normal individuals. Normal **pulmonary artery pressure** (PAP) is 15 to 30 mmHg and is equal to right ventricular systolic pressure. Normal diastolic PA pressure is 8 to 15 mmHg, and the mean PA pressure is 10 to 20 mmHg.

The pulmonary artery pressure waveform is similar to that seen in systolic arterial pressure monitoring. The systolic phase of the waveform results from blood entering the pulmonary artery from right ventricular contraction. As right ventricular ejection ends, pressure in the pulmonary artery then falls. When the right ventricular pressure drops below the pressure in the pulmonary artery, the pulmonic valve closes. Closure of the pulmonic valve allows a slight backflow of blood, causing a dicrotic notch, or incisura, on the pressure waveform. Pressure in the pulmonary artery then falls gradually as blood flows through the pulmonary arteries and pulmonary veins into the left atrium and left ventricle. The lowest point, or nadir of this pressure wave, in late diastole, is

Table 9–3	Right Ventricular Pressure (RVP)
Abnormal Low Pressures	**Abnormal High Pressures**
Fluid volume deficit/hypovolemia	Right ventricular failure/infarction
Right ventricular failure from ischemic heart disease	Pulmonary hypertension
Transducer placement above the level of the phlebostatic axis	Chronic left ventricular failure
	Pulmonary infarction
	A/V septal defects
	Pulmonic stenosis

Pulmonary Artery Pressure (PAP)

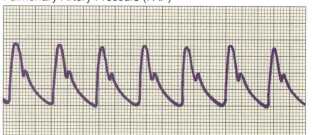

termed the end-diastolic PA pressure. The PA pressures that are most often measured are the peak systolic pressure, the mean PA pressure, and the end-diastolic PA pressure. It is not unusual to see a small (approximately 5 mmHg) gradient in peak systolic pressure between the right ventricle and the pulmonary artery.

The PA diastolic pressure reflects the resistance of the pulmonary vascular bed and, to a limited degree, the left ventricular end-diastolic pressure (LVEDP). The PA diastolic pressure theoretically, and under absolutely normal conditions, is an indirect measure of left ventricular pressure because the pulmonary vascular system, left atrium, and open mitral valve allow equalization of pressure from the left ventricle back to the tip of the PA catheter. See Figure 9-23 ■, which illustrates the pulmonary artery waveform and Table 9–4.

Pulmonary Artery Wedge Pressure

After introduction of the PA catheter into the PA, the catheter tip with the inflated balloon can be advanced until it lodges in a PA branch that is of equal or lesser diameter. When the balloon "wedges" in the PA branch, the forward flow of blood through the affected PA branch is stopped forming **pulmonary artery wedge pressure (PAWP).** This creates a static column of blood from that PA branch, through the left atrium, through the open mitral valve during diastole, and the left ventricle. Thus, the PAWP more closely measures left atrial and left ventricular end-diastolic pressure than the PA diastolic pressure because balloon inflation halts blood flow past the catheter tip and thereby decreases the influence of pulmonary vascular resistance on the pressure reading. Normal PAWP is 8 to 12 mmHg.

The pulmonary artery waveform is similar to that of the left atrium, but is damped and somewhat delayed. A normal PAWP waveform should show *a* waves, *c* waves, and *v* waves. The electrical

pulmonary artery wedge pressure (PAWP) *measures left atrial and left ventricular end-diastolic pressure, normal range is 8 to 12 mmHg.*

Table 9–4	Pulmonary Artery Pressure (PAP)
Abnormal Low Pressures	**Abnormal High Pressures**
Fluid volume deficit/hypovolemia	Primary pulmonary abnormalities (pulmonary hypertension, pulmonary embolism, ARDS) with or without left ventricular involvement
Acute/chronic right ventricular failure	Acute/chronic left ventricular failure
Transducer placement above the level of the phlebostatic axis	Mitral stenosis
	Transducer placement below the level of the phlebostatic axis
	Physiological increases in intrathoracic pressure (coughing, vomiting, seizure)
	Mechanical increases in intrathoracic pressure (positive pressure ventilation, positive end-expiratory pressure, continuous positive airway pressure)

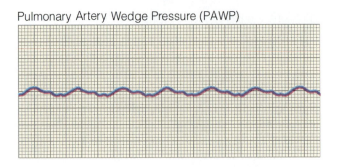

Pulmonary Artery Wedge Pressure (PAWP)

and mechanical events that generate these waves are the same as those that generate the right atrial waveform, except that the PAWP waveform reflects activity from the left side of the heart. The *a* wave is caused by left atrial contraction, and the *v* wave corresponds to bulging of the mitral value into the left atrium during late systole. The *c* wave is due to bulging of the mitral valve into the left atrium after systole.

Following measurement of the PAWP, the balloon is deflated and the PA waveform is again seen. When the PAWP is to be measured, the balloon is inflated, floated slightly forward until it wedges, and then the PAWP waveform is seen. After measuring the required parameters, the balloon is deflated and the catheter withdrawn slightly. The balloon should remain deflated at all times except when measuring PAWP as described earlier. See Figures 9-24 ■ and 9-25 ■, which illustrate pulmonary artery wedge waveforms and Table 9–5.

Complications of PA Catheterization

Pulmonary artery catheterization and monitoring is a relatively safe procedure. However, complications are possible. The most frequently encountered complications include the following:

★ *Pneumothorax.* Pneumothorax is a recognized complication of central line placement. Typically, PA catheter introducers are inserted into the subclavian vein or internal jugular vein. The patient's anatomy can sometimes make introducer insertion very difficult. This is particularly true in patients who are obese or who have slightly altered vein anatomy. The needle or introducer can inadvertently puncture the lung during insertion, resulting in an apical pneumothorax. Post-placement chest X-rays should always be obtained in order to identify a possible pneumothorax.

★ *Ventricular dysrhythmias.* Insertion of the PA catheter frequently causes ventricular dysrhythmias. As the catheter is advanced through the heart, it can irritate the endocardium causing premature ventricular contractions (PVCs) or, in some cases, ventricular tachycardia. Most dysrhythmias stop when the catheter is advanced into the pulmonary artery.

■ **Figure 9-25** Pulmonary artery wedge pressure.

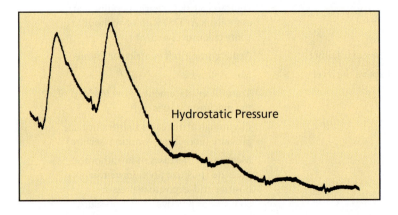

Hydrostatic Pressure

Table 9–5	Pulmonary Artery Wedge Pressure (PAWP)
Abnormal Low Pressures	**Abnormal High Pressures**
Fluid volume deficit/hypovolemia	Fluid volume overload
Transducer placement above the level of the phlebostatic axis	Mitral stenosis
Constrictive cardiomyopathies	Acute/chronic left ventricular failure
	Cardiac tamponade
	Constrictive pericarditis
	Transducer placement below the level of the phlebostatic axis
	Physiological increases in intrathoracic pressure (coughing, vomiting, seizure)
	Mechanical increases in intrathoracic pressure (positive pressure ventilation, positive end-expiratory pressure, continuous positive airway pressure)

★ *Infection.* Contamination of the PA catheter, insertion site, or pressure monitoring equipment can cause systemic infection and sepsis. Because of this, it is important to pay special attention to sterile technique during manipulation of the PA catheter.

★ *Pulmonary artery rupture.* Although rare, pulmonary artery rupture can result from catheterization of the pulmonary artery. Rupture can occur during insertion or manipulation of the catheter. It can also result from overinflation of the balloon. If the catheter has advanced too far distally into a small PA, normal inflation of the balloon can cause tearing or rupture.

Abnormalities in PA Catheter Pressures

An abnormality in one of the many physiological parameters measured with the PA catheter can be an early indicator of a serious disease process or processes. As a rule, measurement of all hemodynamic pressures is most accurate when obtained at the end of expiration. Changes in intrathoracic pressure during inspiration can impair many of the physiological parameters, reducing the accuracy of the readings. (See Figure 9-26 ■.) Most hemodynamic monitoring systems have alarms that alert critical care personnel when selected physiological parameters exceed predetermined limits.

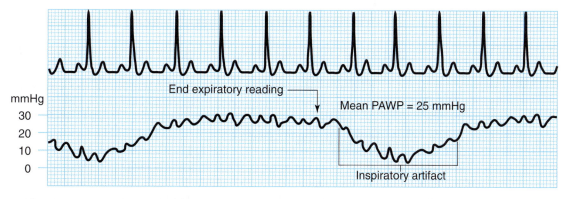

■ Figure 9-26   Respiratory variance.

Abnormalities in the RA waveform usually affect the *a* wave or the *v* wave. An increase in the size of the *a* wave is usually caused by impaired atrial emptying during atrial contraction. This is seen in tricuspid stenosis and right ventricular failure. An elevation in the *v* wave is usually due to incompetence of the tricuspid valve, resulting in regurgitation of blood back into the right atrium during right ventricular contraction.

An elevation in PA pressure usually indicates left ventricular failure, mechanical ventilation, and increased pulmonary vascular resistance. Causes of increased pulmonary vascular resistance include primary pulmonary hypertension, pulmonary embolism, and acute respiratory distress syndrome (ARDS).

Abnormalities in the PAWP waveforms are more common than right atrial waveform abnormalities because left ventricular dysfunction and mitral valve disease are much more common than right ventricular dysfunction or tricuspid valve disease. Pressure changes caused by disorders in the left side of the heart are transmitted back through the pulmonary veins to the tip of the PA catheter. These are reflected as changes in the PAWP waveform.

Elevated PAWP is usually due to left ventricular dysfunction or an increase in circulating blood volume. Mitral stenosis causes large *a* waves while mitral regurgitation causes large *v* waves. Increases in both right and left ventricular diastolic pressures may indicate pericardial tamponade or constrictive pericarditis.

CARDIAC OUTPUT DETERMINATION

The cardiac output (CO) is an important parameter to monitor in the critically ill or injured patient. CO is the volume of blood ejected by the heart in 1 minute and is the function of stroke volume (SV) and heart rate (HR). In the normal state, the CO of the right ventricle and the left ventricle are identical.

Systemic or pulmonary blood flow can be measured by one of two methods: the Fick method and the thermodilution method. With the direct Fick method, oxygen consumption is measured simultaneously with determination of the arteriovenous oxygen difference across the lungs. The Fick principle states:

$$Q\,(L/min) = \frac{O_2 \text{ consumption (mL/min)}}{\text{Arteriovenous oxygen difference (mL/min)}}$$

The cardiac output is calculated by dividing O_2 consumption by the arteriovenous O_2 difference across the lungs (estimated pulmonary venous O_2 content − pulmonary arterial O_2 content). This calculation provides a measure of pulmonary blood flow (Q_p).

Fick method Standard technique for measuring CO in pulmonary blood flow.

The direct **Fick method** is the standard technique for CO measurement. With the direct Fick method, all variables are measured. The indirect Fick method is a noninvasive method for the determination of CO that is based on the substitution of CO_2 rather than O_2 into the Fick equation as follows:

$$CO = VCO_2 \text{ [ml/min]}/(CO_{2art} - CO_{2ven}) \text{ [mL/L]}$$

Expired CO_2 can be used instead of O_2 to make this calculation. In the modern critical care unit, cardiac output is most commonly measured by the thermodilution technique. To achieve this, a thermistor is mounted 4 cm from the tip of the PA balloon-flotation catheter. The catheter is positioned so that the catheter tip and thermistor are located in the pulmonary artery. Cold or room temperature dextrose solution or saline is injected into the proximal port of the PA catheter into the right atrium. When injected, the solution passes a temperature probe in the system and enters the right atrium. The solution flows through the right side of the heart and past the thermistor. The change in temperature as measured at the thermistor is integrated mathematically. The resulting integral is inversely proportional to the volume flow rate past the thermistor. This results in a cardiac output measurement (actually a pulmonary blood flow measurement). Several cardiac output readings are required to obtain a final measurement because of the number of physiological variables. Three consecutive measurements are usually adequate if they vary by 10% or less. The thermodilution technique is less effective when cardiac output is low. In contrast, the Fick method is most dependable when the cardiac output is low and the arteriovenous oxygen difference is large.

HEMODYNAMIC PARAMETERS

The PA catheter is able to generate a large number of hemodynamic measurements. Some are measured while others are calculated. The following discussion will address the more common hemodynamic parameters used in modern critical care.

Body Surface Area

The body surface area is a much better indicator of body size than either height or weight alone. It is a factor in many hemodynamic parameters making it simpler to compare persons of varying sizes and weights:

$$\text{Body surface area (m}^2) = \sqrt{\frac{[\text{Height (cm)} \times \text{Weight (kg)}]}{3,600}}$$

Cardiac Index

To compare persons of varying body weights and sizes, oxygen consumption and cardiac output are commonly divided by the body surface area. This results in a measurement called the **cardiac index** (**CI**) that is expressed in [(liters/minute)/meters^2]. In physiological measurements, the abbreviation Q is often used to indicate cardiac output instead of CO:

$$\text{Cardiac index [(L/min)/m}^2] = \text{Cardiac output (L/min)/Body surface area (m}^2)$$

cardiac index (CI)
compares O_2 consumption and CO of different people.

Central Venous Pressure

The CVP was presented earlier in the discussion of venous pressure monitoring. The CVP can also be measured with the PA catheter through the proximal port, which is normally situated in the vena cava or right atrium. In the normal state, the CVP should be equal to right atrial pressure. The RAP should be the same as the right ventricular end-diastolic pressure (RVEDP) provided there is no obstruction between the right atrium and the right ventricle.

$$\text{CVP} = \text{Right atrial pressure} = \text{Right ventricular end-diastolic pressure}$$

Pulmonary Capillary Wedge Pressure

In the normal state, the pulmonary capillary wedge pressure should be the same as the left atrial pressure (LAP). The LAP should be the same as the left ventricular end-diastolic pressure (LVEDP) provided there is no obstruction between the left atrium and the left ventricle:

$$\text{PCWP} = \text{Left atrial pressure} = \text{Left ventricular end-diastolic pressure}$$

Pulmonary artery capillary wedge pressure provides important information about the left side of the heart.

Stroke Volume Index

The **stroke volume index** (**SVI**) is the amount of blood ejected by the ventricles during one contraction. It can be easily measured with the PA catheter:

$$\text{SVI} = \text{Cardiac index/Heart rate}$$

stroke volume index (SVI)
the amount of blood ejected by the ventricles during one contraction.

Systemic Vascular Resistance

Systemic vascular resistance (SVR) refers to the resistance to blood flow offered by all of the systemic vasculature, excluding the pulmonary vasculature. This is sometimes referred as total peripheral resistance (TPR). SVR is therefore determined by factors that influence vascular resistance in individual vascular beds. Mechanisms that cause vasoconstriction increase SVR, and those that cause vasodilation decrease SVR. Although SVR is primarily determined by changes in blood vessel diameters, changes in blood viscosity can also affect SVR.

SVR can be calculated using the cardiac output (CO), mean arterial pressure (MAP), and central venous pressure (CVP). Using this formula, the SVR is measured in dyne/sec/cm^{-5}:

$$SVR = (MAP - CVP) \div CO$$

Normal SVR (using this formula) is 900 to 1,200 dyne/sec/cm^{-5}. Because CVP is normally near 0 mmHg, the calculation is often simplified to:

$$SVR = MAP \div CO$$

When using this formal calculation, the SVR is measured in Woods' units (1 Woods' unit equals the approximate SVR of a normal person). Normal SVR using this formula is ≈1 Woods' unit.

Systemic Vascular Resistance Index

The systemic vascular resistance index (SVRI), except the pulmonary circulation, is a measure of the vascular resistance caused by the entire systemic circulation. It is proportional to the pressure gradient from the aorta to the right atrium. (A factor of 80 is required for unit conversion.)

$$SVRI = (\text{Mean arterial pressure} - \text{Right atrial pressure}) \times 80 / \text{Cardiac index}$$

SVR is dependent on peripheral resistance, preload, and cardiac output—three components of cardiovascular performance. Calculating SVR is helpful in determining the origin of low perfusion, or shock, states. Table 9–6 lists causes of SVR abnormalities, and Table 9–7 lists indicators for determining shock state using the SVR and CO.

Pulmonary Vascular Resistance

The pulmonary vascular resistance (PVR) is the resistance to flow offered by the pulmonary vasculature from the pulmonary artery to the left atrium. The formula is:

$$\text{PVR (dyne/sec/cm}^{-5}) = (\text{Mean pulmonary artery pressure} - PCWP) \times 80$$

Normal is 100 to 200 dyne/sec/cm^{-5}.

Table 9–6	Causes of Systemic Vascular Resistance Abnormalities	
Causes of Increased Systemic Vascular Resistance		**Decreased Systemic Vascular Resistance**
Vasopressive medications		Antihypertensive medication administration
Catecholamine release		Increased parasympathetic tone
Aortic stenosis		Vasovagal reaction
Activation of the sympathetic nervous system		Distributive shock (neurogenic, septic, anaphylactic)

| Table 9–7 | Determining Shock State by CO and SVR |

Type of Shock State	Cardiac Output	Systemic Vascular Resistance
Cardiogenic	Decreased	Increased
Distributive (septic warm phase)	Increased	Decreased
Distributive (septic late phase)	Decreased	Decreased
Neurogenic (spinal)	Normal	Decreased
Anaphylactic	Normal to decreased	Decreased
Hypovolemic/hemorrhagic	Normal to decreased	Increased
Obstructive	Decreased	Increased

Pulmonary Vascular Resistance Index

The pulmonary vascular resistance index (PVRI) is the resistance to flow offered by the pulmonary vasculature from the pulmonary artery to the left atrium divided by the cardiac index. Because the PCWP is equal to the LAP, the pressure gradient across the lungs can be expressed as (PAP − PCWP):

$$PVRI = (PAP - PCWP) \times 80/Cardiac\ index$$

Pulmonary vascular resistance (PVR) is the calculation of right-sided afterload, or the resistance the right ventricle must overcome to eject blood through the pulmonic valve and into pulmonary circulation for reoxygenation. Also generally speaking, as the PVR continues to rise, the output from the right ventricle falls. PVR abnormalities are listed in Table 9–8.

SYSTEMIC OXYGEN TRANSPORT

Oxygen content is the total amount of oxygen in the blood that is available to the cells. Most of the oxygen (95% to 97%) is reversibly bound to hemoglobin in the form of oxyhemoglobin. The amount of oxygen bound to hemoglobin is reflected in the arterial oxygen saturation. A small amount of oxygen (3% to 5%) is dissolved in the plasma. This component of oxygen transport is determined by the partial pressure of oxygen (PaO_2) as measured in a blood gas sample.

The physiological parameters presented thus far in this chapter have strictly addressed blood flow. However, blood flow is useless if the blood is inadequately oxygenated or if carbon dioxide and other waste products are not being removed. Respiratory gas transport and measurement were discussed in Chapter 7. Many of the respiratory physiological parameters can be integrated into data obtained from hemodynamic monitoring that will provide essential

Table 9–8	Abnormalities in Pulmonary Vascular Resistance
Increased Pulmonary Vascular Resistance	**Decreased Pulmonary Vascular Resistance**
Pulmonary hypertension	Pulmonary vasodilation
COPD (inducing pulmonary HTN)	
Pulmonary embolism	
Positive end-expiratory pressure	
Pulmonic stenosis	

information regarding oxygen delivery, oxygen uptake, oxygen extraction ratio, and mixed venous oxygen saturation.

Oxygen Delivery

Oxygen delivery is the rate of oxygen transport in arterial blood. It is a function of the cardiac output and the arterial blood oxygen concentration. Arterial oxygen delivery (DO_2) can be defined by the following equation where Hb is hemoglobin and SaO_2 is the arterial oxygen saturation. The 1.34 term (mL/g) is the amount of oxygen that can be bound by a single gram of hemoglobin. For the oxygen delivery equation, the factor 1.34 has been multiplied by 10 (13.4) to convert units of measure.

$$DO_2 = \text{Cardiac index} \times 13.4 \times \text{Hb} \times SaO_2$$

Mixed Venous Oxygen Saturation

The saturation of oxygen in the pulmonary artery (SvO_2) can be constantly monitored with a specialized PA catheter. Alternatively, the oxygen saturation in PA blood can be measured by taking a sample of blood from the distal port of the catheter (located in the PA). Blood obtained from the PA is referred to as mixed venous blood as there is some mingling of oxygenated blood with the un-oxygenated blood being transported. The SvO_2 varies inversely with the amount of oxygen extracted from the peripheral microcirculation:

$$SvO_2 = 1/O_2 \text{ extraction}$$

Oxygen Uptake

The oxygen uptake (VO_2) is the rate of oxygen uptake by the systemic microcirculation. It is a product of the cardiac output and the difference in oxygen concentration between arterial and mixed venous blood.

$$VO_2 = \text{Cardiac index} \times 13.4 \times \text{Hb} \times (SaO_2 - SvO_2)$$

Oxygen Extraction Ratio

The oxygen extraction ratio (O_{2ER}) reflects the amount of oxygen taken up from the systemic microcirculation. It is equivalent to the ratio between O_2 delivery and O_2 uptake. This ratio is usually multiplied by 100 and expressed as a percentage.

$$O_{2ER} = (VO_2/DO_2) \times 100$$

CLINICAL INTEGRATION

The role of the pulmonary artery catheter has come under some scrutiny in recent years. The catheter is quite expensive as is the measuring equipment required to support it. In a critical self-appraisal, many researchers have looked at the PA catheter in order to determine whether it really impacted the patient's survival and length of ICU stay. It is clear that many patients, especially those on multiple medications for pressure support, do indeed benefit from PA catheter monitoring. However, the relatively uncomplicated ICU patient can often be managed without placement of a PA catheter.

The PA catheter provides significant information about the performance of the right and left sides of the heart. Using this information, in conjunction with other parameters such as oxygen transport, it is often possible to determine the underlying pathophysiological process involved.

Heart failure occurs when cardiac output falls. In right heart failure, the right ventricle is inefficient as a forward pump. This causes pooling of blood in the systemic venous circulation. Physi-

Table 9–9	Summary of Hemodynamic Indices	
Type of Index	**Calculation of Index**	**Normal Index Values**
Cardiac index (CI)	CO/BSA	$2.5–4.0$ L/min/m^2
Stroke volume index (SVI)	SV/BSA	$33–47$ mL/beat/m^2
Systemic vascular resistance index (SVRI)	$\dfrac{(MAP - RA)}{CI} \times 80$	$1600–2400$ dyne/sec/cm^{-5}/m^2
Pulmonary vascular resistance index (PVRI)	$\dfrac{(PAMP - PAWP)}{CI} \times 80$	$50–270$ dyne/sec/cm^{-5}/m^2

ological parameters that are typically seen during PA monitoring of right heart failure include a decreased CI, decreased RAP, and an elevated PVRI. With left heart failure, the left heart is inefficient as a forward pump and blood pooling occurs in the pulmonary vascular system. Physiological parameters seen with PA monitoring of left heart failure include a decreased CI, an elevated PCWP, and an elevated SVRI. In cardiogenic shock, the heart is unable to meet the physiological demands of the body, resulting in inadequate tissue perfusion. PA monitoring of the cardiogenic shock patient will often reveal a decreased CI, elevated CVP, an elevated SVRI, and a low VO$_2$. Cardiogenic shock can be distinguished from heart failure because of a fall in the oxygen delivery. This results in inadequate tissue perfusion, the hallmark of shock.

Hypotension is an abnormally low arterial blood pressure. Blood pressure is a function of cardiac output and peripheral vascular resistance. Hypotension can result from inadequate fluid within the circulatory system (hypovolemia), from failure of the heart to maintain normal cardiac output (cardiogenic), or from dilation of the peripheral vasculature (distributive). The following PA profiles can help determine the underlying physiological process when confronted by a hypotensive patient:

Hypovolemia	**Cardiogenic**	**Distributive**
Decreased CI	Decreased CI	Increased CI
Decreased CVP	Elevated CVP	Decreased CVP
Elevated SVRI	Elevated SVRI	Decreased SVRI

Shock should be considered if the oxygen uptake (VO$_2$) levels start to decline. This may be one of the earliest indicators of shock. To correct the situation, evaluate the physiological parameters and begin necessary treatment.

A summary of the hemodynamic indices is given in Table 9–9.

PLACEMENT OF A PULMONARY ARTERY CATHETER

In the late 1960s and early 1970s, Drs H. J. C. Swan and William Ganz developed a device (the pulmonary artery catheter) that could measure left ventricular pressures—beyond that of central venous monitoring—at the patient's bedside. Previous to this invention, the only way that ventricular pressures could be assessed was with a left ventriculography, which was only performed in the cardiac catheterization suite.

The pulmonary artery catheter is a long device that measures 110 cm in length. Its balloon-tipped, flow-directed catheter is also a multiple-lumen device that can be used simultaneously as a hemodynamic monitoring line, allowing concurrent administration of intravenous fluids and medications. Each lumen of the PA catheter has a port that opens in a different section of the cardiopulmonary anatomy, and these ports have specific purposes.

Starting with the most distal aspect of the pulmonary artery catheter, the distal port is where the monitoring of the wedge pressure is done. The distal tip has a small balloon that, when inflated, allows the tip of the device to occlude a small pulmonary artery vessel, and the pressure sensor in the tip of the

PA catheter can then calculate the pressure between the catheter's tip and the left side of the heart (pulmonary capillary wedge pressure). The balloon inflation port is equipped with a special 3-cc syringe that will only inject 1.5 cc into the distal balloon. The red-capped thermistor port connects a cardiac output monitor to an internal temperature probe located at the distal tip of the PA catheter. It gives a continuous reading of the patient's core temperature, and is used for the calculation of cardiac output.

The next port moving proximally opens into the right ventricle. This port, when present, allows for medication administration, and on some types of PA lines it also allows for the insertion of a ventricular pacing wire should the patient be in need of intracardiac pacing. The most proximal port on the PA line is the CVP port, which opens into the right atrium and is used for determining central venous pressure.

There is also a universal color scheme in use for identifying the different ports of the PA catheter. Again, starting distally, the line that has the balloon and sensor for floating wedge pressures is red. The next proximal port, the one used for medication administration (that exits into the right ventricle), is clear. Finally, the line with the port used for determining the central venous pressure in the right atrium is blue. Being familiar with all aspects of the pulmonary artery catheter (location of ports, function of lines, and color scheme) will assist the critical care paramedic in efficiently monitoring and using the PA line in critical patients during transport.

The PA catheter has the capability of being advanced through the right atrium and ventricle and into the pulmonary artery. By advancing the catheter past the pulmonic valve and into the pulmonary artery, the critical care paramedic has the ability to "see" pulse pressures within the pulmonary artery. During diastole, pressures within the pulmonary artery and vein, a static column of blood, give the provider a picture of left-sided preload. Because of this, the PA catheter is beneficial for the critical care paramedic in assessing left ventricular pressures and function. The types of patients that the critical care paramedic will most likely see a PA line inserted into are those in need of ongoing significant management, such as patients with ARDS and those with multisystem organ dysfunction syndrome (MODS).

INDICATIONS

★ Diagnosis of shock states and shock types
★ Diagnosis of high-pressure vs. low-pressure pulmonary edema
★ Assessment of vascular tone
★ Assessment of myocardial contractility, including the determination of cardiac output
★ Assessment of intravascular fluid balance
★ Analysis of mixed venous oxygen saturation
★ Monitoring and management of complicated AMI
★ Assessment of hemodynamic response to therapies
★ Management of MODS and/or severe burns
★ Management of hemodynamic instability after cardiac surgery

INSERTION OF THE PULMONARY ARTERY CATHETER

Placement of a PA catheter is very similar to the placement of a central venous catheter, requiring venipuncture and the use of a catheter-over-guidewire technique for placement. The major difference in placing a PA catheter results from its exceptional length. Because the catheter is 110 cm in length, it requires that an introducer be placed initially, and the PA catheter is advanced through the introducer. The introducer, usually a size 8 or 9 French, single-lumen central venous catheter, provides central vascular access and an additional port for intravenous fluid administration. Sites of placement of introducers and PA catheters are similar to central venous catheters, and include internal jugular, subclavian, and femoral veins (although femoral veins, due to their distal location, are commonly not recommended).

Following normal technique, the introducer is successfully placed, and the PA catheter is threaded through the introducer and advanced into the right atrium. Once the distal tip of the

PA catheter is in the RA, the distal balloon is inflated with 1.5 cc of air with the supplied syringe, and then advanced through the tricuspid valve and into the right ventricle (RV). It continues to be advanced through the pulmonic valve into the pulmonary artery, with the balloon still inflated, until the PA catheter "wedges" itself into a branch of the pulmonary artery. When this occurs, right- to left-sided blood flow is blocked and backpressure from the pulmonary vein and left atrium (left preload) is exerted on the tip of the catheter. Generally speaking, as the left ventricle fails (a drop in ejection fraction), there will be a greater amount of blood left in the ventricle, which will then transmit greater pressure into the atrium and eventually into the pulmonary veins. This is why the wedged pressure can give an indication as to the efficiency of the left ventricular activity.

PREPARATION FOR HEMODYNAMIC MONITORING

The placement of an arterial, central venous, or pulmonary artery catheter is a means to obtain and measure hemodynamic pressures within the cardiovascular system. To generate waveforms and their corresponding pressures, the critical care paramedic needs to understand the process of the monitoring setup and placement of the monitoring setup. Setting up a hemodynamic monitoring system includes the following steps:

1. Priming the flush system
2. Connection of the transducer to the monitor
3. Placement of the transducer
4. Zeroing the pressure system to atmospheric pressure
5. Calibration of the pressure system

PRIMING THE FLUSH SYSTEM

The flush system used for hemodynamic monitoring is a high-pressure, low-volume system used to maintain patency of the catheter being monitored. The flush system contains a one-way valve that, when closed, requires pressures greater than the pressures within the catheter being monitored in order to maintain patency. For example, if an arterial catheter is being monitored on a patient with a systolic blood pressure of 180 mmHg, the flush system must be under pressures of greater than 180 mmHg to overcome the patient's blood pressure and flush the catheter system. The use of a pressure infusion bag is helpful to accomplish this. The steps for priming the flush system are as follows:

1. Gather equipment:
   a. 250 to 500 cc 0.9% normal saline solution (some systems may still use heparinized saline per local protocols)
   b. Flush administration setup
2. Tighten all connections within the flush administration set.
3. Expel all air from the flush bag:
   a. Spike the medication administration port of the solution bag with an 18-gauge needle and invert the solution bag; squeeze the air from the solution bag and remove the needle; discard the needle in an approved sharps container.
4. Spike the flush bag and partially fill the drip chamber with solution from the IV bag.
5. Prime the remainder of the flush administration set by releasing the one-way valve to allow flush solution to flow free. Flush all sideports and replace vented caps with supplied nonvented caps at all sideports.
6. Inspect the flush system for air bubbles; if bubbles are visualized, continue to flush the administration set while inverting the set at the level of the transducer.

7. Connect the flush administration set to the catheter being monitored.

    a. Flush the administration set while connecting it to the catheter to eliminate the introduction of air to the catheter.

8. Apply a pressure infuser bag to flush solution; inflate to 300 mmHg.

CONNECTION OF THE TRANSDUCER TO THE MONITOR

Once the flush administration set is primed and connected to the catheter being monitored, the critical care paramedic is now capable of obtaining waveform and pressures within that particular catheter. The next step is to connect the catheter to a monitoring system that will generate a waveform and corresponding pressures. Within the flush administration set is a transducer, or computer chip, that recognizes pressure influences and relays the information through a connecting cable to a monitor for measurement. The transducer contains a pigtail connector that attaches the communicating cable to the monitor being used. If the flush setup at the requesting facility is incompatible with the transport monitoring equipment, the transducer from the critical care paramedic's flush administration setup can be added to the existing flush administration set. By flushing the added transducer, the critical care paramedic can utilize the flush system already connected to the monitored catheter, without the delay in transport that would be necessary if the entire system had to be switched out.

Once the transducer communicating cable connects the flush system transducer and the monitor, the critical care paramedic will be able to visualize the respective waveform of the invasive catheter being monitored. Although the transport monitoring equipment will recognize an invasive catheter and its waveform, it cannot measure its corresponding pressures. A prompt such as "Not Zeroed" or "Not Calibrated" should appear on the screen of the monitor, indicating to the critical care paramedic that the monitor needs further communication with the flush system's transducer before it can generate measurable pressures from the invasive catheter. Correct placement of the transducer and zeroing of the transducer accomplish this.

TRANSDUCER LEVELING AND ZEROING OF THE TRANSDUCER

To get the most accurate pressures within the waveform of any invasive line, the transducer of the flush system must be in a fixed position relative to the system being monitored (the cardiovascular system). The transducer must be placed at a level corresponding to the right atrium in order to provide the most accurate measurements. The phlebostatic axis, located at the fourth intercostal space, midaxillary line, is the approximate level of the right atrium. Placement of the transducer at the phlebostatic axis is best accomplished initially while the patient is supine. Once this is established, the transducer is ready to be zeroed to atmospheric pressure. By turning the transducer OFF to the patient, by way of a stopcock proximal to the transducer, the waveform of the invasive catheter will be lost. Opening the sideport of the shut-off stopcock just utilized and removing the end cap of the sideport will allow the monitor to eliminate any real or perceived atmospheric pressure interference, and the lost waveform will be brought to a "zero" pressure reference line. By depressing the appropriate button on the monitor, which allows the monitor to reset at zero, for a few seconds, the monitor will signal to the critical care paramedic that the invasive pressure catheter has been "zeroed" and is ready to generate not only waveforms, but measurable pressures. Place the end cap back on the sideport and turn the stopcock back to the sideport and open to the patient. Flush the pressure administration line to maintain patency, and observe for the resumption of the waveform and a measurable, accurate pressure.

Keep in mind that zeroing the catheter without the transducer positioned at the phlebostatic axis will result in a correct waveform and an *incorrect* pressure value. If the transducer is above the level of the phlebostatic axis, the monitor will read an inaccurately *low* pressure as pressure is shifted away from the transducer. Conversely, if the transducer is below the level of the phlebostatic axis, the monitor will read an inaccurately *high* pressure, since more pressure is being placed on the transducer due to its location below the right atrium.

It is known that pressure inaccuracies of 0.75 mmHg can occur with catheter position changes of 1 cm above or below the phlebostatic axis. For example, let's say a patient with an arterial catheter is receiving vasoactive drugs for hypotension. A transducer that is placed 30 cm (13 inches) below the phlebostatic axis may produce systolic pressures more than 22 mmHg higher than actual pressures, and titration of vasoactive drugs may not be done when it actually should be. While zeroing the transducer with the patient supine is recommended initially, the critical care paramedic can continue to obtain accurate pressure readings throughout transport as long as the transducer remains in a position that is *dependent on* patient positioning. What this means is that if the transducer is in a fixed position while the patient is supine, and then the patient positioning subsequently changes, an inaccurate pressure reading will occur. For example, if the transducer is zeroed in a supine position, and then the patient is placed in a semi-Fowler's position during flight for patient comfort, the monitored pressures will be inaccurate. If the patient's positioning changes after transducer positioning, the transducer must be rezeroed as previously described after it has been repositioned to the phlebostatic axis. This is not a hard process, but an extremely important one that the critical care paramedic must remember with hemodynamic monitoring.

CALIBRATION OF THE TRANSDUCER WAVEFORM

When the transducer is connected to the critical care transport monitor, it is internally calibrated to the type of catheter and transducer being utilized. If the critical care monitoring equipment has two invasive pressure inputs, the critical care paramedic will need to utilize the appropriate steps of calibrating the unit for both the arterial catheter and the central venous or pulmonary artery catheter. Most monitors on the market currently, once they recognize that an invasive catheter is being monitored, will display waveforms in a default scale, respective of the input to which the connecting cable is attached. The critical care paramedic can rescale the waveform by using the procedure outlined in the manual that accompanies the type of monitoring equipment in use. Most pressure monitoring equipment will also allow the critical care paramedic to change from systolic/diastolic pressure readings to mean pressure readings if central venous pressures are being measured. Finally, the monitoring unit should also allow the critical care paramedic to label or name the waveform on the monitor oscilloscope (ART/CVP/PA/ICP) for documentation purposes.

COMPLICATIONS OF INVASIVE CATHETERS

Despite continuous assessment and care of invasive catheters, complications arise, and the critical care paramedic must be prepared to intervene if complications occur. Although most complications can be routinely corrected, complications of invasive catheters do pose risk of limb loss and, rarely, life threats. (See Table 9–10.)

Complications related to the placement of the introducer are similar to central venous catheter placement and were discussed earlier. Bleeding and ventricular irritability are frequently seen. Pneumothorax and myocardial laceration by the guidewire are less common and can be serious. Complications associated with the advancement of the PA catheter include coiling of the catheter within the right atrium or ventricle, valvular damage to the tricuspid or pulmonic valves, and pulmonary arteriole hemorrhage or infarction if the distal balloon is left inflated. Ventricular irritability and dysrhythmia may also occur during insertion of the PA line as the tip of the catheter passes through the right ventricle. Inflating the distal balloon while it is in the right atrium and leaving it inflated for the duration of the placement procedure can minimize coiling of the PA catheter. Unfortunately, the inflated balloon, while it will assist in directing the PA catheter through the valves of the right heart (tricuspid and pulmonic), also increases the risk for valvular damage to the right heart valves. The risk can be minimized by preprocedure evaluation for the presence of vegetations on the valves, or tricuspid and/or pulmonic valvular insufficiency. This can be accomplished by transthoracic echocardiography (TTE). Additionally, by slowly advancing the catheter through the individual valves and into the respective heart and pulmonary structure, the risk of valvular damage and right ventricular irritation is decreased. Deflation of the distal balloon once placement of the PA catheter is completed can minimize potential pulmonary

Table 9–10 | Complications of Invasive Catheters

Complications	Possible Causes	Interventions
Loss of waveform	Disconnection of communicating cable	Reconnect communicating cable to transducer, monitor; zero transducer at phlebostatic axis.
	Disconnection of flush system from invasive catheter	Control bleeding at catheter site by attaching syringe to invasive catheter; clear flush system or air, blood prior to reconnecting to invasive line; zero transducer at phlebostatic axis.
	Kinking of catheter	Repositioning maneuvers (placing patient supine, semirecumbent if central venous catheter, or extending extremity if arterial catheter); flush system to ensure patency.
	Stopcock positioning OFF to patient or transducer	Check all stopcocks to ensure that stopcocks are OFF to sideports of flush system; flush system to ensure patency.
	Waveform scaled incorrectly	Rescale.
	Clotting of waveform	Remove end cap at most proximal sideport; attach 10-cc syringe; turn stopcock OFF to transducer and attempt to aspirate. If blood return is present, turn stopcock OFF to patient, flush sideport to clear blood, replace end cap and turn stopcock OFF to sideport; observe for resumption of waveform; If no blood return is obtained or if waveform does not return, contact medical direction.
Dislodgement of catheter	Accidental	If complete dislodgement of catheter, apply direct pressure for no less than 10 minutes at insertion site (more if patient is receiving anticoagulant therapy); apply sterile, occlusive dressing over insertion site; contact medical direction.

infarction and hemorrhage. Continued inflation of the distal balloon is *only* indicated during insertion of the PA catheter. Once successfully positioned into a branch of the pulmonary artery, the PA catheter balloon can be inflated intermittently to obtain a PCWP waveform and reading. If the PA catheter happens to migrated further into the PA arteriole than desired, positioning the patient on the left side, flushing the catheter, or pulling the catheter back 1 to 2 cm may assist in removing the deflated catheter tip from a wedged position, and thus allow perfusion around the catheter to continue. (See Table 9–11.) The final component of PA catheters, waveforms, was discussed earlier in this chapter.

The PA waveform should be monitored continuously during care of the patient with a PA catheter in place, because it gives the critical care paramedic information as to where the distal tip of the catheter is located. Ideally, the critical care paramedic should avoid moving or manipulating PA catheters during transport. If the critical care paramedic does not have the ability to monitor the PA waveform during transport, the critical care paramedic can use a reference point to monitor the PA catheter during transport. By visualizing the markings on the PA catheter in relationship to its insertion position relative to the introducer, the critical care paramedic can monitor for the potential changes in its position. As a rough estimate, a PA catheter placed in the internal jugular or subclavian vein is normally positioned at the 45- to 55-cm mark on the PA catheter. A PA catheter placed in the femoral vein is normally positioned at the 65- to 75-cm mark.

The PA waveform should be monitored continuously during care of the patient with a PA catheter in place, because it gives the critical care paramedic information as to where the distal tip of the catheter is located.

INTRA-AORTIC BALLOON PUMP (IABP)

Intra-aortic balloon counterpulsation provides mechanical circulatory support for the failing heart. (See Figure 9-27 ■.) The intra-aortic balloon pump (IABP) consists of a 30-cm polyurethane balloon attached to the end of a large-bore catheter. The device is inserted into the femoral artery in

Table 9–11 Complications of Pulmonary Artery Catheters

Complications	Possible Causes	Intervention
Unable to obtain PCWP waveform	Ruptured balloon	Attempt to inflate distal balloon ×2; if unable to inflate balloon, use PA diastolic pressure to reflect PCWP pressure; contact medical direction.
	PA catheter tip migrated back in pulmonary artery	Attempt repositioning maneuvers (left side lying) while flushing catheter; contact medical direction. DO NOT ATTEMPT TO ADVANCE THE CATHETER.
	Balloon inflated over distal tip of PA catheter ("superwedge")	Remove balloon syringe from port; ensure balloon port is open and allow air to passively deflate; inflate with 0.8–1.2 cc air and observe for PCWP waveform.
Continuous PCWP waveform	PA catheter tip migrated forward into pulmonary artery branch	Attempt repositioning maneuvers (left side lying) while flushing catheters; if unsuccessful, contact medical direction.
	Balloon inflated continuously	Attempt to withdraw from balloon with syringe. If this deflates the balloon, clamp the line to retain negative pressure within the balloon. If this does not work, remove balloon syringe from port; ensure balloon port is open and allow air to passively deflate.
Dampening of waveform	Air in transducer/flush system	Observe for air in flush system; if present, turn proximal stopcock OFF to patient, open side port, and clear flush system of air; close side port, turn ON to patient, and zero transducer at phlebostatic axis.
	Blood clot at distal tip of catheter or within transducer/flush system	Observe for blood in the flush system; if present, flush the system free of blood and zero the transducer at phlebostatic axis; if clot is suspected at distal tip of catheter, attach 10-cc syringe to side port of flush system and attempt to aspirate for blood return; flush system and observe for resumption of PA waveform; if no waveform present, contact medical direction.
Ventricular irritability Observation of right ventricular (RV) waveform	Distal tip migrated back into right ventricle	Observe for change in PA catheter reference point (point where PA catheter enters introducer). If patient is hemodynamically stable, contact medical direction; if patient is hemodynamically unstable, pull PA catheter back until RA waveform is observed or until ventricular irritability ceases; contact medical direction.

the groin with the balloon wrapped tightly around the catheter. The balloons are sized based on the patient's height. Once inserted, the catheter is advanced up the femoral artery into the aorta. It is positioned so that the distal tip of the catheter lies just beyond the origin of the left subclavian artery. Once in place, the balloon wrapping is released, which allows periodic inflations of the balloon.

The intra-aortic balloon is rapidly inflated with 35 to 40 mL of helium at the onset of each diastolic period when the aortic valve closes. (See Figure 9-28A ■ and B ■.) The balloon rapidly deflates at the beginning of ventricular systole just before the aortic valve opens. Inflation of the balloon increases the peak diastolic pressure and displaces intravascular blood toward the periphery. This increase in diastolic pressure increases the mean arterial pressure and thus increases blood flow toward the periphery. Coronary blood flow occurs during diastole. Because of this, coronary blood flow should increase with inflation of the balloon. However, it is important to point out that the IABP only increases coronary blood flow in hypotensive patients. It does not increase coronary blood flow in normotensive patients. Deflation of the intra-aortic balloon also reduces the end-diastolic pressure, thus reducing the impedence to blood flow when the aortic valve opens at the beginning of systole. This effectively decreases ventricular afterload and enhances ventricular stroke volume.

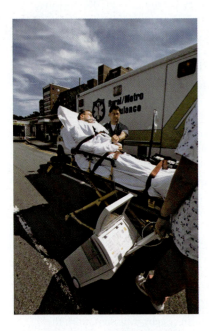

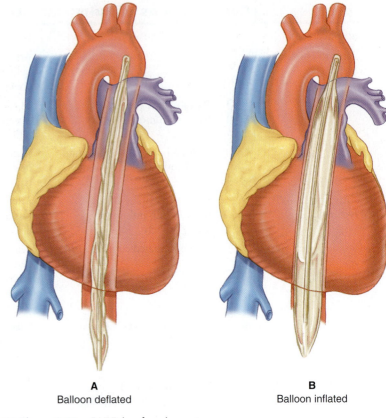

A	B
Balloon deflated	Balloon inflated

■ **Figure 9-28** IABP in place in aorta.

In the nonsurgical setting, the primary indication for intra-aortic balloon counterpulsation is acute myocardial infarction complicated by cardiogenic shock. It is also used for unstable angina that is refractory to other treatment modalities. Most commonly, the IABP is used before and after cardiac bypass and before and after cardiac transplantation. In fact, it is becoming common practice to use the IABP as a bridge to cardiac transplantation. Critical care paramedics will most frequently encounter an IABP in patients being transferred to a tertiary care facility for cardiac surgery and definitive care.

The IABP is a bulky device that inflates and deflates the intra-aortic balloon based on the cardiac cycle. The pump can be adjusted so that it provides counterpulsation with every beat (1:1), every other beat (1:2), or less frequently (i.e., 1:3, 1:4). In addition, the inflation volume is adjustable. (See Figure 9-29 ■.) Although it can be a lifesaving device, the IABP is difficult to insert and has a high complication rate. Some studies indicate that complication rates range from 15% to 45% with serious complications occurring in 5% to 10% of patients. The most common complications are leg ischemia and infection. With leg ischemia, removal of the device is usually sufficient to restore blood flow to the affected leg. The balloon can sometimes migrate up and down the aorta. If it migrates too far inferiorly, it can occlude the renal arteries leading to acute renal ischemia and possibly renal failure. If it slides too far superiorly, it can damage the great vessels or malfunction.

Transport of patients with IABPs in place should be avoided. However, large ground transport units with a stable 110-volt AC power supply can be used to move patients in situations where the transferring physician feels that the risks associated with transfer are outweighed by the benefits of the transfer. IABP settings initiated at the transferring hospital should be maintained unless directed otherwise by the transferring physician or your medical direction physician.

All crew members should be familiar with the basic operations of the intra-aortic balloon pump.

MECHANICAL CIRCULATORY SUPPORT

Selected patients with significant myocardial injury may benefit from a ventricular assist device (VAD). The VAD is a pump that is used to enhance cardiac output in patients where the IABP fails

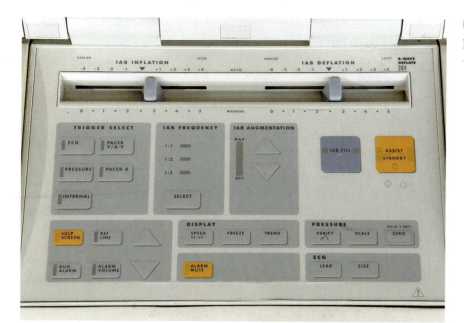

■ **Figure 9-29** IABP control panel. (© *Craig Jackson/In the Dark Photography*)

to provide adequate circulatory support. The VAD is most commonly used following cardiopulmonary bypass surgery. The devices are either pulsatile or nonpulsatile pumps that are placed in parallel with the right ventricle, left ventricle, or both ventricles. These devices may be used short term in patients with left ventricular failure who are expected to recover from myocardial infarction or surgical procedures. Unfortunately, many patients cannot be weaned from a VAD. Long-term devices are still highly experimental and are used as a bridge to cardiac transplantation. In the future, it is hoped that these devices may provide an alternative method of permanent cardiac support.

VADs require an external power source. These can be quite bulky for units used in the critical care unit. Experimental devices utilize power packs that are worn on a belt allowing the patient some freedom of movement. Transport of patients with a VAD must be tailored to the type of device utilized and the requirements of the power source. Always consult with personnel at the transferring hospital. Often, a VAD technician or advanced practice nurse will accompany these patients.

Summary

Hemodynamic monitoring plays a major role in modern critical care. Virtually all major physiological parameters can be monitored using the pulmonary artery catheter, central venous pressure monitor, or arterial pressure catheter. Modern critical care monitoring equipment contains the necessary hardware and software for physiological monitoring. These devices can measure the common physiological parameters and can calculate derived measurements. It is essential that critical care paramedics be intimately familiar with these monitoring devices. In most situations, critical care paramedics will not be called on to establish these monitors. However, they will be expected to continue these monitors during transport in order to provide a seamless record of the critical care patient's hemodynamic status.

Review Questions

1. Name five invasive ways to evaluate hemodynamic status.
2. Why does the critical care provider need to be intimately familiar with hemodynamic monitoring?

3. Most PA lines have three ports. Explain the function of these ports in a distal to proximal order.

4. Explain the purpose for, and the function of, the phlebostatic axis.

5. What would be three potential problems if your patient displayed low CVP, diminished CO, and elevated SVR?

6. If during flight, the patient with a PA line consistently exhibits a wedged waveform on the monitor, despite the cuff being deflated, what should the critical care paramedic do?

7. Name three reasons why the hemodynamic waveform might be lost in a patient with ongoing hemodynamic monitoring?

8. What is meant by the complication of a "superwedge" and how is it avoided?

9. Why might the CI be a better gauge of left ventricular function than the CO?

10. Under what situation should the critical care paramedic withdraw the PA line back to a right atrial waveform?

See Anwers to Review Questions at the back of this book.

Case Study Follow-Up

The following questions pertain to the case study that opened the chapter. Please refer to it in order to respond to these questions. The answers with a brief rationale are provided at the back of this book.

1. Given the case study information, calculate the following values for the patient:
   a. Mean arterial pressure (MAP)
   b. Stroke volume (SV)
   c. Systemic vascular resistance (SVR)
   d. Pulmonary vascular resistance (PVR)
   e. Cardiac index (CI)

2. Given the above information, the critical care paramedic would assess this patient's primary cause of dyspnea and hypoxia to be:
   a. cardiac in origin.
   b. noncardiac in origin.

During transport, this patient becomes even more restless and agitated despite sedation. Assessment by the critical care paramedic reveals:

- Heart rate: 126/minute
- Respiratory rate: 24/minute
- Blood pressure: 140/88 mmHg
- Pulse oximetry: 85%
- Temperature: 37.4° C (99.3° F)
- Pulmonary artery pressure: 54/30 mmHg
- Pulmonary artery wedge pressure: 24 mmHg
- Lungs sounds: Diminished with scattered crackles
- Heart tones: Distant, rapid, regular

3. Given the new assessment findings, calculate the following values for the patient:
   a. Mean aterial pressure (MAP)
   b. Stroke volume (SV)
   c. Systemic vascular resistance (SVR)
   d. Pulmonary vascular resistance (PVR)

4. Given the changes in physical assessment and pressure findings, you would expect the critical care paramedic to:
   a. continue monitoring, given the patient's history of heart disease.
   b. administer vecuronium (Norcuron).

c. administer furosemide, 40 mg intravenously; administer morphine sulfate 4 mg intravenously; and consider the initiation of intravenous nitroglycerine at 10 mcg/min.

d. Increase oxygenation and wean dopamine.

Further Reading

Bledsoe BE, Porter RS, Cherry RA. *Paramedic Care: Principles & Practice,* 2nd ed. Upper Saddle River, NJ: Pearson Prentice Hall, 2005.

Braunwald E *et al. Harrison's Principles of Internal Medicine,* 15th ed. New York: McGraw-Hill, 2001.

Hudak CM, Gallo BM, Morton PG. *Critical Care Nursing: A Holistic Approach,* 7th ed. Philadelphia: Lippincott-Raven, 1998.

Marino PL. *The ICU Book,* 2nd ed. Philadelphia: Lippincott Williams & Wilkins, 1998.

Roberts JR, Hedges JR. *Clinical Procedures in Emergency Medicine,* 3rd ed. Philadelphia: Saunders/Harcourt Brace, 1998.

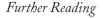

ECG Monitoring and Critical Care

Bob Page, AAS, NREMT-P, I/C

Objectives

Upon completion of this chapter, the student should be able to:

1. Describe how to attach ECG leads to display leads MCL-1 and MCL-6. (p. 248)
2. Describe the management priorities of those patients at risk for complete heart block. (p. 250)
3. Describe simple criteria for determining left versus right bundle branch block. (p. 250)
4. Using a simple chart, determine the presence of fascicular block. (p. 250)
5. Describe the clinical significance of bifascicular blocks. (p. 252)
6. Using leads MCL-1 and MCL-6, differentiate wide-complex tachycardia as either ventricular tachycardia or bundle branch block. (p. 257)
7. Describe criteria for Wolff-Parkinson-White syndrome. (p. 258)
8. Describe the assessment, management, and ECG findings of hyperkalemia and other electrolyte abnormalities. (p. 261)
9. Describe the clinical significance of prolonged QT syndrome. (p. 264)
10. Describe the diagnosis of and clinical implications of a right ventricular infarction. (p. 266)
11. Describe the procedure and lead placement for acquiring a 15-lead ECG. (p. 266)

Key Terms

Case Study

You are called to transport a patient from a rural community hospital to a cardiac tertiary care center. The transport will be by ground and the patient is a direct admission to the CCU. Your patient is a 50-year-old attorney who collapsed into cardiac arrest in the courtroom. He was resuscitated with an AED and transported to the local hospital by BLS ambulance. He has been given three nitro tablets with some relief. Aspirin was also given and a heparin drip has been started. However, he still has some chest discomfort. The hospital 12-lead ECG shows a normal sinus rhythm with a left bundle branch block. The QT interval is within normal limits.

You decide to place the pacer/defibrillator pads on the patient as a precautionary measure. Immediately upon departure you administer 4 milligrams of morphine IV for the patient's chest pain. About 10 minutes into transport, the patient complains of nausea. You are about to administer Zofran when the patient slumps and becomes unresponsive. A quick look at the monitor in lead MCL-1 reveals a wide-complex tachycardia of ventricular tachycardia-type morphology. The patient still has a pulse. With the pads already connected, you perform synchronized cardioversion and convert him back into a sinus rhythm. The patient regains consciousness after a few minutes and again complains of nausea. The Zofran is administered and the patient says he feels a little better. No further medications are administered and patient remains stable for the rest of the transport.

Upon arrival at the tertiary care center, the patient is reevaluated by a cardiologist and ultimately taken to the cardiac catheterization lab where significant occlusion is found and relieved in his left anterior descending (LAD) coronary artery. The patient remains stable throughout his hospital stay and is released to the cardiac rehabilitation unit.

INTRODUCTION

This case illustrates the importance of 12- and 15-lead ECG assessment and the value of monitoring patients in **modified central lead 1 (MCL-1),** which is essentially a bipolar version of lead V1. The cardiac patient who is having an acute coronary syndrome is capable of a number of lethal dysrhythmias—some easy to see (ventricular fibrillation and asystole)—other complex and deceiving for a single-lead II analysis. The critical care provider should be adept at monitoring and interpreting multiple leads for this information. This chapter will focus on understanding assessment findings and developing a monitoring plan for the critical care patient. It is

modified central lead 1 (MCL-1) *a bipolar version of lead V_1. With ECG monitor set to Lead III or V_1, electrode placement is RA (white), LA (black), and LL (red), at the right side, 4th intercostal space.*

Prehospital critical care ECG monitoring should be customized for the condition being treated. It should be a part of your diagnostic arsenal.

designed to give the critical care provider the information needed to be proactive in knowing "what to look for" in a variety of situations.

MONITORING LEADS

In the critical care environment, careful assessment of the baseline 12-lead and 15-lead ECG is imperative to determine patient risk for the transport. In addition, different leads should be selected for monitoring while en route. Whenever possible, the entire 12-lead ECG should remain attached to the patient and ready to record when something changes.

For years, students in health care professions have been taught to monitor patients in lead II. Thus, it didn't take long for this to become a "standard" of sorts. At the time, that was the only lead for which criteria for "naming" the various rhythms had been published. However, rhythm interpretation is based on the P-QRS complex relationships. In all fairness, lead II does give a great look at these relationships. For normal sinus rhythms, sinus tachycardia, and atrioventricular (AV) blocks, lead II is acceptable. However, when the heart rate becomes either fast or slow and the QRS complex becomes narrow or wide, the accuracy of lead II wanes.

It has been consistently shown that leads V1 and V6 (or their bipolar equivalents, MCL-1 and MCL-6) are the best leads for differentiating wide QRS rhythms. The morphology of the QRS complexes as displayed in these leads has been shown to be invaluable in differentiating ventricular tachycardia from supraventricular tachycardia with aberrant conduction. However, recent studies have shown that lead V1 may be even better than MCL-1 in that QRS morphology differed between V1 and MCL-1 in 40% of patients with ventricular tachycardia. Because of this, the American Heart Association does not recommend MCL-1 for diagnosing wide QRS complex tachycardia. However, if you do not have a 12-lead monitor, the MCL-1 lead is better than anything else available. In addition, other findings such as the presence of AV dissociation, QRS width, QRS axis, and the presence of fusion or capture beats can be often be better observed in these leads as well. Multiple-lead monitoring is better than single-lead monitoring, and obtaining a 12-lead ECG during the dysrhythmia is most helpful.

It is important to point out that monitoring in multiple leads is not a new idea. Cardiologists, intensive care nurses, some paramedics, and other critical care providers have always known this. The need for other leads is patient based and reflects common sense. If you choose to monitor the heart, you monitor for changes. In lead II, a change is all you will see. If you monitor in a diagnostic lead, such as V1, MCL-1 (V1) or **modified chest lead 6** (**MCL-6**) (V6), you will see the change and know exactly what it is or isn't. In other words, if a critical patient needs to be monitored, it is a good idea to monitor in a lead that can more clearly identify potentially serious complications.

Modified Chest Lead I is sometimes called the **Marriott lead** or the gold mine lead. To monitor MCL-1 (Figure 10-1 ■):

modified chest lead 6 (MCL-6) *same as V6 on 12-lead. Set monitor to Lead III, rotate LL (red) electrode wire (LL) to the 5th IC space, mid-axillary, left side.*

Marriott lead *same as MCL-1, also know as the "Gold Mine Lead."*

★ Place the RA lead (white) on the right upper arm and the LA (black) lead on the left upper arm.

★ Place the LL (red) lead on the fourth intercostal (IC) space, right side of sternum.

★ Place your monitor in lead III.

★ Or simply choose lead V1 on the 12-lead ECG.

In lead II, the P, QRS, and T waves are usually upright. This is because the positive electrode is inferior to the heart, and the normal electrical flow is downward, making the complexes appear to be positive. (See Figure 10-2 ■.)

In lead MCL-1 (V1), the P waves are usually upside down (but can be biphasic or up), QRS is normally negatively deflected, and the T waves can also be negative or positive. The positive electrode for MCL-1 is located level with or above the atria. Thus, in a normal electrical flow, the impulse is moving away from the electrode causing the negative deflection. (See Figure 10-3 ■.)

Benefits of MCL-1

★ P waves may be easier to see.

★ Looks at the ventricles (an eyewitness).

★ Bundle branch blocks are easy to identify.

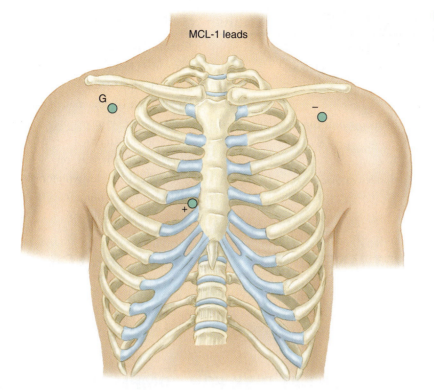

MCL-1 leads

G — +

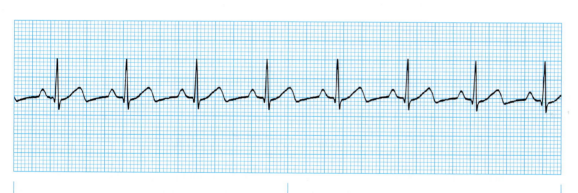

■ **Figure 10-2** ECG lead II strip.

Risks of MCL-1

★ It is not a true V1.

★ Some discrepancy is seen in the morphology of wide-complex tachycardia between V1 and MCL-1.

To monitor MCL-6 (V6 on the 12-lead ECG):

★ Leave the cardiac monitor in lead III.

★ Rotate red electrode wire (LL) to the fifth IC space, midaxillary on the left side (V6 lead).

★ Or simply choose lead V6 on the 12-lead ECG.

Benefits of MCL-6

★ Essentially the same as MCL-1.

★ May be used when dressing is applied to anterior chest (i.e., immediately post-op cardiac surgery) or with anterior chest trauma.

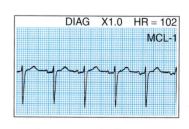

DIAG X1.0 HR = 102
MCL-1

■ **Figure 10-3** ECG lead MCL-1 strip.

Table 10-1	Pretransport ECG Evaluation
Risk Factor	**Conditions to Look For**
Complete heart block	Fascicular blocks
	Bundle branch blocks
	Two or more combination of single blocks
Hemodynamic compromise	Right ventricular infarction
	BBB with QRS duration > 170 ms
	Left ventricular hypertrophy
Sudden cardiac death	Any of the above plus symptomatology
	Prolonged QTc syndrome
	Acute coronary syndrome

PRETRANSPORT EVALUATION OF THE ECG

Before leaving the pickup site, the critical care provider should carefully investigate the 12- and 15-lead ECG for risk factors of various conditions that could occur in transport. The risk factors shown in Table 10–1 must be considered if preparation is to be made for the prevention and management of conditions as they arise.

THE PATIENT AT RISK FOR COMPLETE HEART BLOCK

sinoatrial (SA) blocks
conduction blocks occurring in the SA node and include sinus arrest, sinus pause, and sinus block.

atrioventricular (AV) blocks *conduction blocks that occur in the AV node and include 1st degree and both 2nd degree blocks.*

interventricular (IV) blocks *conduction blocks that occur in the interventricular pathways and include fascicular and bundle branch blocks.*

hemiblock *a block of one of the two fascicles of the left-bundle-branch system.*

left-anterior hemiblock
anterior hemi-fascicular block of the left bundle branch, effectively causes a pathological left-axis deviation.

Generally speaking, when a patient has two separate blocks from any category, he is considered high risk for complete heart block. The three categories include:

★ **Sinoatrial (SA) blocks:** sinus arrest, sinus pause, or sinus block
★ **Atrioventricular (AV) blocks:** traditional first-degree, second-degree type 1 and type 2
★ **Interventricular (IV) blocks:** fascicular blocks, bundle branch blocks

AXIS DEVIATION/HEMIBLOCKS (FASCICULAR BLOCKS)

A marked axis deviation often indicates the presence of a hemiblock. A **hemiblock** is best defined as a block of one of the two fascicles of the left bundle branch system. (See Figure 10-4 ■.) Note that there is a right bundle branch and a left bundle branch that divides into two separate fascicles, or what this book refers to as *hemi-fascicles*. These hemi-fascicles—known as the left anterior and the left posterior—and the right bundle branch make up a trifascicular system.

Impulses can travel in three ways to the ventricles:

★ Right bundle branch
★ Left-posterior hemi-fascicle
★ Left-anterior hemi-fascicle

Blocks in this system can be a precursor to complete heart block. Information on the presence of hemiblock can help the critical care provider determine which patients are at risk for developing complete heart block. Determining the axis is about 98% of the task of detecting the presence of a hemiblock. A hemiblock can also help determine the severity of the patient's acute problem.

LEFT-ANTERIOR HEMIBLOCK

A **left-anterior hemiblock** occurs when the anterior hemi-fascicle of the left-bundle-branch system becomes blocked, thereby causing, in effect, a pathological left-axis deviation. Other clues to a left-anterior hemiblock are a small Q wave in lead I and a small R wave in lead III. A hemiblock can have

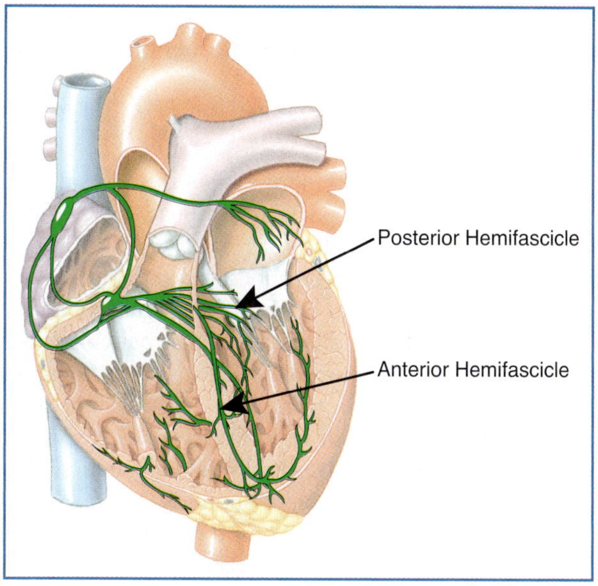

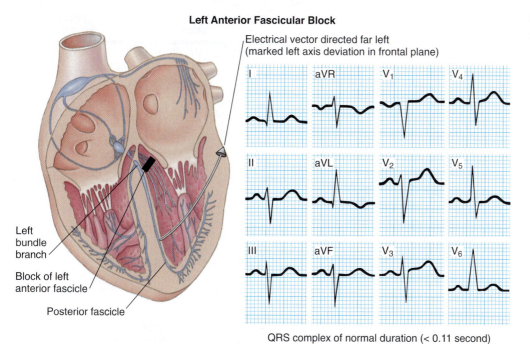

■ **Figure 10-4**
Hemifascicles.

Posterior Hemifascicle

Anterior Hemifascicle

a narrow QRS complex. Thus, a wide complex (>0.12 second) is not the only indicator of an intra-ventricular conduction deficit.

The left-anterior hemi-fascicle is made up of living cardiac conduction system (CCS) cells. In other words, they need a steady blood supply. The LAD branch of the left coronary artery provides blood supply for the anterior hemi-fascicle. Note that the left-anterior hemi-fascicle, is long and thin and is the more common of the hemiblock. (See Figure 10-5 ■.) An anterior hemiblock alone is usu-ally well tolerated by an asymptomatic patient and generally requires no treatment. However, in the setting of an acute myocardial infarction (AMI), an anterior hemiblock may indicate a more serious condition. As discussed earlier, impulses normally travel via three paths to the ventricles. Thus, with an anterior hemiblock, only two are available. This difference has been attributed to an occlusion of a feeder artery that branches off the coronary artery proximally. (See Figure 10-5.) Furthermore,

■ **Figure 10-5**   Left-anterior fascicle hemiblock.

Left Anterior Fascicular Block

Electrical vector directed far left
(marked left axis deviation in frontal plane)

Left bundle branch

Block of left anterior fascicle

Posterior fascicle

I aVR V₁ V₄

II aVL V₂ V₅

III aVF V₃ V₆

QRS complex of normal duration (< 0.11 second)
in all leads. S wave > R wave in leads II, III,
and aVF (marked left axis deviation)

studies have suggested that a person with a conduction-system problem, such as a hemiblock in the setting of an AMI, has a mortality rate four times higher than someone without such a problem.

LEFT-POSTERIOR HEMIBLOCK

left-posterior hemiblock
posterior fascicular block of the left-bundle branch, effectively causes a pathological right-axis deviation.

A **left-posterior hemiblock** occurs when the posterior fascicle of the left-bundle branch system is blocked. For practical purposes, in a patient with cardiovascular symptomatology, a right-axis deviation is indicative of a left-posterior hemiblock. Other clues include small R waves in lead I and small Q waves in lead III. The critical care paramedic should also inspect for the presence of right-ventricular hypertrophy as evidenced by jugular vein distention (JVD), pedal edema, and patient history. However, because the critical care paramedic is targeting the worst condition, posterior hemiblock should be assumed in the patient with signs and symptoms of a myocardial infarction. The posterior hemiblock is worse than the anterior hemiblock. Note that the posterior hemi-fascicle is thicker than the anterior hemi-fascicle, thus having more cells and needing a richer supply of blood. (See Figure 10-5.) Dead cells do not conduct impulses. To maintain constant perfusion of these fascicles, a redundant blood supply is required from two different coronary arteries: the right coronary artery and the circumflex. If both coronary arteries are blocked, then an extensive coronary occlusion has occurred. In one study of 3,160 patients with AMI, only 70 had posterior hemiblocks. Of those, 14% died before they left the hospital. Of the remaining patients who were followed, 63% had persistent cardiac problems, 22% developed congestive heart failure (CHF), 13% had another MI, and the last 2% died within 20 days to 24 months. In other words, a posterior hemiblock with an MI is a serious sign. In such circumstances, it may be necessary to combat both conduction problems and, possibly, hypotension/cardiogenic shock. (See Figure 10-6 ■.)

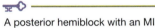

A posterior hemiblock with an MI is a serious sign.

CLINICAL SIGNIFICANCE OF A HEMIBLOCK

The clinical significance of a hemiblock can be summarized as follows:

★ Mortality rate is four times higher for patients having an AMI with a hemiblock than those without a hemiblock.

■ Figure 10-6 Left-posterior fascicle hemiblock.

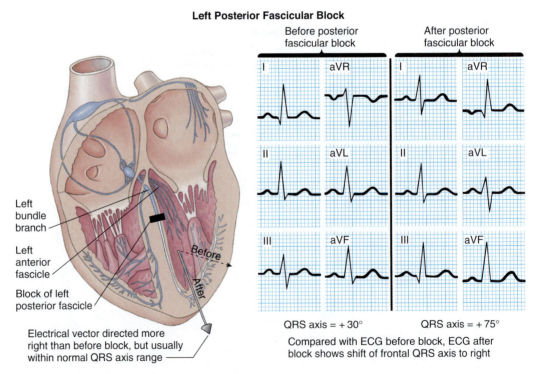

Left Posterior Fascicular Block

Before posterior fascicular block

After posterior fascicular block

I   aVR   I   aVR

II   aVL   II   aVL

III   aVF   III   aVF

QRS axis = +30°   QRS axis = +75°

Compared with ECG before block, ECG after block shows shift of frontal QRS axis to right

Left bundle branch

Left anterior fascicle

Block of left posterior fascicle

Before

After

Electrical vector directed more right than before block, but usually within normal QRS axis range

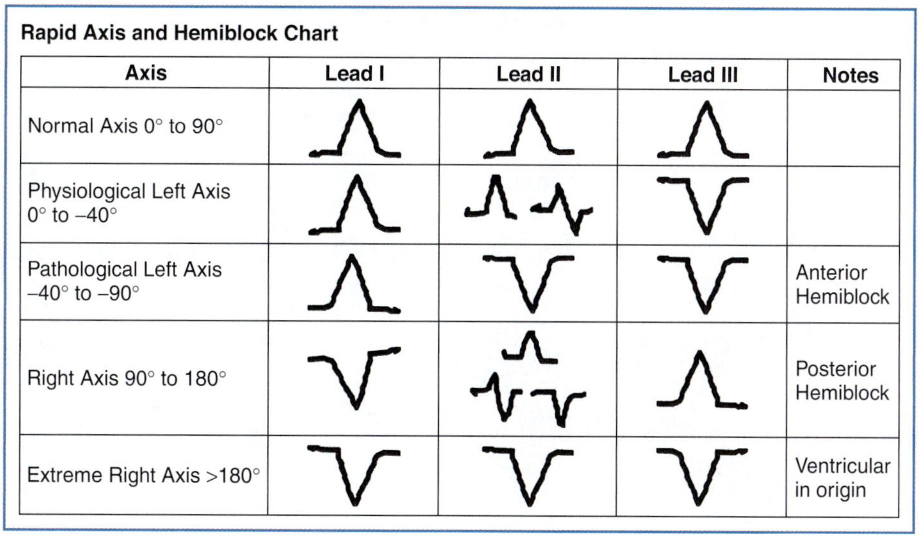

Rapid Axis and Hemiblock Chart

Axis	Lead I	Lead II	Lead III	Notes
Normal Axis 0° to 90°				
Physiological Left Axis 0° to −40°				
Pathological Left Axis −40° to −90°				Anterior Hemiblock
Right Axis 90° to 180°				Posterior Hemiblock
Extreme Right Axis >180°				Ventricular in origin

■ **Figure 10-7** Rapid axis and hemiblock.

★ Risk factor for complete heart block; if another block is present with a hemiblock, the patient is at high risk for complete heart block.

★ In the setting of an AMI, can indicate proximal artery occlusion.

RAPID AXIS AND HEMIBLOCK DETERMINATION

Rapid Axis and Hemiblock Chart

It has been said that one should never commit to memory what can be written down. The rapid axis and hemiblock chart is designed to quickly allow the clinician to determine the presence of axis deviation and hemiblock. (See Figure 10-7 ■.) The chart can be used in two ways. If a three-lead monitor or other machine that does not provide axis information is being used, the following method applies. Look at leads I, II, and III on the 12-lead. Determine whether the QRS complex is more positively or negatively deflected in each lead. Compare your findings to the rapid axis and hemiblock chart to identify the axis and hemiblock. If a 12-lead machine is being used and provides the numerical angle, use this information.

Calculated Axis Angle

Recall that the 12-lead machine can calculate the axis information accurately. (See Figure 10-8 ■.) The number to look for is the R axis or QRS axis. With this information available, the rapid axis and hemiblock chart can be used to identify the axis deviation. For example, suppose that the machine shows an R axis of −53; the chart shows that −53 is in the range of −40 to −90: a pathological left-axis deviation and an anterior hemiblock. This number represents the exact geometrical axis angle based on the hexaxial system.

BUNDLE BRANCH BLOCKS

A **bundle branch block** (BBB) is a block of either the right or left bundle branch system. (See Figures 10-9 ■ and 10-10 ■.) A working knowledge of bundle branch blocks will help the clinician determine the following:

1. Who is at risk for hemodynamic compromise?
2. Who is at risk for complete heart block?

Vent. rate	64	BPM
PR interval	192	ms
QRS duration	82	ms
QT/QTc	398 / 404	ms
P–R–T axes	46 −53 63	

■ **Figure 10-8** ECG description chart.

bundle branch block (BBB) *block of either the right or left bundle branch system, associated with an MI, congenital defects, ischemic tissue, or RF ablation.*

■ Figure 10-9   Right bundle branch block.

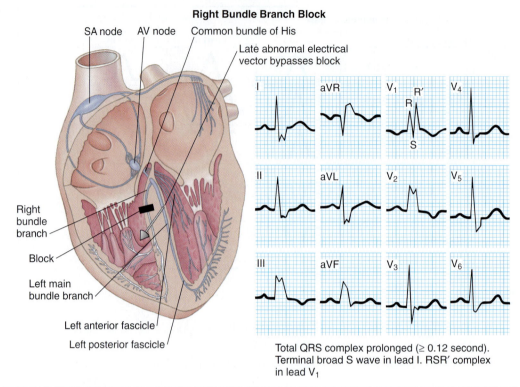

Right Bundle Branch Block

SA node   AV node   Common bundle of His

Late abnormal electrical vector bypasses block

Right bundle branch

Block

Left main bundle branch

Left anterior fascicle

Left posterior fascicle

Total QRS complex prolonged (≥ 0.12 second). Terminal broad S wave in lead I. RSR′ complex in lead V_1

■ Figure 10-10   Left bundle branch block.

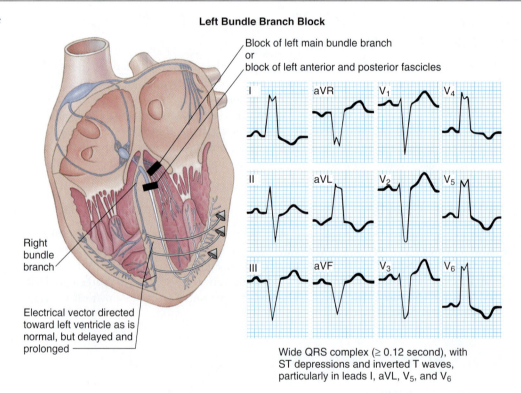

Left Bundle Branch Block

Block of left main bundle branch
or
block of left anterior and posterior fascicles

Right bundle branch

Electrical vector directed toward left ventricle as is normal, but delayed and prolonged

Wide QRS complex (≥ 0.12 second), with ST depressions and inverted T waves, particularly in leads I, aVL, V_5, and V_6.

WHAT HAPPENS DURING A BUNDLE BRANCH BLOCK?

A block of one of the fascicles of the bundle branch system can be caused by myocardial infarction (old or new), congenital defects, or ischemic tissue. In a few cases, people may have acquired a BBB secondary to a procedure known as RF (radio-frequency) ablation. This procedure is performed to destroy cells (which happen to be part of the bundle branch) that cause ectopy or dangerous rhythms such as ventricular tachycardia. Some BBBs only occur during fast heart rates and can

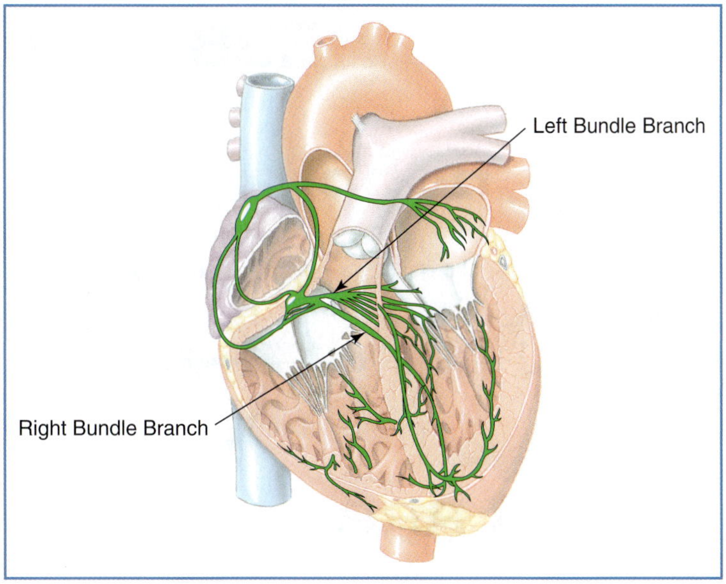

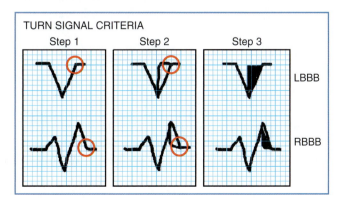

■ **Figure 10-11** Bundle branch anatomy.

Left Bundle Branch

Right Bundle Branch

have defined "start and stop" rates. Nonetheless, a bundle branch block represents an increased risk for developing complete heart block, hemodynamic compromise, and, of course, sudden death when associated with an MI due to the proximal occlusion of the LAD coronary artery.

As the impulse coming from the AV node travels down the bundles, it reaches the tissue that is blocked on one side. The impulse stops on that side. The other side proceeds to depolarize as normal. (See Figure 10-11 ■.) The wave of depolarization eventually works its way across to the blocked side, causing a delayed depolarization. As you might guess, the ventricles contract out of sync. The more diseased the muscle, the longer it will take to completely depolarize the heart. If the total time to depolarize the ventricles is longer than 120 ms or 0.12 second, then criteria is met for a bundle branch block.

Since the left side has two fascicles and the right side has just one, a left bundle branch block has a higher mortality rate. It is important for the acute care provider to understand bundle branch blocks and be able to rapidly identify and differentiate left from right. Furthermore, a left bundle branch block makes it almost impossible to diagnose ST segment elevation as an MI.

THE "TURN SIGNAL CRITERIA" FOR BUNDLE BRANCH BLOCKS

The turn signal criteria were first suggested by Mike Taigman in his book *Taigman's Advanced Cardiology (In Plain English)*. These criteria are incredibly accurate and have been proven clinically.

MCL-1 (V1) (or any of the precordial leads) can be used to detect bundle branch blocks. This lead looks across the ventricles and can see both bundle branches, thereby acting as an eyewitness to an accident. To run MCL-1 (V1), leave your lead select in lead III, and place the red electrode in the fourth intercostal space to the right of the sternum. To diagnose bundle branch blocks, use the turn signal criteria. (See Figure 10-12 ■.) Note, however, that this method works only in lead

TURN SIGNAL CRITERIA
Step 1   Step 2   Step 3

LBBB

RBBB

■ **Figure 10-12** Turn signal criteria. (1) Find and circle and the J point. (2) Draw a line back toward the complex in the direction of the terminal deflection. (3) Shade in the triangle, or arrowhead. If the arrowhead points up, it is a right bundle branch block (RBBB). If it points down, it is a left bundle branch block (LBBB).

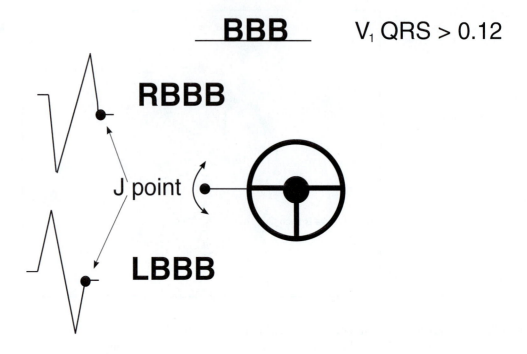

MCL-1 (V1) or the precordial leads and that the QRS must be >0.12 second to 20 ms, or three small squares on the ECG paper. To use the system:

1. First, determine that the QRS complex is consistently greater than 0.12 second throughout the ECG. Again, you can do this best by viewing the QRS duration in MCL-1 or the precordial leads.

2. Second, view the QRS of V1 (or MCL-1). It lies immediately over the right ventricle and provides the best view of the superior aspect of the interventricular septum.

3. Third, identify the J point of the QRS—the junction between the end of the QRS and the beginning of the ST segment.

4. Finally, draw a horizontal line from the J point to an intersecting line of the QRS, or to the beginning of the QRS. This will produce a triangle pointing either up or down. If the triangle points up, it indicates a right bundle branch block (RBBB). (If you push up on a vehicle's turn signal, the signal lights indicate a right turn.) If the triangle points down, it indicates left bundle branch block (LBBB). (If you pull down on a vehicle's turn signal, the signal lights indicate a left turn.) (See Figure 10-13 ■.) Figure 10-14 ■ shows a right bundle branch block. Note the RSR'complex and the positive terminal deflection in lead MCL-1 (V1). The QRS duration is 144 ms. Figure 10-15 ■ illustrates a left bundle branch block. Note the negative terminal deflection in lead V1 (MCL-1). The QRS complex is 144 ms. Also note that lead I shows a notched R wave, another indicator of a left bundle branch block.

RATE-DEPENDENT BUNDLE BRANCH BLOCKS

A major reason to monitor in MCL-1 is to spot a rate-dependent bundle branch block when it occurs. Atrial fibrillation and atrial flutter can develop this condition as heart rate increases. Normally, atrial contraction (referred to as "atrial kick") can account for up to 25% of cardiac output. Thus, decreasing cardiac output due to the lack of an atrial kick, at a certain rate, can result in ischemia and can lead to a bundle branch block. Care should be taken not to mistake this for ventricular tachycardia (VT) because therapy for VT could cause a rapid demise of the patient. Recognize the criteria for BBB (RSR',

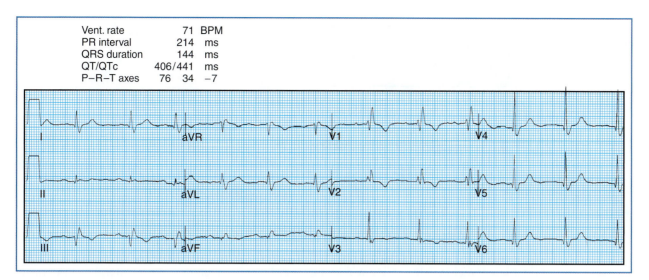

Vent. rate	71	BPM
PR interval	214	ms
QRS duration	144	ms
QT/QTc	406/441	ms
P–R–T axes	76 34 −7	

■ **Figure 10-14** ECG of right bundle branch block.

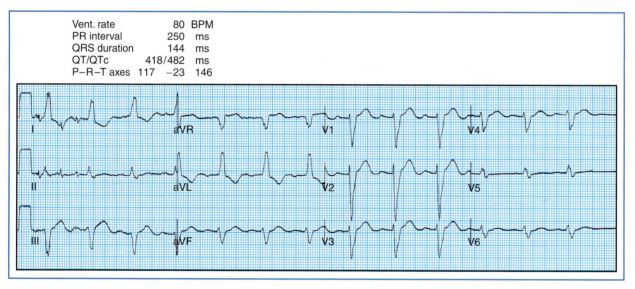

Vent. rate	80	BPM
PR interval	250	ms
QRS duration	144	ms
QT/QTc	418/482	ms
P–R–T axes	117 −23 146	

■ **Figure 10-15** ECG of left bundle branch block.

or QRS complex) rapidly. Look carefully for an irregular rhythm. That would be a tipoff for A-fib (atrial fibrillation) and therefore BBB when the complex turns wide.

For critical care monitoring in MCL-1, here are a couple of simple criteria: If you see an RSR' complex that is more than 120 ms wide, it is diagnostic for RBBB (and not VT). Similarly, if you see a QRS complex that is wider than 120 ms, it is diagnostic for a LBBB (and not VT). These criteria are specific for lead MCL-1 (V1). Lead II in these cases would be the wrong lead to be monitoring.

WIDE-COMPLEX TACHYCARDIA: SINGLE-LEAD MORPHOLOGY FOR VT

Wide-complex tachycardia is one of the most challenging ECG situations facing critical care paramedics. However, using established criteria, one can determine the cause of wide-complex tachycardia using a single ECG lead.

Figure 10-16 Ventricular tachycardia: QRS positive in MCL-1 (V1), with three variables.

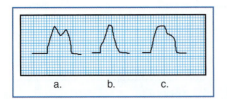

a.   b.   c.

LEAD MCL-1 (V1) MORPHOLOGY CRITERIA

If MCL-1 (V1) is an upright complex (Figure 10-16 ■), it will have these characteristics:

1. Taller left peak than right ("BIG mountain little mountain")
2. Single upright peak ("steeple sign")
3. Single peak with a slur ("fireman's hat")

Lead MCL-1 (V1) morphology has a 94% diagnostic accuracy if it looks like one of these examples. Thus, if they look like this in wide-complex tachycardia, treat for VT. If the morphology does not meet any of these criteria, try examining lead V6.

If MCL-1 (V1) is a negative deflection (Figure 10-17 ■), it will have these characteristics:

1. Fat "R" wave (The R wave is more than 40 ms, one little square wide.)
2. Slurring or notching to the initial downstroke (Q or S wave)

Figure 10-17 Ventricular tachycardia: QRS negative in MCL-1 (V1).

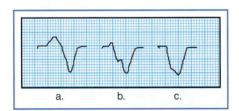

a.   b.   c.

If it meets this criterion, treat as VT. If it does not or you are unsure, go to V6. (See Figure 10-18 ■.)

1. A predominantly negative complex (QS complex) (when you get to this point) is VT.
2. Rare cases show a fat Q wave in a biphasic complex.

Figure 10-18 Lead V6 (MCL-6) morphology criteria.

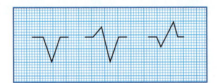

SOME TIPS ABOUT MONITORING

With your advanced knowledge of using different leads, it is important that you set your machine up correctly to monitor the patient. If you have a monitor that will display several leads or channels at once, select leads V1 and V6 and monitor those leads continuously. (See Figure 10-19 ■.) For quick reference, a wide-complex tachycardia that has a predominately positive deflection in lead MCL-1 and a mostly negative deflection in lead MCL-6 (V6) is most likely VT!

PREEXCITATION SYNDROMES

Wolff-Parkinson-White syndrome (WPW) *pre-excitation syndrome characterized by errant excitation of the Bundle of Kent, causing early depolarization.*

One renowned dysrhythmia, **Wolff-Parkinson-White (WPW) syndrome,** is caused by the presence of an accessory conduction pathway. In WPW, the impulse from the atria does not travel through the AV node to the ventricles. Instead it takes an accessory pathway commonly known as the bun-

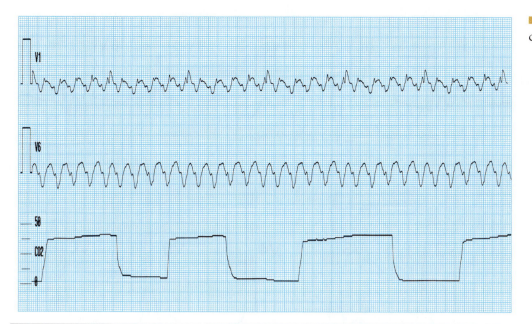

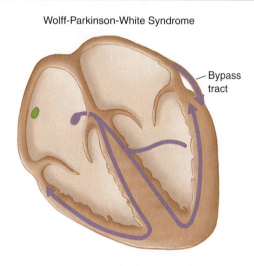

Wolff-Parkinson-White Syndrome

Bypass tract

■ **Figure 10-20** Wolff-Parkinson-White bypass tract.

dle of Kent. By bypassing the AV node, there is nothing to slow the impulse to the ventricles. (See Figure 10-20 ■.) The result is a preexcitation of the ventricles, which causes them to depolarize and contract before they have time to completely fill. This preexcitation syndrome results in a classic ECG finding of delta waves and short PR interval (less than 120 ms). (See Figure 10-21 ■.) The accessory pathway is unreliable and will allow impulses to pass from the ventricles back to the atria causing it to depolarize, thus completing a reentry pathway. The result could be a very fast tachycardia that can quickly become hemodynamically unstable.

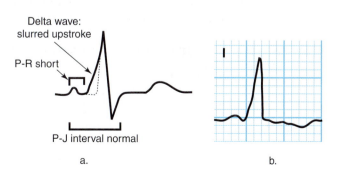

Delta wave: slurred upstroke

P-R short

P-J interval normal

a.

b.

■ **Figure 10-21** Delta wave of Wolff-Parkinson-White.

Preexcitation Syndromes **259**

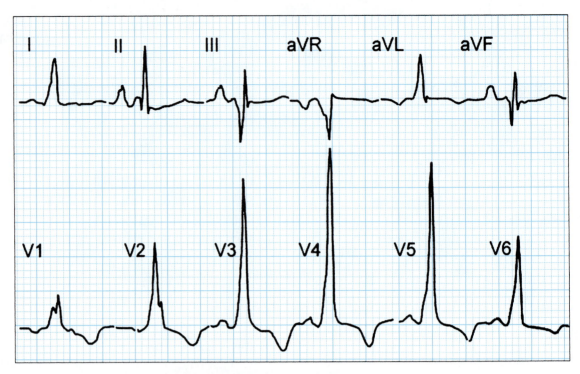

Figure 10-22 12-lead of Wolff-Parkinson-White.

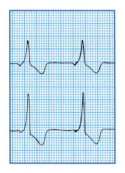

Figure 10-23 Delta waves characteristic of Wolff-Parkinson-White.

It is important to note again that the best leads to appreciate WPW's "delta waves" are the anterior/lateral leads of a 12-lead (leads V4-V6, I, aVL). (See Figure 10-22 ■.) Notice that lead II offers little or no help in recognition. Unfortunately, this is a common occurrence.

Remember that WPW can occur in almost any supraventricular rhythm and frequently occurs with atrial fibrillator and can lead to a serious tachydysrhythmia. (See Figure 10-23 ■.)

MANAGEMENT OF WPW WHEN THE EJECTION FRACTION IS ABOVE 40%

Antidysrhythmics effective in the treatment of WPW when the ejection fraction is greater than 40% include procainamide and amiodarone. Avoid adenosine, beta-blockers, calcium channel blockers, and digoxin. Adenosine, while listed as a contraindication in some guides, has been used in electrophysiology labs to *induce* WPW for mapping and ablation purposes.

MANAGEMENT OF WPW WHEN THE EJECTION FRACTION IS BELOW 40%

As the heart rate increases with WPW, the ventricular filling time falls, thus decreasing ventricular filling. This can lead to a reduced ejection fraction. Patients will tolerate a falling ejection fraction based upon their underlying health status. When patients with WPW start to decompensate, emergent synchronized cardioversion is indicated. In less severe cases, there may be a role for a trial of an antidysrhythmic such as procainamide first. Regardless, when the patient decompensates, emergency countershock is indicated.

LOWN-GANONG-LEVINE

Lown-Ganong-Levine syndrome (LGL) *pre-excitation syndrome characterized by possible existence of intra- and/or para-nodal fibers that bypass all or part of the (AV) node.*

The **Lown-Ganong-Levine syndrome (LGL)** is another type of preexcitation syndrome similar to WPW. However, in LGL, there is a different accessory tract called *James's fibers*. These fibers are actually an aberrant continuation of the posterior internodal tract. They serve to electrically connect the atria to the bundle of His. Thus, atrial impulses bypass the AV node resulting in preexcitation and tachycardia. Clinically, LGL is characterized by a short PR interval and a normal QRS (no delta wave).

ECG AND ELECTROLYTES

Electrolytes are extremely important to the body's electrical system. (See Figure 10-24 ■.) They are responsible for the heart's polarity changes that are picked up by the ECG machine. (See Table 10–2.) Most criteria for interpreting electrolyte changes are based on the assumption of homeostasis, the normal electrolyte ranges for an individual. The electrolytes potassium and calcium have

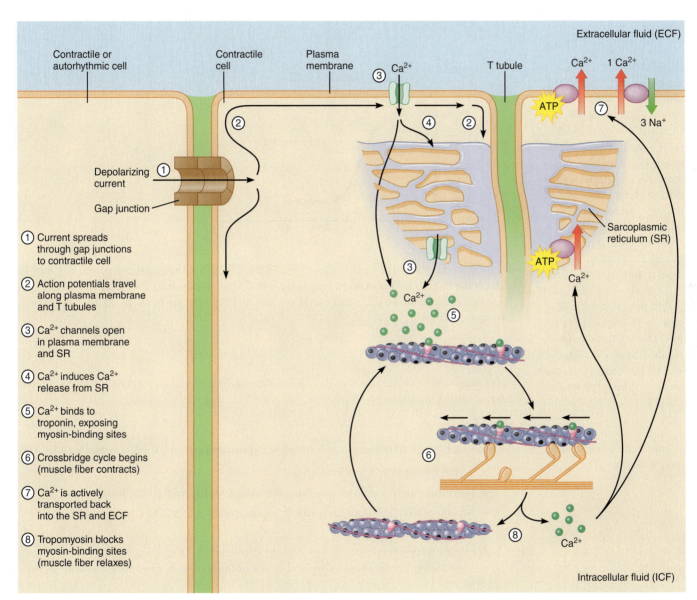

■ Figure 10-24   Excitation—contraction coupling in cardiac muscle. Cardiac muscle is excited by the spread of depolarizing current through gap junction. The depolarization triggers the opening of calcium channels in the plasma membrane and sarcoplasmic reticulum. Calcium binds to troponin, enabling the crossbridge to occur. To terminate contraction, calcium is pumped out of the cytosol into the sarcoplasmic reticulum and interstitial fluid. *(Fig. 14-13, p. 430, from* Principles of Human Physiology, *2nd ed., by William J. Germann and Cindy L. Stanfield. Copyright © 2005 by Pearson Education, Inc. Reprinted by permission.)*

Table 10–2 | Pacemaker Cell Action Potential

Autorhythmic cell potential change	Ion channel gating	Ion movement
Pacemaker potential		
Initial period of spontaneous depolarization to subthreshold	Funny channels open	Sodium moves in, potassium moves out
Latter period of spontaneous depolarization to threshold	T-type calcium channels open	Calcium moves in
Rapid depolarization phase of action potential	L-type calcium channels open	Calcium moves in
Repolarization phase of action potential	Potassium channels open	Potassium moves out

Source: Table 14–1, p. 428, from *Principles of Human Physiology*, 2nd ed., by William J. Germann and Cindy L. Stanfield. Copyright © 2005 by Pearson Education, Inc. Reprinted by permission.)

■ **Figure 10-25** The cardiac action potential. An action potential recorded from a ventricular muscle cell. P_{Na} increases during phase 0 (green) and decreases during phase 1 (yellow). P_{Ca} increases and P_K decreases during phase 2 (orange) and then P_{Ca} decreases and P_K increases during phase 3 (purple). During phase 4 (blue), all ion channels are in their resting state (P_K high, P_{Ca} and P_{Na} low). *(Fig. 14-12, p. 428, from* Principles of Human Physiology, *2nd ed., by William J. Germann and Cindy L. Stanfield. Copyright © 2005 by Pearson Education, Inc. Reprinted by permission.)*

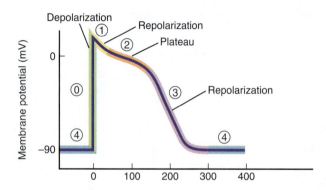

hypokalemia *abnormally low potassium.*

strong influences over the cardiac cycle. (See Figure 10-25 ■.) Abnormalities sometimes may be seen on the ECG. It is important to note that an ECG is not a substitute for blood studies to determine the actual serum level. These criteria are designed as guidelines to aid in discovering possibly covert conditions.

POTASSIUM (K⁺)

Potassium is an important cation in the cardiac impulse. Abnormalities in potassium levels can have adverse cardiac effects.

Hypokalemia

An abnormally low level of potassium is known as **hypokalemia** and has the following characteristics:

★ Serum levels below 3.5 to 5 mEq/L
★ Most commonly caused by vomiting, diarrhea, diuretics, and gastric suctioning
★ Accompanied by hypomagnesemia, or low magnesium, which has the same ECG characteristics
★ Muscle weakness and polyuria as common signs and symptoms
★ Digitalis toxicity resulting in hypokalemia, causing serious dysrhythmias (torsade de pointes)
★ Atrial flutter, heart blocks, and bradycardia

ECG changes are associated with potassium abnormalities. Figure 10-26 ■ illustrates hypokalemia-induced ECG changes including:

★ ST segment depression
★ T waves flattened or joined with U waves

- ★ U waves getting larger than the T waves as the potassium level falls
- ★ QT interval appearing to lengthen as T combines with U
- ★ Increasing PR interval

Needed actions for worsening hypokalemia include:

- ★ Monitor the ECG.
- ★ Increase dietary intake of potassium.
- ★ Begin careful parenteral potassium replacement.

Hyperkalemia

Abnormally elevated potassium, a condition known as **hyperkalemia,** has the following characteristics (Figure 10-27 ■):

- ★ Serum levels above the normal range
- ★ Most commonly caused by renal failure
- ★ Possible sinus node failure at 7.5 mEq/L
- ★ VF, or asystole, at 10 to 12 mEq/L

ECG changes associated with hyperkalemia include:

Mild cases (<6.5 mEq/L):

- ★ Tall, tented, peaked T waves with a narrow base (QTc still normal)
- ★ Best seen in leads II, III, V2, and V4
- ★ Normal P waves

Moderate cases (<8 mEq/L):

- ★ Widening QRS
- ★ Broad S wave in V leads
- ★ Left-axis deviation
- ★ ST segment is gone, contiguous with the peaked T wave
- ★ Flattening and diminishing P wave

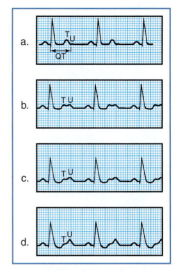

■ **Figure 10-26**
Hypokalemia-induced ECGs. (a) shows normal serum potassium levels (3.5 to 5.0 mEq/L); (b) shows about 3.0 mEq/L; (c) shows 2.0 mEq/L; and (d) shows 1.0 mEq/L.

hyperkalemia *abnormally elevated potassium.*

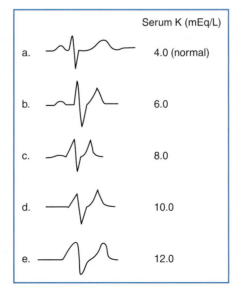

■ **Figure 10-27**
Hyperkalemia ECG patterns.

Severe cases (> 8 mEq/L).

★ P waves disappear

★ Sine waves

Management of Hyperkalemia

★ Stabilize excitable membranes with calcium chloride or calcium gluconate.

★ Cause intracellular ion-shift with sodium bicarbonate, insulin and glucose, beta blocker, or albuterol.

★ Remove it from the body with dialysis, Kayexalate.

Critical Care ECG Tip: Wide-complex tachycardia in renal patient = hyperkalemia!

■ **Figure 10-28** Calcium-related ECG patterns. (a) shows normal QT interval within a range of 0.32 to 0.39 sec for heart rate of 80; (b) shows hypocalcemia, a QT interval below normal range; and (c) shows hypocalcemia, a QT interval above normal range.

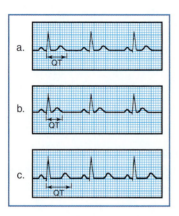

CALCIUM

Figure 10-28 ■ illustrates characteristic calcium-related ECG patterns. On the ECG, hypercalcemia is suggested by a shortened QT interval (QTc for heart rate). Hypocalcemia is suggested by a prolonged QT Interval (QTc for heart rate).

EFFECTS OF DRUGS ON QT INTERVAL

QT interval *an indirect measure of ventricular repolarization.*

corrected QT interval (QTc) *QT interval adjusted for current heart rate.*

The **QT interval** is an indirect measure of ventricular repolarization. Acute increases in the QT interval can be observed in multiple clinical situations and can be associated with an increased risk of syncope and sudden death from *torsade de pointes*–type ventricular tachycardia. Clinical situations that may lead to QT prolongation include initiation, increased dosage or overdosage of QT-prolonging drugs, ischemia/infarction, electrolyte disorders, sudden decreases in heart rate, and acute neurologic events.

From an electrophysiological standpoint, the QT interval represents the time from the start of depolarization of the ventricles to the end of ventricular repolarization. This is functionally the refractory period. The QT interval is measured from the start of the QRS complex to the end of the T wave. This distance is done on the vital signs part of the 12-lead ECG. Note on the 12-lead the QT/QTc interval: The QT is the measurement; the QTc represents the **corrected QT interval (QTc)** for the current heart rate. (See Figures 10-29 ■ and 10-30 ■.) It is determined in the following formula:

Vent. rate		81	BPM
PR interval		194	ms
QRS duration		100	ms
QT/QTc	446/512		ms
P–R–T axes	71	−48 71	

$$QT_c = \frac{QT}{\sqrt{R - R'}}$$

■ **Figure 10-29** Example of QT measurement.

where QTc is the QT interval corrected for rate, the RR is the interval from the onset of one QRS until the next (measured in seconds). In other words, QTc equals the QT interval divided by the

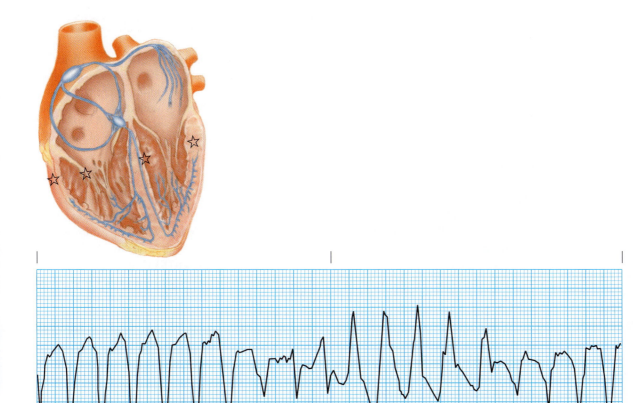

■ Figure 10-30   Torsades de pointes.

square root of the respiratory rate (RR) interval. To determine whether a QT is prolonged, refer to Table 10–3.

Some medications that the patient takes or that we give can also prolong QT intervals. These include amiodarone, procainamide, haloperidol, erythromycin, droperidol, and some tricyclic antidepressants. The critical care provider should carefully evaluate QT intervals and understand what can and cannot be determined from it.

Table 10–3	QTc Interval	
Heart Rate	**R-R Interval**	**QTc and Range**
40	1500	460 (410–510)
50	1200	420 (380–460)
60	1000	390 (350–430)
70	860	370 (330–410)
80	750	350 (320–390)
90	670	330 (300–360)
100	600	310 (280–340)
120	500	290 (260–320)
150	400	250 (230–280)
180	330	230 (210–250)
200	300	220 (200–240)

WHO IS AT RISK FOR HEMODYNAMIC COMPROMISE?

The critical care provider must be on the lookout for conditions that place the patient at risk for hemodynamic compromise. Such conditions could cause rapid decompensation of the patient's blood pressure if vasoactive medications are given. Monitoring the patient's blood pressure is a must—but is not predictive of which patients' BP will drop before it happens. The electrocardiogram can offer proven criteria that are useful in predicting these conditions.

RIGHT VENTRICULAR INFARCTION

right ventricular infarction (RVI) *tissue damage to the right ventricle that can affect systemic preload, causing decreased cardiac output and cardiogenic shock.*

The right ventricle, responsible for the heart's preload, receives its blood supply from the right coronary artery, which also feeds the inferior and posterior walls. Whenever damaged, the right ventricle can dramatically affect the blood available for the left ventricle to pump. The cardiovascular system can compensate for the reduction in preload by increasing peripheral vascular resistance through vasoconstriction. The patient with **right ventricular infarction (RVI)** can be normotensive or hypotensive on presentation. Clinicians should be aware that nitrates might cause a precipitous drop in blood pressure in the setting of an AMI. This is secondary to nitroglycerin's effect on the preload. The right ventricle is involved in an inferior MI approximately 50% of the time.

Specialized ECG leads can be used to more effectively evaluate the right ventricle. Lead V4R looks at the right ventricle. The 15-lead ECG, and lead V4R in particular, can be helpful in discovering the presence of RVI. (See Table 10–4.)

In addition to 15-lead ECG evidence, the following clinical triad of signs and symptoms provides further clues for the condition:

★ Jugular vein distention (JVD)

★ Hypotension, either presenting or following nitroglycerin administration

★ Clear lung sounds

It is important for the clinician to assess for the conditions before giving nitrates or morphine. Patients with RVI frequently require fluids in larger quantity than you would expect to give an MI patient. Some cases have required up to 1 L or more initially in order to restore an adequate blood pressure. An RVI presents with ST segment elevation in Lead V4R. (See Figure 10-31 ■.) Reciprocal changes will not be seen, owing to the small size of the ventricle and the fact that it is across the septum from a reciprocal lead. Before administering any nitrate or vasoactive drug, the acute-care provider should assess for lung sounds. A 1-liter IV bag with large tubing should be established with an isotonic solution, such as normal saline.

ACQUIRING THE 15-LEAD ECG

Most standard 12-lead machines do not have the extra leads to run the posterior and right ventricular leads. To acquire the 15-lead ECG, follow these steps (Figures 10-32 ■ and 10-33 ■):

1. Run the initial 12-lead ECG as usual.

2. Place an electrode pad on the midclavicular line at the fifth intercostal space on the right side of the patient—the same as V4 on the left side.

Table 10–4	Indications for Running a 15-Lead ECG
• Normal 12-lead ECG.	
• ECG evidence of an acute inferior infarction.	
• ST depression in Leads V1 to V4, suggesting posterior infarction.	

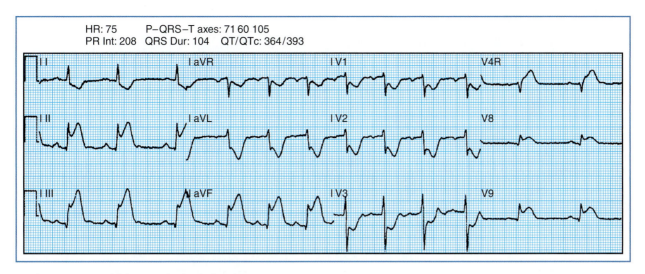

HR: 75   P–QRS–T axes: 71 60 105
PR Int: 208   QRS Dur: 104   QT/QTc: 364/393

■ Figure 10-31   Right ventricular infarction.

3. On the back, place an electrode pad in the fifth intercostal space, midscapular line, that is, the lead V8 (posterior) position. This lead aligns with lead V4 on the front of the patient's chest at the same height.

4. Place another electrode between V8 and the spine in the same intercostal space; this is the lead V9 (posterior) position.

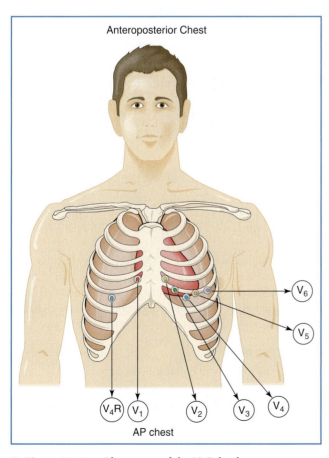

■ Figure 10-32   Placement of the V4R lead.

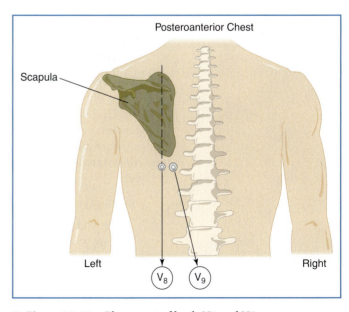

■ Figure 10-33   Placement of leads V8 and V9.

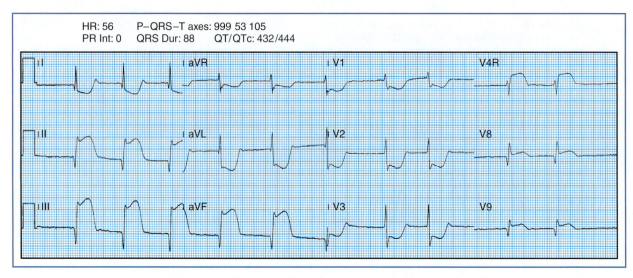

HR: 56   P–QRS–T axes: 999 53 105
PR Int: 0   QRS Dur: 88   QT/QTc: 432/444

■ Figure 10-34   Right ventricular infarction.

5. Remove the electrode wires for leads V4, V5, and V6.

6. Attach the V4 wire to the V4R lead placement.

7. Attach the V5 wire to the lead V8 placement and the V6 wire to the lead V9 placement.

8. Run a second 12-lead ECG with the new lead placements.

9. Label the second 12-lead ECG to reflect the new leads: V4 as V4R, V5 as V8, and V6 as V9. (See Figure 10-34 ■.)

CLINICAL IMPLICATIONS: HEMODYNAMIC ISSUES

HEMODYNAMICS 101: CO (cardiac output) = HR (Heart rate) × SV (Stroke volume)

Preload: Volume and pressure on LV

Afterload: Vascular tone

Contractility: Inotropic state

If the QRS duration is >120 ms (0.12 sec) (three little boxes), then at the least a BBB exists. The ventricles, being out of sync have reduced preload.

If the QRS is >170 ms, then the ejection fraction is 50% at the MOST. The ejection fraction is the percentage of blood ejected with each heart contraction. Healthy people at rest and awake normally have an ejection fraction between 60% and 75%. A lowered ejection fraction results from *reduced contractility* because it takes so much time to depolarize; the contraction is also slow and weak.

What Does This Mean to the Critical Care Provider?

1. Before you give a med (other than O_2) make sure you determine the presence or absence of bundle branch block.

2. If the QRS is wider than 170 ms and you are going to give a vasoactive drug such as nitroglycerin, REMEMBER:

   a. Don't use NTG without an IV Line.

   b. Before giving nitroglycerin, always check ALL lung fields (especially posterior lobes).

c. ALWAYS have plan "D" ready:

    i. Plan D is actually the drug dopamine (Intropin) or other pressor.

    ii. The dose for contractility support (inotropic) is 5 mcg/kg/min then titrated.

Colorado Down and Dirty Dopamine Dose Ditty

Take the weight in pounds / 10 then subtract 2. This gives you the pump setting in mL/hr or gtts/min for dopamine at 5 mcg/kg/min with in bag concentration of 1,600 mcg/mL.

Example: The patient says he weighs 100 kg. Therefore, the patient weighs 220 lbs. That would be 220 /10, which is 22 minus 2 leaves 20. Set your pump at 20 mL/hr!

Now look at the 12-lead ECGs shown in Figures 10-35 ■ through 10-38 ■ and read them for the risk factors mentioned in this chapter: risk for sudden death dysrhythmias, risk for heart block, and risk for hemodynamic compromise.

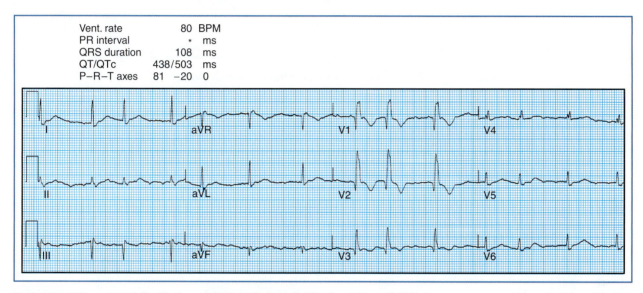

Vent. rate	80	BPM
PR interval	*	ms
QRS duration	108	ms
QT/QTc	438/503	ms
P–R–T axes	81 −20 0	

■ **Figure 10-35** Atrial fibrillation, right bundle branch block, prolonged QT.

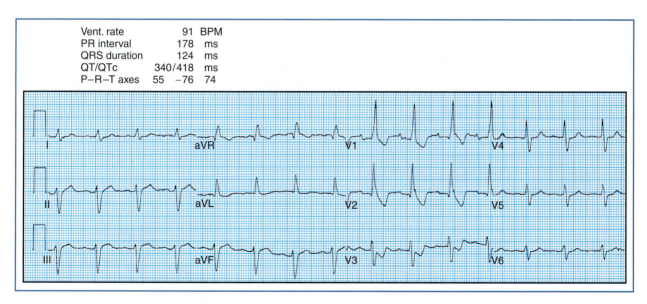

Vent. rate	91	BPM
PR interval	178	ms
QRS duration	124	ms
QT/QTc	340/418	ms
P–R–T axes	55 −76 74	

■ **Figure 10-36** Normal sinus rhythm, pathological left axis, anterior hemiblock, right bundle branch block.

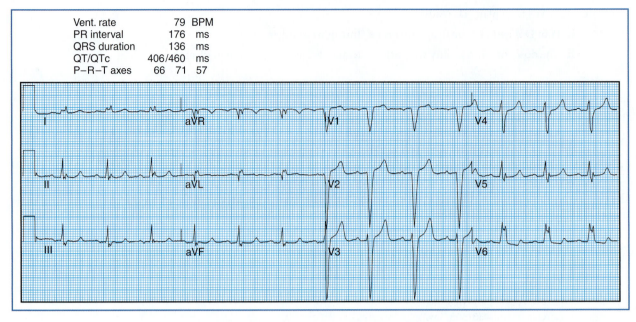

Vent. rate	79	BPM
PR interval	176	ms
QRS duration	136	ms
QT/QTc	406/460	ms
P–R–T axes	66 71 57	

■ Figure 10-37 Normal sinus rhythm, left bundle branch block.

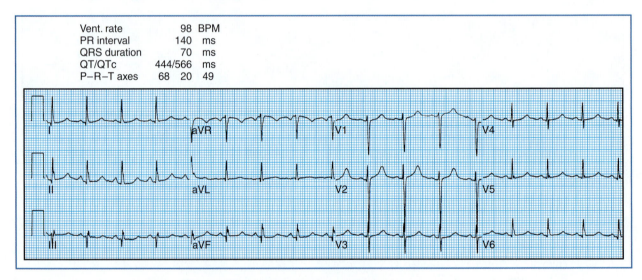

Vent. rate	98	BPM
PR interval	140	ms
QRS duration	70	ms
QT/QTc	444/566	ms
P–R–T axes	68 20 49	

■ Figure 10-38 Normal sinus rhythm, prolonged QT.

Summary

In the critical care patient, 12-lead and 15-lead ECGs are very important to understanding the potential for arrest or serious complication. By reading these ECGs, the clinician can prepare for and rapidly intervene after conditions occur. All critical care personnel must be competent in multiple-lead monitoring and complex 12- and 15-lead ECG interpretation. This goal is best attained through continued practice.

Review Questions

1. Discuss the importance of multiple-lead monitoring in critical care transport medicine.
2. What is the advantage of MCL-1 and MCL-6 as monitoring leads?
3. Detail risk factors for complete heart block.
4. Describe how to determine the QRS axis and whether or not axis deviation exists.
5. List the ECG findings associated with:

   - Left-anterior hemiblock
   - Right-anterior hemiblock
   - Left bundle branch block
   - Right bundle branch block

6. List the clinical significance of the hemiblocks and bundle branch blocks.
7. Differentiate between the underlying causes of wide-complex tachycardia.
8. Discuss the importance of the 12- and 15-lead ECG in right ventricular infarctions.
9. Describe how to obtain a 15-lead ECG with a standard 12-lead machine.

See Answers to Review Questions at the back of this book.

Further Reading

Chan TC, Brady WJ, Harrigan RA, Ornato JP, Rosen P. *ECG in Emergency Medicine and Acute Care.* Saint Louis, MO: Mosby, 2005.

Drew BJ, Cardiff RM, Funk M, *et al.* "AHA Scientific Statement: Practice Standards for Electrocardiographic Monitoring in Hospital Settings: An American Heart Association Scientific Statement from the Councils on Cardiovascular Nursing, Clinical Cardiology, and Cardiovascular Disease in the Young: Endorsed by the International Society of Computerized Electrocardiology and the American Association of Critical-Care Nurses." *Journal of Cardiovascular Nursing,* Vol. 20, No. 2 (2005): 76–106.

Drew BJ, Scheinman MM. "ECG Criteria to Distinguish between Aberrantly Conducted Supraventricular Tachycardia and Ventricular Tachycardia: Practical Aspects for the Immediate Care Setting." *Pacing and Clinical Electrophysiology,* Vol. 18, (1995): 2194–2208.

Page B. *12-Lead ECG for Acute and Critical Care Providers.* Upper Saddle River, NJ: Pearson Prentice Hall, 2005.

Phalen T. *The 12-Lead ECG in Acute Myocardial Infarction.* Saint Louis, MO: Mosby, 1996.

Critical Care Pharmacology

Tim Duncan, RN, CCRN, CEN, CFRN, EMT-P,
and Randall W. Benner, M.Ed., MICP, NREMT-P

Objectives

Upon completion of this chapter, the student should be able to:

1. Discuss why it behooves the critical care paramedic to have a solid understanding of a drug's mechanism of action. (p. 273)
2. Define the role of critical care pharmacology. (p. 274)
3. Understand the difference between pharmacodynamics and pharmacokinetics. (p. 275)
4. Describe the factors that can affect the administration of critical care pharmacologic agents. (p. 275)
5. Understand how derangements in normal cellular activity may influence the response that medications exert on the body (p. 275).

Key Terms

agonists, p. 274
antagonists, p. 274
bioavailability, p. 275
biotransformation, p. 275

chronotope, p. 276
drug toxicity, p. 275
half-life, p. 275
inotropic, p. 276

pharmacodynamics, p. 275
pharmacokinetics, p. 275
pharmacology, p. 275

Case Study

You are summoned for a 35-year-old male patient who presents to the ED with acute dyspnea and hypoxia. His pertinent medical history includes poorly controlled asthma and tobacco use. Since the weather conditions make it impossible to fly to the outlying hospital, you and your partner utilize your system's ground transport critical care unit for patient transfer.

On arrival at the requesting hospital 48 minutes later, the critical care paramedic finds the patient in a high Fowler's position, he is slightly confused, and is occasionally combative to your attempts at physical assessment. Vitals signs include heart rate, 135; respiratory rate, 40; blood pressure, 190/104; and SpO_2, 77%. The patient is unable to complete sentences, and lungs sounds are greatly diminished with inspiratory and expiratory wheezing. The critical care transport team has opted to electively intubate the patient to better manage his onset of acute respiratory failure, but the accepting pulmonologist at the destination hospital refuses to allow nasotracheal intubation. Given this presentation, the critical care team has to determine what pharmacology would be best for the following points:

★ Best initial agent for the induction needed to facilitate intubation

★ Best agent to maintain proper sedation and paralysis for the long transport

★ Best agent to consider for the bilateral wheezing, and if the patient is refractory to this, what else could be considered given the patient's age, history, and physical condition

INTRODUCTION

As critical care interventions have advanced into the 21st century, so too has critical care pharmacology. The critical care paramedic faces a tremendous task in staying current with new pharmacologic treatments in the care of the critically ill or injured patient. While understanding the principles of pharmacology and drug pharmacokinetics is important, the understanding of drug pharmacodynamics in the critical care patient is essential.

As a critical care paramedic, you cannot become complacent and rely exclusively on charts or pocket references to guide your drug therapy during patient management. Books and charts cannot interpret the special circumstances that are part of every patient encounter in critical care, nor can they offer all the differential approaches to drug therapy that may be required. This is not to say that having a reference immediately available is inappropriate, just that relying solely on a reference chart to make your drug therapy decisions is not the intended purpose of these guides. Proper patient management will only occur when the critical care provider understands the pathophysiology behind the patient's condition, understands the physiological actions of the drugs (pharmacodynamics), and can then apply this knowledge to provide the appropriate pharmacologic care to the patient. A reference chart or book should be used to augment this decision-making process.

To aid in the learning process, the information contained within this chapter is presented in a logical, concise, and easy-to-read format. It will take, however, an investment of time on the part of the reader to comprehend and apply the information. One word of caution is essential. Do not simply try to "memorize" drug indications, side effects, contraindications, and so forth. Information learned by rote memory is commonly lost due to a lack of use, or in the stress of an emergency cannot be recalled. Instead, take the time to thoroughly understand how a drug works. If you are familiar with how a drug works in the body, the indications, contraindications, and side effects become obvious. Thus the only thing left to memorize is the specific drug dose—and there is no shortcut to memorizing drug doses. Then, as you read through other chapters of the book, refer

Proper patient management will only occur when the critical care provider understands the pathophysiology behind the patient's condition, understands the physiological actions of the drugs, and can apply this knowledge to provide the appropriate pharmacologic care to the patient.

back to this one for more information about specific drugs that you will be using in the critical care environment. These drugs are integral to the successful management of a critical patient, and any one of them has the potential to help, or harm, your patient.

This chapter will cover many of the pharmacologic agents commonly used in a critical care transport setting, both as emergent treatments for changes in the hemodynamic stability of the patient, or as ongoing treatment for specific disease processes commonly encountered. Note, however, that the information in this chapter is not intended to be used as medical directives nor to supersede the medical directives supplied by the critical care paramedic's medical director.

Additionally, as medical treatment modalities change, so do the pharmacologic agents used in patient management. Although this chapter includes many agents used in the critical care transport setting, it focuses on those agents that are considered customary by national standards (or trends) in the management of critical patients. Ultimately, it is the sole responsibility of the critical care provider to become intimately familiar with the pharmacologic agents used in his respective system.

CRITICAL CARE PHARMACOLOGY

For years, prehospital care providers had a somewhat limited scope of practice regarding the types of pharmacologic agents that they could administer. But now as paramedics progress to the critical care realm, medical directives have expanded to include agents above and beyond typical advanced cardiac life support (ACLS) agents or those drugs used for the emergent treatment of pulmonary disorders or alterations in mental status.

The ongoing (and not just emergent) treatment of cardiovascular, neurologic, pulmonary, and infectious disease processes is now within the scope of practice for the critical care paramedic. Having a clear understanding of the major physiological body systems and knowing how a particular medication may or may not work are added responsibilities that the critical care paramedic must accept.

Above and beyond the traditional EMT-Paramedic scope of practice, you will be responsible for probably twice as many *additional* medications than you were as a prehospital provider. As mentioned previously, understanding the drug effects, side effects, indications, and contraindications is of vital importance for the critical care paramedic. And this topic, critical care pharmacology, is often one of the most challenging hurdles to overcome when progressing from a prehospital paramedic to a critical care transport paramedic.

DIFFERING INFLUENCES ON CRITICAL CARE DRUG THERAPY

agonists *drugs that stimulate receptor sites inhibit in order to cause an effect.*

antagonists *drugs that block receptor sites in order to inhibit a certain cellular function.*

For all intents and purposes, the administration of drugs by the critical care paramedic is done to *alter* cellular activity—not to make a cell do something it cannot do. Beyond the research that is done by medical and biological experts regarding DNA and RNA manipulation, the critical care paramedic is using pharmacology to alter cellular activity by manipulating the cellular receptor sites that are specifically targeted by a drug. **Agonists** are drugs that stimulate the receptor sites on the cells in order to cause an effect, whereas **antagonists** are drugs that block the receptor sites in order to inhibit a certain cellular function. The alteration of cellular activity in turn affects the action of the tissue and organ system it is part of, culminating in the desired clinical effect. For example, the critical care provider may administer a drug to the patient to increase or decrease the heart rate (by altering cardiac conduction cell activity), but the provider cannot administer a drug that will make the cardiac muscle cells suddenly become a functional part of the conduction system. This perspective illustrates why it is important for the critical care paramedic to *understand the cellular effects* of the drugs being used, not just simply look for some clinical effect after the drug is given. Being able to understand pharmacology this way requires an appreciation of the pharmacokinetics and pharmacodynamics of the drugs.

First, **pharmacology** refers to the study of drugs and how they relate to altering the body's activities. Within this field of study there are two areas that the critical care paramedic should be familiar with after completing paramedic education: pharmacokinetics and pharmacodynamics. As a reminder, **pharmacokinetics** is the study of what the body does to a drug. Or, in other words, after administration how the body breaks down the drug and absorbs it for distribution systemically, how the drug is transported, how the drug is inactivated by the body, and, finally, how it is eliminated. **Pharmacodynamics** is the study of what the drug does to the body, that is, its ability to alter cellular and tissue activity in order to achieve some clinical response.

Both pharmacodynamic and pharmacokinetic activities will change from patient to patient and situation to situation. For example, the administration of a narcotic analgesic to a patient with a complaint of lumbar back pain may result in a very different response than the administration of the same drug at the same dosage to the agitated patient with multisystem organ failure who requires ventilator assistance. Influences on the drug action include the metabolic, hemodynamic, and elimination capabilities of the patient and, as such, these capabilities determine how effective or ineffective a particular agent will be in a given situation.

The metabolic status of the critically ill patient may be significantly altered based on cellular perfusion status. As end-cell perfusion is decreased, the ability to transport a drug to the cellular receptor sites is delayed. Furthermore, metabolic changes may delay breakdown of a drug at the receptor sites, causing an increase in the **half-life** of the drug which is the time it takes the body to eliminate one-half of the medication from the bloodstream. This lengthening of the drug's half-life can cause an accumulative effect (an effect that lasts longer than anticipated) that is detrimental to overall patient care. An example of this would be a patient with poor metabolic status who receives a neuromuscular blockade (paralytic) for airway control during transport. Because of the deranged metabolic status of the patient, he may remain chemically paralyzed for hours after administration of the drug, exposing the patient to the complications of chemical paralysis (tissue breakdown, deep venous thrombosis formation, and so on).

Hemodynamic status may also influence the effects of medications. If a patient is febrile and hyperdynamic, the drug may be metabolized more rapidly and more profoundly, hence shortening its half-life. In contrast, a medication administered through a peripheral IV in a patient who is hypoperfusing, has a decreased cardiac output, or has poor peripheral perfusion may have a decreased or slower than expected action or effect.

A final factor in medication considerations is the **bioavailability** of a drug. The bioavailability of a drug refers to the rate and extent to which a drug is circulating through the blood stream, and has access to its site of action, since many drugs bind with protein molecules in the blood stream rendering then inactive while bound. An altered responsiveness may occur in a burn patient due to the disturbance in serum protein levels. Other patients, such as those with renal or hepatic failure, will need to be managed carefully to prevent **drug toxicity** (harmfully high levels of drug in the bloodstream) due to inadequate **biotransformation** of the drug into inactive metabolites for clearance from the body. Antibiotic toxicity is prevalent in patients with renal failure, so peak and trough levels are commonly drawn to prevent "overdosing."

What these various effects mean is that the critical care paramedic must have a good working knowledge of the patient's condition in order to properly assess what pharmacologic agents should be used. Then, beyond recognizing what drug is indicated, the critical care paramedic must "forecast" what he believes the effect of the drug will be given any alteration in the patient's hemodynamic, metabolic, or elimination systems. If there is a grave disturbance in any of these, commonly the dose needs to be altered, or an alternative drug with a differing mechanism of action (but same clinical response) must be chosen.

CARDIOVASCULAR DRUGS

When the cardiovascular system is in *extremis,* pharmacologic agents are often employed to restore blood pressure, to increase myocardial contractility, or to produce other desired changes in hemodynamic pressures. A logical thought process on the part of the critical care paramedic must be used in deciding which agent to administer.

pharmacology *the study of drugs, and how they relate to altering the body's activities.*

pharmacokinetics *the study of how the body absorbs, distributes, transports, inactivates, and eliminates a drug.*

pharmacodynamics *the study of what a drug does to the body as it alters cellular and tissue activity in order to achieve a clinical response.*

Both pharmacodynamic and pharmacokinetic activities will change from patient to patient and situation to situation.

half-life *the time in which it takes one-half of a particular drug to be eliminated from the blood/body.*

bioavailability *free, unbound state of a drug molecule, making it capable of exerting an action.*

drug toxicity *harmful levels of a drug in the blood stream.*

biotransformation *method by which a drug changes into inactive metabolites for elimination from the body.*

Beyond recognizing what drug is indicated, the critical care paramedic must "forecast" what he believes the effect of the drug will be given any alteration in the patient's hemodynamic, metabolic, or elimination systems.

A common clinical situation encountered in critical care medicine is hypotension. To elevate the patient's blood pressure, you must first assess what factors are causing the disturbance. For example, does the patient simply need an increase in the heart rate (positive **chronotropic** effect) to elevate cardiac output and raise the mean arterial pressure? Patients who are volume depleted (decreased central venous pressure) or acidotic will not respond as anticipated due to the altered physiological environment. Will an **inotropic** agent (one that causes the myocardium to contract more forcefully) strengthen the stroke volume of each contraction, thereby raising cardiac output and blood pressure? Or could it be that the patient needs an agent that will directly increase afterload by way of alpha stimulation to the peripheral vasculature? As the critical care team can see in this one instance of clinically inadequate systolic perfusion pressure, numerous components may play a role in the disturbance. Because all of these aforementioned components can be altered pharmacologically in the patient, it takes a thorough assessment of hemodynamic function to determine in which direction to proceed.

The opposite may occur also in the patient. The patient you are caring for may be in need of antihypertensive agents that will directly dilate peripheral vasculature (both at the venous and arterial levels). This may be warranted so as to increase the volume of blood the vessels can hold without causing an undue pressure increase in the vascular bed. The end result is a diminishment of the patient's preload pressure with a reflective drop in systolic pressure.

Beta-blocking agents such as labetalol and metoprolol produce negative inotropic and chronotropic effects, which translates into lower myocardial metabolic demands (from the decrease in myocardial workload). In the presence of acute myocardial infarction, sympathetic tone is elevated, which results in an increase in myocardial oxygen consumption (MVO_2), causing a further extension of tissue ischemia and necrosis. Beta-blockers decrease MVO_2 by reducing inotropy and chronotropy, which can result in a smaller infarction size, decreased morbidity and mortality, and diminished likelihood of re-infarction in the acute phase.

In any instance of hemodynamic alteration, the critical care paramedic must perform a thorough history and physical exam of the patient in order to determine what agent is best. Failure to do so will unequivocally lead to errors in management and, because many of the drugs used by the critical care paramedic affect the autonomic nervous system, an error in judgment can be a fatal one to the patient.

ANTIHYPERTENSIVES

When blood pressure rises, the cardiac system must work harder to "push" the blood through the increased resistance, resulting in elevated metabolic demands to the heart and increasing the risk for both myocardial and systemic ischemic events. In such cases, antihypertensive agents are needed to help decrease myocardial workload and reduce the chance of end-organ damage in the clinically hypertensive patient.

Although antihypertensive agents act in different ways, the goal is constant: Decrease systemic arterial pressures. By doing so, cardiac output and end-organ perfusion are improved (including cerebral perfusion). If hypertension is allowed to continue unabated, the patient has higher myocardial oxygen needs and is at grave risk for end-organ dysfunction.

DIRECT VASODILATORS

NITROPRUSSIDE SODIUM (NITROPRESS, NIPRIDE)

Classifications   CARDIOVASCULAR AGENT; ANTIHYPERTENSIVE AGENT; VASODILATOR, NONNITRATE

- ★ *Actions:* Through direct relaxation of vascular smooth muscle in the venous and arterial vasculature, there is a resultant decrease in systolic and diastolic pressures, as well as left ventricular preload and afterload.

- ★ *Indications:* Hypertensive emergency, especially in those patients with neurologic changes, such as hypertensive encephalopathy. It can also be used as adjunctive therapy in treatment of cardiogenic shock by decreasing left ventricular afterload (however, it is less commonly used for this purpose).

★ *Contraindications:* Clinically significant hypotension, known allergy, lactation.

★ *Side Effects:* Since the medication lowers blood pressure, accidental hypotension (which may be profound) can occur. Others include flushing, nausea, and vomiting (these are also usually related to hypotension). Finally, thiocyanate toxicity as evidenced by blurred vision, tinnitus, confusion, hyperreflexia, and seizures.

★ *Dosage: Adult dose:* 0.5–10 mcg/kg/min infusion. *Pediatric dose:* Same as adult dose. This medication is supplied in 50-mg vials for reconstitution.

★ *Special Considerations:* Start at low dose and titrate every 5–10 minutes until the desired blood pressure is obtained. Monitor the blood pressure closely, at least every 5 minutes. Use cautiously with patients with renal or hepatic dysfunction due to diminished clearing, and administer the drug in a light-resistant container because it is converted to thiocyanate. It is intended for short-term administration (less than 72 hours) because infusions greater than 72 hours are associated with increased risk for thiocyanate toxicity. Nitroprusside must be protected from light and should be wrapped in foil immediately after preparation.

NITROGLYCERIN IV (TRIDIL, NITROSTAT I.V.)

Classifications   CARDIOVASCULAR AGENT; VASODILATOR, NITRATE

★ *Actions:* Through direct relaxation of vascular and coronary smooth muscle, there is a resultant decrease in systolic and diastolic blood pressure as well as improvement of blood flow through the coronary arteries. The enhanced coronary perfusion coupled with the drop in cardiac workload results in enhanced oxygen and blood supply to ischemic cardiac tissue.

★ *Indications:* Direct vasodilation of systemic and coronary blood vessels aids in the treatment of hypertension, ischemic chest pain, acute myocardial infarction, and acute cardiac load reduction.

★ *Contraindications:* Preexisting hypotension, known hypersensitivity.

★ *Side Effects:* Possible hypotension, patients usually complain of headaches and palpitations. Reflexive tachycardia, flushing of the skin, and methemoglobinemia.

★ *Dosage: Adult dose:* 5–50 mcg/min administered as a constant infusion. *Pediatric dose:* Not yet established. The drug is commonly supplied in 25- and 50-mg bottles for infusion or 50-mg vials for reconstitution in glass bottle.

★ *Special Considerations:* Titrate every 5–10 minutes to obtain desired response of blood pressure and/or chest pain. Monitor blood pressure closely, at least every 5 minutes, for development of hypotension. As needed, nitroglycerin is compatible with heparin and lidocaine.

NESIRITIDE (NATRECOR)

Classifications   CARDIOVASCULAR AGENT; ATRIAL NATRIURETIC PEPTIDE HORMONE

★ *Actions:* B-type natriuretic peptide (recombinant); this drug binds to vascular receptor sites so as to cause vascular smooth muscle relaxation. The dilation of veins and arteries decreases preload and afterload, creating a more favorable hemodynamic environment for a failing heart to pump within.

★ *Indications:* Treatment of acutely decompensated congestive heart failure, especially if refractory to more conservative therapy such as nitroglycerin, furosemide, and morphine administration. The vasodilatory properties of this drug allow for maximum cardiac performance.

- ★ *Contraindications:* Clinical hypotension, valvular stenosis, restrictive or obstructive cardiomyopathies, and cardiac tamponade. In these aforementioned conditions, the resulting drop in blood pressure may be exaggerated.

- ★ *Side Effects:* As with other antihypertensives, the patient may experience hypotension. There may also be the emergence of cardiac dysrhythmias such as atrial fibrillation, ventricular tachycardia, or atrioventricular (AV) conduction delays. Finally, angina pectoris, headache, and palpitations are reported.

- ★ *Dosage: Adult bolus dose:* 2 mcg/kg IV push over 60 seconds with a *maintenance infusion* of 0.01 mcg/kg/min infusion. *Optimal pediatric dose:* Not yet established. The drug comes supplied in 1.58-mg vials for reconstitution.

- ★ *Special Considerations:* Use cautiously with pregnant or actively lactating patients. Additionally, nesiritide binds with heparin, so do not administer through any heparin-coated catheters (nor should this drug be administered through the same IV port as other medications). Monitor vital signs and cardiac rhythm closely.

HYDRALAZINE HYDROCHLORIDE (APRESOLINE, ALAZINE)

Classifications   CARDIOVASCULAR AGENT; VASODILATOR, NONNITRATE; ANTIHYPERTENSIVE AGENT

- ★ *Actions:* Direct arteriolar vasodilation by unknown mechanism, resulting in drop of systolic and diastolic blood pressure. Has little effect on venous blood vessels. Degree of hypotensive effect may be limited to sympathetic mediated reflexes such as elevation of cardiac output.

- ★ *Indications:* Rapid-acting vasodilator is effective in treatment of acute hypertensive emergency; front-line agent in pregnancy-induced hypertension and preeclampsia. Can also be used in short-term treatment of congestive heart failure (CHF) or unexplained pulmonary hypertension.

- ★ *Contraindications:* Coronary artery disease, mitral valve disease, preexisting hypotension, myocardial infarction (MI), hypersensitivity, or persistent tachycardia.

- ★ *Side Effects:* Drug-induced hypotension, dizziness, headache, tachycardia, angina pectoris, nausea/vomiting, decreased hematocrit and hemoglobin.

- ★ *Dosage: Adult dose:* 5–40 mg IV push slowly over 1–2 minutes; may repeat as needed to achieve control of blood pressure. *Pediatric dose:* Not yet established. The drug is supplied in 20-mg vials for injection.

- ★ *Special Considerations:* Monitor vital signs and cardiac rhythm closely (every 5 minutes until stabilized and then every 15 minutes thereafter). Exercise caution when administering the drug concurrently with beta-blockers for compounded BP effects.

NICARDIPINE HYDROCHLORIDE (CARDENE, CARDENE I.V.)

Classifications   CARDIOVASCULAR AGENT; CALCIUM CHANNEL BLOCKER; ANTIHYPERTENSIVE AGENT

- ★ *Actions:* Calcium entry blocker that inhibits the influx of calcium ions into cardiac muscle and smooth muscle, thus affecting contractility. More selectively affects vascular smooth muscle than cardiac muscle; relaxes coronary vascular smooth muscle with little or no negative inotropic effect.

- ★ *Indications:* Rapid-acting vasodilator is effective in treatment of acute hypertensive emergency. Significantly decreases systemic vascular resistance. Can be used alone or with beta-blockers for chronic or stable angina. Can also be used either alone or with other antihypertensives for essential hypertension.

- ★ *Contraindications:* Hypersensitivity to nicardipine; advanced aortic stenosis; lactation.

- *Side Effects:* Drug-induced hypotension, palpitations, and tachycardia. It may also cause vertigo, headache, fatigue, anxiety, paresthesias, nervousness, nausea/vomiting, decreased hematocrit and hemoglobin.
- *Dosage: Adult dose:* Constant infusion of 5 mg/hr initially, increase dose by 2.5 mg/hr every 15 minutes for severe hypertension. Max dose is 15 mg/hr. *Pediatric dose:* 1–3 mcg/kg/min in children 9 days old to 10 years. The drug comes packaged in 2.5 mg/mL for intravenous use.
- *Special Considerations:* Monitor vital signs and cardiac rhythm closely (every 5 minutes until stabilized and then every 15 minutes thereafter). Exercise caution when administering the drug concurrently with other drugs that affect the hemodynamic stability of the patient. Also use cautiously in patients with CHF, hepatic impairment, and pregnancy.

FENOLDOPAM MESYLATE (CORLOPAM)

Classifications CARDIOVASCULAR AGENT; ANTIHYPERTENSIVE AGENT; VASODILATOR, NONNITRATE; DOPAMINE AGONIST AGENT

- *Actions:* Rapid-acting vasodilator that is a dopamine-like receptor agonist. Exerts hypotensive effects by decreasing peripheral vascular resistance while increasing renal blood flow and diuresis.
- *Indications:* Rapid-acting antihypertensive agent that decreases both systolic and diastolic pressures. It can be used for short-term management of severe hypertension (less than 48 hours).
- *Contraindications:* Known hypersensitivity to fenoldopam, also contraindicated for concomitant use with beta-blockers.
- *Side Effects:* Known side effects include headache, nervousness, vertigo, hypotension, tachycardia, T-wave inversion, flushing, postural hypotension, palpitations, dysrhythmias to include bradycardia, heart failure, and possible MI. It also may increase creatinine, BUN, and glucose levels.
- *Dosage: Adult dose for severe hypertension:* 0.025–0.3 mcg/kg/min by continuous infusion. The dose may be increased by 0.05–0.1 mcg/kg/min increments every 15 minutes (normal dosage range is 0.01–1.6 mcg/kg/min). *Pediatric dose:* Not established. The drug comes packaged in 10 mg/mL or 2.5 mg/mL vials for mixing with normal saline (NS) or D_5W.
- *Special Considerations:* Use with caution in patients with asthma, hepatic cirrhosis, portal hypertension, or variceal bleeding. Also safety and efficacy in children is not yet established.

CENTRAL-ACTING ANTIHYPERTENSIVES

CLONIDINE HYDROCHLORIDE (CATAPRES, DIXARIL)

Classifications CARDIOVASCULAR AGENT; CENTRAL NERVOUS SYSTEM (CNS) AGENT; ANALGESIC

- *Actions:* Stimulates alpha-adrenergic receptors in CNS, resulting in inhibition of sympathetic vasomotor centers and decreased nerve impulses, causing drop in systolic and diastolic blood pressure and bradycardia; minimal effect on venous pressure. Also inhibits renin release from the kidneys.
- *Indications:* Emergent treatment of hypertensive emergency without intravenous access. Excellent results have been obtained with patients in acute ethanol and opiate withdrawal syndrome with or without hypertension. Can be used alone or with diuretic (or other) antihypertensive agents.

- *Contraindications:* Preexisting hypotension, diminished mental status of patient, known hypersensitivity.

- *Side Effects:* Postural hypotension from the antihypertensive effects, possible bradycardia or tachycardia, angioedema, weakness, and somnolence.

- *Dosage: Adult dose:* Usually 0.1–0.2 mg orally or sublingually. If desired blood pressure control is not achieved, the drug may be repeated once. *Pediatric dose for emergent situations:* 5–10 mcg/kg per day, divided over 8–12 hours. The drug is commonly supplied in tablets that are 0.1 mg each.

- *Special Considerations:* As with any antihypertensive agent, monitor the blood pressure and cardiac rhythm closely. This drug is also associated with rebound hypertension. Administration of this drug is also associated with lowering the patient's mental status, so monitor the airway closely.

ACE INHIBITORS

ENALAPRIL (VASOTEC I.V.)

Classifications   CARDIOVASCULAR AGENT; ANGIOTENSIN-CONVERTING ENZYME INHIBITOR; ANTIHYPERTENSIVE AGENT

- *Actions:* Angiotensin-converting enzyme (ACE) catalyzes the conversion of angiotensin I to angiotension II, which is a potent vasoconstrictive substance. As such, the inhibition of ACE by this drug decreases levels of angiotension II, which leads to a drop in blood pressure from inhibited vasoconstrictive stimulation. It is also known to lower the pulmonary capillary wedge pressure (PCWP).

- *Indications:* Used in the management of mild to moderate hypertension. This drug can be used in combination therapy for acute CHF (with furosemide) or in acute myocardial infarction because the drug's effects decrease both preload and afterload to the heart.

- *Contraindications:* Preexisting hypotension, cardiogenic shock, and known hypersensitivity.

- *Side Effects:* Hypotension or postural hypotension. The patient may also experience reflexive tachycardia with heart palpitations. Finally, the patient may display angioedema, nausea/vomiting, alterations in kidney function and hyperkalemia.

- *Dosage: Adult dose:* 1.25 mg slow IV push over 5 minutes; may repeat every 6 hours. *Pediatric IV dose:* 5–10 mcg/kg every 8 hours. Enalapril comes supplied as 1.25-mg vial for injection.

- *Special Considerations:* Use cautiously with patients with renal impairment or renal artery stenosis, on diuretic therapy, or undergoing dialysis. As with other antihypertensives, monitor the blood pressure and cardiac rhythm closely. Also, serial lab values should be monitored so that potassium levels can be watched closely for hyperkalemia.

BETA BLOCKERS

ESMOLOL HYDROCHLORIDE (BREVIBLOC)

Classifications   AUTONOMIC NERVOUS SYSTEM AGENT; BETA-ADRENERGIC ANTAGONIST (SYMPATHOLYTIC)

- *Actions:* Beta-adrenergic blockade resulting in decreases in chronotropic (heart rate), dromotropic (conduction rate), and inotropic (contractility) effects on myocardium. It has a rapid onset (<5 minutes) and very short half-life. It inhibits the agonist effect of catecholamines by competitive binding at beta-adrenergic receptor sites.

- *Indications:* Hypertensive emergency, hypertension associated with aortic aneurysms, antidysrhythmic for treatment of supraventricular tachycardias such as paroxysmal supraventricular tachycardia (PSVT). It can also be used to blunt the transient adrenergic response to stress in susceptible patients, such as pre- or post-surgery.

- *Contraindications:* Cardiac failure, hypotension, AV heart block greater than first degree, sinus bradycardia, or moderate to severe CHF.

- *Side Effects:* Hypotension (which is usually dose related), bradycardia, development of an AV conduction defect, bronchospasm, headache, dizziness, confusion, and nausea/vomiting.

- *Dosage: Adult loading dose IV:* 500 mcg/kg/min for 1 minute followed by a maintenance infusion of 50 mcg/kg/min, which can be increased every 5–10 minutes to a max of 300 mcg/kg/min. The maintenance dose is usually 25 mcg/kg/min infusion. *Pediatric dose:* Not yet established. The drug is supplied in 10-mg vials for injection, and 250-mg vials for dilution for maintenance infusions.

- *Special Considerations:* Use cautiously with patients who have a history of asthma, emphysema, CHF, or kidney dysfunction. Monitor vital signs and cardiac rhythm closely. If a heart block, bradycardia, or hypotension ensues, discontinue infusion immediately. Do not administer Brevibloc in higher doses than recommended.

LABETALOL HYDROCHLORIDE (NORMODYNE, TRANDATE)

Classifications AUTONOMIC NERVOUS SYSTEM AGENT; ALPHA ADRENERGIC AGONIST AND BETA-ADRENERGIC ANTIAGONIST; ANTIHYPERTENSIVE AGENT

- *Actions:* A nonselective beta-blocking agent somewhat similar to Brevibloc, it slows sinoatrial [SA] discharge, AV conduction, and lessens ventricular inotropy, and also causes alpha blockade effects which result in vasodilation and a diminishment in peripheral resistance. Labetolol has a longer half-life and longer duration of action than that of esmolol.

- *Indications:* Hypertensive emergencies, especially in hypertension-induced neurologic emergencies with resultant increased intracranial pressure (intracranial hemorrhage, traumatic brain injury).

- *Contraindications:* Bronchial asthma, bradycardia, hypotension, heart block beyond first degree, and uncontrolled cardiac failure.

- *Side Effects:* Due to its beta-blocking effects, bradycardia, hypotension, and cardiac dysrhythmias are often seen. The patient may also experience bronchospasm, and this drug is associated with dizziness, fatigue, nausea, and vomiting. Finally, this drug may precipitate CHF in the susceptible patient.

- *Dosage: Adult bolus dose:* 20 mg IV push slowly over 2 minutes; may repeat 40–80 mg IV push every 10 minutes until desired effect is achieved or until a maximum dose of 300 mg total has been reached. The maintenance infusion is started at 2 mg/min and titrated to desired effect. *Pediatric dose:* Not established. The drug is supplied in 100-mg vials.

- *Special Considerations:* Monitor vital signs and cardiac rhythm closely for the development of excessive hypotension, bradycardia, or conduction defects. Use cautiously as well in patients with a history of chronic obstructive pulmonary disease (COPD) or bronchospasms.

VASOPRESSOR AGENTS

When fluid resuscitation proves inadequate or inappropriate to maintain end-organ perfusion and adequate hemodynamics, the administration of vasopressor agents may be necessary to increase afterload, blood pressure, and distal capillary bed perfusion. Though the following pharmacologic

When fluid resuscitation proves inadequate or inappropriate to maintain end-organ perfusion and adequate hemodynamics, the administration of vasopressor agents may be necessary to increase afterload, blood pressure, and distal capillary bed perfusion.

agents constrict peripheral veins and arteries to maximize preload and afterload, they are not without their risks or side effects.

The utilization of vasopressor agents is often a "risk/benefit" dilemma for the critical care paramedic. If given, systemic blood pressure will ideally rise, increasing end-cell perfusion; however, it may also increase heart rate and myocardial workload (especially in those patients with acute or preexisting cardiac problems), increasing the risk for cardiac ischemia and cardiac dysrhythmias. The critical care paramedic must weigh the risks and benefits of administering vasopressor agents, and be confident prior to their use that intravascular volume needs have been met. Finally, with the administration of these agents the critical care paramedic should preferentially administer them through an established central line (if an established line is available), to decrease the incidence of peripheral extravasation of medication with resultant tissue necrosis that is more commonly seen in peripheral line administration.

VASOPRESSORS/SYMPATHOMIMETICS

DOPAMINE HYDROCHLORIDE (INTROPIN, DOPASTAT)

Classifications   AUTONOMIC NERVOUS SYSTEM AGENT (SYMPATHOMIMETIC); ALPHA- AND BETA-ADRENERGIC AGONIST

★ *Actions:* As a precursor to epinephrine, dopamine acts as a beta- and alpha-adrenergic stimulant, resulting in increased cardiac contractility and myocardial workload, as well as peripheral vasoconstriction (both venous and arterial). Its dose-dependent effect on dopaminergic receptors in mesenteric and renal vascular beds has been documented, but is undergoing closer scrutiny in more current literature.

★ *Indications:* To correct hemodynamic imbalance in hypoperfusion syndromes due to causes other than volume deficit. More specifically, cardiac dysfunctions due to MI or CHF, poor perfusion states from sepsis or neurologically induced vasodilation, or renal failure. In all situations, however, intravascular volume must be assured to be normal.

★ *Contraindications:* Pheochromocytoma, uncontrolled tachycardia, ventricular irritability, hypertension, or hypoperfusion from volume depletion.

★ *Side Effects:* Side effects are common to those seen with other sympathomimetic agents such as tachycardia, hypertension, ventricular irritability, angina, anxiety, decreased peripheral perfusion. Due to the alpha effects, tissue necrosis may occur if the IV line infiltrates.

★ *Dosage:* Although the dose-dependent response of dopamine has come under closer scrutiny in more current literature, the following doses are still generally believed to have the following effects. The dose range employed should be consistent with the patient's needs:

– *Adult dopaminergic (renal) dose:* 2–5 mcg/kg/min
– *Adult beta agonist (cardiac) dose:* 5–15 mcg/kg/min
– *Adult alpha agonist (vasopressor) dose:* >15 mcg/kg/min

Pediatric dose: Starts at 5 mcg/kg/min. In either the adult or child, the dose can be titrated up to a max of 50 mcg/kg/min as needed for the desired response. However, at this dose, the effect is primarily alpha stimulation. Dopamine comes supplied as 40 mg/mL, 80 mg/mL, and 160 mg/mL vials, but is most commonly premixed in either 1600- or 3200-mcg concentrations.

★ *Special Considerations:* Use cautiously with children and in patients with occlusive vascular disease (or other types of peripheral vascular insufficiency). Careful monitoring of the patient is warranted, being especially alert to signs of cardiac compromise (angina, ischemia, and so on).

DOBUTAMINE HYDROCHLORIDE (DOBUTREX)

Classifications AUTONOMIC NERVOUS SYSTEM AGENT (SYMPATHOMIMETIC); BETA-ADRENERGIC AGONIST (SYMPATHOMIMETIC); CATECHOLAMINE

★ *Actions:* Synthetically derived agent that enhances cardiac output by beta-1 receptor stimulation, and myocardial alpha-adrenergic receptor stimulation. The net result is enhancement in cardiac output, which is balanced by a drop in PCWP and peripheral resistance. So cardiac effectiveness is enhanced, but the perfusion pressures remain relatively constant.

★ *Indications:* Short-term treatment of cardiac dysfunction secondary to poor cardiac contractility, such as decompensating cardiomyopathy and congestive heart failure.

★ *Contraindications:* Preexisting hypertension, tachycardia, acute coronary syndrome with ventricular irritability, and idiopathic hypertrophic subaortic stenosis. Also avoid use in patients with known history of hypersensitivity to sympathomimetic amines.

★ *Side Effects:* Tachycardia, hypertension, cardiac dysrhythmia, anginal pain, anxiety, decreased peripheral perfusion, and tissue necrosis if infiltration occurs. The patient may also complain of nausea/vomiting.

★ *Dosage: Adult and pediatric dose:* 2.0–20 mcg/kg/min, titrated to desired hemodynamic response. Dose of 40 mcg/kg/min has been given for up to 72 hours without documented decrease in effectiveness. The medication comes supplied in a 12.5 mg/mL vial for dilution.

★ *Special Considerations:* Start at lowest dose and titrate to desired effect. Do not administer as IV bolus (infusion only), and monitor vital signs and cardiac rhythm closely. Finally, also monitor the IV patency so as to avoid medication infiltration.

PHENYLEPHRINE HYDROCHLORIDE (NEO-SYNEPHRINE)

Classifications AUTONOMIC NERVOUS SYSTEM AGENT (SYMPATHOMIMETIC); ALPHA-ADRENERGIC AGONIST (SYMPATHOMIMETIC); EYE AND NOSE PREPARATION; MYDRIATIC; DECONGESTANT

★ *Actions:* Potent, synthetic, direct-acting sympathomimetic with strong alpha-adrenergic and weak beta-adrenergic cardiac stimulant actions. Elevates systolic and diastolic pressures through arteriolar constriction; also constricts capacitance vessels and increases venous return to heart. Produces little or no CNS stimulation.

★ *Indications:* Maintain BP during anesthesia and to treat vascular shock. Commonly used antihypertensive in critical care/intensive care units.

★ *Contraindications:* Coronary artery disease, severe hypertension, and ventricular tachycardia.

★ *Side Effects:* Side effects are common to those seen with other sympathomimetic agents such as tachycardia, hypertension, ventricular irritability, angina, and anxiety. Tissue necrosis may occur if the IV line infiltrates.

★ *Dosage: Adult dose:* 0.1–0.18 mg/min until the blood pressure stabilizes; then administer 0.04–0.06 mg/min for maintenance. *Pediatric dose:* Not established for hypotension. The drug is supplied in a 10 mg/mL concentration for dilution into NS or D_5W.

★ *Special Considerations:* Use cautiously in patients with hyperthyroidism, diabetes mellitus, known myocardial disease, cerebral arteriosclerosis, and bradycardia.

NOREPINEPHRINE BITARTRATE (LEVARTERENOL, LEVOPHED, NORADRENALINE)

Classifications AUTONOMIC NERVOUS SYSTEM AGENT (SYMPATHOMIMETIC); ALPHA- AND BETA-ADRENERGIC AGONIST

★ *Actions:* Alpha-adrenergic receptor stimulant, resulting in direct peripheral venous and arterial constriction. This drug is considered to be a very potent vasoconstricting agent.

★ *Indications:* To help restore normal perfusion states in patients with certain types of hypoperfusion etiologies where vasopressor tone is lost. Most commonly this is vasodilatory shock secondary to sepsis. It also has been used for hypotension associated with sympathectomy, spinal cord injury, and poliomyelitis.

★ *Contraindications:* Because of its vasoconstrictive effects, administration to patients with preexisting hypertension should be avoided. Furthermore, hypotension from hypovolemia should be corrected with fluids rather than a vasopressor.

★ *Side Effects:* Decreased renal perfusion, tachycardia, hypertension, cardiac dysrhythmia, and decreased peripheral perfusion. Also severe tissue necrosis will occur if medication infiltrates (use central line if possible).

★ *Dosage: Adult dose:* Initially 0.5–1.0 mcg/min; titrate up to 30 mcg/min as needed to obtain desired hemodynamic effect. The typical therapeutic dose range is 8–12 mcg/min. *Pediatric dose:* Start at 0.01 mcg/min/min and titrate as needed. It is rarely used in pediatrics. This drug can be supplied in 0.25 mg/mL or 1 mg/mL vials for dilution.

★ *Special Considerations:* Monitor BP every 5–15 minutes, assess urinary output, monitor for tachycardia or cardiac rhythm changes and IV patency. Cautiously use this drug in patients with hyperthyroidism and/or heart disease. Extravasation can cause significant tissue sloughing.

EPINEPHRINE HYDROCHLORIDE (ADRENALINE CHLORIDE)

Classifications AUTONOMIC NERVOUS SYSTEM AGENT (SYMPATHOMIMETIC); ALPHA- AND BETA-ADRENERGIC AGONIST; BRONCHODILATOR

★ *Actions:* Marked alpha- and beta-adrenergic stimulation, resulting in cardiac stimulation, bronchodilation, and vascular bed constriction. Epinephrine can cross the placental barrier, but does NOT cross the blood–brain barrier. This drug imitates all actions of normal sympathetic stimulation except those that occur in the facial arteries and sweat glands.

★ *Indications:* This is an extremely flexible drug that finds a multitude of uses in emergency medicine (in both the arrested and nonarrested patient). Epinephrine is the frontline agent for arrest rhythms (ventricular fibrillation, pulseless ventricular tachycardia, pulseless electrical activity (PEA) and asystole). It can also be used for acute hypotensive shock states not responsive to dopamine. Finally, epinephrine is used for the management of bronchoconstriction in asthma and correction of the pulmonary and vascular disturbances seen in anaphylactic shock.

★ *Contraindications:* Contraindications are somewhat dependent on the desired clinical use of the drug, and need to be interpreted individually. But, generally speaking, in the nonarrested patient, epinephrine should be avoided in those patients with preexisting hypertension or tachycardia, acute coronary syndrome, ischemic chest pain, narrow-angle glaucoma, and advancing age. In the arrested patient, there are no clinical contraindications other than any known hypersensitivity and allergy issues.

★ *Side Effects:* Consistent with sympathomimetic agents, the patient may display tachycardia, hypertension, palpitations, cardiac dysrhythmias (including life-threatening ventricular dysrhythmia), tissue necrosis with infiltration, and transient elevations in blood glucose levels.

★ *Dosage:* The following outlines typical dosage regimes for the *adult* patient:
  – Anaphylaxis: 0.1–0.5 mg SQ/IM or IV

- Arrest rhythms: 1.0 mg IVP as needed every 3–5 minutes
- Refractory bradycardia: 2–10 mcg/min infusion
- Refractory hypotension: 1–4 mcg/min infusion, titrating to desired effect

  The *pediatric* dosing regime is as follows:
- Anaphylaxis: 0.01 mcg/kg SQ/IM or IV
- Arrest rhythms: 0.01 mg/kg initial dose, 0.1 mg/kg subsequent doses IV push every 3–5 minutes
- Infusion: 0.1–1.0 mcg/min infusion

Epinephrine is supplied in two concentrations. The 1:1000 concentration (1 mg/1 mL) is used when the epinephrine is being administered either SQ/IM, ET, or is being mixed for an infusion. The 1:10,000 concentration of epinephrine (1 mg/10 mL) is used for intravenous bolus administration.

★ *Special Considerations:* May be given by IV, IM, SQ, IO, or intracardiac routes so ensure you are using the correct concentration of epinephrine for the route chosen. Protect epinephrine from light (whether still packaged or being used as a constant infusion). And, as always, monitor the patient's vital signs and cardiac rhythm, and assess the IV site frequently to assure patency.

VASOPRESSIN INJECTION (PITRESSIN)

Classifications HORMONE AND SYNTHETIC SUBSTITUTES; PITUITARY (ANTI-DIURETIC)

★ *Actions:* Polypeptide hormone extracted from animal posterior pituitaries. Possesses antidiuretic (ADH) properties, but when administered at a much higher dose, it has the additional property of causing vascular smooth muscle contraction, which elevates systemic vascular resistance.

★ *Indications:* Antidiuretic to treat diabetes insipidus, and can be used for transient polyuria from ADH deficiency (related to head injuries or to neurosurgery). It also finds use as vasoconstrictor agent in cardiac arrested patients with ventricular fibrillation; however, it should not be used concurrently with epinephrine (a single dose of vasopressin can be considered an alternative to the initial dose of epinephrine). It may also be used as a vasopressor in hemodynamically unstable vasodilitory shock refractory to more traditional therapy.

★ *Contraindications:* Known hypersensitivity to the drug or any of its components. In addition, for perfusing patients avoid use with concurrent chronic nephritis, advanced arteriosclerosis, or ischemic heart disease. In the arrested patient, no other contraindications exist.

★ *Side Effects:* Bronchoconstriction; pallor; nausea and abdominal cramping; angina, hypertension, or dysrhythmias; respiratory congestion to include rhinorrhea, irritation, mucosal ulceration and pruritus, and postnasal drip.

★ *Dosage:* It is particularly desirable to give a dose not much larger than sufficient to elicit the desired physiological response. In the perfusing patient with appropriate indications, administer 10 units of the drug intravenously. In the arrested patient, a single dose of 40 units is given IV push. The drug is supplied 20 units/mL for injection.

★ *Special Considerations:* Vasopressin should be used with caution in patients who are either pregnant or who have coronary artery disease. Additionally, use cautiously in the presence of epilepsy, migraine, asthma, heart failure or any condition in which a rapid addition to extracellular water may be detrimental to an already overburdened system.

ANTIDYSRHYTHMICS

Ischemic cardiac tissue, as a result of hypoxia or decreased perfusion due to poor cardiac function, may place the critical care patient at risk for life-threatening electrical dysrhythmias, including ventricular tachycardia and ventricular fibrillation. The administration of antidysrhythmic agents may be necessary to maintain normal cardiac conduction to maximize cardiac contractility and cardiac output. Antidysrhythmic agents are usually classified into classes based on their characteristics. (See Table 11–1.) Drugs in each class have a similar mechanism of action. (See Figure 11-1 ■.)

Generally, drugs of this category exert their action on the refractory period (phase 4) of the cardiac cycle, thus inhibiting the likelihood of dysrhythmias originating from changes in automaticity or reentry mechanisms. (See Figure 11-2 ■.)

Keep in mind also that electrolyte imbalances can be the cause of the dysrhythmia, and the critical care paramedic must correct electrolyte imbalances prior to the administration of antidysrhythmic agents (because *all* antidysrhythmic agents have as their most serious side effect, prodysrhythmic capabilities). Magnesium and potassium levels are probably the two most important electrolytes to monitor and correct, but sodium and bicarbonate levels also need to be closely observed.

LIDOCAINE HYDROCHLORIDE (XYLOCAINE, DILOCAINE)

Classifications   CARDIOVASCULAR AGENT; ANTIDYSRHYTHMIC CLASS IB; CENTRAL NERVOUS SYSTEM AGENT; ANESTHETIC, LOCAL

★ *Actions:* Suppresses automaticity of ischemic ectopic foci without affecting conduction through the cardiac tissue. It is also thought to raise the ventricular fibrillation threshold. It is also used as an induction agent for blunting intracranial pressure (ICP) elevations with rapid-sequence intubtion (RSI) and endotracheal intubation (although the efficacy has been questioned). Finally, it can be used as a local anesthetic where its effects are prompt and long lasting.

★ *Indications:* Management of acute ventricular dysrhythmias such as ventricular tachycardia, ventricular fibrillation, PVCs, and wide-complex tachycardia of unknown etiology.

★ *Contraindications:* Known hypersensitivity, Stokes-Adams syndrome, ventricular ectopy in the presence of bradycardia, and severe conduction abnormalities without pacemaker availability.

Table 11–1 | Antidysrhythmic Classes

Drug Class	Channel Effect	Repolarization Time	Drug Examples
IA	Causes sodium blockade with marked inhibitory effect	Prolongs repolarization	Procainamide, Quinidine
IB	Rapid sodium channel blocker with inhibitory effect	Shortens repolarization	Lidocine, Phenytoin
IC	Sodium blockade with strong inhibitory effect	Repolarization unchanged	Flecainide, Propafenone
II	Inhibit depolarization and indirect closure of Ca^{2+} channels	Repolarization unchanged	Labetalol, Esmolol
III	Blocks outward potassium channels to prolong potential	Significantly prolongs repolarization	Amiodarone, Bretylium
IV	Inhibit inward calcium channel in AV nodal tissue	Repolarization unchanged	Verapamil, Diltiazem
IV-like	Indirect calcium antagonist to inhibit AV nodal channels	Repolarization unchanged	Adenosine, ATP

Class I effect
Sodium channel blockade

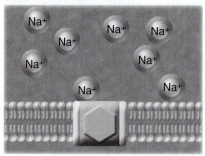

Class II effect
Noncompetitive alpha- and beta-blockade

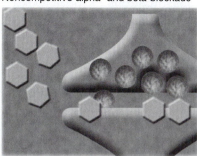

Class III effect
Potassium channel blockade

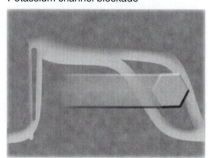

Class IV effect
Calcium channel blockade

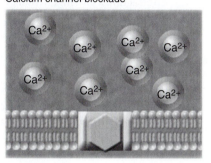

■ Figure 11-1 Vaughan Williams classification of antidysrhythmic drugs.

★ *Side Effects:* Anxiety, seizures with higher doses, hypotension, bradycardia, cardiac dysrhythmia, nausea/vomiting, drowsiness, and generally mild paresthesias.

★ *Dosage: Adult dose via intravenous bolus:* 1.0–1.5 mg/kg over 3 minutes. The repeat dose is given 5–15 minutes later at usually half the initial dose in perfusing patients. Arrested patients can receive the same dose as the initial upon repeat. The maximum dose in either instance is 3 mg/kg total. The initiation of the maintenance infusion following correction of the ventricular abnormality is 1–4 mg/min. *Pediatric dose:* Administration of lidocaine is 0.5–1.0 mg/kg per bolus, with a maintenance infusion of 20–50 mcg/kg/min, titrating to desired effect. Due to its varied uses, lidocaine comes prepared in a multitude of concentrations to include 1%, 2%, 4%, 10%, and 20% vials.

★ *Special Considerations:* Use cautiously in patients with renal or hepatic dysfunction; in these patients reduce the maintenance infusion by 50% and monitor for accidental overdosage (worsening of CNS findings). As with other medications, reassess the patient's vital signs and cardiac monitor following administration.

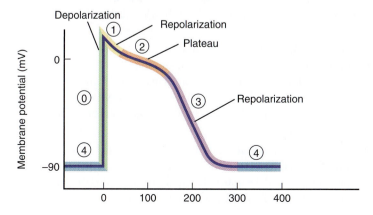

■ Figure 11-2 The cardiac action potential. An action potential recorded from a ventricular muscle cell. P_{Na} increases during phase 0 (green) and decreases during phase 1 (yellow). P_{Ca} increases and P_K decreases during phase 2 (orange) and then P_{Ca} decreases and P_K increases during phase 3 (purple). During phase 4 (blue), all ion channels are in their resting state (P_K high, P_{Ca} and P_{Na} low). *(Fig. 14-12, p. 428, from* Principles of Human Physiology, *2nd ed., by William J. Germann and Cindy L. Stanfield. Copyright © 2005 by Pearson Education, Inc. Reprinted by permission.)*

PROCAINAMIDE HYDROCHLORIDE (PRONESTYL, PROCAN)

Classifications   CARDIOVASCULAR AGENT; ANTIDYSRHYTHMIAS CLASS IA

★ *Actions:* Depresses conduction velocity through the myocardium (atria, AV node, and Purkinje system), and prolongs the refractory period of the atria. This results in depression of ectopic ventricular sites, but also causes a negative inotropic and dromotropic effect to the heart.

★ *Indications:* Ventricular dysrhythmias, such as ventricular tachycardia refractory to more popular agents (amiodarone, lidocaine). It can also be used to help maintain normality of the conduction system following conversion of atrial or junctional dysrhythmias.

★ *Contraindications:* Known drug allergy, myasthenia gravis, blood dyscrasias, AV conduction blocks, torsades de pointes, asymptomatic premature ventricular contractions, patients with digitalis toxicity, and hypotension.

★ *Side Effects:* Because this drug causes a negative inotropic effect, exercise caution in patients with border-line hypotension. Also, exercise caution with hepatic or renal impaired patients so as to avoid toxicity of the drug. Because of the negative dromotropic activity, it may also precipitate conduction defects in the myocardial tissues.

★ *Dosage: Adult dose:* 20 mg/min loading infusion to a max dose of 17 mg/kg is initiated until a recognized endpoint is reached (abolishment of ectopy, hypotension ensues, QRS or QT lengthens, or the max dose is given). The maintenance infusion of procainamide should conversion occur is 1–4 mg/min, titrating to effect. *Pediatric administration* is not recommended. The drug is supplied as 1 gm/mL vials for dilution.

★ *Special Considerations:* Monitor the blood pressure and cardiac rhythm closely. Remember to watch for the endpoints of administration mentioned above.

AMIODARONE HYDROCHLORIDE (CORDARONE, PACERONE)

Classifications   CARDIOVASCULAR AGENT; ANTIDYSRHYTHMIAS CLASS III

★ *Actions:* Structurally related to thyroxine, this drug blocks sodium and potassium channels at rapid pacing frequencies, increasing duration of action potential and refractory periods, as well as alpha- and beta-adrenergic blockade. This drug can result in increased PR and QT intervals, as well as vascular smooth muscle relaxation with IV administration. The smooth muscle relaxation results in decreased vascular resistance (afterload), which in turn promotes a slight elevation in the cardiac index.

★ *Indications:* Initial treatment of ventricular dysrhythmias, including ventricular tachycardia and ventricular fibrillation. It can also be used for atrial dysrhythmias such as atrial fibrillation, atrial flutter, and PSVT (refractory to other antidysrhythmics).

★ *Contraindications:* Known hypersensitivity to the drug, certain cardiac dysrhythmias such as sinus bradycardia and second- or third-degree heart blocks. Also avoid use in cardiogenic shock and severe CHF.

★ *Side Effects:* Given the effects of the drug, hypotension, bradycardia, AV blocks, and ventricular dysrhythmias may occur. Pulmonary toxicity (including ARDS, alveolitis, pneumonitis, and interstitial pulmonary fibrosis). Anorexia, nausea, vomiting, and constipation have also been associated with the drug, as has photosensitivity to sunlight. Finally, the patient may acquire hyperthyroidism or hypothyroidism with continued administration of the drug.

★ *Dosage: Adult dose:* Dose for perfusing ventricular dysrhythmias is 150 mg bolus IV over 10 minutes (15 mg/min), followed by 1 mg/min infusion over 6 hours, which is then followed by 0.5 mg/min over the next 18 hours. The maintenance infusion can continue for up to 2–3 weeks at 0.5 mg/min. If the patient has a nonperfusing ventricular tachycardia or ventricular fibrillation, the 150-mg IV bolus may be repeated once at 300 mg after 5–15 minutes. *Pediatric dose:* 5 mg/kg IV/IO by rapid bolus. Maximum dose is 15 mg/kg. Amiodarone comes packaged in vials containing a concentration of 50 mg/mL ampules.

★ *Special Considerations:* Attempt to correct hypokalemia or hypomagnesemia (if present) prior to the administration of the therapy. Also protect from light unless otherwise directed.

ATROPINE SULFATE (ATROPINE)

Classifications AUTONOMIC NERVOUS SYSTEM AGENT; ANTICHOLINERGIC (PARA-SYMPATHOLYTIC); ANTIMUSCARINIC AGENT

★ *Actions:* Anticholinergic agent that blocks muscarinic responses to acetylcholine, whether excitatory or inhibitory. Net effects include action to smooth muscle, cardiac muscle, exocrine glands, urinary bladder, and a depressant action to the SA and AV nodes of the heart.

★ *Indications:* Since this drug inhibits vagal tone, it is primarily used in emergency medicine to remove excessive parasympathetic tone to vagally induced bradycardia and bronchoconstriction. It can also be used for GI disorders, to produce mydriasis and cycloplegia before refraction, and to help dry oral secretions and blunt vagal tone when performing an RSI procedure.

★ *Contraindications:* Known hypersensitivity to belladonna alkaloids. But in an emergency cardiac situation (i.e., asystole, symptomatic bradycardia), or organophosphate poisoning, no other absolute contraindications exist.

★ *Side Effects:* Side effects occur secondary to its anticholinergic properties, and include cardiac palpitations, tachycardia, dry mouth, dilated pupils, and possible anxiety.

★ *Dosage: Adult dose:* 0.5–1.0 mg IVP every 3–5 minutes to a max dose of 0.04 mg/kg for significant cardiovascular instability. The dose for organophosphate poisoning is higher, at 2–3 mg IV push (IVP), and should be given until sufficient abatement of the cholinergic influence has been removed. *Pediatric dose:* 0.01–0.03 mg/kg IVP. If given via endotracheal tube, the dose should be doubled for both adults and pediatrics. The drug is commonly supplied in a syringe of 1 mg/10 mL.

★ *Special Considerations:* Too small a dose may result in paradoxical slowing of the heart rate, increased intraocular pressure, and an unreliable pupillary assessment following administration; it may precipitate ventricular dysrhythmias or increase the infarction size when used in an MI patient for bradycardia. As such, caution should be used when administering to a patient with any type of cardiovascular disease. Monitor heart rate and cardiac rhythm closely. The use of multiple anticholinergic agents in the same patient may result in an additive effect.

ADENOSINE (ADENOCARD, ADENOSCAN)

Classifications CARDIOVASCULAR AGENT; ANTIDYSRYTHMIC CLASS IV-LIKE

★ *Actions:* A naturally occurring substance that blocks K^+ channels in the cardiac conductive system. Its effects include slowing conduction through AV pathways while interrupting reentry pathways through the AV node, restoring normal sinus rhythm in PSVT.

★ *Indications:* Supraventricular tachycardias, including PSVT that are hemodynamically stable in presentation, but unresponsive to conservative therapy (vagal maneuvers).

★ *Contraindications:* AV heart blocks more significant than first degree since worsening of the block may occur. Also sick sinus syndrome (without the presence of a functioning artificial pacemaker).

★ *Side Effects:* Transient (but short-lasting) first-, second-, or third-degree heart blocks; sustained ventricular tachycardia, ventricular fibrillation, facial flushing, palpitations, and anxiety.

★ *Dosage:* Initial bolus of 6 mg rapid IVP followed by 10–20 cc normal saline flush to speed drug to core circulation. Dose may be repeated twice at 12 mg rapid IVP, to a maximum of 30 mg. *Pediatric dose:* Not universally recognized, but when used it is commonly given in a dose range of 0.05–0.1 mg/kg rapid IVP. Supplied in both 3 mg/mL and 6 mg/2 mL preparations.

★ *Special Considerations:* Monitor heart rate and cardiac rhythm closely. Administer oxygen and provide emotional support during administration. If this drug is used on a patient currently taking carbamazepine (Tegretol) or dipyridamole (Persantine), the drug dose may be potentiated. Theophylline and related drugs may reduce the effectiveness of adenosine. In either instance, contact medical direction.

MAGNESIUM SULFATE (EPSOM SALT)

Classifications   GASTROINTESTINAL AGENT; LAXATIVE, SALINE; REPLACEMENT SOLUTION; ANTICONVULSANT

★ *Actions:* An essential element for muscle contraction; decreases the sensitivity of the motor end-plate to acetylcholine and decreases the excitability of the motor nerve terminals.

★ *Indications:* Ventricular tachydysrhythmias refractory to other antidysrhythmics; also used as a tocolytic agent in the patient with preterm labor; finally it can be used in acute bronchospasms that remain refractory to more traditional frontline agents. It acts as a laxative when given orally.

★ *Contraindications:* Heart block, renal disease, and toxemia of pregnancy in patients when delivery is imminent (within 2 hours).

★ *Side Effects:* Hypotension, tachycardia, respiratory depression (maternal and neonatal), flushing, CNS depression, and diaphoresis.

★ *Dosage:* 1–2 g diluted in 100–250 mL D_5W, and administered over 10–20 minutes (higher doses often needed for torsade de pointes. *Pediatric dose:* 25–50 mg/kg IV or IM. It commonly is supplied in vials of 4 mEq/mL (5 g).

★ *Special Considerations:* Administer slowly and monitor vital signs and cardiac rhythm closely. Be alert for orthostatic blood pressure changes. If long-term administration is warranted, also monitor deep tendon reflexes and have calcium gluceptate or calcium gluconate available for administration as needed.

DILTIAZEM (CARDIZEM, CARDIZEM LYO-JECT, CARDIZEM I.V.)

Classifications   CARDIOVASCULAR AGENT; CALCIUM CHANNEL BLOCKER; ANTI-HYPERTENSIVE AGENT

★ *Actions:* Calcium channel blocker; primary action to slow conduction velocity through SA and AV nodes. Also decreases myocardial contractility and decreases peripheral vascular resistance.

★ *Indications:* Atrial fibrillation/flutter with rapid ventricular response; supraventricular tachycardias refractory to frontline agents such as adenosine.

★ *Contraindications:* Since this drug will slow the heart rate and drop the blood pressure, contraindications naturally include hypotension, bradycardia, and AV heart blocks greater than first degree without a functioning ventricular pacemaker. Known hypersensitivity to the drug also serves as a contraindication.

★ *Side Effects:* Given the effects of diltiazem in blocking calcium movement, cardiovascular effects typically dominate. Hypotension, bradycardia, heart block, CHF, and occasionally peripheral edema may be observed.

★ *Dosage: Adult bolus dose:* 0.25 mg/kg IVP over 2 minutes; if no response the dose may be increased to 0.35 mg/kg IVP over 2 minutes. If a maintenance infusion is warranted, it should be run at 5–15 mg/min. *Pediatric dose:* Not yet established. The drug is commonly supplied as 5 mg/mL vials.

★ *Special Considerations:* Do NOT mix with intravenous beta-blocker administration; monitor vital signs and cardiac rhythm and blood pressure closely for bradycardia or hypotension. This drug is not recommended for infusion over 24 hours.

PROPRANOLOL HYDROCHLORIDE (INDERAL, APO-PROPRANOLOL)

Classifications   AUTONOMIC NERVOUS SYSTEM AGENT; BETA-ADRENERGIC ANTAG-ONIST (SYMPATHOLYTIC); ANTIHYPERTENSIVE AGENT; ANTIARRHYTHMIC CLASS II

★ *Actions:* This drug is also a beta-blocker agent that is similar to labetalol, but has more prominent beta-2-adrenergic blocking activity. The drug also provides direct membrane-stabilizing action on cardiac cells to provide a positive stabilizing effect to prevent/suppress cardiac dysrhythmias.

★ *Indications:* Cardiac ventricular dysrhythmia primarily, ventricular tachycardia, and occasionally ventricular fibrillation. It can also be used for supraventricular tachycardias refractory to frontline agents, and those patients with prolonged QT syndrome, especially in pediatric populations.

★ *Contraindications:* Because of its beta-2 blocking effects, this drug should not be used with patients who have severe asthma or other COPD disorders. Nor should it be used with bradycardia, hypotension, or acute CHF because it will only worsen the clinical condition of the patient.

★ *Side Effects:* From its antagonizing effect on beta-adrenergic receptor sites in the myocardium, this drug may precipitate hypotension, bradycardia, AV heart blocks, bronchospasm, decreased inotropy, and CHF.

★ *Dosage: Adult dose:* 1–3 mg slow IVP; may repeat in 2 minutes if no response, then administer every 4 hours as needed. *Pediatric dose:* 0.01 mg/kg IVP up to 1 mg slow IVP when indicated. Commonly supplied in 1 mg/mL vials for injection.

★ *Special Considerations:* Do not give more than 1 mg/min IVP because it may potentiate many of its side effects. Use cautiously with   patients with chronic lung diseases as well, even if asymptomatic.

CARDIOPROTECTANTS

Many patients with acute myocardial infarction die every year due to sudden cardiac arrest, which is generally defined as death within 2 hours of the onset of cardiac symptoms. Those who survive a myocardial infarction, they may still have residual effects of cardiac dysfunction for years due to the infarction size and decreased contractility. The administration of cardioprotectant agents decreases mortality, decreases infarction size, and decreases risk for re-infarction when administered appropriately.

The administration of cardioprotectant agents decreases mortality, decreases infarction size and decreases risk for re-infarction when administered appropriately.

ASPIRIN (ACETYLSALICYLIC ACID, A.S.A.)

Classifications   CENTRAL NERVOUS SYSTEM AGENT; ANALGESIC; SALICYLATE; ANTI-PYRETIC

★ *Actions:* Inhibits platelet aggregation by decreasing the synthesis of blood coagulation factors VII, IX, and X (which mediate platelet aggregation). It also is thought to inhibit the action of vitamin K.

★ *Indications:* Reduction of morbidity and mortality of patients with acute cardiovascular insult, including acute MI and stroke; decrease risk of cardiovascular insult with patients with stable angina and TIA.

★ *Contraindications:* Allergy to salicylates, bleeding tendencies, severe anemia, recent history of surgery, history of GI bleed. Aspirin should also be avoided in pregnant females.

★ *Side Effects:* Hypersensitivity reactions, including anaphylaxis; bleeding, GI upset, thrombocytopenia, nausea and vomiting.

★ *Dosage: Adult dose:* 162 mg (two baby aspirin) for 30 days from diagnosis of acute MI. For prophylaxis purposes, 81–325 mg daily if diagnosis of acute coronary syndrome (ACS) is made, or 30 days after acute MI. *Pediatric dose:* Although a child dose is available for its anti-inflammatory, antipyretic, and analgesic actions, a pediatric dose for a suspected ACS is not established. Aspirin is supplied in multiple strengths, to include 81-, 165-, 325-, and 500-mg tablets and capsules. Coated aspirin products should not be used in the emergency setting as they delay establishment of therapeutic drug levels.

★ *Special Considerations:* Screen carefully before administration for risks factors that may precipitate hemorrhage, and monitor the patient closely for an allergic reaction.

METOPROLOL TARTRATE (LOPRESSOR, NOROMETOPROL)

Classifications   AUTONOMIC NERVOUS SYSTEM AGENT; BETA-ADRENERGIC ANTAGONIST (SYMPATHOLYTIC); ANTIHYPERTENSIVE AGENT

★ *Actions:* Another beta-1-specific adrenergic blockade agent that decreases the inotropic, chronotropic, and dromotropic properties of myocardial muscle. The net result is a drop in blood pressure mediated by a diminished cardiac output.

★ *Indications:* Myocardial preservation during acute myocardial infarction; decreases infarction size, risk of sudden cardiac death, and the potential risk for re-infarction. It may also be used for the management of mild to severe hypertension in isolation or in concert with a thiazide. One off-label use of this drug is in the management of CHF as well.

★ *Contraindications:* Similar to other beta-blocking agents discussed earlier, this drug should be avoided in patients with AV heart blocks greater than first degree, those with preexisting bradycardia, hypotension, moderate to severe left ventricular failure, and known hypersensitivity.

★ *Side Effects:* Hypotension, bradydysrhythmias (including heart blocks), bronchospasm in higher doses, hypoglycemia, and dizziness.

★ *Dosage: Adult dose:* 5 mg slow IVP can be used as an initial dose, and repeated up to three times in 5-minute intervals. The ongoing maintenance dose is usually 25–100 mg by mouth daily. *Pediatric dose:* the drug is avoided in children so there is no specific pediatric dose. The drug is available in preparations of 5 mg/mL ampules, and orally as 25-, 50-, and 100-mg tablets.

★ *Special Considerations:* Use cautiously with acute inferior wall MI, or acute MI with SA/AV nodal involvement. In such cases a complete heart block may result. Monitor the vital signs and cardiac rhythm closely.

INOTROPIC AGENTS

Patients with acute congestive heart failure and poor cardiac contractility may require a "boost" to increase peripheral perfusion and decrease preload and afterload by increasing stroke volume and heart rate. The administration of inotropic agents in these patients assists the diseased myocardium to pump more efficiently to increase end-organ perfusion. By increasing cardiac output, the patient can better perfuse end organs, especially the liver and kidneys, so that other agents being administered will perform more efficiently.

MILRINONE LACTATE (PRIMACOR)

Classifications   CARDIOVASCULAR AGENT; INOTROPIC AGENT

★ *Actions:* Inhibits peak III cyclic AMP isoenzyme in cardiac and vascular muscle, resulting in elevation of cyclic AMP and a release of calcium. This results in a direct inotropic effect (increased contractility) and direct arterial vasodilation with little chronotropic activity.

★ *Indications:* Short-term treatment of acute congestive heart failure, usually with patients taking digitalis and diuretics. In therapeutic doses, this drug can increase cardiac output and drop PCWP and SVR without increasing myocardial oxygen demand.

★ *Contraindications:* Hypotension, severe aortic/pulmonic valve obstruction. As with any other drug, if known hypersensitivity exists, the drug is not to be administered.

★ *Side Effects:* Cardiac dysrhythmias, including ventricular and supraventricular dysrhythmias, hypotension, chest pain, cardiac ischemia, and thrombocytopenia.

★ *Dosage:* A loding dose of 50 mcg/kg can be given IVP slowly over 10 minutes to achieve a therapeutic level. Afterward a maintenance infusion should be initiated at 0.375–0.75 mcg/kg/min. *Pediatric dose:* Not established. The drug is supplied as a 1 mg/mL vial for injection and as a 200 mcg/mL premix for infusion.

★ *Special Considerations:* Given the drug's mechanism of action, the provider should monitor vital signs, urinary output, and cardiac rhythm closely. Be careful not to administer furosemide (Lasix) through the Y-site of the administration set infusing this drug because precipitation will occur. Long-term management should include daily monitoring of platelet count.

INAMRINONE LACTATE (INOCOR)

Classifications   CARDIOVASCULAR AGENT; INOTROPIC AGENT

★ *Actions:* Inhibits peak III cyclic AMP isoenzyme in cardiac and vascular/muscle, resulting in direct inotropic effect and direct arterial vasodilation. This drug acts slightly different than digitalis and beta-adrenergic stimulants. It enhances contractility and cardiac output while simultaneously dropping ventricular preload and PCWP and SVR.

★ *Indications:* Short-term treatment of acute congestive heart failure, usually in patients taking digitalis and diuretics. Inamrinone promotes hemodynamic improvements in patients with CHF from ischemic heart disease.

★ *Contraindications:* Hypersensitivity to the drug or to bisulfites, preexisting hypotension, and the presence of uncorrected aortic/pulmonic valve obstruction. The drug should also be avoided in patients with uncorrected hypokalemia or dehydration.

★ *Side Effects:* The patient may complain of pain, tenderness, or muscular stiffness near the site of injection following drug administration. There may also be a local inflammatory reaction. Systemically, there may be hypotension or drug-induced thrombocytopenia.

★ *Dosage: Adult dose:* Like many other drugs, this drug requires a loading dose to rapidly elevate blood levels to a therapeutic range. The recommended dose of 0.75 mcg/kg slow IVP over 2–3 minutes should achieve this. The maintenance infusion can be run at 5–10 mcg/kg/min. *Pediatric dose:* A loading dose of 3–4.5 mg/kg in divided doses can be given with a maintenance infusion of 0.01 mg/kg/min. The drug is commonly supplied in 5 mg/mL vials.

★ *Special Considerations:* Do not mix with furosemide or dextrose-containing solutions. Monitor vital signs for hypotension and the cardiac rhythm closely for dysrhythmias (terminate administration if either occurs). The drug may become hepatotoxic, and long-term use should include platelet count monitoring daily.

ANTICOAGULANT/ANTIPLATELET AGENTS

When perfusion is under stress due to the formation of a thrombus or embolism, the critically ill patient may require the administration of anticoagulant agents to prevent new clots from forming or an existing clot from enlarging. Note, however, that such agents don't dissolve blood clots. Anticoagulants are also given to certain people at risk for forming blood clots, such as those with artificial heart valves or who have atrial fibrillation.

Another category of drugs for use in patients with clinical consequences of a newly formed thrombus is the fibrinolytics. During the normal hemostatic response of the body to vascular injury, a local thrombosis is created. Under normal conditions, the formed thrombus is confined to the immediate area of injury and does not obstruct distal flow of blood. Under pathologic conditions however, the thrombus can propagate into the otherwise normal blood vessel and inhibit blood flow. Abnormal thrombosis can occur in any vessel at any location in the body. The principal clinical syndromes that result are acute myocardial infarction, deep venous thrombosis, pulmonary embolism, acute nonhemorrhagic stroke, and acute peripheral arterial occlusion.

The fibrinolytic agents available today work by converting plasminogen to the natural fibrinolytic agent plasmin. Plasmin lyses a clot by breaking down the fibrinogen and fibrin contained in a clot. With the thrombus dissolved, blood flow through the vessel is again restored.

In patients with acute MI who fit the administration criteria, early administration of a fibrinolytic agent reduces mortality and is associated with improved short- and long-term clinical outcomes. From a pathophysiological perspective, the restoration of blood flow through an occluded coronary artery reduces infarct size and minimizes the extent of myocardial damage, preserves left ventricular function, reduces morbidity, and prolongs survival.

HEPARIN SODIUM (HEPALEAN)

Classifications   BLOOD FORMERS, COAGULATORS AND ANTICOAGULANTS

★ *Actions:* An anticoagulant agent that inhibits reactions that lead to the clotting of blood and the formation of fibrin clots by blocking the conversion of prothrombin to thrombin and fibrinogen to fibrin. The drug does not dissolve existing clots, but can prevent clot extension and inhibit new clot formation.

★ *Indications:* For prophylaxis and treatment of pulmonary embolism in patients with new onset of atrial fibrillation with embolization, for diagnosis and treatment of acute and chronic consumptive coagulopathies (disseminated intravascular coagulation), for prevention of clotting in arterial and cardiac surgery, and for prophylaxis and treatment of peripheral arterial embolism.

★ *Contraindications:* Known hypersensitivity, severe thrombocytopenia, active bleeding, bleeding tendencies (hemophilia, purpura, and so on), recent surgery, blood dyscrasias, advanced liver and kidney disease, severe hypertension, and suspected intracranial hemorrhage.

★ *Side Effects:* Numerous side effects have been documented with the administration of heparin, of these the most clinically significant include spontaneous hemorrhaging, thrombocytopenia, chest pain, anaphylactoid reactions, and bronchospasm.

★ *Dosage: Adult dose:* The loading dose for administration ranges from 5000 to 7500 units IVP. A maintenance infusion of heparin is then needed, but is based on partial thromboplastin time (PTT) levels. The dose usually is then 1000 to 2000 units/hr by continuous infusion. *Pediatric loading dose:* 50 units/kg IVP with a maintenance infusion of 50–100 units/kg IVP every 4 hours continuously. Heparin is supplied in vials containing 5000 units or 10,000 units.

- *Special Considerations:* Monitor PTT levels frequently, especially after rebolus or adjustment to continuous infusion. Monitor the platelet count frequently and avoid any unnecessary venipunctures or arterial punctures. Apply direct pressure to any venipuncture site for at least 5 minutes; monitor closely for any unexplained hemorrhaging syndromes or potential intracranial or internal bleeds. Protamine sulfate is a drug that can be used as an antagonist to accidental heparin overdosing, but its use should be guided by PTT levels as well.

ENOXAPARIN (LOVENOX)

Classifications BLOOD FORMERS, COAGULATORS AND ANTICOAGULANTS; LOW-MOLECULAR-WEIGHT HEPARIN

- *Actions:* A low-molecular-weight heparin that has antithrombotic properties. Does not affect PT, but can affect thrombin time and activated thromboplastin time.
- *Indications:* As an effective anticoagulation agent, this drug can be used as an antithrombotic agent following surgery, as a prevention modality for deep venous thrombosis (DVT) postoperatively, and in the management of patients with diagnosis of ACS and pulmonary emboli.
- *Contraindications:* Drug hypersensitivity, active major bleeding, hemorrhage disorders, recent surgery, blood dyscrasias.
- *Side Effects:* Possible mild or severe allergic reaction, hemorrhage, thrombocytopenia, ecchymosis, and anemia. Some patients have also reported dyspnea with drug administration.
- *Dosage: Adult dose for DVT prophylaxis:* 30 mg subcutaneous b.i.d. *Adult dose for ACS:* 1 mg/kg subcutaneously. It may be repeated in the hospital every 12 hours for 2–8 days. *Pediatric dose:* Not established.
- *Special Considerations:* Unlike heparin, no antagonist is available. Given its mechanism, monitor for bleeding and avoid unnecessary invasive procedures. Assess PTT level prior to administration, and use cautiously in patients with uncontrolled hypertension and GI disease.

WARFARIN SODIUM (COUMADIN SODIUM, PANWARFIN)

Classifications BLOOD FORMERS, COAGULATORS AND ANTICOAGULANTS; ORAL ANTICOAGULANT

- *Actions:* An anticoagulant agent that indirectly interferes with blood clotting by depressing hepatic synthesis of vitamin K-dependent coagulation factors. The drug does not dissolve existing clots, but can prevent clot extension and inhibit new clot formation.
- *Indications:* For prophylaxis and treatment of DVT and its extension, pulmonary embolism; treatment of atrial fibrillation with embolization. Also used as an adjunct in the treatment of coronary occlusion, cerebral transient ischemic attacks (TIAs), and as a prophylactic in patients with prosthetic cardiac valves.
- *Contraindications:* Known hypersensitivity, patients with hemorrhagic tendencies, vitamin C or K deficiency, hemophilia, coagulation factor deficiencies, blood dyscrasias; active bleeding; open wounds, active peptic ulcer, esophageal varices, extreme diastolic hypertension, cerebral vascular disease; pericarditis with acute MI; severe hepatic or renal disease.
- *Side Effects:* Numerous side effects have been documented with the administration of warfarin, which may include a life-threatening hemorrhage from any tissue or organ. Less common side effects may include abdominal pain and cramping, diarrhea, fatigue, fever, fluid retention, lethargy, liver damage, nausea.

- ★ *Dosage: Adult dose:* The dosage must be individualized for each patient based upon numerous parameters including the baseline PT or INR. *Pediatric dose:* Not routinely administered to this population.
- ★ *Special Considerations:* Numerous drugs have been cited in the literature that alter the expected response of warfarin, so consulting a compatibility drug chart is recommended. In addition, cautious drug use should be considered in patients with the following: alcoholism, menstruation, lactation, debilitation, carcinoma, CHF, collagen diseases, hepatic and renal insufficiency, pancreatic disorders, vitamin K deficiency, hypothyroidism, hyperlipidemia, hypercholesterolemia, and hereditary resistance to warfarin therapy.

EPTIFIBATIDE (INTEGRILIN)

Classifications   CARDIOVASCULAR AGENT; ANTITHROMBOTIC AGENT; ANTIPLATELET ANTIBODY; GLYCOPROTEIN IIB/IIIA INHIBITOR

- ★ *Actions:* Reversibly inhibits platelet aggregation by preventing the binding of fibrinogen, Von Willebrand factor to glycoprotein IIb/IIIa (GPIIb/IIIa). Drug is immediately effective after IV use.
- ★ *Indications:* Treatment of acute coronary syndrome, with or without emergent coronary intervention; treatment of those undergoing coronary intervention, including stenting.
- ★ *Contraindications:* Active pathologic bleeding within 30 days; history of bleeding abnormalities; history of AV malformation, intracranial bleeding, brain tumor; history of recent trauma that increases risk of bleeding; uncontrolled hypertension with systolic BP > 200 mmHg. The drug is also contraindicated if known hypersensitivity exists.
- ★ *Side Effects:* Bleeding, including life-threatening hemorrhage, anemia, and thrombocytopenia.
- ★ *Dosage:* Initial IV bolus of 180 mcg/kg upon diagnosis in the adult patient for ACS. A maintenance infusion is then inititated at 2 mcg/kg/min for 72–96 hours (or until hospital discharge). *Pediatric dose:* not established. The drug is commonly supplied in 10 mL and 100 mL vial containers as a 0.75 mg/mL.
- ★ *Special Considerations:* Monitor for bleeding; use cautiously in patients with renal insufficiency/failure. Use with caution in patients receiving oral anticoagulants or NSAID medications.

ABCIXIMAB (REOPRO)

Classifications   BLOOD FORMERS, COAGULATORS AND ANTICOAGULANTS; ANTI-THROMBOTIC AGENT; ANTIPLATELET AGENT; GLYCOPROTEIN IIB/IIIA INHIBITOR

- ★ *Actions:* Inhibits platelet aggregation by preventing the binding of fibrinogen, Von Willebrand factor to glycoprotein IIb/IIIa receptor sites of platelets.
- ★ *Indications:* Inhibition of platelet aggregation during coronary intervention (PCTA, intracoronary stenting) in patients at high risk for coronary reocclusion.
- ★ *Contraindications:* Active pathologic bleeding within 30 days; history of bleeding abnormalities; history of AV malformation, intracranial bleeding, brain tumor; history of recent trauma that increases risk of bleeding.
- ★ *Side Effects:* Bleeding, including life-threatening hemorrhage; cardiac dysrhythmias, including bradycardia, AV blocks, and atrial fibrillation. Also may precipitate hypotension and hematemesis.
- ★ *Dosage: Adult dose:* Initial IV bolus of 0.25 mg/kg given 10–60 minutes prior to the start of the intervention, followed by continuous infusion of 10 mg/min for 12 hours

after intervention. For patients undergoing intervention within 24 hours, the dosage schedule is 0.25 mg/kg IV bolus followed by continuous infusion at 10 mg/min for 18–24 hours. *Pediatric dose:* Not established. The drug is supplied in 5 mL vials (2 mg/mL) for injection.

★ *Special Considerations:* Monitor for bleeding, and use cautiously in patients weighing <75 kg, older adults, history of GI disease, and PTCA procedures that lasts >70 minutes. Do not shake vial.

TIROFIBAN HYDROCHLORIDE (AGGRASTAT)

Classifications   BLOOD FORMERS, COAGULATORS AND ANTICOAGULANTS; ANTI-PLATELET AGENT; GLYCOPROTEIN IIB/IIIA INHIBITOR

★ *Actions:* Inhibits platelet aggregation at glycoprotein IIb/IIIa receptor sites of platelets. Since this inhibits platelet aggregation, it also inhibits thrombotic events during ACS management.

★ *Indications:* Combination therapy with heparin sodium for acute coronary syndrome, with or without emergent cardiac intervention (PCTA).

★ *Contraindications:* Active pathologic bleeding within 30 days; history of bleeding abnormalities; history of AV malformation, intracranial bleeding, brain tumor; history of recent trauma that increases risk of bleeding.

★ *Side Effects:* Bleeding, including life-threatening hemorrhage, vasovagal reaction, vertigo, bradycardia, anemia, thrombocytopenia.

★ *Dosage: Adult dose:* Initially 0.4 mcg/kg/min for 30 minutes, then followed by a 0.1 mcg/kg/min continuous infusion. *Pediatric dose:* Not established.

★ *Special Considerations:* Use cautiously with patients with platelet count less than 150,000 mm^3; monitor for bleeding and exercise caution when using this drug in the presence of other fibrinolytic agents or drugs that cause hemolysis.

CLOPIDOGREL BISULFATE (PLAVIX)

Classifications   BLOOD FORMERS, COAGULATORS AND ANTICOAGULANTS; ANTI-PLATELET AGENT

★ *Actions:* Inhibits platelet aggregation by selectively preventing the binding of adenosine diphosphate (ADP) to its receptor on platelets. The consequence is a prolongation of bleeding time due to inhibition of clotting.

★ *Indications:* Reduction of MI (secondary prevention), lower risk of stroke and vascular death in clients with atherosclerosis; to improve outcome of patients with acute coronary syndrome and acute MI undergoing percutaneous coronary angioplasty (PCTA); for use with aspirin in combination therapy with patients with acute coronary syndrome not undergoing PCTA.

★ *Contraindications:* Hypersensitivity, active pathologic bleeding (ulcer, intracranial bleeding), lactating mothers.

★ *Side Effects:* Life-threatening bleeding, including intracranial hemorrhage, possible hypertension, syncope, palpitations.

★ *Dosage: Adult dose:* For recent MI, stroke, or peripheral artery disease, 75 mg daily PO. For ACS with (or without) intervention 300 mg initially and then 75 mg daily. *Pediatric dose:* Not established. Drug is prepared as a 75-mg tablet to be taken orally.

★ *Special Considerations:* Monitor for bleeding; avoid unnecessary invasive procedures. Use with caution in patients receiving other drugs that may induce gastrointestinal hemorrhage. Moderate concern for hepatic impairment.

FIBRINOLYTICS

TENECTEPLASE RECOMBINANT (TNKASE)

Classifications   BLOOD FORMERS, COAGULATORS AND ANTICOAGULANTS; FIBRINOLYTIC ENZYME

★ *Actions:* A single-bolus fibrinolytic agent that has been approved by the U.S. Food and Drug Administration for the treatment of acute MI. Drug works by stimulating the body's own clot-dissolving mechanism by activating plasminogen, a naturally occurring substance secreted by endothelial cells in response to injury to the artery walls that contributes to clot formation. When TNKase activates plasminogen, it converts it into plasmin, which breaks down the fibrin mesh that binds the clot together. The clot then dissolves, restoring blood flow to the heart. (See Figure 11-3 ■.)

★ *Indications:* ECG-documented acute myocardial infarction.

★ *Contraindications:* Active internal bleeding, history of stroke, CNS surgery within past 2 months, neoplasm, AV malformations, severe uncontrolled hypertension (SBP > 180, DBP > 110).

★ *Relative Contraindications:* Recent major surgery, for example, coronary artery bypass graft, obstetrical delivery, organ biopsy, previous puncture of noncompressible vessels, cerebrovascular disease. Recent gastrointestinal or genitourinary bleeding. Recent trauma. Hypertension with a systolic BP ≥ 180 mmHg and/or diastolic BP ≥ 110 mmHg. High likelihood of left heart thrombus, for example, mitral stenosis with atrial fibrillation. Acute pericarditis and subacute bacterial endocarditis. Hemostatic defects, including those secondary to severe hepatic or renal disease. Severe hepatic dysfunction, pregnancy, and hemorrhagic ophthalmic conditions.

★ *Side Effects:* Bleeding, including hemorrhage; intracerebral hemorrhage; reperfusion dysrhythmias, cholesterol embolization (rare).

★ *Dosage: Adult dose:* Given over 5 seconds via IVP:
   - <60 kg = 30 mg
   - 60–70 kg = 35 mg
   - 70–80 kg = 40 mg
   - 80–90 kg = 45 mg
   - >90 kg = 50 mg

   Pediatric dose: Not established. This drug comes supplied as 50-mg vials that need reconstitution.

■ **Figure 11-3**   Basic action of fibrinolytic drugs.

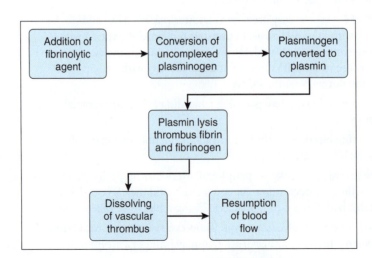

- *Special Considerations:* Screen carefully for contraindications and relative contraindications prior to administration. Continuously monitor vital signs and cardiac rhythm; obtain baseline neurologic assessment and reassess every 15 minutes; monitor closely for evidence of internal bleeding. Ensure direct pressure to any venipuncture sites for a minimum of 5 minutes if bleeding occurs. Do not administer any other medication through TNKase line; to be used in combination with heparin sodium therapy.

RETEPLASE RECOMBINANT (RETAVASE, rt-PA)

Classifications   BLOOD FORMERS, COAGULATORS AND ANTICOAGULANTS; FIBRI-NOLYTIC ENZYME

- *Actions:* Recombinant plasminogen activator similar to t-PA, catalyzing endogenous plaminogen to generate plasmin; degrades fibrin and promotes the lysis of thrombus formation.
- *Indications:* Thrombolysis of coronary clot during active MI to reduce mortality and/or incidence of CHF.
- *Contraindications:* Similar to tenecteplase, and includes active internal bleeding, history of stroke, CNS surgery within past 2 months, neoplasm, AV malformations, severe uncontrolled hypertension.
- *Side Effects:* Anemia, bleeding, intracerebral hemorrhage, reperfusion dysrhythmias.
- *Dosage: Adult dose:* 10 units IVP over 2 minutes; repeat dosage after 30 minutes (total of 20 U). *Pediatric dose:* Not established. Drug is supplied in a 10-unit vial for reconstitution.
- *Special Considerations:* Stop concomitant heparin if bleeding develops. Monitor bleeding sites.

ALTEPLASE RECOMBINANT (ACTIVASE, t-PA, ACTILYSE)

Classifications   BLOOD FORMERS, COAGULATORS AND ANTICOAGULANTS; FIBRI-NOLYTIC ENZYME

- *Actions:* Similar to tenecteplase and reteplase in that it is a recombinant tissue plasminogen activitor that stimulates plasmin release for clot lysis. This is the only fibrinolytic agent approved by the FDA for the treatment of acute MI, acute ischemic stroke, and acute pulmonary embolism.
- *Indications:* Similar to tenecteplase, to also include acute ischemic stroke and acute pulmonary embolism.
- *Contraindications:* Active internal bleeding, history of stroke, CNS hemorrhage within past 2 months, recent trauma, AV malformation, bleeding disorders, and uncontrolled hypertension.
- *Side Effects:* Again, side effects are similar to other fibrinolytic agents and include internal and superficial hemorrhage.
- *Dosage: Adult dose:* Depends on reason for administration, weight of the patient, and is given over a specific amount of time:
  - *Acute MI*
    - For weight ≥ 65 kg: 15 mg IVP over 2 minutes, followed by 50 mg IV over next 30 minutes, followed by 35 mg IV over next 60 minutes
    - For weight < 65 kg: 15 mg IVP over 2 minutes, followed by 0.75 mg/kg IVP over the next 30 minutes, followed by 0.5 mg/kg IVP over the next 60 minutes

– *Ischemic Stroke*
- 0.9 mg/kg IV (maximum dose = 90 mg), with 10% of dose given as bolus over 1 minute

– *Pulmonary Embolism*
- 100 mg IV over 2 hours

Alteplase is supplied as a 100-mg vial for reconstitution.

★ *Special Considerations:* See tenecteplase. Additional considerations include the need to obtain a non-contrast CT in order to rule out hemorrhagic stroke prior to t-PA administration. Patients with signs/symptoms of stroke must receive t-PA within 3 hours of onset of symptoms. A spiral chest CT or VQ lung scan is required prior to administration of t-PA with suspicion of acute pulmonary embolism.

NEUROLOGICAL DRUGS

The administration of agents in the patient with new onset seizure disorder, breakthrough seizure, or *status epilepticus* (continuous seizure) is to preserve brain function by inhibiting the abnormal electrical impulses in the brain.

The administration of agents in the patient with new onset seizure disorder, breakthrough seizure, or *status epilepticus* (continuous seizure) is to preserve brain function by inhibiting the abnormal electrical impulses in the brain, which then controls the motor effects of the seizure. Failure to do so will allow the seizure to continue unabated. This places the patient at great risk for cellular ischemia (due to increased metabolic demands), cellular damage (rhabdomyolysis from tonic-clonic muscle movements), and all the sequelae that occur during seizure activity (injury, long bone and vertebral fractures, aspiration, airway loss).

ANTIEPILEPTICS

PHENYTOIN SODIUM (DILANTIN)

Classifications   CENTRAL NERVOUS SYSTEM AGENT; ANTICONVULSANT, HYDANTOIN

★ *Actions:* Phenytoin is an antiepileptic that is chemically similar to barbiturates, and is thought to act in the motor cortex, where the spread of seizure activity is inhibited. It stabilizes the seizure threshold caused by excessive stimulation, and has been used on occasion as treatment for digitalis toxicity. It also has antidysrhythmic properties beneficial for ventricular dysrhythmias with QT prolongation.

★ *Indications:* Treatment of tonic-clonic or complex partial seizure activity, whether new onset or breakthrough in presentation. Also useful for seizure control that occurs during or after neurosurgery.

★ *Contraindications:* Allergy to phenytoin, hypoglycemic seizures, cardiac dysrhythmias such as bradycardias and heart blocks, and Adams-Stokes syndrome (sick-sinus syndrome).

★ *Side Effects:* Numerous side effects are associated with this drug, many of which are relatively benign in a critical setting. More significant findings may include various neurologic symptoms such as ataxia, slurred speech, confusion, CNS depression, and nystagmus. The patient may also display hypotension with rapid administration, gingival hyperplasia with prolonged use, and tissue necrosis if the IV infiltrates.

★ *Dosage: Adult loading dose:* Typically 10–15 mg/kg slow IVP over 30 minutes or a single 1000-mg loading dose, followed by a maintenance dose of 4–8 mg/kg slow IVP. For digitalis toxicity, a dose of 3–5 mg/kg slow IVP can be considered. *Pediatric dose:* 15–20 mg/kg slow IVP. IV dilantin is supplied in 50 mg/mL vials.

★ *Special Considerations:* Do not give faster than 50 mg/min; monitor for vital signs, especially blood pressure and cardiac rhythm; use cautiously in patients with hepatic or renal disease. Therapeutic drug levels occur at 10–20 ng/dL. Not compatible with dextrose-containing IV solutions.

PHENOBARBITAL SODIUM (LUMINAL, BARBITAL, SOLFOTON)

Classifications   CENTRAL NERVOUS SYSTEM AGENT; ANTICONVULSANT; SEDATIVE-HYPNOTIC; BARBITURATE

★ *Actions:* Long-lasting anticonvulsant drug in the barbiturate class of agents. Inhibition of impulse transmission in the cerebral cortex via the ascending reticular activating system (ARAS). The net effect is CNS depression and hypnotic effects. Controls the spread of seizures by raising the threshold for motor cortex stimuli.

★ *Indications:* Treatment of tonic-clonic and complex partial seizures. Used primarily for new onset seizures in the pediatric population. Can also be used for eclampsia and as a sedative for highly anxious states.

★ *Contraindications:* Allergy to barbiturates. Significant hepatic, respiratory, or renal disease, and significant hypotension.

★ *Side Effects:* Sedation, bradycardia, hypotension, respiratory depression, nystagmus, confusion, ataxia, and somnolence.

★ *Dosage: Adult dose:* 100–250 mg slow IVP over 5 minutes (rapid administration worsens side effects). *Pediatric dose:* 10–20 mg/kg also given via slow IVP over 5 minutes. The drug is packaged in a multitude of forms, but can commonly be found in 65 mg/mL and 130 mg/mL vials for IV use.

★ *Special Considerations:* Monitor vital signs and cardiac rhythm closely. Be prepared to assist with ventilations if respiratory depression occurs; use cautiously with elderly patients and with patients with hepatic and renal failure.

FOSPHENYTOIN SODIUM (CEREBRYX)

Classifications   CENTRAL NERVOUS SYSTEM AGENT; ANTICONVULSANT, HYDANTOIN

★ *Actions:* Parenteral prodrug to phenytoin that converts to phenytoin after administration; hence, its action is similar to that of phenytoin.

★ *Indications:* See phenytoin. Used primarily when oral agents cannot be given or adequately absorbed.

★ *Contraindications:* See phenytoin; also includes hypersensitivity to hydantoin products.

★ *Side Effects:* See phenytoin.

★ *Dosage: Adult loading dose:* 15–20 mg PE/kg (PE = phenytoin equivalents), IVP slowly. A maintenance infusion is necessary, and should be given at 4–6 mg PE/kg/day IVP slowly. *Pediatric dose:* Not yet established. The drug comes supplied as 75 mg/mL ampules (equivalent to 50 mg phenytoin).

★ *Special Considerations:* Do not give any faster than 100–150 mg PE/min, and keep refrigerated prior to administration. Monitor vital signs for hypotension and bradycardia; and monitor the ECG for emergence of dysrhythmias. Use with caution on patients with impaired hepatic, renal, or pulmonary function.

MISCELLANEOUS NEUROLOGIC DRUGS

Cerebral perfusion pressure is the difference between mean arterial pressure (MAP) minus the intracranial pressure (ICP). Or in formula form: CPP = MAP − ICP. When ICPs increase, cerebral perfusion is altered and over time the risk for long-term disability may arise if intracranial swelling is not addressed. In the acute phase, ICP may rise so high from the edema that the brain starts to herniate through the foramen magnum, which is often a grave condition. The use of mannitol can aid in the reduction of swelling at the cerebral level, and serves to decrease ICP regardless of the cause (tumor, trauma, infectious causes, or medical/trauma-induced cerebral tissue edema).

When intracranial pressures increase, cerebral perfusion is altered and over time the risk for long-term disability may arise if intracranial swelling is not addressed.

Corticosteroids (dexamethasone and methylprednisolone) are sometimes used to help prevent inflammation, particularly with tumors and infection (meningitis).

MANNITOL (OSMITROL)

Classifications   ELECTROLYTIC BALANCE AND WATER BALANCE AGENTS; DIURETIC, OSMOTIC

★ *Actions:* Hyperosmolar agent that draws interstititial fluid into the intravascular space. This then increases the amount of fluid passing through the kidneys (enhances glomerular filtration rate), which decreases the reabsorpition of sodium and thus promotes water loss. Onset of action: 15 minutes to decrease intracerebral pressure.

★ *Indications:* Acute traumatic or atraumatic brain injury with evidence of increased intracranial pressure or herniation syndrome (Cushing's reflex).

★ *Contraindications:* Hypotension in the trauma patient, severe dehydration, acute pulmonary edema, anuria, history of allergy.

★ *Side Effects:* Given the drug's mechanism of action, obvious side effects would include hypotension, dehydration, acidosis, and electrolyte imbalances. If the patient has poor renal function, he may become edematous, have hypertension, experience headaches, and complain of nausea and vomiting.

★ *Dosage: Adult dose:* For elevations in intracranial or intraocular pressure, the adult patient should receive 1.5–2 g/kg IVP over 30–60 minutes. *Pediatric dose:* Not established for ICP problems. Drug is supplied in 20% vials containing 200 g for injection.

★ *Special Considerations:* Use cautiously with patients with actual or suspected blood loss, hypotension, or dehydration. Monitor urinary output closely after administration, and be alert for transient hypertension. Caution should be used in patients with poor left ventricular function and those with renal disease or insufficiency.

METHYLPREDNISOLONE (SOLU-MEDROL, MEDROL)

Classifications   HORMONE AND SYNTHETIC SUBSTITUTES; CORTICOSTEROID, GLUCOCORTICOID; ANTI-INFLAMMATORY

★ *Actions:* Intermediate-acting synthetic glucocorticoid used for its anti-inflammatory and immunosuppressive properties. Also alters the body's immune response to a variety of stimuli.

★ *Indications:* To decrease inflammation and swelling; for treatment of acute bronchospasm; and can be used as an anti-inflammatory agent for chronic inflammatory diseases.

★ *Contraindications:* Suspected fungal infections, known hypersensitivity.

★ *Side Effects:* Edema, hypokalemia, hypotension, hypertension, elevated blood glucose, CHF, delayed wound healing, and possible hypokalemia. The patient may become dependent with long-term use.

★ *Dosage:* Methylprednisolone was once recommended as a treatment for acute spinal cord injury. More recent evidence has shown it to be ineffective and associated with multiple complications. Now it is only a treatment *option* for acute spinal cord injuries. If used for acute spinal cord injury, the recommended *adult dose* is 30 mg/kg IV over 10–20 minutes, followed by 5.4 mg/kg/hr for 23 hours after bolus. For acute bronchospasm: 40–125 mg IVP over 2 minutes. *Pediatric dose:* 1–2 mg/kg IVP over 2 minutes. Drug is supplied as 40-mg, 125-mg, and 1-g vials for injection purposes.

★ *Special Considerations:* Monitor vital signs closely, especially with spinal cord bolus (may cause hypertension). Also use caution with Cushing's syndrome, GI ulcerations, diabetic patients, and those with psychotic tendencies. This may also cause a steroid-like glucose release, resulting in hyperglycemia in the nondiabetic patient.

DEXAMETHASONE (DECADRON, HEXADRYL, DEXASONE)

Classifications HORMONE AND SYNTHETIC SUBSTITUTES; CORTICOSTEROID; GLUCOCORTICOID

- ★ *Actions:* A glucocorticoid used for its potent anti-inflammatory properties; able to cross the blood–brain barrier for use with acute increases in intracranial pressure (less common).
- ★ *Indications:* Adrenal insufficiency concomitantly with a mineralocorticoid; inflammatory conditions, allergic states, collagen diseases, hematologic disorders, and addisonian shock. Also palliative treatment of neoplastic disease, short-term therapy in acute rheumatic disorders and GI diseases, and as a diagnostic test for Cushing's syndrome and for differential diagnosis of adrenal hyperplasia and adrenal adenoma.
- ★ *Contraindications:* Allergy to the drug, systemic fungal infections, acute infections, tuberculosis, and varicella. Also if the patient is known to be allergic to this drug or it preservatives.
- ★ *Side Effects:* Edema, hypokalemia, hypotension, hypertension, elevated blood glucose, CHF, delayed wound healing, and possible hypokalemia.
- ★ *Dosage: Adult dose:* 1–2 mg/kg as a single dose then 1–1.5 mg/kg tapered dose over 4–6 hours. *Pediatric dose:* 0.5–1.0 mg/kg as a loading dose. Dexamethasone is supplied as 4 mg/ml vials for injection.
- ★ *Special Considerations:* Monitor vital signs closely, be alert for signs of CHF, and use cautiously in patients with renal disease and cirrhosis. Also use carefully in patient with GI ulceration history, diabetes, seizure disorders, and psychiatric disorders.

NIMODIPINE (NIMOTOP)

Classifications CARDIOVASCULAR AGENT; CALCIUM CHANNEL BLOCKER

- ★ *Actions:* Calcium channel blocker causing smooth muscle relaxation, with greater effect on cerebral arteries than on other arteries in the body due to its ability to bind specifically to cerebral tissue.
- ★ *Indications:* Improvement of neurologic deficits due to vasospasm after atraumatic subarachnoid hemorrhage.
- ★ *Contraindications:* Lactation, known hypersensitivity.
- ★ *Side Effects:* Hypotension, tachycardia, ECG abnormalities, GI bleeding, peripheral edema.
- ★ *Dosage: Adult dose:* 60 mg PO or NG every 4 hours within 96 hours of subarachnoid hemorrhage; continued for 21 consecutive days. *Pediatric dose:* Not established. Drug is packaged as a 60-mg capsule.
- ★ *Special Considerations:* Monitor vital signs and cardiac monitor closely, be cautious when administering this drug with other calcium channel blockers.

PULMONARY DRUGS

In a patient in acute respiratory distress due to bronchoconstriction, hypoxia and hypercapnia become major concerns. Additionally, acute agitation, cardiac ischemia, and organ dysfunction may occur as a result of the failing pulmonary system. The critical care paramedic must attempt to reverse this bronchoconstriction in order for oxygen and carbon dioxide exchange to take place, decreasing the risk of hypoxic changes. The administration of sympathomimetic agents allows for bronchodilation, and, with supplemental oxygen administration, increases oxygen delivery to the cells.

Acute agitation, cardiac ischemia, and organ dysfunction may occur as a result of the failing pulmonary system.

If the patient is breathing inadequately, nebulizing a drug is basically worthless.

Many of the following drugs may be given as a nebulized treatment; however, to nebulize a drug it must be understood that it will only be effective if the patient is breathing adequately and is able to ventilate the lower airways to deposit the medication where the bronchiole smooth muscle is located. If the patient is breathing inadequately, nebulizing a drug is basically worthless. Naturally, the medication could be ventilated with ventilation support, but if the patient still has significant bronchoconstriction this may fail as well. For this patient, the use of a parenteral sympathomimetic bronchodilator may be warranted.

SYMPATHOMIMETIC AEROSOLS

ALBUTEROL (PROVENTIL, VENTOLIN)

Classifications AUTONOMIC NERVOUS SYSTEM AGENT (SYMPATHOMIMETIC); BETA-ADRENERGIC AGONIST (SYMPATHOMIMETIC); BRONCHODILATOR

★ *Actions:* This drug is considered to be a beta-2-specific agent, promoting relaxation of bronchiole smooth muscle, but it still has a small degree of beta-1 and alpha properties. The net result is bronchodilation as well as tachycardia, vasoconstriction, and beta cell stimulation in the pancreas.

★ *Indications:* Acute bronchospasm in COPD processes and in acute asthma. It may also be used emergently for the treatment of hyperkalemia, because its beta-adrenergic properties aid in the release of insulin, shifting potassium from the extracellular to intracellular sites.

★ *Contraindications:* Excessive tachycardia, cardiac dysrhythmia (especially tachycardic ones), preexisting hypertension.

★ *Side Effects:* Given its sympathomimetic actions, side effects are consistent with evidence of enhanced sympathetic tone. These findings include tachycardia, hypertension, cardiac dysrhythmia, anxiety, palpitations, nausea/vomiting, and dilated pupils.

★ *Dosage: Adult dose:* 2.5 mg mixed with 3–5 mL saline and nebulized as needed to reverse bronchoconstriction. *Pediatric dose:* 1.25 mg, which is also mixed with 3–5 mL saline and nebulized. The drug comes supplied as a 2.5 mg/0.5 mL vial.

★ *Special Considerations:* Monitor vital signs and cardiac monitor closely. Ensure the patient's tidal volume is great enough that he can entrain the medication deep into the pulmonary tree. If not, consider using an in-line nebulizer with bag-value ventilation or the use of parenteral medications.

IPRATROPIUM BROMIDE (ATROVENT)

Classifications AUTONOMIC NERVOUS SYSTEM AGENT (SYMPATHOMIMETIC); ANTICHOLINERGIC (PARASYMPATHOLYTIC); BRONCHODILATOR

★ *Actions:* Cholinergic blocking agent, chemically related to atropine, that antagonizes the action of acetylcholine, causing bronchial smooth muscle relaxation by decreasing intracellular cyclic GMP.

★ *Indications:* To treat bronchoconstricter in patients with COPD and acute bronchospasm not resolved by albuterol aerosol. Also used as a maintenance therapy for long-standing COPD disorders.

★ *Contraindications:* Hypersensitivity to atropine or ipratropium. It should also not be the primary (first-line) agent administered for reversal of acute bronchospasms.

★ *Side Effects:* Due to abolishment of vagal tone, there may be tachycardia, palpitations, nervousness, dry mouth, and headache.

★ *Dosage: Adult dose:* 500 mcg (unit dose vial) every 4–6 hours. If using a metered-dose inhaler (MDI), administer 2 inhalations every 4 hours. *Pediatric dose (3–12 years old):*

125–250 mcg nebulized, or 1–2 inhalations from an MDI. For inhalation purposes the drug comes prepared in an 18 mcg/inhalation MDI. For nebulization use a 0.02% solution.

★ *Special Considerations:* May be given simultaneously with albuterol as Combivent; monitor vital signs and cardiac monitor closely.

LEVALBUTEROL HYDROCHLORIDE (XOPENEX)

Classifications AUTONOMIC NERVOUS SYSTEM AGENT (SYMPATHOMIMETIC); BETA-ADRENERGIC AGONIST (SYMPATHOMIMETIC); BRONCHODILATOR

★ *Actions:* Chemically related to albuterol, this drug has a higher specificity for beta-2 receptor sites with a longer duration of action than albuterol. Decreases airway resistance, facilitates mucous drainage, and increases vital capacity.

★ *Indications:* Similar to albuterol in the treatment or prevention of reversible bronchoconstriction in susceptible patients.

★ *Contraindications:* Hypersensitivity to levalbuterol or albuterol, children less than 6 years of age, and pregnant females.

★ *Side Effects:* Nervousness, palpitations, dry mouth, headache, and tachycardia.

★ *Dosage: Adult dose:* 0.63–1.25 mg every 6–8 hours as needed by nebulization. *Pediatric dose (between 6 and 11 years old):* Administer 0.31–0.63 mg every 6–8 hours by nebulization. Supplied as 0.31 mg/3 mL, 0.63 mg/3 mL, 1.25 mg/3 mL concentrations.

★ *Special Considerations:* As with other inhaled beta-2 agonists, be cautious with patients who have cardiovascular disease (CVD), coronary artery disease (CAD), dysrhythmias, convulsive disorders, hyperthyroidism, and diabetes. Additionally, ensure the patient can inhale deeply enough to ventilate the bronchioles for maximum effect.

SYMPATHOMIMETICS (INJECTION)

TERBUTALINE (BRETHAIRE, BRETHINE, BRICANYL)

Classifications AUTONOMIC NERVOUS SYSTEM AGENT (SYMPATHOMIMETIC); BETA-ADRENERGIC AGONIST (SYMPATHOMIMETIC); BRONCHODILATOR

★ *Actions:* Specific beta-2 receptor stimulant, resulting in bronchodilation and relaxation of peripheral vasculature; also produces uterine muscle relaxation.

★ *Indications:* Acute bronchospasm unresponsive to nebulizer therapy or in patients when inhaled nebulization is not feasible due to degree of bronchoconstriction. It can also be used as a tocolytic agent to treat preterm labor.

★ *Contraindications:* Known hypersensitivity, severe hypertension, CAD, lactating mothers, and concurrent digitalis toxicity.

★ *Side Effects:* Sympathomimetic findings to include tachycardia, hypertension, nervousness, palpitations, nausea, and vomiting.

★ *Dosage: For patients > 12 years old:* Administer 0.25 mg subcutaneously initially, repeat every 15–30 minutes up to 0.5 mg in 4 hours if unresponsive. *For patients < 12 years old:* Administer 0.005–0.01 mg/kg (max 0.4 mg) every 15–20 minutes for two doses. The drug is commonly supplied as 1 mg/mL ampules for injection.

★ *Special Considerations:* Monitor vital signs and cardiac monitor closely. Although the drug could be inhaled, the critical care paramedic should opt for the more beta-2-specific medications previously mentioned. Other considerations that pertain to beta-2-specific drugs apply here as well.

CORTICOSTERIODS

HYDROCORTISONE SODIUM (A-HYDROCORT, SOLU-CORTEF)

Classifications SKIN AND MUCOUS MEMBRANE AGENT; ANTI-INFLAMMATORY; HORMONE AND SYNTHETIC SUBSTITUTES; CORTICOSTEROID; CORTICOSTEROID, GLUCOCORTICOID; CORTICOSTEROID, MINERALOCORTICOID

★ *Actions:* Short-acting synthetic steroid with both immunosuppressive and anti-inflammatory actions. Primarily used for its anti-inflammatory properties.

★ *Indications:* For the pulmonary patient, it is used to help with the long-term management of acute bronchospasm caused by COPD and asthma.

★ *Contraindications:* Allergy to agent or preservatives used in manufacturing, idiopathic thrombocytopenic purpura, psychosis, Cushing's syndrome, acute hepatic dysfunction, and children < 2 years old.

★ *Side Effects:* Similar to previously mentioned steroidal medications, to include hypertension, hyperglycemia, flushing, tachycardia, anaphylactoid reactions, weight gain, mental disturbance, thrombocytopenia, and muscle wasting.

★ *Dosage: Adult dose:* 100 mg IVP every 6 hours is considered a standard dose. *Pediatric dose (>2 years old):* Administer 1–2 mg/kg IVP. Drug is supplied in multiple forms, to include 100-mg, 250-mg, 500-mg, and 1-g vials for injection.

★ *Special Considerations:* Monitor vital signs closely, and use cautiously in diabetics, children, hepatitis, convulsive disorders, hypothyroidism, gastritis, CHF, hypertension, and renal insufficiency.

NEUROMUSCULAR BLOCKERS

The administration of neuromuscular blockade, or paralytics, is an adjunct that is widely used in the task of obtaining and protecting an airway on the critical care patient.

During transport, the maintenance of an airway is essential for the critical care paramedic. The administration of neuromuscular blockade, or paralytics, is an adjunct that is widely used in the task of obtaining and protecting an airway on the critical care patient. Moreover, the administration of neuromuscular blocking agents helps to decrease oxygen demands, intracranial pressure, and risk for aspiration. Paralytic agents, when used in conjunction with sedation agents, allow for muscular flaccidity and suppression of the gag reflex when the need for a more controlled endotracheal intubation procedure is required.

Depolarizing neuromuscular blocking agents have a rapid onset with a short half-life. This makes them particularly useful as a primary induction agent for intubation. If endotracheal intubation is unsuccessful, the agent will metabolize quickly, and spontaneous respirations will return within minutes. Drugs of this kind will be discussed first.

SUCCINYLCHOLINE CHLORIDE (ANECTINE, QUELICIN, SUCOSTRIN)

Classifications AUTONOMIC NERVOUS SYSTEM AGENT (SYMPATHOMIMETIC); SKELETAL MUSCLE RELAXANT, DEPOLARIZING

★ *Actions:* Neuromuscular blockade that combines with cholinergic receptors of the motor end-plate to produce depolarization, observed as fasciculations. Onset of flaccid paralysis is rapid (less than 1 minute) and lasts 4–6 minutes.

★ *Indications:* Adjunct to facilitate endotracheal intubation when employing an RSI procedure.

★ *Contraindications:* Personal or familial history of malignant hyperthermia, skeletal muscle myopathies (myasthenia gravis). Use cautiously with pediatric patients, patients with burns, and patients after acute traumatic events because hyperkalemia may develop as a result of rhabdomyolysis.

- *Side Effects:* Respiratory paralysis, malignant hyperthermia, muscular fasciculations, rhabdomyolysis, increased intracranial pressure, increased intragastric pressure.
- *Dosage: Adult dose:* Dependent on the specific need of the patient. The adult dose is 1.0–1.5 mg/kg IVP. *Pediatric dose:* 1.0–2.0 mg/kg IVP. The drug is supplied in vials containing 2 mg/mL.
- *Special Considerations:* Prepare for endotracheal intubation immediately after administration; if intubation is unsuccessful, ventilatory assistance is required. Maintain eye care to avoid corneal abrasions. Refrigerate until utilized because drug has a shelf life of 30 days after removal from refrigeration.

Nondepolarizing neuromuscular blocking agents are commonly used after successful endotracheal intubation is accomplished. Since the patient will be under the care of the critical care team for a while, there is still a concern for accidental extubation due to patient dislodgement. The administration of a nondepolarizing neuromuscular agent will assist in decreasing these risks for a longer period of time than depolarizing agents. Additionally, risks for aspiration are decreased, as are intracranial pressures and metabolic needs. Nondepolarizing agents generally have a longer onset of action (making them less desirable for immediate paralysis in a critical patient), but have a longer half-life (making them more desirable for long-term paralysis for airway and mechanical ventilation control).

VECURONIUM (NORCURON)

Classifications   AUTONOMIC NERVOUS SYSTEM AGENT; SKELETAL MUSCLE RELAXANT, NONDEPOLARIZING

- *Actions:* Nondepolarizing neuromuscular blocking agent that acts by competing for cholinergic receptor sites at motor end-plates (resulting in paralysis). It is approximately one-third more potent than pancuronium and has a shorter half-life. Of patients receiving this drug, 95% have recovery in 45–65 minutes after administration.
- *Indications:* For airway maintenance and to enhance ventilatory management of the intubated patient. Especially useful in patients with kidney disease, history of asthma, or diminished cardiac reserve.
- *Contraindications:* Other than known hypersensitivity, none in the emergency setting.
- *Side Effects:* Similar to succinylcholine, but without the fasciculating side effects.
- *Dosage: Adult dose:* As with other paralytic agents, different doses exist depending on desired result:
  - *Defasciculating dose:* 0.01 mg/kg IVP
  - *Paralyzing dose:* 0.08–0.10 mg/kg IVP; may repeat every 1–2 hours

  Pediatric dose: 0.1 mg/kg IVP, and may repeat every 1–2 hours. The medication is supplied as 10-mg vials for reconstitution.
- *Special Considerations:* Vecuronium should not be used in dosages greater than 0.01 mg/kg IVP prior to intubation. Train-of-four testing or peripheral nerve testing is beneficial. Maintain meticulous eye care (lubrication) for prolonged paralysis. The use of vecuronium must be accompanied with either a sedative or analgesic, to decrease cardiovascular side effects.

PANCURONIUM BROMIDE (PAVULON)

Classifications   AUTONOMIC NERVOUS SYSTEM AGENT; SKELETAL MUSCLE RELAXANT, DEPOLARIZING, NONDEPOLARIZING

- *Actions:* Similar to vecuronium, but produces little histamine release or ganglionic blockade and thus does not precipitate bronchospasm or hypotension.
- *Indications:* Similar to vecuronium to include facilitating intubation and to provide long-term paralysis to patients receiving mechanical ventilation.

- *Contraindications:* Known hypersensitivity, extreme tachycardia.
- *Side Effects:* Also similar to vecuronium, although cardiovascular side effects may be more pronounced and include increased pulse rates and ventricular ectopy.
- *Dosage: Adult dose:* 0.04–0.10 mg/kg IVP. *Pediatric dose:* 0.04–0.1 mg/kg IVP. Drug is supplied as 2 mg/mL vials.
- *Special Considerations:* Similar to vecuronium. Use with caution in debilitated patients; those with severe pulmonary, renal, or hepatic disease; and patients with neuromuscular disorders.

ROCURONIUM BROMIDE (ZEMURON)

Classifications   AUTONOMIC NERVOUS SYSTEM AGENT; SKELETAL MUSCLE RELAXANT, DEPOLARIZING, NONDEPOLARIZING

- *Actions:* Another nondepolarizing agent with actions similar to vecuronium, but with limited cardiovascular side effects.
- *Indications:* Used as an adjunct to general anesthesia to facilitate rapid-sequence intubation. Can also be used to provide skeletal muscle relaxation during surgery or mechanical ventilation.
- *Contraindications:* Known hypersensitivity to rocuronium.
- *Side Effects:* Similar to vecuronium, with fewer cardiovascular side effects.
- *Dosage: Adult dose:* Dependent on desired need:
  - Rapid-sequence induction: 0.6 mg/kg IVP
  - Maintenance paralysis: 0.1–0.2 mg/kg IVP every 1–2 hours
  - Continuous infusion: 0.01–0.012 mg/kg/min; train-of-four nerve stimulation testing must be done with continuous infusion

  Pediatric dose (>2 years old): 0.6 mg/kg IVP. Drug is supplied in vials containing 10 mg/mL.
- *Special Considerations:* Similar to vecuronium; includes maintenance of meticulous eye care (lubrication) for prolonged paralysis. The use of rocuronium must be accompanied with either a sedative or analgesic.

CISATRACURIUM BESYLATE (NIMBEX)

Classifications   AUTONOMIC NERVOUS SYSTEM AGENT; SKELETAL MUSCLE RELAXANT, NONDEPOLARIZING

- *Actions:* Cisatracurium is a neuromuscular blocking agent with intermediate onset and duration of action compared with other nondepolarizing agents. It binds competitively to cholinergic receptors on the motor end-plates of neurons, antagonizing the action of acetylcholine to induce paralysis.
- *Indications:* Consistent with the nondepolarizing class of paralytics, this can be used adjunctively for general anesthesia to facilitate tracheal intubation by providing muscle relaxation. Can also be used during mechanical ventilation in the intubated patient.
- *Contraindications:* Hypersensitivity to cisatracurium or other related agents.
- *Side Effects:* Cardiovascular side effects include bradycardia, hypotension, and flushing of the skin. May also precipitate bronchospasm in the susceptible patient.
- *Dosage: Adult dose:* Commonly 0.15–0.20 mg/kg IVP. For maintenance of paralysis in the adult, an infusion of 1–3 mcg/kg/min can be administered. *Pediatric dose (≥2 years old):* For intubation, 0.1 mg/kg. The pediatric infusion dose is 1–2 mcg/kg/min.

The drug comes supplied in 2 mg/mL and 10 mg/mL preparations for intravenous use.

★ *Special Considerations:* Electrolyte imbalances, burn patients, neuromuscular diseases (e.g., myasthenia gravis), older adults, renal function impairment, and pregnancy.

ANALGESICS

Pain can be a major contributor to the consumption of oxygen in the critically ill or injured patient. The administration of analgesics decreases patient response to pain, decreases metabolic demands, and may increase oxygen supply for utilization by ischemic cells and tissues. As such, the critical care provider must be thoroughly knowledgeable about common analgesic agents used in critical care medicine. (See Table 11–2.)

The administration of analgesics decreases patient response to pain, decreases metabolic demands, and may increase oxygen supply for utilization by ischemic cells and tissues.

NARCOTIC ANALGESICS

HYDROMORPHONE HYDROCHLORIDE (DILAUDID, DILAUDID-HP)

Classifications   CENTRAL NERVOUS SYSTEM AGENT; NARCOTIC (OPIATE) AGONIST

★ *Actions:* Semisynthetic derivative structurally similar to morphine but with 8–10 times more potent analgesic effect. Has more rapid onset and shorter duration of action than morphine and is reported to have less hypnotic action and less tendency to produce nausea and vomiting.

★ *Indications:* Moderate to severe pain, such as trauma, medical, or surgical pain. Can also be used to control a persistent nonproductive cough.

Table 11–2	Opoid Dosage Equivalency Comparison
Drug Name	**Equivalent Single Dose**
Narcotic Agents	
• Morphine	5 mg
• Codeine	30–60 mg
• Fenatyl	0.05–0.1 mg
• Hydrocodone	10 mg
• Hydromorphone	0.6–0.7 mg
• Meperidine	25–50 mg
• Methadone	5 mg
Mixed Agonists/Antagonists	
• Buprenorphine	0.2 mg
• Butorphanol	1.5 mg
• Dezocine	25 mg
• Ketorolac	30 mg
• Pentazocine	30 mg
Other	
• Tramadol	50 mg

- *Contraindications:* Known hypersensitivity to hydromorphone. Intolerance to opiate agonists; lactation. Use with caution in intra-abdominal and intracranial pathologies prior to diagnosis.
- *Side Effects:* As with other narcotic agents, hydromorphone may cause respiratory depression, hypotension, bradycardia, or reflex tachycardia. Nausea, vomiting, and constipation have also been reported as well as CNS findings of euphoria, vertigo, sedation, and drowsiness.
- *Dosage: Adult dose:* For moderate to severe pain, 1–4 mg IVP every 4–6 hours as needed. *Pediatric dose:* 0.015 mg/kg every 4–6 hours. Drug is supplied in 1 mg/mL, 2 mg/mL, 4 mg/mL, and 10 mg/mL preparations.
- *Special Considerations:* Respiratory conditions, possible ICP elevations, supraventricular tachydysrhythmias, liver and renal diseases, hypothyroidism, and those patients with Addison's disease. Naloxone can be used as an antagonist in cases of overdose or toxicity.

MORPHINE SULFATE (DURAMORPH, MS CONTIN)

Classifications   CENTRAL NERVOUS SYSTEM AGENT; ANALGESIC; NARCOTIC (OPIATE) AGONIST

- *Actions:* A naturally occurring narcotic analgesic; a derivative of the opium poppy. After injection, causes feelings of euphoria and well-being, altering reactions to pain; has mild vasodilation properties to include decreasing preload and afterload; also decreases myocardial oxygen consumption.
- *Indications:* Moderate to severe pain; mild to moderate congestive heart failure; myocardial chest pain.
- *Contraindications:* Allergy to opiates; decreased level of consciousness, hypotension, increased intracranial pressure, respiratory depression, convulsive disorder, ingested poisoning, undiagnosed intra-abdominal and intracranial conditions.
- *Side Effects:* Respiratory depression, hypotension, localized allergic reaction with intravenous administration, nausea/vomiting, constipation, addiction with long-term use.
- *Dosage: Adult dose:* 2–10 mg IVP slowly over 1–2 minutes; repeat every 1 hour as needed. *Pediatric dose:* 0.05–0.1 mg/kg IVP (maximum dose 15 mg), and may be repeated every 1–4 hours as needed. Supplied as 2-mg, 4-mg, 8-mg, and 10-mg syringes.
- *Special Considerations:* Monitor vital signs and cardiac rhythm closely; be prepared to assist with ventilations or tracheal intubation if respiratory depression occurs; action is potentiated when used in combination with sedatives, hypnotics, or barbiturates. Antagonist: Naloxone (Narcan) 2 mg IVP. *Pediatric dose:* of naloxone is 0.01 mg/kg IVP.

MEPERIDINE HYDROCHLORIDE (DEMEROL)

Classifications   CENTRAL NERVOUS SYSTEM AGENT; NARCOTIC (OPIATE) AGONIST

- *Actions:* Synthetic opiate with actions on opiate receptor sites of the brain similar to morphine. Related low, medium, and high doses of the drug mirror similar analgesic responses as the prototype morphine.
- *Indications:* Moderate to severe pain, such as trauma, medical, or surgical pain. Has minimal to no antidiarrheic or antitussive actions.
- *Contraindications:* Known hypersensitivity to meperidine, seizure disorders, and intra-abdominal and intracranial pathologies prior to diagnosis.

- *Side Effects:* Akin to those of morphine; however, localized reaction may be more severe. Meperidene tends to cause more euphoria than morphine.
- *Dosage: Adult dose:* 25–100 mg slow IVP over 1–2 minutes every 3–4 hours. *Pediatric dose:* 0.5–1.0 mg IVP over 1–2 minutes; repeated at 3- to 4-hour intervals. Drug is supplied as 25-mg, 50-mg, 75-mg, and 100-mg syringes.
- *Special Considerations:* Respiratory conditions, possible ICP elevations, supraventricular tachydysrhythmias, liver and renal diseases, hypothyroidism, and those patients with Addison's disease. Narcan can be used as an antagonist in cases of overdose or toxicity.

FENTANYL CITRATE (SUBLIMAZE, DURAGESIC)

Classifications   CENTRAL NERVOUS SYSTEM AGENT; ANALGESIC; NARCOTIC (OPIATE) AGONIST

- *Actions:* Narcotic analgesic approximately 10 times more potent than morphine, and is also more prompt in onset with a less prolonged duration of action.
- *Indications:* For analgesic purposes similar to morphine; however, this drug is particularly useful as an adjunct for endotracheal intubation during RSI procedures.
- *Contraindications:* Similar to morphine. Also avoid use in patients receiving monoamine oxidase inhibitor drugs (MAOIs) within previous 14 days, patients with myasthenia gravis, and during active labor and delivery. Drug should also be avoided with known or suspected hypersensitivity.
- *Side Effects:* Similar to morphine with euphoria, vertigo, delirium. Can also cause bradycardia and hypotension. Nausea, vomiting, and constipation have been reported, as has muscle rigidity (especially in pediatrics).
- *Dosage: Adult dose:* 25–200 mcg slow IVP over 1–2 minutes. *Pediatric dose:* 1–2 mcg/kg IVP over 1–2 minutes. Drug is supplied in 100-mcg ampules.
- *Special Considerations:* Use cautiously with head injuries (if at all), older and debilitated patients, COPD, bradydysrhythmic patients, and patients with severe pulmonary, renal, or hepatic diseases.

NARCOTIC AGONISTS-ANTAGONISTS

NALBUPHINE HYDROCHLORIDE (NUBAIN)

Classifications   CENTRAL NERVOUS SYSTEM AGENT; ANALGESIC; NARCOTIC (OPIATE) AGONIST-ANTAGONIST

- *Actions:* Synthetic opioid agonist-antagonist analgesic with actions on opiate receptor sites similar to morphine. This drug's analgesic action will relieve moderate to severe pain with a low potential for dependence.
- *Indications:* Moderate to severe pain; may also be used to slow labor process in obstetric patient. In hospital it is used for both preoperative analgesia and supplemental operative analgesia.
- *Contraindications:* Allergy to nalbuphine. Prolonged use during pregnancy may result in neonatal withdrawal, so it should be avoided.
- *Side Effects:* Similar to morphine in its CNS, cardiovascular, and respiratory depression effects. May interfere with subsequent narcotic dosing and anesthesia.
- *Dosage: Adult dose:* 5–10 mg IVP every 3–6 hours as needed. *Pediatric dose:* 0.1–0.15 mg/kg every 3–6 hours. Supplied as 10-mg and 20-mg ampules.
- *Special Considerations:* Similar to morphine. Use cautiously in patients with history of long-term use of narcotics because withdrawal symptoms may occur.

NON-STEROIDAL ANTI-INFLAMMATORY AGENTS

KETOROLAC TROMETHAMINE (TORADOL, ACULAR)

Classifications CENTRAL NERVOUS SYSTEM AGENT; NONSTEROIDAL ANTI-INFLAMMATORY DRUG (NSAID); ANALGESIC; ANTIPYRETIC

★ *Actions:* Inhibits synthesis of prostaglandins and is a peripherally acting analgesic. Ketorolac does not have any known effects on opiate receptors.

★ *Indications:* The short-term (up to 5 days in adults) management of moderately severe acute pain that requires analgesia at the opioid level. It is not used for minor or chronic painful conditions.

★ *Contraindications:* Known hypersensitivity to ketorolac; individuals with complete or partial syndrome of nasal polyps, angioedema, and bronchospastic reaction to aspirin or other NSAIDs; during labor and delivery; patients with severe renal impairment or at risk for renal failure due to volume depletion; patients with risk of bleeding; active peptic ulcer disease; or in combination with other NSAIDs.

★ *Side Effects:* Adverse effects include drowsiness, vertigo, possible headache, GI distress to include nausea and vomiting. Increasing the dose of drug beyond recommendations will not provide better efficacy, but may result in increasing the risk of developing serious adverse events.

★ *Dosage: Adult dose:* 30 mg IVP if under 65 years of age. In those patients who are over 65, renally impaired, or weigh less than 50 kg, a single dose of 15 mg can be given. Both populations can be redosed every 6 hours to a max of 120 mg or 60 mg, respectively. *Pediatric dose (2–16 years old):* Single dose of 0.5 mg/kg to a max of 15 mg can be administered. Supplied as 15 mg/mL and 30 mg/mL for injection purposes.

★ *Special Considerations:* May increase methotrexate levels and toxicity; may also increase lithium levels and toxicity.

SEDATIVES AND HYPNOTICS

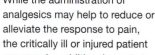

While the administration of analgesics may help to reduce or alleviate the response to pain, the critically ill or injured patient may require additional agents to alleviate the responses to stress and anxiety that his condition is causing.

While the administration of analgesics may help to reduce or alleviate the response to pain, the critically ill or injured patient may require additional agents to alleviate the responses to stress and anxiety that his condition is causing. Intubation and mechanical ventilation, ICU psychoses, and other situations where pain may not be a factor may indicate the need for the administration of sedatives or hypnotics. As the critical care paramedic's scope of practice expands in response to the myriad of critical patients who utilize the service, the administration of sedatives or hypnotics will increase in frequency in the critical care transport setting.

BENZODIAZEPINES

MIDAZOLAM HYDROCHLORIDE (VERSED)

Classifications CENTRAL NERVOUS SYSTEM AGENT; BENZODIAZEPINE ANTI-CONVULSANT; SEDATIVE-HYPNOTIC

★ *Actions:* Short-acting benzodiazepine with hypnotic, sedative, and amnestic properties. Drug acts on GABA receptor sites in the central nervous system where it increases GABA activity to induce calming, skeletal muscle relaxation, and sleep with higher doses.

★ *Indications:* Sedation due to general anxiety, as an adjunct to endotracheal intubation; for sedation in ventilated patient and to suppress acute seizure activity.

★ *Contraindications:* Hypotension, decreased level of consciousness, hypoperfusion, alcohol intoxication, narrow-angle glaucoma.

- *Side Effects:* Hypotension (may be profound), tachycardia or bradycardia, respiratory depression, altered level of consciousness.
- *Dosage: Adult dose:* Commonly 1.0–2.5 mg slow IVP over 1–2 minutes. *Pediatric dose:* 0.05–0.2 mg/kg slow IVP over 2–3 minutes. Drug is supplied as 2-mg, 5-mg, and 10-mg vials for parental injection.
- *Antagonist:* Flumazenil (Romazicon) 0.2 mg IVP as needed up to 1 mg. *Pediatric dose:* 0.01 mg/kg IVP up 0.05 mg/kg or 1 mg. Use with caution in benzodiazepine dependence.
- *Special Considerations:* Monitor vital signs and cardiac rhythm closely; administer fluid bolus for hypotension. Be prepared to assist with ventilations or endotracheal intubation; use cautiously with elderly and pediatric patients; may be given intramuscularly; potentiated with combination therapy of analgesics.

DIAZEPAM (VALIUM)

Classifications   CENTRAL NERVOUS SYSTEM AGENT; BENZODIAZEPINE ANTICON-VULSANT; ANXIOLYTIC

- *Actions:* Benzodiazepine derivative, similar actions as midazolam on the CNS.
- *Indications:* Similar to midazolam and is often the agent of choice for status epilepticus.
- *Contraindications:* Hypersensitivity to diazepam, severe depression to either the pulmonary or cardiovascular systems.
- *Side Effects:* Similar to other benzodiazepines, to include CNS depression, respiratory depression, and cardiovascular depression. It has a slightly longer half-life, so side effects may be more pronounced and long lasting.
- *Dosage: Adult dose:* Commonly 2–10 mg slow IVP as an initial dose, which may repeat every 1–2 hours as needed. *Pediatric dose:* 0.5–2.0 mg slow IVP as needed. Supplied in 5-mg and 10-mg vials.
- *Special Considerations:* As with midazolam and other benzodiazepines, the dose should be given slowly, no faster than 1 mg/min intravenously or by IM if necessary. A non–oil-based formulation of the drug, Diastat, can be used for rectal administration as needed. Flumazenil can be used as antagonist.

LORAZEPAM (ATIVAN)

Classifications   CENTRAL NERVOUS SYSTEM AGENT; ANXIOLYTIC; SEDATIVE-HYPNOTIC; BENZODIAZEPINE

- *Actions:* Benzodiazepine with properties similar to midazolam, but it is the most potent of the available benzodiazepine agents. Effects include antiolysis, sedation, and skeletal muscle relaxation.
- *Indications:* Similar to midazolam; commonly used for management of anxiety disorders.
- *Contraindications:* Consistent with other benzodiazepine agents, to include hypersensitivity.
- *Side Effects:* Similar to other benzodiazepine agents.
- *Dosage: Adult dose:* 0.5–2.0 mg slow IVP (average single dose is 2–4 mg), every 1–2 hours as needed in the acute situation. *Pediatric dose:* 0.03–0.05 mg/kg slow IVP up to 4 mg. Supplied as 2-mg vials.
- *Special Considerations:* Similar to midazolam; must be refrigerated before administration. Flumazenil can be used as an antagonist medication.

HYPNOTICS

PROPOFOL (DIPRIVAN)

Classifications CENTRAL NERVOUS SYSTEM (CNS) AGENT; GENERAL ANESTHESIA; SEDATIVE-HYPNOTIC

★ *Actions:* Sedative-hypnotic in fat emulsion; action is unknown but is thought to slow impulses in limbic system.

★ *Indications:* Sedative used for induction for conscious sedation procedures, such as closed reduction of fractures and dislocations; also as an adjunct for endotracheal intubation and for sedation for mechanical ventilation.

★ *Contraindications:* Allergy to propofol and its additives; allergy to eggs.

★ *Side Effects:* Hypotension, altered level of consciousness, respiratory depression, bradycardia, tachycardia, pain at injection site, and acalculous cholecystitis with prolonged use.

★ *Dosage:* Based on age and need:
  – For induction: 2–2.5 mg/kg slow IVP over 1 minute
  – Maintenance dosage: 6–12 mg/kg/hr continuously
  – Pediatric dosage (≥3 years old): 2.5–3.5 mg/kg IVP over 1 minute
  – Pediatric maintenance: 7.5–18 mg/kg/hr continuously
  Supplied as 10 mg/mL vials.

★ *Special Considerations:* Monitor vital signs and cardiac rhythm closely; be prepared to assist with ventilations or intubate; fluid bolus may be required for hypotension; with continuous infusion, patient should be allowed to "wake up" daily to assess level of consciousness, and finally analgesia may be needed additionally, because propofol has no analgesic properties.

NONBARBITURATE HYPNOTIC

ETOMIDATE (AMIDATE)

Classifications CENTRAL NERVOUS SYSTEM AGENT; GENERAL ANESTHESIA

★ *Actions:* A nonbarbiturate hypnotic that causes few changes in hemodynamics after administration. It is both a rapid-acting and short-lived drug (100-second period of hypnosis per 0.1 mg/kg dose). The mechanism of action is unknown, but it is thought to work at the limbic system.

★ *Indications:* Induction agent for endotracheal intubation or anesthesia.

★ *Contraindications:* Known allergy, pregnancy, adrenocortical function suppression.

★ *Side Effects:* Respiratory depression, bronchospasm, bruxism, vein irritation, and muscle tightening.

★ *Dosage: Adult and pediatric dose (>10 years old):* 0.1–0.3 mg/kg IVP over 1 minute. Drug is supplied in 2 mg/mL vials for injection.

★ *Special Considerations:* Monitor level of consciousness, respiratory rate, and vital signs closely; be prepared to assist with ventilations as needed; rapid administration of etomidate will exacerbate side effects. Etomidate has no analgesic effects, and must be used in combination therapy if that effect is desired.

NARCOTIC/BENZODIAZEPINE ANTAGONISTS

Rarely will the critical care paramedic need to reverse the effects of analgesics or sedatives when their actual effects are greater than their desired effects. While the administration of antagonist agents will reverse the effect of specific agents, the risk of immediate withdrawal in the patient with long-term narcotic or sedative use (or abuse) carries its own unique set of risks. For example, the critical care paramedic is transporting an elderly patient with a COPD history and decreased level of consciousness. After the administration of an antagonist agent, the patient becomes tachycardic, hypertensive, and begins to display seizure activity. Further investigation by the critical care paramedic reveals the use of benzodiazepines by the patient for an unknown period of time. Now that the antagonist has been administered with subsequent seizure due to rapid withdrawal, the critical care paramedic CANNOT utilize benzodiazepines to control seizure, because those receptor sites are "blocked" by the antagonist. The critical care paramedic should weigh each circumstance individually, and weigh the risk and benefits of reversing the effects of a specific agent.

NALOXONE HYDROCHLORIDE (NARCAN)

Classifications   CENTRAL NERVOUS SYSTEM AGENT; NARCOTIC (OPIATE) ANTAGONIST

★ *Actions:* Analogue of oxymorphone. A "pure" narcotic antagonist, essentially free of agonistic (morphine-like) properties. Used to block opiate receptor sites and reverse effects of narcotic administration or overdose. It produces no significant analgesia, respiratory depression, or miosis when administered in the absence of narcotics.

★ *Indications:* Complete or partial reversal of narcotic depression including respiratory depression induced by natural and synthetic narcotics. Drug of choice when nature of depressant drug is not known and for diagnosis of suspected acute opioid overdosage.

★ *Contraindications:* Other than known allergy, none in the emergency setting.

★ *Side Effects:* Hypertension, tachycardia, ventricular dysrhythmias; risks of abrupt withdrawal symptoms in long-term narcotic users and abusers.

★ *Dosage: Adult dose:* Initial dose ranges from 0.4 to 2.0 mg IVP, IM, or SQ every 2–3 minutes up to 10 mg. *Pediatric dose:* 0.01 mg/kg IV, IM, or SQ every 2–3 minutes as needed. The drug comes prepared in 0.4 mg/mL and 2 mg/mL vials or syringes for injection.

★ *Special Considerations:* Be prepared for rapid withdrawal symptoms, including agitation, rhythm disturbances, pulmonary edema, and cardiovascular collapse.

FLUMAZENIL (MAZICON, ROMAZICON)

Classifications   CENTRAL NERVOUS SYSTEM AGENT; BENZODIAZEPINE ANTAGONIST

★ *Actions:* Benzodiazepine antagonist used to block GABA receptor sites in the brain; used to reverse effects of benzodiazepine administration or overdose.

★ *Indications:* Antagonizes the effects of benzodiazepine on the CNS, including sedation, impairment of recall, and psychomotor impairment. Does not reverse the effects of opioids.

★ *Contraindications:* Allergy to flumazenil, history of long-term benzodiazepine use (for example, seizure disorders).

★ *Side Effects:* Hot flashes, pain at injection site, agitation; breakthrough seizures, elevated CNS response, anxiety.

★ *Dosage: Adult dose:* 0.2 mg IVP every 1 minute as needed up to 1.0 mg total dose. *Pediatric dose:* As needed, is 0.01 mg/kg IVP (up to 0.2 mg) every 1 minute up to

1.0 mg total. If the effects of the sedative outlast the response from flumazenil, repeated doses can be administered.

★ *Special Considerations:* Monitor vital signs and cardiac rhythm closely; be prepared for rapid withdrawal symptoms; if seizures occur phenobarbitol is the drug of choice for seizure resuppression. Flumazenil should NOT be used for routine benzodiazepine overdose—instead supportive measures (ventilation) should be provided.

ANTIBIOTICS AND ANTIFUNGALS

The administration of antibiotics or antifungals is often an important part of care for critically ill or injured patients. While their presentation to a specific hospital may not be infected or infectious in nature, their exposure to various organisms while hospitalized puts them at risk for infection. Many patients are on specific antibiotics for specific organisms, while others may be on broad-spectrum antibiotics when organism type has not been identified or if multiple organisms have been identified.

The critical care paramedic will be responsible for monitoring antibiotics and antifungals while en route to the receiving hospital.

The critical care paramedic will rarely initiate these medications during transport, but many of them will already be established by the sending facility, so the critical care paramedic will be responsible for monitoring them while en route to the receiving hospital. This section is to help provide a basic familiarization of the medications for these purposes for the critical care paramedic.

CEFAZOLIN SODIUM (ANCEF, KEFZOL, ZOLICEF)

Classifications   ANTI-INFECTIVE; ANTIBIOTIC; CEPHALOSPORIN, FIRST-GENERATION

★ *Actions:* Cephalosporin-type bactericidal agent with action against both gram-positive and gram-negative bacteria.

★ *Indications:* Antibiotic therapy of choice in trauma patient with skin or soft-tissue injury.

★ *Contraindications:* Allergy to cephalosporin group of antibiotics.

★ *Side Effects:* GI symptoms (nausea, vomiting, diarrhea), Stevens-Johnson syndrome.

★ *Dosage: Adult dose:* Usually 1 gm/50 mL IV over 15–30 minutes every 8 hours. *Pediatric dose:* Commonly 25 mg/kg IV divided in 3 doses over 15–30 minutes every 8 hours. Supplied as 500-mg and 1-g vials.

★ *Special Considerations:* Monitor for allergic reaction; use cautiously with patients with penicillin allergy.

CEFTRIAXONE SODIUM (ROCEPHIN)

Classifications   ANTI-INFECTIVE; ANTIBIOTIC; CEPHALOSPORIN, THIRD-GENERATION

★ *Actions:* Broad-spectrum cephalosporin-type bactericidal agent with action against gram-positive, gram-negative, aerobic, and anaerobic organisms. Ceftiaxone can cross the blood–brain barrier.

★ *Indications:* Otitis media, septicemia, meningitis, postoperative infection, preoperative prophylaxis.

★ *Contraindications:* Allergy to cephalosporin group of antibiotics.

★ *Side Effects:* GI symptoms (nausea, vomiting, diarrhea), leukopenia, pain at injection site.

★ *Dosage: Adult dose:* 1–2 g/100 mL IV daily. *Pediatric dose:* Usually 50–75 mg/kg IV daily. Drug is supplied as 500-mg and 1-g vials.

★ *Special Considerations:* Monitor for allergic reaction; use cautiously with patients with penicillin allergy; reconstituting with 1% Xylocaine with IM injection decreases pain at injection site.

IMIPENEM-CILASTATIN SODIUM (PRIMAXIN)

Classifications   ANTI-INFECTIVE; BETA-LACTAM ANTIBIOTIC

- ★ *Actions:* Broad-spectrum carbopenem-type antibiotic with action against gram-positive, gram-negative, aerobic, and anaerobic organisms.
- ★ *Indications:* Broad-spectrum antibiotic therapy for organisms resistant to frontline antibiotic therapy.
- ★ *Contraindications:* Allergy to imipenem and its additives, especially lidocaine.
- ★ *Side Effects:* GI symptoms (nausea, vomiting, diarrhea), leukopenia, and pain at injection site.
- ★ *Dosage: Adult dose:* 250–500 mg/100 mL over 1 hour every 6–8 hours. *Pediatric dose:* 10–15 mg/kg every 6 hours. Drug is supplied as 500-mg and 750-mg vials.
- ★ *Special Considerations:* Monitor for allergic reaction; use cautiously on patients with impaired renal function.

VANCOMYCIN HYDROCHLORIDE (VANOCIN)

Classifications   ANTI-INFECTIVE; ANTIBIOTIC

- ★ *Actions:* Antibiotic agent with action against gram-positive, gram-negative, aerobic, and anaerobic organisms, including methicillin-resistant *Staphylococcus aureus* (MRSA).
- ★ *Indications:* Broad-spectrum antibiotic therapy for organisms resistant to frontline antibiotic therapy, including MRSA.
- ★ *Contraindications:* Allergy to drug or its additives.
- ★ *Side Effects:* Nephrotoxicity, pseudomembranous colitis, ototoxicity, neutropenia, drug fever, and pain at injection site.
- ★ *Dosage: Adult dose:* 0.5–1 g IV over 1 hour, every 12 hours. *Pediatric dose:* 10 mg/kg IV over 1 hour every 6 hours. The dose should be adjusted for patients with renal impairment, the elderly, and is based on peak and trough drug levels. Vancomycin is supplied as 500-mg and 1-g vials.
- ★ *Special Considerations:* Monitor for allergic reaction; monitor IV site for irritation, infiltration.

GENTAMICIN SULFATE (GARAMYCIN)

Classifications   ANTI-INFECTIVE; AMINOGLYCOSIDE

- ★ *Actions:* Aminoglycoside-type antibiotic with action against infections in the central nervous, respiratory, and gastrointestinal systems. Also used for septicemia.
- ★ *Indications:* Antibiotic therapy for severe infections in an individual system or systemic bacteremia; used most commonly in a pediatric critical care setting.
- ★ *Contraindications:* Allergy to gentamycin or aminoglycoside family of agents.
- ★ *Side Effects:* Nephrotoxicity (increased BUN, creatinine levels), neurotoxicity (tinnitus, hearing loss, muscle twitching, convulsion), confusion, urticaria, drug fever, nausea, vomiting, and joint pain.
- ★ *Dosage: Adult loading dose:* 1.5–2.0 mg/kg IV over 1–1.5 hours. Maintenance infusion is 3–5 mg/kg/day IV in divided doses. *Pediatric dose:* 6–7.5 mg/kg/day IV in divided doses, usually every 8 hours. The dose should be adjusted for patients with renal impairment, the elderly, and is based on peak and trough drug levels. Supplied in 10 mg/mL and 40 mg/mL vials.
- ★ *Special Considerations:* Monitor for allergic reaction; monitor IV site for irritation or infiltration.

CLINDAMYCIN HYDROCHLORIDE (CLEOCIN, DALACIN)

Classifications   ANTI-INFECTIVE; ANTIBIOTIC

★ *Actions:* Bactericidal agent with action against anaerobic bacteria such as enterococcus, staphylococcus, and streptococcus bacteria.

★ *Indications:* Antibiotic therapy for severe infections (especially septicemia) caused by certain anaerobic organisms. Used most commonly in a pediatric critical care setting.

★ *Contraindications:* Allergy to clindamycin or lincomycin.

★ *Side Effects:* GI effects (colitis, diarrhea, abdominal pain), metallic taste, rash.

★ *Dosage: Adult dose:* 300–900 mg IV over 1 hour in 2, 3, or 4 equal doses. *Pediatric dose:* 20–40 mg/kg/day IV over 1 hour in 3 or 4 equal doses. Drug is supplied as 150 mg/mL vials.

★ *Special Considerations:* Monitor for allergic reactions. If diarrhea or GI symptoms occur, discontinue infusion.

AMPICILLIN/SULBACTAM SODIUM (UNASYN)

Classifications   ANTI-INFECTIVE; ANTIBIOTIC; AMINOPENICILLIN

★ *Actions:* Penicillin-class antibiotic with action against many gram-postitive, gram-negative and anaerobic organisms. The sulbactam component aids in treatment of resistant strains.

★ *Indications:* Antibiotic therapy for variety of infectious conditions including respiratory, urinary tract, and postoperative infections.

★ *Contraindications:* Allergy to Unasyn and penicillin group agents.

★ *Side Effects:* GI symptoms (diarrhea, abdominal distention, flatulence), rash, facial swelling, candidiasis, fatigue.

★ *Dosage: Adults dose:* 1.5–3.0 g (ampicillin equivalent)/100 mL IV over 30 minutes every 6 hours. *Pediatric dose (>40 kg):* Full adult dosage in 50–100 mL IV over 30 minutes. *Pediatric dose (<40 kg):* 300 mg/kg/day in 50–100 ml IV over 30 minutes. Supplied as 1.5-g and 3.0-g vials.

★ *Special Considerations:* Monitor for allergic reactions.

FLUCONAZOLE (DIFLUCAN)

Classifications   ANTI-INFECTIVE; ANTIBIOTIC; ANTIFUNGAL

★ *Actions:* An antifungal agent with action against Candida and Cryptococcus fungal infections.

★ *Indications:* Treatment of candidemia, disseminated candidiasis, fungal pneumonia, and cryptococcal meningitis.

★ *Contraindications:* Allergy to fluconazole or the azole class of antifungals.

★ *Side Effects:* Nausea, headache, skin rash, diarrhea, and liver damage (rare).

★ *Dosage: Adult loading dose:* 200–400 mg/100 mL IV over 1 hour. The maintenance dose is 100–200 mg/100 mL IV over 1 hour daily. *Pediatric loading dose:* 6–12 mg/kg/50 mL IV over 1 hour, with maintenance of 3–6 mg/kg/50 mL IV over 1 hour. Drug is supplied as 100-mg vials.

★ *Special Considerations:* Monitor for allergic reaction; use cautiously in patients with renal impairment.

DIURETICS

When fluid volume excess proves problematic, with resultant increased left preload pressures and the risk for left ventricular failure looming, the administration of diuretics may prove beneficial to reduce intravascular volume and decrease myocardial workload.

FUROSEMIDE (LASIX)

Classifications   ELECTROLYTIC BALANCE AND WATER BALANCE AGENTS; DIURETIC, LOOP

- ★ *Actions:* Loop diuretic that blocks reabsorption of sodium and water in renal tubules, causing profound diuresis.
- ★ *Indications:* Treatment of fluid volume excess due to intrinsic or extrinsic hypervolemia, or due to a failing left ventricle with resultant pulmonary edema. It can also be used for mild impairment of renal perfusion, and in the treatment of acute CHF.
- ★ *Contraindications:* Allergy to furosemide, anuria, hypotension, and dehydration. Monitor closely in patients with sulfa allergy. Also the drug will not be beneficial to patients with renal failure.
- ★ *Side Effects:* Cramping, diarrhea, nausea, vomiting, tinnitus, vertigo, headache, leukopenia, anemia, urticaria, rash, and hypokalemia. If diuresis is profound, the patient may become dehydrated.
- ★ *Dosage: Adult dose:* 1 mg/kg (usual single dose of 40–80 mg) slow IVP over 1–2 minutes. *Pediatric dose:* 1 mg/kg slow IVP when needed. Drug is supplied in 10 mg/mL vials or prefilled syringes.
- ★ *Special Considerations:* Monitor vital signs and cardiac rhythm closely. Also monitor the serum electrolytes because furosemide-induced dehydration may cause cardiac disturbances.

BUMETANIDE (BUMEX)

Classifications   ELECTROLYTIC BALANCE AND WATER BALANCE AGENTS; DIURETIC, LOOP

- ★ *Actions:* Loop diuretic that blocks reabsorption of sodium and water in the renal tubules, causing profound diuresis. The drug causes a diuresis that is 40 times greater than furosemids, but with a shorter half-life.
- ★ *Indications:* Edema that is associated with acute CHF; hepatic or renal diseases. May be considered for combination therapy with a potassium-sparing diuretic.
- ★ *Contraindications:* Allergy to bumetanide, anuria, hypotension, dehydration, hepatic coma, and patients with a high BUN. Monitor closely in patients with sulfa allergy.
- ★ *Side Effects:* Cramping, diarrhea, nausea, vomiting, tinnitus, vertigo, headache, leukopenia, anemia, urticaria, rash, hypokalemia.
- ★ *Dosage: Adults dose:* Typically 0.5–2.0 mg slow IVP over 1–2 minutes. Repeat at 4- to 5-hour intervals to a max allowance of 10 mg per day. *Pediatric dose:* 0.015–0.1 mg/kg every 6–24 hours to a max of 10 mg/day.
- ★ *Special Considerations:* Monitor vital signs and cardiac rhythm closely. Like the patient receiving furosemids, monitor electrolytes regularly as well. In those patients with furosemide allergy, bumetanide can be substituted at a 40:1 ratio (40 mg furosemide = 1 mg bumetanide).

H$_2$ BLOCKERS/PROTON PUMP INHIBITORS

The enteral administration of nutrition for the critical patient has been shown to aid in the healing process, so the proper function of the gut is important. However, development of stress ulcers and gastrointestinal bleeding is very prevalent in the critically ill and injured patient. As such the prevention of an ulcer is a high priority in the critical care setting, because it decreases the risk of bleeding dyscrasias, and allows the continued use of the enteral route for nutritional intake. Agents that decrease the production of digestive acids aid in the prevention of stress ulcer formation and allow the critical care practitioner to utilize the digestive system for feedings.

RANITIDINE HYDROCHLORIDE (ZANTAC)

Classifications   GASTROINTESTINAL AGENT; ANTISECRETORY (H$_2$-RECEPTOR ANTAGONIST)

★ *Actions:* Potent H$_2$-receptor antagonist that inhibits basal gastric acid secretion.

★ *Indications:* Treatment of ulcer disease, GI bleeding, and prophylaxis to decrease risk of stress ulcer. Also used for short-term management of duodenal ulcers and long-term maintenance therapy following active ulceration healing.

★ *Contraindications:* Allergy to ranitidine or its additives.

★ *Side Effects:* Cardiac dysrhythmia (bradycardia with rapid IVP), nausea, vomiting, rash, reversible mental confusion in the elderly. May also cause constipation.

★ *Dosage: Adult dose:* 50 mg/50 mL IVP over 15–30 minutes every 6–8 hours. *Pediatric dose:* 2–4 mg/kg/day in divided doses. Supplied as 50 mg/mL vials.

★ *Special Considerations:* Monitor vital signs and cardiac rhythm closely. Use cautiously in the elderly and the critically ill (while monitoring for mental status changes). Use cautiously in patients with hepatic and renal impairment.

CIMETIDINE (TAGAMET)

Classifications   GASTROINTESTINAL AGENT; ANTISECRETORY (H$_2$-RECEPTOR ANTAGONIST)

★ *Actions:* H$_2$-receptor antagonist, with minimal H$_1$ effects, that inhibits basal gastric acid secretion in the stomach. Also indirectly reduces pepsin secretion.

★ *Indications:* Treatment of GI ulcer disease, GI bleeding, and prophylaxis to decrease risk of stress ulcer.

★ *Contraindications:* Allergy to cimetidine or its additives. Safety in children less than 16 years old not established.

★ *Side Effects:* Cardiac dysrhythmias with rapid IV bolus, nausea, vomiting, rash, drowsiness, reversible mental confusion in the elderly, and reversible impotence.

★ *Dosage: Adult dose:* 300 mg/50 mL IV over 15–30 minutes every 6–8 hours. *Pediatric dose:* Parenteral administration is 20–40 mg/kg/day in divided doses. Drug is supplied in 300-mg vials.

★ *Special Considerations:* Monitor vital signs and the cardiac rhythm closely. Use cautiously in the elderly and the critically ill while monitoring for mental status changes. Use cautiously in patients with renal impairment.

FAMOTIDINE (PEPCID)

Classifications   GASTROINTESTINAL AGENT; ANTISECRETORY (H$_2$-RECEPTOR ANTAGONIST)

★ *Actions:* Structurally similar to cimetidine, it is a potent competitive H$_2$-receptor antagonist in gastric parietal cells where it inhibits basal gastric acid secretion.

- *Indications:* Treatment of ulcer disease, GI bleeding, and for prophylaxis therapy to decrease risk of stress ulcers.

- *Contraindications:* Known allergy to famotidine or its additives.

- *Side Effects:* Cardiac dysrhythmias, nausea, vomiting, rash, dizziness or drowsiness, reversible mental confusion in the elderly, and increased BUN and serum creatinine.

- *Dosage: Adult dose:* 10–20 mg/10 mL slow IVP over at least 2 minutes every 12 hours. *Pediatric dose:* 0.5 mg/kg every 8–12 hours to a max of 40 mg in one day. Famitodine is supplied in 10 mg/mL vials.

- *Special Considerations:* Monitor vital signs and cardiac rhythm closely. Use cautiously in the elderly and critically ill while monitoring for mental status changes. Use cautiously in patients with renal impairment.

ANTIEMETICS

Vomiting in the critically ill or injured patient is not just a situation of discomfort. Aspiration, electrolyte imbalances, and increased intrathoracic and intracranial pressures are a few of the problems that can occur as a result of vomiting. The administration of antiemetic agents can decrease the adverse effects caused by the physiology of vomiting, thus decreasing the complications.

> The administration of antiemetic agents can decrease the adverse effects caused by the physiology of vomiting, thus decreasing the complications.

PROMETHAZINE HYDROCHLORIDE (PHENERGAN, HISTANTIL, PHENAZINE, PHENCEN)

Classifications   GASTROINTESTINAL AGENT; ANTIEMETIC; ANTIVERTIGO AGENT; PHENOTHIAZINE

- *Actions:* Phenothiazine derivative with antipsychotic, H_1-receptor blocking, and vomiting center blocking properties. Unlike other phenothiazine agents, this drug is relatively free of extrapyramidal adverse effects (except at high doses).

- *Indications:* Treatment of nausea and vomiting associated with disease processes, or as a result of different medication administration. It can be used also as an antiemetic agent in those patients who are nauseated or become nauseated with flight.

- *Contraindications:* Allergy to promethazine, stenosing peptic ulcer, patients in a comatose state, bladder neck obstruction, and narrow-angle glaucoma. Not intended for children less than 2 years.

- *Side Effects:* Extrapyramidal symptoms (torticollis, oculogyric crisis, tongue protrusion, convulsive seizures, altered mental status) with high doses or rapid intravenous administration. CNS depression, respiratory depression, and cardiovascular depression. Also urticaria, leukopenia, and dry mouth.

- *Dosage: Adult dose:* 12.5–25 mg slow IVP every 4–6 hours; may give 25–50 mg IM if necessary. *Pediatrics dose (>2 years old):* 0.25–0.5 mg/kg slow IVP every 4–6 hours, or 12.5-25 mg IM.

- *Special Considerations:* Monitor vital signs and the level of consciousness continuously. Also watch the cardiac rhythm, and be prepared to assist with ventilations as needed. Treat extrapyramidal side effects with diphenhydramine (Benadryl) 12.5–25 mg slow IVP as needed.

PROCHLORPERAZINE (COMPAZINE)

Classifications   PSYCHOTHERAPEUTIC AGENT; PHENOTHIAZINE; GASTROINTESTINAL AGENT; ANTIEMETIC

- *Actions:* Like other phenothiazines, it exerts an antiemetic effect through a depressant action on the chemoreceptor trigger zone (CTZ) for vomiting in the CNS.

- *Indications:* Treatment of nausea and vomiting associated with disease processes, or as a result of different medication administration. Also can be used for psychotic disorders and anxiety.

- *Contraindications:* Do not use in comatose states or in the presence of large amounts of CNS depressants (alcohol, barbiturates, narcotics).

- *Side Effects:* Extrapyramidal symptoms (torticollis, oculogyric crisis, tongue protrusion, convulsive seizures, altered mental status), hypotension or hypertension, tachycardia, urticaria, leukopenia, dry mouth, respiratory depression.

- *Dosage: Adult dose:* 2.5–10 mg slow IVP over 1-2 minutes. Repeat every 6–8 hours to a max of 40 mg/day. *Pediatric intravenous dose:* Not established. Supplied in 10-mg vials.

- *Special Considerations:* As with other antiemetics that exert a depressant action to the CNS, monitor vital signs, level of consciousness, and cardiac rhythm closely. Be prepared to assist with ventilations as needed. If extrapyramidal side effects become manifested, treat with diphenhydramine (Benadryl) 12.5–25 mg slow IVP as needed.

ONDANSETRON HYDROCHLORIDE (ZOFRAN)

Classifications   GASTROINTESTINAL AGENT; ANTIEMETIC; SEROTONIN 5-HT$_3$-RECEPTOR ANTAGONIST

- *Actions:* Ondansetron is a selective 5-HT$_3$-receptor antagonist. While ondansetron's mechanism of action has not been fully characterized, it is not a dopamine-receptor antagonist. Serotonin receptors of the 5-HT$_3$ type are present both peripherally on vagal nerve terminals, and centrally in the CTZ.

- *Indications:* Treatment of nausea and vomiting associated with disease processes, or as a result of different medication administration.

- *Contraindications:* Allergy to ondansetron or its additives.

- *Side Effects:* Hypotension, tachycardia, constipation, elevated liver enzymes, depressed CNS activity.

- *Dosage: Adult dose:* 4 mg slow IVP over 2–5 minutes every 4–6 hours. *Pediatric dose (≥2 years old):* 0.1 mg/kg slow IVP every 4–6 hours. Drug is supplied in 4 mg/mL vials.

- *Special Considerations:* Monitor vital signs and cardiac rhythm closely. Use cautiously in elderly patients and patients with renal impairment.

MISCELLANEOUS PHARMACOLOGIC AGENTS

While rare, the critical care paramedic may transport those patients with overwhelming sepsis, where supportive and antibiotic therapy are not enough to maintain homeostasis. The administration of drotrecogin alfa is indicated for the septic patient when sepsis-induced disseminated intravascular coagulation (DIC) is a concern.

DROTRECOGIN ALFA (XIGRIS)

Classifications   IMMUNOMODULATOR; RECOMBINANT HUMAN ACTIVATED PROTEIN C

- *Actions:* Recombinant form of exogenous activated protein C, an anti-imflammatory mediator that exerts an antithrombotic effect by inhibiting factors Va and VIIIa.

- *Indications:* Indicated for the reduction of mortality in adult patients with severe sepsis (sepsis associated with acute organ dysfunction) who have a high risk of death.

★ *Contraindication:* Active internal bleeding, recent hemorrhagic stroke (within 3 months), recent intracranial/intraspinal surgery (within 2 months), trauma with an increased risk of life-threatening bleeding, presence of an epidural catheter.

★ *Side Effects:* Bleeding, including hemorrhage and intracranial hemorrhage.

★ *Dosage: Adult dose:* 24 mcg/kg/hr by continuous infusion for 96 hours. *Pediatric dose:* Not established. Drug is supplied in 5-mg and 20-mg vials.

★ *Special Considerations:* Monitor closely for bleeding. Should it occur, discontinue infusion and transfuse with fresh frozen plasma or cryoprecipitate.

Summary

Of all the new disciplines that the critical care paramedic will face in his or her new role, the discipline of pharmacology may be the most comprehensive. The agents available to the critical care team will be more extensive, as will the responsibility to fully understand all of the actions and reactions of each individual agent. The prehospital and interfacility critical care transport settings have widened immensely with this "extension" of critical care medicine, and it is incumbent on the critical care paramedic to meet these new challenges.

Additional Case Studies

1. *A 60-year-old male is being transported to an interventional cardiac catheterization lab for emergent cardiac catheterization. His initial ECG upon arrival to the requesting facility showed hyperacute ST segment elevation in leads V1–V4, with reciprocal changes in leads II, II, and AVF.*

   Treatment at the requesting facility included aspirin, 162 mg PO; heparin, 7500 units IVP; followed by continuous heparin infusion at 1200 units/hr, and nitroglycerin by continuous infusion at 40 mcg/min. The patient received his first dose of retaplase 15 minutes prior to the arrival of the transport crew. Current vital signs include heart rate, 68; BP, 126/60; respiratory rate, 18; and pulse oximetry of 99% on 4 lpm by nasal cannula. The patient continues to have chest pain rated as 5 on a 1–10 scale.

   Given the above information, what is your diagnostic impression?

   During the transport, the second dose of reteplase (Retavase) is administered. Ten minutes following that, the patient starts complaining of slight dyspnea and lightheadedness. Vital signs show heart 45 with a wide-complex QRS morphology, BP is 100/50, respiratory rate 20, and pulse oximetry 96%.

   The critical care paramedic's next pharmacologic intervention would be to administer what agent?

   Five minutes later, the patient develops acute dyspnea with audible rales. His vital signs reveal heart rate, 110; BP, 190/100; respiratory rate, 30; and pulse oximetry, 84%. Emergent treatment would include what?

2. *A 45-year-old with a history significant for tobacco abuse and hypertension presents to a community hospital with severe headache. The patient's medication history is noncontributory, and he is allergic to morphine. Vital signs are heart rate, 50; BP, 226/114; respiratory rate, 18; pulse oximetry, 99% on room air; Glasgow Coma Scale (GCS), 15.*

   The critical care paramedic is called to transport this patient for neurologic evaluation. He has an intravenous infusion of 0.9% normal saline in place, has received clonidine 0.1 mg PO, and nalbuphine

5 mg IVP for complaints of headache. Based on CT scan evaluation, the working diagnosis is acute sub-arachnoid hemorrhage.

Based on the above information, which intervention would the critical care paramedic complete first?

a. Administer clonidine (Catapres) 0.1 mg PO.
b. Administer labetolol (Normadyne) 20 mg slow IVP.
c. Begin nitroprusside (Nipride) at 0.5 mcg/kg/min and titrate to decrease blood pressure to 160 systolic.
d. Administer fentanyl (Sublimaze) 100 mcg IVP for complaints of headache.

During transport, the patient's condition rapidly deteriorates to find him with the following assessment findings: heart rate, 44; BP, 188/100; respiratory rate at 16 by bag-valve-mask assistance; pulse oximetry, 100%; GCS 4, with decerebrate posturing.

After establishing airway control, the critical care paramedic would administer what hyperosmolar medication?

The decision is made to initiate the RSI protocol in order to secure the airway more definitively.

Following this procedure and after ensuring that the endotracheal tube is properly placed, and vecuronium (Norcuron) has been given for continued paralysis, the critical care paramedic must then consider the administration of

a. analgesics, such as morphine sulfate or fentanyl (Sublimaze).
b. benzodiazepines, such as midazolam (Versed) or lorazepam (Ativan).
c. both of the above.
d. neither of the above.

See Answers to Review Questions at the back of this book.

Further Reading

Bledsoe BE, Clayden DE. *Prehospital Emergency Pharmacology, 6th ed.* Upper Saddle River, NJ: Pearson Prentice Hall, 2005.

Koda-Kimble MA, Young LY, Kradjan WA, Cuglielmo JB. *Handbook of Applied Therapeutics.* Philadelphia, PA: Lippencott William & Wilkins, 2002.

Mistovich JJ, Benner RW, Margolis GS. *Prehospital Advanced Cardiac Life Support.* Upper Saddle River, NJ: Pearson Prentice Hall, 2004.

RxList Inc. http://www.rxlist.com.

Shannon MT, Wilson BA, Stang CL. *Health Professional's Drug Guide.* Upper Saddle River, NJ: Pearson Prentice Hall, 2004.

Spratto GR, Woods AL. *PDR Nurse's Drug Handbook, 2004 Edition.* Clifton Park, NY: Thomson Delmar Learning.

Interpretation of Lab and Basic Diagnostic Tests

Bryan E. Bledsoe, DO, FACEP

Objectives

Upon completion of this chapter, the student should be able to:

1. Discuss the importance of laboratory and basic diagnostic testing in critical care transport. (p. 328)

2. Describe how normal laboratory values are established. (p. 328)

3. Define the terms *specificity* and *sensitivity* as they pertain to medical testing. (p. 329)

4. List the elements of a complete blood count and discuss what any abnormal readings may indicate. (p. 331)

5. List the elements of a coagulation panel and discuss what any abnormal readings may indicate. (p. 334)

6. Describe calculation of the International Normalized Ratio (INR). (p. 334)

7. Discuss the significance of the D-dimer assay. (p. 335)

8. Describe why electrolytes are measured in milliequivalents per liter. (p. 336)

9. Describe the anion gap, how is it calculated, and what is its clinical significance? (p. 336)

10. List the elements of an electrolyte panel and discuss what any abnormal readings may indicate. (p. 336)

11. List the elements of a renal function panel and discuss what any abnormal readings may indicate. (p. 337)

12. Describe the importance of blood glucose testing in modern emergency care. (p. 340)

13. List the elements of a lipid panel and discuss what any abnormal readings may indicate. (p. 340)

14. List the five most frequently used cardiac markers. (p. 342)
15. Detail the timing of cardiac marker elevations after a myocardial infarction. (p. 342)
16. Discuss the importance of isoenzymes in CK and LDH testing. (p. 342)
17. List the elements of a liver function panel and discuss what any abnormal readings may indicate. (p. 344)
18. Describe the role of serologic testing in critical care transport. (p. 344)
19. Discuss the importance of accurate blood banking in emergency care. (p. 345)
20. Describe common endocrine function tests encountered in critical care transport. (p. 346)
21. Briefly describe how bacteria are identified and isolated. (p. 347)
22. List the elements of a urinalysis and discuss what any abnormal readings may indicate. (p. 347)
23. Discuss the importance of toxicological testing in critical care transport. (p. 347)
24. Discuss the role of diagnostic imaging in medicine and briefly describe the following:
    * ★ X-rays (p. 349)
    * ★ Fluoroscopy (p. 349)
    * ★ CT (CAT) scanning (p. 349)
    * ★ Ultrasonography (p. 349)
    * ★ Nuclear medicine (p. 349)
    * ★ Magnetic resonance imaging (MRI) (p. 349)
    * ★ Positron emission tomography (PET) (p. 349)
25. Describe common physiological tests encountered in medicine. (p. 349)
26. List the elements of an arterial blood gas panel and discuss what any abnormal readings may indicate. (p. 350)

Key Terms

ABO typing, p. 345
arterial blood gas, p. 350
blood banking, p. 345
blood urea nitrogen (BUN), p. 337
B-natriuretic peptide (BNP), p. 344
cholesterol, p. 341
Coombs' test, p. 346
creatine kinase (CK or CPK), p. 342
creatinine, p. 337
critical values, p. 328
CT (CAT) scanning, p. 349
D-dimer, p. 335
electrolytes, p. 336
erythrocyte sedimentation rate (sed rate), p. 332

glycohemoglobin, p. 340
Gram stains, p. 347
HDL, p. 341
hematology, p. 331
International Normalized Ratio (INR), p. 334
laboratory tests, p. 328
laboratory values, p. 328
lactic dehydrogenase (LD or LDH), p. 342
LDL, p. 342
Le Système International d'Unités, p. 330
lipoproteins, p. 341
magnetic resonance imaging (MRI), p. 349
medical imaging, p. 348
myoglobin, p. 344

normal reference values, p. 328
partial thromboplastin time (PTT), p. 334
positron emission tomography (PET), p. 349
prothrombin time (PT), p. 334
reticulocyte count, p. 332
sensitivity, p. 329
specificity, p. 329
triglycerides, p. 341
troponins, p. 344
ultrasound, p. 349
urinalysis, p. 347
VLDL, p. 342
X-rays, p. 349

Case Study

Your critical care transport unit is called to transfer a critically ill patient from a community hospital to a large teaching hospital. The transport time is approximately 90 minutes. The patient is a 57-year-old male scheduled for a liver transplant. Thus far, a donor organ has not become available and the patient's condition is deteriorating. Because of this, the patient is being transferred to the teaching hospital where he will be nearby as soon as a donor liver becomes available.

You go to the ICU. The patient is resting quietly in bed—obviously jaundiced. Multiple IV infusions are being administered and the patient is not on a ventilator. The nurse hands you the chart. You take a brief look at the admission history and physical and flip through the physicians' and nurses' notes and come to the laboratory. There are numerous studies in the chart with numerous abnormal readings. First, you note the comprehensive metabolic panel.

- ★ Glucose (174 mg/dL)
- ★ Calcium (4.4 mEq/L)
- ★ Albumin (3.2 g/dL)
- ★ Total protein (5.1 g/dL)
- ★ Sodium (141 mEq/L)
- ★ Potassium (5.1 mEq/L)
- ★ CO_2 (12 mEq/L)
- ★ Chloride (96 mEq/L)
- ★ BUN (blood urea nitrogen) (101 mg/dL)
- ★ Creatinine (2.1 mg/dL)
- ★ ALP (alkaline phosphatase) (741 U/L)
- ★ ALT (alanine amino transferase) (886 U/L)
- ★ AST (aspartate amino transferase) (1512 U/L)
- ★ Bilirubin (3.1 mg/dL)

His CBC was normal except for mild anemia. You note that his coagulation panel is markedly abnormal:

- ★ PT (45.2 seconds)
- ★ PTT (71.4 seconds)
- ★ INR (3.6)

Your partner notices the abnormal coagulation tests and asks if the patient is on heparin. You point out that the abnormal test results are due to the liver failure (the liver makes the coagulation elements) and not heparin or warfarin (Coumadin).

Following your assessment, the patient is moved to the ambulance and does well during transport. He has some delirium that you feel is probably due to his liver failure. You deliver him to the transplant unit at the teaching hospital where he remains for another 2 weeks. A donor liver was never found and the patient subsequently died of fulminant liver failure.

INTRODUCTION

As a critical care paramedic, a great deal of your transports will be between health care facilities. Usually, patients are transferred to more advanced levels of care. On most occasions, certain diagnostic and laboratory tests have been conducted in the transferring facility prior to transport. These tests provide valuable information about the patient. Because of this, the critical care paramedic must have a basic understanding of common lab tests routinely encountered during interfacility transfer.

Diagnostic tests can be divided into three general categories: laboratory tests, medical imaging, and physiological testing. There may be significant overlap among these categories based on the hospital department responsible for performing the tests. Some tests are formally interpreted by a physician while others are not. Unfortunately, the transcribed interpretation may not be available for a day or so after the test and unavailable at the time of critical care transport. However, with emergency or "stat" tests, the consultant may provide a preliminary or initial interpretation until the formal interpretation is available.

In this chapter we will detail common diagnostic tests and their significance in critical care transport. It is important to point out that there are thousands of tests available and this chapter cannot possibly address each.

LABORATORY TESTS

laboratory tests *specific studies or assays performed on various body tissues.*

Laboratory tests are specific studies or assays performed on various body tissues. Common tissues include blood, serum, urine, stool, spinal fluid, and many more. For each test a normal reference value (or range) is established based on a survey of a healthy population. Any abnormal value is one that falls outside of the reference range. With certain tests a "panic value" or "critical value" has been determined in order to alert health care practitioners about potentially life-threatening laboratory values.

Laboratory tests are often divided into various categories based on the substance being tested and the part of the lab responsible for the test. These categories include hematology, chemistry, microbiology, serology, and pathology.

LABORATORY VALUES

laboratory values *analysis of a specimen in comparison with a set of controls and known parameters.*

normal reference values *nationally established parameters based upon a large number of lab tests conducted over several years, affected by gender and age.*

When a laboratory test is ordered, the specimen is collected and prepared for analysis. During analysis the specimen is compared with known **laboratory values** (controls) and a result is obtained. This result may be quantitative (a numerical value is provided) or qualitative (a simple yes/no answer is provided).

Normal reference values are usually established nationally based on a large number of lab tests conducted over several years. These are published periodically in the *New England Journal of Medicine*. For many tests, a normal curve (or Gaussian distribution) is determined by statistical analysis. A cutoff point is determined—usually 2 standard deviations from the mean or the average. (See Figure 12-1 ■.) By using this method, 95% of the population tested is considered normal. The remaining 5% would be abnormal. Another, and perhaps better, method of establishing normal values is the percentile ranking system. With this system, all values are ranked, and a percentage given for each value in relation to the other values. The value in the middle (the median) is the 50th percentile. Thus, 50% of the scores are either higher or lower than the median.

Each local lab will confirm these normals in their population and, in some cases, will alter slightly the normal reference range. The major physiological variables that affect normal reference values are sex and age. Any test result that falls outside of the normal range is considered abnormal. Life-threatening values are often flagged as "panic values" or **critical values.**

critical values *life-threatening values or "panic" values.*

It is important to remember that some "normal" lab values may in fact be abnormal for the patient in question. This is particularly true for pregnant women and children. Always keep this con-

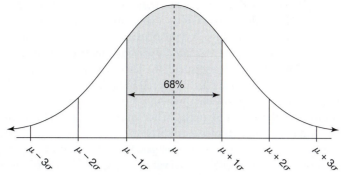

68% confidence level (1 standard deviations from the mean)

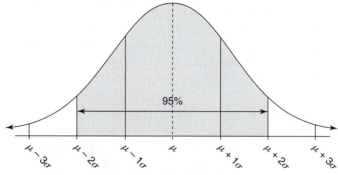

95% confidence level (2 standard deviations from the mean)

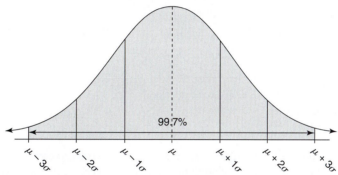

99.7% confidence level (3 standard deviations from the mean)

μ = mean
σ = standard deviation

sideration in mind when dealing with these populations. Many labs will publish addendum normal values for special populations.

The terms *specificity* and *sensitivity* are often used in relation to laboratory testing. The **specificity** of a test is a measure of how well it detects a disease. If a test is 100% specific, it will identify the disease in question in 100% of patients who have the disease. A test with a high specificity has few false-positives. However, few, if any, tests are 100% specific because multiple factors can affect the test. For example, a test is developed that is supposed to detect the SARS virus. The test is administered to 255 patients *without* SARS. Of these, the test is negative in 230 of the cases. The specificity is 230/255 or 90%. People who have the disease and test positive are called true-positives. People who do not have the disease and test negative are called true-negatives. People who test positive, yet do not have the disease, are called false-positives. People who test negative, yet who have the disease are called false-negatives.

The **sensitivity** of a test is the degree to which a test detects disease without yielding a false-negative result. No test is 100% sensitive. A test with high sensitivity has few false-negatives. For

specificity *the measure of how well a test detects a disease without yielding a false-positive result. (High specificity = low false-positives)*

sensitivity *the degree to which a test detects disease without yielding a false-negative result. (High sensitivity = low false-negatives)*

example, we have developed a test that detects the human form of "mad cow disease" known as Creutzfeldt-Jakob disease (CJD). The test is administered to 45 patients who are known to have the disease. Of these, the test is positive in 36 of the cases. The sensitivity is 36/45 or 80%.

Laboratory values are usually reported in metric system values. However, because the quantity of tested material can be so small, the terms *picogram (pg)* or *nanogram (ng)* are more frequently encountered. Electrolytes are measured in *milliequivalents (mEq)*. There has been an international trend to switch to a more comprehensive form of the metric system called **Le Système International d'Unités** (abbreviated SI units). The biggest changes have been to report concentrations as an amount per volume (moles or millimoles per liter). For some laboratory tests, the numbers remain the same although the unit has changed. Glucose readings have traditionally been expressed in milligrams per deciliter with normal values being 70–100 mg/dL. With the SI system, glucose is established in millimoles per liter with normal values being 3.9–5.6 mmol/L. The United States has been slow to switch to the SI system, but it is commonly used in EMS systems in Canada, the United Kingdom, and Australia.

Most laboratory specimens are collected in standardized transport media. Blood is usually collected in sealed tubes that contain a vacuum. When punctured, the vacuum only allows a certain amount of blood to enter the tube. Some tubes contain preservatives and others contain anticoagulants. Each type of laboratory test requires a specific type of blood tube. Although the colors and

Le Système International d'Unités a comprehensive form of the metric system that deals in more precise measurements (abbreviated SI units) than standard metric.

Table 12–1 | CBC Values

Measurement	Meaning	Normal	High Values	Low Values
Hemoglobin	Amount of hemoglobin present in blood	Men: 13.0–18.0 g/dL Women: 12–16 g/dL	–Smokers	–Anemia –Blood loss –Overhydration
Hematocrit	Percentage of RBCs in the plasma	Men: 37–49% Women: 36–46%	–Dehydration –Polycythemia	–Overhydration –Anemia –Blood loss
WBC	Number of white blood cells per cubic millimeter of blood	$4,500$–$11,000/mm^3$	–Infection –Leukemia –Steroids	–Viral infection –Immunodeficiency
RBC	Number of red blood cells per cubic millimeter of blood	Men: 4.5–5.3 million/mm^3 Women: 4.1–5.1 million/mm^3	–Polycythemia –High altitudes	–Bone marrow suppression –Abnormal loss/suppression of erythrocytes
MCV	Mean corpuscular volume (size of RBC)	Men: 78–100 μm^3 Women: 78–102 μm^3	–Folic acid deficiency –Vitamin B_{12} deficiency –Alcoholism	–Iron-deficiency anemia –Lead poisoning
MCH	Mean corpuscular hemoglobin (amount of hemoglobin present in one cell)	25–35 pg	–Folic acid deficiency –Vitamin B_{12} deficiency	–Iron-deficiency anemia –Thalassemias
MCHC	Mean corpuscular hemoglobin concentration (the proportion of each cell occupied by hemoglobin)	31–37%	–Folic acid deficiency –Vitamin B_{12} deficiency	–Iron-deficiency anemia –Thalassemias
RDW	Red blood cell distribution width (calculated from the MCV and RBC)	11.5–14.0%	–Iron deficiency –Thalassemia minor	

types can vary by hospital the most commonly used system is the following system, in which tubes are usually filled in a particular order to ensure the most accurate test:

1. Blood cultures (yellow top)
2. Nonadditive tubes (red top)
3. Coagulation tubes (light blue top)
4. Serum separator tubes (tiger top)
5. Heparin tubes (green top)
6. EDTA tubes (lavender top)
7. Oxalate fluoride (gray top)

HEMATOLOGY

The testing and study of blood and its various elements is called **hematology.** Today, virtually all hematological studies are automated. The most commonly ordered hematological test is the complete blood count (CBC), which is usually performed automatically by a cell counter. Common values found on a CBC are detailed in Table 12–1. The types of white blood cells present are usually measured and this measurement is referred to as the *differential.* (See Figure 12-2 ■.) Formerly, these were measured by microscope—but are now measured by machine. Table 12–2 details the

hematology *the testing and study of blood and its various elements.*

■ **Figure 12-2**   White blood cells. (*Ed Reschke/Peter Arnold, Inc.*)

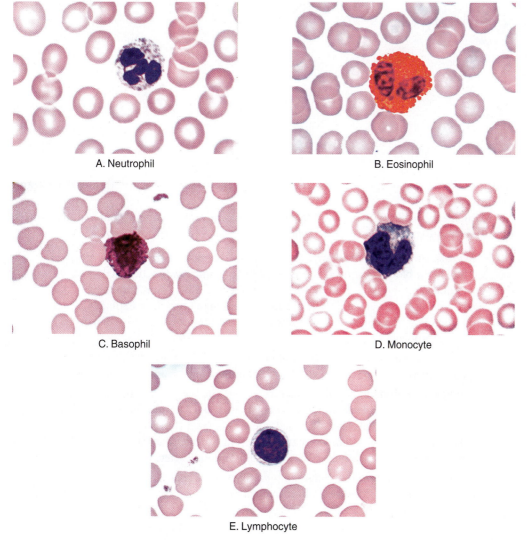

A. Neutrophil

B. Eosinophil

C. Basophil

D. Monocyte

E. Lymphocyte

Table 12-2	WBC Differential				
Measurement	Meaning	Normal*	High Values	Low Values
Bands or stabs†	Percentage of young or immature neutrophils	0–5%	–Bacterial infection –Severe stress	–Typhoid –Tularemia –Brucellosis –Cancer –Bone marrow depression
PMNs or segs	Percentage of segmented or mature neutrophils	45–70%	–Bacterial infection –Severe stress	–Typhoid –Tularemia –Brucellosis –Cancer –Bone marrow depression
Eosinophils	Percentage of eosinophils present	0–8%	–Allergies –Parasites	–Corticosteroid therapy
Basophils	Percentage of basophils present	0–3%	–Leukemia –Not well understood	–Corticosteroid therapy –Allergic reactions
Lymphocytes	Percentage of lymphocytes present	16–46%	–Viral infections –Leukemia	–AIDS –Autoimmune disease
Monocytes	Percentage of monocytes present	4–11%	–Tuberculosis –Protozoan infections –Leukemia	

* Percentage should add up to 100%.

† Bands/stabs may not be counted on automated machines.

WBC differential. Figure 12-3 ■ shows development of the various blood cells through the various cell lines.

Many specialized hematology tests are available—some more commonly ordered than others. Among the more common tests are the following:

reticulocyte count
measures less mature types of RBCs in the bloodstream; a function of bone marrow production.

★ *Reticulocyte count.* A **reticulocyte count** is a measurement of the less mature types of RBCs in the bloodstream and is a measure of bone marrow function. A normal reticulocyte count in an adult is 0.5–2.5% of the total RBC count. Increased reticulocyte counts are indicative of a more rapid than usual increase in RBC production by the bone marrow. A low reticulocyte count is indicative of a bone marrow problem.

★ *Peripheral blood smear.* A peripheral blood smear is a test in which a thin layer of blood is placed on a microscope slide and examined for various abnormalities.

erythrocyte sedimentation rate (sed rate) *a nonspecific hematologic test that can point to various problems. An elevated sed rate is associated with pregnancy, autoimmune disease, and inflammation, as well as diagnostic for temporal arteritis.*

★ **Erythrocyte sedimentation rate (sed rate)** A sed rate is a nonspecific test, but can point to various problems. Normally the sed rate is 0–17 mm/hr for men and 1–25 mm/hr for women. An elevation in sed rate is associated with pregnancy, autoimmune disease, and inflammation. A sed rate greater than 60 mm/hr with associated temporal headache is diagnostic for temporal arteritis.

★ *Serum folic acid, serum B_{12}, and serum iron.* These tests are ordered to aid in determination of deficiencies in folic acid, vitamin B_{12}, or iron and are thus helpful in diagnosing the type of anemia present.

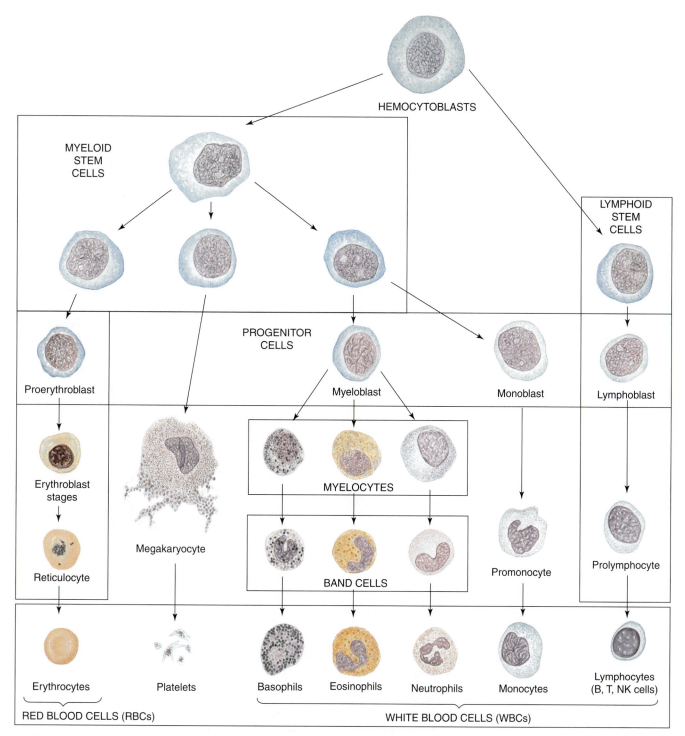

HEMOCYTOBLASTS

MYELOID STEM CELLS

LYMPHOID STEM CELLS

Proerythroblast

PROGENITOR CELLS

Myeloblast

Monoblast

Lymphoblast

Erythroblast stages

MYELOCYTES

Megakaryocyte

BAND CELLS

Promonocyte

Prolymphocyte

Reticulocyte

Erythrocytes

Platelets

Basophils

Eosinophils

Neutrophils

Monocytes

Lymphocytes (B, T, NK cells)

RED BLOOD CELLS (RBCs)

WHITE BLOOD CELLS (WBCs)

■ **Figure 12-3**   The origins and differentiation of blood cells. Hemocytoblast divisions give rise to myeloid and lymphoid stem cells. Lymphoid stem cells produce the various classes of lymphocytes. Myeloid stem cells produce progenitor cells, which divide into various classes of blood cells. (*Fig. 12-7, p. 346, from* Essentials of Anatomy & Physiology, *2nd ed., by Frederic H. Martini, Ph.D. and Edwin F. Bartholomew, M.S. Copyright © 2000 by Frederic H. Martini, Inc. Published by Pearson Education, Inc. Reprinted by permission.*)

Figure 12-4 Medical lab shorthand for complete blood count.

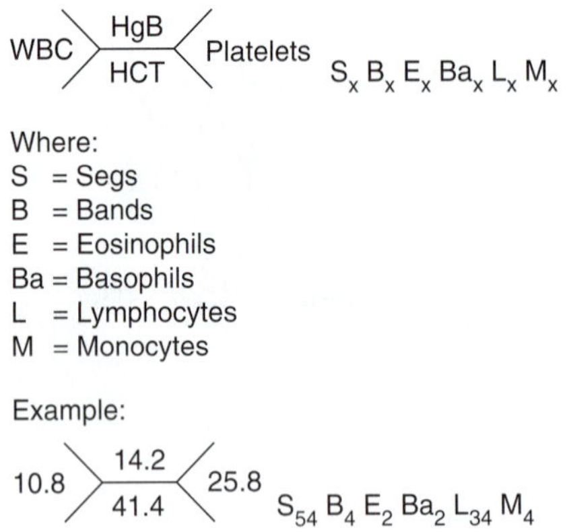

$$WBC \diagdown \frac{HgB}{HCT} \diagdown Platelets \quad S_x \, B_x \, E_x \, Ba_x \, L_x \, M_x$$

Where:
S = Segs
B = Bands
E = Eosinophils
Ba = Basophils
L = Lymphocytes
M = Monocytes

Example:

$$10.8 \diagdown \frac{14.2}{41.4} \diagdown 25.8 \quad S_{54} \, B_4 \, E_2 \, Ba_2 \, L_{34} \, M_4$$

The final component of the CBC is the platelet count and mean platelet volume. Platelets are not intact cells, but are fragments of cells important in blood clotting. The average number of platelets present in an adult ranges from 150,000 to 350,000/mm^3. An abnormal elevation in platelets is called thrombocytosis and is associated with tumors and following splenectomy. A fall in platelets is called thrombocytopenia and is associated with viral infections, AIDS, and lupus. Sometimes, the cause is unknown (idiopathic thrombocytopenia).

Most CBCs will be printed out on a form from the lab. Sometimes, in charting, the physician will record the CBC. Figure 12-4 ■ shows a typical CBC in physician charting. The differential is usually written with the segs and bands (granulocytes) on the left and the lymphocytes and other cells (agranulocytes) on the right. An increase in the number of segs and bands indicates a probable bacterial infection and is referred to as a *left shift*. (See Table 12–3.) The term *right shift* is less frequently used and indicates an increase in lymphocytes and a possible viral infection.

Table 12–3	Differential Shifts in Disease					
Shift	Segs (%)	Bands (%)	Eosinophils (%)	Basophils (%)	Lymphocytes (%)	Monocytes (%)
None	61	3	4	1	26	5
Left	65	10	3	1	17	4
Right*	30	2	4	2	58	4

* Infrequently used (slang).

COAGULATION TESTS

prothrombin time (PT) *prothrombin is factor II in the coagulation cascade, produced by the liver and essential to normal blood coagulation.*

partial thromboplastin time (PTT) *the PTT, also called the activated partial thromboplastin time. Used to detect coagulation disorders and monitor heparin therapy.*

International Normalized Ratio (INR) *the INR reports PT in a more standardized form, comparing it to a preestablished control.*

The process of coagulation is essential to homeostasis. The body must maintain the fine balance between hemorrhage and thrombus formation. Common coagulation tests encountered in critical care transport include the following:

★ **Prothrombin time (PT).** Prothrombin is factor II in the coagulation cascade. It is produced by the liver and is essential to normal blood coagulation. (See Figure 12-5 ■.) The PT is specific for measuring the effectiveness of the coumarin type of anticoagulants (i.e., warfarin [Coumadin]). The PT is usually reported in seconds.

★ **Partial thromboplastin time (PTT).** The PTT, also called the activated partial thromboplastin time, is used to detect coagulation disorders in the intrinsic pathway of the coagulation cascade. It is also used to monitor heparin therapy.

★ **International Normalized Ratio (INR).** The INR is now frequently used to report the PT in a more standardized form. The INR compares the PT to a preestablished control. In the normal person not on anticoagulants, the PT and the control should be the same resulting in a ratio of 1.0. With warfarin therapy, the goal is to maintain the INR at 1.5–2.5 (1.5–2.5 times the control).

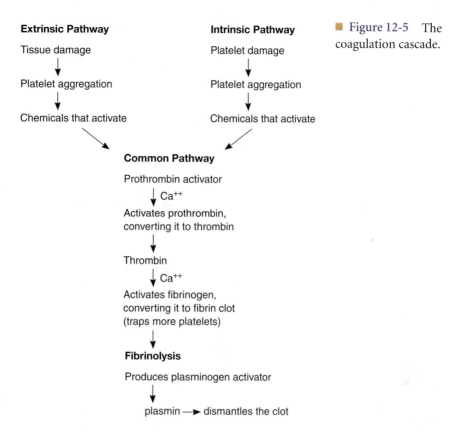

Figure 12-5 The coagulation cascade.

These tests are detailed in Table 12–4. Less frequently encountered coagulation tests include the following:

★ *Factor VIII.* Factor XII is used for the diagnosis of classic hemophilia (hemophilia A).

★ *Factor IX.* Factor IX is used for the diagnosis of Christmas disease (hemophilia B).

★ *von Willebrand Factor (vWF).* vWF is used to diagnose von Willebrand disease, the most common inherited bleeding disorder. Unlike hemophilia, it is not sex linked.

★ *Fibrinogen.* Fibrinogen is factor I and is responsible for the formation of fibrin in blood coagulation. A low fibrinogen is often due to disseminated intravascular clotting (DIC) and is due to a pathologic overstimulation of the coagulation process.

★ *Fibrin split products.* Fibrin split products measure the products that result from the breakdown of a fibrin clot by the enzyme plasmin. These are found in DIC.

★ *D-dimer screen.* The **D-dimer** is the degradation products of cross-linked fibrin. D-dimer screening has proven helpful in diagnosing abruptio placenta, DIC, deep venous thrombosis (DVT), and pulmonary embolism.

D-dimer *the degradation products of cross-linked fibrin.*

Table 12–4	Common Coagulation Tests				
Test	**Meaning**	**Normal**	**High Values**	**Low Values**	**Treatment**
PT	Prothrombin time	11.2–13.2 seconds	–Liver cirrhosis –Low vitamin K levels –DIC	Not clinically significant	Treatment for elevated PT is to administer vitamin K and withhold warfarin. In severe cases fresh frozen plasma may be administered.
PTT	Partial thromboplastin time	22.1–34.1 seconds	–Heparin therapy –Hemophilia	Not clinically significant	Treatment for an elevated PTT is to decrease heparin dose or administer protamine. In severe cases fresh frozen plasma may be administered.

★ *Thrombin time.* The thrombin time is the time it takes blood to clot when thrombin is added. If a clot does not form, there is a fibrinogen deficiency.

★ *Plasminogen assay.* Plasminogen is an inactive precursor of plasmin. The test is used in the diagnosis of DIC.

CHEMISTRIES

Chemistry testing is commonly performed in medicine. These tests are often run in panels that contain tests that provide similar information (i.e., liver function panel). These chemistries are usually measured on a sophisticated machine capable of analyzing numerous substances. In this discussion, we will detail the most commonly encountered chemistry tests in critical care transport.

ELECTROLYTES

electrolytes *chemical substances that take on an electrical charge when dissolved in water.*

Electrolytes are chemical substances that take on a charge when dissolved in water. The four most commonly measured electrolytes are sodium, potassium, chloride, and bicarbonate. Less commonly measured electrolytes are calcium, magnesium, and phosphate. Sodium, chloride, and bicarbonate are the principal elements in the extracellular fluid. Potassium, magnesium, and phosphate are the principal elements of the intracellular fluid.

Electrolytes are measured in milliequivalents per liter instead of milligrams because milligram units only measure the weight of the chemical element, not chemical activity. The standard of equivalents is based on how many grams of an element or compound liberate or combine with 1 gram of hydrogen. A *milliequivalent* is 1/1000 of an equivalent. Table 12–5 details this relationship.

Electrolytes that take on a positive charge are called *cations* and include sodium, potassium, magnesium, and calcium. Electrolytes that take on a negative charge are called *anions* and include chloride, bicarbonate, and phosphate. There must be a constant balance between the positively and negatively charged ions. This is referred to as *chemical electrical neutrality.* Thus, when the concentration of one of the electrolytes changes, other electrolytes shift to maintain chemical electrical neutrality. For example, when metabolic acids are introduced into the body, bicarbonate ions (HCO_3^-) are utilized as buffers. When the bicarbonate ions are eliminated, a negative ion deficit is left. To maintain chemical electrical neutrality, chloride ions (Cl^-) are shifted out of the cells to maintain electrical chemical neutrality. While most electrolytes are easily measured, some are not. When cations and anions in the serum are measured, there appears to be a deficit in the number of anions, which is referred to as the *anion gap.* This gap is made up of unmeasured anions such as organic acids, sulfates, and phosphates. To calculate the anion gap, add the measured cations and subtract the measured anions. The difference in the anion gap is usually about 12–14 mEq.

$$(Na^+ + K^+) - (Cl^- + HCO_3^-) = \text{Anion gap}$$
$$(140\,\text{mEq} + 4\,\text{mEq}) - (103\,\text{mEq} + 27\,\text{mEq}) = \text{Anion gap}$$
$$144\,\text{mEq} - 130\,\text{m Eq} = 14\,\text{mEq}$$

The anion gap is important in that it is increased in certain metabolic acidosis states. Thus, an increase in the anion gap helps identify the type of metabolic acidosis present.

Table 12–5	Conversion of Milligrams to Milliequivalents	
Measurement of Weight	**Measurement of Chemical Activity**
23 mg sodium (Na^+)	1 mEq
39 mg potassium (K^+)	1 mEq
36 mg chloride (Cl^-)	1 mEq
30 mg bicarbonate (HCO_3^-)	1 mEq

The most frequently occurring cations include:

★ *Sodium (Na⁺)*. Sodium is the most prevalent cation in the extracellular fluid. It plays a major role in regulating the distribution of water because water is attracted to and moves with sodium. In fact, it is often said that "water follows sodium." Sodium is also important in the transmission of nervous impulses. An abnormal increase in the relative amount of sodium in the body is called *hypernatremia,* while an abnormal decrease is referred to as *hyponatremia.*

★ *Potassium (K⁺)*. Potassium is the most prevalent cation in the intracellular fluid. It is also important in the transmission of electrical impulses. An abnormally high potassium level is called *hyperkalemia,* while an abnormally low potassium level is referred to as *hypokalemia.*

★ *Calcium (Ca²⁺)*. Calcium has many physiological functions. It plays a major role in muscle contraction as well as nervous impulse transmission. An abnormally increased calcium level is called *hypercalcemia,* while an abnormally decreased calcium level is called *hypocalcemia.* About half of the calcium in the serum is loosely associated with proteins. The other half (which is the metabolically active portion) is called *ionized calcium.* The usual methods for measuring calcium measure the total calcium level (bound + free). Ionized calcium is measured when other factors complicate the interpretation of the normal serum calcium test. For example, if the levels of binding proteins are increased or decreased (for example, in the presence of abnormal amounts of albumin or immunoglobulins), the amount of serum calcium will appear to be increased or decreased, because it is the free calcium that is regulated hormonally by the body. In these circumstances, ionized calcium is a more reliable measure of calcium levels.

★ *Magnesium (Mg²⁺)*. Magnesium is necessary for several biochemical processes that occur in the body and is closely associated with phosphate in many processes. An abnormally increased magnesium level is called *hypermagnesemia;* an abnormally decreased magnesium level is called *hypomagnesemia.*

The most frequently occurring anions include:

★ *Chloride (Cl⁻)*. Chloride is an important anion. Its negative charge balances the positive charge associated with the cations. It also plays a major role in fluid balance and renal function. Chloride has a close association with sodium.

★ *Bicarbonate* (HCO_3^-). Bicarbonate is the principal buffer of the body. This means that it neutralizes the highly acidic hydrogen ion (H^+) and other organic acids.

★ *Phosphate* (HPO_4^-). Phosphate is important in body energy stores. It is closely associated with magnesium in renal function. It also acts as a buffer, primarily in the intracellular space, in much the same manner as bicarbonate.

Many other compounds carry negative charges. Among these are some of the proteins, certain organic acids, and other compounds.

The status of the electrolytes can provide a great deal of information about the patient's condition. Table 12–6 details the common electrolytes and their associated abnormal states.

RENAL FUNCTION TESTS

Chemical indicators of renal function are often measured in conjunction with normal electrolytes because renal function plays an important role in electrolyte balance. The two most common renal function tests are the blood urea nitrogen (BUN) and creatinine. (See Table 12–7.)

★ **Blood Urea Nitrogen (BUN).** The BUN measures the amount of urea nitrogen in the blood. Urea is a waste product of protein metabolism and exclusively cleared by the kidneys. Thus, the BUN is an indicator of renal function.

★ **Creatinine.** Creatinine is a waste product derived from skeletal muscle and a good indicator of renal function.

blood urea nitrogen (BUN) *measures the amount of urea nitrogen in the blood (a waste product of protein metabolism), an indicator of renal function.*

creatinine *a waste product derived from skeletal muscle, associated with renal function.*

Table 12–6 | Electrolytes

Test	Meaning	Normal	High Values	Low Values
Na^+	Sodium	135–145 mEq/L	*Hypernatremia* –Dehydration –Excess saline administration –Exchange transfusion with stored blood –Impaired renal function	*Hyponatremia* –Overhydration –Sodium loss (vomiting, diarrhea, sweating, GI suctioning) –Increased renal sodium loss (diuretics, DKA, Addison's disease, renal disease)
K^+	Potassium	3.5–5.0 mEq/L	*Hyperkalemia* –Renal failure –Excess K^+ replacement –Massive tissue damage –Associated with metabolic acidosis	*Hypokalemia* –Diuretics –Inadequate intake –Large steroid doses –Associated with metabolic alkalosis
Cl^-	Chloride	100–108 mEq/L	*Hyperchloremia* –Increased Na^+ level –Decreased HCO_3^- levels –Renal failure	*Hypochloremia* –Vomiting –Gastric suction –Diarrhea –Diuretic use
HCO_3^-	Bicarbonate*	24–30 mEq/L	*Base excess metabolic alkalosis* –Loss of gastric contents –Diuretic use	*Base deficit metabolic acidosis* –Consumption of bicarbonate –Loss of bicarbonate –Increase in serum chloride level
Mg^{2+}	Magnesium	1.4–1.9 mEq/L	Hypermagnesemia	Hypomagnesemia
Ca^{2+}	Calcium	4.3–5.3 mEq/L	*Hypercalcemia* –False rise due to dehydration –Hyperparathyroidism –Malignant tumors –Immobilization –Thiazide diuretics –Vitamin D intoxication	*Hypocalcemia* –Hypoparathyroidism –Chronic renal disease –Pancreatitis –Massive blood transfusions –Severe malnutrition –False decrease due to low albumin levels
Free Ca^{2+}	Ionized calcium	4.3–5.3 mEq/L	–Hyperparathyroidism –Metastatic bone tumor –Milk-alkali syndrome –Multiple myeloma –Paget's disease –Sarcoidosis –Tumors producing a PTH-like substance –Vitamin D intoxication	–Hypoparathyroidism –Malabsorption –Osteomalacia –Pancreatitis –Renal failure –Rickets –Vitamin D deficiency
PO_4^-	Phosphate	1.8–2.6 mEq/L	*Hyperphosphatemia* –Hyperparathyroidism –Renal failure –Increased growth hormone –Vitamin D intoxication	*Hypophosphatemia* –Hyperparathyroidism –Diuresis – Malabsorption/malnutrition –Carbohydrate loading –Antacid abuse

* In some labs bicarbonate is referred to as CO_2. This is actually CO_2 combining power and an indirect measurement of bicarbonate (usually 1–2 mEq different).

Table 12-7 Renal Function Indicators

Test	Meaning	Normal	High Levels	Low Levels
BUN	Blood urea nitrogen (renal function)	8–25 mg/dL	–Renal disease –Renal damage –Dehydration –Shock –CHF –GI bleeding –High protein diets	–Overhydration –Increased ADH secretion
Creatinine	Creatinine (renal function)	Men: 0.6–1.4 mg/dL Women: 0.6–1.1 mg/dL	–Kidney disease –Renal toxic medications	–Low muscle mass –Muscle atrophy

★ BUN/creatinine ratio. The BUN/creatinine ration is a calculation that helps determine the cause of an abnormal BUN. Creatinine is only changed by renal dysfunction, whereas there are multiple causes for changes in the BUN. (See Table 12–8.)

The BUN and creatinine are often included along with sodium, potassium, chloride, bicarbonate, and glucose in what is called a basic metabolic panel (BMP). Figure 12-6 ■ details the common charting nomenclature for a BMP.

There are several less common renal function tests. Whereas the BUN and creatinine are the most frequently encountered, the following tests may also be encountered:

★ Creatinine clearance. The creatinine clearance is a timed test that is used to determine the glomerular filtration rate—a good indicator of renal function. It involves measuring the urine volume, urine creatinine and serum creatinine:

$$\frac{\text{Urine creatinine} \times \text{Urine volume}}{\text{Plasma creatinine} \times \text{time}} = \text{Creatinine clearance rate (mL/min/1.72 m}^2 \text{ BSA)}$$

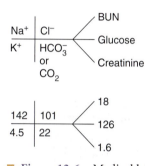

■ Figure 12-6 Medical lab shorthand for basic metabolic panel (BMP).

Table 12-8 BUN/Creatinine Ratio

BUN/Creatinine Ratio	Meaning	Cause	Treatment
>10:1	Extrinsic disease	*Prerenal Causes* –Decreased renal refusion (hypovolemia, CHF) –Increased urea load (GI bleed, corticosteroids) *Postrenal Causes* –Obstruction (prostate) –Kidney stone	Treat underlying cause: –Hydration –Kidney stone removal –Foley catheter
10:1	Renal disease	–Normal –Chronic renal failure –Decreased urea load (low-protein diet, liver failure) –Inhibited creatinine secretion due to medications –Dialysis	–Remove offending medications –Dialysis (if severe)

where BSA stands for body surface area.

★ *Serum osmolality.* The serum osmolality rises in dehydration and falls in overhydration. It is useful in several diagnostic schemes including the diagnosis of nonketotic hyperosmolar coma.

★ *Uric acid.* Uric acid is the end product of purine metabolism and comes from both dietary and body proteins. An elevated uric acid is seen in gout (but is not diagnostic).

TESTS OF GLUCOSE METABOLISM

Glucose is one of the three energy sources for the body (the others being proteins and lipids). Ultimately, proteins and lipids are broken down to glucose or other sugars to be utilized by the cell. In addition, glucose is the principal energy source used by the brain. Because of this, it is very important to monitor glucose levels. An abnormally high level of glucose in the plasma is referred to as *hyperglycemia*, while a lower than normal level of glucose in the plasma is referred to as *hypoglycemia*.

The most common blood glucose monitor is the finger-stick method routinely used by diabetics and EMS. This method determines the glucose level in whole blood. Lab tests usually determine the glucose level in plasma (serum). The differences in the two are detailed in Table 12–9.

Diabetics are most vulnerable to alterations in glucose levels. The closer they maintain their glucose levels to normal, the fewer complications they tend to develop. The ability of the diabetic patient to regulate his glucose levels can be monitored over time with a test called **glycohemoglobin** or *hemoglobin A1C.* With prolonged hyperglycemia, the RBCs will remain saturated with glucose in the form of glycohemoglobin. By measuring the percent saturation we can get an indicator of the patient's blood glucose control for the last 3 to 4 months. People without diabetes will normally have a hemoglobin A1C between 4% and 6%. Diabetics should strive to keep their hemoglobin A1C at less than 7%. Glycosylated hemoglobin is a better measurement because it actually measures the three components of hemoglobin (A1A, A1B, and A1C). A level of 7.5% or less indicates good diabetic control, whereas a level of 7.6% to 8.9% indicates fair diabetic control. A level of 9.0% or greater suggests poor diabetic control.

When glucose is not available, the body begins to utilize fats and proteins for energy. As a result of these, ketones (acetoacetic acid, acetone, and beta-hydroxybutyric acid) are produced. A simple test will detect the presence of ketones. It is usually reported as negative if no ketones are detected and rated on a scale of 1+ to 4+. This test is useful in the diagnosis of diabetic ketoacidosis, severe malnutrition, and similar states.

glycohemoglobin *the amount of glucose bound to hemoglobin; indicates recent regulation of glucose levels in diabetic patients.*

TESTS OF LIPID METABOLISM

Lipids are one the three energy sources for the body (the others being proteins and carbohydrates). Ultimately, lipids are broken down to glucose or other sugars to be utilized by the cell. An increase in the amount of lipids in the blood is termed *hyperlipidemia*.

Table 12–9	Blood Glucose Normals	
Source	**Timing**	**Normals (mg/dL)**
Whole blood	Average before meals	80–120
Whole blood	Average at bedtime	100–140
Plasma	Average before meals	90–130
Plasma	Average at bedtime	110–150

There are two major classes of lipids: cholesterol and triglycerides. In addition, we can measure specific lipoproteins. Lipoproteins are not lipids, but the proteins that transport lipids in the plasma. (See Table 12–10.)

★ **Cholesterol.** Cholesterol is an important lipid in that it is required for production of bile salts, which are necessary for digestion. In addition, the cholesterol molecule forms the framework for many of the steroid hormones. Cholesterol is derived from saturated fats in the diet (of animal origin) and is combined with fatty acids by the liver. Numerous medications have been developed to help lower serum lipid. These either bind cholesterol in the bowel to prevent absorption (cholestyramine) or reduce production in the liver (statins).

★ **Triglycerides.** Triglycerides are the most abundant of the lipids and are derived from both plant and animal fats and oils. Excess triglycerides, an energy source, are stored in the adipose tissues.

★ **Lipoproteins.** As mentioned above, lipoproteins are not lipids, but specialized proteins that transport the lipids in the serum. These proteins are classified by their molecular weight:

★ *High-density lipoproteins (HDL).* The cholesterol component of **HDL** is usually measured. Normally, about 20% of the cholesterol is HDL cholesterol. Low levels of

cholesterol *an important lipid for digestion; required for production of bile slats.*

triglycerides *the most abundant of the lipids; derived from both plant and animal fats and oils.*

lipoproteins *specialized proteins that transport the lipids in the blood serum.*

HDL *high-density lipoproteins, a component of cholesterol.*

Table 12–10	Lipids and Lipoproteins		
Test	**Normal**	**High Levels**	**Low Levels**
Cholesterol	Desirable: <200 mg/dL	–Cause often unknown	–Hyperthyroidism
	Borderline high: 200–239 mg/dL	–Dietary	–Severe liver damage
	High: ≥240 mg/dL	–Hereditary	–Malnutrition
		–Pregnancy	
		–Pancreatic problem	
Triglycerides	Desirable: <150 mg/dL	–Dietary	–Malnutrition
	Borderline high: 150–190 mg/dL	–Hereditary	–Medications
	High: 200–499 mg/dL	–Pregnancy	
	Very high: ≥500 mg/dL	–Pancreatitis	
		–Alcohol abuse	
HDL	*Positive cardiac risk factor:*	–Medications	–Tobacco use
	HDL <35 mg/dL	–Moderate alcohol intake	–Diabetes mellitus
	Total cholesterol to HDL ratio:	–Exercise	–Menopause
	Men > 5.0	–Weight loss	–Obesity
	Women > 4.5		
	Negative cardiac risk factor:		
	HDL > 60 mg/dL		
LDL	<160 mg/dL	–High-fat diet	–Advanced liver disease
		–Hyperthyroidism	–Malnutrition
		–Nephrotic syndrome	
		–Diabetes mellitus	
		–Familial lipid disease	
VLDL	10–31 mg/dL	–Diabetes mellitus	
		–Obesity	
		–Hepatic oversecretion	

HDL cholesterol are associated with an increased risk of cardiovascular disease. (Thus, it is often called "good cholesterol.") HDL cholesterol is usually measured.

LDL *low-density lipoproteins, transport cholesterol in the plasma.*

★ Low-density lipoproteins (LDL). **LDL** carries cholesterol in the plasma and is associated with an increased risk of atherosclerosis and coronary artery disease. (Thus, it is often called "bad cholesterol.") LDL can be calculated if triglyceride levels are less than 400 mg/dL.

$$\text{LDL cholesterol} = \text{Total cholesterol} - (\text{HDL cholesterol} + \text{VLDL})$$

VLDL *very-low-density lipoproteins; transports triglycerides and cholesterol.*

★ Very-low-density lipoproteins (VLDL). **VLDL** primarily transports triglycerides although it does transport some cholesterol. It can be calculated by dividing the triglyceride level by 5.

$$\text{VLDL} = \text{Triglycerides}/5$$

Thus,

$$\text{LDL cholesterol} = \text{Total cholesterol} - [\text{HDL cholesterol} + (\text{triglycerides}/5)]$$

The ratio of total cholesterol to HDL (total divided by HDL) is used as a risk factor for coronary artery disease and atherosclerosis. The desirable ratio is 4.5 for women and 5.0 for men.

CARDIAC ENZYMES AND MARKERS

The measurement of enzymes and markers associated with cardiac disease is an important aspect of medical practice—especially emergency medicine and critical care transport. Numerous tests are used to help diagnose and classify cardiac disease.

When cells are damaged, enzymes within those cells are leaked into the circulatory system. While these enzymes may not be tissue specific, various forms of the enzymes (called *isoenzymes*) can be tied to a specific tissue type.

The most frequently encountered cardiac enzymes and markers include the following (see Table 12–11):

creatine kinase (CK or CPK) *isoenzymes important in energy utilization.*

★ **Creatine kinase (CK or CPK).** Creatine kinase (formerly called creatinine phosphokinase) is important in energy utilization. Almost all CK comes from muscle tissue, but it can be separated into three different isoenzymes:

CK-I (BB): Produced primarily in the brain and in selected smooth muscle.

CK-II (MB): Primarily produced in the heart

CK-III (MM): Primarily produced in skeletal muscle

An elevated CK may be caused by various factors such as an IM medication injection or skeletal muscle trauma. But, when the isoenzymes are isolated, then the source of the elevation is known. CK is the first enzyme to elevate after acute myocardial infarction and is increased in 90% of infarctions. (See Figure 12-7 ■.)

Time sequence after myocardial infarction:

– Begins to rise in 4–6 hours

– Peaks at 24 hours

– Returns to normal in 3–4 days

lactic dehydrogenase (LD or LDH) *enzyme found in heart muscle, skeletal muscle, liver, erythrocytes, kidney, and some types of tumors.*

★ **Lactic dehydrogenase (LD or LDH).** LDH is found in heart muscle, skeletal muscle, liver, erythrocytes, kidney, and some types of tumors. It is increased in more than 90% of myocardial infarctions. However, it can be increased in diseases of any of the above organs or hemolysis. There are five LDH isoenzymes:

LDH_1: Heart, erythrocytes, renal cortex

LDH_2: Reticuloendothelial system

LDH_3: Lung tissue

LDH_4: Placenta, kidney, pancreas

LDK_5: Skeletal muscle, liver

Table 12–11   Cardiac Enzymes and Markers

Test	Meaning	Normal	High Levels	Low Levels
CK	Creatine kinase	Men: 60–100 U/L Women: 40–150 U/L Isoenzymes: –CK-I (BB): 0–1% –CK-II (MB): <3% –CK-III (MM): 95–100%	–Muscle disease –Exercise –IM injections –Shock –Tumors	Not clinically significant
CK-MB	Creatine kinase (MB fraction)	<10 U/L: MI improbable 10–12 U/L: inconclusive >12 U/L: MI probable	–Cardiac damage	Not clinically significant
LDH	Lactate dehydrogenase	Adult: 40–90 U/L Isoenzymes: –LDH_1: 17–27% –LDH_2: 21–28% –LDH_3: 18–28% –LDH_4: 5–15% –LDH_5: 5–15%	–Anemias elevate LDH_1 and LDH_2 –Pulmonary embolism elevates LDH_3 –Liver damage elevates LDH_4 and LDH_5 –MI causes reversal of LDH_1 and LDH_2 ratio	Not clinically significant
Myoglobin	Myoglobin	50–120 mcg/dL	–Rhabdomyolysis –Myocardial infarction –IM injections –Strenuous exercise	Not clinically significant
Troponin	Troponin	*Troponin I:* <6 ng/mL >1.5 ng/mL (MI) *Troponin T:* > 0.1–0.2 ng/mL (MI)	–Myocardial necrosis	Not clinically significant
BNP	B-natriuretic peptide	5–100 pg/dL	–Abnormal ventricular function –Congestive heart failure	Not clinically significant

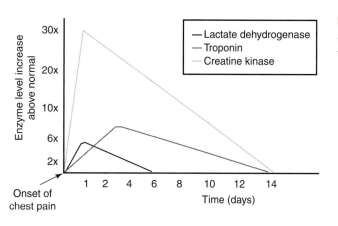

■ **Figure 12-7** Cardiac enzyme changes associated with myocardial infarction.

Reversal of the LDH_1/LDH_2 ratio is characteristic of an acute myocardial infarction, with 80% to 85% sensitivity.

Time sequence of LD after myocardial infarction:

- Begins to rise in 24 hours

- Peaks in 3 days

- Returns to normal in 8–9 days

myoglobin *hemeprotein found in striated muscle; contains iron, stores oxygen, gives muscle its red color.*

★ **Myoglobin.** Myoglobin is found in striated muscle and contains iron. It stores oxygen and gives muscle its red color. Damage to skeletal or cardiac muscle releases myoglobin into the circulation. Myoglobin rapid assay kits are available that allow testing in the prehospital critical care, and emergency department settings.

Time sequence after myocardial infarction:

- Rises fast (2 hours) after MI

- Peaks at 6–8 hours

- Returns to normal in 20–36 hours

- False-positives are seen with skeletal muscle injury and renal failure.

troponins *contractile proteins of the myofibril.*

★ Troponin I, T, and C. The **troponins** are the contractile proteins of the myofibril. The cardiac isoforms are very specific for cardiac injury and are not present in serum from healthy people. Troponin I is the form frequently assessed. There is a new form (Troponin L) that may be detected earlier. Troponin rapid assay kits are available that allow testing in the prehospital, critical care, and emergency department settings.

Time sequence after myocardial infarction:

- Rises 4–6 hours after injury

- Peaks in 12–16 hours

- Stays elevated for up to 10 days

B-natriuretic peptide (BNP) *peptide found in the ventricles of the heart, increases when ventricular filling pressures are high; can be used to detect CHF.*

★ **B-natriuretic peptide (BNP).** BNP is a peptide found in the ventricles of the heart. Levels increase when ventricular filling pressures are high. It can be used to detect congestive heart failure.

TESTS OF LIVER FUNCTION

The liver plays a significant role in metabolism and the production of various substances required by the body. It is also the major processor of potentially toxic substances. Various tests have been established to evaluate liver function. These are detailed in Table 12–12.

Bilirubin results from the breakdown of old or damaged red blood cells and occurs primarily in the liver. An enzyme, glucuronyl transferase, transforms or conjugates bilirubin making it water soluble and ready for excretion. It is then excreted into the intestine as bile salts. Once in the intestines, bacteria break down the bilirubin into urobilinogen.

When assayed, bilirubin is reported as total bilirubin, conjugated bilirubin, and unconjugated bilirubin. Unconjugated bilirubin is due to an excess breakdown of red blood cells or an increase in free bilirubin in the bloodstream. An increase in conjugated, or direct, bilirubin is due to obstruction of the biliary tract. An elevation in bilirubin results in jaundice.

There are numerous enzymatic processes in the liver. Many of these can be assayed and these can help determine the nature of a problem. Certain enzymes (amylase and lipase) are specific for pancreatic function. An elevation in either of these two enzymes is associated with pancreatitis.

SEROLOGIC TESTING

Serologic testing is a broad area of laboratory analysis and includes such things as blood banking, identification of antibodies against infectious disease, and autoimmunity studies. Serologic tests can be either specific or nonspecific depending on the test and the method employed.

Table 12–12 | Tests of Liver/Pancreatic Function

Name	Meaning	Normal	High Levels	Low Levels
Total Bilirubin	Total bilirubin	0.1–1.0 mg/dL	See indirect and direct entries below	Not clinically significant
Indirect bilirubin	Unconjugated bilirubin	0.1–1.0 mg/dL Mean = 0.5 mg	–Sickle cell disease –Autoimmune disease –Hemorrhage –Drug toxicity	Not clinically significant
Direct bilirubin	Conjugated bilirubin	0.0–0.4 mg/dL Mean = 0.1 mg/dL	–Obstructive jaundice –Gallstones –Congenital biliary tract abnormalities –Medications	Not clinically significant
ALP	Alkaline phosphatase	Men: 45–115 U/L Women: 300–100 U/L	–Bone abnormality –Liver abnormality –Eclampsia	–Scurvy –Genetic defects –Excessive vitamin D intake
GGT	Gamma-glutamyl transferase	Men: 1–94 U/L Women: 1–70 U/L	–Liver disease –Alcohol use	Not clinically significant
Ammonia	Ammonia	10–80 mcg/dL	–Liver failure –Reye's syndrome	Not clinically significant
ALT	Alanine transaminase (formerly SGPT)	Men: 10–55 U/L Women: 7–30 U/L	–Severe hepatitis –Cirrhosis –Mononucleosis	Liver failure
AST	Aspartate transaminase (formely SGOT)	Men: 10–40 U/L Women: 9–25 U/L	–Myocardial infarction –Hepatitis	Liver failure
Aldolase	Aldolase	0–7 U/L	–Muscular disorders	Not clinically significant
Amylase	Amylase	53–123 U/L	–Pancreatitis –Pancreatic trauma	Pancrestic destruction
Lipase	Lipase	3–19 U/L	–Pancreatitis –Pancreatic trauma	Not clinically significant

BLOOD BANKING

Blood banking is an important aspect of serologic testing. Because transfusion reactions can be severe—even fatal—there are numerous checks and balances in blood bank procedures. In addition, donor blood is routinely tested for the presence of infectious diseases such as HIV, hepatitis, syphilis, and cytomegalovirus.

Several tests are routinely performed that must match prior to the administration of blood. These include:

★ **ABO typing.** The ABO typing determines which of the four blood groups a patient or sample has. These are Type A, Type B, Type AB, or Type O. These are often referred to as the major antigens.

★ *Rh factor.* A second test is the Rh factor (name derived from the Rhesus monkey). A person will either have (Rh-positive) or not have (Rh-negative) the Rh antigen.

blood banking *routine tests that include ABO typing, Rh factor and direct Coombs test (RBC antibody screening).*

ABO typing *the ABO typing determines which of the four blood groups a sample belongs to.*

★ *Direct Coombs' test.* The **Coombs' test,** also called the RBC antibody screen, is used to screen blood for crossmatching, to check for hemolytic transfusion reactions, and to assess for hemolytic disease of the newborn.

★ *Indirect Coombs' test.* The indirect Coombs', also called the antibody screening test, is used to detect various antibodies present in the blood.

MICROBIOLOGICAL SEROLOGIC TESTS

There are an ever-increasing number of tests that can be used to detect the presence of an infectious disease. A summary of these is detailed in Table 12–13.

ENDOCRINE TESTS

Many endocrine tests are available. However, these rarely play a role in emergency medicine. The most commonly encountered endocrine tests in critical care transport are probably the thyroid tests and cortisol. These are detailed in Table 12–14.

MICROBIOLOGY

The study of organisms that cannot be easily seen without magnification is referred to as *microbiology.* In medicine, microbiology plays an important role in identifying bacteria, viruses, and other organisms responsible for infection.

Table 12–13 Common Microbiological Serologic Tests

Test	Organism	Comments
VDRL	Syphilis	Screening test
RPR	Syphilis	Screening test
FTA-ABS	Syphilis	Confirmatory test
MHA-TP	Syphilis	Confirmatory test
HBsAg	Hepatitis B virus	Confirms presence of hepatitis B virus
Anti-HAV	Hepatitis A	Measures antibodies to hepatitis A
Anti-HCV	Hepatitis C	Measures antibodies to hepatitis C
HIV	AIDS	Measures either antibodies or antigens for the AIDS virus
CMV	Cytomegalovirus	Screening for cytomegalovirus
Monospot	Mononucleosis	Screening test for mononucleosis

Table 12–14 Common Endocrine Testing

Test	Meaning	Normal	High Values	Low Values
Cortisol	Adrenocortical function	5–25 mcg/dL	–Cushing's syndrome –Pituitary tumors	–Addison's disease
TSH	Thyroid-stimulating hormone (released by pituitary)	0.5–5.0 µU/mL	–Thyroid failure –Pituitary tumor	–Hyperthyroidism –Pituitary failure
Total T_4	L-Thyroxine	4.5–10.9 mcg/dL	–Hyperthyroidism	–Hypothyroidism
T_3	Triiodothyronine	60–181 ng/dL	–Hyperthyroidism	–Hypothyroidism
Free T_4	Free thyroxine	0.8–2.7 ng/dL	–Hyperthyroidism	–Hypothyroidism

Bacteria are identified through several methods. First, a microscope slide of the suspected bacteria is prepared. Then, a series of stains, referred to as **Gram stains,** are applied. Bacteria are then classified as gram positive or gram negative depending whether they take the stain. In addition, the shape is determined. Finally, various biochemical tests are used to identify the bacteria. Bacterial cultures can also be used to determine which antibiotics are effective in treating the infection. This is referred to as culture and sensitivity testing.

Specific body areas and secretions can be cultured including whole blood. Cultures of the urine, vagina, throat, nose, and stool are common. Infections that fail to respond to standard antibacterial therapy are cultured.

> **Gram stains** *bacteria identified with various stains and then classified as gram positive or gram negative (whether they take the stain(s) or not).*

URINALYSIS

Urine testing (**urinalysis**) is routinely performed and the urine can provide a great deal of information about the patient. Most urine testing is automated. However, chemical reagent strips are available that can be used in even the most austere settings for urine testing. Normal urinalysis typically reports the following information:

> **urinalysis** *urine test designed to detect medication/drug use, blood, infection, pH, density, protein, glucose, ketones, bilirubin, nitrites, and other formed elements.*

★ *Color.* Normally urine is light yellow to amber in color. Several things, such as medication use, the presence of blood, or the presence of infection can discolor the urine.

★ *pH.* The pH of the urine ranges from 5 to 9 and depends on the patient's diet and other factors. Changes in pH are typically associated with infection.

★ *Specific gravity.* The specific gravity compares the density of urine with water. Water has a density of 1.000. Urine can be as dilute as water but is typically more concentrated.

★ *Protein.* Little protein should be found in the urine. The presence of protein is associated with renal disease, preeclampsia, and other infections.

★ *Glucose.* Glucose is not normally present in the urine. Glucose in the urine (glycosuria) is usually associated with diabetes.

★ *Ketones.* Normal urine should not contain ketones (the end products of fatty acid metabolism). The presence of ketones is associated with several conditions including diabetic ketoacidosis, malnutrition, and dieting.

★ *Bilirubin.* Bilirubin is not usually found in the urine and, when found, is indicative of liver disease such as hepatitis.

★ *Occult blood.* Blood in the urine is abnormal and can be associated with trauma, kidney stones, tumors, and certain urinary tract infections.

★ *Nitrites.* The presence of nitrites indicates infection with bacteria.

★ *Leukocyte esterase.* Normally, white blood cells are not found in the urine. However, when the urine is infected, white blood cells are often present. The leukocyte esterase test checks for the presence of white blood cells and indicates urinary tract infection (UTI).

★ *Urobilinogen.* Urobilinogen is conjugated bilirubin and indicates liver disease.

In addition to the chemical tests just listed, the urine is usually spun in a centrifuge and the sediment examined under the microscope for the presence of crystals, casts, white blood cells, and red blood cells. (See Table 12–15.)

TOXICOLOGY

Toxicological testing is now available for almost any substance. However, these tests are often sophisticated and not readily available on an emergent basis. However, several rapid screens have been developed that can be used at the bedside and in the ambulance. These drug screens are referred to

Table 12–15 | Urinalysis Findings

Test	Meaning	Normal	High Levels	Low Levels
pH	Acidity of the urine	5–9 (mean of 6)	–UTI –Bicarbonate use	–Acidosis
Specific gravity	Concentration of urine	Adult: 1.001–1.035 Child: 1.001–1.018	–Dehydration –Increased ADH secretion	–Overhydration
Protein	Presence of protein in the urine	Negative	–Renal disease –Preeclampsia/PIH	Not clinically significant
Sugar	Presence of sugars in the urine	Negative	–Diabetes –Stress	Not clinically significant
Ketone	Presence of ketones in the urine	Negative	–Malnutrition –DKA –Dieting	Not clinically significant
Nitrites	Indicative of infection	Negative	–UTI	Not clinically significant
Leukocyte esterase	Indicative of infection	Negative	–UTI	Not clinically significant
Bilirubin	Indicative of liver problems	Negative	–Liver disease	Not clinically significant
Urobilinogen	Indicative of liver problems	0.1–1.0 Ehrlich U/dL	–Liver disease	Not clinically significant
Microscopic crystals	Presence of crystals	Variable	–Gout	Not clinically significant
Microscopic casts	Usually abnormal when present	Variable	–Cancers	Not clinically significant
Microscopic WBCs	Minimally present	<4–5 per HPF*	–UTI	Not clinically significant
Microscopic RBCs	Minimally present	<2–3 per HPF*	–Trauma –Infection –Kidney stones	Not clinically significant

* HPF, high-power microscopic field.

as *triage screens* and usually screen for opiates, benzodiazepines, THC (marijuana), cocaine, amphetamines, barbiturates, and other popular substances.

Toxicological testing is also used to measure the amount of therapeutic medications in the system. This is particularly important for medications that have a low therapeutic index (i.e., digitalis, lithium, aminoglycoside antibiotics).

IMAGING

medical imaging *use of technology to electronically visualize the body.*

Some of the most amazing developments in modern medicine have occurred in the realm of diagnostic **medical imaging.** Once limited to simple X-rays, radiologists now have numerous diagnostic modalities available to aid them. It is not within the scope of this chapter to address these in detail. However, we will present a brief overview of each:

★ *X-rays.* **X-rays** still play a major role in diagnostic imaging. X-rays are electromagnetic radiation with a very short wavelength and are capable of penetrating most body tissues. A photographic plate (X-ray film) is placed on the opposite side of the patient from the X-ray tube. Images are then recorded on the film for interpretation. The densities of the tissue can be seen on the X-ray. These include air (blackish), fat (dark gray), water (lighter gray), and bone (whitish). X-rays remain the primary examination tool for bones and as a screening tool for the chest. Dyes that resist radiation can be administered to help highlight certain structures. These dyes, referred to as contrast dyes, are available in various forms depending on the organ or tissue being imaged.

★ *Fluoroscopy.* Fluoroscopy is a form of X-ray where the patient is examined using real-time imaging. This is used for specialized procedures and special tests such as gastrointestinal studies.

★ *Computed tomography.* Computed tomography, also called **CT (CAT) scanning,** uses focused X-ray beams to examine various body areas. These beams are reconstructed by the computer to give a high-quality view of the area in question. CT scans typically consists of multiple sequential images or "cuts" that allow for detailed examination.

★ *Ultrasonography.* The use of **ultrasound** does not expose the patient to potentially harmful radiation. With ultrasound, sound waves are transmitted into the area of interest. Some of these waves pass through while denser tissues reflect the waves back to the transducer of the machine. Here they are reconstructed to form an image of the object in question. Ultrasound plays an important role in obstetrics, gynecology, and certain abdominal problems (gallbladder, renal). Ultrasound can also be used to measure blood flow in cases of suspected arterial or venous obstruction.

★ *Nuclear medicine.* Nuclear medicine studies involve the administration of a low dose of a radioisotope and then measuring the movement of the isotope with a nuclear medicine camera. These tests are useful in determining how well an organ or gland is functioning. Scanning of the heart and bones are common nuclear medicine procedures.

★ **Magnetic resonance imaging (MRI).** The MRI is able to provide high-quality images of body areas without the use of ionizing radiation. All body tissues contain water. By exposing these tissues to a strong magnetic field, the atoms in the water molecule will align while in the magnetic field, allowing for the production of an image. MRI is excellent for nervous tissue (brain, spinal cord) as well as soft tissues and joints. The effects of bone seen on CT are minimized with MRI scanning.

★ **Positron emission tomography (PET).** PET scanning is becoming an important component of diagnostic imaging. Unlike most of the other imaging modalities, PET scanning can tell about organ function, especially in the brain. It can be used to diagnose depression, schizophrenia, stroke, epilepsy, migraine headaches, Parkinson's disease, dementia, and similar illnesses that are often hard to diagnose.

X-rays *electromagnetic radiation with a very short wavelength, capable of penetrating most body tissues.*

CT (CAT) scanning *use of focused x-ray beams to examine various body areas.*

ultrasound *diagnostic sound waves transmitted into an area of specific interest.*

magnetic resonance imaging (MRI) *high-quality magnetic images of body areas without the use of ionizing radiation.*

positron emission tomography (PET) *imaging modalities capable of observing organ function, especially in the brain.*

These diagnostic tests are usually interpreted by a physician who specializes in diagnostic imaging, that is, a radiologist. These interpretations are usually with the patient's chart. Some interpretations are arrived at by sending the digital images to the radiologist at a different location (teleradiology).

Critical care paramedics should become somewhat proficient at recognizing major abnormalities on X-rays—especially long bone films. Chest X-rays (CXR) are quite difficult to read and require considerable practice and experience. (See Figures 12–8 ■ through 12–10 ■.)

PHYSIOLOGICAL TESTS

Various types of physiological tests are used in the diagnosis and treatment of disease. These tests are often classified by the hospital department that conducts them (i.e., respiratory therapy, electrodiagnostics). Common tests include pulmonary function testing, arterial blood gas analysis,

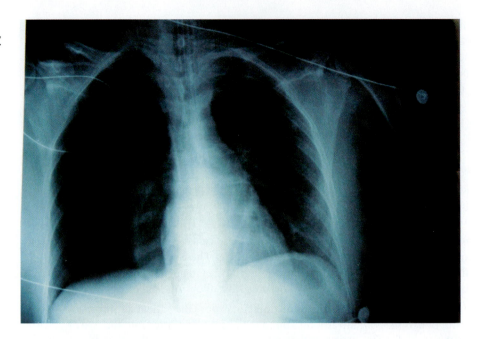

■ **Figure 12-8** Chest X-ray of pneumothorax. *(Edward T. Dickinson, MD)*

arterial blood gas *dissolved gases in the arterial circulation. Generally consists of: pH, pCO_2, pO_2, HCO_3^-, oxygen saturation, and hemoglobin.*

stress testing, specialized electrocardiographic imaging, and numerous others. Electrocardiographic imaging is discussed in Chapters 9 and 10.

Arterial blood gas analysis is particularly important in the critical care setting, and the critical care paramedic must have a good understanding of this. The arterial blood gas generally consists of the following variables:

★ *pH.* The pH simply reflects the hydrogen-ion concentration of the arterial blood. The greater the concentration, the lower the pH. It is important to remember that pH is a logarithmic relationship. A change in units reflects a 10-fold change in hydrogen-ion concentration. (See Figure 12-11 ■.)

$$pH = \log \frac{1}{[H^+]}$$

■ **Figure 12-9** Chest trauma. *(Kathy Altergott, BSN, MBA, CRA. Banner Good Samaritan Medical Center, Phoenix, AZ)*

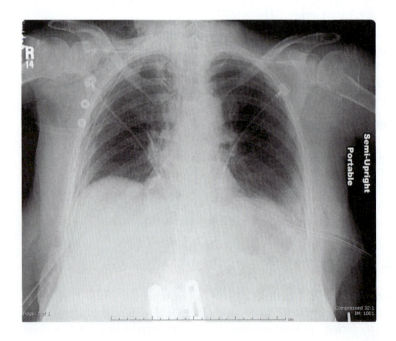

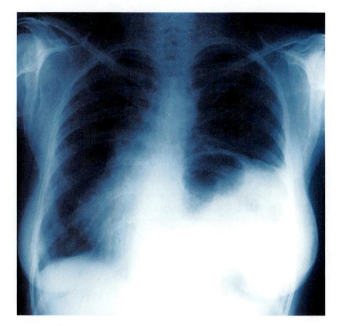

■ **Figure 12-10** X-ray of the chest, front view, in a patient with a traumatic diaphragmatic hernia. The post-trauma left diaphragmatic hernia is indicated by the presence of the stomach, small intestine, and colon in the left pulmonary compartment, the ascension of the left diaphragmatic cupola, and an air fluid level. *(© Chris Barry/PhototakeUSA)*

★ *pCO₂*. The partial pressure of carbon dioxide reflects the amount of carbon dioxide present in the arterial system. Carbon dioxide is transported in the serum although some is combined with water to form carbonic acid (H_2CO_3).

★ *pO₂*. The partial pressure of oxygen in the blood reflects the amount of oxygen dissolved in the serum. Most (approximately 98%) oxygen is transported by hemoglobin. However, there is a direct, yet complex, relationship between pO_2 and hemoglobin saturation.

★ HCO_3^-. The bicarbonate ion is one of the principal metabolic buffers. Abnormalities in the amount of bicarbonate present tell a great deal about any acid–base derangements. An excess of bicarbonate ion is called a *base excess* while a decreased amount of bicarbonate is called a *base deficit*.

★ *Oxygen saturation (SaO_2)*. The oxygen saturation provides information concerning the percentage of hemoglobin that is saturated with oxygen. This should be identical to

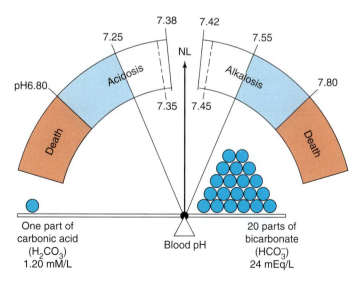

■ **Figure 12-11** Arterial blood gas changes.

readings obtained though the use of pulse oximeters. This reading is important because most oxygen is transported bound to hemoglobin.

★ *Hemoglobin.* Most arterial blood gas units will provide a spot hemoglobin reading because anemia can affect oxygen transport. This should correspond to any measurements obtained during the complete blood count.

Oftentimes, critically ill patients will have undergone multiple arterial blood gas readings, especially if the patient is on a ventilator. In these cases, the readings may be displayed sequentially or graphically by the hospital information system. (See Tables 12–16 through 12–19.)

Table 12–16 | Arterial Blood Gas Analysis

Test	Meaning	Normal	High Levels	Low Levels
pH	Acidity of the blood	7.35–7.45	–Alkalosis	–Acidosis
pCO_2	Partial pressure of CO_2 in the blood	35–45 mmHg	–Respiratory acidosis –Hypoventilation	–Respiratory alkalosis –Hyperventilation
pO_2	Partial pressure of oxygen in the blood	80–100 mmHg	–Over-oxygenation –Hyperventilation	–Hypoxia –Hypoventilation
HCO_3^-	Bicarbonate-ion concentration	24–30 mEq/L	–Base excess –Metabolic alkalosis –Bicarbonate ingestion	–Base deficit –Metabolic acidosis –Increased serum chloride
SaO_2	Percentage of hemoglobin saturated with oxygen	95–100%	Not clinically significant	–Hypoxia –Hypoventilation
Hgb	Amount of hemoglobin present	12–18 g/dL	–Dehydration –Polycythemia	–Overhydration –Anemia –Hemorrhage

Table 12–17 | Distinguishing Acid–Base Imbalances

Abnormality	pH Value	Physiological Cause	Physiological Compensation
Respiratory acidosis	<7.35	↑ $PaCO_2$	↑ HCO_3^-
Respiratory alkalosis	>7.45	↓ $PaCO_2$	↓ HCO_3^-
Metabolic acidosis	<7.35	↓ HCO_3^-	↓ $PaCO_2$
Metabolic alkalosis	>7.45	↑ HCO_3^-	↑ $PaCO_2$

Table 12–18 Acid–Base Derangements

Derangement	Cause	Clinical Signs/Symptoms
Respiratory acidosis	*Hypoventilation* –COPD –Airway obstruction –Respiratory arrest –CNS depression –Atelectasis –Pneumonia –Pulmonary edema –Chest wall trauma	*Initially:* ↑ Heart rate ↑ Respirations *Later:* ↓ Respirations ↓ Blood pressure Altered mental status Dysrhythmias Somnolence Coma
Respiratory alkalosis	*Hyperventilation* –Anxiety –Fever –Asthma (early) –Pneumothorax (early) –Chest wall pain –Mechanical ventilation (excessive) –Salicylate intoxication (early)	↑ Heart rate ↑ Respirations Anxiety Dry mouth ↑ Sweating Carpopedal spasms Confusion
Metabolic acidosis	*Net acid gain* –Shock –DKA –Poisoning (cyanide, others) –Renal failure –Diarrhea	↑ Heart rate ↑ Respirations ↓ Blood pressure Weakness Abdominal pain Nausea Vomiting Malaise Headache Confusion
Metabolic alkalosis	*Net acid loss* –Severe vomiting –NG suctioning –Steroid usage –Excessive bicarbonate dosing –Diuretic therapy	↓ Respirations Nausea Vomiting Diarrhea Altered mental status Seizures

Table 12–19 | Mixed Acid–Base Disorders

Mixed Acid–Base Disorder	Possible Clinical Causes
Mixed acidosis	–Respiratory arrest (respiratory acidosis)
	–Cardiac arrest (metabolic acidosis)
Mixed alkalosis	–Vomiting (metabolic alkalosis)
	–Bicarbonate administration (metabolic alkalosis)
	–Hyperventilation (respiratory alkalosis)
Respiratory acidosis and metabolic alkalosis	–Vomiting (metabolic alkalosis)
	–Bicarbonate administration (metabolic alkalosis)
	–Overzealous diuresis (metabolic alkalosis)
	–Hypoventilation (respiratory acidosis)
	–COPD (respiratory acidosis)
Respiratory alkalosis and metabolic acidosis	–Excessive ventilation (respiratory alkalosis)
	–Renal failure (metabolic acidosis)

Summary

Critical care paramedics, especially during interhospital transport, will have access to laboratory and diagnostic studies initiated and/or completed at the transferring hospital. These data can provide a significant amount of information about the patient and his condition. Because such data will be frequently encountered, critical care paramedics must be familiar with the normal as well as the abnormal results of these tests. Any information is helpful in patient care and laboratory and diagnostic data should not be overlooked.

Review Questions

1. Discuss the importance of laboratory and diagnostic tests in emergency medicine.
2. Distinguish between the following:
   a. true-positives
   b. true-negatives
   c. false-positives
   d. false-negatives
3. Distinguish the sensitivity and specificity of a test.
4. Describe common elements of a complete blood count.
5. Describe the common substances assayed in a basic metabolic panel.
6. Describe the major cardiac enzymes and cardiac markers used in the diagnosis of heart disease.

See Answers to Review Questions at the back of this book.

Further Reading

Corbett JV. *Laboratory Tests and Diagnostic Procedures with Nursing Diagnoses,* 6th ed. Upper Saddle River, NJ: Pearson Prentice Hall, 2004.

Vaughn G. *Understanding & Evaluating Common Laboratory Tests.* Upper Saddle River, NJ: Pearson Prentice Hall, 1999.

Introduction to Trauma

Allan Bulkley, NREMT-P, FP-C, RN, Flight Paramedic

Objectives

Upon completion of this chapter, the student should be able to:

1. Describe some of the main points regarding the epidemiology of trauma in the United States. (p. 359)
2. Discuss the costs of modern trauma care. (p. 359)
3. Describe the history of trauma care and trauma systems in the United States. (p. 361)
4. Describe the basic structure of a regional trauma system in the United States. (p. 362)
5. Discuss the categories for trauma facilities in the United States and the characteristics and limitations of each. (p. 362)
6. Discuss the importance of injury prevention in modern society. (p. 363)
7. Discuss the application of the Haddon matrix to trauma prevention programs. (p. 363)
8. Describe the utility and basis for common trauma scoring systems. (p. 364)
9. Describe the physics and biomechanics of trauma. (p. 367)
10. Describe the initial assessment and priorities during resuscitation of the trauma patient. (p. 368)
11. Describe general considerations for transport of a severely traumatized patient. (p. 369)

Key Terms

Case Study

A helicopter EMS crew is alerted to a scene flight at a location approximately 40 nautical miles (20-minute flight) from their base. As the pilot checks weather and readies the aircraft, the critical care paramedic contacts the communications center to obtain grid coordinates and the nature of the call. The only information that the communication center is able to provide is that the crew is being summoned to pick up "a man who fell into a gorge."

A few minutes after liftoff, the flight paramedic makes radio contact with the incident commander who relays that the patient is still trapped on a ledge approximately 50 feet below the top of a cliff, and that the county high-angle rescue team is setting up a rope system in order to extricate the patient. The flight paramedic notifies the incident commander of the crew's estimated time of arrival, and confirms that a safe landing zone (LZ) has been secured.

After the pilot has landed the helicopter, the flight paramedic and flight nurse exit the aircraft with their stretcher, their critical care monitor/defibrillator, and their "scene bag." The flight crew is led at the LZ by a fire officer in a pickup truck to a trail that leads to the top of a gorge. Here they find a large group of rescue workers assembled near the edge of the cliff.

The flight paramedic and flight nurse are led to the EMS commander, who briefs them on the situation: "The patient is a seventeen-year-old male who was part of a group of kids that were jumping from the top of the gorge into a deep pool in the creek at the bottom of the gorge. Witnesses tell us that he tried to stop himself after he started running towards the edge of the cliff, but momentum and loose soil caused his feet to slide out from under him and he went over the cliff, feet first. His friends say that on the way down he struck the back of his head on an outcropping before falling into the pool. His friends pulled him out of the pool onto the ledge. Right now we have a paramedic and his EMT partner down there with the patient, working with members of the rope team. They are trying to get the patient packaged so that the rope team can haul him up."

Just then the paramedic who is with the patient calls the EMS commander on the radio, and asks to speak to the flight paramedic: "We have a seventeen-year-old male patient with a severe head injury. His mental status alternates between combativeness and unresponsiveness. We have also witnessed some intermittent seizure activity. Right now he is breathing well, but he is difficult to assess and impossible to package due to his combativeness. We would like for you to hike down the trail to where we are to help us manage this patient and get him ready for extrication."

The flight crew finds the patient loosely immobilized on a spine board, which is already strapped into a Stokes basket. After the initial assessment and rapid trauma assessment, the flight paramedic determines that the patient is breathing rapidly but adequately, is moving all of his extremities, and appears to have no severe injuries other than a very bloody depressed area at the junction of the right temporal, occipital, and parietal regions. He has strong radial pulses at a rate of about 65. His last blood pressure, taken several minutes ago, was 180/110. The patient is very agitated, and is fighting every effort to properly immobilize him. He has a Glasgow Coma Score of 7 (M:3, V:3, EO:1).

The flight paramedic and flight nurse both agree that the patient needs to be paralyzed and intubated for several reasons. First, because of the patient's combativeness, he will need to be well sedated for the extrication and the flight. Second, because of the severe head injury, there is a concern that the patient could lose the ability to protect his own airway, or that his respiratory effort will become insufficient. Third, paralysis and intubation will allow the use of controlled hyperventilation to manipulate carbon dioxide levels and help manage any acute increases in intracranial pressure, if necessary. Finally, paralysis and intubation will allow for initiation of a propofol infusion, which is a very favorable medication for patients with increased intracranial pressure.

The paramedic on scene established two IVs prior to the flight crew's arrival, but they were both accidentally pulled out in the chaos of trying to restrain the combative patient. As the flight paramedic assesses the patient's airway and readies the intubation equipment, monitoring devices, oxygen, manual suction, and rescue airway devices, the flight nurse establishes an intraosseous line in the patient's right proximal tibia using an IO device. The flight nurse draws up and administers 40 mg of etomidate, 180 mg of succinylcholine, and 5 mg of Versed.

The flight paramedic positions himself and the patient for the intubation, and instructs one of the EMTs to maintain manual in-line stabilization of the neck throughout the intubation. He signals to his partner that he is ready, and she administers the sedative and paralytic agents nearly simultaneously.

After about 30 seconds, the patient is completely flaccid and the paramedic attempts to visualize the glottis. Because of the manual in-line stabilization, the vocal cords appear very anterior and are difficult to visualize clearly, and the flight paramedic struggles with placing the endotracheal tube. His partner hands him the gum elastic bougie, which he easily passes into the glottis by sliding it along the anterior side of the pharynx. He then slides the 8.0 ETT over the bougie stylet, and the patient is intubated quickly. The crew verifies placement with auscultation and capnometry, secures the ETT, and replaces the cervical collar. They then administer 50 mg of rocuronium and 5 mg of Versed in order to maintain sedation and paralysis throughout the extrication. They recheck the patient's vital signs, which are virtually unchanged. They tape the small capnometry device to the patient's head blocks, and instruct the EMT from the rope rescue team who will accompany the patient up the cliff to ventilate the patient with the bag-valve-mask (BVM) unit at a rate that will maintain the end-tidal CO_2 ($ETCO_2$) at around 35–45 mmHg. The patient is secured to the backboard and Stokes basket, and the IV bag is put under pressure from an inflatable pressure infuser and secured to the patient.

The crew then hikes back up the trail to rendezvous with the patient and rope rescue team at the top of the gorge. When the patient arrives at the top of the cliff, the crew reassesses the patient and ETT placement, and helps to carry the patient up the trail to the waiting ambulance. Once inside the ambulance, the flight crew reassesses the patient again. The patient is still paralyzed, and is ventilating easily with the BVM. SpO_2 is in the upper 90s, and $ETCO_2$ is being maintained around 35 mmHg. BP is now 190/110, and the heart rate is 60. Radial pulses are strong and his skin is warm and pink.

The crew arrives at the LZ to find that the pilot has already started the aircraft and is waiting to help load the patient. The communication center had notified the pilot and the flight paramedic by pager that the destination of choice is a level II trauma center that is about an 18-minute flight away. There are several level I facilities in the state, but the level II facility is the closest by several minutes, and the flight paramedic knows that the level II facility does have 24/7 neurosurgical coverage. The page he received from the communications center also advised him that the destination facility has been alerted and their trauma team has been activated.

As the helicopter lifts off, the flight paramedic readies the transport ventilator as the flight nurse prepares a propofol infusion. The initial ventilator settings are set while the flight paramedic closely watches the capnograph on the monitor and the pressure readings on the ventilator for any early signs of tension pneumothorax or ETT displacement or obstruction. The flight nurse initiates a propofol infusion at 10 mg/min, and slowly titrates upward to maintain deep sedation and favorable cerebral hemodynamics, while avoiding hypotension. She also administers 1 gram of Rocephin IV to help protect from meningitis due to the obviously open skull fracture. A loading dose of 1 g of Dilantin is also initiated, due to the possibility of seizures.

During transport, the flight paramedic notes that the patient's heart rate has become bradycardic (50–55) and the systolic blood pressure has risen to 195, in spite of the patient receiving a large continuous infusion (35 mg/min) of propofol. He also notices increased bleeding and for the first time sees brain tissue beginning to protrude from the hole in the skull. Recognizing the signs of cerebral herniation, he increases tidal volume to 800 cc. The peak airway pressure is still well within acceptable limits for a young, healthy patient at 25 mmHg, and after several minutes the patient's $ETCO_2$ is down to 30 mmHg and his heart rate has begun to rise into the 60s. The crew briefly discusses the option of administering a mannitol bolus or infusion, but they are now only about 10 minutes from the receiving facility, and the patient seemed to respond well to the increase in minute volume. They decide to wait and let the receiving neurosurgeons make the decision on whether to administer mannitol.

INTRODUCTION

Whereas a common question used to be "Can EMS personnel safely perform that intervention?" that question is being posed less and less frequently as numerous systems have shown that properly trained paramedics can safely perform many relatively advanced medical procedures, such as rapid-sequence intubation, central venous access, mechanical ventilation, and invasive hemodynamic monitoring.

Trauma is a surgical disease.

The current controversy, then, is not so much whether paramedics are *capable* of performing advanced interventions, but rather, whether paramedics *should* perform advanced interventions. This is especially true in the case of the trauma patient, because much of the current research continues to indicate that victims of severe trauma are best served by early surgical intervention, as little else has been consistently shown to improve outcomes in these patients.

The less frequently a prehospital skill is used, the more frequently it must be practiced.

However, this does not mean that the care that a severely traumatized patient receives early in the course of his medical treatment is unimportant. What it means is that the critical care paramedic has a responsibility to use his or her more finely tuned assessment and clinical decision-making skills in addition to—or, in many cases, instead of—their more advanced interventional capabilities. Although this is a textbook written for the critical care paramedic, competent prehospital and interfacility care of the trauma patient relies mostly on basic patient management techniques. *It is at least as important to know when not to perform a given intervention as it is to know how to perform it.*

When it comes to the management of critical trauma patients, faster transport is generally considered better. Every intervention, whether basic or advanced, must be aimed at securing the patient's vital systems and providing adequate supportive care and rapid transport to the appropriate tertiary facility. As much of the necessary care as possible should be done en route; pretransport management should be limited to securing the airway, controlling severe bleeding (even those interventions are sometimes best done en route), and ensuring appropriate immobilization of suspected or known spinal injuries.

Certain procedures, such as rapid-sequence intubation (RSI), central IV line placement, and advanced pharmacologic intervention (mannitol, propofol, and so forth) may benefit certain patients, but should usually only be used when more basic, necessary care has been carried out and has been ineffective in maintaining the patient's basic physiological functions. Generally speaking, the more "advanced" or "invasive" an intervention, the more risk it carries. Often the more advanced interventions are not well supported by research. Therefore, the need for the more advanced interventions generally has to be quite pressing in order to satisfy the risk benefit analysis that is the core of competent clinical decision making.

In our case study, the flight crew was called to transport a severely head-injured patient directly from the scene of injury to a tertiary facility. Head injuries account for most cases of severe trauma, and a patient such as this would be fairly typical for a critical care paramedic who works for an HEMS service. Though the transport team did perform several advanced interventions during the prehospital phase of the transport, everything that was done prior to transport was done with the intention of either securing the airway or packaging the patient for safe transport—both undeniably crucial objectives. No time was wasted performing unnecessary assessment or intervention, and the more advanced procedures were only carried out when it was reasonably anticipated that the simpler approaches would be ineffective or unsafe.

EPIDEMIOLOGY AND COST OF TRAUMA

In the United States, trauma is *the* leading cause of death for *all* persons under the age of 44, and is the fifth leading cause of death in all ages. (See Table 13–1.) Each year trauma kills more people than AIDS, cancer, or heart disease. Trauma is the leading cause of death in children in the United States.

In a typical year, approximately 150,000 Americans die from trauma. In the United States, more than 400 people—50 of whom are children—die of an injury every day. Well over twice as many Americans die from trauma every year than died in the entire Vietnamese conflict. Approximately 90,000 of these deaths annually are due to unintentional injury, with the rest resulting from violence.

The most common causes of trauma deaths vary by age, but by far the single most prevalent cause of trauma-related deaths is the motor vehicle crash (MVC); this makes the MVC the number one cause of death in the United States. Approximately 1 in 70 Americans will eventually die from an MVC of some type. In addition to deaths, MVCs cause more than 500,000 hospitalizations per year, and are the most common cause of major central nervous system trauma, which is arguably the most devastating type of survivable injury. It is important to note that a full half of all motor vehicle crashes involve alcohol. Firearms and falls are the next most common cause of injury. (See Figure 13-1 .)

Alarmingly, intentional injuries (homicide and suicide) account for more than 50,000 deaths per year. Our society appears to be becoming more violent; even though by most accounts the annual number of homicides has fallen during the past several decades, the number of aggravated assaults has actually risen markedly. The drop in the number of deaths from physical assault can probably be attributed in large part to the development of more organized and effective trauma care in the United States, not a declining rate of violence.

As staggering as the numbers are, the number of annual deaths from trauma truly represents only the tip of the iceberg, in terms of the magnitude of the problem. This is because, even though tens of thousands of Americans die from trauma each year, the vast majority of trauma patients do survive their injuries, and are left living with the physical and emotional effects of the incident for the rest of their lives. Many victims require expensive medical care and rehabilitative therapy, and a large percentage of major trauma victims are never able to return to fully functional status. Annually, about 1.5 million people are injured seriously enough to require hospitalization, but survive to be discharged. Tens of thousands of these people suffer temporarily or permanently debilitating disabilities that cost society billions of dollars annually in rehabilitation and other care costs. In 1994 the total cost of injury was estimated at $224 billion, a figure that includes direct medical costs, rehabilitation costs, and lost wages. This is a staggering figure even when compared to other major causes of death, such as cardiovascular disease or cancer.

Trauma is a particularly costly disease not only in terms of dollars, but also because of its cost in terms of the number of years of productive life lost (YPPL). This figure is calculated by subtracting the age at death from 65, the average retirement age. Other diseases (cancer, heart disease) account for more total years of life lost (YLL), but because those diseases primarily affect older people, they do not account for as many *productive* years lost. In the case of permanent disability instead of death, the younger trauma victim will cost society much more in rehabilitation, care, insurance costs, and lost wages than will an older person who is left debilitated because of a stroke. The most tragic and costly aspect of the trauma epidemic is the fact that trauma is most likely to affect those persons who have the most potential to contribute positively to society.

None of these figures, of course, can even begin to quantify what trauma costs society in terms of the incredible physical and emotional pain that it clearly causes.

Trauma is the leading cause of death in the United States for all persons under the age of 44.

Most trauma patients survive their injuries—sometimes with a lifetime disability.

Table 13–1 | Leading Causes of Death, United States, 2002, All Races, Both Sexes

Age Groups

Rank	<1	1–4	5–9	10–14	15–24	25–34	35–44	45–54	55–64	>65	All
1	Congenital Anomalies	Unintentional Injury	Unintentional Injury	Unintentional Injury	Unintentional Injury	Unintentional Injury	Unintentional Injury	Malignancies	Malignancies	Heart Disease	Heart Disease
2	Short Gestation	Congenital Anomalies	Malignancies	Malignancies	Homicide	Suicide	Malignancies	Heart Disease	Heart Disease	Malignancies	Malignancies
3	SIDS	Homicide	Congenital Anomalies	Suicide	Suicide	Homicide	Heart Disease	Unintentional Injury	Chronic Respiratory Disease	Cerebrovascular Disease	Cerebrovascular Disease
4	Maternal Complication	Malignancies	Homicide	Congenital Anomalies	Malignancies	Malignancies	Suicide	Liver Disease	Diabetes Mellitus	Chronic Respiratory Disease	Chronic Respiratory Disease
5	Placenta	Heart Disease	Heart Disease	Homicide	Heart Disease	Heart Disease	HIV/AIDS	Suicide	Cerebrovascular Disease	Influenza and Pneumonia	Unintentional Injury
6	Unintentional Injury	Influenza and Pneumonia	Benign Neoplasms	Heart Disease	Congenital Anomalies	HIV/AIDS	Homicide	Cerebrovascular Disease	Unintentional injury	Alzheimer's Disease	Diabetes Mellitus
7	Respiratory Distress	Sepsis	Sepsis	Chronic Respiratory Disease	Chronic Respiratory Disease	Diabetes	Liver Disease	Diabetes Mellitus	Liver Disease	Diabetes Mellitus	Influenza and Pneumonia
8	Sepsis	Chronic Respiratory Disease	Chronic Respiratory Disease	Cerebro-vascular Disease	HIV/AIDS	Cerebrovascular Disease	Cerebrovascular Disease	HIV/IDS	Suicide	Nephritis	Alzheimer's Disease
9	Circulatory System Disease	Perinatal Period	Influenza and Pneumonia	Influenza and Pneumonia	Cerebrovascular Disease	Congenital Anomalies	Diabetes Mellitus	Chronic Respiratory Disease	Nephritis	Unintentional injury	Nephritis
10	Intrauterine Hypoxia	Benign Neoplasms	Cerebrovascular Disease	Sepsis	Diabetes	Liver Disease	Chronic Respiratory Disease	Viral Hepatitis	Sepsis	Sepsis	Sepsis

Source: Centers for Disease Control and Prevention

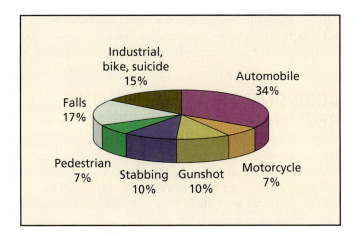

■ Figure 13-1 Breakdown of trauma in the United States.

HISTORY AND OVERVIEW OF TRAUMA SYSTEMS

Historically, both the public and the health care communities have viewed trauma as being very different from other disease processes, in that traumatic injury was always seen as the result of accidental or unavoidable events. An "accident," by definition, is a random event that is difficult or impossible to predict or prevent. Because of this view, little was done to attempt to organize trauma care or develop the system approach to trauma that has since shown to be very beneficial.

Once the medical community began to view trauma as a distinct disease that could be studied, managed, and prevented, the way was paved for the development of regional trauma systems; this development, for the most part, paralleled the growth of EMS in this country.

The concept of trauma as a distinct disease that requires a "system approach" did not begin to come into wide acceptance until after a white paper, titled *Accidental Death and Disability: The Neglected Disease of Modern Society*, was published in 1966 by the National Academy of Science and the National Research Council. This landmark publication helped alert the public and the medical community to the magnitude of the trauma epidemic, and ultimately helped to convince Congress to pass the Highway Safety Act (1966), which required each state to develop highway safety programs and suggested funding for EMS system development. The Emergency Medical Services Systems Act followed in 1973; this legislation was amended twice in the late 1970s, and offered funding and a detailed outline for states to follow in the development of their own EMS systems. In 1981 the responsibility for the continued development of EMS systems was transferred from the federal government to the individual states, and federal funding was significantly decreased. In 1990, however, the Trauma Care Systems Planning and Development Act was passed and provided funding and guidance for the development of comprehensive trauma systems, to include EMS, trauma system, and research initiatives.

The military approach to trauma care has had a huge influence on the development of civilian trauma systems. In each of the major military conflicts of the 20th century, battlefield mortality rates among seriously injured combatants fell significantly when compared to the previous conflict, despite more accurate and lethal weaponry being employed. The single theme that can be easily identified over and over again in military trauma care philosophy is the idea that seriously injured soldiers must be treated by qualified surgical personnel as early as possible. Appropriate triage and rapid patient transport are the central components of this philosophy, and they led to the heavy utilization of medical evacuation (Medevac) helicopters and forward location of field surgical hospitals in the Korean, Vietnam, and subsequent conflicts. The apparent success of this approach was mirrored somewhat by the experience of so-called early trauma centers in Maryland and Illinois, and they set the stage for the very ideas of the "Golden Hour" and rapid transport.

In 1960, the earliest dedicated, civilian, trauma-specific care was being provided at the University of Maryland in Baltimore, and the first dedicated trauma unit was opened by Cook County Hospital in Chicago, Illinois, in 1966. In 1971 Illinois began operating the first statewide trauma system, and the State of Maryland followed in 1977. Though the efforts were preliminary, they were

Research has shown that trauma patients have better outcomes when they are treated at actual trauma centers, which deal with trauma day in, day out.

well organized and by most accounts quite successful. Much research on trauma care was carried out at both institutions—most notably in Baltimore—and both systems served as models for the development of trauma care systems throughout the rest of the country.

COMPONENTS OF A STATE OR REGIONAL TRAUMA SYSTEM

trauma system *combined triage and transport protocols, referral guidelines, transfer agreements, education, consultation, research and injury prevention programs; designed to assist EMS, hospitals, physicians, and tertiary centers in providing patient access to appropriate care.*

The American College of Surgeons' Committee on Trauma publishes guidelines and provides accreditation of regional trauma centers, as do most states. Numerous components must be considered when developing a regional **trauma system,** one of the central ideas being that enough serious trauma cases must be available so as to maintain a high level of expertise among the specialists at the receiving trauma centers.

The four levels of trauma center accreditation as outlined by the American College of Surgeons (ACS) are:

Level I. Offers comprehensive trauma care, from initial evaluation (and often transport) to rehabilitation. Can manage any type of patient and offers many specialized services, such as burn, neurologic, and cardiovascular surgical subspecialists. Level I centers must maintain a predetermined number of available operating rooms, resuscitation areas, and ICU beds. They remain active in planning and research, and are usually located at university medical centers. An important point is that the Level I center must receive a predetermined number of severe trauma patients annually.

Level II. Can appropriately manage most seriously injured patients, but lacks some surgical subspecialties. May not focus as much on research and education as a Level I facility, but still must adhere to rigorous staff educational and credentialing requirements.

Level III. Often located in community hospitals, these centers provide expert initial resuscitation and stabilization but lack much of the surgical specialty and intensive care that is available at the larger centers.

Level IV. This designation has been implemented to help guide the very rural center in the development of standardized plans for the initial management and rapid transfer of the trauma patient.

It is important to note that "trauma center" designation may vary significantly from state to state, because some states award the designation whether or not the facilities have been evaluated by the ACS as meeting their criteria. For instance, Level I and II centers, per the ACS criteria, must have neurosurgical capability 24 hours a day. This may not be true, however, of Level II centers per some state criteria. It is important for the critical care paramedic to know what trauma centers exist within their service area, and to have an idea of what each specific hospital's capabilities are.

Trauma systems are more than trauma centers; they are systems meant to provide a framework within which EMS services, community hospitals, referring physicians, and tertiary centers can all work together to provide rapid access to appropriate care. Triage and transport protocols, referral guidelines, transfer agreements, education, consultation, and research and injury prevention programs are all integral components of the successful, well-designed trauma system.

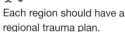

Each region should have a regional trauma plan.

The central focus of a trauma system is to ensure that trauma patients reach appropriate care as rapidly as possible. In theory, the decision to transfer a patient from a local facility (or the field) to a tertiary facility should be quite easy to make: Either the first facility has the resources to appropriately manage the patient, or it doesn't. In reality, however, the waters surrounding the decision tend to be muddied with political, financial, logistical, and clinical issues. Instead of being transferred now, can the severely injured patient just wait a few minutes at the local facility until his surgeon and anesthetist can come in from home? Should the patient being transferred be sent out immediately with local EMS resources, or should she wait a little longer at the referring facility for the regional critical care transport team to arrive? By placing predetermined transfer criteria in effect, trauma systems attempt to make the decision-making process simple and objective and answer as many of these questions as possible ahead of time.

INJURY PREVENTION

Death following trauma proceeds via a trimodal distribution. The first group (approximately 50% of trauma deaths) dies immediately or within several minutes of the injury. Causes of death include massive injury to the brain, heart, great vessels, and upper spinal cord. The vast majority of patients in this category cannot be saved. The second group (approximately 30% of trauma deaths) dies within several hours of their injury (usually within the first 4 hours). Causes of death in this group include brain hemorrhage or clots, hemothorax or pneumothorax, abdominal bleeding, and fractures (pelvic/long bone). Although these injuries are life threatening, they are treatable. The third group (approximately 20% of trauma deaths) dies within days to weeks of their injury. Causes of death in this group include infection and multiple-organ failure. (See Figure 13-2 ■.)

Death from trauma follows a trimodal distribution: immediate, hours, and days.

It is quite apparent according to these statistics that even the best-designed trauma system, with the fastest and most highly trained paramedics delivering their patients to the most technologically advanced trauma centers staffed with the most talented surgeons, can do nothing at all to help a full 50% of potential trauma deaths. These victims can only be saved by preventing the injury in the first place.

Regardless of the care available, some trauma patients cannot be saved.

Several epidemiologists worked to change the concept of trauma as resulting from random, unpredictable "accidents." The most notable by far was William Haddon, who served as the first director of the National Highway Traffic Safety Administration. Haddon worked to refine the idea that illnesses and injuries were the result of interaction between the *agent* (the car involved in a crash, for instance), the *environment* (wet roads and darkness, for example), and the *host* (the driver of the car). His *Haddon matrix* has become the classic model used for the explanation and illustration of the method of transmission of communicable disease, and has been widely used in the development of programs for infectious disease control. The matrix also works well to illustrate the preventability of trauma deaths. The core concept of the **Haddon matrix** as it applies to injury prevention is the thought that the energy transfer that causes trauma is predictable, and can be prevented in many cases by manipulating the environment, the agent, or the host's behavior. (See Figure 13-3 ■.)

Haddon matrix *applied theory about injury prevention. The core concept is that the energy transfer that causes trauma is predictable, and can be prevented in many cases by manipulating the environment, agent, the host's behavior, or a combination of these.*

While the concepts of Haddon's work can easily be applied to injury prevention, actual implementation is more difficult.

Injury prevention efforts are usually described as being either active or passive, from the point of view of the host (the potential victim). An active intervention is one that involves an action by the host that will reduce the likelihood of exposure to energy. Buckling a seat belt, putting on a helmet, and carefully scanning for traffic before crossing the street are all examples of active interventions. Passive interventions are those strategies that do not involve any action on the part of the host. Roadway design and traffic signs, automotive air bags, and safety rails are all examples of passive interventions. Passive interventions are inherent in the design of the environment, and are generally considered much more reliable than active interventions.

Injury prevention is always a better expenditure of money than treatment.

In many cases, active interventions only work reliably when they are mandated by law, and only when the laws are enforced reliably. In states with motorcycle helmet laws for instance, the incidence

Injury prevention (child car seats, seat belts, air bags, crumple zones, and so on) has been more effective in reducing trauma morbidity and mortality than post-injury trauma care.

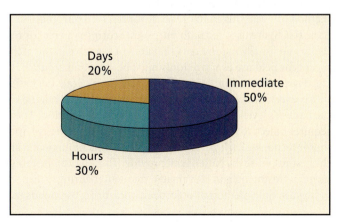

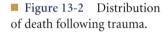
■ Figure 13-2 Distribution of death following trauma.

Figure 13-3 Haddon's matrix as applied to ground ambulance collision.

Haddon's Matrix	Human	Vector/Vehicle	Physical/Social Environment
Pre-Event Activity	Braking Experience Education Attitude toward safety Radio distraction Partner distraction	Weight Vehicle design Passengers Vehicle safety equipment	Sun Driver distractions Road hazards Road design Road surface
Event Activity	Personal protective equipment Reaction time	Vehicle safety equipment Personal protective equipment	Road detour Road surface
Post-Event Activity	Education Evaluation Accident review	Automated crash notification system Black box	EMS response Weather report Police report

of severe brain injury secondary to motorcycle crashes is significantly lower than in states where wearing a helmet is optional. Compliance with seat belt laws, however, is marginal in many areas because the laws are fairly difficult to enforce.

Engineering interventions are aimed either at the behavior of the host or, more commonly, at changing the environment or agent in a way that will reduce the likelihood of energy transfer to the host. For instance, anti-lock brakes make car crashes less likely, and air bags protect the host if a crash does occur; these are passive engineering interventions. Installing a system that will not allow a car to be shifted into drive until the drivers' seat belt is buckled is an example of an active engineering intervention.

EMS and critical care transport services can have a positive effect on injury prevention by participating in safety campaigns and public awareness programs. These programs work most effectively when coupled with legislation and enforcement. For instance, laws that require infant car seats are most effective when combined with public education efforts to teach the importance and proper use of the infant car seats.

TRIAGE AND TRAUMA SCORING SYSTEMS

Many trauma scoring systems have been developed. We will outline some of the systems that are pertinent to trauma care. Generally, a given scale is meant to serve as either a triage tool or as a method of stratifying injury severity for research purposes. Some scales, such as the Glasgow Coma Scale (GCS) are used for both purposes. Scoring systems for research purposes tend to be rather in depth and usually require data that are not available in the prehospital phase, while scoring systems meant for field use as triage tools must be valid and accurate, yet easy to use.

First published in 1974, the Glasgow Coma Scale is a basic and useful scoring tool with which nearly every clinician is familiar. When properly applied, the GCS provides an objective analysis of the patient's level of consciousness and cerebral function. The GCS is very easy to apply, because it requires objective evaluation of only three parameters: eye opening, best verbal response, and best motor response. Each parameter is graded on a numerical scale, and requires the clinician to elicit the best response the patient can provide. The GCS can be rapidly figured early in the course of prehospital treatment, and reevaluated frequently during transport and on arrival at the hospital, providing a simple method of objectively measuring the trends in the patient's neurologic status. (See

Infants and Toddlers			Children and Adult		
Eye opening	Spontaneous	4	Eye opening	Spontaneous	4
	To voice	3		To Voice	3
	To pain	2		To Pain	2
	None	1		None	1
Best verbal response	Smiles, interacts	5	Best verbal response	Oriented	5
	Consolable	4		Confused	4
	Cries to pain	3		Inappropriate words	3
	Moans to pain	2		Incomprehensible words	2
	None	1		None	1
Best motor response	Normal spontaneous movement	6	Best motor response	Obeys commands	6
	Localizes pain	5		Localizes pain	5
	Withdraws to pain	4		Withdraws (pain)	4
	Abnormal flexion	3		Flexion (pain)	3
	Abnormal extension	2		Extension (pain)	2
	None	1		None	1

■ **Figure 13-4** Glasgow coma scale.

Figure 13-4 ■.) Many references suggest that trauma patients with a GCS < 13 should be evaluated at a Level I or Level II trauma center.

The original Trauma Score (TS) included four physiological parameters (respiratory rate, respiratory expansion, systolic blood pressure, capillary refill) and the GCS. It had a range from 1 to 16 points. Patients with a score of 12 or less were deemed to be seriously injured and required specialized trauma care. The TS was revised in 1989 and became the Revised Trauma Score. Two of the physiological parameters (respiratory expansion and capillary refill) were dropped. The range of the RTS is 0 to 12. Patients with a score of 11 or less are deemed to require specialized trauma care. The RTS is easy to calculate and has been shown to be an accurate and reliable predictor of trauma severity. (See Table 13–2.)

The **Revised Trauma Score** (**RTS**) is a triage tool that requires evaluation of three easy-to-measure parameters: respiratory rate, systolic blood pressure, and the GCS. The RTS assigns a numeric value to each of the parameters with the total score being between 0 and 12. The lower the score, the more severely injured the patient. The RTS is easy to calculate and has been shown to be an accurate and reliable predictor of trauma severity. Like the GCS, the RTS can be used as a scoring tool to help determine which patients require evaluation at a trauma facility.

While the RTS is most commonly used in the prehospital setting, a weighted form of the scale is used to predict patient outcomes following trauma. With the weighted RTS, greater emphasis is placed on the GCS. The range for the weighted RTS is 0 to 7.8408. Higher scores are associated with a better prognosis.

The **Pediatric Trauma Score** (**PTS**) is a version of the Trauma Score that is extensively modified to take into account the different normal vital sign ranges, developmental levels, and increased

Revised Trauma Score (RTS) *triage tool that requires evaluation of respiratory rate, systolic blood pressure, and the result of the Glasgow Coma Score.*

Trauma scoring systems, such as the RTS, are much better predictors of who needs trauma center care than mechanism of injury criteria.

Pediatric Trauma Score (PTS) *modified version of the trauma score accounting for pediatric differences in normal vital sign ranges, developmental levels, and increased physiological reserve, as compared to adults.*

Table 13–2	Revised Trauma Score		
Glasgow Coma Scale Score	Systolic Blood Pressure (mmHg)	Respiratory Rate (breaths/min)	Coded Value
13–15	>89	10–29	4
9–12	76–89	>29	3
6–8	50–75	6–9	2
4–5	1–49	1–5	1
3	0	0	0

Table 13–3	Pediatric Trauma Score (Example)		
	Coded Value		
Patient Characteristics	+2	+1	−1
Weight (kg)	>20	10–20	<10
Airway	Normal	Maintained	Unmaintained
Systolic BP (mmHg)	>90	50–90	<50
Central nervous system	Awake	Obtunded	Coma
Open wound	None	Minor	Major
Skeletal trauma	None	Closed	Open, multiple

physiological reserve that children possess compared to adults. The parameters evaluated by the PTS include the size (in kilograms) of the patient, the airway status, systolic blood pressure, central nervous system status (awake or unconscious), skeletal system (any obvious open or closed fractures), and cutaneous system. This system takes into account the fact that children are difficult to assess using "adult" neurologic criteria, and also that children are more likely to be victims of multiple trauma than are adults. A child with a PTS of ≤8 (or an RTS < 11) should be transported to a pediatric trauma center. (See Table 13–3.)

Abbreviated Injury Scale (AIS) *developed to collect detailed data on the types and severity of injuries suffered by victims of motor vehicle crashes.*

The **Abbreviated Injury Scale (AIS)** is a severity scale that was developed jointly by the American Medical Association, the American Association for Automotive Medicine, and the Society of Automotive Engineers in order to collect detailed data on the types and severity of injuries suffered by victims of motor vehicle crashes. The AIS requires detailed assessment of seven anatomical regions: the head and face, the neck, the chest, the spine, the abdominal and pelvic organs, the extremities and pelvic girdle, and the integument. Each region receives a score from 1 to 6, with 1 being a very minor injury and 6 being an unsurvivable one. The score for each region is assigned based on the potential for death to be caused by the specific, most severe injury suffered in that region. (See Table 13–4.)

Injury Severity Score (ISS) *scoring system calculated retrospectively by adding the squares of the highest of the seven Abbreviated Injury Scale (AIS) scores (score of 1 to 75).*

A much more comprehensive scoring system used for patient stratification is the **Injury Severity Score (ISS),** which is calculated retrospectively by adding the squares of the highest of the seven Abbreviated Injury Scale scores. The ISS results in a numerical score of 1 to 75, with 1 indicating a very minor, isolated injury, and 75 indicating multiple severe, unsurvivable injuries. The ISS is used extensively by trauma registries for data collection and research purposes. Patients with an ISS > 15 are deemed to require specialized trauma care, whereas patients with an ISS of 15 or less are considered to have non–life-threatening injuries. (See Table 13–5.)

The Trauma Score, Injury Severity Score, Age Combination Index (TRISS) method combines the physiological measurements of the RTS with the anatomical components of the ISS, along with the patient's age, to attempt to provide a comprehensive and accurate indication of the overall severity and survivability of a given patient's injuries. The TRISS score is used primarily by trauma registries and is impractical for clinical use.

Table 13–4	Abbreviated Injury Score
Injury	**AIS Score**
1	Minor
2	Moderate
3	Serious
4	Severe
5	Critical
6	Unsurvivable

Table 13–5	Injury Severity Score		
Region	Injury Description	AIS	Square Top Three
Head and Neck	Cerebral Contusion	3	9
Face	No Injury	0	
Chest	Flail Chest	4	16
Abdomen	Minor Contusion of Liver	2	
	Complex Rupture Spleen	5	25
Extremity	Fractured femur	3	
External	No Injury	0	___
	Injury Severity Score:		**50**

RESEARCH IN TRAUMA MANAGEMENT

Because it was only fairly recently that trauma came to be viewed as a preventable disease with predictable patterns and identifiable risk factors, relatively little research has historically been conducted on the topic as a whole.

Research in trauma generally falls into one of two very broad categories: research into the efficacy of new or existing techniques for managing trauma patients, and epidemiological research, the primary purpose of which is to gather information that will allow for development or evaluation of injury prevention programs.

The critical care paramedic has a responsibility to attempt to remain abreast of new developments and thinking in trauma care. The principles of evidenced-based medicine must be used when evaluating whether or not to institute new or change existing patient management techniques. Interventions that seem to make perfectly good sense and appear to produce favorable results are sometimes later shown to be quite ineffective or even harmful upon close scientific scrutiny.

EMS and critical care transport agencies should track data related to patient outcomes, based on types of patients and the treatment they received during transport. Setting up such a system can be a labor-intensive endeavor, but the information gathered is invaluable to the quality assurance process and should help guide training and protocol development programs. At the very least, agencies should participate closely in receiving hospitals' research programs in order to allow for evaluation of the efficacy of given patient management techniques.

EMS personnel should play a role in trauma research.

BIOMECHANICS OF TRAUMA AND MECHANISM OF INJURY

Trauma results from acute exposure to an energy source in a quantity sufficient to cause physical damage to the cells of the body. Kinetic energy, thermal energy, electrical energy, and radiation energy are examples of sources of energy that may cause injury. Kinetic injury is by far the most common cause of trauma deaths in the United States.

The term *mechanism of injury* refers to the actual, immediate physical cause of the injury. The term is usually used when describing an assessment of how kinetic energy was likely transmitted through the body, and which organ systems were likely affected. The *biomechanics of trauma* is a term often used interchangeably with mechanism of injury, though it may actually have a slightly different definition in that the *biomechanics of trauma* explains the physical RESULTS of the mechanism of injury. In other words, the mechanism of injury is what happened outside the body; the biomechanics of trauma is the study of what happens inside the body, as a result of the mechanism of injury.

The most important basic concepts to keep in mind when assessing the mechanism of injury are the anatomy of the area affected by the trauma, and Newton's first law of motion, which states that "An object at rest will remain at rest, and an object in motion will remain in motion, until acted upon by an outside force."

Newton's first law explains common blunt trauma and acceleration/deceleration injuries. If a patient is traveling in a car at 60 mph, and the car suddenly stops when it strikes a bridge abutment, the victim's body will remain traveling at 60 mph until it is acted upon by an "outside force," such as the steering wheel, windshield, or seat belt. The patient's brain and internal organs will do the same; they will continue traveling at the same speed until they strike the inside of the skull or thoracic wall.

A detailed lesson of the biomechanics of trauma is well beyond the scope of this chapter, and the mechanisms of injury that correspond to specific injury patterns will be reviewed in the sections that cover those injuries. Evaluation of the mechanism of injury is invaluable to the formulation of the plan of care. Even sophisticated imaging and assessment tools do not reduce the importance of mechanism of injury consideration. If the receiving trauma surgeon or ED physician doesn't know the mechanism of injury, she won't know what type of injuries to suspect or which assessment method to use. What good is a CT scanner or ultrasound machine if the physician doesn't know which part of the body to look at?

GENERAL APPROACH TO THE TRAUMA PATIENT

The critical care paramedic should approach the trauma patient in the same manner that every clinician should approach every potentially critical patient: cautiously, expeditiously, and with the intention of rapidly identifying and managing life-threatening injuries.

Courses such as prehospital trauma life support and basic trauma life support courses teach a systematic framework for the approach and management of the trauma patient in the prehospital setting. Regardless of the course or reference, however, the priorities for management of the trauma patient in the prehospital setting are universal and clear. They include:

1. Safety of the rescuer(s)
2. Safety of the victim(s)
3. Management of airway and/or respiratory system compromise
4. Management of life-threatening hemorrhage
5. Protection/prevention of actual or potential spinal cord injury
6. Rapid transport to an appropriate facility
7. Maintenance of body temperature
8. Pain control
9. Other

On any trauma scene, your first priority is your safety and that of your fellow rescuers.

In the prehospital environment, scene safety is the first and most important factor to consider when approaching a trauma patient. The domestic, roadside, and industrial environments all hold numerous threats to safety that must be evaluated and dealt with before the patient can be. Upon approaching the patient, a general idea of the mechanism of injury and the potential injuries should be formulated.

The very first step of the actual patient assessment involves speaking to the patient to determine airway patency, adequacy of breathing, mental status, and chief complaint(s). A large amount of information concerning a patient's overall status can be gathered simply by introducing yourself to the patient, asking him what happened and what is bothering him, and then listening closely. If the patient can speak coherently, then you have—for the immediate time being, anyway—a noncritical patient with intact ABCs. If the patient is not coherent, then you immediately move to assess and secure the airway and respiratory status, and determine the level of consciousness.

At this time a rapid physical exam should take place, which includes assessment of respiratory rate and effort, pulse quality and rate, skin color/temperature, extremity movement/response to painful stimuli, and a formulation of a general impression of how "sick" the patient looks. With trauma, hemorrhagic shock can often be quantified. (See Table 13–6.) This can and should be completed in a matter of seconds, and preparation for the movement of the critical patient should be under way. The patient is immobilized and moved rapidly to the transport vehicle, where interventions and a more detailed physical exam, including vital signs, cardiac monitoring, and venous access, occur while en route to the receiving facility.

Table 13-6 | Hemorrhagic Shock Classification

	Class I	Class II	Class III	Class IV
Degree of hemorrhage	Very mild	Mild	Moderate	Severe
Blood volume loss	<15 %	15–25 %	26–39 %	>40 %
Cardiovascular	HR normal or mildly increased, normal pulses, normal BP	Tachycardia, peripheral pulses may be decreased, normal BP	Significant tachycardia thready peripheral pulses, decreased BP	Severe tachycardia thready CENTRAL pulses, significantly decreased BP
pH	Normal	Normal	Metabolic acidosis	Significant acidosis
Respiratory	RR normal	Tachypnea	Moderate tachypnea	Severe tachypnea
CNS	Slightly anxious	Irritable, confused, or combative	Irritable, lethargic, or diminished pain response	Lethargic, coma
Skin	Warm, pink, capillary refill brisk	Cool extremities, mottled, delayed capillary refill	Cool extremities, mottled or pallor, prolonged capillary refill	Cold extremities, pallor or cyanosis
Kidneys	Normal urine output	Oliguria, increased specific gravity	Oliguria, increased BUN	Anuria

The primary difference between the critical care paramedic and the "street" paramedic is that the critical care paramedic specializes in the interfacility transport of critical patients who require therapies or interventions not usually implemented or performed in the field. The management priorities when transporting a trauma patient from a referring facility are identical to those when transporting from a prehospital scene; however, in most cases, immediately life-threatening injuries have been managed or controlled by the time the critical care paramedic has arrived to transport the patient to the next level of care.

In a setting such as this, the critical care paramedic (critical care paramedic) has a list of tasks that must be completed in order to prepare the patient for safe transport.

First, the critical care paramedic must get a report on the patient; the transporting critical care paramedic must understand, at a minimum, the mechanism of injury, what the suspected or known injuries are, and what has been done to manage the patient thus far. Known medication allergies are a critical part of the history as well. This exchange often takes place between the critical care paramedic and the referring physician or nurses while the critical care paramedic is performing his own assessment, which should focus on confirming the critical elements of patient preparation that should have been relayed by the referring staff. In some cases, much of the report may be given while the critical care paramedic is en route to the referring facility.

The next task is to perform a rapid, cursory patient assessment that focuses on ensuring that all critical elements of patient management and preparation have been performed, such as ensuring appropriate ETT placement and appropriate intravenous access, ensuring that appropriate medications or blood products are available during transport, ensuring that the patient is properly immobilized if indicated, and so on. Time is of the essence in this stage of the transport, and a rapid clinical evaluation can usually provide all the information needed to decide whether or not the patient is ready for transport. For instance, clear, equal breath sounds, combined with good oxygen saturation and normal end-tidal CO_2 levels, tell you all you really need to know about the ETT placement and oxygenation/ventilation status; there is probably no need to go searching through the paperwork right now to find the most recent arterial blood gas values or to bother finding a light box to inspect the chest X-ray for ETT placement. It is much more efficient and usually just as safe and effective to confirm these things clinically, and then focus your attention on the next priority on the list.

As in the prehospital setting, a judgment must be made as to whether to perform interventions before or during transport, although often for different reasons. For instance, if there is some concern over whether or not a patient's airway will become compromised during transport, it may be desirable for many reasons to simply perform an intubation in the ED prior to departure. On the other hand, there may be good reasons for not doing so, as well. Many factors are involved in such decisions, and protocols, on-line medical direction, and strong clinical decision making should all be consulted in such cases.

After the critical interventions have been confirmed, the patient is placed on the transport monitor, medications are switched to the transport IV pumps, and doses/infusion rates are double-checked. The transport ventilator may be hooked to the patient at this point (or the patient may be ventilated with a BVM and the ventilator attached once in the transport vehicle). At this time the patient assessment is ongoing, pain status is addressed, and the plan of care is formulated. One team member may consult with medical direction or the receiving facility if necessary, while the other completes the patient-preparation tasks. Significant time in this phase may be able to be saved if the referring facility knows exactly what the transport team needs to complete before the patient can be transported; this can be achieved through the development of a strong working relationship with referral facilities. Patient packaging must always consider the importance of keeping the trauma patient warm, even in moderate weather. It may be advisable to take a little extra time to ensure that the patient is packaged neatly, and that monitor leads, oxygen tubing, IV lines, ventilator circuits, and so on, are all packaged and secured as neatly as possible. IV line ports should be readily accessible.

Finally, the patient is moved to the transport stretcher and then to the transport vehicle. The patient is, of course, closely monitored throughout the transport, and managed per the plan of care, which is guided by agency protocols and/or transport orders from the referring physician.

Summary

It has been the primary intention of this chapter to emphasize the immense scope of the trauma epidemic and to reinforce the importance of relatively basic care and rapid transport of the severely traumatized patient. We also hoped to introduce or reinforce the importance of the systems approach to the management of the trauma patient, and we introduced some of the history of trauma system development as well as the basic workings of a typical trauma system. Some of the basic tools used in evaluation and stratification of trauma patients were also presented; these are all things with which every critical care paramedic should be familiar.

We briefly described the role of the critical care paramedic as it relates to the care of the trauma patient. We reviewed the importance of considering the mechanism of injury when assessing the trauma patient, as well as the basic considerations and techniques of assessment, packaging for transport, and general management of the victim of major trauma. We cannot overemphasize that the general assessment and management priorities of the severely traumatized patient remain consistent and relatively simple, no matter what level of training the clinician possesses. Other chapters will cover specific injuries and conditions in much detail, as well as the assessment and management techniques for those specific injuries.

Review Questions

1. List several components of a typical trauma system.
2. Explain the magnitude of trauma as a disease process in the United States.
3. What are several ways in which an organized trauma response can reduce mortality and morbidity in a severe trauma patient?
4. Describe some trauma scoring systems.
5. What is a primary difference between a Level I and Level II trauma center?
6. What are the priorities when assessing and managing a victim of severe trauma?

7. How does the critical care paramedic differ from the traditional paramedic, in terms of his abilities and priorities when managing the victim of major trauma?

8. Describe specific considerations for transport of a severely traumatized patient in the interfacility setting.

See Answers to Review Questions at the back of this book.

Further Reading

American College of Surgeons Committee on Trauma. *Advanced Trauma Life Support for Doctors,* 7th ed. Chicago, IL: Author, 2004.

Brain Trauma Foundation. *Guidelines for Prehospital Management of Traumatic Brain Injury.* New York: Author, 2002.

Centers for Disease Control and Prevention. http://www.cdc.gov.

Gawande A. "Casualties of War—Military Care for the Wounded from Iraq and Afghanistan." *New England Journal of Medicine,* Vol. 351, No. 24 (2004): 2471–2475.

Harris AR, Thomas SH, Fisher GA, Hirsch DJ. "Murder and Medicine: The Lethality of Criminal Assault, 1960–1999." *Homicide Studies,* Vol. 6 (2002): 128–166.

Holleran RS. *Air and Surface Patient Transport: Principles and Practices,* 3rd ed. St Louis, MO: Mosby, 2003.

Hubble MW, Hubble JP. *Principles of Advanced Trauma Care.* Clifton Park, NY: Thomson Delmar Learning, 2002.

Knight RL. "The Glasgow Coma Scale: Ten Years After." *Critical Care Nurse,* Vol. 6 (1988): 65–71.

Moore EE, Feliciana DV, Mattox KL. *Trauma,* 5th ed. New York: McGraw-Hill, 2004.

National Academy of Sciences and National Research Council. *Accidental Death and Disability. The Neglected Disease of Modern Society.* Washington, DC: National Academies Press, 1966.

National Association of Emergency Medical Technicians and American College of Surgeons Committee on Trauma. *Prehospital Trauma Life Support,* rev. 5th ed. St. Louis, MO: Mosby, 2003.

Trauma.org. [Available at: http://www.trauma.org]

Walls RM. *Manual of Emergency Airway Management,* 2nd ed. Philadelphia: Lippincott Williams & Wilkins, 2000.

Wang H, Davis D, Wayne M, Delbridge T. "Prehospital RSI: What Does the Evidence Show?" Paper presented at 2004 NAEMSP Annual Meeting.

Winkler JV, Rosen P, Alfey EJ. "Prehospital Use of the Glasgow Coma Scale in Severe Head Injury." *Journal of Emergency Medicine,* Vol. 2 (1984): 1–6.

Neurologic Trauma

Donald J. Perreault, Jr., RN, BSN, CCRN, EMT

Objectives

Upon completion of this chapter, the student should be able to:

1. Understand the mechanism underlying the progression of secondary injuries after central nervous system (CNS) trauma. (p. 374)
2. Develop neurologic assessment skills. (p. 375)
3. Identify diagnostic tests and imaging used in the treatment of CNS-injured patients. (p. 376)
4. Discuss the role of autoregulation in the maintenance of normal cerebral perfusion pressure and cerebral blood flow. (p. 379)
5. Identify the basic concepts of intracranial pressure monitoring, as well as equipment and techniques utilized. (p. 384)
6. Discuss the role of pharmacologic agents in reducing intracranial pressure in the management of head and spinal injury patients. (p. 392)

Key Terms

autoregulation, p. 379
cerebral perfusion
  pressure (CPP), p. 379
coma, p. 378

external auditory meatus
  (EAM), p. 384
hydrocephalus, p. 383
ICP waveform, p. 385

intracranial pressure
  (ICP), p. 379
Monroe-Kellie
  hypothesis, p. 379
tentorium cerebelli, p. 381

Case Study

Your helicopter is called on to perform a transfer from an emergency department in a small community hospital to a tertiary care facility in a nearby city. Your patient is an 18-year-old male who was the driver of a small car that collided with a tree head-on at a high rate of speed. The patient was unrestrained, and was found unconscious by local EMS crews. He could not be intubated in the field, and was transferred to the closest facility for stabilization.

Upon arrival, you assess the patient. He is intubated, chemically paralyzed, and sedated. There is obvious soft-tissue trauma to the face, and a hard cervical collar remains in place. He has bilateral large-bore intravenous lines with a keep-vein-open (KVO) infusion of normal saline in each. The ED nurse gives you a report as you prepare the patient for transfer.

The patient arrived in full spinal immobilization, and was being manually ventilated with a bag-valve mask. There was no obvious trauma apart from the facial lacerations. His initial vital signs were a pulse rate of 65 in a sinus rhythm, a blood pressure of 182/100 mmHg, and an oxygen saturation of 100% with effective manual ventilation. According to EMS, he had agonal respirations on scene. Prior to the administration of paralytic agents, the patient did not open his eyes to painful stimulus and had no verbal response. A brisk sternal rub elicited decerebrate posturing. His pupils were 5 mm and sluggishly reactive bilaterally. The patient was given 100 mg of IV lidocaine, 5 mg of IV midazolam, and 100 mg of IV succinylcholine, at which point he was successfully intubated with an 8.0 mm endotracheal tube (ETT).

The CT scan revealed bilateral pulmonary contusions, but no further injury to the rest of his thorax, abdomen, pelvis, or osseous cervical spine. His head CT was remarkable for cerebral contusions in both frontal lobes, with an apparent contrecoup contusion to the occipital lobe and small punctate hemorrhages deep in the white matter of the basal ganglion. The patient is to be transferred to a tertiary care facility with an experienced neurosurgical service for management of his closed head injury.

You connect the patient to your ventilator and transfer him to the aircraft. You program the ventilator to the following settings:

- ★ Assist-control ventilation
- ★ $FiO_2 = 1.0$
- ★ $V_T = 600$ mL
- ★ Rate $= 12$/minute
- ★ Pressure support $= 10$ cm/H_2O
- ★ PEEP $= 5$ cm/H_2O

In addition, you attach an end-tidal CO_2 monitor to ensure that the patient is receiving optimal ventilation. The initial reading is 42. You adjust the ventilator to a rate of 14, and the patient's CO_2 corrects to 33. En route, the patient becomes tachycardic and begins to trigger the ventilator with a tachypneic pattern of spontaneous respiration. You administer an additional 5 mg of midazolam as well as 100 mcg of IV fentanyl. The remainder of the transport is uneventful.

Four days later, you check in on the patient in the ICU. Shortly after his arrival at the receiving facility, neurosurgeons inserted a fiber-optic intracranial pressure (ICP) bolt monitor into his brain parenchyma and received an initial reading of 30 mmHg. He was given IV mannitol to help reduce his ICP. Central venous access and an arterial line were also established. The patient was placed on a propofol infusion for sedation, which has been lifted every 2 hours since his arrival to evaluate his neurologic status. His exam has remained the same.

Within the last 24 hours, the patient's ICP waveform has changed to reflect a P_2 wave, which has become elevated over the P_1 wave. He is receiving 100 grams of IV mannitol every 6 hours to help combat cerebral edema. In spite of this, his ICP is sustained above 25 mmHg with frequent spikes as high as 50. He is placed on an IV neosynephrine infusion to help maintain a cerebral perfusion pressure (CPP) of greater than 60 mmHg. He has also required intermittent boluses of 23.4% sodium chloride to help maintain his ICP. CT scans reveal diffuse cerebral edema.

One week later, the patient's cerebral edema appears to have resolved via CT. He no longer requires pharmacologic intervention to maintain an adequate CPP. His ICP has not spiked above 20 for several days, and the ICP bolt is discontinued. The patient is weaned from the propofol infusion, and after an additional 2 days, he is found to have pupils that are fixed at midpoint bilaterally. He has no spontaneous respiratory effort, no corneal, cough, or gag reflexes, and no motor response to painful stimuli. The patient's family is uncertain about how to proceed, and an MRI is obtained to help provide further prognostic indication. The MRI reveals large regions of hypoperfused, infarcted tissue, as well as hyperdense signal in the white matter that is highly suspicious for diffuse axonal injury (DAI). The patient meets all criteria for brain death. The family is presented with the information and makes the decision to pursue withdrawal of care and organ donation.

INTRODUCTION

Injuries to the central nervous system (CNS) can be both devastating and highly complex. Significant neurologic trauma can occur even in the presence of relatively low-energy mechanisms of injury, and almost always results in substantial mortality and morbidity. Moreover, neurologic injuries are difficult to manage in that there is often significant secondary injury that can occur in the first few hours and days after the primary injury as the result of the loss of autoregulatory function, histopathologic changes, and edema. The prognosis of neurotrauma patients is often difficult to predict, but almost invariably entails a lengthy and frustrating recovery. According to the Centers for Disease Control and Prevention, from an epidemiological standpoint, approximately 1.5 million traumatic brain injuries (TBIs) are sustained in the United States each year. Of these, 50,000 are fatal, 230,000 result in survivable hospitalizations, and 80,000 to 90,000 will face long-term disability. The estimated cost of TBI in the United States in 1995 was $56.3 billion. Approximately 11,000 new spinal cord injuries (SCIs) occur annually in the United States, and roughly 190,000 Americans currently live with some form of paralysis as the result of SCI. The total cost of SCI in America is roughly $7 billion annually.

DIAGNOSIS OF CNS TRAUMA

The diagnosis of CNS trauma requires an adequate history, clinical examination, and the use of diagnostic imaging and other modalities.

THE CLINICAL EXAM

Despite all of the technologic advancement in critical care medicine, the most definitive and valuable indicator of neuropathology continues to be the clinical exam. EMS personnel should already be familiar with basic neurologic assessment. However, the critical care paramedic (CCP) who practices a sophisticated neurologic examination is in possession of an extremely valuable and sensitive diagnostic tool that can be employed even in the most austere setting. The findings of a detailed neuro exam are a window into the location of CNS lesions.

Critical care paramedics who experience lengthy transport times should perform a neurologic examination on the critical care neuro patient at least every 2 hours, unless otherwise contraindicated, and whenever clinically appropriate in addition. It is not necessary to assess individual cranial nerves in great detail during transport; however, the critical care paramedic should have a working understanding of the anatomy and physiology of the CNS, as well as the implications of aberrant findings on exam.

The Glasgow Coma Score is an excellent starting point for the neurologic exam. However, it is only one piece of a much larger picture. (See Figure 14-1 ■.)

Infants and Toddlers			Children and Adult		
Eye opening	Spontaneous	4	Eye opening	Spontaneous	4
	To voice	3		To voice	3
	To pain	2		To pain	2
	None	1		None	1
Best verbal response	Smiles, interacts	5	Best verbal response	Oriented	5
	Consolable	4		Confused	4
	Cries to pain	3		Inappropriate words	3
	Moans to pain	2		Incomprehensible words	2
	None	1		None	1
Best motor response	Normal spontaneous movement	6	Best motor response	Obeys commands	6
	Localizes pain	5		Localizes pain	5
	Withdraws to pain	4		Withdraws (pain)	4
	Abnormal flexion	3		Flexion (pain)	3
	Abnormal extension	2		Extension (pain)	2
	None	1		None	1

■ Figure 14-1 Glasgow Coma Scale.

DETAILED NEURO ASSESSMENT
The Conscious Patient

★ If the patient does open his eyes, does he regard the examiner and track her movement?

★ Assess extraocular movement in all extremes of the visual field, noting abnormal findings including nystagmus or gaze restriction.

★ Cover each eye and assess for visual field deficit by asking the patient to look at your nose. Move your wiggling fingers into each of his four visual quadrants and ask him to identify when he can see them in his peripheral vision.

★ Ask the patient about the presence of visual changes. These can include numerous subjective complaints, such as blurred vision, diplopia (double vision), the perception of "floaters," or spots of light floating across the visual field, and loss of vision, either transient or ongoing, in any aspect of his visual field.

★ Assess facial symmetry.

★ Ask the patient to stick out his tongue and say "ah." Look for tongue deviation to one side or the other, as well as bilateral rise of the soft palate.

★ Ask the patient the standard questions of orientation. Be aware, however, that patients may be able to successfully answer these questions but can still be confused. Be alert to strange behavior, affect, repetitive questioning, or other indications of confusion.

★ Assess speech for clarity.

★ Ask the patient to hold out his arms at shoulder height with his palms facing upward, and to close his eyes. This simultaneously assesses for motor weakness and a pronator drift. If unilateral weakness is detected, it can be further evaluated by other motor strength assessments. Pronator drift is specific to the cerebellum, and occurs when there is a loss of visual input to help maintain proprioception. One of the hands will invert, and will sink downward.

★ Cerebellar ataxia can be assessed further in a nonambulatory patient by asking her to point her finger to her own nose, and then to reach out and touch your extended index finger in sequence. As you move your finger about to different positions, assess the patient for the inability to accurately localize your finger in space.

★ Hand grasps are a subjective indicator of basic, gross motor strength, and are not the most sensitive indicator of weakness. Be aware also of other limiting factors when assessing motor strength, such as pain, injury, or old deficit. Also, the grasp reflex is an infantile reflex that may reemerge in patients with substantial neurologic compromise, and must not be mistaken for purposeful movement or the ability to follow commands.

★ Assess motor strength in the legs by asking the patient to lift them against resistance.

★ Ask the patient about paresthesias or other sensory abnormalities.

The Unresponsive Patient

★ If the patient is not responsive, has he been chemically paralyzed? If so, this greatly reduces the efficacy of your neurologic exam, because even cranial nerves are affected by chemical paralysis.

★ If the patient does not open his eyes, lift the lids and see if there is a gaze preference, a disconjugate gaze, or strange eye movement noted? Repetitive or "roving" eye movements may be indicative of seizure activity.

★ Flick your hand toward the patient's face to elicit a reflexive blink. Do they "blink to threat"?

★ Is there overt seizure activity? Any repetitive behavior or focal movement is suspicious for seizure activity.

★ Attempt to elicit a motor response with a brisk sternal rub. Patients who do not give an appropriate response to this should also be assessed by applying nail bed pressure to each extremity.

★ Assess the Babinski reflex by stroking the plantar surface of the foot with a rigid object. The correct technique is performed by using a rigid object and performing a J-shaped scratch or rub in a single smooth motion, starting toward the heel on the lateral aspect of the foot's plantar surface and tracing a line upward and medially along the ball of the foot from the first to fifth toes. Toes that splay outward are a positive, and therefore abnormal, finding, except in children less than 1 year of age. The normal response would be an inward curling of the toes, toward the plantar surface of the foot. Toes that do not respond at all are not considered to be a "positive" (abnormal) finding.

★ Assess for clonus by holding the plantar surface of the foot and rapidly dorsiflexing the ankle (assuming other injuries do not contraindicate this). If rhythmic jerking occurs, clonus is present, and may indicate a seizure state or other abnormal tone.

★ If the patient is not sedated or chemically paralyzed, does he have spontaneous respirations?

★ Touch the surface of each eyeball with a sterile wisp of gauze and assess for a blink. This tests the presence or absence of a corneal reflex, and should be done bilaterally.

★ Insert a rigid tonsil tip suction catheter into the patient's oropharynx and assess both sides for the presence of a gag reflex.

★ Determine if the patient coughs on his endotracheal tube, or if he has a cough reflex in response to deep tracheal suctioning.

★ Is there cerebrospinal fluid (CSF) drainage from the ears, nose, or from a surgically placed drain? If so, this holds a severe potential for infection.

DIAGNOSTIC IMAGING AND PROCEDURES

X-RAYS

Although skull X-rays can be useful in assessing facial fractures and penetrating injury, they are rarely used today. Orthopedic injuries of the spine are generally evaluated with X-rays in addition to other imaging techniques.

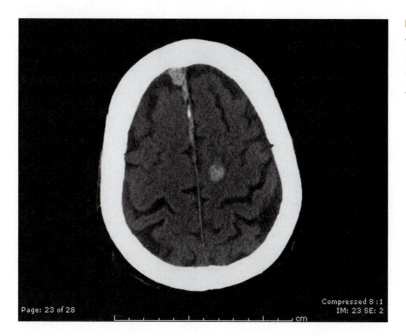

■ Figure 14-2 CT of head with traumatic brain injury. *(Kathy Altergott, BSN, MBA, CRA. Banner Good Samaritan Medical Center, Phoenix, AZ)*

COMPUTED TOMOGRAPHY (CT) SCAN

CT scans have become the standard for acute diagnostic imaging in the presence of neurologic injury. A CT scan is a sensitive indicator of osseous injury, and can detect the presence of blood and changes in tissue density. It is a quick and noninvasive procedure and is of great value in determining the treatment needs of acute patients. (See Figure 14-2 ■.)

MAGNETIC RESONANCE IMAGING (MRI)

The MRI has greater specificity and sensitivity than the CT scan when evaluating soft-tissue changes. However, MRI takes considerably longer to perform than a CT scan, and can be more distressing to the alert patient. Also, patients with certain types of prosthetic implants, pacemakers, or past injury with metallic objects cannot undergo MRI because of the affinity of these objects for the powerful magnet. (See Figure 14-3 ■.)

LUMBAR PUNCTURE

A lumbar puncture involves the insertion of a needle into the subarachnoid space of the lumbar spine below the terminal end of the spinal cord (L4-L5). It allows for a one-time pressure evaluation, as well as collection of CSF for laboratory analysis. This procedure is contraindicated when elevated intracranial pressure (ICP) is suspected.

ELECTROENCEPHALOGRAM (EEG)

This is a device that consists of numerous wires that record brain wave activity. Electroencephalograms are intended to document seizure activity, states of consciousness, and similar brain electrical emission.

HEAD TRAUMA

One of the most essential concepts in neuroscience critical care is that the primary injury sustained by a trauma patient is often only the beginning. Having a high index of suspicion and treating preventively for secondary injury is vital to the reduction of overall morbidity and the preservation of neurologic function.

Figure 14-3 Nuclear magnetic resonance (NMR) image of a crosssection of the head of a person suffering from a subdural hematoma, a condition involving the loss of blood into the space between the brain and skull. Image contrast has been enhanced by prior injection of a gadolinium compound (Gd-DPTA). The blood (indicated by the 2 elongated white areas on left side of brain) builds up and cannot escape; the increased intercranial pressure could endanger life. *(Photo Researchers, Inc.)*

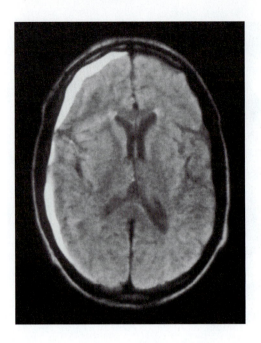

coma *state in which a patient has had no meaningful response to external stimuli for a significant period of time.*

Critical care paramedics should have a working understanding of the terminology used to identify levels of consciousness and neurologic function. Many of these terms are used incorrectly in popular media, and misconceptions may occur among persons who are not educated properly on their meaning. Remember that the reticular activating system is responsible for maintaining our levels of waking consciousness. The term **coma** refers to a state in which a patient has no meaningful response to external stimuli, and implies that this state is ongoing for a significant period of time. The transient unconsciousness that may accompany a concussion is not generally regarded as a "coma." Comatose patients may have nonpurposeful motor responses to noxious stimuli, but they will not react purposefully with any verbal output, motor response, or eye opening response.

Another term that the critical care paramedic should become familiar with is *persistent vegetative state*. This state can be somewhat confusing in that patients may appear awake, with open eyes and the capacity to withdraw from painful stimuli. However, patients in a persistent vegetative state are not clinically or legally regarded to have any higher cognitive function such as thought, purpose, and intent.

On the opposite end of the spectrum from the coma is the state of being "locked in." Lesions that are localized to the brainstem may entirely eliminate a patient's ability to speak, breathe, or move anything but their eyes. Even extraocular movements may be severely affected. However, if the reticular activating system is preserved and the cortex is spared, the patient may in fact have all of their higher cognitive function intact. They literally become a thinking, feeling brain that is "locked in" their own nonfunctional body. Locked-in patients maintain full awareness of their environment, and can hear, see, and understand everything going on around them.

Because the cardiac centers of the brain are well protected, deep in the brainstem, widespread cortical destruction and damage to deeper structures may not necessarily result in cardiac death. A patient may continue to have a heartbeat, and can yet be completely brain dead. Brain death is regarded to be a state of true clinical death. Patients who are determined to be brain dead may even have organs procured for donation while their heart is still capable of beating. However, critical care providers must understand that these patients are actually deceased when brain death is declared. Patients who are brain dead must not be chemically influenced by any medication. They will have pupils that are fixed and nonreactive, generally at the midpoint, and will not have corneal reflexes. They will also lose their occulovestibular reflex. Motor responses will be gone, although decerebration may still occur in the extremities. The patient will also be apneic. Although not a requirement, the absence of brain wave activity on an EEG or the lack of brain perfusion as assessed through cerebral angiography may augment the diagnosis of brain death.

From a histological perspective, neurons are among the most sensitive cells in the body with regard to the potential damage inflicted by hypoperfusion. The neurons of the CNS require a tremendous amount of oxygen and glucose to ensure proper functioning, and have very little reserve to compensate for an interruption in that supply.

Cerebral perfusion pressure (CPP) is a measure of the efficacy of brain perfusion. It is calculated by subtracting the **intracranial pressure** (ICP) from the mean arterial pressure (MAP). A CPP of less than 60 mmHg is suggestive of hypoperfusion in adults, and a CPP of less than 40 mmHg indicates hypoperfusion in pediatric populations under 10 years of age.

To ensure that the brain maintains adequate perfusion in spite of fluctuation in the CPP, the brain's vasculature is capable of **autoregulation,** a process of vasoconstriction and vasodilation that controls cerebral blood flow (CBF). If the CPP rises, the cerebral arterial system vasoconstricts in order to decrease CBF. Decreased CPP results in vasodilation to improve CBF and ensure adequate perfusion. This autoregulatory mechanism, however, is unable to compensate for a CPP lower than 60 mmHg or greater than 160 mmHg. Other causes of autoregulatory impairment include head injury and certain vasoactive medications. Patients who suffer from chronic hypertension develop autoregulatory mechanisms that are accustomed to elevated blood pressure. Therefore, autoregulation within this population may be too impaired to respond appropriately to hypotension relative to the patient's MAP, even if numerically they appear normotensive when compared to the average patient.

If autoregulation is overwhelmed in the presence of decreased CPP, cerebral ischemia and tissue death occur. Decreased CPP is generally the result of an increased ICP from direct injury or advancing secondary injury, or from systemic hypotension from comorbid injuries. Frequently, both of these mechanisms can be found in the multisystem trauma patient. The clinical picture of a traumatically injured patient with elevated ICP due to head injury and decreased MAP subsequent to other injuries inducing hypovolemia is quite common. As cerebral ischemia progresses, the hypoperfused, injured brain tissue begins to swell. This results in a further elevation of ICP and further reduction of CPP. (See Figure 14-4 ■.)

The brain's arterial system also responds to changing levels of serum carbon dioxide (PCO_2), and, to a lesser extent, serum hypoxia (PO_2). Hypercapnia causes cerebral vasodilation, which results in increased CBF and further elevates ICP. Hypocapnia, which can be achieved by therapeutic hyperventilation, will reduce ICP by causing vasoconstriction. However, vasoconstriction also results in local hypoperfusion resulting in further ischemia. (See Figure 14-5 ■.)

Histopathologic changes also occur on a cellular level: As anaerobic metabolism replaces aerobic metabolism in ischemic cells, lactate and other damaging acids are produced. The number of calcium ions and oxidating free radicals that cause further cellular damage also increase.

cerebral perfusion pressure (CPP) *measures efficacy of brain perfusion, determined by subtracting the intracranial pressure from the mean arterial pressure. Represented in formula as: MAP−ICP = CPP.*

intracranial pressure (ICP) *the pressure within the cranial vault.*

autoregulation *inherent ability of the arterial system within the brain to adjust in attempts to maintain adequate cerebral perfusion, despite changes in systemic pressure.*

1. Normal ICP 0–10 mmHg.

2. Increase in volume shows little change in pressure due to compensation.

3. Maximum compensation.

4. Small volume increase results in large pressure increase. Compliance is lost.

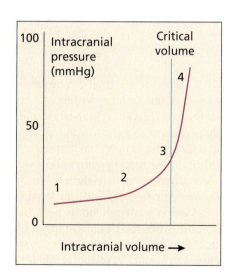

■ **Figure 14-4** Intracranial pressure volume curves.

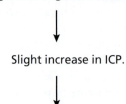

Figure 14-5 Traumatic brain injury.

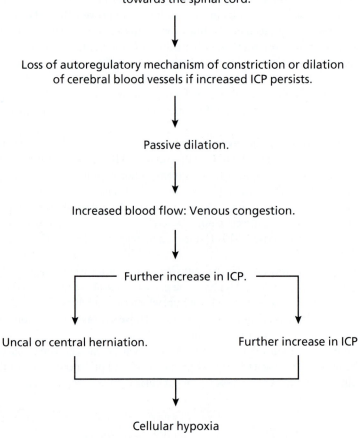

- Trauma
- Cerebral edema
- Hydrocephalus (following surgery, infection, hypoxia, SAH)
- A space-occupying lesion (e.g., abscess)

↓

Slight increase in ICP.

↓

Attempt at regulation of ICP by decreased blood flow to head, movement of CSF towards the spinal cord.

↓

Loss of autoregulatory mechanism of constriction or dilation of cerebral blood vessels if increased ICP persists.

↓

Passive dilation.

↓

Increased blood flow: Venous congestion.

↓

Further increase in ICP.

Uncal or central herniation.   Further increase in ICP

↓

Cellular hypoxia
+
Death

Cerebral edema itself can be subdivided into two etiological categories. Cytotoxic edema occurs when intracellular swelling results from tissue insult or a sudden accumulation of intracellular fluid, such as can occur in severe and rapidly achieved hyponatremia. The anaerobic metabolism that occurs in response to ischemia causes individual brain cells to become deficient in ATP, which is essential for proper functioning of the sodium-potassium (Na-K) pump of active transport. When the Na-K pump fails, sodium accumulates within the cell, causing the intracellular fluid to become hypertonic in relation to the extracellular fluid. Water then rushes into the cell to maintain the concentration gradient, causing the cell to swell.

Vasogenic edema tends to be more localized, and is caused by an increase in interstitial fluid. It occurs when local lesions or insult causes increased vascular permeability within the capillaries that form the blood–brain barrier, resulting in the leakage of proteins into the interstitium. This creates an osmotic gradient that then pulls fluid from the intravascular space, resulting in interstitial edema.

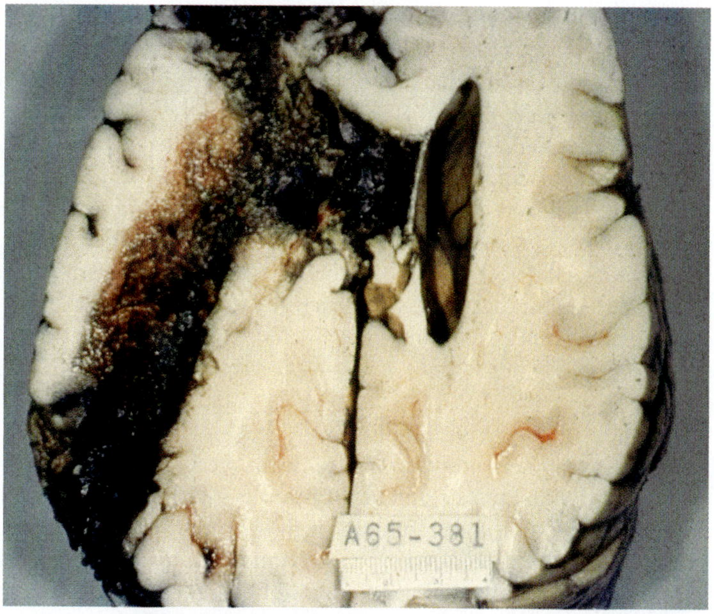

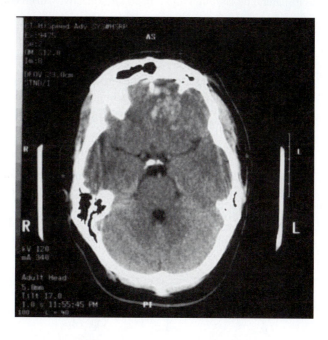

■ **Figure 14-6A** Bullet injury to the brain.

■ **Figure 14-6B** CT of cerebral contusion. *(Edward T. Dickinson, MD)*

The relationship between space-occupying lesions and intracranial pressure is defined by the **Monroe-Kellie hypothesis.** This doctrine states that there are three substances within the fixed space of the intracranial vault as defined by the skull and dura mater: brain tissue, blood, and CSF. If one of these substances accumulates as the result of pathology, there must be a compensatory reduction in one or both of the other components. Otherwise, there will be an increase in ICP. (See Figure 14-6 ■ .)

Normal ICP ranges from 0 to 10 mmHg. ICP values greater than 10 mmHg are considered elevated, and values greater than 20 mmHg are generally treated in the critical care setting. Transient spikes occur in healthy individuals for a variety of reasons, including sneezing, coughing, or straining at defecation. However, the ICP resolves almost immediately to its normal level after these activities cease. The damage caused by elevated ICP is defined by three factors: the amount of pressure achieved, the duration of the elevation, and the speed with which the elevation occurred. For example, while sneezing, a healthy individual's ICP may rise to 40 mmHg; however, this elevation lasts for no more than a second or two before returning to normal, and no damage

Monroe-Kellie hypothesis *the intracranial vault is a fixed space that contains brain tissue, blood, and cerebrospinal fluid. Volume expansion of any (or all) of these components will increase ICP unless the volume of one of the other components is reduced.*

is incurred. Patients with slow-growing tumors may have elevated ICP for quite some time and may be largely asymptomatic. Patients with a similar ICP value that is achieved rapidly as the result of an acute intracranial hemorrhage may be in immediate danger of herniation or other severe secondary injury.

One of the earliest compensatory mechanisms that occur within the cranial vault in response to cerebral edema and elevated ICP is the compression of the low-pressure venous system. If cerebral edema is allowed to progress unchecked, it will begin to displace the brain away from the expanding mass, a process known as *mass effect*. This ultimately causes the movement of brain tissue into anatomical defects and spaces that offer less resistance, as well as compression of specific regions of the brain against fixed structures within the skull's architecture, creating predictable *herniation syndromes*. (See Figure 14-7 ■.)

TENTORIAL (UNCAL) HERNIATION

tentorium cerebelli *section of dura mater invaginated into the cranial vault, forming a barrier between the cerebrum and the cerebellum, and defined by the posterior fossa.*

Tentorial (uncal) herniation is a syndrome that occurs above the **tentorium cerebelli** whereby a unilateral mass lesion causes a shift of the brain in a lateral vector away from it. The medial edge of the temporal lobe, or *uncus*, herniates through the tentorial hiatus. If untreated, this can ultimately lead to central herniation. Some common signs and symptoms include a depressed level of consciousness (LOC) from compression of components of the reticular activating system in the midbrain, as well as ipsilateral ptosis, pupil dilation, and nonreactivity from compression of the occulomotor nerve.

CENTRAL TENTORIAL HERNIATION

Central tentorial herniation occurs when either diffuse or midline lesions push the midbrain and diencephalon downward through the tentorial hiatus. In addition to a depressed LOC, the patient may have impaired eye movements, as well as bilaterally constricted pupils that eventually become fixed at midpoint.

SUBFALCINE HERNIATION

Subfalcine herniation is an early form of lateral herniation that occurs when the midline of the brain is pushed laterally underneath the falx cerebri. It is commonly known as *midline shift*. Signs

■ Figure 14-7 Anatomic basis of herniation syndromes. An expanding supratentorial mass lesion may cause brain tissue to be displaced into an adjacent intracranial compartment, resulting in (1) cingulated herniation under the falx, (2) downward transtentorial (central) herniation, (3) uncal herniation over the edge of the tentorium, or (4) cerebellar tonsillar herniation into the foramen magnum. Coma and ultimately death result when (2), (3), or (4) produces brainstem compression.

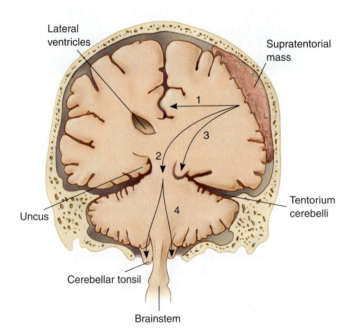

and symptoms of this herniation syndrome depend on the degree of shift and the speed with which it develops.

TONSILLAR HERNIATION

Posterior fossa lesions and severe supratentorial lesions producing central tentorial herniation may result in the herniation of the cerebellar tonsils through the foramen magnum at the base of the skull. Some degree of upward herniation may also initially occur. Tonsillar herniation will ultimately result in brainstem compression, leading to cardiopulmonary arrest.

Hydrocephalus is a term used to describe the abnormal accumulation of cerebrospinal fluid in the brain. The etiological origin of hydrocephalus may vary, and its severity depends on the volume of CSF accumulated, as well as the speed with which it developed. Rarely, hydrocephalus may be caused by hypersecretory tumors of the choroid plexus. More commonly, hydrocephalus occurs when circulation throughout the subarachnoid space is obstructed by a space-occupying lesion such as a tumor or edema, or when the arachnoid villi are occluded and overwhelmed, such as by blood in a subarachnoid hemorrhage. As dictated by the Monroe-Kellie hypothesis, CSF accumulation can cause local mass effect and a dangerous elevation of ICP. (See Figure 14-8 ▪.)

hydrocephalus describes the abnormal accumulation of cerebrospinal fluid in the brain.

Diabetes insipidus, or DI, is an endocrine disorder that may result from compression of or damage to the hypothalamus or posterior pituitary gland, and may be a sign of advanced central herniation. Essentially the neuroendocrine structures responsible for the release of antidiuretic hormone (ADH) are impaired. The result is a deficiency of ADH, which renders the body incapable of conserving water. The patient will present clinically by dumping large volumes of dilute urine. Although the patient appears to be well hydrated because of his high urine output, he in fact becomes severely dehydrated. Failure to correct DI with hormone replacement can cause hypovolemia, hemodynamic instability, and severe hypernatremia.

Syndrome of inappropriate antidiuretic hormone (SIADH) is the opposite of DI, in that the production of ADH is excessive, resulting in the retention of water by the kidneys. The patient will void only small amounts of highly concentrated urine. Clinically, such patients are at risk for severe fluid volume overload, as well as dilutional hyponatremia. Abnormally low serum osmolality can exacerbate cerebral edema.

Cerebral salt-wasting syndrome is a somewhat mysterious but well-documented complication of brain insult whereby patients lose excessive sodium in their urine. Unlike SIADH, it does not involve ADH secretion, and in fact its etiology is uncertain. However, significant hyponatremia may result if exogenous salt and other medications promoting sodium reabsorption are not administered.

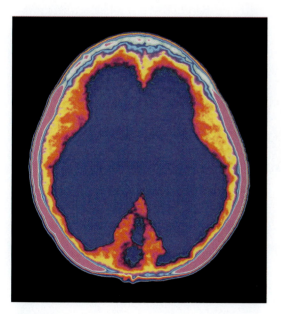

▪ **Figure 14-8** Hydrocephalus. Colored computed tomography (CT) scan of an axial (horizontal) section through the brain of a child with hydrocephalus (water on the brain). The fluid-filled ventricles (purple) have been enlarged by the excessive production, or blockage in the circulation, of the cerebrospinal fluid (CSF) that fills the spaces in and around the brain and spinal cord. (*Photo Researchers, Inc.*)

INTRACRANIAL PRESSURE MONITORING

ICP monitoring is an important tool in the critical care setting that helps to ensure optimal management of the head-injured patient. ICP monitoring devices must be inserted by an experienced neurosurgeon and carefully maintained by the critical care team. Several types are in use, each offering its own advantages and disadvantages.

VENTRICULOSTOMY AND EXTRAVENTRICULAR DRAIN (EVD)

external auditory meatus (EAM) *external landmark, a.k.a. the "ear canal." Visually correlates with the level of the lateral ventricles within the brain.*

This is a technique whereby a fluid-filled catheter is inserted into one of the ventricles of the brain, typically the lateral ventricle of the patient's nondominant side. The catheter is connected to a pressure transducer, which is maintained at the level of the **external auditory meatus (EAM),** a reliable external landmark that correlates with the level of the lateral ventricles within the brain. The transducer records an ICP waveform on a monitor. This technique is generally regarded as the standard for ICP monitoring; however, it also holds the greatest risk of complication. (See Figure 14-9 ■.)

★ *Advantages:* The EVD's greatest advantage is that CSF can be drained into a sterile collection bag from the ventricular system to allow for reduction in ICP. It also allows quick and easy access to the CSF for sampling.

★ *Disadvantages:* The EVD catheter itself travels through a hole in the skull and directly into the ventricular system, creating a vulnerable route for infection. The insertion procedure is highly invasive and can be difficult to achieve if the ventricles are compressed by intracranial pathology. The catheter can easily break or become dislodged. Occasionally the catheter is rendered useless when clogged by clotted blood or pieces of gray matter. External CSF leakage from the site of the insertion is another possible complication. Because the transducer is pressure dependent, it must be maintained at the level of the EAM at all times in order to ensure accurate readings. Thus, it must be continually checked and repositioned when the patient's position changes. The EVD's drainage system is also pressure dependent, and thus there is a risk of overdrainage of CSF from the ventricles in the event that the open system is lowered (or dropped) below the EAM.

■ **Figure 14-9** Major types of intracranial pressure monitoring. Coronal section of the brain shows potential sites for placement of the monitoring devices.

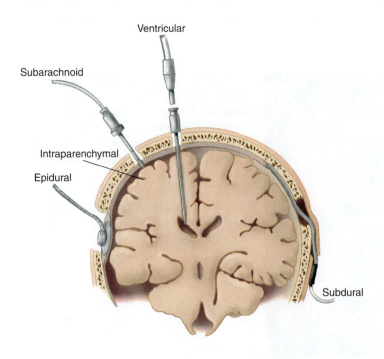

Ventricular

Subarachnoid

Intraparenchymal

Epidural

Subdural

FIBER-OPTIC BOLT

This device can be placed into a variety of areas of the brain, but is generally inserted directly into the parenchyma. It records a pressure waveform based on pressure waves transmitted through the brain tissue itself and is perhaps the most commonly used device in patients with cerebral edema subsequent to head trauma.

★ *Advantages:* Can be placed quickly and easily, regardless of anatomical changes related to edema or similar injury. It has a relatively lower risk of infection than EVD, and does not require repositioning to ensure accurate readings. There is less "baseline drift," or change in the measurement accuracy of the bolt, than with other types of ICP monitoring devices.

★ *Disadvantages:* The fiber-optic bolt can be easily damaged, and must be calibrated properly upon initial insertion, because it cannot be recalibrated after the procedure is complete. It does not allow access to CSF for ICP management or sampling. The bolt becomes increasingly inaccurate as time passes.

SUBARACHNOID SCREW

No longer in common use.

★ *Advantages:* Quick and easy placement that does not entail parenchymal involvement.

★ *Disadvantages:* Less accurate than other devices, particularly in the setting of markedly elevated ICP. It requires frequent leveling, similar to the EVD, but provides no access to CSF. The potential for external CSF leakage and infection remains.

THE ICP WAVEFORM

The **ICP waveform** is generated by the pulsations created by the cardiovascular system, which translate through the cerebrospinal fluid into the brain parenchyma via the choroid plexus. The waveform itself appears similar to an arterial line waveform and is, in fact, the result of arterial pulsation.

There are three primary components of the waveform. The first of these, P_1, is formed by each systolic arterial pulsation hitting the choroid plexus. In the healthy patient, P_1 should be the highest portion of the ICP waveform. P_2, the second waveform component, can be variable in size, and is reflective of the compliance present within the brain. P_3 follows P_2, and is reflective of the closing of the semilunar valves in the cardiac cycle. It is similar to the dichrotic notch on the arterial line waveform.

In the normal ICP waveform, P_1 should be the highest component, followed by P_2 and then P_3, in a pattern reminiscent of a descending staircase. (See Figure 14-10 ■.) When brain compliance is impaired, however, as in the case of intracranial hypertension or cerebral edema, P_2 may become elevated over P_1.

In addition to assessment of the components of the waveform and their relationship to one another, the waveform itself must be assessed to determine if the ICP value given is accurate. As with A-line and central line tracings, ICP wave tracings can be dampened or altered for a variety of reasons, producing falsely high or low numbers.

Patients who have undergone neurosurgical bone flap removal for ICP management may have abnormally muted waveforms that are lacking in clear P waves. This is an expected finding based on the changes in brain compliance caused by the absence of a portion of the skull.

ICP waveform
representation of the pulsations created by the cardiovascular system, translated through CSF into the brain parenchyma via the choroid plexus.

THE EXTRAVENTRICULAR DRAIN

This is an extremely valuable tool for ICP monitoring and management. However, EVDs that are operated by poorly trained or inexperienced personnel hold the potential for significant detriment to the patient.

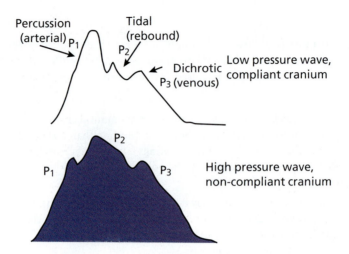

Figure 14-10 Intracranial pressure changes.

Percussion (arterial) P₁

Tidal (rebound) P₂

Dichrotic P₃ (venous)

Low pressure wave, compliant cranium

P₁ P₂ P₃ High pressure wave, non-compliant cranium

- **P1: Percussion wave**: sharp peak, constant amplitude reflects pulse.
- **P2: Tidal wave**: shape and amplitude variable, ends on dichrotic notch; indicates cerebral compliance
- **P3: Dichrotic wave**: immediately following the dichrotic notch

As ICP increases, the amplitude of the pulse pressure wave increases.

Most EVDs consist of a flexible catheter that extends into the patient's ventricle, which is then tunneled under the scalp for a short distance and sutured in place. It is then covered with a sterile, bio-occlusive dressing. Critical care transport providers should always ensure that the catheter is properly sutured prior to patient transfer, because the catheter can become easily dislodged.

The catheter travels a short distance until it attaches to a three-way stopcock. This stopcock is critical for determining whether the drainage portion is in the "open" or "closed" position. The catheter should also be securely fastened to the stopcock to ensure that no break in the sterile, enclosed system occurs. This is typically accomplished with suture thread.

Also connected to the stopcock is the pressure recording system. A piece of tubing filled with preservative-free saline travels back to the transducer, which is held at the EAM at all times. The transducer is then connected to a wire that will translate the measured ICP values and waveform onto the monitor. Beneath the transducer, a syringe filled with preservative-free saline allows the tubing to be flushed to clear debris that might occlude the drainage system. Although this design is very similar to an arterial line setup, it should NEVER be connected to a bag of IV fluid.

Directly across from the EVD catheter, the drainage system attaches to the stopcock. This consists of a length of semirigid plastic tubing that extends back to a collection burette. At the base of the burette, an additional stopcock allows the burette to be periodically opened so that its contents may drain into a collection bag. This stopcock should remain closed at all times to allow regular documentation of the volume of CSF drained into the burette, typically performed every 2 hours or so. Leaving the stopcock in an open position will allow CSF to drain directly into the bag, making accurate measurement impossible.

Above all else, it is essential to remember that the EVD provides a gravity-dependent, open pathway between the patient's ventricular system and the environment. The critical care paramedic must always be cognizant of the fact that changes in the patient's or the device's positioning will have implications both on the measured ICP and the rate of drainage of CSF into the collection system. Here are some general guidelines:

★ Always confirm the prescribed level at which the drain is to be maintained in relation to the EAM, as well as whether or not the drain is to be maintained in an open or closed position. The level of the drain is determined by where the drain's opening into the collection chamber will be held, which determines how quickly CSF will drain and at what relative pressure. It is commonly held from 15 cm above the EAM to 10 cm below, depending on the patient's requirements.

★ If the drain is to be kept closed, confirm the order dictating the circumstances whereby it should be opened. Often, drains that are closed will be opened to drain CSF in the event of a sustained ICP of greater than 20 mmHg.

★ If the drain is to be kept open, be aware that it cannot accurately measure an ICP in this position. Therefore, the ICP must be periodically spot-checked by closing the drain. Generally, the frequency of ICP value measurement will be ordered, but should also be performed at any time when the patient's condition warrants it, such as during an acute change in mental status.

★ If the drain is kept in the open position and is not turned off to the transducer, a waveform and ICP value will continue to be recorded. Although this is not as accurate a measurement as a "closed" ICP, it can be an early indicator of pathologic change or device failure even when not "spot-checking." Thus, the EVD should not be turned off to the transducer under normal circumstances.

★ If the drain is to be maintained in an open position, it MUST be closed to prevent excessive drainage of CSF any time the patient is repositioned at all. Always maintain the EVD in a closed position during patient transfer until the patient is in a stable position that will allow the drain to be reliably set at its prescribed level.

★ Regardless of drain position, the transducer should always be maintained at the level of the EAM in order to record an accurate pressure. Again, the drain must be closed and a reliable waveform apparent on the monitor in order for the device to measure ICP.

★ Be alert to sudden increases in drainage, or changes in the character of the drainage. CSF is typically a clear, somewhat straw-colored fluid. In the presence of intraventricular or subarachnoid blood, the drainage will be blood tinged or may even appear as frank blood. Turbid or cloudy CSF may be indicative of infection. Always determine the baseline appearance of the CSF prior to transport—a sudden change in the character of the CSF may be indicative of further acute pathology.

PROCEDURES

OPENING AND CLOSING THE DRAINAGE SYSTEM

★ Don appropriate body substance isolation (BSI) gear. Nonsterile gloves are adequate.

★ Hold the drainage catheter secure to ensure that it is not pulled or damaged during device manipulation.

★ Turn the stopcock upward to maintain the system in a position open to both drainage and pressure monitoring.

★ Turn the stopcock off to the drainage system to reposition the drain or the patient, or to record an ICP.

★ Ensure that the drain is left in the prescribed position after all manipulation is complete.

BALANCING THE TRANSDUCER

★ Don appropriate BSI gear.

★ Hold a leveling device next to the transducer. Several types are available, including carpentry-type levels and laser devices.

★ Place the other end of the level or laser dot onto the patient's external auditory meatus.

★ Change the height of the transducer to ensure that it is in line with the leveling device.

ZEROING THE MONITOR

★ Don appropriate BSI gear.

★ Turn the catheter's stopcock off to the drainage system.

★ Turn the stopcock between the collection burette and the collection bag upward. There is a small fluid-filled opening to the right of the transducer with a dead-end cap on it. Unscrew this cap, thereby making the transducer open to the air.

★ Press the "zero" button on your monitor and wait until the recorded value is zero.

★ Replace the cap, and turn all stopcocks back to their appropriate position.

★ Ensure that the recorded values and waveform seem clinically appropriate.

EMPTYING THE COLLECTION BURETTE

★ Don appropriate BSI gear.

★ Turn the stopcock on the EVD catheter off to the drainage system. Failure to do so may result in unwanted and unrecorded drainage of CSF during this procedure.

★ Record the CSF present within the collection burette.

★ Open the stopcock between the burette and collection bag and allow the CSF to passively drain.

★ When drainage is complete, return all stopcocks to their original positions.

EMPTYING THE COLLECTION BAG

★ The EVD collection system is a closed, sterile system, which helps to decrease the risk of infection. However, periodically, the collection bag must be emptied as it fills with CSF. Typically, this action should only be performed when the bag is completely full to reduce the chances of introducing infection into the closed system. It may be prudent, however, for the critical care paramedic to empty a partially filled system prior to transport, to reduce the risk of dislodging or puncturing the bag.

★ The base of the bag should have some sort of cap or connection for drainage. After determining the type of connection, have all supplies ready to perform the drainage procedure.

★ Don appropriate BSI gear. Nonsterile gloves are acceptable.

★ Remove any protective caps and swab the area with Betadine. If the cap is removed, it should be placed on a sterile surface.

★ Open the drainage system and remove the CSF from the bag. This is often accomplished by removing a cap and screwing in a Luer-Lok-type attachment, which is connected to a length of tubing and a vacuum collection bag.

★ After drainage is complete, swab the area again, and replace the protective cap securely.

FLUSHING THE COLLECTION SYSTEM

Note: This is a potentially dangerous procedure, and should only be performed by trained individuals as a last resort to maintain collection system patency.

★ Don appropriate BSI gear.

★ Record and drain any CSF present in the collection burette.

★ Turn the stopcock on the EVD catheter off to the catheter itself, so that no open portal exists between the catheter and the rest of the system.

★ Gently pull the "pigtail"-like device on the pressure transducer. This opens a plastic valve within the transducer that allows fluid to be pushed through it.

- There should be a preconnected syringe filled with preservative-free saline just beneath the pressure transducer.
- While holding the transducer's valve open, gently depress the syringe's plunger and flush several cc's of saline through the system.
- Watch carefully to ensure that fluid is being flushed into the collection burette.
- If resistance is met, do not force the plunger. The system must be evaluated by a neurosurgeon.
- After the tubing is flushed, release the pigtail valve and drain the accumulated material in the collection burette.
- Turn all stopcocks back to their appropriate positions and reevaluate the recorded waveform and ICP.
- Failure to close the stopcock to the EVD catheter will result in the flushing of saline directly into the ventricles of the patient's brain. It is absolutely imperative that the critical care provider ensures this stopcock is in the proper position prior to flushing the drainage system.

TROUBLESHOOTING THE EVD

CESSATION OF DRAINAGE

Cessation of drainage in the EVD may indicate occlusion in the CSF drainage system, but may also be an expected finding in the setting of overdrained or effaced ventricles. If no drainage is noted for a period of time, the collection burette may be quickly lowered below its prescribed level to assess for the presence of CSF drainage. The collection system may also be carefully flushed to determine the presence of occlusion. A lack of drainage may indicate the need for intervention by a neurosurgeon.

ABSENCE OF WAVEFORM

Ensure that the entire system is leveled and zeroed properly. Ensure that the three-way stopcock at the end of the EVD catheter is turned off to the collection burette, but not to the line connected to the pressure transducer.

GROSSLY ABNORMAL OR NEGATIVE ICP VALUES

The most important cause to rule out is overt pathologic change. Sudden spikes in ICP may well be the result of further disease progression. Ensure that the system is leveled and zeroed properly, and that the stopcocks are set appropriately for ICP recording. Ensure that the system is draining to rule out the presence of catheter occlusion. Negative values may indicate an improperly calibrated monitoring device or "overdrained" ventricles.

ABNORMAL WAVEFORM

Again, this may be the result of pathologic changes or of equipment maladjustment and improper calibration.

TROUBLESHOOTING THE FIBER-OPTIC BOLT

The fiber-optic bolt is commonly utilized for ICP measurement in trauma patients since it can be easily inserted and is not dependent on ventricular size. In the absence of hydrocephalus, the lateral ventricles are often obscured and effaced in patients with significant cerebral edema. Thus, EVDs are often of little use in these patients, and may be extremely difficult to place. The ICP bolt is also easily transported, and is not dependent on positioning for accurate measurement. Critical care paramedics must take care with the device, however, because it can easily be broken. Once inserted, the device requires little maintenance, with the exception of periodically zeroing the monitor to which it connects. Again, it should be covered with a sterile, bio-occlusive dressing. As with all graphic monitoring devices, accuracy should be determined by the morphology of the waveform, as well as by the patient's clinical presentation.

ADDITIONAL MONITORING DEVICES

Because cerebral perfusion pressure is so heavily dependent on mean arterial pressure, patients undergoing ICP monitoring should ideally have an arterial line in place to allow for continuous blood pressure monitoring. Central venous access is also ideal, preferably in the subclavicular or internal jugular veins to allow for accurate central venous pressure monitoring.

A number of experimental monitors on the market today are designed to augment CPP monitoring. One of the more proven devices is the Licox ™ Brain Oxygen Saturation Monitor, manufactured by Integra Neuroscience. This device is inserted concurrently with a fiber-optic ICP bolt. In addition to recording the ICP and CPP, the Licox monitor allows for accurate assessment of the actual oxygen saturation of the brain tissue itself. Jugular bulbs are occasionally inserted to assess mixed venous oxygen saturation in the jugular vein, to determine how much oxygen the brain is extracting from the blood perfusing it.

These additional therapeutic modalities offer exciting potential for the future of head injury management.

SURGICAL MANAGEMENT OF HEAD TRAUMA

The fragile nature of the brain restricts the degree of surgical intervention that can be performed to manage head injury without causing further detriment. The most easily managed traumatic lesions, from a surgical perspective, are those that are localized and relatively superficial. Deeper or more diffuse injuries are often deemed surgically inaccessible.

★ *Skull fractures.* Depressed skull fractures can be surgically elevated and secured. Nondisplaced fractures are not generally intervened upon.

★ *Subdural hematoma (SDH).* SDHs are generally evacuated through burr holes, which are small holes placed in the skull in the area of the hematoma so that the clot can be drained out with a vacuum.

★ *Epidural hematoma (EDH).* Clots from EDH can also be evacuated by similar means to that of SDH.

★ *Intraparenchymal hemorrhage (IPH).* IPH tend to be deep and nonoperable.

★ *Cerebral contusion.* These types of contusions are also generally nonoperable since they tend to be diffuse lesions, unless lobectomy is performed.

★ *Hemicraniectomy with bone flap removal.* A hemicraniectomy is a procedure that is essentially designed to reverse the Monroe-Kellie hypothesis. A segment of the skull of variable size is removed completely from the patient's head in order to decompress the cranial vault and prevent secondary crushing injury from edema by allowing the brain tissue room to swell. The scalp is then sutured closed over the defect. Because bone is living tissue, it is generally implanted into the abdominal wall to allow continued perfusion until it can be reimplanted via cranioplasty at a later time. This treatment modality works best with focal lesions and edema, but can be employed for more diffuse lesions as well, as in the case of severe cerebral edema, and is occasionally radical enough to involve both sides of the skull. Obviously, the critical care paramedic must take great care to protect the portion of the head without the bone flap from injury. (See Figure 14-11 ■.)

★ *Lobectomy.* A lobectomy is a radical procedure that is sometimes performed in the setting of severe cerebral edema and intracranial hypertension, or occasionally in the event of an irreparably contused local segment of the brain. An entire lobe, most

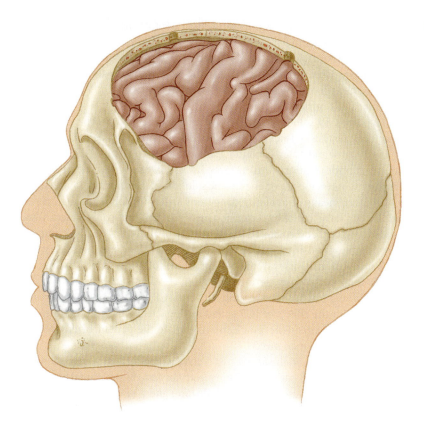

commonly one of the temporal lobes, is excised and removed from the brain. This is generally done with an overlying bone flap removal to allow sparing of the remaining brain in the setting of severe edema.

BEDSIDE MANAGEMENT OF INTRACRANIAL HYPERTENSION

Elevated ICP can cause rapid damage to brain structures, and can be difficult to combat in the presence of severe edema or other injury. However, the critical care paramedic can do several things to manage elevated ICP and help to reduce patient morbidity.

Prior to initiating transport, the critical care paramedic should determine if there is any restriction present on the patient's positioning. The presence of a cervical collar does not necessarily preclude a patient from being maintained in a semi-Fowler's position. Elevating the head of the bed is a simple, rapid intervention that can have an immediate impact on the patient's ICP. If the patient is to be maintained supine in full spinal immobilization, the critical care providers should remember that this restriction only applies to patients with regard to the immobilization device itself. In other words, nothing prevents the critical care providers from elevating the entire patient and backboard by placing bulky material or pillows underneath the top of the backboard, maintaining the linear spinal alignment but elevating the patient's head nonetheless. If the patient is secured properly on the backboard, the entire board can be elevated in a sort of "reverse Trendelenburg" position to help decrease ICP.

ICP is also very dependent on the venous outflow tracts of the venous sinus drainage system. These low-pressure vessels are compressed early in the pathologic changes of intracranial hypertension. Any impedance to the outflow of venous blood from the brain by compression of the veins in the neck may have a significant impact on the ICP. This impedance can be relieved by ensuring that the head and neck are in a neutral alignment, and that cervical collars are not excessively tight. Extreme flexion of the limbs can also contribute to elevated ICP.

An elevated body temperature may occur in response to the stress of injury, infection, or even as the direct result of hypothalamic compression. Fevers can potentiate further secondary insult by increasing the basal metabolic demand, and therefore the oxygen consumption requirements, of an already stressed patient.

Elevated blood glucose has also been proven to occur in response to the stress of severe brain injury. Hyperglycemia is detrimental to the head-injured patient, and is a poor prognostic indicator. Thus, head-injured patients should receive frequent blood glucose monitoring and should be maintained at a normoglycemic level.

Hypotonic IV solutions and free water can be rapidly absorbed by edematous brain tissue, causing an exacerbation and worsening of the edema. Thus, providers must take care to avoid administering any dextrose and water-containing solutions that are not rendered isotonic by the addition of 0.9% sodium chloride solution. Also, intravenous admixtures should never be mixed in dextrose with water solution unless the use of an isotonic solution such as normal saline is absolutely contraindicated.

Another means of avoiding dangerous spikes in ICP is through careful handling of patients with known intracranial hypertension and poor cerebral compliance. Manipulation of the patient should be limited and clustered together so as to allow elevated ICP ample time to resolve between spikes. For example, if the patient requires endotracheal suctioning, try to coordinate with the patient's neuro exam. This way, the patient is able to return to his baseline in between insults, rather than having a persistently elevated ICP from repeated stimulation.

Suctioning can have a dramatic effect on ICP, but is obviously necessary to ensure airway patency. To blunt the effects of ICP spikes during suctioning secondary to hypoxia and hypercarbia, the critical care paramedic should preoxygenate the patient briefly with 100% oxygen before all planned suctioning maneuvers.

There was a time in the recent past when therapeutic hyperventilation was the standard of care in the EMS setting for all patients suffering from suspected intracranial hypertension. The reason for this is that hypercapnia causes cerebral vasodilation and a resultant increase in CBF, thus increasing ICP. Hyperventilating a patient will reduce his ICP dramatically. However, research has shown that the resultant hypocapnia will not only decrease ICP, but cause hypoperfusion (and therefore ischemia) secondary to vasoconstriction as well. Furthermore, it has been demonstrated that this effect is temporary, and becomes less effective as it continues to be used. Thus, it is no longer recommended that critical care paramedics routinely hyperventilate their patients to reduce ICP. Permutations of this technique are still valuable for temporary intervention, however, as in the case of ETT suctioning. It can also be utilized under dire circumstances in the setting of impending herniation when more definitive intervention is at hand but not immediately available. It is believed that the optimal PCO_2 for patients with intracranial hypertension is in the range of 30 to 35 mmHg, slightly but not dramatically hypocapnic.

Although it has been common practice to use permissive hypotension in modern EMS, one must be sure the patient has an adequate mean arterial pressure to overcome any increased intracranial pressure to ensure cerebral perfusion.

HYPOTHERMIA

The role of therapeutic hypothermia in brain-injured patients is now being actively explored. This technique was initially developed to improve survival rates after successful resuscitation from cardiac arrest. It has been demonstrated that a reduction in the body core temperature may decrease the progression of cerebral edema after brain injury occurs, thereby reducing ICP and improving outcome. Therapeutic hypothermia is achieved through a variety of passive and invasive techniques, and to varying extents. Research continues to analyze the benefit of therapeutic hypothermia in brain-injured patients, as well as the safest and most effective means of achieving it. This technique may eventually become significant in the prehospital environment as it continues to be developed. However, extensive evidence-based research needs to be conducted before this protocol can be considered a standard of care.

Hypoxia and hypercapnia in the prehospital setting have been associated with increased mortality and should be avoided.

PHARMACOLOGIC INTERVENTION FOR HEAD TRAUMA

Elevated ICP subsequent to cerebral edema is most effectively controlled by the reduction of brain tissue mass. This is primarily accomplished by the administration of medications that reduce the volume of edema fluid within the brain tissue. In cases where medical therapy alone is inadequate, surgical intervention may be required. This can include the insertion of extraventricular drains to allow the reduction of CSF, allowing for greater room for increasing brain tissue mass, in accordance with the Monroe-Kellie hypothesis. This intervention may not always be appropriate, particularly in situations where diffuse edema causes an effacement of the ventricular system and reduction in the size of CSF-filled space. In these more advanced cases, surgical removal of brain tissue may be required to provide adequate space for brain tissue swelling while attenuating the concomitant increase in intracranial pressure that would otherwise result.

MANNITOL

Mannitol is an osmotic diuretic medication made from the sugar alcohol of mannose. When administered intravenously, it has a powerful diuretic effect that pulls intracellular fluid from the brain and decreases cerebral edema, and therefore ICP. Although potentially deleterious in the already hypotensive patient because of its diuretic effects, mannitol is among the first-line agents given to combat intracranial hypertension, specifically in the case of suspected or impending herniation. It is typically given in an IV bolus dose of approximately 1 g/kg, although it is most commonly administered in rounded doses of 50 to 100 g.

Because mannitol has a high tendency to crystallize, it must be administered with an in-line filter to prevent the infusion of precipitate. Crystallization can occur near or below room temperature, and the formation of large crystals can render a dose of mannitol useless. These crystals can be reincorporated into solution form through gentle and even heating of the container if necessary, as through an increase in ambient storage temperature or through the application of heating pads. However, mannitol containers should be regularly evaluated for crystallization and stored appropriately at a temperature of approximately 18°–30° C (65°–85° F) to prevent this complication from interrupting patient care. Mannitol can be given approximately every 6 hours. Because it is a diuretic, it may serve to dehydrate the patient significantly, and thus serum osmolality should be monitored.

Mannitol readily crystallizes and sometimes must be heated to restore the crystals to solution.

HYPERTONIC SALINE

Infusions or bolus doses of sodium chloride with concentrations greater than that which is isotonic with plasma (0.9%) have also been proven to create a powerful osmotic draw to reduce ICP. Hypertonic saline also decreases the inflammation of the cells lining the lumens of blood vessels, improving cerebral blood flow. Research demonstrates that it may reduce histopathologic and neurohormonal changes that contribute to secondary injury after TBI, and may even offer a boost to the immune system. Hypertonic saline helps to elevate the mean arterial pressure without requiring the large volumes that isotonic fluid resuscitation necessitates.

BARBITURATE COMA

Potent barbiturates such as pentobarbital and thiopental may be given for some cases of intracranial hypertension that are refractory to less aggressive management. A state of coma is induced in the patient that is deep enough to eliminate all motor and sensory responses, including reflexive and cranial nerve function. The patient should be monitored with a continuous EEG and therapy is titrated to brain wave activity. This technique is somewhat dated, and its efficacy has been debated, particularly since the induction of a coma state for a prolonged period carries a high risk of side effects. Chief among these is the profound vasodilatory effect of barbiturates and the subsequent hypotension that often accompanies it. This requires aggressive monitoring and management to ensure that adequate MAP and CPP are maintained.

In addition to the reduction of cerebral edema and ICP, pharmacologic agents may further be required to increase CPP through an elevation of the mean arterial pressure. This commonly requires the administration of vasopressor agents such as norepinephrine and phenylephrine. Patients with invasive ICP monitoring devices or known CSF leaks should also be receiving prophylactic broad-spectrum antibiotics such as nafcillin or vancomycin. Neurosurgical patients are generally maintained on steroids such as dexamethasone to reduce postoperative edema, although this is somewhat disputed in the literature and may not be the standard of care in all areas. Corticosteroids can lead to elevated blood glucose levels, which must then be tightly controlled, because even moderate hyperglycemia has been shown to increase morbidity in the brain-injured population. Finally, analgesics, sedatives, and paralytics are also commonly required in the head injured population.

ACUTE SPINAL CORD INJURIES

Acute spinal cord injury (SCI) may result from a wide variety of injury mechanisms and often coexists with other forms of trauma. Histopathologic injury of the spinal cord is as diverse in origin and type as in the cerebrum. Like brain tissue, the spine may be concussed, contused, infarcted, or subject to edema and compression. Injury may be complete or incomplete, and early management is targeted toward the prevention of secondary injury progression in the form of hypoxia and edema.

Complete injury is manifested by the total loss of motor and sensory function below the site of the injury. Depending on the level of the spinal cord lesion, autonomic function may also be impaired. (See Figure 14-12 ■.)

Partial cord syndromes are predictable patterns of deficit based on incomplete injury to the spinal cord in specific physiologically significant regions.

ANTERIOR CORD SYNDROME

Injury to the anterior portion of the spinal cord, often from a traumatically herniated disk, causes the loss of pain and temperature sensation below the level of the lesion, with sparing of touch, vibration, and position sense. There may be incomplete or total loss of motor function.

CENTRAL CORD SYNDROME

This syndrome occurs when the center portion of the spinal cord is damaged, generally as the result of hematoma formation, infarction, or hypoxia. It is most often noted with hyperextension injuries, and

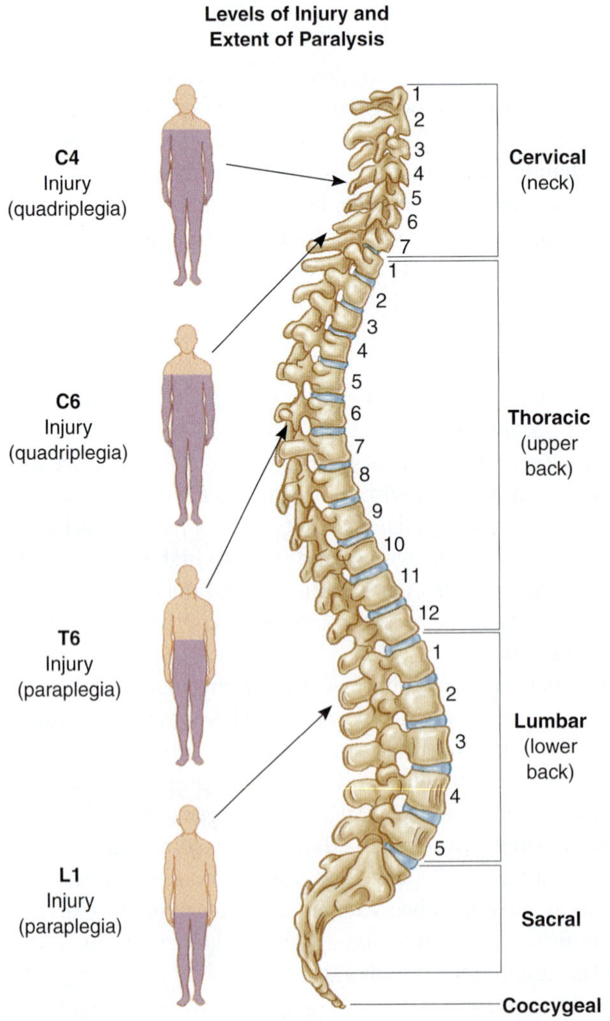

High-dose corticosteroids for acute spinal cord injury are NOT a standard of care, and the risks tend to exceed any possible benefits.

■ Figure 14-12 Spinal injury levels.

Levels of Injury and Extent of Paralysis

C4 Injury (quadriplegia)

C6 Injury (quadriplegia)

T6 Injury (paraplegia)

L1 Injury (paraplegia)

Cervical (neck)

Thoracic (upper back)

Lumbar (lower back)

Sacral

Coccygeal

may or may not have overlying osseous injury to the spinal column. The syndrome manifests by motor and sensory deficits, which are more severe in the upper extremities than in the lower extremities.

BROWN-SEQUARD SYNDROME

Brown-Sequard syndrome is caused by lateral injury to one-half of the spinal cord in the horizontal plane. In the trauma patient, this relatively rare phenomenon tends to be most commonly seen with penetrating injuries. It is manifested by the presence of motor weakness and the loss of light touch, vibratory, and position sense on the ipsilateral side of the lesion, and contralateral loss of pain and temperature sensation. Motor loss will be greater on the ipsilateral side.

SPINAL SHOCK

Spinal shock is a temporary phenomenon that may persist for several days or even weeks following SCI, and is clinically distinct from *neurogenic shock*. It presents as a loss of motor, sensory, and reflexive function below the level of the injury. The patient will be incontinent of urine and feces. Unlike neurogenic shock, there are no direct hemodynamic consequences.

NEUROGENIC SHOCK

Neurogenic shock is typically seen in patients with SCI above the level of T6. It causes interruption of the sympathetic autonomic nervous fibers that connect to the brain, resulting in unopposed parasympathetic stimulation. The result is a loss of vascular tone, the loss of the body's ability to autoregulate blood pressure, resulting in hypotension, and deceleration of the heart rate. The capacity for diaphoresis is also lost below the level of the lesion. Thus, the classic picture of a patient in neurogenic shock is one who is hypotensive and bradycardic, with flushed, warm, dry skin below the level of the lesion and cool, clammy skin above. Neurogenic shock will typically resolve over time.

AUTONOMIC DYSREFLEXIA (AD)

Autonomic dysreflexia is a dangerous process caused by the aberrant response of an impaired sympathetic autonomic nervous system (SANS) to stimuli. The most common cause is stimulation of the stretch receptors in the viscera of the bowel or bladder, as in urinary retention or fecal impaction. However, cutaneous stimuli may also cause AD. The result is a dramatic increase in sympathetic tone, which can cause a severe hypertensive crisis. Bradycardia, as well as peripheral vasodilation and diaphoresis above the level of the lesion, may also occur. Hypertension may become symptomatic with the patient complaining of a headache and visual changes.

The initial treatment of AD involves the correction of the precipitating factor. Where protocol allows, this may include assessment for urinary retention and possible insertion of a urinary catheter into patients who lack bladder catheterization or the changing of an indwelling catheter to a clean one when obstruction is suspected. Critical care providers should also be aware that fecal impaction may be a precipitating cause. Appropriately trained providers may perform a rectal exam and manual disimpaction if necessary, but it is unlikely that this procedure will be appropriate in the critical care transport setting, and thus these patients should be brought to a practitioner who can perform the appropriate intervention in a timely fashion. If reversal of AD does not occur following correction of the precipitating agent, then further pharmacologic intervention may be indicated to prevent injury caused by hypertension and sympathetic overstimulation.

DIAGNOSIS OF SCI

One of the most critical diagnostic evaluations of SCI is the patient's physical exam. Patients should be evaluated for pain and point tenderness on the spine, bony crepitus or "step-offs," paresthesias, and other motor and sensory changes, as well as assessment of the Babinski reflex. More sophisticated sensory exams will assess different elements of the spine's sensory tracts, such as light touch and pain. The presence of any motor or sensation below the level of a suspected lesion is suggestive of incomplete injury. Even in the absence of these indicators, all SCI should be treated aggressively to improve functional prognosis and decrease the risk of secondary injury. Some SCIs may become remarkably better with treatment, and they can always be made worse by careless handling and lack of proper immobilization. (See Figures 14-13 ■ and 14-14 ■.)

It is a fundamental tenet of basic trauma life support to protect the spine of any trauma patient with sufficient mechanism or complaint of injury by immobilizing him. All patients with spinal cord injury or the potential thereof must continue to be immobilized and log rolled carefully until their injuries are deemed stable or nonexistent. Most patients with potential spinal cord injury will undergo radiologic examination with X-rays and potentially CT scan to rule out the presence of osseous injury. These exams are not sensitive for soft-tissue or ligamentous injury, however. Thus, in the presence of a sufficient mechanism of injury, negative radiologic findings in the osseous spine do not preclude the need for continued precaution. Often, patients will be maintained in a soft C-collar until their soft tissue can be evaluated by careful clinical exam or MRI.

Immobilization is initially accomplished through the familiar means of mechanical stabilization with cervical collar, cervical immobilization device, and long backboard. Patients may have the head of their beds elevated if their injuries are limited to the cervical spine and the injuries are deemed stable enough. Not all spinal column fractures will be treated immediately, but many patients do require surgical stabilization. Patients with cervical spine injuries may require the placement of a HALO-type vest stabilization device.

Another option for surgical treatment of SCI is decompression of the spinal cord in the presence of edema. By removing some of the osseous mass of the vertebrae, the spinal cord is given room to swell, hopefully with a subsequent reduction in compression-induced secondary injury. The critical care paramedic can expect that any patient who has undergone spinal surgery for acute SCI will have strict stabilization protocols that must be adhered to during transport.

PHARMACOLOGIC MANAGEMENT OF SCI

The standard of practice has been to administer high-dose intravenous corticosteroids to reduce the inflammatory processes that occur after SCI to decrease the effects of secondary injury. The overall benefit of this therapy has been debated considerably in the literature, and has not been supported

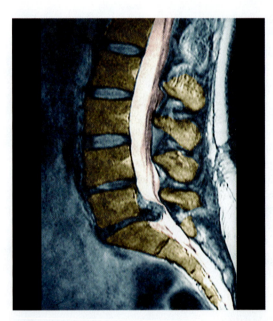

■ Figure 14-13   Herniated disc. Colored magnetic resonance imaging (MRI) scan of a sagittal (side) section through the lower spine of a patient suffering from a herniated disc. The central part (blue, lower center) of one of the discs that separate the bones (vertebrae, brown) of the spine has been forced through a weakened area of the disc, and is protruding into the spinal cord (pink/white, top center to bottom right). *(Zephyr/Photo Researchers, Inc.)*

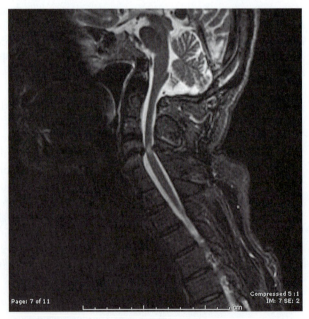

■ Figure 14-14   Cervical spinal cord injury. *(Kathy Altergott, BSN, MBA, CRA. Banner Good Samaritan Medical Center, Phoenix, AZ)*

by large randomized controlled studies, and the risks outweigh any benefits. However, it is still used in the care of SCI in some areas, and should therefore be familiar to critical care paramedics. It is generally accepted that high-dose steroid therapy is most effective when initiated shortly after the injury. Although a number of drugs have been tested, methylprednisolone, or Solu-Medrol, remains the most commonly utilized. (See Figure 14-15 ■.)

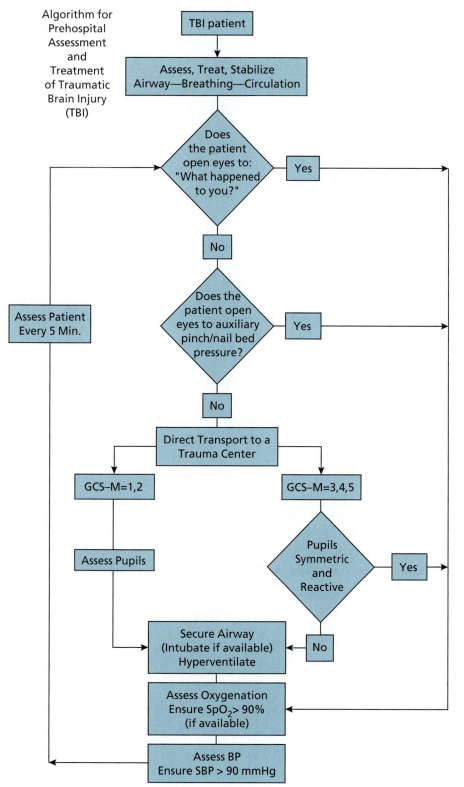

■ **Figure 14-15** Prehospital algorithm traumatic brain injury. *(Reproduced with permission of the Brain Trauma Foundation)*

Experimental dosages and regional protocols may vary somewhat. However, Solu-Medrol is typically given in an initial bolus of 30 mg/kg IV over 15 minutes, followed by a maintenance infusion of 5.4 mg/kg per hour for 23 hours. There is a period of "rest" between the bolus and maintenance doses wherein no Solu-Medrol is given, typically 45 minutes.

In the acute phase of injury, other pharmacologic agents such as vasopressors, analgesics, and sedatives may be required.

Summary

Traumatic injury to the central nervous system is a leading cause of death and disability. The brain and spinal cord are highly susceptible to secondary injury that may occur hours or days after the initial injury. To prevent the progression of secondary injury, it is essential that patients with CNS trauma be carefully monitored and aggressively treated by vigilant care providers.

Review Questions

1. What are the physiological criteria for determining brain death?
2. What is cerebral perfusion pressure and how is it determined?
3. At what range of CPP can autoregulation occur?
4. What is the effect of carbon dioxide on cerebral vasculature? What is the ideal PCO_2 for a patient with elevated ICP and cerebral edema?
5. Define cytoxic cerebral edema and its cause.
6. Define vasogenic edema and its cause.
7. What does the Monroe-Kellie hypothesis state?
8. What is the range for normal ICP values?
9. Which anatomical structure within the brain does the external auditory meatus (EAM) landmark?
10. In the ICP waveform of a normal brain, which waveform component should be the highest?
11. What position must the stopcock connecting the external ventricular drain (EVD) to its collection system be in to allow for accurate ICP measurement?
12. What position should the stopcock be in when moving patients?
13. Why should hypotonic intravenous fluids not be used as infusions or admixture diluents for patients at risk for cerebral edema?
14. At what level of the spinal column can a spinal cord injury be expected to cause neurogenic shock?
15. What is the most common cause of autonomic dysreflexia in the patient with spinal cord injury?

See Answers to Review Questions at the back of this book.

Further Reading

American Association of Critical Care Nurses. *Core Curriculum for Critical Care Nursing,* 5th ed. Philadelphia: W. B. Brace, 1998.

Arbour R. "Intracranial Hypertension." *Critical Care Nurse,* Vol. 24, No. 5 (2004): 19–32.

Bledsoe BE, Porter RS, Cherry RA. *Paramedic Care: Principles and Practice: Trauma Emergencies,* 2nd ed. Upper Saddle River, NJ: Pearson Prentice Hall, 2006.

Bledsoe BE, Wesley AK, Salomone JP. "Position Statement: High-Dose Steroids for Acute Spinal Cord Injury in Emergency Medical Services." *Prehospital Emergency Care,* Vol. 8, No. 3 (2004): 313–316.

Brain Trauma Foundation. *Guidelines for the Prehospital Management of Traumatic Brain Injury.* New York: Author, 2000.

Devinsky O, Feldmann E, Weinreb HJ, Wilterdink JL. *The Resident's Neurology Book.* Philadelphia: F. A. Davis, 1997.

Doyle J, Davis D, Hoyt DB. "The Use of Hypertonic Saline in the Treatment of Traumatic Brain Injury." *Journal of Trauma: Injury, Infection, and Critical Care,* Vol. 50 (2001): 367–383.

Hugenholtz H, et al. "High-Dose Methylprednisolone for Acute Closed Spinal Cord Injury—Only a Treatment Option." *Canadian Journal of Neurological Sciences,* 29 (2002): 227–235.

Lindsay KW, Bone I, Callander R. *Neurology and Neurosurgery Illustrated,* 3rd ed. Edinburgh, Scotland: Churchill-Livingstone, 1997.

McCutcheon EP, Selassie AW, Gu JK, Pickelsimer EE. "Acute Traumatic Spinal Cord Injury, 1993–2000: A Population-Based Assessment of Methylprednisolone Administration and Hospitalization." *Journal of Trauma: Injury, Infection, and Critical Care,* Vol. 56, No. 5 (2004): 1076–1083.

Miller MT, et al. "Initial Head Computed Tomography Scan Characteristics Have a Linear Relationship with Intracranial Pressure after Trauma." *Journal of Trauma: Injury, Infection, and Critical Care,* Vol. 56, No. 5 (2004): 967–973.

Sarrafzadeh AS, et al. "Secondary Insults in Severe Head Injury: Do Multiply Injured Patients Do Worse?" *Critical Care Medicine,* Vol. 29, No. 6 (2001): 1116–1123.

Shiozaki T, et al. "Efficacy of Moderate Hypothermia in Patients with Severe Head Injury and Intracranial Hypertension Refractory to Mild Hypothermia." *Journal of Neurosurgery,* Vol. 99 (2003): 47–51.

Valadka AB, et al. "Relationship of Brain Tissue PO_2 to Outcome after Severe Head Injury." *Critical Care Medicine,* Vol. 26, No. 9 (1998): 1576–1581.

Thoracic Trauma: Assessment and Management

Lee Richardson, NREMT-P, CCEMT-P, FP-C

Objectives

Upon completion of this chapter, the student should be able to:

1. Identify common and life-threatening thoracic injuries based on anatomy and mechanism of injury. (p. 402)
2. Explain the physiology of ventilation. (p. 403)
3. Integrate the relationship between anatomy, kinematics, and assessment findings to identify specific thoracic injuries. (p. 403)
4. Describe general treatment modalities for the following thoracic injuries:
    A. Tension pneumothorax (p. 404)
    B. Hemothorax (p. 405)
    C. Pneumothorax (both open and closed) (p. 410)
    D. Flail chest (p. 412)
    E. Blunt and penetrating cardiac injuries including:
        i. Pericardial tamponade (p. 413)
        ii. Myocardial rupture (p. 415)
        iii. Myocardial contusion (p. 416)
    F. Aortic rupture (p. 415)
    G. Pulmonary contusions (p. 416)
    H. Diaphragmatic rupture (p. 417)
    I. Tracheal and bronchial rupture (p. 417)
    J. Esophageal perforation (p. 418)
5. Identify and differentiate between patients who require stabilization and rapid transport versus on-the-scene assessment and management.
6. Discuss ongoing maintenance care for chest tubes and the various drainage systems that may be present. (p. 407)

Key Terms

Case Study

It is another hot summer day when Medic 14 is dispatched to Universal Steel on an "unknown medical emergency." Upon arrival at the plant, the paramedics are met by a company security guard who leads them to the patient. The patient is located just outside one of the large smelters. He is lying on the ground in the shade. The scene is safe so paramedics approach the patient and begin their assessment.

The patient is a muscular 36-year-old male who works in the smelter. He is wearing a long-sleeve shirt and heavy steel-toed boots. His supervisor is with him and states that he thinks the patient got overheated. The smelter is indeed hot. The outside temperature is nearly 100 degrees and the temperature in the smelter building is probably 140 degrees.

Paramedics begin their assessment. The patient is pale and diaphoretic. He is alert but slow in responding to commands. His pulse rate is 152, his blood pressure is 92/80 mmHg, and his respiratory rate is 30 breaths per minute. A rapid trauma assessment was unremarkable for obvious trauma. The paramedics have trouble evaluating both breath sounds as well as heart tones due to the extreme noise from the steel factory. With help from several of the steelworkers, the patient is moved to the ambulance stretcher and then to the ambulance where the paramedics have left the air-conditioning running.

Once in the ambulance, they close the doors to keep the unit cool. One paramedic starts an IV of normal saline and begins to infuse it wide open. The other paramedic places a nonrebreather mask and begins to administer oxygen at 100%. Paramedics remove the patient's heavy clothing and as they are applying the ECG electrodes, they notice a small adhesive bandage over the patient's right lateral chest. As they begin a more detailed assessment of the patient's chest, they remove the bandage to discover what appears to be a small soft-tissue injury that looks like a puncture wound in his right axillary area. There is no obvious bleeding or air escaping.

After the IV is flowing, the paramedics repeat the vital signs. The pulse rate is 160 per minute and thready. The blood pressure is 88/80 mmHg. Because the patient's hypotension appears to be worsening, paramedics start a second IV of normal saline and administer it wide open. Just before they are going to begin transport to the hospital, the back doors of the ambulance are opened by the factory nurse. She just found out about the incident and came to tell the paramedics that about 30 minutes ago the patient had come to the nurse's office complaining that a piece of steel had struck him on the chest. She stated she had evaluated the wound and decided it was superficial. She cleaned the wound, applied an antibacterial ointment and adhesive bandage, and had the man return to work.

The paramedics quickly reassess the patient. His pulse rate is 160 per minute and his blood pressure 86/80. His respirations are 32. His mental status has declined and he now responds only to verbal stimuli. Upon auscultation of breath sounds and heart tones, breath sounds are equal but diminished due to the patient's respiratory rate and depth; his heart tones appear to be somewhat muffled.

Because pericardial tamponade is suspected, the patient is emergently transported to the closest hospital. There, the emergency physician performs a pericardiocentesis and withdraws nearly 100 milliliters of unclotted blood. The patient immediately improves. His heart rate slows to 120 per minute, his blood pressure increases to 118/86 mmHg, and his mental status improves.

The hospital does not have cardiovascular surgery capabilities, and the patient requires a pericardial exploration and possible window. So the critical care transport crew is summoned to transfer the patient 30 miles to the receiving hospital. The transport goes uneventfully and no additional pericardiocentesis is required. The patient is taken to the operating room where the penetrating injury is repaired and a small pericardial window placed. He tolerates the procedure well and is discharged 5 days later.

INTRODUCTION

Transporting patients with thoracic injuries can present a demanding and sometimes challenging task for the critical care paramedic. It is estimated that one in four trauma deaths (25%) is directly due to thoracic injuries. Thoracic trauma is a contributing factor in an additional 25% of trauma patients who die from their injuries.

The harsh reality is that many of these patients do not have to succumb to their injuries. It simply takes an astute clinician to rapidly identify and intervene. Although thoracic trauma is a leading cause of trauma deaths (second only to central nervous system injuries) in North America, statistics show that the vast majority (90% of blunt trauma and 70% to 85% of penetrating trauma) can be managed without surgery. Furthermore, only a small number of patients (less than 10% of blunt trauma and 15% to 30% of penetrating trauma) require thoracotomy. In the pediatric population, with the exception of pulmonary contusions, the mortality rate is 50% or higher. Mechanisms of injury (MOIs) for thoracic trauma include motor vehicle crashes (MVCs), falls, sports injuries, crush injuries, stab wounds, and gunshot wounds. This high death rate is attributed to serious injuries to vital thoracic structures. By understanding the severity of the injury, the MOI, management concerns of specific thoracic injuries, and the unique challenges associated with transporting these patients, especially in the air, the critical care paramedic can anticipate potential complications and be ready to promptly manage them. Thoracic injuries that are missed or go unrecognized until the patient is in *extremis* due to incomplete or inaccurate assessment techniques will be deadly.

Thoracic injuries can have a high mortality rate if not recognized and aggressively treated.

It is assumed that the student has a thorough knowledge of the following topics prior to beginning this chapter: anatomy and physiology of the thorax, assessment and management of the different types of thoracic injuries, understanding of flight physiology specifically relating to thoracic trauma complications, and general transportation considerations for patients with thoracic trauma.

PATHOPHYSIOLOGY

Multiple processes are involved in the act of breathing. These include mechanics of ventilation, neurochemical control of respiration, and the pathophysiology of specific injuries. Thoracic trauma can be either blunt or penetrating in nature. The biggest difference in these two is the associated injury patterns. Blunt injuries are those where the forces are spread over a larger area; the actual injuries occur from forces such as compression and shearing.

Penetrating trauma injuries are those where the forces are limited to a very small area and actually penetrate the thoracic cavity. The most common causes of penetrating trauma include stab wounds, gunshot wounds, and falls onto sharp objects. With penetrating injuries, any structure or organ in the thoracic cavity may be injured. Most often the organs injured are those that are in the direct path of the penetrating object.

Thoracic injuries can produce hypoxia, hypercarbia, and acidosis. Tissue hypoxia results from inadequate delivery of oxygenated blood to the tissue cells. This can result from hypoperfusion (typically hypovolemia) or decreased oxygenation of the red blood cells (RBCs) (such as occurs with ventilation/perfusion mismatch caused by pulmonary contusions, hematomas, or alveolar collapse). Hypercarbia results from decreased ventilation, which is typically a result of changes in intrathoracic pressure relationships and/or depressed levels of consciousness. Acidosis (typically metabolic) is secondary to anaerobic metabolism created by the inadequately oxygenated cells (hypoperfusion). Based on the MOI (specifically rapid-deceleration), anatomy, and clinical assessment, the critical care paramedic should have a high index of suspicion for specific injuries, such as pneumothorax, pericardial tamponade, flail chest, pulmonary contusions, and aortic disruption, and be ready to intervene quickly.

GENERAL MANAGEMENT

The overall management for a patient who has sustained thoracic trauma is to identify and correct the underlying problem. It cannot be emphasized enough that the critical care paramedic must have good assessment skills as well as a comprehensive understanding of anatomy and pathophysiology in order to rapidly identify the specific injury, halt its progression, and begin aggressive treatment. The general management of thoracic trauma is to provide generalized supportive care while trying to identify the underlying cause. Generalized management includes ensuring the patient has a patent airway, adequate oxygenation, ventilation, perfusion, and body temperature while identifying and correcting the underlying cause.

INITIAL ASSESSMENT AND MANAGEMENT

The initial assessment of the thoracic trauma patient is no different than with any other critically ill or injured patient. Once you have determined that the scene is safe for you to enter, you should follow a systematic assessment approach, giving particular attention to life-threatening and potentially life-threatening conditions first. You should always start with the basics—observation, palpation, and auscultation—then work your way down to specifics:

★ Airway maintenance with cervical spine protection if needed

★ Breathing and ventilation

★ Circulation with bleeding control

★ Mental status (assess neurologic deficits)

The critical care paramedic must ensure that life-threatening or potentially life-threatening thoracic injuries are not missed. The best way to do this is to remove all clothing and perform a detailed exam. This will facilitate complete patient evaluation. This concept has been used for years by paramedics and is based on the fact that "you cannot fix something if you don't know it's there." Once you have completed your examination, the patient should be covered with blankets to prevent hypothermia. Another way to prevent hypothermia is to increase the temperature of the environment (i.e., ED, MICU, or aircraft). Because hypothermia is an inherent problem in most trauma patients, administration of warmed (102° F) fluids and blood should be used during resuscitation efforts.

DETAILED EXAM/HISTORY

As with any critically ill/injured patient, addressing the ABCDEs and managing any potential or actual life threats found should be the first priority in the care of the patient who has sustained thoracic trauma. Once this is complete and proper resuscitative efforts are well established, a more detailed exam and patient history may be addressed if time allows. Typically this detailed exam consists of reevaluation of the initial assessment and then a detailed head-to-toe examination of the patient. A complete and detailed exam and history are necessary to ensure that all injuries and preexisting diseases are identified and appropriately managed to minimize any potential complications. A detailed examination will also allow the critical care paramedic to monitor patient trends. A complete and ongoing neurologic exam should be performed, especially if the patient receives pharmacologic agents that alter the ability to accurately assess the patient such as sedatives, analgesics, and paralytic agents. Obtain radiological and laboratory studies if time allows. (Do not delay treatment/transportation to obtain these.)

PATIENT HISTORY

Although in a large number of patients the MOI will be very obvious, every effort must be made to obtain as much information as possible regarding the circumstances surrounding the incident. Initial management as well as definitive care is dictated by things such as preexisting disease processes, MOI in patients sustaining thoracic trauma, and the duration and severity of the injury.

The thoracic injuries discussed in the following pages have been categorized into life threatening and potentially life threatening, but it is always important to remember that *any* chest injury can be potentially life threatening.

MANAGEMENT OF LIFE-THREATENING INJURIES

TENSION PNEUMOTHORAX

In trauma, a leak can develop in the lung. This may be due to a rib fracture, blunt or penetrating injury, or barotrauma. **Tension pneumothorax** results from an accumulation of air within the pleural space of the hemithorax, increasing the pressure within. This condition is characterized as progressive air accumulation under pressure, wherein the flap of the injured lung acts as a one-way valve and air is allowed to enter the pleural space on inspiration but not allowed to escape on expiration. (See Figure 15-1 ■.) Ventilation is severely compromised due to the increases in intrapleural pressure with each breath. This will lead to collapse of the ipsilateral lung and a mediastinal shift to the opposite side, leading to compression of the contralateral lung. Perfusion becomes inadequate because of decreased venous return to the heart as a result of the increased pressure and mediastinal shifting of the thoracic structures.

Typical symptoms of a patient with a tension pneumothorax include severe and increasing respiratory distress, dyspnea, and possibly cyanosis. Altered mental states such as anxiety and agitation may also be seen due to the profound hypoxia and hypercapnia. Clinical signs and symptoms of shock will be present (i.e., systolic BP < 90 mmHg); breath sounds may either be decreased or absent on the affected side and, in later progression, both sides. Tracheal deviation away from the affected side (toward the unaffected side) as the intrathoracic pressure increases is seen. (This is a very ominous and late sign.) Additionally, jugular vein distention may also be present. (*Note:* May not be present if patient is hypovolemic.) The presence of subcutaneous air in the tissues of the neck and/or chest wall may also be seen. It should be emphasized that a very careful assessment of breath sounds (and heart tones) should occur prior to transport, because auscultation during transport, especially if by air, will be very difficult if not impossible. Because of this, constant observation/assessment of the patient's chest excursion is a very important aspect of management.

Management of Tension Pneumothorax

This condition must be promptly identified and treated, because it is truly a life-threatening emergency. Needle decompression of the affected side is the most common method of relieving a tension pneumothorax. This may be all that is required and the patient may or may not require chest tube (tube thoracostomy) placement later. A single chest tube will usually suffice for pneumothorax, hemothorax, or hemopneumothorax. In addition to relief of the tension, adequate management of the patient's oxygenation and ventilation status must be continued as well as fluid resuscitation.

Apprehension, agitation

Increasing cyanosis, air hunger (ventilation severely impaired)

Possible subcutaneous emphysema

Shock; skin cold, clammy

Distended neck veins

Trachael displacement toward uninjured side

Hyperresonant percussion note, breath sounds ↓ or absent

Here is a summary of pleural decompression: Identify the location for the procedure to be performed. This is normally the 2nd or 3rd intercostal space (ICS) in the midclavicular line but may also be placed in the 4th or 5th ICS midaxillary line but this site is not preferred for relief of tension pneumothorax. Using a large-bore (10- to 14-gauge) over the needle IV catheter, place the needle onto the rib below the identified location, slide the needle upward over the top of the rib making sure to keep the needle in contact with the superior portion of the rib and into the pleural space. Pay particular attention to see if there is a rapid release of air once the needle pierces the pleural space. Reassess the patient for signs of improvement. Note that current standards do not require the addition of a one-way "flutter valve" on chest decompression catheters. The critical care paramedic should be vigilant in continuing to monitor the patient for the need to perform additional decompressions.

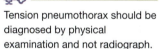

Tension pneumothorax should be diagnosed by physical examination and not radiograph.

MASSIVE HEMOTHORAX

Similar to the tension pneumothorax, a massive **hemothorax** can be caused by either blunt or penetrating trauma or can be a result of nontraumatic causes such as lung cancer or a leaking AV malformation. Injuries to intrathoracic organs or lacerations to major vessels will cause rapid accumulation of blood and fluid in the pleural cavity, which can result in severe respiratory and hemodynamic compromise. (See Figure 15-2 ■.) Hypovolemic shock may also be present because the uninjured lung can offer little or no resistance to a large amount of blood accumulating in the pleural space. This will eventually lead to compression and/or collapse of the ipsilateral lung. If severe enough mediastinal shifting occurs, the result will be compression of the contralateral lung. When this happens the patient will sustain a significant ventilation perfusion imbalance.

Assessment findings of a patient with a massive hemothorax include the following: Due to the decrease in blood volume, the patient will exhibit signs and symptoms of hypovolemic shock including altered mental status, increased heart rate, decreased blood pressure (this is a late finding), and other signs of peripheral vasoconstriction such as delayed capillary refill and pale, cold, clammy

hemothorax *rapid accumulation of blood and fluid in the pleural cavity which can result in severe respiratory and hemodynamic compromise.*

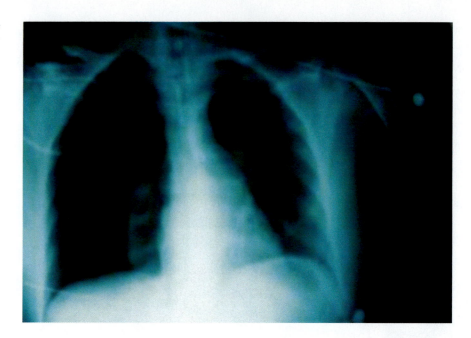

■ **Figure 15-2** Chest X-ray of tension pneumothorax. *(Edward T. Dickinson, MD)*

skin. Breath sounds will be decreased or absent on the affected side and chest wall expansion will be decreased also. Note that, unlike a tension pneumothorax or pericardial tamponade, the patient with a massive hemothorax will have a midline trachea (usually) and the jugular veins will be flat. (See Table 15–1.)

Management of Massive Hemothorax

Two major issues exist, the first of which is airway and ventilation management. This includes administration of high-flow, high-concentration oxygen, possibly endotracheal intubation and tube thoracotomy. The second is administering fluids to maintain adequate perfusion until the source of bleeding can be controlled. The critical care paramedic must monitor fluid administration very carefully and be cognizant of the fact that excessive fluid administration, especially in penetrating injuries, can be detrimental. If the critical care paramedic is faced with prolonged transport times, isolated thoracic trauma, conflicting religious beliefs, or difficulty in obtaining cross-matched

Table 15–1	Comparison of Tension Pneumothorax, Hemothorax, and Pericardial Tamponade		
Symptoms	**Tension Pneumothorax**	**Massive Hemothorax**	**Pericardial Tamponade**
Primary presenting symptom	Difficulty breathing, then shock	Shock, then difficulty breathing	Shock
Pulse Rate	Rapid	Rapid	Rapid
Systolic BP	Low	Low	Low
Neck Veins	Usually distended	Usually flat	Usually distended
Breath Sounds	Decreased or absent on side of injury	Decreased or absent on side of injury	Normal or diminished bilaterally
Heart Sounds	Audible	Audible	Muffled
Percussion of the chest	Hyperresonant	Dull	Normal
Trachea	Deviated	Midline or deviated	Midline
Chest Symmetry	Asymmetrical	Symmetrical	Symmetrical
Pulsus paradoxus	Yes	No	Maybe

blood, autotransfusion may be the best modality until more definitive care can be provided. With autotransfusion, blood from the chest is run through a filter device (Cell Saver) and readministered to the patient intravenously.

The decision to perform surgical intervention (thoracotomy) is based on multiple factors such as the amount of initial chest tube drainage, the patient's hemodynamic status, volume of fluid resuscitation required and the patient's response to it, location of the injury, and the rate of volume loss (typically >200 mL/hr). If a chest tube is placed, the critical care paramedic must carefully monitor the amount of drainage, both initially and ongoing. If blood loss exceeds 1,000 mL the chest tube should be clamped and constant evaluation for possible ventilatory compromise should be performed.

Placement and Care of Chest Tubes

In your work as a critical care paramedic you will often encounter chest tubes. In some systems, critical care paramedics may be taught how and allowed to insert chest tubes. Chest tubes may be indicated for the treatment of a significant pneumothorax (>20%), hemothorax, hemo/pneumothorax, or hemo- or pneumomediastinum. The trend seems to be much more conservative in placement of chest tubes because many pneumothoraces will heal without drainage. Placement of chest tubes can cause significant inflammation in the pleura causing scarring. However, this scarring can actually be beneficial and decreases the likelihood of recurrent spontaneous pneumothoraces. Patients who suffer multiple or recurrent pneumothoraces usually require chest tube placement versus needle decompression because their pleurae do not seal properly. (See Figure 15-3 ■.)

Here is a summary of the tube thoracostomy procedure:

★ Gather all required equipment and supplies.

– Open the chest tube insertion tray maintaining strict sterile technique.

– Don personal protective equipment (PPE) including eye/face protection.

– Preload a syringe with lidocaine solution.

– Prepare suture materials. Attach needle holder to suture.

In thoracic trauma, when the source of bleeding cannot be controlled, administer only enough fluid to maintain a systolic blood pressure of 80 mmHg.

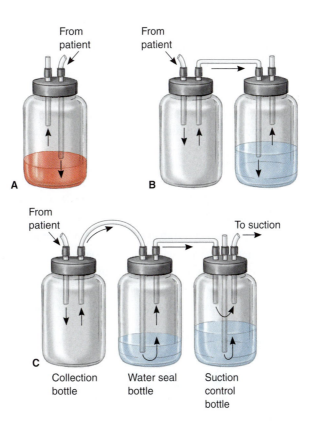

From patient

From patient

A

B

From patient

To suction

C

Collection bottle

Water seal bottle

Suction control bottle

■ **Figure 15-3** Chest tube drainage systems. A. Single bottle system. B. Double bottle system. C. Triple bottle system.

- Secure a large Kelley clamp to the proximal end of the tube (unless using the trocar technique).
- If the patient is hemodynamically stable, consider conscious sedation with careful titration of a short-acting narcotic and benzodiazepine. However, use of a local anesthetic often is adequate. If the patient is unstable, do not waste time with these procedures.

★ Place the patient in a 30°–60° reverse Trendelenburg position if not contraindicated.

★ Identify the intended insertion site (this is clinician and injury specific).

- Prepare insertion site with antiseptic solution and placement of sterile drapes.
- If anesthetic is being used, prepare equipment and anesthetize the area surrounding the insertion site including the skin, subcutaneous tissue, muscle, and periosteum. Using a 5-mL syringe with a small (25-gauge) needle, inject a SQ wheal of lidocaine at the site of insertion. Then using a 10-mL syringe with a larger needle (20 gauge), advance the needle while aspirating until you get either air or pleural fluid, then inject the lidocaine into the deep tissues as well as the tract while withdrawing, making sure to provide a generous injection to the rib periosteum SQ and surrounding tissues.

★ Make a 3- to 4-cm transverse incision over the inferior aspect of the rib below the insertion site. This is typically the fifth or sixth rib in the midaxillary line (this is the standard site) or in the 2nd or 3rd lateral ICS midclavicular line (superior portion of the anterior axillary lobe).

★ Use a curved hemostat to puncture the intercostal muscles and parietal pleura immediately superior to the rib border, avoiding damage to the underlying lung using an opening and closing technique to form a tunnel until the pleural space is penetrated. Then, slide a finger over the clamp to maintain the formed tract.

★ Perform a digital examination to assess the location and to evaluate pulmonary adhesions. Sweep the finger in all directions, and feel for the diaphragm and possible intra-abdominal structures. To avoid losing the desired tract, keep the finger in place until the tube is inserted.

★ Insert the chest tube alongside the finger, using a clamp on the tube, if desired.

★ Direct the chest tube posteriorly and inferiorly, and insert it until it is at least 5 cm beyond the last hole of the tube.

★ Attach the chest tube to a seal device and suction. If a water seal set-up is used, look for respiratory variation and bubbling of air through the water seal. Also document the amount of blood or other fluids that may drain. If the seal device used is of the unidirectional valve design, attach suctioning and monitor for drainage. (See Figure 15-4 ■.)

★ Suture the site, and secure the tube. (See Figure 15-5 ■.) A variety of anchoring and closure techniques exist, all of which are probably equivalent. Cover the site with Vaseline-impregnated gauze, and apply a suitable dressing.

★ Follow-up chest radiography is required to confirm tube placement and lung reexpansion, but transport should not be delayed to accomplish this.

★ Comprehensive assessment of the system to ensure it is "closed" should be performed immediately after tube placement. The following is the recommended technique for evaluating/managing the underwater-seal drainage system (Figure 15-6 ■):

- Tape all connections and possibly the chest tube to the chest wall.

■ **Figure 15-4** Chest tube valve.

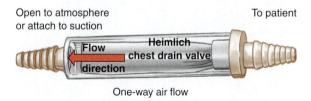

Open to atmosphere or attach to suction

To patient

Flow direction

Heimlich chest drain valve

One-way air flow

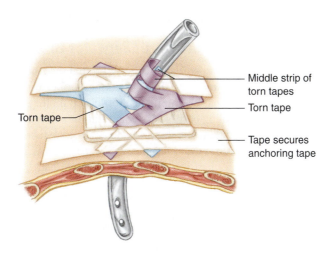

To skin on one side of tube

Wide tape — To wrap around chest tube

To skin on other side of tube

Half length of tape torn into 3 pieces

Middle strip of torn tapes

Torn tape

Torn tape

Tape secures anchoring tape

■ **Figure 15-5** Securing the chest tube.

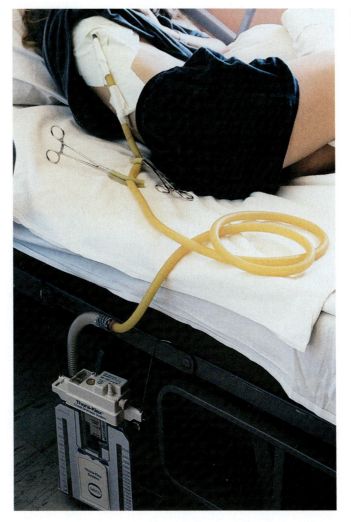

■ **Figure 15-6** Padded hemostat or plastic tube clamp is used for clamping chest tube.

The trend in management of pneumothoraces is to monitor small injuries and use smaller tubes where drainage is needed.

– Ensure there are no kinks in the tube or system components.
– Maintain appropriate fluid levels in both the underwater seal chamber as well as the suction chamber.
– Continuous reassessment of the patient for signs of hypoxia and developing tension pneumothorax should be performed.
– Clamping of chest tubes should be avoided unless specifically indicated (i.e., >1,000 cc of blood return).

Troubleshooting Closed Underwater Drainage Systems

The critical care paramedic should be aware that the amount of suction applied to the chest tube is determined by the water level in the suction chamber and not the amount of suction applied by the suction unit. The goal is a minimal amount of bubbling. Excessive bubbling can cause rapid evaporation loss. Bubbling occurs during expiration and indicates air removal from the pleural space. The critical care paramedic should evaluate the long tube of the underwater-seal chamber for fluctuations. Fluctuations indicate a patent "closed" system. Fluctuations will stop once the lung is re-expanded or if the chest tube becomes kinked or obstructed. Continuous bubbling on inspiration and expiration indicates an "open" system.

The critical care paramedic must quickly find and correct any leaks to avoid possible deterioration in the patient's condition. Some clinicians have been taught to "strip" the chest tube if it becomes visibly obstructed with clots or tissue. Stripping is associated with increased negative pleural pressure, which could cause further damage to the fragile lung tissue. Usually, using an alternating hand-over-hand technique of squeezing the tubing will create enough pressure to unobstruct the tubing. The patient should be placed in a position to promote the best expansion of the unaffected lung. This can be accomplished by placing the unaffected side down with the head of the bed elevated (if not contraindicated), which provides the best ventilation/perfusion match, or the semi-Fowler's position, which typically provides both a position of comfort as well as good chest expansion. Patients should be given analgesia to treat pain associated with chest tube insertion and maintenance.

OPEN PNEUMOTHORAX (SUCKING CHEST WOUND)

sucking chest wound
external penetration of the chest wall allowing air to enter the pleural cavity.

An open pneumothorax is caused when a penetration in the chest wall occurs, allowing air to enter the pleural cavity. If the diameter of the wound is larger than the diameter of the trachea and airways, then air will move through the chest wound rather than through the airways. A **sucking chest wound** will result in equalization of atmospheric and pleural pressure. This equalization results in loss of the negative intrathoracic pressure, which will lead to respiratory compromise. When air enters the pleural cavity, collapse of the injured lung and eventually a mediastinal shift to the collateral or unaffected side may occur. This shift in conjunction with the loss of normal negative intrathoracic pressure produces decreased venous return to the heart leading to cardiac insufficiency. Typical MOIs for open pneumothorax are gunshot wounds and stab wounds.

Assessment findings of a patient with an open pneumothorax include respiratory distress characterized by dyspnea, tachypnea, and grunting as air enters and leaves the pleural cavity through the chest wall defect. The critical care paramedic may actually hear a sucking noise during respiration. Signs of shock may also be present secondary to the intermittent obstruction in venous return.

Management of Open Pneumothorax

Asherman chest seal
commercial device commonly used to mitigate effects of sucking chest wounds.

Primary treatment is to prevent further air entry into the thoracic cavity. This can be accomplished with either a commercial device, such as an **Asherman chest seal,** or with the use of an occlusive dressing that is taped only on three of four sides. (See Figure 15-7 ■.) Both of these create a type of one-way valve that allows air to escape from the chest cavity but prevents air from entering on inspiration.

The critical care paramedic should constantly reassess the patient for signs of developing tension pneumothorax caused by sealing the wound. If this develops simply remove the occlusive dressing to relieve the pressure. If this does not correct the problem, then the critical care paramedic should manage the patient as described earlier. Most patients with this type of thoracic injury will require chest tube placement to treat the lung injury. The critical care paramedic should constantly

On inspiration, dressing seals
wound, preventing air entry

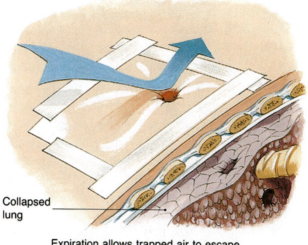

Collapsed
lung

Expiration allows trapped air to escape
through untaped section of dressing

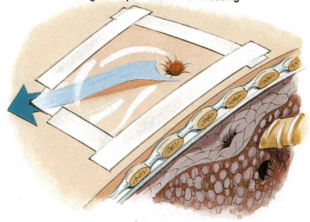

reassess the patient's oxygenation and ventilation status and immediately secure the airway with an ET tube if deterioration occurs. In addition, maintaining intravenous access is also imperative as a route for volume administration as well as medication administration.

FLAIL CHEST

By definition, a **flail chest** is three or more ribs broken in two or more places. (See Figure 15-8 ■.) Flail chest is usually a result of blunt trauma, such as MVCs or falls, and typically involves either anterior or lateral ribs. (Posterior ribs have more protection from muscles and the scapula.) These fractures cause a separation of the rib cage and loss of stability of the chest wall. The classic sign seen with flail chest is a movement known as paradoxical motion. Paradoxical movement occurs during respiration. During normal ventilation the diaphragm moves inferiorly and the intercostal muscles elevate and separate the ribs. Intrathoracic pressure decreases, allowing the greater atmospheric pressure to equalize and thus inflating the lungs. This is known as the "bellows" function. Paradoxical movement affects this function, which causes inadequate ventilation and oxygenation. With paradoxical motion the flail segment moves opposite of the rest of the rib cage. The critical care paramedic must be cognizant of the fact that paradoxical movement is not typically appreciated and may not be seen except in cases of severe flail, so frequent reassessment is mandatory. Combine a flail segment with the underlying pulmonary contusion, which will cause progressive respiratory insufficiency, instability, pain and muscle spasms caused by the rib fractures, and the

flail chest *defined as 3 or more ribs broken in 2 or more places.*

Management of Life-Threatening Injuries **411**

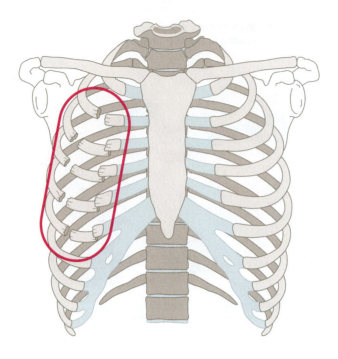

■ **Figure 15-8** Flail chest occurs when three or more adjacent ribs fracture in two or more places.

patient will experience hypoventilation and subsequent hypoxia and hypercapnia. Other clinical findings might include increasing respiratory distress, with grunting, cyanosis, severe chest pain on the affected side and the use of accessory muscles. (See Figure 15-9 ■.)

Management of Flail Chest

The critical care paramedic must perform a good assessment of the patient with flail chest to determine how compromised the patient is. A patient who is in *extremis* (severe respiratory distress or respiratory failure) must have an ET tube placed immediately and mechanical ventilation begun. The critical care paramedic should opt to use a bag-valve mask (BVM) to ventilate the patient if their transport ventilator does not have the ability to recognize a developing tension pneumothorax (i.e., peak airway pressures). Recent studies have demonstrated that facial continuous positive

■ **Figure 15-9** Physical findings of flail chest.

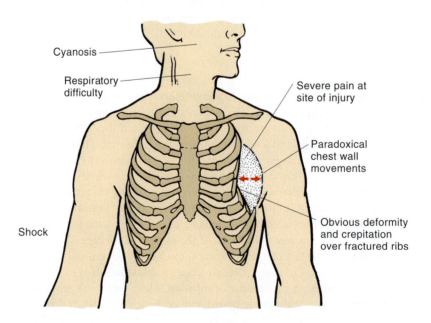

Cyanosis

Respiratory difficulty

Severe pain at site of injury

Paradoxical chest wall movements

Shock

Obvious deformity and crepitation over fractured ribs

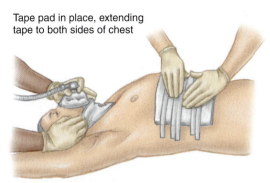

Tape pad in place, extending
tape to both sides of chest

Intubation and positive pressure
ventilation is the best stabilization

■ **Figure 15-10**   Stabilizing
flail chest.

airway pressure (CPAP) can be an effective prehospital treatment for flail chest. The flail segment
should be externally stabilized to prevent further complications. This can be accomplished by several means including gentle pressure to the segment with a pillow or large trauma dressing or, if not
contraindicated, placing the patient with the injured side down. (See Figure 15-10 ■.)

PERICARDIAL TAMPONADE

Pericardial tamponade is a condition caused by accumulation of blood in the pericardial space between the pericardial sac and the heart itself. (See Figure 15-11 ■.) Tamponade can be caused by either penetrating or blunt trauma. The hemodynamic effect of cardiac tamponade depends largely on
the amount of accumulation in the sac. The pericardial sac usually contains between 20 and 50 mL of
pericardial fluid. A rapid accumulation of 150 to 200 mL may be fatal. If the accumulation is slower,
then the pericardium can stretch enough to hold up to 2 liters of blood or fluid without significant
hemodynamic compromise. Hemodynamic compromise is caused by a decrease in diastolic filling

pericardial tamponade
*hemodynamic compromise
resulting in decreased cardiac
output, as a result of blood
accumulation in the pericardial
space between the pericardial
sac and the heart itself.*

■ **Figure 15-11**   Physical
findings of cardiac
tamponade.

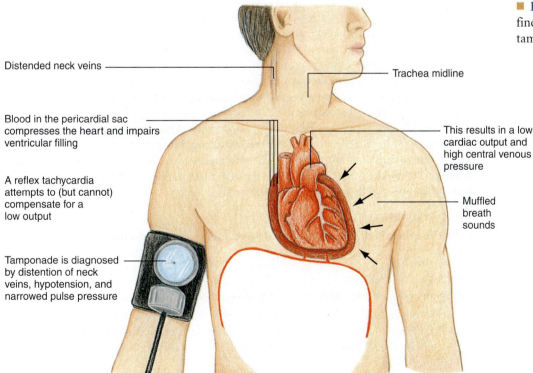

Distended neck veins

Trachea midline

Blood in the pericardial sac
compresses the heart and impairs
ventricular filling

This results in a low
cardiac output and
high central venous
pressure

A reflex tachycardia
attempts to (but cannot)
compensate for a
low output

Muffled
breath
sounds

Tamponade is diagnosed
by distention of neck
veins, hypotension, and
narrowed pulse pressure

pressure due to increased intrapericardial pressure. When the diastolic filling decreases, stroke volume and cardiac output both fall and central venous pressure increases. Once enough blood occupies the pericardial space to cause hemodynamic compromise, the patient will present with signs of decreased cardiac output such as altered mental status, cool, clammy skin, tachycardia, and falling blood pressure. High venous pressure may also be evident by the presence of jugular vein distention (JVD) if the patient is not hypovolemic. A cardinal sign of tamponade is **Beck's triad,** which is JVD, diminished or muffled heart sounds, and decreased blood pressure. The critical care paramedic must be able to distinguish between normal and muffled heart tones. However, this may prove difficult in the field setting or during transport. Another potential sign is *pulsus paradoxus. Pulsus paradoxus* is a fall in systolic blood pressure greater than 15 mmHg during normal inspiration.

Here is the procedure for measuring *pulsus paradoxus:*

★ Place BP cuff on patient and inflate to a level above the systolic blood pressure.

★ Instruct the patient to breathe as normally as possible.

★ Slowly deflate the BP cuff while auscultating the blood pressure.

★ Note the first Korotkoff sound, which, with cardiac tamponade, will occur during expiration as well as the manometer reading associated with the first sound.

★ Continue to deflate the cuff until Korotkoff's sounds are audible during both inspiration and expiration.

★ Record the difference (mmHg) between the first and second sound. This is *pulsus paradoxus.*

A procedure that is gaining momentum as the standard of care in both the ED and the field is the use of noninvasive ultrasound (echocardiogram). This procedure is very rapid and fairly simple to perform and interpret, making it a very good diagnostic adjunct for pericardial tamponade evaluation. The critical care paramedic must use some caution regarding the accuracy of ultrasound, because it has been reported that there is up to 5% incidence of false-negatives. The critical care paramedic should strongly consider a pericardial tamponade in a trauma patient who continues to deteriorate despite use of the most aggressive treatment modalities.

Management of Pericardial Tamponade

This is another true emergency for which the critical care paramedic must appropriately manage the patient's airway and ensure adequate oxygenation and ventilation. The next most important intervention is the rapid administration of volume to improve filling pressures. This will in turn improve, although temporarily, cardiac output until a more definitive intervention can be made (i.e., pericardiocentesis). A **pericardiocentesis** is a procedure in which a needle is placed into the pericardial sac and blood or fluid is withdrawn. A significant improvement in the patient's condition may be seen with the removal of as little as 20 mL of blood. Pericardial blood can be identified because it will not clot because it has been defibrinated by heart motion. Pericardiocentesis can be challenging for the critical care paramedic to perform during transport, particularly in flight due to the confined environment and turbulence. Note also that performing a pericardiocentesis should not be delayed to perform other diagnostics in the hemodynamically compromised patient.

Here is a summary of how to perform a pericardiocentesis:

★ Prepare all equipment and supplies.

★ Place patient with his head elevated 60 degrees if not contraindicated.

★ Prep the skin using an antiseptic solution.

★ Don PPE.

★ Prepare a 50-cc syringe with a three-way stopcock and a 3-inch cardiac needle.

★ Ideally, you should attach one end of an alligator clip to the proximal portion of the needle (closest to the syringe or hub of a sheathed needle) and the other end to the V1 lead for the ECG machine. If the patient is unstable or is in the prehospital setting, do not waste time with this technique.

★ Another technique that can be utilized in the hospital setting is the use of 2D or 3D echocardiogram to guide needle placement and aspiration of the fluid.

Beck's triad *diminished or muffled heart sounds, jugular venous distension, and decreased blood pressure. In the presence of pulsus paradoxus, this triad is presumptive for pericardial tamponade.*

pericardiocentesis *insertion of a specialized needle into the pericardial sac as a means of aspirating blood or other fluids.*

Pericardiocentesis is best deferred to the emergency department or surgery.

- ★ Continuously monitor the 3-lead or 12-lead ECG, vital signs, pulse oximetry, capnography, and any other invasive lines during needle aspiration, fluid withdrawal, and withdrawal of the needle. Auscultate both heart and breath sounds prior to and immediately after the procedure.
- ★ Insert the needle using the subxiphoid approach at a 30-degree angle providing negative pressure on the syringe until the pericardial fluid is aspirated. Alternatively, the left parasternal approach may also be used but is not considered the site of choice.
- ★ Place the fluid into a container to determine if the fluid clots or not.
- ★ Withdraw the needle slowly following the same path as entry.
- ★ Monitor for bleeding at the site as well as recurrence during transport.
- ★ Treat any dysrhythmias per advanced cardiac life support (ACLS) standards.
- ★ Hemoglobin, hematocrit, and coagulation studies should be performed and monitored.

The critical care paramedic must be cognizant of the fact that a pericardiocentesis is typically only a technique to buy time until definitive care can be provided (i.e., pericardial window with constant drainage until fluid output decreases to an acceptable level).

AORTIC RUPTURE

Where the critical care paramedic can save lives is by rapid assessment to identify potential or actual aortic injuries. A failure to identify and rapidly treat aortic injuries results in mortality rates between 25% and 40%. An actual **aortic rupture** can be caused by either blunt or penetrating injuries, and rupture is associated with an overall 90% mortality rate (long-term survival is only about 10%). Approximately 80% to 90% of patients with traumatic aortic rupture die immediately after the injury is sustained. The critical care paramedic should be very suspicious for shearing injuries of the aorta when confronted with a significant MOI (particularly rapid deceleration). Other clinical findings of aortic injuries include severe chest and back (usually midscapular) pain and dyspnea (if conscious). The patient may also experience hypertension in the upper extremities, which can be caused by periaortic hematomas, partial aortic occlusion, or stretching of the cardiac plexus; a harsh systolic murmur will be heard on auscultation along the precordium. Assessment of the chest X-ray, if one has been done (prior to interfacility transport), will suggest findings that should raise the critical care paramedic's index of suspicion for an aortic injury. These include widening of the superior mediastinum, a loss of the aortic knob shadow, fractures of the first two sets of ribs, depression of the left mainstem bronchus, deviation of the trachea to the right (make sure it is not a technique or patient positioning issue), pleural capping, and possible deviation of the gastric tube in the esophagus if in place. In addition, you may or may not see signs of external chest trauma.

aortic rupture *lethal injury with high potential for immediate exsanguination; associated with blunt and/or penetrating chest trauma.*

Aortic rupture, even in the best surgical hands, has a high mortality rate.

Management of Aortic Rupture

Basically, the only treatment for these patients is rapid transport to a definitive care facility that can intervene surgically. The critical care paramedic should recognize this fact and ensure that the ABCs of trauma resuscitation are addressed because it will be impossible to prevent death if the rupture occurs during transport.

MYOCARDIAL RUPTURE

Myocardial rupture is the most lethal of all thoracic injuries and always occurs as a result of major blunt force trauma such as is sustained in MVCs. To date, there are few cases of survival of patients sustaining nonpenetrating myocardial rupture. Almost all involved male patients who were involved in MVCs. The clinical presentation of patients who sustain myocardial rupture is usually cardiopulmonary arrest.

myocardial rupture *the most lethal of all thoracic injuries, occurs as a result of major blunt force trauma.*

Management of Myocardial Rupture

The critical care paramedic must use good assessment skills to determine if the arrest has a treatable cause. In most cases of blunt trauma arrests, if the patient is found without vital signs, resuscitation efforts should probably be withheld.

MANAGEMENT OF POTENTIALLY LIFE-THREATENING INJURIES

MYOCARDIAL CONTUSION

myocardial contusions *a result of severe blunt force trauma, the heart is compressed between the sternum and the spinal column, resulting in a "bruised heart."*

Simply stated this is a "bruised heart". **Myocardial contusions** are sustained when the heart is compressed between the sternum and the spinal column as a result of severe blunt force trauma. (See Figure 15-12 ■.) Typical MOIs include MVCs, falls, and actual blows to the chest. Patients sustaining myocardial contusions may be asymptomatic or they may present with all of the signs and symptoms of an acute coronary syndrome (ACS). The extent of the injury is directly related to the size of the contusion and can range from small areas of petechiae to large contusions that produce necrosis of the myocardial muscle. Bleeding and edema occur at the site of the injury and can be a factor also. The critical care paramedic should have a high index of suspicion based on the patient's MOI and clinical assessment/presentation. In addition to the symptoms just described, patients sustaining myocardial contusions may also present with sinus tachycardias and cardiac dysrhythmias, particularly ventricular ectopy. The critical care paramedic should evaluate the patient's 12-lead ECG as soon as possible for ST segment abnormalities because patients who have abnormal initial ECGs are at the greatest risk of complications.

Myocardial contusion may behave like acute coronary syndrome.

Management of Myocardial Contusions

Essentially, patients sustaining myocardial contusions should be assessed and treated similarly to a patient experiencing ACS; that is, ABCs, oxygen, large-bore IV access and possibly the administration of antidysrhythmic agents. Recent studies question the efficacy of both critical care monitoring and lengthy hospital admission of patients sustaining simple myocardial contusions.

PULMONARY CONTUSIONS

pulmonary contusions *an area of "bruised lung" resulting from blunt force trauma to the thoracic wall, most commonly seen in conjunction with flail segments.*

Simply stated this is a "bruised lung." **Pulmonary contusions** are sustained by blunt force thoracic trauma and are commonly seen in conjunction with flail chests. The most dangerous complication associated with pulmonary contusions is systemic hypoxia and hypercapnia. These occur as a result of intra-alveolar hemorrhage and edema, which occur as a result of the traumatic forces causing injury to the lung parenchyma. The specific mechanism is that the alveolar-capillary integrity is either diminished or totally lost and both interstitial hemorrhage and edema result, which in turn

■ **Figure 15-12** Myocardial contusion most frequently affects the right atrium and ventricle as they collide with the sternum.

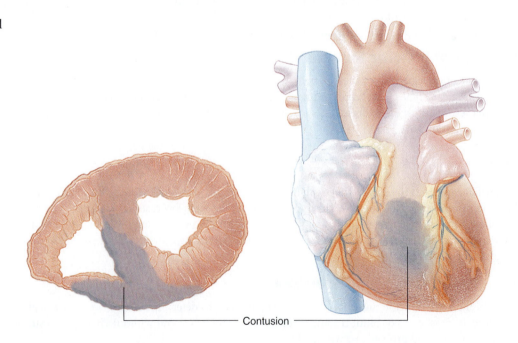

Contusion

causes decreased lung compliance and ventilation/perfusion imbalance. Typical assessment findings of significant pulmonary contusions include dyspnea and tachypnea. The patient may also present with anxiety and tachycardia induced by either a hypoxic state or physiological stress of the injury. On auscultation of the chest, the critical care paramedic will discover rales and/or rhonchi at the injury site. Chest X-rays will show the maximum changes between 48 and 72 hours postinjury. Last, the critical care paramedic should have a high index of suspicion if he has a patient whose oxygen saturation fails to improve despite aggressive oxygen therapy.

Management of Pulmonary Contusions

The primary treatment for severe pulmonary contusions is ensuring that the patient has adequate ventilation and fluid restriction. In addition, the patient should have very aggressive pulmonary toilet. Positive-pressure ventilation via a correctly placed ET tube is indicated if the patient's pO_2 is lower than 60 mmHg on room air or 80 mmHg on supplemental oxygen. Fluid restriction is recommended to reduce edema unless needed for resuscitation. The use of steroids (corticosteroids) is currently somewhat controversial, but may be used by some trauma surgeons based on their experience with their use.

DIAPHRAGMATIC RUPTURE

Diaphragmatic rupture occurs as a result of severe blunt or penetrating injury to the abdomen or lower thorax, creating a defect in the diaphragm. A commonly seen result is, if the diaphragm is injured during contraction, a large avulsion-type tear will occur. Most diaphragmatic injuries occur on the left side because of the protection afforded by the liver on the right. Once the integrity of the diaphragm has been compromised, the contents of the abdominal cavity will be pushed (herniated) into the thoracic cavity, causing compression of the ipsilateral lung and displacement of structures that lie in the mediastinal space. This sets up a myriad of potential complications including cardiopulmonary insufficiency and herniated viscera compression, which can cause either gastric or intestinal obstruction and/or ischemia, and ultimately gangrene can set in.

Clinical findings of a patient with a diaphragmatic injury vary greatly. Depending on the severity of the injury, the patient may be asymptomatic or may be in severe distress. The patient might be experiencing pain in the chest and/or abdomen with a common finding being radiation to the shoulder. Additional common signs indicating severe diaphragmatic injury include dyspnea and cyanosis. One of the most common findings on assessment is the presence of bowel sounds in the chest. While this is a very obvious sign, the critical care paramedic must be cognizant of the fact that a paralytic ileus may also accompany the injuries, making these sounds absent. Breath sounds will typically be greatly decreased or absent on the side of the injury, there may be a mediastinal shift to the unaffected side, and the abdomen will be markedly scaphoid.

Management of Diaphragmatic Rupture

The management of this injury is primarily supportive in nature, specifically aggressive oxygenation and ventilation, and routine resuscitation measures such as fluid administration while rapidly transporting the patient to definitive care, which, in this case, is surgical intervention.

TRACHEOBRONCHIAL DISRUPTION

Tracheobronchial disruption occurs most commonly as a result of blunt force trauma but can also be caused by penetrating trauma. Air will pass from the airways into the pleural space or even the mediastinal space through the tear in the trachea. Complications depend on the injury site and can include pneumothorax and pneumomediastinum, which causes mediastinal emphysema. Because of the tracheobronchial cartilage's ability to hold the lumen of the airway open, initial management of the airway may be fairly easy. Once the injury progresses, the patient will exhibit signs of deterioration including hemoptysis, severe dyspnea, and subcutaneous and/or mediastinal emphysema. The critical care paramedic should have a high index of suspicion of a tracheobronchial injury if the patient has a significant MOI and has either a pneumothorax with a persistent air leak or one that will not reexpand after chest tube placement. In some cases a tension pneumothorax may be the first sign seen.

Pulmonary contusions are more common in children because of the elasticity and resilience of their thoracic skeleton.

diaphragmatic rupture *a defect in the diaphragm that occurs as a result of severe blunt or penetrating injury to the abdomen or lower thorax.*

tracheobronchial disruption *thoracic injury, most commonly from blunt force trauma; allows air to pass from the trachea and/or bronchii into the pleural or mediastinal space.*

Management of Tracheobronchial Disruption

This injury will challenge the critical care paramedic's airway management skills. Rapid placement of an appropriately sized ET tube with placement being below the level of the injury and rapid transport to definitive care for emergency bronchoscopy are the treatments of choice. Placement of chest tube(s) should also be the standard of care. The critical care paramedic should rely on both his experience and the patient's clinical presentation to help make the decision whether to place the chest tube prior to transport or whether the patient can be safely transported and the chest tube placed after arrival at the tertiary facility.

ESOPHAGEAL PERFORATION

esophageal perforation *tear or rupture of the esophagus.*

Boerhaave syndrome *an esophageal perforation that can lead to leakage of gastric contents into the mediastinal space. It can have a high mortality rate.*

Esophageal perforation leads to leakage of gastric contents into the mediastinal space. This is usually referred to as **Boerhaave syndrome** and has a high mortality rate. This can lead to complications such as mediastinitis, severe sepsis, and massive fluid loss (hypovolemia). The most common MOI for this injury is iatrogenic instrumentation, but it can also be caused by penetrating trauma, blunt trauma, and ingestion of a foreign body. The clinical presentation of a patient experiencing an esophageal perforation will depend greatly on the location of the injury. Findings may include chest pain, dyspnea, hematemesis, dysphagia, fever, subcutaneous emphysema, and shock.

Management of Esophageal Perforation

The definitive care for a patient with an esophageal perforation is surgery. The critical care paramedic should ensure that the patient receives the appropriate supportive care needed during transport including IV fluids, administration of antibiotics, and careful placement of either an orogastric or nasogastric tube.

Summary

Caring for and transporting a patient who has sustained thoracic trauma will be one of the most challenging things a critical care paramedic will do. Effective and safe management and transportation requires the critical care paramedic to have a good understanding of the anatomy and physiology associated with the contents of the thoracic cavity as well as the ability to perform a detailed clinical exam to both identify and intervene in patients with life-threatening thoracic injuries. This includes anticipating both the patient's potential needs during transport and making appropriate plans to have all of the necessary equipment and resources available.

The critical care paramedic must also be familiar with the various unique pieces of equipment that may be used to treat patients with significant thoracic injuries and have the ability to perform, or at the very minimum assist with, specific procedures such as tube thoracotomy (chest tube placement) and pericardiocentesis as well as safely transport these devices if necessary. The critical care paramedic should maintain a high index of suspicion based on the patient's clinical presentation and the MOI. Specific interventions, especially aggressive airway management, based on the specific injury may reduce the mortality and morbidity of these injuries.

Review Questions

1. Detail the most serious thoracic trauma conditions likely to be encountered in critical care practice.
2. Discuss the adverse effects thoracic trauma has on the body's physiological processes.
3. Describe the pathophysiology and treatment of tension pneumothorax.
4. Describe the pathophysiology and treatment of massive hemothorax.

5. Describe the pathophysiology and treatment of flail chest.

6. Describe Beck's triad.

7. Discuss the pathophysiology and management of pericardial tamponade.

8. What are the common, yet non-life-threatening, thoracic injuries encountered in critical care practice.

9. Describe the management of chest tubes and chest tube drainage systems during initial care transport.

See Answers to Review Questions at the back of this book.

Further Reading

American College of Surgeons Committee on Trauma: Thoracic Trauma. *Advanced Trauma Life Support Student Course Manual.* Chicago: Author, 1997.

Campbell J. *Basic Trauma Life Support,* 5th ed. Upper Saddle River, NJ: Pearson Prentice Hall, 2003.

National Association of EMTs, NAEMT, Thoracic Trauma. *Pre-Hospital Trauma Life Support Student Manual.* St. Louis, MO: Mosby, 2003.

Chapter 16

Abdominal and Genitourinary Trauma

Scott R. Snyder, B.S., NREMT-P, CCEMT-P

Objectives

Upon completion of this chapter, the student should be able to:

1. Describe the anatomy and physiology of the organs and structures that are of concern in abdominal trauma. (p. 423)
2. Discuss and differentiate the pathophysiology of specific abdominal injuries. (p. 428)
3. Discuss imaging and laboratory studies available to aid in the identification of intra-abdominal injury. (p. 432)
4. Discuss the management of intra-abdominal injury. (p. 440)
5. Describe the anatomy and physiology of the organs and structures that are of concern in genitourinary trauma. (p. 441)
6. Discuss and differentiate the pathophysiology of specific genitourinary injuries. (p. 443)
7. Discuss imaging studies available to aid in the identification of genitourinary injury. (p. 447)

Key Terms

Case Study

It is 2 A.M., and your critical care transport team is activated to respond to a rural community hospital to transport a victim of a motor vehicle collision to the Level 1 trauma center you are based at for evaluation of a possible intra-abdominal injury. You receive the information from dispatch and note that it is a facility you have been to before, and remember it as a small three-bed emergency department staffed by an attending physician and a nurse. The facility is about a 45-minute flight from the trauma center. You and the flight nurse go to the crew room, retrieve the refrigerated drugs and blood, and head out to the helipad and meet up with the pilot. Together, the three of you perform the preflight check, and then take off. When airborne, you use the on-board cell phone to call the transferring ED and talk to the attending physician. She informs you that the patient has not arrived at the ED yet, but she activated your crew after receiving a report from EMS providers at the scene who indicated that they were going to be transporting a trauma patient with abdominal pain. This small, rural emergency department is underequipped to handle trauma patients, and the physicians are in the habit of calling for critical care transport early, based on the reports they receive from the field providers.

Upon arrival at the transferring facility, you are presented with a 38-year-old female who is conscious, alert, and a bit anxious. She arrived at the ED about 5 minutes prior to your arrival. She was the unbelted driver of a car that struck a utility pole, and she states she slid forward into the steering column. The EMS providers on scene had taken pictures of the car, and you shuffle through a stack of pictures that clearly show significant damage to the front end of the vehicle, a deformed lower half of the steering wheel, an intact windshield, and a broken utility pole. The EMS providers, who are all basic EMTs, had found the patient conscious and alert at the time of their arrival, complaining of abdominal pain. They administered 100% oxygen via a nonrebreather mask (NRM), applied a cervical collar, extricated the patient with a KED, placed her on a spine board, and transported her to the ED.

You and your partner immediately note that she is conscious, alert, and oriented, protecting her airway and breathing about 20 times a minute. A quick reach down to her wrist reveals a strong, rapid radial pulse. You note that her skin is cool, slightly pale, and dry. A physical exam reveals a large bruise across the upper quadrants of her abdomen, extending to her left flank. She is guarding her upper left quadrant, and has pain with palpation. She also reports pain with palpation of her epigastric area, and you note that her right and lower quadrants are benign. All other physical exam findings are normal. You perform a FAST exam with your portable ultrasound unit and easily identify blood in the splenorenal space. You look up at your partner, motion to the ultrasound unit screen, and he gives you a nod indicating he understands. The attending physician asks if you would like her to place a central venous catheter; you think of the 45-minute flight back to the trauma center and take her up on the offer. The ED nurse reports that the patient's vital signs are:

★HR = 122
★RR = 20 and regular
★BP = 106/62
★SpO$_2$ = 100% on 10 lpm via NRM

Your partner has started a peripheral IV in the A/C area just in case the central line attempt fails, and starts a normal saline drip. "I'm going to set this at KVO," she reports. "No need to dump fluid in her right now." Considering the BP of 102 systolic and the intra-abdominal bleed, you agree. You place the patient on your cardiac monitor and automated blood pressure cuff, and hear the attending say "You're going to feel some pressure . . ." as she advances the probe needle. "We're in" she says, and proceeds to complete the subclavian catheterization. By the time she has finished securing the central line, you and your partner have identified and confirmed that the blood you are going to administer is O$^-$, and are ready to attach the blood administration set to the central line, and set the flow rate for 2 cc/min. The ED nurse inserts a Foley catheter, and you note the immediate return of clear, yellow urine. She then inserts a nasogastric tube. The ED nurse reports that she has performed a glucose check and ABG with a portable analyzer and the results are:

★ pH = 7.34
★ PO$_2$ = 96%
★ PCO$_2$ = 34 mmHg
★ HCO^3 = 21
★ BG = 102 mg/dL

In addition, she reports that she dipped the patient's urine with a reagent strip and there was no blood present. You tell the pilot that you are just about ready to leave, and he goes outside to prepare the helicopter. Your partner gathers all of the patient records, and you tell her that you have the scene pictures in your pocket; you know that the trauma team will appreciate those.

The patient is moved to the transport stretcher, and the four of you wheel her out to the landing pad, where the pilot is waiting with open doors. The patient is loaded into the cabin, and the pilot proceeds to start up the ship. You place a headset on the patient, adjust her volume, and ask her how she's feeling. "A bit overwhelmed" she says, with a grimace. You reach down and hold her hand as the engines power up prior to takeoff. You note the patient's vital signs.

★ HR = 118
★ RR = 20 and regular
★ BP = 104/60
★ SpO$_2$ = 100% on 15 lpm via NRM

While en route, you call the attending in the emergency department at your facility and give him the patient report, then complete an uneventful transport to the trauma center. After evaluation in the emergency department, the patient goes immediately to surgery where a splenectomy is performed, and a perforated small bowel is identified and repaired.

INTRODUCTION

Both abdominal and genitourinary trauma present a unique problem for the critical care transport team in that a devastating, life-threatening injury may often remain occult until the very late stages of hemorrhagic shock. The critical care paramedic must appreciate the mechanism of injury, have a high index of suspicion, and frequently reevaluate the patient with abdominal or genitourinary trauma. This chapter will review the anatomy and physiology, pathophysiology, assessment, and management of both systems.

ABDOMINAL TRAUMA

Abdominal trauma is a major cause of death. As with any body cavity injury, it is difficult, if not impossible, to control bleeding from an internal injury without surgery. Abdominal trauma can be difficult to diagnose until the patient is in the later stages of shock. Because of this, the critical care paramedic must look for clues, which are often subtle, that indicate abdominal trauma.

ANATOMY AND PHYSIOLOGY

The abdominal cavity is divided into three spaces: the *peritoneal space*, the *retroperitoneal space*, and the *pelvic space*. (See Figure 16-1 ■.) Organs and structures located within the peritoneal space include the stomach, proximal duodenum, ascending colon, transverse colon, sigmoid colon, liver, gallbladder, and spleen. Retroperitoneal organs include the kidneys, ureters, distal duodenum, descending colon, and pancreas. The urinary bladder, rectum, and urethra are located in the pelvic space. In the female, the ovaries and fallopian tubes are also located in the pelvic cavity. Superficially, the abdomen is divided by horizontal and vertical lines, which cross at the umbilicus to form the four quadrants. The critical care paramedic should already be familiar with the organs located in the four abdominal quadrants. (See Figure 16-2 ■.)

The peritoneal space is lined with a serous membrane, the parietal peritoneum, which is continuous with the visceral peritoneum covering the abdominal organs. The portions of the digestive tract located within the peritoneal space are suspended by the mesentery, which is continuous with both the visceral and parietal membranes. Thus, the visceral peritoneum, parietal peritoneum, and mesentery form a large, continuous sheet of serous membrane that lines the peritoneal space, and also serves to cover (and suspend) the peritoneal organs.

Abdominal trauma is a major cause of death. As with any body cavity injury, it is difficult, if not impossible, to control bleeding from an internal injury without surgery.

The critical care paramedic must look for clues, which are often subtle, that indicate abdominal trauma.

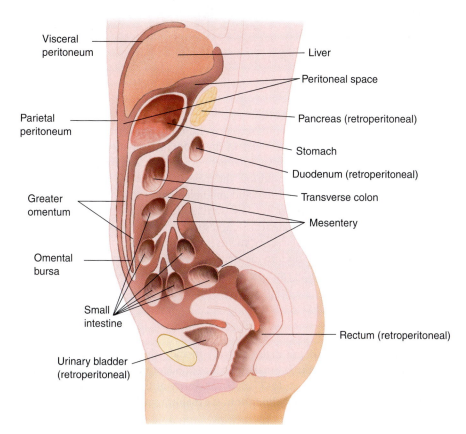

■ Figure 16-1 Peritoneal and retroperitoneal anatomy.

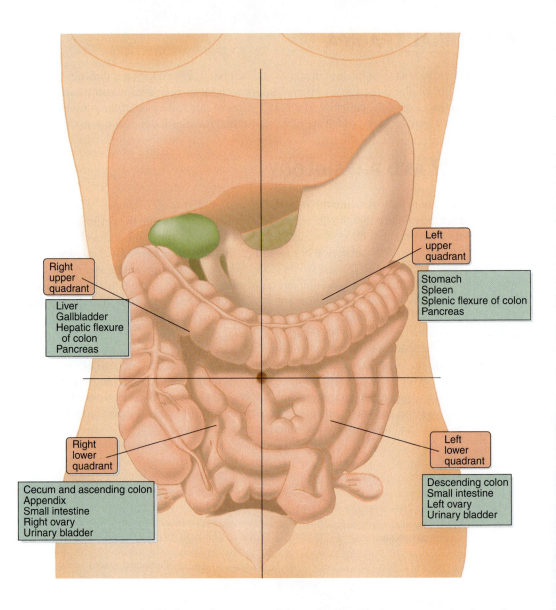

■ **Figure 16-2** Abdominal quadrants.

Right upper quadrant

Liver
Gallbladder
Hepatic flexure
  of colon
Pancreas

Left upper quadrant

Stomach
Spleen
Splenic flexure of colon
Pancreas

Right lower quadrant

Cecum and ascending colon
Appendix
Small intestine
Right ovary
Urinary bladder

Left lower quadrant

Descending colon
Small intestine
Left ovary
Urinary bladder

The mesentery is a double layer of serous membrane connected by loose connective tissue that extends inferiorly from the posterior wall of the abdominal cavity. This space between the double layer serves as a conduit for the vast vascular network, nerves, and lymphatic structures to and from the large and small intestines. In addition, the mesentery acts as a supportive structure for the digestive tract, preventing the movement and entanglement of the intestines.

The greater and lesser omentum are similar double-layer membranes hanging from the greater and lesser curvatures of the stomach, respectively. The greater omentum in effect lies over and conforms to the abdominal viscera, and its rich supply of adipose tissue provides padding, protection, and insulation to the underlying structures. The lesser omentum lies in the space between the liver and stomach, providing an access route for blood vessels entering the liver and support for the stomach.

DIGESTIVE TRACT

Abdominal components of the digestive tract include the very distal esophagus after passing through the diaphragm, stomach, small intestine (duodenum, jejunum, and ileum), large intestine (colon), and rectum. (See Figure 16-3 ■.) The majority of the stomach lies in the upper left quadrant of the abdomen, immediately inferior to the diaphragm, between the level of vertebrae T7 and

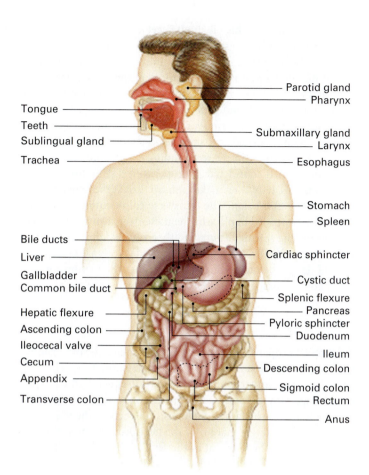

Parotid gland
Pharynx
Tongue
Teeth
Sublingual gland
Submaxillary gland
Larynx
Trachea
Esophagus

Stomach
Spleen
Bile ducts
Liver
Cardiac sphincter
Gallbladder
Cystic duct
Common bile duct
Splenic flexure
Hepatic flexure
Pancreas
Ascending colon
Pyloric sphincter
Ileocecal valve
Duodenum
Cecum
Ileum
Appendix
Descending colon
Sigmoid colon
Transverse colon
Rectum
Anus

L3. The exact size and extension can be variable between individuals and meals. The stomach receives food from the upper GI tract via the esophagus, and empties through the pyloric sphincter into the duodenum. The stomach is divided into four regions: the cardia, fundus, body, and pylorus. The esophagus enters the stomach at the cardia, so named due to its proximity to the heart located just across the diaphragm. The fundus lies superior to the gastroesophageal junction, and comes into contact with the abdominal surface of the diaphragm. The largest of the four regions is the body, which extends from the fundus to the pylorus, the region that connects to the duodenum via the pyloric sphincter. The stomach has a rich vascular supply consisting of the left gastric artery and branches of the splenic and common hepatic arteries. These arteries together comprise the three branches of the celiac artery, which itself branches off the abdominal aorta.

The digestive functions of the stomach are carried out by chemical and mechanical means. The churned food, called chyme, exits the stomach through the pyloric sphincter and enters the small intestine, where further digestion and up to 90% of nutrient absorption will take place. The small intestine ranges in length from 15 to 25 feet, with a diameter of 1 to 1.5 inches. It is located in every abdominal quadrant and takes up the majority of space in the peritoneal cavity. As such, it is frequently injured when the abdomen is subjected to traumatic insult. Recall also that the small intestine is suspended in place by the mesentery and protected by the greater omentum.

The duodenum is the shortest segment of the small intestine, measuring approximately 10 inches long, and is "C-shaped." The majority of it is located in the retroperitoneal cavity. In addition to chyme from the stomach, it receives digestive secretions from the pancreas and gallbladder to both aid in digestion and lower the pH of the chyme. The duodenum reenters the peritoneal cavity just before its transition with the jejunum. The jejunum is approximately 8 feet long, and is the site of the bulk of digestion and absorption within the small intestine. The most distal segment of the small intestine is the ileum, which is about 8 feet in length. The ileocecal valve at its terminus regulates the flow of material from the small intestine into the first segment of the large intestine, the cecum.

The large intestine, from its beginning at the ileocecal valve, runs a horseshoe-shaped route around the small intestine to its terminus at the anus. It is responsible for the resorption of water, electrolytes, and some vitamins from the intestinal contents. The large intestine has an overall length of about 5 feet, and is divided into the cecum, colon, and rectum. The colon is further divided into the ascending, transverse, and descending colon.

The cecum is a small, expandable pouch that receives material from the ileum and begins the process of fecal collection. The ascending colon, while covered on its anterior surface by the parietal peritoneum, is considered a retroperitoneal structure. It ascends the right posterolateral wall of the abdominal cavity, then makes a sharp turn at the hepatic flexure below the liver, and transitions into the transverse colon. The transverse colon curves anteriorly to reenter the peritoneal cavity, where it is suspended in place by the mesentery. The transverse colon transitions into the descending colon at the splenic flexure and then travels inferiorly along the left posterolateral wall of the abdominal cavity. Transition to the sigmoid colon takes place at the level of the iliac fossa with the sigmoid flexure before ending at the rectum. The rectum forms the lasts 6 inches of the digestive tract, and is a storage area for fecal material prior to defecation.

ACCESSORY ORGANS

The accessory organs of the digestive tract include the liver, gallbladder, and pancreas. The liver lies in the upper right quadrant of the abdomen within the peritoneal cavity and is the largest organ in the abdominal compartment. As such, it is frequently the recipient of traumatic forces. The inferior rib cage provides some bony protection to the liver. The falciform ligament bisects the liver, dividing it into the left and right lobes, and anchors the liver to the posterior and anterior abdominal walls. The inferior margin of the falciform ligament thickens to form the ligamentum teres, which is actually the remnant of the fetal umbilical vein. The liver is encapsulated in a tough, fibrous layer that is itself covered with a layer of visceral peritoneum. The hepatic artery provides the liver's enormous blood supply, which is about 25% of cardiac output. Venous return is via the hepatic vein, which deposits blood into the inferior vena cava. In addition to a rich arterial supply, the liver receives all venous blood exiting the digestive system through the hepatic portal vein. The hepatic portal vein, hepatic artery, nerves, lymphatic structures, and the hepatic bile ducts pass through the hilus.

The liver's functions can be divided into three categories: metabolic regulation, hematologic regulation, and bile synthesis and secretion. In addition to monitoring circulating levels of carbohydrates, fats, and amino acids, the liver removes old or damaged red blood cells from circulation and synthesizes plasma proteins. Bile, produced to aid in the digestion of fats, is produced in the liver, stored in the gallbladder, and excreted into the duodenum.

The gallbladder is located on the posterior surface of the liver and stores and concentrates bile produced in the liver prior to secretion into the duodenum. When needed, bile exits the gallbladder through the cystic duct, which joins the common hepatic duct from the liver to form the common bile duct that terminates at the duodenum. The pancreatic duct shares this terminus, and the hepatopancreatic sphincter controls the secretion of bile and pancreatic juice into the duodenum.

The pancreas is a retroperitoneal structure that is about 6 inches in length. The head of the pancreas is tucked into the C-shaped fold of the duodenum, and its body and tail extend back into the abdominal cavity toward the spleen, coming to a point at, and adhering to, the posterior abdominal wall. The pancreatic duct carries digestive enzymes and buffers secreted by the pancreas to the duodenum. The pancreas also secretes insulin, glucagon, and somatostatin from specialized cells located in the islets of Langerhans. As such, it has both endocrine and exocrine functions.

OTHER ABDOMINAL STRUCTURES

The spleen, the body's largest lymphoid organ, lies in the upper left abdominal quadrant and is approximately 5 inches long. It sits just inferior to the diaphragm, protected by the inferior margin of the left rib cage. The spleen removes abnormal blood cells from circulation and stores B and T cells ready to combat antigens detected in the circulating blood. As such, the spleen receives a significant blood supply via the splenic artery. Approximately 5% of circulating blood volume is filtered through the spleen every minute. The splenic vein returns blood to the inferior vena cava. Blood vessels, nerves, and lymphatic structures entering and exiting the spleen travel through the hilus.

The abdomen also has a rich vascular network. (See Figure 16-4 ■.) The abdominal aorta travels inferiorly along the left lateral spinal column, bifurcating in the pelvis at the level of the sacrum to form the common iliac arteries. Numerous branches of inferior and superior mesenteric arteries, themselves branches of the aorta, supply the bowel with blood. The mesenteric, splenic, gastroepiploic, and gastric veins all join the hepatic portal vein to divert venous blood flow from the bowel, spleen, and stomach to the liver prior to deposition in the inferior vena cava.

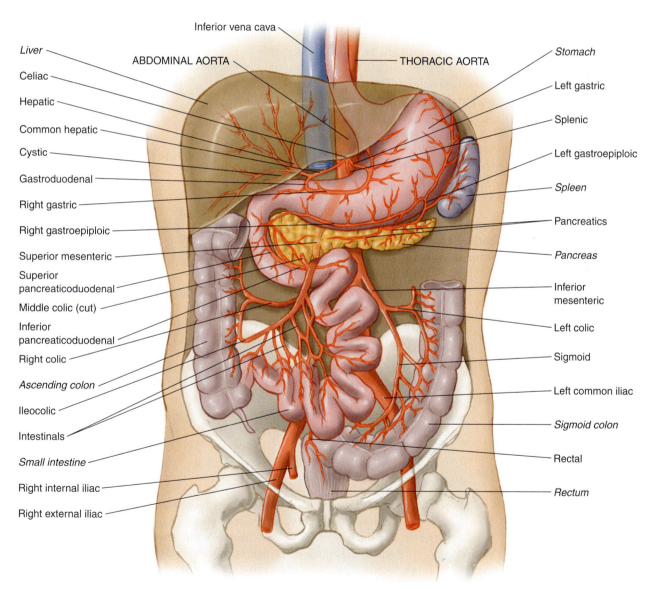

■ **Figure 16-4** The abdominal arteries.

PATHOPHYSIOLOGY

While it may be an admittedly simplistic way to consider it, abdominal trauma can be divided into two types: blunt and penetrating. Patients may, and very often do, suffer both blunt and penetrating traumatic insult. What both classifications of abdominal trauma have in common is that outward signs of injury may not be immediately apparent due to the lack of skeletal structures protecting the abdominal compartment. This results in an unobstructed pathway for the transmission of energy from the vehicle of trauma to the intra-abdominal organs.

Many factors contribute to the high mortality associated with abdominal trauma, including time from incident to arrival at an emergency department, facility type, and severity of injury. The golden rule in trauma care has always been the "Golden Hour," during which every attempt is made to deliver a trauma patient to the operating table to ensure the highest chance of survival. While recent academic scrutiny has failed to find any historical data to support this specific claim, what is clear is that patients who suffer intra-abdominal trauma will experience a decreased risk of mortality the sooner they arrive at an emergency department. The emergency department of choice would be a Level 1 trauma center that is staffed, has the ability, and is prepared to treat the patient. In addition, intra-abdominal trauma patients seldom have a single injury to a single organ. More often, multiorgan and/or multisystem trauma is involved, which significantly increases mortality.

Blunt trauma is the most common mechanism of injury seen in the United States.

Blunt trauma is the most common mechanism of injury seen in the United States. The solid abdominal organs are particularly susceptible to the extreme, diffuse pressure extremes that accompany many blunt mechanisms of injury; as such, they account for a high percentage of blunt abdominal injuries. The abdominal organs most frequently injured in blunt trauma, in order from highest incidence of injury to lowest are:

- ★ Liver
- ★ Spleen
- ★ Large intestine
- ★ Small intestine

Penetrating trauma typically affects the hollow organs because they occupy a vast majority of the space in the abdominal cavity, and penetrating injury energy transfer tends to be very localized. Gunshot and stab wounds account for the vast majority of these penetrating injuries. Gunshot wounds tend to injure, in descending order:

- ★ Small bowel
- ★ Mesentery structures
- ★ Liver
- ★ Colon
- ★ Diaphragm

With stab wounds, the order of frequency is slightly different (again in descending order of occurrence):

- ★ Liver
- ★ Colon
- ★ Small bowel
- ★ Stomach

In cases of penetrating trauma, local wound exploration will be performed by a surgeon to determine if the insult simply penetrates the anterior or posterior fascia and does not enter the peritoneum, in which case the patient is often discharged home. This does not suggest, however, that wound exploration should take place in the field. Treatment and transport decisions should still be made accordingly. Digital exploration is discouraged, because wound exploration is a surgical procedure requiring proper lighting, instruments, asepsis, and ability.

Although specific intra-abdominal organ injury may have common presentation findings, collectively they commonly have one of more of the following general findings:

- ★ Abdominal pain
- ★ Hypoperfusion (hemorrhagic shock)
- ★ **Devascularization** (loss of blood supply to a part or organ of the body)

SPECIFIC ABDOMINAL ORGAN INJURIES

LIVER

The liver, being the largest solid organ in the abdomen, is extremely vulnerable to both blunt and penetrating mechanisms of injury. The liver's tough, fibrous outer capsule can split when subjected to the introduction of energy via trauma mechanisms, resulting in "fracturing" of the organ. The significant blood flow, up to 25% of cardiac output, and its dense vascular anatomy combine to contribute to severe hemorrhage when the liver is injured. It has been shown that up to 60% of liver trauma patients present to the emergency department unstable, reflecting the trend toward hemodynamic instability from these injuries. About 80% of liver injuries are secondary to penetrating trauma, with blunt trauma responsible for the remaining 20%.

Liver injuries are categorized according to the American Association for the Surgery of Trauma (AAST) Liver Injury Scale, on which they are assigned a grade of I through VI. Familiarization with this scale by the critical care paramedic is important because this information may be in the report given to the critical care team prior to transport.

- ★ *Grade I and II injuries* are subcapsular hematomas that are nonexpanding and represent less than 50% of surface area, or are lacerations of the capsule that are at most bleeding lightly with a depth of less than 3 cm or length of less than 10 cm. These injuries account for 70% to 80% of all liver injuries.

- ★ *Grade III injuries* start to get more serious, and include hematomas involving greater that half of the liver surface area and lacerations deeper than 3 cm.

- ★ *Grade IV–VI injuries* are increasingly more severe, with a grade VI resulting in total avulsion of the liver from the hepatic artery and vein, a devastating injury with an extremely high mortality secondary to exsanguination.

While the overall mortality associated with liver injury is less than 10% and grade IV or higher liver injuries occur in less than 6% of all injuries, the importance of identifying liver injury and anticipating the potential for exsanguination cannot be overstated. As a highly vascular organ, the liver may hemorrhage significantly, and the potential outcome associated with unrecognized injury can be disastrous.

The liver, being the largest solid organ in the abdomen, is extremely vulnerable to both blunt and penetrating injury.

GALLBLADDER

Due to the protected location of the gallbladder, injuries to it, the bile duct, and the cystic duct almost never present as isolated injuries. Factors that predispose individuals to a biliary injury include gallbladder distention and alcohol abuse. Penetrating trauma is a common cause of gallbladder injuries, but compression injuries sustained when it is crushed between the liver and spine account for the majority of trauma. Due to a lack of specific symptomatology, diagnosis of a biliary injury on clinical grounds alone can prove quite challenging, if at all possible.

Due to the protected location of the gallbladder, injuries to it, the bile duct, and the cystic duct almost never present as isolated injuries.

SPLEEN

The spleen is the second most commonly injured abdominal organ in blunt trauma, with motor vehicle collisions (MVCs) the most frequent mechanism of injury. It is important to remember, however, that mechanisms sufficient to cause splenic injury can be so unimpressive that a patient may have no recall of a "traumatic" incident. In addition, delayed rupture of the spleen occurs in approximately 5% of blunt trauma splenic injuries, with most cases (80%) presenting within 2 to 3 weeks of injury.

The spleen is the second most commonly injured abdominal organ in blunt trauma, with motor vehicle collisions the most frequent mechanism of injury.

Splenic injuries are categorized according to the AAST Spleen Injury Scale, on which they are assigned a grade of I through V:

★ *Grade I injuries* include small subcapsular hematomas and shallow capsular lacerations.

★ *Grade II injuries* include hematomas involving up to 50% of surface area, and capsular lacerations up to 3 cm and hemorrhaging.

★ *Grade III injuries* are subcapsular hematomas covering greater than 50% of surface area or are expanding, and lacerations greater than 3 cm or involving trabecular blood vessels in the spleen parenchyma.

★ *Grade IV injuries* include ruptured, hemorrhaging interparenchymal hematomas and deep lacerations resulting in devascularization of greater than 25% of the spleen.

★ *Grade V injuries* are those that completely shatter or devascularize the spleen.

STOMACH

Stomach injury secondary to blunt trauma is an extremely rare event, accounting for about 1% of all blunt intra-abdominal injuries.

Stomach injury secondary to blunt trauma is an extremely rare event, accounting for about 1% of all blunt intra-abdominal injuries. Most often, gastric rupture occurs when a full stomach is subjected to a compressive force, as in the case of the abdomen coming into contact with a steering wheel in an MVC. The stomach is injured much more frequently in penetrating injuries, with mechanisms that include gunshot and stab wounds. Along with stomach involvement, remember that these penetration injuries may also involve other structures such as the colon, liver, spleen, small intestine, pancreas, and omentum.

DUODENUM

Because of its intimacy with other organs, duodenal injuries almost never occur in isolation.

Located in the retroperitoneal space next to the head of the pancreas, the duodenum is well protected, and as a result accounts for a rather low percentage (3% to 5%) of all abdominal injuries. Because of its intimacy with other organs, duodenal injuries almost never occur in isolation. Other organs commonly injured in decreasing frequency include the liver, pancreas, small intestine, and colon. Duodenal rupture is usually contained within the retroperitoneal space, and patients often initially present asymptomatic. A high index of suspicion based on appreciation of mechanism of injury is usually required to suspect a duodenal injury.

JEJUNUM AND ILEUM

Overall, penetrating trauma accounts for the vast majority of small bowel injury. About 80% of gunshot wounds and 30% to 50% of stab wounds include small bowel insult. Blunt trauma most often results in injury to the proximal jejunum and terminal ileum as the small bowel is torn away from the ligament of Trietz and cecum both of which are sturdily anchored to the abdominal wall. The mesenteric vasculature is often also involved, contributing to intra-abdominal hemorrhage. In addition, bowel contents, including digestive enzymes and partially digested chyme, can spill into the peritoneal cavity, resulting in gastrointestinal contamination, possible infection, autodigestion, and eventual peritonitis. Bowel evisceration occurs when the abdominal wall is violated, allowing abdominal contents, most often mesentery and small bowel, to protrude through the insult to the extra-abdominal environment. Slashing-type injuries secondary to an assault with a knife or other sharp object are frequent causes of injuries that result in evisceration.

PANCREAS

With the pancreas located in a protected area deep within the peritoneal cavity, pancreatic trauma is uncommon, accounting for about 7% of all traumatic abdominal injuries. When it is injured, 70% to 75% of the time it is secondary to penetrating trauma. When blunt trauma is the mechanism of injury, the midbody of the pancreas is often crushed against the vertebral column by a crushing force to the anterior thoracic and abdominal wall, as when the driver of a car collides with a steering wheel. More than 90% of patients with pancreatic insult have concomitant injury to an additional abdominal organ, with the mean number of additional injuries being about three per patient.

The three organs most likely to be injured along with the pancreas are the liver, stomach, and abdominal vascular structures. In addition to the threat of hemorrhage, the disruption of the exocrine pancreas tissue can lead to the leaking of digestive enzymes within the retroperitoneal space and subsequent autodigestion of surrounding tissue.

LARGE INTESTINE

The colon and rectum account for 5% of all intra-abdominal injuries, and almost 96% of injuries to these structures are secondary to penetrating trauma. Gunshot wounds are the most frequent cause of colon and rectal injury, with stab wounds accounting for less than 10% of all injuries. Blunt force trauma accounts for 3% to 10% of all traumatic colorectal injuries. Colorectal trauma is often also complicated by the introduction of fecal material into the abdominal or pelvic compartments, resulting in peritonitis and sepsis. Mortality from colon injury is between 2% and 12%.

VASCULAR INJURIES

The abdominal cavity and viscera are rich in large vascular structures that circulate a significant quantity of blood. As such, injury to abdominal vascular structures is associated with some of the highest mortality rates of abdominal injuries; between 30% and 60% combined. Individually, injuries to the aorta have a 50% to 70% mortality, iliac artery 40% to 53%, inferior vena cava 30% to 53%, portal and splenic veins 40% to 70%, and iliac vein 38%. Ninety-seven percent of abdominal vascular injuries are secondary to penetrating trauma. Blunt trauma can occur to abdominal vasculature in a variety of ways. The mobile small bowel and colon often avulse branches off the fixed superior mesenteric artery when subjected to rapid deceleration injuries. Aortic injuries can occur when the aorta is crushed against spine by pressure applied to the abdomen from an improperly worn seat belt. In these cases, the intimal layer of the aorta is typically lacerated, resulting in a thrombus formation.

The mortality associated with the larger vascular structures of the abdomen can be quite high. Because the abdominal compartment is able to expand and accommodate a significant amount of blood, outward evidence of massive internal bleeding can be occult; the care provider must suspect intra-abdominal bleeding secondary to the mechanism of injury and clinical exam findings suggesting developing hypovolemic shock.

ASSESSMENT OF THE ABDOMINAL INJURY

Assessment of the abdominal trauma patient, as with all trauma patients, needs to take place rapidly, with initial attention paid to the airway, breathing, and circulatory status of the patient. Whether providing initial care at the scene of an accident, or transferring a patient from an ED to a tertiary care facility, a sincere effort must be made by the critical care paramedic to record an accurate history of the events resulting in injury. If the critical care team arrives at a care facility after the emergency crew that provided prehospital care has left, you may wish to inquire if they can return although this is rarely, if ever, done. They are in the best position to provide answers to any questions regarding the scene that you may need. If at all possible, get to the source of information; do not rely on second, third, or fourth parties to provide descriptions of the scene and the mechanism of injury.

If the critical care team is performing an interfacility transfer, the physicians, nurses, paramedics, and technicians at the transferring facility should provide you with a full patient report at the time of your arrival. The results of all studies performed should be reported and made available for review and transport with the patient. (Refer to Chapter 6, "Patient Assessment and Preparation for Transport," for more information regarding this.)

With the pancreas located in a protected area deep within the peritoneal cavity, pancreatic trauma is uncommon, accounting for about 7% of all traumatic abdominal injuries.

Gunshot wounds are the most frequent cause of colon and rectal injury.

Kehr's sign *blood in the peritoneum that irritates the diaphragm and causes referred pain in the shoulder as nerve impulses travel to nerve roots in the lower cervical spine.*

Cullen's sign *blood in the abdomen that has tracked to the umbilicus through the ligamentum teres, resulting in periumbilical bruising.*

Grey Turner's sign *retroperitoneal bleeding that causes bruising to the flank.*

Even though the patient's abdomen may have already been assessed by the initial care providers, the critical care paramedic should complete another abdominal assessment on his own. Remember that, many times, the initial assessment may not yield indications of an injury that is progressing. By the time you arrive, the patient is typically in better lighting, and injury findings not present initially may now be readily evident.

Be sure to not only inspect and palpate the anterior abdomen, but to closely assess the lateral and posterior aspects as well.

A multitude of diagnostic modalities are used to evaluate the abdomen and genitourinary tract, including laparotomy, diagnostic peritoneal lavage, sonography, and radiograph.

laparotomy *a surgical incision into a cavity of the abdomen.*

Even though the patient's abdomen may have already been assessed by the initial care providers, the critical care paramedic should complete another abdominal assessment on his own. Remember that, many times, the initial assessment may not yield indications of an injury that is progressing. By the time you arrive, the patient is typically in better lighting, and injury findings not present initially may now be readily evident.

Fully expose the abdomen prior to beginning your exam. Inspect the abdomen for any obvious signs of trauma, including abrasions, bruising, penetrating injuries, lacerations, bruising, deformity, or contusions. After palpation, the abdomen should be auscultated to assess the presence and quality of bowel sounds. If conditions on a scene prevent any likelihood of appreciating bowel sounds, do not belabor the fact. Palpation should be performed to assess for tenderness, guarding, rigidity, masses, pulsations, or crepitus of the lower ribs. Tenderness or signs of trauma in the upper right quadrant suggest liver injury, while the same findings in the upper left quadrant are consistent with injury to the spleen. Likewise, fractured ribs increase the likelihood of injury to the spleen or liver. In addition, pain to the left shoulder unsupported by mechanism or signs of injury in an abdominal trauma patient may indicate a splenic injury. This occurs when blood in the peritoneum irritates the diaphragm, resulting in referred pain in the shoulder as the nervous impulse travels to the nerve roots in the lower cervical spine (a condition known as **Kehr's sign**). Periumbilical bruising (**Cullen's sign**) indicates blood in the abdomen, often from the liver, that has tracked to the umbilicus through the ligamentum teres, the remnant of the fetal umbilical vein. Bruising to the flanks (**Grey Turner's sign**) can be indicative of retroperitoneal bleeding. Important to remember, though, is that the last two aforementioned findings are more indicative of an older injury, so their presence suggests a mechanism that occurred some time prior.

Be sure to not only inspect and palpate the anterior abdomen, but to closely assess the lateral and posterior aspects as well. Roll the patient over (maintaining in-line immobilization as necessary), and ensure that you have an unobstructed view and adequate lighting. Do not make the mistake of rushing through the exam; be deliberate, systematic, and thorough every time. Too many injuries go unrecognized in part because of incomplete abdominal exams.

Any tenderness upon palpation, guarding, or the presence of a significant mechanism of injury should raise the index of suspicion for intra-abdominal injury, as it represents a common physical finding. A large percentage of traumatic abdominal injury cases may have no initial complaint or outward signs of injury during the initial assessment, but use this information as a baseline to compare the numerous reassessments that should be performed while en route to the receiving facility. Even then, many injuries will remain occult and not be diagnosed or suspected until CT, sonography, or diagnostic peritoneal lavage is performed.

SCREENING EXAMS FOR ABDOMINAL INJURY

A multitude of diagnostic modalities are used to evaluate the abdomen and genitourinary tract, including laparotomy, diagnostic peritoneal lavage, sonography, and radiograph. No test is perfect for every patient, and each must be used after consideration of the physical exam, patient stability, and assessment findings. The results of these exams can be utilized by the critical care paramedic when the patient is undergoing an interfacility transfer. Always inquire as to any screening exams performed, their results, and if you are able, review the studies yourself. Copies of all results and films should be included in the patient's records and be transferred to the receiving facility with the patient. (See Figure 16-5 ■.)

LAPAROTOMY

Laparotomy (the surgical opening of the abdomen) is considered the "gold standard" therapy for intra-abdominal injury because it allows an unparalleled assessment of the abdomen and retroperitoneum, is definitive, and allows for immediate injury repair. Given that a majority of intra-abdominal injuries can be managed nonoperatively, not every patient who presents as such should

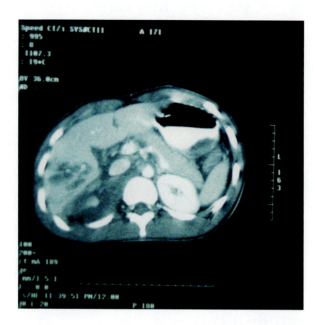

■ **Figure 16-5** CT of abdominal injury. (*Edward T. Dickinson, MD*)

receive it. Laparotomy is usually reserved for those patients who present with hemodynamic instability, penetrating abdominal injury, peritoneal findings, gross blood in the abdomen, intraperitoneal free air, and CT findings that suggest the necessity for surgical repair. In hemodynamically stable patients, less invasive methods of assessing the abdomen such as CT, sonography, and diagnostic peritoneal lavage are usually considered.

Obviously, because laparotomy is an involved surgical procedure, the critical care transport teams will not be performing this procedure in the field. Rather, the critical care team is likely to transport a patient who has already undergone emergent laparotomy for abdominal trauma or one who is in need of this procedure if the referring facility is unable to address the problems found. In such a case, the critical care paramedic should expect to receive a report on injuries diagnosed, any repair procedures performed, and any other information that the surgeon feels is important for the team to be aware of.

DIAGNOSTIC PERITONEAL LAVAGE

Diagnostic peritoneal lavage (DPL) involves the insertion of a catheter into the peritoneal cavity to assess for the presence of blood. First introduced in 1965, it has an impressive history of 97% accuracy, a record that is equaled by few other diagnostic exams in medicine.

The procedure is performed by inserting a catheter into the peritoneal space by either the open or closed technique. In the open technique, a small incision is made through the abdominal fascia, muscle, and peritoneum just below the umbilicus, and then a catheter is passed through. In the closed method, a trochar is used to puncture the fascia, muscle, and peritoneum, and the catheter is then advanced off the needle via the Seldinger technique (although the open technique is preferred, because it minimizes the risk of injury to the abdominal contents). Once the catheter is in place, a syringe is used to attempt aspiration of any gross blood. Aspiration of 10 mL of blood is considered positive, and the patient will often receive an explorative laparotomy. If no blood is aspirated, 1 L of normal saline is infused into the peritoneal cavity, allowed to diffuse for 5–10 minutes, and then removed. This can often be accomplished by simply lowering the IV bag to the floor and allowing gravity to aid draignage. The fluid is then inspected in a laboratory and considered positive if:

★ There are more than 100,000 RBC/mm^3 for blunt trauma or 5,000 RBC/mm^3 for penetration wounds.

★ There are more than 500 WBC/mm^3.

diagnostic peritoneal lavage (DPL) *technique for ascertaining the presence of blood in the abdomen via insertion of a catheter into the peritoneal cavity, then aspirating fluids for examination.*

★ Bile or an amylase greater than serum amylase is present, or if bacteria, fecal matter, or food particles are present.

Indications for DPL include a history of trauma and suspicion of intra-abdominal injury. Relative contraindications include pregnancy and previous abdominal surgery. While DPL is rapid and sensitive, it is not specific. All a DPL really reveals is that there is blood in the abdomen; the site and severity of the hemorrhage remain unknown. It has often been lamented that DPL results in the identification of minor, normally inoperative injuries that result in unnecessary laparotomies. In addition, while DPL enjoys a relatively low complication rate, it has limitations. There may be complications secondary to the insertion of the needle or catheter, it cannot determine if a patient is continuing to bleed, and it is ineffective for identifying retroperitoneal hemorrhage.

A DPL should only be performed by a surgeon who will be making surgical decisions about the patient. The role of DPL in critical care transport is limited, because the technology for peritoneal fluid evaluation has not caught up with critical care transport requirements for small, light, and easily portable units. The critical care paramedic could be educated on the skill needed to perform DPL in the field, thereby having the 50-mL sample ready for evaluation promptly at the time of arrival, but this is not yet the case. It is more likely that a critical care transport team may be asked to finish a lavage that was started prior to their arrival. In cases of transport from a facility that has performed a DPL, knowledge of the results could aid in decision making prior to and during transport. (See Figure 16-6 ■.)

SONOGRAPHY

Sonography is the use of inaudible sound (or ultrasound) to produce an image of an organ or tissue. The ultrasonic echoes are recorded as they strike the tissues of various densities. **Focused assessment with sonography for trauma (FAST)** is an ultrasound assessment designed to detect blood in the pericardium or abdomen secondary to traumatic injury. It is quickly becoming an important tool in the emergency department because, as the acronym implies, the study is fast (performed in 3–4 minutes by experienced examiners), is accurate (96% to 98% accuracy at detecting fluid in the peritoneal cavity), rather inexpensive, is without complications since it is noninvasive, and is repeatable as often as necessary.

The FAST exam involves the assessment of four areas of a supine patient. First, the pericardium is assessed for fluid via a sagittal view from the subxiphoid area. (See Figure 16-7 ■.) Second, a sagittal view of the abdomen from the right midaxillary line between the 11th and 12th ribs is used to

sonography *inaudible sounds (ultrasonic echoes) that are recorded as they strike the tissues of various densities in order to produce an image of an organ or tissue.*

focused assessment with sonography for trauma (FAST) *ultrasound assessment designed to detect blood in the pericardium or abdomen, secondary to traumatic injury.*

■ **Figure 16-6** Diagnostic peritoneal lavage. *(Edward T. Dickinson, MD)*

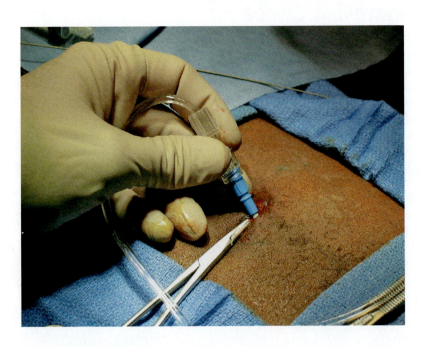

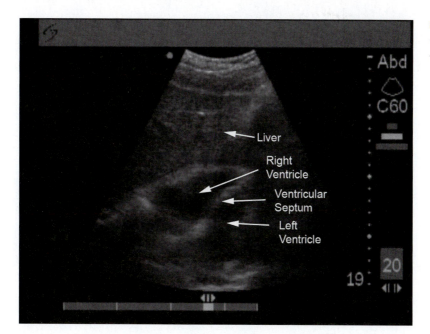

evaluate the hepatorenal space, or Morrison's pouch, for blood. (**Morrison's pouch** is the recess of the peritoneal cavity that lies between the liver in front and the kidney and adrenal behind.) (See Figure 16-8 ■.) Third, a sagittal view of the abdomen from the left midaxillary line between the 10th and 11th ribs is used to assess the spleen and kidney and assess the splenorenal space for blood. (See Figures 16-9 ■ through 16-11 ■.) Fourth, it provides a coronal view superior to the pubis symphysis that is utilized to assess the pelvis for blood. (See Figure 16-12 ■.)

FAST can be considered an initial diagnostic modality for use in the abdominal trauma patient, and can be performed easily during the detailed physical exam. FAST does have its limitations, chief among them an inability to reveal small amounts of blood (<200 mL), and false-negative results have been reported in instances of diaphragmatic rupture (in which intra-abdominal blood traversed the injured diaphragm, resulting in hemoperitoneum and a negative FAST exam).

Morrison's pouch *the hepatorenal space, a recess of the peritoneal cavity that lies between the liver in front and the kidney and adrenal behind.*

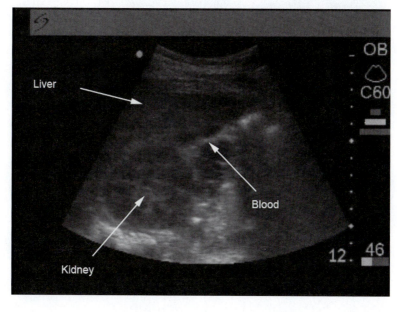

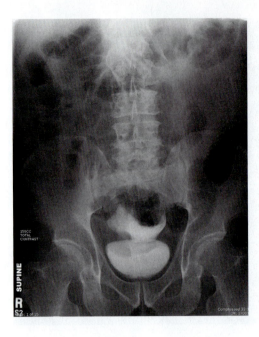

Figure 16-9 X-ray of bladder rupture. Note extravasation of dye into abdominal cavity. *(Kathy Altergott, BSN, MBA, CRA. Banner Good Samaritan Medical Center, Phoenix, AZ)*

FAST has been shown to have a sensitivity for the presence of hemoperitoneum between 73% and 88%, a specificity between 98% and 100%, and is accurate 96% to 98% of the time.

Overall, FAST has been shown to have a sensitivity for the presence of hemoperitoneum between 73% and 88%, a specificity between 98% and 100%, and is accurate 96% to 98% of the time. Perhaps more impressive, it has been shown that the level of accuracy is independent of the level of the practitioner performing the study. Ultrasound technicians have results equal to those of ED physicians and trauma surgeons. This suggests that with proper training and frequent use, it could be adapted to the critical care transport environment with success. Another factor making ultrasound a very real possibility in critical care transport medicine is the handheld ultrasound units, which are now readily available and arguably affordable.

In summation of this assessment technique, it has been shown that aeromedical transport teams can be successfully educated on performing FAST assessments in the field. However, they are yet unable to perform a complete exam while in flight (or en route with ground units) secondary to the time restraints, limited personnel, and the dynamic environment in an aircraft or ground unit. As such, if the critical care paramedic has the opportunity to utilize handheld ultrasound, it

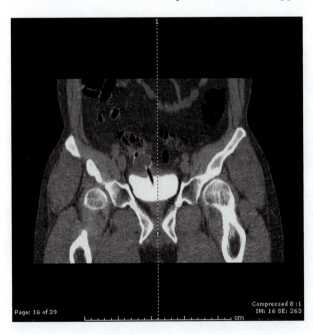

Figure 16-10 CT scan of bladder rupture. *(Kathy Altergott, BSN, MBA, CRA. Banner Good Samaritan Medical Center, Phoenix, AZ)*

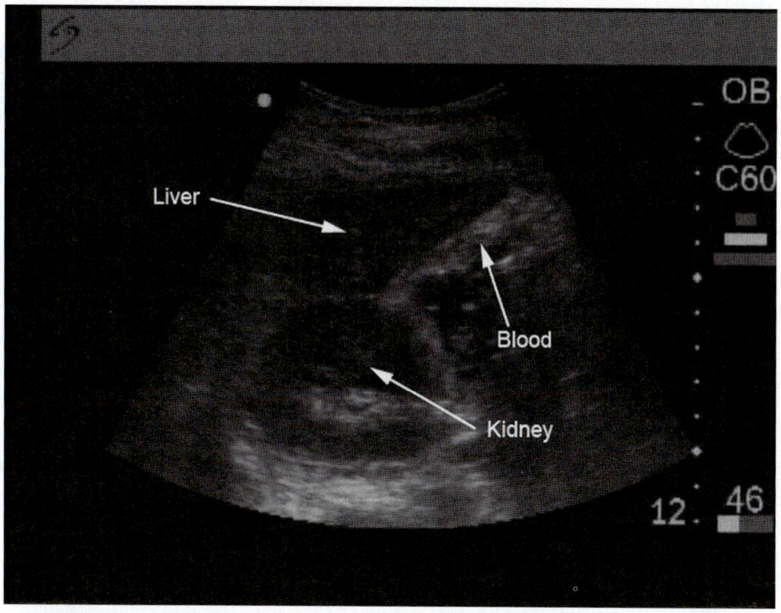

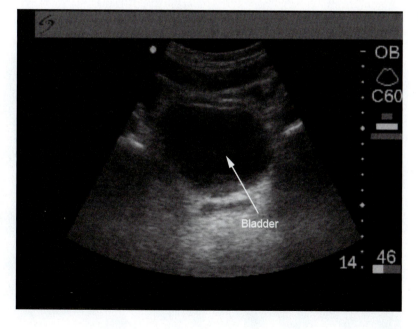

■ Figure 16-11 FAST ultrasound (sagittal view). *(David Spear, MD)*

should be done prior to transport. Remember also that the critical care paramedic is not necessarily going to alter specific treatment modalities based on the FAST exam results. While the critical care transport team should obtain as much information as possible, the key is rapid transport for surgical intervention.

COMPUTED TOMOGRAPHY

Computed tomography (CT), a process by which transverse planes of tissues are swept by a pinpoint radiographic beam allowing the construction of a computerized image, provides an excellent modality to screen for specific abdominal injury in the stable trauma patient who may not require operative management of his intra-abdominal injuries. It is also indicated in patients with altered sensorium secondary to pharmacologic or traumatic etiologies.

computed tomography (CT) *a process by which transverse planes of tissues are swept by a pinpoint radiographic beam allowing the construction of a computerized image.*

■ Figure 16-12 FAST ultrasound (coronal–above symphysis). *(David Spear, MD)*

CT's great advantage over the DPL technique is that it allows for a specific diagnosis, particularly solid organ injuries. It also allows for a greater number of intra-abdominal trauma patients to be managed nonoperatively after the diagnosis has been made. In addition, it can (unlike DPL) diagnose retroperitoneal injuries. CT does, however, tend to miss injuries that do not result in the introduction of blood or other fluids into the abdominal cavity. Injuries to the pancreas, diaphragm, empty urinary bladder, and small bowel and mesenteric injuries are often underdiagnosed.

However, the more critically injured a patient is, the greater the danger due to treatment delays created by obtaining a CT scan. Currently in unstable patients, a greater emphasis is placed on the immediate performance of a DPL, or in transporting the patient to the operating room for an exploratory laparotomy. This trend may change, however, with the availability of more advanced helical or spiral CT machines. This newer technology can reduce the scanning time to as little as 5 minutes, reducing the risk of worsening hemodynamic instability during the exam.

Evaluation of a CT requires the services of a radiologist to identify the finer injury patterns that can appear on CT. At a minimum though, the critical care paramedic can be taught how to identify frank blood and obvious organ insult on a CT result, allowing for a better understanding of patient pathology and a patient's particular needs with regard to transport and management.

RADIOGRAPHY

Although every trauma patient with a suspected abdominal injury should receive a pelvic and chest X-ray, they are of limited use in the blunt abdominal trauma patient. A radiograph can detect free air in the abdomen and a diaphragmatic rupture, but it cannot detect hemoperitoneum, hollow organ injury, solid organ injury, or vascular injury. There is limited use though in penetrating trauma to rule out the presence of a missile. (See Figure 16-13 ■.)

At best though, common radiograph findings in abdominal trauma can be suggestive for abdominal and genitourinary injuries, but not definitive. Fractured ribs can raise the index of suspicion for liver, spleen, and renal injury, while pelvic fractures can increase the risk of urinary and vascular injuries.

All critical care team members should be familiar with ABG and blood chemistry values and be able to not only interpret the results, but also understand their relationship to the patient's clinical condition and usefulness in diagnosis and management.

PERTINENT LAB VALUES

The critical care paramedic will frequently be presented with labs results on arrival at a transferring facility. In addition, portable blood analyzers are available for critical care use, allowing for arterial blood gas (ABG) and blood chemistry determination on all patients. All critical care team members

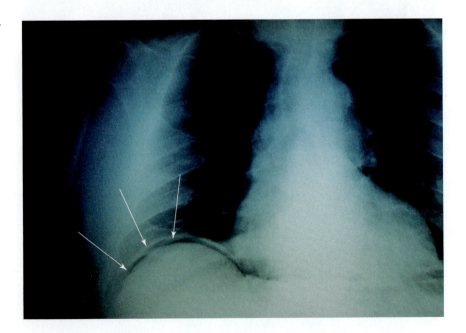

■ Figure 16-13 KUB X-ray with free air. (*Edward T. Dickinson, MD*)

should be familiar with ABG and blood chemistry values and be able to not only interpret the results, but also understand their relationship to the patient's clinical condition and usefulness in diagnosis and management. The following components of each have some value in the evaluation of the patient with abdominal trauma.

ABG

Serum pH indicates the acid–base status. Metabolic acidosis with a high lactate level indicates that anaerobic metabolism is taking place secondary to tissue hypoperfusion. In other words, your patient is in shock, regardless of the blood pressure. In addition, PO_2 and PCO_2 are invaluable information to help determine the oxygenation and ventilation status of your patient.

Blood Chemistry

It is important to remember that most blood chemistry changes that occur secondary to abdominal trauma do not occur acutely. Rather, numerous hours or even days, are required for many values to change.

A liver function test, consisting of an ASP (SGOT), GTT/alkaline phosphatase, and ALT (SGPT) may be elevated in liver trauma or incidences of "shock liver." Particularly in crushing injuries, there can be a transient increase in serum bilirubin secondary to the lyses of red blood cells. Bilirubin will not be elevated in acute liver trauma, but will rise at a rate of approximately 0.8–1.0 per day in liver failure.

The serum lactate is a good indicator of the perfusion status of tissue, especially tissue in the GI tract. An elevated lactate level indicates that VO_2 (the rate of oxygen uptake by tissues from the microcirculation) does not meet the metabolic demand.

Serum amylase and lipase are not reliable indicators for pancreatic trauma, with a positive predictive value of about 10%. A rising serum amylase and lipase indicate a need for further, more sensitive studies of the pancreas. In cases of normal serum amylase after blunt trauma there is a 95% likelihood of no injury to the pancreas. In small bowel injury, the serum amylase will rise independent of lipase.

Low or decreasing serial hemoglobin/hematocrit (H&H) values after a traumatic mechanism of injury to the abdomen are an indication of intra-abdominal bleeding.

Leukocyte levels above 15,000 u/L is considered suggestive but not diagnostic for traumatic injury when a mechanism of injury has been identified. Any stress on the body, physical or psychological, can result in an elevated WBC count, so it's extremely nonspecific and has questionable value. In addition, the WBC count could have been elevated prior to the traumatic event.

An HCG screen to rule out pregnancy should be performed on every female trauma patient of childbearing age to ensure that there is only one patient who requires treatment and not two.

BUN/creatinine will gradually increase in patients who have sustained renal trauma and have limited or no kidney function.

A finger-stick, or similarly rapid, glucose determination should be made on every patient as soon as the ABCs have been addressed, because traumatic events often occur secondary to hypoglycemia.

Urinalysis

Evaluation of the urine for blood is required in trauma patients to assess for hematuria secondary to GU insult. Determination of gross blood can be made clinically by direct observation of the urine after catheterization. Urine reagent strips are useful for a rapid assessment of the urine.

Sublingual Capnometry

Sublingual capnometery is an assessment modality that is gaining support in the trauma and critical care environments. An electrode is placed under the tongue to evaluate the sublingual PCO_2. Because the sublingual mucosa is embryologically and anatomically continuous with the intestinal mucosa, evaluation of the sublingual PCO_2 is, in effect, an evaluation of the visceral PCO_2. Because the gut is among the first tissue to be affected by decreasing tissue perfusion, monitoring of its PCO_2 can alert the care provider very early in the development of shock. Of special interest in abdominal trauma, insult to the bowel results in elevated PCO_2 levels. Sublingual capnometry can therefore

sublingual capnometry
an electrode is placed under the tongue to evaluate the sublingual PCO_2, (essentially the visceral PCO_2); an early diagnostic marker for shock.

help identify subclinical cases of blunt abdominal trauma. Some concern is surfacing, however, with the use of this technique in pediatric populations with accidental malfunction or detachment of the electrode with subsequent aspiration.

MANAGEMENT

The end point for the management of life-threatening abdominal, for that matter all, trauma is surgical care by a trauma team. The role of the critical care paramedic is to correct all immediate life-threatening injuries and provide rapid, safe transport to a trauma center. While airway control and ventilation are, for all intents and purposes, straightforward in isolated abdominal trauma, the identification and control of intra-abdominal hemorrhage is not.

As discussed, intra-abdominal injury can be occult. The critical care paramedic must continuously reassess the trauma patient for signs and symptoms of developing shock secondary to intra-abdominal hemorrhage. While it is impossible to control intra-abdominal bleeding with the typical "direct pressure, elevate, pressure point" modality, shock as a syndrome can be treated. The key is to recognize developing hypovolemic shock and prevent decompensation to eventual cardiovascular collapse.

After securing the airway and ensuring proper ventilation, the patient's circulatory status should be addressed. Initiation of large-bore peripheral access is appropriate, but the establishment of two sites is more desirable. Ideally, and especially in cases of developing or severe hypovolemic shock, central venous access should be established. Central lines placed in large vessels such as the femoral, subclavian, or internal jugular veins offer many advantages over peripheral IVs, including the ability to rapidly administer blood or fluid products. In addition, the larger vessels utilized in central venous access are not as susceptible to vascular collapse in shock as are the peripheral. Note that the external jugular (as opposed to the internal jugular) vein is considered a peripheral and not a central site for IV access due to its smaller lumen diameter. Finally, if it has not been done yet, the critical care paramedic should obtain venous blood samples immediately after successful venous cannulation.

Volume administration in trauma is a subject that is undergoing constant reevaluation after recent academic scrutiny and research. This subject is covered in more depth in Chapter 8, but the recent trend in volume resuscitation suggests that providers should avoid the blind administration of 1–2 L of a crystalloid solution that was the standard of care for hypotensive trauma patients. The critical care paramedic should endeavor to achieve a blood pressure of about three-quarter's of the patient's normal blood pressure. This can be achieved by administering 250 cc fluid boluses of a crystalloid solution until a blood pressure of 75–80 mm/Hg is obtained. It has been fairly well established that this practice of **permissive hypotension** (or the allowance of a lower systolic pressure to maintain perfusion to the heart, brain, lungs, and kidneys during the initial phases of trauma resuscitation) results in less bleeding in patients with uncontrolled hemorrhage. This is not to suggest that the administration of large volumes of crystalloid should never occur though. Many trauma patients lose large volumes of blood that must be replaced rapidly to even reach any threshold of hemodynamic stability, and in such cases administration of 2–3 L of crystalloid may be warranted to keep systolic BP at 75–80 mmHg.

Because infusions of large volumes of crystalloids can lead to hemodilution, the administration of whole blood or packed RBCs should be considered, if available. While there is no clear point at which the literature suggests transitioning from fluid to blood, it is acceptable (if not prudent), to start administration as soon as it is obvious that a patient has lost large quantities of blood volume. Ideally, typed and cross-matched blood should be administered, but the critical care paramedic will more frequently administer type-specific or O⁻ blood in the acute emergency. Recently, synthetic fluids with oxygen-carrying capacity have been introduced, but have not been employed in mainstream medicine as of yet. They are of special interest to critical care transport because, unlike blood, they do not require refrigeration.

Placement of a **Foley catheter,** which is inserted into the urethral meatus for bladder drainage, should also occur prior to transport after urethral injury has been ruled out. This will allow the conscious patient to void his bladder throughout the transport, and allow the critical care paramedic to evaluate urine output, color, and consistency. Before placing a Foley, it is important to ensure there is no blood at the urethral meatus, which is indicative of possible urethral trauma.

The end point for the management of life-threatening abdominal, and for that matter all, trauma is surgical care by a trauma team.

permissive hypotension *purposeful maintenance of a lower systolic pressure that will maintain perfusion to the heart, brain, lungs, and kidneys during the initial phases of trauma resuscitation, without "popping the clot."*

Volume administration in trauma is a subject that is undergoing constant reevaluation after recent academic scrutiny and research.

Foley catheter *A large diameter tube attached to a metered drainage bag; inserted into the urethral meatus for bladder drainage and to measure urine output.*

After addressing the airway, breathing, circulation, and immobilization needs, few other true treatments for abdominal injuries exist. Bowel evisceration can be treated by covering the exposed bowel with a moist, sterile dressing taking care not to put too much pressure on the viscera, which can further complicate already potentially impaired perfusion. Penetrating objects in the abdomen should be treated like all penetrating objects: They should not be removed, but rather secured in place and kept stable during transport. The patient should be kept warm.

GENITOURINARY TRAUMA

Genitourinary trauma can occur from both blunt and pentetrating trauma. In most instances of external genitalia injuries, the finding may be graphic but are not usually life-threatening with proper management. Trauma to the urinary septem may be more severe since numerous internal organs may be damaged. This section will further review the anatomy and physiology, pathophysiology, assessment, and management of genitourinary trauma.

ANATOMY AND PHYSIOLOGY

URINARY SYSTEM

The kidneys are located in the retroperitoneal space lateral to the spinal column between the 12th thoracic and 3rd lumbar vertebrae, each about 4 inches in length. The left kidney typically sits a bit higher in the abdominal cavity than does the right. A layer of collagen fibers called the renal capsule covers the outer surface of the kidney and offers some protection from injury. Some of these collagen fibers extend out and attach to the renal fascia, which itself is connected posteriorly to the deep fascial layers surrounding the abdominal muscles of the posterior abdominal wall. Between the renal capsule and the renal fascia is a layer of adipose tissue. Together, the renal capsule, adipose layer, and renal fascia serve to suspend and protect the kidneys.

The kidneys receive 20% to 25% of total cardiac output via the renal artery, a branch of the abdominal aorta. The renal vein returns blood to the inferior vena cava. All blood vessels, lymphatic structures, and the ureters travel through the hilus when entering or exiting the kidney.

The kidney's major roles include the regulation of fluid and electrolytes, urine formation, waste product removal, red blood cell production, and homeostasis. Failure of the renal system will lead to death without appropriate and timely intervention.

Once the urine is produced in the kidneys, the ureters drain the urine in an inferior direction where the ureters enter the bladder on its posterior side. The urinary bladder is an expandable, muscular reservoir for urine located in the pelvic cavity. Its exact position is different between men and women due to differences in reproductive anatomy. In men, the inferior urinary bladder sits between the rectum and symphysis pubis; in women, it sits inferior to the uterus and anterior to the vagina. When full, the urinary bladder distends and can extend well into the lower abdominal quadrants. The urethra exits the bladder at the neck, and travels to the terminus of the external genitalia. (See Figure 16-14 ■.) The female urethra is about 1–1.5 inches in length, terminating at the vaginal vestibule. The male urethra is about 7–8 inches in length, terminating at the tip of the penis. In the male, the urethra is divided into three parts: the prostatic urethra, the membranous urethra, and the penile urethra. The prostatic urethra passes through the prostate gland, the membranous urethra travels through the urogenital diaphragm, and the penile urethra travels the length of the penis. There are functional differences between these divisions that are of no consideration in trauma.

REPRODUCTIVE SYSTEM: GENITALIA

The female reproductive system consists of the ovaries, fallopian tubes, uterus, and vagina. (See Figure 16-15 ■.) The ovaries are small, paired organs that are located near the lateral walls of the pelvic cavity. They are secured in place in the pelvic cavity by the suspensory and ovarian ligaments.

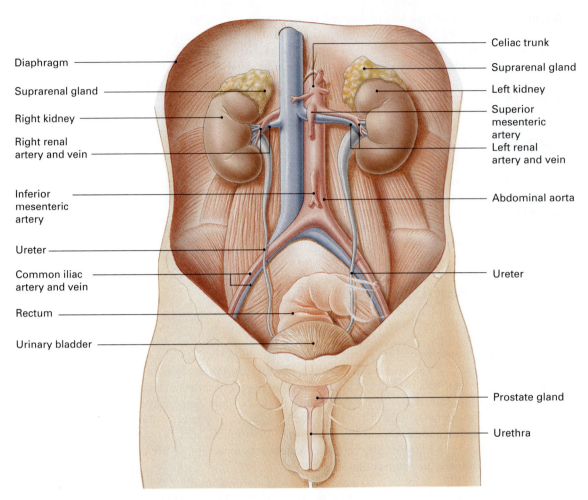

Diaphragm

Suprarenal gland

Right kidney

Right renal
artery and vein

Inferior
mesenteric
artery

Ureter

Common iliac
artery and vein

Rectum

Urinary bladder

Celiac trunk

Suprarenal gland

Left kidney

Superior
mesenteric
artery

Left renal
artery and vein

Abdominal aorta

Ureter

Prostate gland

Urethra

■ **Figure 16-14**   The urinary system.

The two primary functions of the ovaries are the production of ova and secretion of hormones. After puberty, the ovary releases an ovum every 28 days as a result of hormonal changes influenced by the ovarian cycle. The ovum then travels through the fallopian tube to the uterus.

The fallopian tube is a hollow, muscular tube about 5 inches in length. It is divided into three parts: the infundibulum, the ampulla, and the isthmus. The most distal part of the fallopian tube, the infundibulum, has a number of finger-like projections termed fimbriae, whose wave-like motion creates a current in the intra-abdominal fluid of the pelvic cavity that encourages the released ovum to travel into the fallopian tube. The ovum then travels through the ampulla and isthmus, which opens up into the uterus.

The nongravid uterus is a small, hollow, pear-shaped organ about 3 inches long and 2 inches wide that lies on the superior aspect of the urinary bladder, anterior to the rectum. It is held in place in the pelvic cavity by the uterosacral, the broad, and the round ligaments, and receives a rich blood supply provided by the uterine artery. It is divided into four parts: the superior fundus, the body, the isthmus, and inferior cervix. The uterus serves as the "organ of pregnancy," providing protection and support for a developing fetus.

The cervix houses the cervical canal, which enters into the vaginal canal. The vaginal canal is an elastic yet muscular tube that extends about 3 inches to the vestibule of the external genitalia. The vagina receives its blood supply via the vaginal artery, which originates from the uterine artery. The vagina is the birth canal, and is able to stretch and accommodate the fetus as it is expelled from the uterus during labor. In addition, it is a passageway for menstrual blood flow, and receives the penis during intercourse.

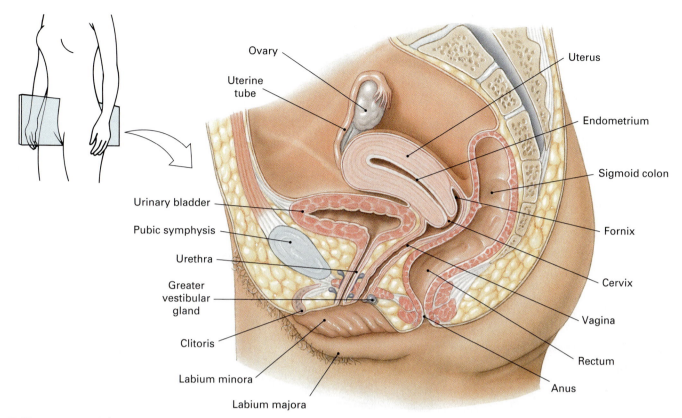

Figure 16-15 The components of the female reproductive system. *(Fig. 20-8, p. 556, from* Essentials of Anatomy & Physiology, *2nd ed., by Frederic H. Martini, Ph.D. and Edwin F. Bartholomew, M.S. Copyright © 2000 by Frederic H. Martini, Inc. Published by Pearson Education, Inc. Reprinted by permission.)*

The male reproductive system consists of the testes, epididymis, ductus deferens, seminal vesicle, ejaculatory duct, prostate gland, urethra, and penis. (See Figure 16-16 ■.) The testes are the site of sperm production, and are housed in the scrotum. The scrotum is a hollow pouch of skin that descends from the inferior base of the penis, anterior to the anus. The testes and its blood vessels, nerves, lymphatic structures, and ductus deferens are all enclosed in the spermatic cord, a tough layer of fascia, muscle, and connective tissue that descends into the scrotum from the pelvic cavity through the inguinal canal.

Immature sperm develop in the epididymis, located on the posterior aspect of the testicle. The epididymus is a coiled, twisted tube that is up to 7 feet long. It transitions into the ductus deferens, which travels through the spermatic cord, joining with the ejaculatory duct. The ejaculatory duct connects the seminal vesicles, located on the inferior surface of the urinary bladder, with the urethra. The seminal vesicles secrete seminal fluid, which accounts for about 60% of the volume of semen. The urethra then travels the length of the penis to the outside environment.

The penis is a tubular organ that conducts urine from the bladder to the outside environment and introduces semen into the female vagina during intercourse. The majority of the body of penis consists of erectile tissue: the corpus spongiosum and the corpus cavernosa. Blood supply to the penis and the erectile tissue is via the dorsal artery.

PATHOPHYSIOLOGY

Injuries to the genitourinary system account for 2% to 5% of all adult trauma, the majority of which is secondary to blunt trauma. Approximately 80% of GU trauma involves the kidney, and 10% involves the bladder. Serious urethral injuries are rare and usually associated with penetrating trauma and pelvic fractures. Rapid deceleration injuries can result in renal pedicle and vascular injuries, and mechanisms include falls from height and motor vehicle collisions. Insult to the GU system is

Injuries to the genitourinary system account for 2% to 5% of all adult trauma, the majority of which is secondary to blunt trauma.

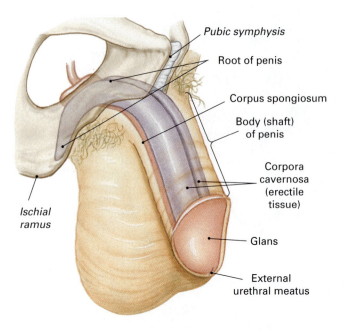

(a) Anterior and lateral view of penis

- Pubic symphysis
- Root of penis
- Corpus spongiosum
- Body (shaft) of penis
- Corpora cavernosa (erectile tissue)
- Glans
- External urethral meatus
- Ischial ramus

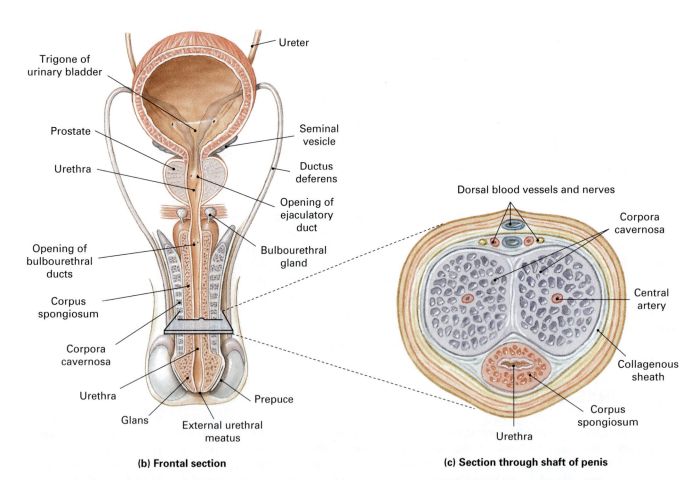

(b) Frontal section

- Trigone of urinary bladder
- Prostate
- Urethra
- Opening of bulbourethral ducts
- Corpus spongiosum
- Corpora cavernosa
- Urethra
- Glans
- External urethral meatus
- Ureter
- Seminal vesicle
- Ductus deferens
- Opening of ejaculatory duct
- Bulbourethral gland
- Prepuce

(c) Section through shaft of penis

- Dorsal blood vessels and nerves
- Corpora cavernosa
- Central artery
- Collagenous sheath
- Corpus spongiosum
- Urethra

■ **Figure 16-16**   The penis. (a) The positions of the erectile tissues. (b) A frontal section through the penis and associated organs. (c) A sectional view through the penis. *(Fig. 20-6, p. 554, from* Essentials of Anatomy & Physiology, *2nd ed., by Frederic H. Martini, Ph.D. and Edwin F. Bartholomew, M.S. Copyright © 2000 by Frederic H. Martini, Inc. Published by Pearson Education, Inc. Reprinted by permission.)*

often overlooked, because injuries are commonly occult and because more than 80% of patients with GU injury will have additional, often life-threatening, injuries elsewhere in the body.

RENAL SYSTEM

KIDNEY

The kidneys are moderately well protected, suspended in an adipose layer within the retroperitoneum, protected by the 11th and 12th ribs. The vast majority (90%) of renal trauma is secondary to blunt force trauma.

Injury to the kidney can be graded according to the AAST Spleen Injury Scale, on which they are assigned a grade of I through V:

★ *Grade I injuries* include small subcapsular hematomas and small contusions with minimal hematuria.

★ *Grade II injuries* include nonexpanding perirenal hematomas confined to the renal retroperitoneum, and lacerations of the renal cortex less than 1 cm in depth and no urinary extravasation.

★ *Grade III injuries* are lacerations to the renal cortex greater than 1 cm in depth, without collection system rupture or urinary extravasation.

★ *Grade IV injuries* include parenchymal lacerations extending through the renal cortex, medulla, and collecting system, and contained injuries to the renal artery and vein.

★ *Grade V injuries* include a completely shattered kidney, or hilar avulsion resulting in renal devascularization.

Renal contusions (grade I and II injuries) include subcapsular hematomas, small surface lacerations, and parenchymal bruising. CT evidence of micro-extravasation of contrast material into the renal parenchyma suggests parenchymal bruising, and a flattening of the renal cortex suggests subcapsular hematoma.

Renal lacerations are divided into two categories; those that extend into the corticomedullary junction or collecting system (grade IV), and those that don't (grade III). The risk of extreme hemorrhage and associated injuries increases significantly with grade IV injuries. CT studies will reveal extravasation of contrast material into the perirenal area or disruption of the renal outline.

Renal ruptures are associated with severe hemorrhage and shock. CT findings include extravasation of contrast material into the perirenal area, severe renal lacerations, and possible renal fragmentation. Rupture that involves the renal pelvis will result in the introduction of urine into the perirenal space.

URETER

Ureteral injuries are rare. They are often the result of penetrating trauma that transects the ureter. Blunt force injury as a result of hyperflexion of the spine results in ureteral rupture at or just below the ureteropelvic junction. Cavitation forces from the passing of a bullet through the pelvic cavity can result in microvascular thrombosis and, over days, necrosis and perforation.

BLADDER

Bladder rupture can be intraperitoneal or extraperitoneal. An intraperitoneal bladder rupture is most often the result of a full bladder and blunt force trauma to the abdomen. Pressure on the full bladder ruptures the bladder dome, spilling urine into the peritoneal cavity. "Seat belt injury," occurring when rapid deceleration results in abdominal and bladder compression as a belted individual is restrained by a seat belt, is a common cause of bladder trauma, especially when the bladder is full. CT or cystogram will reveal extravasation of urine into the bowel above the bladder. Extraperitoneal bladder ruptures are associated with pelvic fracture and occur most often at the bladder neck. CT and cystogram findings include extravasation of contrast material into the pelvic tissue, often described as "flame-like" due to the pattern it produces.

URETHRA

In males, injuries to the urethra can be divided into those that occur to the posterior urethra (prostatic and membranous) and anterior urethra (penile). Posterior urethra injuries are associated with pelvic fractures and additional abdominal, thoracic, and head injuries. Anterior injuries often result secondary to penile fractures and direct force to the penis (falls, straddle injuries). Female urethral injury is rare, and most often occurs secondary to direct pelvic trauma and fractures. Extravasation of contrast material into the surrounding tissue revealed on CT and cystogram are diagnostic for urethral injury.

REPRODUCTIVE

Male

Overall frequency of scrotal injury is low, most likely due to its mobility. Blunt trauma is the most common cause of scrotal injury, with direct blow and impingement against the symphysis pubis the most common mechanisms. Scrotal tissue can also be avulsed secondary to shearing forces. Injury can result in blood accumulation and engorgement of the scrotum, and the testicles themselves can be avulsed, contused, crushed, or dislocated into the inguinal canal.

Penile injuries include penile fractures, hematomas, lacerations, avulsions, and degloving injuries. Vacuum cleaner injuries can cause extensive damage to both the glans and urethra. Penile fractures occur when an erect penis experiences excessive compressive force, resulting in extreme bending, fracturing the engorged corpus cavernosum and injuring the surrounding tissue. A loud, cracking sound is often audible and remembered by the patient. Urethral injury or occlusion due to swelling and developing hematoma are both possible concomitant injuries.

Female

Injuries to the female reproductive structures are rare, but most often involve the external genitalia, vagina, and uterus. Ovarian and fallopian tube injuries are extremely uncommon due to their small size and mobility. When injuries do occur to these structures, they most often include contusions, hematomas, and devascularization injuries. In addition, ovaries, as solid organs, can fracture or shatter. Penetrating trauma is the most frequent cause of injury to the uterus. Devascularization injuries can result secondary to blunt trauma that results in severe movement of the uterus and disruption of its vascular supply.

Injuries to the external genitalia occur as a result of straddle injuries, aggressive consensual sex, sexual assault, and rape. Injury types include hematomas, lacerations, and avulsions.

GU ASSESSMENT

Assessment of the GU system should take place after the assessment of the airway, breathing, and circulation has been performed and only after immediate life threats have been corrected.

The classic triad indicating bladder rupture includes abdominal pain, gross hematuria, and inability to void.

Assessment of the GU system should take place after the assessment of the airway, breathing, and circulation has been performed and any immediate life threats corrected. The abdomen and pelvic regions should be fully exposed for the genitourinary exam. Care must be taken by the examiner to protect the patient's dignity regardless of the patient's level of consciousness. Assessment of the GU system most often takes place in conjunction with an abdominal exam, and should proceed in a systematic fashion to include the anterior, lateral, and posterior abdomen.

Inspection of the flanks to identify obvious trauma such as bruising, abrasions, lacerations, and penetrating injury should take place carefully, methodically, and under appropriate lighting. Grey Turner's sign, bruising on the flanks near ribs 11 and 12, can indicate intra-abdominal or intraperitoneal bleeding. Inspection of the urethra for frank blood should occur if GU trauma is suspected. Palpate the flanks and the inferolateral and inferoposterior wall of the rib cage. Pain or crepitus to the posterior aspects of ribs 11 and 12 suggests rib fracture and potential injury to the kidneys. The pelvic girdle should be assessed for stability, because the presence of pelvic fracture will increase both your suspicion of and the risk of bladder and urethral injury. Palpate the bladder, located in the lower abdominal quadrants. The classic triad indicating bladder rupture includes abdominal pain, gross hematuria, and inability to void. Percussion of the flank can reveal dullness if hemo-retroperitoneum is present, but this would require the examiner to be familiar with the percussive response of a normal flank.

Due to their occult nature, ovarian, fallopian, and uterine injuries will most likely go unrecognized in the emergent situation. A CT exam is the most frequently used diagnostic modality to identify these types of injuries. The clinical exam may reveal vaginal bleeding, more so in cases of uterine rupture, but this alone is not diagnostic for any of these injuries. Vaginal bleeding, depending on the type of insult, can be significant and even life threatening. In such cases, the vaginal and perianal area should be examined closely prior to bulky dressings being applied to the genitalia. With penetrating or blunt trauma, surrounding tissues and organs should be inspected and palpated carefully to rule out concomitant injury. Finally, in all suspected GI/GU trauma, the urethra should be examined closely for blood.

The testicles should be inspected for obvious injuries such as lacerations, abrasions, avulsions, discoloration, or swelling. Penile injuries, as with scrotal injuries, often present with severe pain and obvious bleeding, discoloration, swelling, avulsion, degloving, or amputation. Effort should be made to locate and transport amputated or degloved tissue, because attempts will often be made at reattachment. In all suspected GI/GU trauma, the urethra should be examined closely for blood.

SCREENING EXAMS FOR GENITOURINARY INJURY: IMAGING STUDIES

CYSTOGRAPHY

A retrograde **cystogram** can be useful in the diagnosis of urethral or bladder injury. In this study approximately 300–500 mL of contrast media is infused into the urethra and serial radiographs performed. Any extravasation of contrast from the urethra or bladder indicates perforation.

Plain X-rays cannot detect renal injury or function, so are of limited value in the assessment of the GU patient. X-rays can discover fractures of ribs 10–12, which should increase the index of suspicion for renal trauma.

cystogram *x-ray study used in the diagnosis of urethral or bladder injury; contrast media is placed into the urethra. Any extravasation of contrast from the urethra or bladder seen on serial radiograph indicates injury.*

COMPUTED TOMOGRAPHY

Spiral CT with contrast is the imaging modality of choice for the diagnosis of kidney injury, and is able to show enough detail to allow accurate grading of the renal injury. It is important to evaluate the BUN/creatinine prior to the administration of contrast dye to ensure uncomplicated renal elimination. A CT cystogram can be performed much like a radiographic one.

SONOGRAPHY

Sonography has no real role in the evaluation of genitourinary trauma. Numerous conditions make adequate imaging of anatomical structures difficult, and the test reveals nothing regarding renal function.

PERTINENT LABORATORY VALUES

Blood Chemistry

BUN/creatinine will gradually increase in patients who have sustained renal trauma and have limited or no kidney function. Comparison of the blood urea compared with serum creatinine can aid in the diagnosis of bladder rupture. Both are in urine, and are spilled into the peritoneal cavity when the bladder ruptures. Because urea is a smaller molecule, it is more readily absorbed through the peritoneum, resulting in a disproportionate increase in the serum urea as compared to creatinine.

Urinalysis

Evaluation of the urine for blood is required in trauma patients to assess for hematuria secondary to GU insult. Determination of gross blood can be made clinically by direct observation of the urine after catheterization. Urine reagent strips are useful for a rapid assessment of the urine.

MANAGEMENT

Management of the GU patient by the critical care paramedic is relatively straightforward, because the definitive treatment for serious and life-threatening GU trauma is surgery. Your care will consist primarily of securing the airway, ensuring breathing adequacy and oxygenation, treating shock as needed, and providing rapid and safe transport to the receiving facility. Circulatory considerations for shock are the same as for the GI patient, as discussed earlier.

Vaginal bleeding can be controlled by the application of dressings and direct pressure to the vaginal area. The vaginal canal should never be packed. Penile bleeding can be controlled by applying direct pressure around the circumference of the base of the penis.

Summary

Evaluation of patients who have sustained abdominal trauma, particularly blunt trauma, may pose a significant diagnostic and management problem to the critical care transport team. Trauma produces a spectrum of injury from minor single-organ injury to devastating, multiorgan or even multisystem injury. In addition to a command of anatomy, physiology, and injury pathology, the critical care paramedic must be able to perform a thorough physical exam and take advantage of the diagnostic tools available in today's emergency medicine realm and critical care environment.

Review Questions

1. How would you grade a liver laceration that extended 3 cm into the renal parenchyma, was 6 cm in length, and bleeding actively?

2. A patient presents complaining of lower quadrant abdominal pain after an MVC. His blood chemistry comes back from the lab and you note a serum urea that is disproportionately high compared to creatinine. What diagnostic study should be performed next?

3. Injury to the lower right rib cage should increase the index of suspicion for injury to what solid organ?

4. Where should the ultrasound transducer be placed in order to evaluate for the presence of blood in the hepatorenal space?

5. What is meant by the concept of "permissive hypotension"?

6. What diagnostic study would be best for identifying a urethral or bladder injury?

See Answers to Review Questions at the back of this book.

Further Reading

Bickell WH, Wall MJ, Pape PE, et al. "Immediate versus Delayed Fluid Resuscitation for Hypotensive Patients with Penetrating Torso Injuries." *New England Journal of Medicine,* Vol. 331 (1994): 1105–1109.

Biffel WL, Moore EE. "Diagnostic Peritoneal Lavage." In *Critical Care Secrets,* 3rd ed. Parsons PE, Wiener-Kronish JP, editors. Philadelphia: Hanley & Belfus, 2003.

Bledsoe BE, Porter RS, Cherry RA. *Paramedic Care: Principles & Practices,* 2nd ed. Upper Saddle River, NJ: Pearson Prentice Hall, 2005.

Boulanger BR, Kearney PA, Brenneman FD, Tsuei B, Ochoa J. "Utilization of FAST (Focused Assessment with Sonography for Trauma) in 1999: Results of a Survey of North American Trauma Centers." *American Surgeon,* Vol. 66, No. 11 (November 2000): 1049–1055.

Boulanger BR, McLellan BA. "Blunt abdominal trauma." *Emergency Medicine Clinics of North America*, Vol. 14, No. 1 (February 1996): 151–171.

Dutton RP, MacKensie CF, Scalea TM, et al. "Hypotensive Resuscitation During Active Hemorrhage: Impact on In-Hospital Mortality." *Journal of Trauma*, Vol. 52, No. 6 (2003): 1141–1146.

Heegaard WG, Plummer D, Frascone RJ, Pippert G, Steele D, Dries D. "Ultrasound in Helicopter EMS." *Academic Emergency Medicine*, Vol. 10 (2003): 4492.

Hoff WS, Holevar M, Nagy KK, et al. "Practice Guidelines for the Evaluation of Blunt Abdominal Trauma." *East Practice Management Guidelines Work Group*, 2001.

Holmes JF, Sakles JC, Lewis G, Wisner DH. "Effects of Delaying Fluid Resuscitation on an Injury to the Systemic Arterial Vasculature." *Academic Emergency Medicine*, Vol. 9, No. 4 (2002): 267–274.

Hubble MW, Hubble JP. *Principles of Advanced Trauma Care.* Clifton Park, NY: Thomson Delmar Learning, 2002.

Hudak CM, Gallo BM, Morton PG. *Critical Care Nursing: A Holistic Approach,* 7th ed. Philadelphia: Lippincott-Raven Publishers, 1998.

Levy F, Kelen GD. "Genitourinary Trauma." In *Emergency Medicine: A Comprehensive Study Guide,* 6th ed. Tintinalli JE, Kelen GD, Stapczynski JS, editors. New York: McGraw-Hill, 2004.

Marino PL. *The ICU Book,* 2nd ed. Baltimore, MD: Williams & Wilkins, 1998.

Martini FH, Bartholomew EF, Bledsoe BE. *Anatomy and Physiology for Emergency Care.* Upper Saddle River, NJ: Pearson Prentice Hall, 2002.

Mason PJB. "Abdominal Injuries." In *Trauma Nursing,* 2nd ed. Cardona VD, Hurn P, Mason P, Scanlon A, Veise-Berry S, editors. Phildadelphia: W. B. Saunders, 1994.

Naude GP. "Splenic Injuries." In *Trauma Secrets,* 2nd ed. Naude GP, Bongard FS, Demetriades D, editors. Philadelphia: Hanley & Belfus, 2003.

Naude GP, Van Zyl F. "Gastric Injuries." In *Trauma Secrets,* 2nd ed. Naude GP, Bongard FS, Demetriades D, editors. Philadelphia: Hanley & Belfus, 2003.

Naude JH. "Genitourinary Trauma." In *Trauma Secrets,* 2nd ed. Naude GP, Bongard FS, Demetriades D, editors. Philadelphia: Hanley & Belfus, 2003.

Netter FH. *Atlas of Human Anatomy.* Summit, NJ: Ciba-Geigy Corporation, 1989.

Nguyen DT, Stamos MJ. "Traumatic Injuries to the Small Bowel, Colon, Rectum, and Anus." In *Trauma Secrets,* 2nd ed. Naude GP, Bongard FS, Demetriades D, editors. Philadelphia: Hanley & Belfus, 2003.

Purtill MA, Sabile BE. "Duodenal and Pancreatic Injuries." In *Trauma Secrets,* 2nd ed. Naude GP, Bongard FS, Demetriades D, editors. Philadelphia: Hanley & Belfus, 2003.

Raptopoulos V. "Abdominal Trauma. Emphasis on Computed Tomography." *Radiologic Clinics of North America*, Vol. 32, No. 5 (September 1994): 969–987.

Ryan M, Stella J. "Massive Hemorrhage from Hepatic Laceration with Diaphragmatic Laceration: A Potential Limitation of the FAST Examination: Case Report." *Journal of Trauma*, Vol. 57, No. 3 (September 2004): 633–634.

Scalera TM, Boswell SA. "Abdominal Injuries." In *Emergency Medicine: A Comprehensive Study Guide,* 6th ed. Tintinalli JE, Kelen GD, Stapczynski JS, editors. New York: McGraw-Hill, 2004.

Sole ML, Lamborn ML, Hartshorn JC. *Introduction to Critical Care Nursing,* 3rd ed. Philadelphia: W. B. Saunders, 2001.

Vargas HI. "Liver and Biliary Injuries." In *Trauma Secrets,* 2nd ed. Naude GP, Bongard FS, Demetriades D, editors. Philadelphia: Hanley & Belfus, 2003.

Face/Ear/Ocular/ Neck Trauma

Scott R. Snyder, B.S., NREMT-P, CCEMT-P

Objectives

Upon completion of this chapter, the reader should be able to:

1. Describe basic facial, neck, ocular, and auditory anatomy and physiology. (p. 453)
2. Describe the anatomical zones of the neck. (p. 467)
3. Discuss and differentiate the pathophysiology of facial, neck, ocular, and auditory injuries. (p. 467)
4. Discuss the assessment and management of the patient with a facial injury. (p. 477)
5. Discuss the assessment and management of the patient with an ocular injury. (p. 478)
6. Discuss the assessment and management of the patient with a neck injury. (p. 478)
7. Understand the importance of airway maintenance in the initial management of the patient with facial and/or neck trauma. (p. 480)
8. Discuss the assessment and management of the patient with an auditory injury. (p. 482)

Key Terms

anterior cavity, p. 460
aqueous humor, p. 460
auditory ossicles, p. 458
ciliary body, p. 459
diplopia, p. 470
enophthalmos, p. 470
enucleation, p. 475
eustachian tube, p. 458
glossoptosis, p. 469

Horner's syndrome, p. 476
hyphema, p. 473
lacrimal glands, p. 453
Le Fort system, p. 469
malocclusion, p. 463
optic canal, p. 460
orbit, p. 459
pinna, p. 458
platysma, p. 465

posterior cavity, p. 460
ptosis, p. 470
temporomandibular joint (TMJ), p. 454
vestibulocochlear complex, p. 458
vitreous humor, p. 460
zygomatic bone, p. 454

Case Study

It is a Sunday afternoon, and you and your fellow crew members are enjoying a quiet day in the station quarters of your ground-based, critical care transport service. Your attention is drawn suddenly when the hotline from the dispatch center rings. You turn down the volume on the television, and conversation between you and your nurse partner stops as you both strain to listen in on your supervisor's side of the conversation that is taking place in the office next door. The tone of the conversation quickly suggests that this is indeed a mission, and you see his arm sticking out of the office door, giving you the "thumbs up" as he is busy gathering information.

As you and crew mates have done countless times before, you head over to the refrigerator to gather your drug bags and refrigerated medications while your supervisor, who is the third member of your crew today, heads to the garage to disconnect the AC line from the ambulance, start the engine, and look up a remote address in a neighboring county. "Scene call, MVC with entrapment" your supervisor tells you as he walks by. You gather your equipment, and the grumbling of the diesel engine tells you that the ambulance is ready to go. By the time you get to the ambulance, your supervisor has found the street address and is ready to pull out of the garage. You enter the patient compartment of the ambulance and secure the airway bag to the stretcher then buckle yourself in. Plugging your headset into the on-board communication system, your head comes alive with the chatter on the fire radio. "Confirm entrapment of one patient with severe facial injuries" you hear a responder on scene reporting. Your partner turns and looks at you, and you both smile as she gives the supervisor thumbs up and says, "We're good to go." Your supervisor responds back, "And away we go."

You arrive at the scene some 20 minutes later, and note a midsized sedan with severe front-end damage up against a telephone pole as the critical care ambulance is positioned at a safe position to allow a quick exit from the scene. An on-scene EMS provider greets you and asks you to grab your cot as the patient has just been extricated on a backboard.

After getting your cot and equipment, you make your way to where the patient is back-boarded and introduce yourselves to the paramedic first responder in charge of patient care. You note that there is a mid-30-year-old male fully immobilized with severe facial injuries. The EMT attempting to bag the patient is having a difficult time achieving proper mask seal due to the amount of soft-tissue injury, blood present, and movement by the patient. You start taking the report and listen to lung sounds while your partner goes to the head to perform a primary exam and assess the airway.

The paramedic in charge reports that the patient was the unrestrained driver in a vehicle that struck a light pole at a high rate of speed, resulting in severe damage to his vehicle that trapped him by his lower extremities. The windshield was broken outward, and the steering wheel was intact. He has been mildly combative during the entire period of patient care, and is resisting attempts at assisting his ventilations with a bag-valve mask (BVM).

You and your partner determine that the patient is alert to pain only and is mildly combative. He appears to have a Le Fort II fracture of his midface and has significant soft-tissue injury as well. There is blood in his airway, nares, and right ear canal. Pupils are equal and reactive to light bilaterally. His neck, chest, and abdomen appear atraumatic, lung sounds are clear and equal bilaterally. The diminished level of consciousness, combativeness, and a weak, rapid pulse suggest the development of shock, and you find bilateral femur fractures to confirm your suspicion of additional traumatic injury. Vital signs are:

- ★ HR = 132
- ★ RR = 10 and shallow
- ★ BP = 102/50
- ★ SpO_2 = 95%

You and your partner quickly agree that this patient needs an advanced airway prior to transport, and determine that you will perform rapid-sequence intubation (RSI). You instruct the EMT to suction the airway while the paramedic on scene takes over airway control and does his best to achieve a good mask seal and ventilate the patient with 100% oxygen. You further ask the EMT to squeeze the BVM, allowing the paramedic to use two hands in his attempts at maintaining a mask seal.

As you initiate large-bore IV access, you note that the paramedic is still having difficulty achieving a perfect seal due to the distortion of the facial structures; despite this, however, he has gotten the patient's SpO_2 up to 96%. The EMT bagging is also providing some cricoid pressure. Your partner says to you, "With this kind of facial trauma, we are going to have to do something with the airway before we leave."

Your third crew member, the supervisor, takes care of attaching the patient to your portable equipment while you initiate a second IV and administer a fluid bolus to treat the patient's developing hypovolemic shock. You then draw up the appropriate volumes of etomidate and succinylcholine. Your partner has assembled her intubation equipment, readies an esophageal CombiTube, prepares a cricothyroidotomy tray, and swabs the patient's neck with Betadine. "Just in case," she says.

When you are both ready, you administer the etomidate and then the succinylcholine. When the patient has stopped breathing, you hold in-line stabilization utilizing an inferior approach while your partner attempts the intubation. Because of the blood and soft-tissue damage, your partner initially has some difficulty visualizing the vocal cords. After looking for about 15 seconds, she says "I can't see a thing." "Saturation is still 96%, you still have some time" you say to her. You admire the cool, experienced attitude that she exudes while performing what is surely a difficult intubation.

You are alternating between watching the pulse oximeter and her airway attempt when all of a sudden she exclaims "There we are!" and passes the endotracheal tube. You place your stethoscope on the patient's epigastric zone to ensure the tube is not esophageally placed, and then confirm bilateral breath sounds as BVM ventilations are provided. The capnogram is registering exhaled carbon dioxide, and the pulse oximeter is starting to climb up again. You then reassess the patient while your partner gathers your equipment and ensures that the patient is properly secured to the backboard for transport. You note that the airway is patent, ventilations are adequate, there is no gross external hemorrhage, and no additional trauma is identified. You report that you have bolused about 500 mL of normal saline, and the patient vital signs are now:

- ★ HR = 118
- ★ RR = 20 per minute via BVM
- ★ BP = 112/58
- ★ SpO_2 = 100%
- ★ $EtCO_2$ = 42 mmHg

As you are making your way back to your waiting ambulance with the patient properly secured on your cot, you make sure you tell the EMTs and paramedic on scene that they did a fabulous job, you appreciated their help, and couldn't have done it so smoothly without them. Together, you load the patient into the rear of your ambulance, place him on the portable ventilator, and secure your equipment and yourselves as you prepare for the transport to the regional trauma center about 20 miles away.

INTRODUCTION

As a critical care paramedic, you will often be called on to provide both the initial treatment as well as subsequent transport of patients who have sustained severe maxillofacial and neck trauma. This chapter will provide an overview of the appropriate anatomy, injury pathology, clinical assessment findings, and management of these injuries. While many of the injuries discussed are not in and of themselves life threatening, maxillofacial trauma often accompanies other more potentially life-threatening injuries that can be easily overlooked when confronted with the often dramatic nature of maxillofacial injuries. Although facial trauma is extremely important, the critical care paramedic must not be drawn away by what is most "graphic" and, hence, overlook what is most "life threatening." You should be prepared to treat these injuries while maintaining cervical spine control, airway maintenance, breathing support, hemorrhage control, and any additional interventions necessary. In addition, maxillofacial trauma often has long-term physical and psychological implications for the patient that must be appreciated by the critical care paramedic.

ANATOMY AND PHYSIOLOGY

SOFT TISSUE OF THE FACE

The soft tissue of the face consists of a layer of highly vascularized and innervated skin over a layer of multiple facial muscles. Two major arteries that perfuse this region are the facial and the temporal arteries. The facial artery supplies blood to the lower and middle anterior face, while the temporal artery supplies blood to the superior and anterior face as well as the temporal regions of the scalp. Both vessels are branches of the external carotid artery. Branches of the ophthalmic artery, which originates off the internal carotid artery, supply blood to the soft tissue around the bridge of the nose, orbitals, and central forehead. (See Figure 17-1 ■.)

Innervation of the face is supplied by cranial nerves (CNs) V and VII. The trigeminal nerve (CN V) provides sensory function to the face and controls the muscles of mastication. (See Figure 17-2 ■.) The trigeminal nerve divides into three main branches, each supplying sensation to a specific area of the face. (See Table 17–1.) The facial nerve (CN VII) controls lacrimation, salivation, and the facial muscles. (See Figure 17-3 ■.)

The salivary glands are located within the parenchyma of the maxillofacial region. Specific glands include the parotid, sublingual, and submandibular glands. Salivary secretion is controlled by the autonomic nervous system. Parasympathetic stimulation results in increased secretion and copious saliva production, while sympathetic stimulation results in the secretion of smaller volumes of highly concentrated saliva. This smaller volume is the cause of "dry mouth" associated with sympathetic nervous system activation.

The parotid gland lies over the ramus of the mandible, just superior to the angle of the mandible, anterior to the auditory canal, and inferior to the zygomatic arch. The parotid duct exits the gland then passes over the masseter muscle before draining into the oral cavity by the second upper molar. Another paired gland, the sublingual gland, is located on the floor of the oral cavity at the base of the tongue. It empties into the oral cavity via numerous sublingual ducts located lateral to the lingual frenulum. The submandibular gland, also paired, lies inferior to the angle of the mandible. Numerous submandibular ducts open into the oral cavity posterior to the front teeth on both sides of the distal lingual frenulum.

The **lacrimal glands** are located bilaterally in the superolateral orbital area, and are divided into superior and inferior regions. These glands secrete lacrimal fluid, which moistens and lubricates the

lacrimal glands *glands that secrete lacrimal fluid, which moistens and lubricates the surface of the eye.*

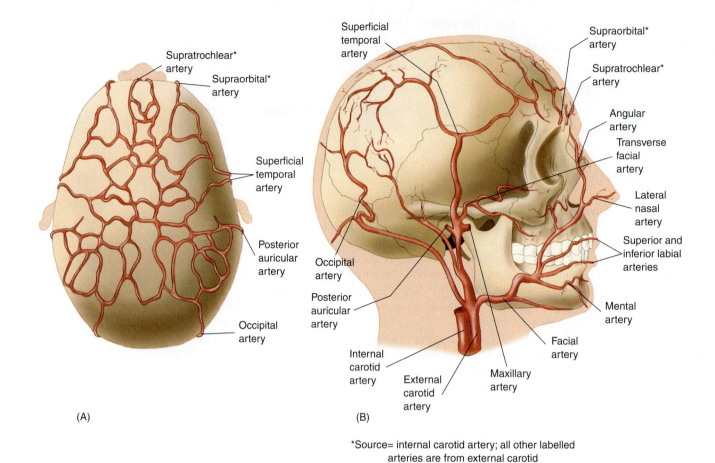

Supratrochlear* artery

Supraorbital* artery

Superficial temporal artery

Posterior auricular artery

Occipital artery

(A)

Superficial temporal artery

Supraorbital* artery

Supratrochlear* artery

Angular artery

Transverse facial artery

Lateral nasal artery

Superior and inferior labial arteries

Mental artery

Occipital artery

Posterior auricular artery

Internal carotid artery

External carotid artery

Maxillary artery

Facial artery

(B)

*Source= internal carotid artery; all other labelled arteries are from external carotid

■ Figure 17-1 Arteries of the face and scalp.

globe of the eye. Lacrimal fluid exits the gland through multiple lacrimal ducts, flows across the globe to the lacrimal papillae and into the lacrimal sac. The lacrimal sac drains into the nasal cavity via the nasolacrimal duct. (See Figure 17-4 ■.)

The soft tissue of the face provides very little protection to the underlying vascular structures and bone.

BONES OF THE FACE

Collectively, the skull is made up of 22 bones, 8 of which form the cranium and 14 of which form the face. The cranium is made up of the ethmoid, sphenoid, frontal, parietal, occipital, and temporal bones, and serves to protect the brain. (See Figure 17-5 ■.) The facial bones include the vomer, mandible, and paired maxillary, palatine, nasal, inferior conchae, zygomatic, and lacrimal bones. These bones provide minimal protection for the airway as well as attachment points for the muscles that control facial expressions and the manipulation of food.

The mandible, the second largest facial bone behind the paired maxillary bones, is the most mobile of the facial bones. This bone is divided into the horizontal body and the ascending ramus, which transition at the mandibular angle. The teeth are embedded in the mandibular body. The condylar process of the mandible articulates with the mandibular fossae of the temporal bone at the **temporomandibular joint** (TMJ), which serves as the hinge joint for the mandible.

Seven cranial and facial bones articulate to form the orbital complex that house and protect each eye. The maxillary bone forms the inferior rim and floor, the **zygomatic bone** forms the lateral rim and wall, and the frontal bone forms the superior rim and wall of each orbit. Proceeding lateral to medial across the posterior wall of the orbit, the zygomatic bone articulates with the sphenoid bone, which constitutes the majority of the posterior wall. The ethmoid bone articulates with

temporomandibular joint (TMJ) *the hinge joint for the mandible; articulation point of the condylar process and the mandibular fossae of the temporal bone.*

zygomatic bone *facial bone that articulates with the frontal bone and maxilla to complete the lateral wall of the orbit.*

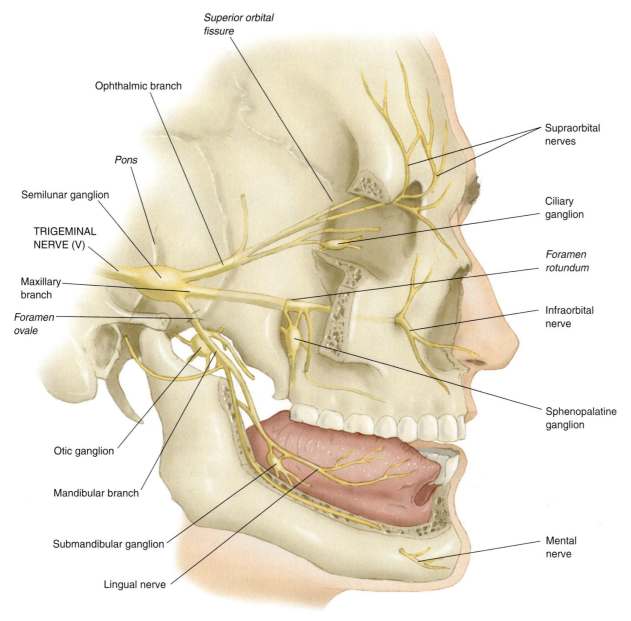

Labels on figure:
- Superior orbital fissure
- Ophthalmic branch
- Pons
- Semilunar ganglion
- TRIGEMINAL NERVE (V)
- Maxillary branch
- Foramen ovale
- Otic ganglion
- Mandibular branch
- Submandibular ganglion
- Lingual nerve
- Supraorbital nerves
- Ciliary ganglion
- Foramen rotundum
- Infraorbital nerve
- Sphenopalatine ganglion
- Mental nerve

■ Figure 17-2   The trigeminal nerve.

Table 17–1	Three Branches of the Trigeminal Nerve (CN V)		
	Ophthalmic Division (V_1)	**Maxillary Division (V_2)**	**Mandibular Division (V_3)**
Origin and Course	Fibers run from face to pons via superior orbital fissure. Cutaneous branch passes through supraorbital foramen.	Fibers run from face to pons via the foramen rotundum. The cutaneous branch passes through infraorbital foramen.	Fibers pass through skull via the foramen ovale. Enters mandible through mandibular foramen. The cutaneous branch passes through the mental foramen.
Function	Transmits sensory impulses from the skin of the anterior scalp, upper eyelid, the nose, nasal cavity mucosa, cornea, and lacrimal gland.	Transmits sensory impulses from nasal cavity mucosa, palate, upper teeth, skin of cheek, upper lip, and lower eyelid.	Transmits sensory impulses from anterior tongue, lower teeth, skin of chin, and temporal region of scalp. Provides motor fibers to, and sensory fibers from, muscles of mastication.

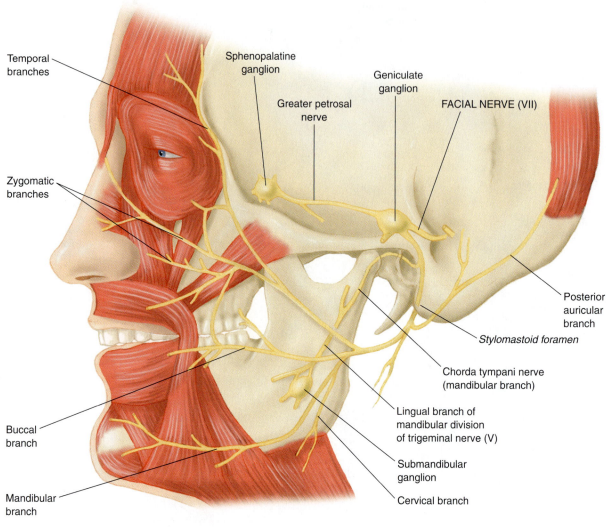

Figure 17-3 The facial nerve.

Figure 17-4 The accessory structures of the eye. The details of the lacrimal apparatus. *(Fig. 10-7b, p. 279, from* Essentials of Anatomy & Physiology, *2nd ed., by Frederic H. Martini, Ph.D. and Edwin F. Bartholomew, M.S. Copyright © 2000 by Frederic H. Martini, Inc. Published by Pearson Education, Inc. Reprinted by permission.)*

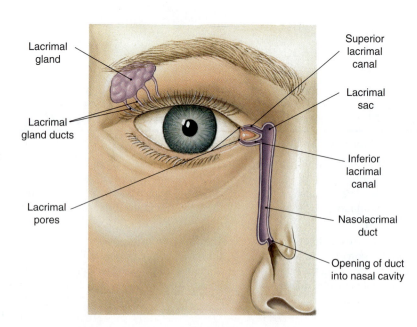

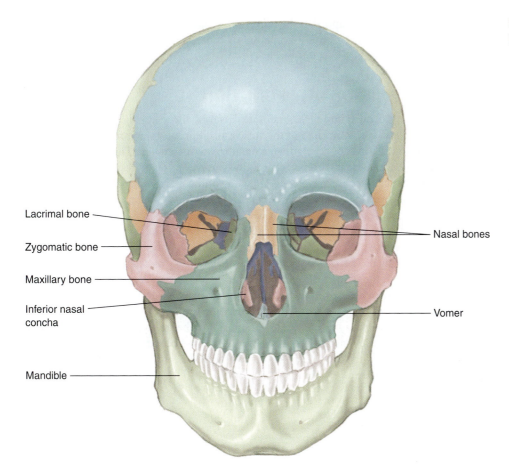

Lacrimal bone

Zygomatic bone

Maxillary bone

Inferior nasal concha

Mandible

Nasal bones

Vomer

the lacrimal bone and the orbital process of the palatine bone to complete the posterior and medial walls of the orbit.

Numerous foramens, fissures, and canals are located in the orbit to allow the passage of nerves and blood vessels. The optic canal, located on the posterior medial wall, allows for the passage of the optic nerve (CN II) and the opthalmic artery into the orbit. The oculomotor (CN III), trochlear (CN IV), opthalmic branch of the trigeminal (CN V), and abducens (CN VI) nerves, as well as the opthalmic vein, all pass through the superior orbital fissure located on the posterior orbital wall. The inferior orbital fissure serves as conduit for sensory nerves entering the skull.

The bones that form the nasal cavities and the paranasal sinuses are collectively known as the nasal complex. The perpendicular plate of the ethmoid bone and the vomer form the nasal septum, which serves as the medial border of the left and right nasal cavities. Portions of the frontal bone, ethmoid bone, and sphenoid bone form the superior border of each cavity. Portions of the maxillary, lacrimal, and ethmoid bones define the lateral borders. The inferior border consists of the maxillary and palatine bones. The inferior, middle, and superior nasal conchae occupy the central portion of the nasal cavity. These conchae, or turbinates, are covered by a layer of pseudostratified, ciliated, columnar epithelium with goblet cells, allowing for the filtering, warming, and humidification of incoming air. The bridge of the nose is formed by the paired nasal bones, which articulate with the maxillary bone. The soft tissue and cartilage of the nose enclose the vestibule, which opens to the outside environment through the nares. Hair in the vestibule allows for the filtering of large particulate matter from incoming air.

The paranasal sinuses are air-filled chambers continuous with the nasal cavities and located within the frontal, ethmoid, sphenoid, and maxillary bones. These sinuses lighten the skull, produce mucus, and allow for resonance during phonation. The frontal sinuses, ethmoid sinuses, and maxillary sinuses are all connected to the nasal cavities by a passageway, or meatus.

Collectively, the nasal cavity and paranasal sinuses serve to protect the lower airway by warming, filtering, and humidifying air entering the upper airway as it passes over the mucociliary carpet.

Particulate matter becomes trapped in the mucus, and ciliated epithelium passes the mucus back to the pharynx, where the mucus can be swallowed or expectorated. Incoming air is humidified and warmed as it passes over the moist mucous layer.

THE EAR AND AUDITORY FUNCTION

The ear is commonly divided into three anatomical regions: the external ear, the middle ear, and the inner ear. The external ear, comprised of the auricle, or **pinna** and the external auditory canal, collects and directs sound waves to the tympanic membrane, or eardrum. The tympanic membrane is a thin, delicate membrane that vibrates from sound waves, and separates the external ear from the middle ear. The structure of the pinna, the "S" shape of the external auditory canal, and the presence of hair and cerumen (wax) along the course of the auditory canal provide some degree of protection for the tympanic membrane.

The middle ear communicates with the nasopharynx via the auditory tube, or **eustachian tube.** This conduit allows for equalization between the middle ear chamber and the atmospheric pressure of the external ear canal. The middle ear contains the **auditory ossicles,** three delicate bones that transmit vibrations of the tympanic membrane to the vestibulocochlear complex located in the inner ear. The **vestibulocochlear complex** is made up of the vestibular complex and the cochlea. The vestibular complex consists of the semicircular canals and the vestibule, which provide information regarding the body's orientation in space and equilibrium. The cochlea houses the auditory sensory receptors and provides the sense of hearing. This complex is housed within the temporal bone, receives its blood supply from the vertebrobasilar system, and is innervated by the vestibulocochlear nerve, CN VIII. (See Figure 17-6 ■.)

pinna *the portion of the ear (auricle) that is visually exposed.*

eustachian tube *the auditory tube; found between the middle ear and the nasopharynx.*

auditory ossicles *three bones in the middle ear that transmit vibrations of the tympanic membrane to the vestibulocochlear complex in the inner ear.*

vestibulocochlear complex *inner ear structure comprised of the vestibular complex (semicircular canals and the vestibule) and the cochlea.*

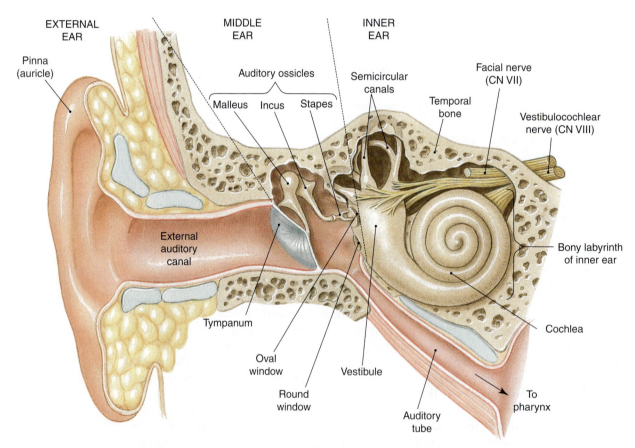

■ Figure 17-6   The anatomy of the ear. The orientation of the external ear, middle ear, and inner ear. *(Fig. 10-19, p. 290, from* Essentials of Anatomy & Physiology, *2nd ed., by Frederic H. Martini, Ph.D. and Edwin F. Bartholomew, M.S. Copyright © 2000 by Frederic H. Martini, Inc. Published by Pearson Education, Inc. Reprinted by permission.)*

THE EYE

Our eyes are elaborate and intricate structures that allow us to detect light, create visual images, and interact with our surrounding environment. They are well protected by the bones of the **orbit,** or eye socket. In addition to the bony structures, the eyelids, eyelashes, and lacrimal apparatus all protect the ocular surface from harm. Frequent blinking of the eyelids keep the surface of the eye well lubricated and free of debris. The conjunctiva is a mucous membrane covering the inner surface of the eyelid and the anterior sclera that serves to keep the eye surface moist. The lacrimal apparatus, consisting of the lacrimal gland, lacrimal ducts, lacrimal sac, and the nasolacrimal duct, produces tears, distributes them across the eye surface, and facilitates tear removal. The cornea is dependent on lacrimal secretions for lubrication as well as oxygenation. Without proper function of the lid and lacrimal apparatus, the cornea can dehydrate, become hypoxic, and will suffer from ischemia or infarction changes. (See Figure 17-7 ■.)

The eye shares the orbit with a number of structures including the extrinsic eye muscles, blood vessels, cranial nerves, and a mass of orbital fat that provides padding and insulation to the globe. The wall of the globe can be divided into three distinct layers, or tunics: the outer fibrous tunic, the middle vascular tunic, and the inner neural tunic. The hollow interior of the eye is divided into the anterior and posterior cavities. (See Figure 17-8 ■.)

The outer layer of the eye, the fibrous tunic, consists of the sclera and the cornea. The sclera, commonly known as the "white of the eye," serves as the attachment site for the six extrinsic eye muscles. The transparent cornea is continuous with the sclera, and covers both the pupil and the iris. Having no vascular supply, the cornea is dependent on the constant washing of lacrimal fluid over its surface for oxygenation, because if the cornea becomes dry, it can also become hypoxic.

The middle layer of the eyeball wall, the vascular tunic, contains the iris, which is the colored, muscular portion that controls the diameter of the pupil and therefore the amount of light entering the eye. The **ciliary body** attaches to the peripheral posterior aspect of the iris, and the ciliary muscles connect to the lens via the suspensory ligaments, holding the lens in place behind the iris and centered on the pupil. In this fashion, all light passing through the pupil passes through the lens on the way to the photoreceptors located on the retina.

The retina, or neural tunic, is the innermost layer of the eye wall. It consists of a pigmented layer and a neural layer that together act as the photoreceptive organ of the eye. An important landmark on the retina is the optic disk. The optic disk is the area where the optic nerve and central retinal vein

orbit   *the bony recess that contains the eye, comprised of the frontal, zygomatic, and temporal bones.*

ciliary body   *muscle group that connects to the lens via the suspensory ligaments; holds the lens in place and divides the eye into the anterior and posterior chambers.*

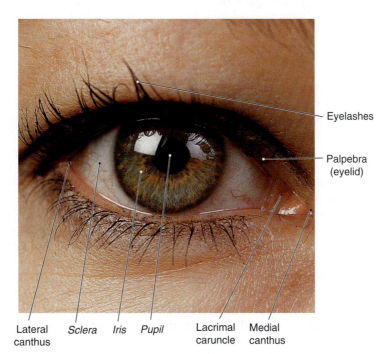

■ **Figure 17-7**   External anatomy of the eye. *(Ralph T. Hutchings)*

Eyelashes

Palpebra (eyelid)

Lateral canthus   *Sclera*   *Iris*   *Pupil*   Lacrimal caruncle   Medial canthus

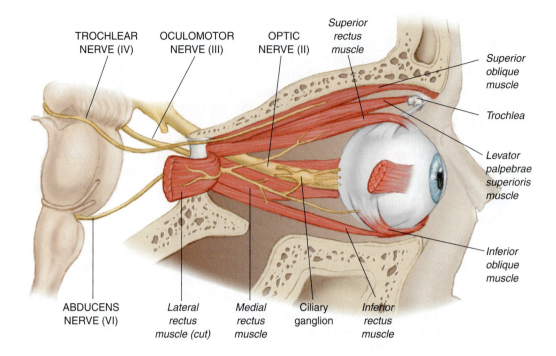

■ Figure 17-8 External muscles and innervation of the eye.

TROCHLEAR NERVE (IV)

OCULOMOTOR NERVE (III)

OPTIC NERVE (II)

Superior rectus muscle

Superior oblique muscle

Trochlea

Levator palpebrae superioris muscle

Inferior oblique muscle

ABDUCENS NERVE (VI)

Lateral rectus muscle (cut)

Medial rectus muscle

Ciliary ganglion

Inferior rectus muscle

leave the eye, and the central retinal artery enters the retina. Because no photoreceptors are located in the optic disk, light striking this area goes unnoticed, resulting in a blind spot in the field of vision.

The ciliary body and lens divide the eye into the anterior and posterior cavities. The **anterior cavity's** borders are the cornea anteriorly and the lens posteriorly. It is further divided into the anterior and posterior chambers, separated by the pupil. **Aqueous humor,** a clear fluid in the anterior cavity, circulates freely between the anterior and posterior chambers through the pupil. The **posterior cavity** is the larger of the two cavities, encompassing all of the area behind the lens. It is filled with a clear, gelatinous fluid known as **vitreous humor.** (See Figure 17-9 ■.)

The muscles and cranial nerves that control eye movement and vision are discussed in the following section on cranial nerves.

anterior cavity *the anterior cornea, separated from the posterior lens by the pupil.*

aqueous humor *a clear fluid in the anterior cavity that circulates freely between the anterior and posterior chambers through the pupil.*

posterior cavity *the larger of the two cavities, encompassing all of the area behind the lens.*

vitreous humor *a clear, gelatinous fluid that fills the posterior cavity.*

optic canal *the passageway for the optic nerve (CN II), from the optic disc to the sphenoid bone.*

THE CRANIAL NERVES

Cranial nerves I through VIII all play a role in sensory or motor function of the face and associated structures, and evaluation of their function can be a valuable tool in forming a differential diagnosis during your physical exam. (See Figure 17-10 ■.) The *olfactory nerve (CN I)* is responsible for our sense of smell. Olfactory receptors located in the roof of the nasal cavity, superior nasal conchae, and superior nasal septum combine to form nerve bundles that penetrate the cribriform plate of the ethmoid bone. These nerve bundles enter the left and right olfactory bulbs, from which the axons of the postsynaptic neurons continue to the cerebrum along the olfactory tracts.

The *optic nerve (CN II)* carries visual information from the eye to the diencephalon. The nerve leaves the eye at the optic disk, passes through the **optic canal,** which is the passage way of the nerve through the sphenoidal bone, and travels through the optic chiasm on its way to the diencephalon.

The *oculomotor nerve (CN III)* enters the orbital through the superior orbital fissure and innervates the intrinsic and four of the six extrinsic eye muscles. The intrinsic eye muscles control pupil diameter and the shape of the lens. Extrinsic muscles control eye movement and include the inferior oblique muscle and the inferior, medial, and superior medial rectus. The levator palpebrae superioris, also innervated by CN III, raises the upper eyelid.

The *trochlear nerve (CN IV)* innervates one of the six extrinsic eye muscles, the superior oblique, which contributes to eye movement. The nerve enters the orbital through the superior orbital fissure of the ethmoid bone.

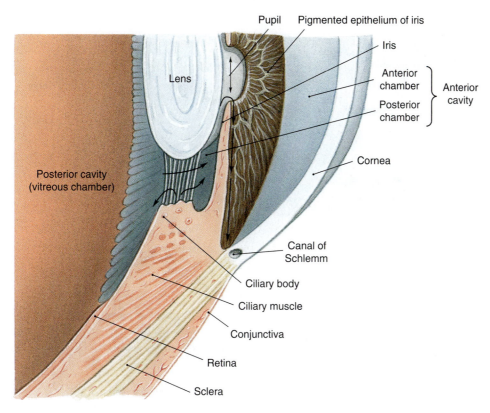

Pupil   Pigmented epithelium of iris

Iris

Lens

Anterior
chamber   } Anterior
Posterior   cavity
chamber

Cornea

Posterior cavity
(vitreous chamber)

Canal of
Schlemm

Ciliary body

Ciliary muscle

Conjunctiva

Retina

Sclera

■ **Figure 17-9** Eye chambers and the circulation of aqueous humor. The lens is suspended between the vitreous chamber and the posterior chamber. Its position is maintained by suspensory ligaments that attach the lens to the ciliary body. Aqueous humor secreted at the ciliary body circulates through the posterior and anterior chambers and is reabsorbed after passing along the canal of Schlemm. *(Fig. 10-12, p. 284, from Essentials of Anatomy & Physiology, 2nd ed., by Frederic H. Martini, Ph.D. and Edwin F. Bartholomew, M.S. Copyright © 2000 by Frederic H. Martini, Inc. Published by Pearson Education, Inc. Reprinted by permission.)*

The *trigeminal nerve (CN V)* has both sensory and motor functions. As suggested by the name, the trigeminal is divided into three major branches, the ophthalmic, maxillary, and mandibular, which exit the cranium at different sites. The ophthalmic branch has purely sensory functions, innervating the nasal cavity and sinuses, various intraorbital structures, and the skin of the forehead, eyebrows, upper eyelids, and portions of the nose. It enters the orbital through the superior orbital fissure. The maxillary branch, also purely sensory, exits the cranium through the foramen rotundum. A branch then enters the orbit through the inferior orbital fissure and follows the infraorbital groove along the floor of the orbit before exiting through the infraorbital foramen to innervate the lower eyelids, cheek, upper lip, and portions of the nose. Deeper divisions of the maxillary branch innervate the teeth, gums, portions of the pharynx, and the palate. The mandibular branch has both motor and sensory functions, and exits the cranium through the foramen ovale. The motor components innervate the muscles of mastication, while the sensory components innervate the anterior portion of the tongue, the mandible, gums, and teeth, as well as the skin of the temple region.

The *abducens nerve (CN VI)* enters the orbit through the superior orbital fissure of the sphenoid bone and innervates the lateral rectus, one of the six extrinsic eye muscles that control eye movement.

The *facial nerve (CN VII)* has both sensory and motor functions. It travels through the internal acoustic canal located in the temporal bone before exiting the cranium through the stylomastoid foramen. The nerve provides sensory information to taste receptors on the distal two-thirds of the tongue, while the motor component innervates the lacrimal, submandibular salivary, and sublingual salivary glands as well as the muscles of facial expression.

The *vestibulocochlear nerve (CN VIII)*, also known as the acoustic or auditory nerve, is a sensory nerve that is divided into the vestibular and cochlear branches. The vestibular branch relays information regarding movement, position, and balance from the sensory receptors in the inner ear to the medulla oblongata and eventually the cerebellum. The cochlear branch relays auditory information from the cochlea in the inner ear to the medulla. Both branches pass through the internal acoustic canal to reach the inner ear and its sensory receptors.

The *glossopharyngeal nerve (CN IX)* has both sensory and motor functions. It exits the cranium via the jugular foramen. Afferent nerve fibers relay sensory information from the proximal

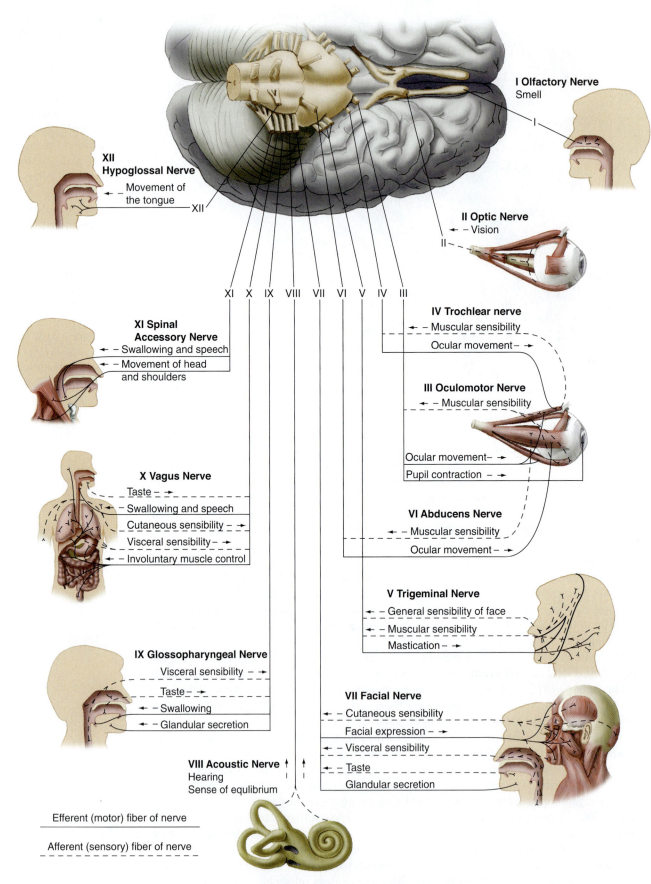

I Olfactory Nerve
Smell

XII Hypoglossal Nerve
← – Movement of the tongue

II Optic Nerve
II – ← – Vision

XI X IX VIII VII VI V IV III

IV Trochlear nerve
← – Muscular sensibility
Ocular movement – →

XI Spinal Accessory Nerve
← – Swallowing and speech
← – Movement of head and shoulders

III Oculomotor Nerve
← – Muscular sensibility
Ocular movement – →
Pupil contraction – →

X Vagus Nerve
Taste – →
– Swallowing and speech
Cutaneous sensibility – →
Visceral sensibility – →
← – Involuntary muscle control

VI Abducens Nerve
← – Muscular sensibility
Ocular movement – →

V Trigeminal Nerve
← – General sensibility of face
← – Muscular sensibility
Mastication – →

IX Glossopharyngeal Nerve
Visceral sensibility – →
Taste – →
← – Swallowing
← – Glandular secretion

VII Facial Nerve
← – Cutaneous sensibility
Facial expression – →
← – Visceral sensibility
← – Taste
Glandular secretion

VIII Acoustic Nerve
Hearing
Sense of equlibrium

Efferent (motor) fiber of nerve

Afferent (sensory) fiber of nerve

■ Figure 17-10   The cranial nerves.

one-third of the tongue, the soft palate, and the pharynx to the medulla. The carotid sinus branch relays information from the carotid sinuses and bodies. Efferent motor nerve fibers innervate the parotid gland and the muscles involved in swallowing.

THE PHARYNX

The pharynx connects all the nose, throat, and mouth to one another, and is divided into three sections: the superior nasopharynx, the oropharynx, and the inferior laryngopharynx (or hypopharynx). The gastrointestinal and respiratory tracts share portions of the pharynx and as such it serves as a common pathway for food, liquid, and air. Important structures in the nasopharynx include the superior, middle, and inferior concha, which increase the surface area of the nasal cavity to facilitate the humidification and warming of inspired air.

The nasal cavity has a significant vascular supply. Anteriorly, the anterior and posterior ethmoid arteries converge to form Kesselbach's plexus. Blood is supplied to the posterior nasal cavity by the sphenopalatine artery.

The oropharynx is separated from the nasopharynx by the soft palate and extends inferiorly to the level of the hyoid bone. The laryngopharynx extends from the hyoid bone inferiorly to the entrance to the esophagus.

THE ORAL CAVITY AND DENTITION

The oral cavity borders include the oropharynx posteriorly, the lips anteriorly, the hard and soft palates superiorly, the floor of the mouth anteriorly, and the cheeks laterally. The tongue is of course the most obvious structure in the oral cavity, and receives blood supply via the lingual artery. The parotid, sublingual, and submandibular ducts open into the oral cavity, and their respective glands secrete copious amounts of saliva when activated by the parasympathetic nervous system.

An adult normally has 32 teeth, with equal distribution between the upper and lower dental arches. Specifically, each arch contains 2 central incisors, 2 lateral incisors, 2 cuspids, or *canines,* 4 bicuspids, or *premolars,* and 6 molars. (See Figure 17-11 ■.) In a perfect set of teeth, all occlusal surfaces of the teeth on the upper dental arch match up with their counterparts on the lower arch. Many adults will normally exhibit some degree of **malocclusion,** which is simply defined as a misfit of the occlusal surfaces of the teeth upon mouth closure.

malocclusion   *a misfit of the occlusal surfaces of the teeth upon mouth closure.*

THE NECK

The anatomy of the neck is unique and of special concern to the critical care paramedic, because it contains many vital structures located in a very small space. Systems represented within the neck include the cardiovascular, musculoskeletal, central nervous, respiratory, digestive, and endocrine systems.

The major vascular structures located in the neck are the carotid arteries and the jugular veins. The common carotid arteries originate from the brachiocephalic artery on the right, and the aorta on the left. They ascend deep in the neck tissue parallel to the trachea before bifurcating at the level of the larynx, forming the external and internal carotid arteries. The carotid sinuses and bodies are located at the carotid bifurcation. Baroreceptors found within the carotid sinuses monitor and control blood pressure, while chemoreceptors within the carotid bodies monitor the PCO_2 and PO_2 concentration of arterial blood. The internal carotid arteries enter the skull through the carotid canals located in the temporal bones and, along with the vertebral arteries, deliver blood to the brain. The internal jugular vein descends lateral to the common carotid artery. Both structures, along with the vagus nerve, are housed in a fascial layer known as the carotid sheath. This sheath is but one of many planes created by the deep cervical fascia, and it provides compartmentalization of the major vascular structures of the neck, limiting external blood loss and reducing the risk of exsanguination should the integrity of any of the vessels be compromised. The external jugular veins descend superficial to the sternocleidomastoid muscle, and drain blood from the face, scalp, and cranium into the subclavian vein posterior to the clavicle. Both the external and internal jugular veins are available for cannulation by the critical care paramedic, with the external jugular the most accessible and most commonly used.

Figure 17-11 Common dental numbering system.

1. 3rd molar (wisdom tooth)
2. 2nd molar (12-yr molar)
3. 1st molar (6-yr molar)
4. 2nd bicuspid (2nd premolar)
5. 1st bicuspid (1st premolar)
6. Cuspid (canine/eye tooth)
7. Lateral incisor
8. Central incisor
9. Central incisor
10. Lateral incisor
11. Cuspid (canine/eye tooth)
12. 1st bicuspid (1st premolar)
13. 2nd bicuspid (2nd premolar)
14. 1st molar (6-yr molar)
15. 2nd molar (12-yr molar)
16. 3rd molar (wisdom tooth)
17. 3rd molar (wisdom tooth)
18. 2nd molar (12-yr molar)
19. 1st molar (6-yr molar)
20. 2nd bicuspid (2nd premolar)
21. 1st bicuspid (1st premolar)
22. Cuspid (canine/eye tooth)
23. Lateral incisor
24. Central incisor
25. Central incisor
26. Lateral incisor
27. Cuspid (canine/eye tooth)
28. 1st bicuspid (1st premolar)
29. 2nd bicuspid (2nd premolar)
30. 1st molar (6-yr molar)
31. 2nd molar (12-yr molar)
32. 3rd molar (wisdom tooth)

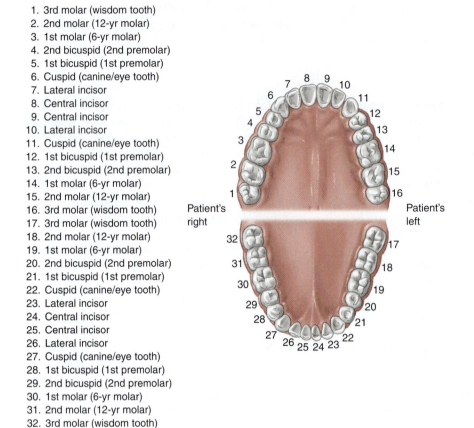

The two major airway structures, located in the neck, are the larynx and the trachea. The larynx, located prominently in the superior anterior neck at the level of C4/C5 to C6, consists of the thyroid and cricoid cartilages, and houses the vocal cords, corniculate and arytenoid cartilages, and the epiglottis. The cricothyroid, or intrinsic, ligament connects the inferior thyroid to the superior cricoid. Unlike the thyroid cartilage, which is incomplete posteriorly, the cricoid cartilage is a complete cartilaginous ring, hence it is called the cricoid ring. (See Figure 17-12 ■.) Cricotracheal ligaments attach the inferior cricoid to the first C-shaped cartilaginous ring of the trachea located at the level of C6. The closed portion of the C-shaped cartilaginous ring protects the anterior and lateral trachea. The posterior tracheal wall is composed of the trachealis muscle, which can be easily manipulated to allow the passage of a food bolus down the esophagus, which is located directly posterior.

The anterior wall of the esophagus is connected to the posterior trachea by the annular ligament, hence the two structures are located in proximity for their entire traverse of the neck. The posterior esophagus lies immediately anterior to the spinal column.

The cervical spine, consisting of the seven cervical vertebrae, is located wholly within the neck and serves to support the head and neck, provide a passageway for the spinal nerves that enter and exit the spinal cord, and protect the spinal cord.

Additional structures in the neck of importance to the critical care paramedic include the thyroid gland, parathyroid glands, cranial nerves IX and X, and the cervical and brachial plexus. The thyroid gland manufactures, stores, and secretes thyroid hormone. It is located inferior to the thyroid cartilage and anterior to the trachea. Two main lobes lie lateral to the trachea and are connected by a small bridge of thyroid tissue called the isthmus. The gland is afforded a significant blood supply from the superior and inferior thyroid arteries. The four parathyroid glands are located on the posterior surface of the thyroid and secrete parathyroid hormone when plasma calcium concentration falls below normal. The carotid sinus branch of the glossopharyngeal nerve, CN IX, traverses the neck as do numerous branches of the vagus nerve as it spreads out to destinations in the pharynx, carotid bodies and sinuses, diaphragm, heart, lungs, and abdominal viscera, among others. The

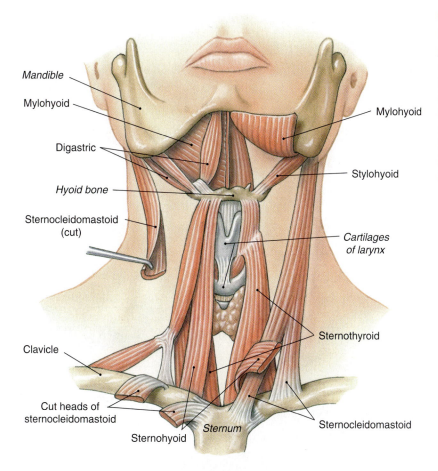

■ **Figure 17-12** Muscles of the anterior neck. *(Fig. 7-12, p. 189, from* Essentials of Anatomy & Physiology, *2nd ed., by Frederic H. Martini, Ph.D. and Edwin F. Bartholomew, M.S. Copyright © 2000 by Frederic H. Martini, Inc. Published by Pearson Education, Inc. Reprinted by permission.)*

Mandible

Mylohyoid

Digastric

Hyoid bone

Sternocleidomastoid (cut)

Clavicle

Cut heads of sternocleidomastoid

Sternohyoid

Mylohyoid

Stylohyoid

Cartilages of larynx

Sternothyroid

Sternocleidomastoid

Sternum

cervical plexus originates bilaterally from spinal nerves C1 through C5, and branches innervate muscles in the neck and account for the entire innervation of the diaphragm via the phrenic nerve. The brachial plexus originates bilaterally from spinal nerves C5 through T1 and provides innervation to the pectoral girdle and arm on their respective sides.

Numerous muscles in the neck serve to hold up and allow movement of the head, assist in respiration if needed, and to some degree protect deep vital structures such as blood vessels located underneath. The critical care paramedic should be familiar with two muscles in particular. The sternocleidomastoid originates at the sternal end of the clavicle and the manubrium, and inserts at the mastoid of the skull. It is an important landmark for procedures such as subclavian and internal jugular vein catheterization. In addition, the neck can be divided into the anterior and posterior triangles using the sternocleidomastoid. (See Figure 17-13 ■.) The **platysma** is a thin, superficial muscle layer located just below the subcutaneous tissue; it is surrounded by the superficial fascial layer. It covers the anterior triangle, and extends into the anteroinferior aspect of the posterior triangle. It effectively covers the neck, originating just inferior of the clavicles in the deep fascia of the upper chest, extending across the neck, and inserting on the mandible and the fascia at the corner of the mouth. Any penetrating trauma that violates the platysma should raise concern for potential damage to the deeper vital structures of the neck.

To aid in the evaluation and management of penetrating neck injuries, the anterior neck is divided into three zones. Zone I extends from the clavicle to the cricoid cartilage, Zone II extends from the cricoid cartilage to the angle of the mandible, and Zone III extends from the angle of the mandible to the base of the skull. (See Figure 17-14 ■.) Table 17–2 lists the anatomical structures located in each zone. As mentioned previously, the neck can also be divided into anterior and posterior triangles. The anterior triangle is the area bordered by the body and sternal head of the sternocleidomastoid, the mandible, and the midline of the neck. The posterior triangle is the area bordered by the body and clavicular head of the sternocleidomastoid, the middle third of the clavicle, and the trapezius muscle.

platysma *a thin, superficial muscle covering mostly the neck; located just below the subcutaneous tissue and surrounded by the superficial fascial layer.*

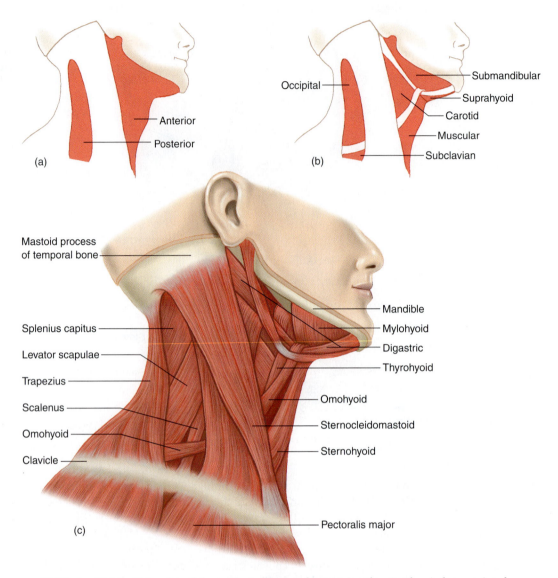

(a)

Anterior
Posterior

(b)

Occipital
Submandibular
Suprahyoid
Carotid
Muscular
Subclavian

(c)

Mastoid process
of temporal bone

Splenius capitus

Levator scapulae

Trapezius

Scalenus

Omohyoid

Clavicle

Mandible
Mylohyoid
Digastric
Thyrohyoid
Omohyoid
Sternocleidomastoid
Sternohyoid

Pectoralis major

■ **Figure 17-13** Triangles of the neck. A. The two larger triangles. B. The six lesser triangles. C. Detailed muscular anatomy.

■ **Figure 17-14** Zones of the neck.

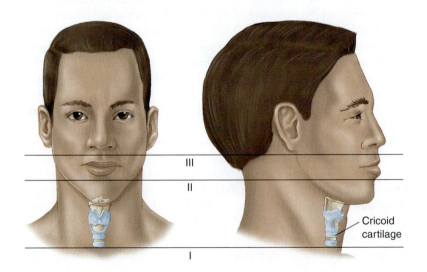

III

II

I

Cricoid cartilage

Table 17–2	Anatomical Zones of the Neck	
Zone	**Location**	**Structures Within**
I	From the thoracic inlet to the cricoid cartilage; defines the base of the neck.	Subclavian vessels, innominate veins, common carotid arteries, jugular veins, aortic arch, trachea, esophagus, lung apices, and cervical spine and cord.
II	From the cricoid cartilage to the angle of the mandible; encompasses the midportion of the neck.	Carotid arteries, vertebral arteries, jugular veins, pharynx, larynx, trachea, esophagus, and cervical spine and cord.
III	From the angle of the mandible to the base of the skull; defines the superior aspect of the neck.	Carotid arteries, jugular veins, salivary glands, parotid glands, esophagus, trachea, cervical spine and cord, and major nerves (cranial nerves IX, X, XI and XII).

PATHOPHYSIOLOGY OF FACIAL INJURIES

SOFT-TISSUE INJURIES

Due to the position and anatomy of the face, soft-tissue injury is perhaps the most common injury that the critical care paramedic can expect to encounter in the critical care environment. More than 50% of facial trauma cases presenting in emergency departments are a result of motor vehicle accidents, with assaults and sports-related injuries making up the majority of remaining cases. The rich vascular supply of the facial soft tissue and scalp ensure that even minor lacerations will bleed impressively at times. This rich vascular supply also allows for rapid wound healing and reduces the incidence of infection. While it is uncommon for facial lacerations to hemorrhage significantly enough to result in hemorrhagic shock, insult to a major vessel such as the facial or temporal artery can result in shock if bleeding is not controlled adequately. When presented with a patient in suspected hemorrhagic shock secondary to a facial trauma, the critical care paramedic should diligently search for and rule out other causes of blood loss. Facial lacerations, avulsions, incisions, and even contusions can result in damage to underlying structures such as cranial nerves, salivary glands, and lacrimal glands that can be identified during a thorough physical exam. (See Figure 17-15 .)

Remember that in addition to shearing, torsional, and frictional forces, compressive forces via blunt trauma can result in lacerations to soft tissue as well. Particular attention must be paid to ensure that there is not a more serious underlying internal injury when assessing these emergencies. In particular, contusions, abrasions, and hematomas should alert the provider that blunt forces were involved and assessment for underlying injury must take place. Common underlying injuries can include fractures and internal hemorrhaging.

Penetrating trauma may also result in a seemingly benign facial insult, and must always be considered when evaluating soft-tissue injuries. (See Figure 17-16 .) Low-velocity (<2,000 ft/sec) gunshot wounds to the face can have a minimal superficial presentation but extensive internal tissue destruction. Stab wounds, lacking the energy of fast-traveling bullets, typically do not result in the extensive internal tissue destruction typical of gunshot wounds. While it is not as common as blunt force trauma, penetrating trauma to the face is associated with a higher incidence of life-threatening airway compromise than is blunt force trauma. In addition, penetrating trauma to the inferior tissue of the face may extend internally into Zone III of the neck and include structures such as the internal carotid, external carotid, and vertebral arteries.

Impaled objects can initially present a particularly challenging dilemma for any health care provider, but a simple rule stands true. Unless it compromises the airway, all penetrating objects are left in place to be removed by a surgeon. Impaled objects frequently impinge or even lacerate arteries, veins, and nerves, and it is not uncommon for an impaled object to tamponade bleeding.

Due to the position and anatomy of the face, soft-tissue injury is perhaps the most common injury that the critical care paramedic can expect to encounter in the critical care environment.

While it is uncommon for facial lacerations to hemorrhage significantly enough to result in hemorrhagic shock, insult to a major vessel such as the facial or temporal artery can result in shock if bleeding is not controlled adequately.

Unless it compromises the airway, all penetrating objects are left in place to be removed by a surgeon.

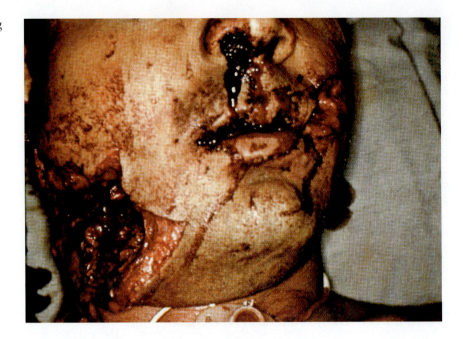

■ **Figure 17-15** A shooting victim with a gaping wound along his jawline and blood pouring from his nose. *(Robert S. Porter)*

Movement or removal of the object can result in further damage to underlying structures and/or allow continued severe hemorrhaging.

Human and animal bites to the face can result in extensive tissue destruction and hemorrhaging as well. Bite wounds to the cheek can be especially extensive and hemorrhage considerably, potentially compromising the airway. Human bites are of particular concern, and even seemingly minor bites can be notoriously deceptive, resulting in infection and tissue deformity. Infection occurs in approximately 10% to 15% of human bites, owing to the fact that human saliva contains up to 100,000,000 organisms/mL, with as many as 190 different species represented. Without proper care, severe complications and even death can occur secondary to animal and especially human bites.

Due to their prominent location, the nasal bones are the most commonly fractured facial bones, followed by the mandible and zygoma.

FACIAL FRACTURES

Due to their prominent location, the nasal bones are the most commonly fractured facial bones, followed by the mandible and zygoma. All of these bones require relatively little force to fracture and frequently present as isolated injuries. Bones that require much more force to fracture include the

■ **Figure 17-16** Penetrating trauma to the neck. *(Edward T. Dickinson, MD)*

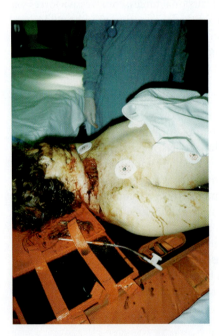

components of the supraorbital ridge and the ramus of the mandible. Any injury to these structures necessitates the ruling out of concomitant, potentially life-threatening injuries including closed head and cervical spine injury.

Nasal injuries commonly occur as a result of motor vehicle collisions or assaults. Nasal fractures often involve only the cartilaginous septum, resulting in deformity, swelling, pain, and minor hemorrhage. If the insult is sufficient to fracture the underlying nasal bones and deeper nasal structures such as the ethmoid bones, significant hemorrhaging can occur if the rich vascular supply of the nasal conchae is disrupted. In such cases, airway obstruction is of concern. In addition, rupture of the cribriform plate of the ethmoid bone can result in basilar skull fracture and torn meninges, exposing the subarachnoid space. Presence of cerebrospinal fluid rhinorrhea can be difficult to appreciate, but is indicative of basilar skull fracture.

The most common sites of mandibular fractures, in descending order of occurrence, are the body, condyle, angle, symphysis, ramus, and coronoid process. Patients with these types of injuries commonly present with malocclusion and limited mandibular mobility. Careful inspecion of the oral cavity should be performed, if possible, to rule out compound fracture. Fractures to the symphysis region, the midline of the mandible between the central incisors, are of particular concern because they can result in **glossoptosis** which is a downward or posterior displacement of the tongue (potentially causing airway compromise), especially when a patient is supine on a spine board.

Temporomandibular joint dislocation occurs when the condylar process of the mandible disarticulates from the mandibular fossae of the temporal bone. Blunt trauma is a common cause, but it can also occur secondary to yawning or seizures. The mandible will present deviated away from the side of a unilateral dislocation, or jutting forward in the case of bilateral dislocation. While the condition is often painful, it seldom results in airway compromise. Treatment is relocation under conscious sedation by a physician.

Zygoma fractures are most often the result of blunt force trauma secondary to assault, motor vehicle collisions, and sports injuries. The most common type of zygoma fracture is a simple fracture of the arch. Isolated zygomatic arch fractures are not a serious life threat. The less common and more serious tripod fracture involves the disarticulation of the zygomatic-frontal suture, fracture of the arch, and fracture of the infraorbital rim. In addition, fractures may extend into the orbital rim. Patients with zygomatic damage present with trismus, subconjunctival hemorrhage, infraorbital anesthesia, difficulty opening the mouth, and flattening of the midface over the fracture site.

Maxillary fractures are classified according to the **Le Fort system** classification. (See Figure 17-17 .) A Le Fort I maxillary fracture is a transverse fracture just superior to the apices of the teeth, through the maxillary sinus and across the nasal septum. It allows movement of the maxilla when the upper teeth are grasped and manipulated. A Le Fort II maxillary fracture (the pyramid fracture), extends superiorly through the infraorbital rims to an apex above the bridge of the nose. It allows movement of the maxilla, infraorbital rims, and nose when manipulated, but not the eyes. A Le Fort III maxillary fracture (the craniofacial dysjunction fracture) is the most serious of the Le Fort fractures. This fracture includes the zygomatic arches, frontozygomatic suture, sphenoid bone, and nasal bone. Simply stated, the facial skeleton is separated from the skull. As the name implies, it allows for movement of the facial structures, including the eyes, when manipulated. Significant force, up to 100 times the force of gravity, is required to fracture the midface, and significant, potentially life-threatening trauma to other systems can be present. Do not allow the dramatic appearance of such injuries to distract from a complete assessment and treatment of these injuries.

Injuries to the face can result in concomitant dentition injury. Teeth can fracture, chip, and be avulsed from the mandible or maxilla. In addition, cases of teeth intruding into the nasal cavity and maxillary sinus after facial trauma have been reported. Care must be taken to account for all teeth, when possible, to reduce the risk of aspiration. To this end, all missing teeth should be considered aspirated until proven otherwise. If possible, intact teeth should be properly cared for, because they can be reimplanted with a high likelihood of success.

Orbital blowout fractures result when a direct blow to the orbit results in an instantaneous increase in intraorbital pressure and subsequent rupture of the orbital floor. With this injury, the maxillary and zygoma bones are most often fractured, but any of the bones comprising the orbit can be involved. In addition, direct blows to the orbital rim can also result in a blowout fracture. Though not always damaged during the insult, one study has reported a 30% increase in the incidence of ruptured globe in conjunction with orbital blowout fractures, suggesting that the globe

glossoptosis *a downward or posterior displacement of the tongue.*

The most common sites of mandibular fractures, in descending order of occurrence, are the body, condyle, angle, symphysis, ramus, and coronoid process.

Le Fort system *classification system for defining maxillary fractures according to structure(s) involved and seriousness.*

Maxillary fractures are classified according to the Le Fort system.

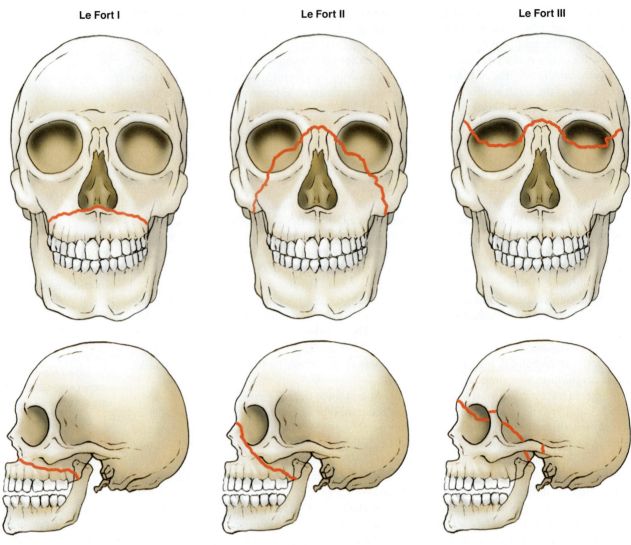

■ **Figure 17-17**   Le Fort facial fracture classification.

diplopia   *double vision.*

enophthalmos   *a posterior displacement of the eye.*

ptosis   *drooping of the eyelid.*

should be examined closely. A restricted upward gaze and **diplopia** (double vision), secondary to entrapment of the inferior rectus muscle, are common findings, and entrapment of the infraorbital nerve can result in anesthesia of the maxillary teeth and upper lip. **Enophthalmos** (a posterior displacement of the eye) may be appreciated, though it may prove difficult to discern secondary to local tissue swelling. (See Figure 17-18 ■.)

Superior orbital fissure syndrome can occur when an orbital fracture involving the superior orbital fissure compresses the oculomotor and ophthalmic branch of the trigeminal nerves, resulting in paralysis of the extraocular muscles, **ptosis,** and periorbital anesthesia. A much more serious variant of this injury, apex syndrome, involves the optic nerve. In addition to the findings consistent with superior orbital syndrome, these patients will also experience decreased visual acuity or blindness. Any patient with these syndromes requires immediate ophthalmic evaluation and intervention to prevent permanent vision loss.

PATHOPHYSIOLOGY OF THE EAR AND AUDITORY INJURIES

EXTERNAL EAR INJURY

The pinna, the visual portion of the ear that is exposed outside of the head, is frequently subjected to trauma. Because of the limited blood supply to the cartilaginous framework of the pinna, it does not hemorrhage significantly when lacerated or avulsed. Unfortunately, this paucity of vasculature

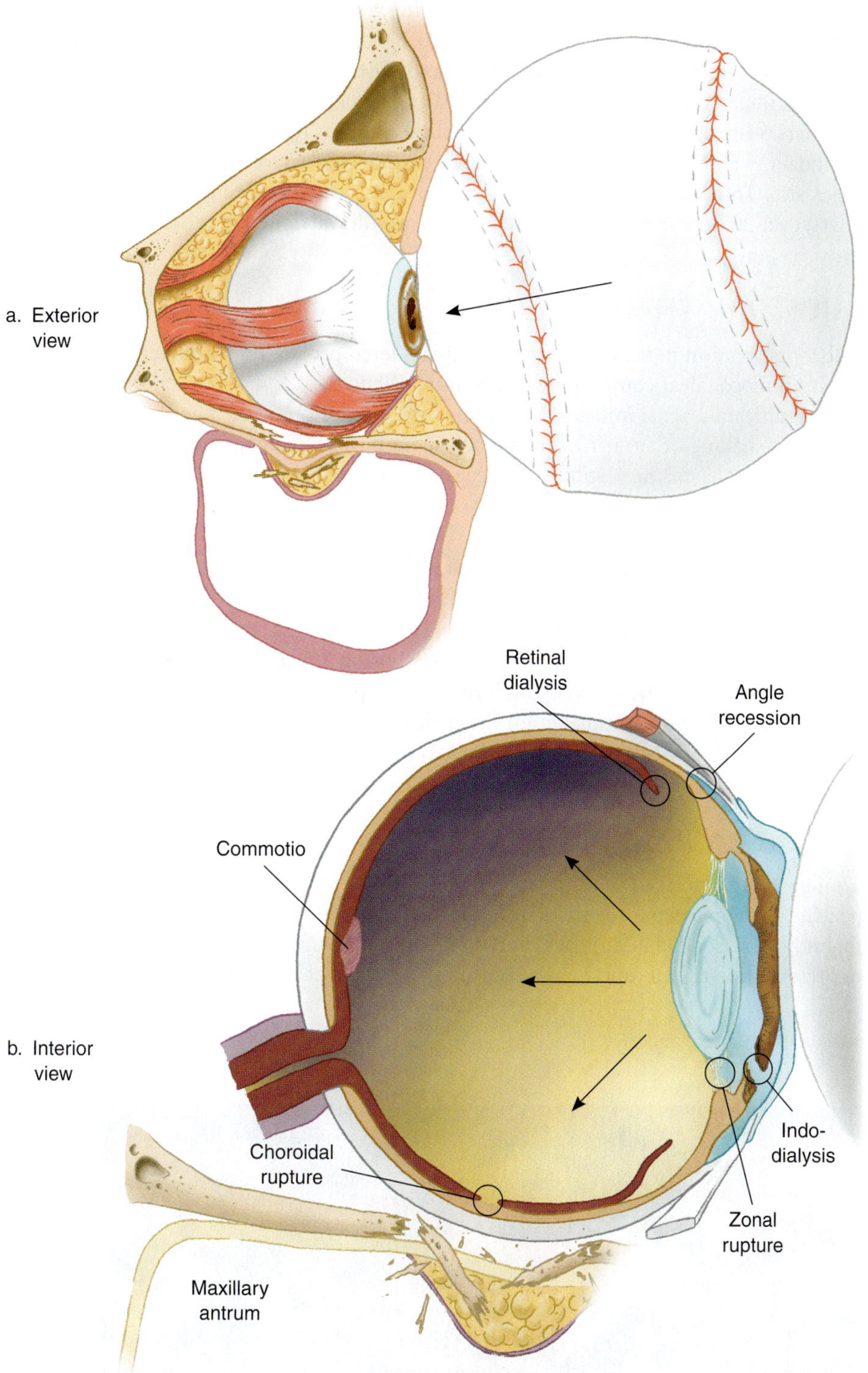

a. Exterior view
b. Interior view
Retinal dialysis
Angle recession
Commotio
Choroidal rupture
Indo-dialysis
Zonal rupture
Maxillary antrum

■ Figure 17-18 Blowout fracture. A. Exterior view. B. Interior view.

can also contribute to necrosis should the perichondrium be sheared from the underlying cartilage, because the cartilage is dependent on the perichondrium for its blood supply. The external ear canal, due to its narrow, winding path and location in the skull, is not often subjected to the forces of trauma and serves to protect the tympanic membrane.

RUPTURED TYMPANIC MEMBRANE

Injuries to the tympanic membrane occur either as a result of direct injury, such as when an object is introduced into the external ear canal and pushed up against the membrane, or indirect injury, such as when rapid changes in pressure rupture the membrane. Explosions, sudden direct blunt trauma to the pinna, and barotrauma from diving are common causes of tympanic membrane rupture. In addition, impact to the anterior mandible can transmit forces through the condyles sufficient enough to fracture the temporal bone and rupture the tympanic membranes. Common signs of tympanic membrane rupture include hearing loss and otorrhea. The tympanic membrane can also be ruptured in cases of basilar skull fracture. Patients with otorrhea and hemorrhagic otorrhea secondary to any insult to the head should be considered to have a basilar skull fracture until proven otherwise. Though isolated tympanic injuries are not life threatening and frequently heal themselves, evaluation in an emergency department is still warranted.

AUDITORY TRAUMA

Due to its location in the inner ear where it is offered protection by the temporal bone, injuries to the vestibulocochlear complex are uncommon. When they do occur, they are frequently associated with significant cranial injuries. Less frequently, disruption of the apparatus can occur secondary to violent shaking or shearing forces resulting in physical damage or dislocation of the vestibulocochlear complex or the vestibulocochlear nerve, CN VIII.

PATHOPHYSIOLOGY OF OCULAR INJURIES

While the orbit does provide adequate protection for the eye, both blunt and penetrating trauma can result in significant globe injury and loss of vision. Once damaged, ocular tissue does not heal or regenerate effectively. The vitreous humor of the posterior chamber, once lost, is not replaced by the body. It is therefore important for the critical care paramedic to be able to differentiate between benign and serious ocular injuries and be familiar with appropriate care.

EYELID LACERATIONS

Though injuries to the eyelid may seem unimpressive, they can include injury to the lacrimal apparatus, tarsal plate, levator muscle, and even the globe itself and should be evaluated by an ophthalmologist. Isolated lid injuries should undergo opthalmological repair within 24 hours of insult to preserve normal lid function and harmony with the lacrimal apparatus. (See Figure 17-19 ■.)

■ Figure 17-19 External eye trauma. *(Ben Ho, MD)*

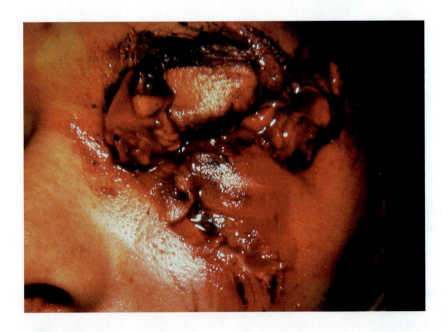

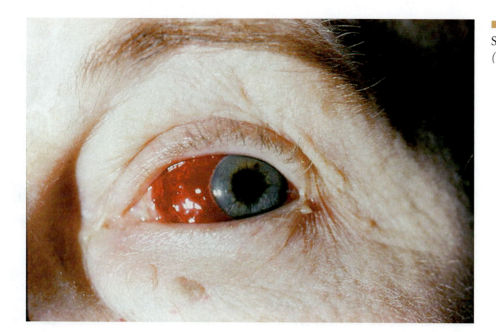

■ Figure 17-20
Subconjunctival hemorhage.
(Ben Ho, MD)

CONJUNCTIVAL INJURIES

A subconjunctival hemorrhage can occur when blunt trauma injures the blood vessels within the conjunctiva. In addition, traumatic asphyxiation, sneezing, coughing, vomiting, or any other maneuver that results in increased pressure can cause rupture of the conjunctival blood vessels. While potentially impressive, subconjunctival hemorrhage is not a serious injury, but does suggest that insult has occurred and additional injuries may be present. There is no treatment for subconjunctival hemorrhages, which typically resolve in 2 to 3 weeks. (See Figure 17-20 ■.)

CORNEAL INJURIES

Corneal abrasions are the most common eye injury evaluated in emergency situations. They result when a foreign body scratches the corneal epithelium, resulting in significant pain, lacrimation, sensation of tearing, and photophobia. Most patients will report a foreign body sensation, and sympathetic movement of the affected eye under a closed lid will often result in increased pain. Possible foreign bodies include dust, dirt, glass, and metal. Contact lenses, if left in too long, can also cause corneal abrasions, and often have a bacterial component to the insult as well. The critical care paramedic should ensure that all unconscious patients who are undergoing interfacility transfer have had contact lenses removed. Diagnosis of corneal abrasion is made with the application of fluorescein and illumination with an ultraviolet or Wood's lamp. (See Figure 17-21 ■.)

The critical care paramedic should ensure that all unconscious patients who are undergoing interfacility transfer have had contact lenses removed.

HYPHEMA

A **hyphema** is a collection of blood in the anterior chamber, and is often the result of blunt trauma to the globe. The bleeding is most commonly a result of torn vessels of the peripheral iris but can also result secondary to lens and retina detachment. The condition is more easily appreciated with the patient sitting upright, because blood will pool dependently in the inferior anterior chamber. With the patient lying supine, blood may not be recognized as readily as it disperses throughout the anterior chamber. Small hyphemas may not be recognized easily, and identification of microhyphemas requires the use of a slit lamp. Hyphema is a potential threat to a patient's vision, and evaluation by an ophthalmologist is required. (See Figure 17-22 ■.)

hyphema *a collection of blood in the anterior chamber of the eye.*

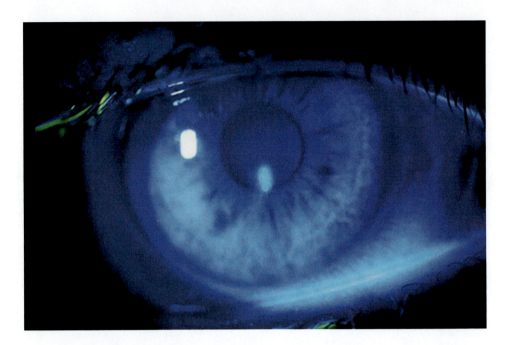

■ **Figure 17-21** Corneal abrasion. *(Ben Ho, MD)*

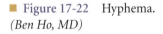

Globe rupture is a serious injury with a high risk for loss of vision, and is always considered a serious ophthalmalogical emergency and always requires surgical intervention.

OCULAR GLOBE RUPTURE

Globe rupture is a serious injury with a high risk for loss of vision, and is always considered a serious ophthalmalogical emergency and always requires surgical intervention. Posterior chamber injury and loss of vitreous humor is associated with a higher frequency of vision loss than are injuries to the anterior chamber. Luckily, the orbit provides a significant amount of protection to the posterior globe. Globe rupture should be suspected whenever there is a history of penetrating or significant blunt trauma. Common penetrating objects include writing instruments, fishhooks, knives, darts, and needles. In addition, any patient who suffers acute eye injury while in the presence of heavy machinery, a power saw, metal grinders, metalworking, or any other situation of high-energy metal-to-metal contact should be considered high risk for globe insult. It is important for the critical care paramedic to remember that globe rupture may initially be insidious, and not readily apparent. More often, decreased visual acuity, an irregular pupil, flattening of the globe, and sub-

■ **Figure 17-22** Hyphema. *(Ben Ho, MD)*

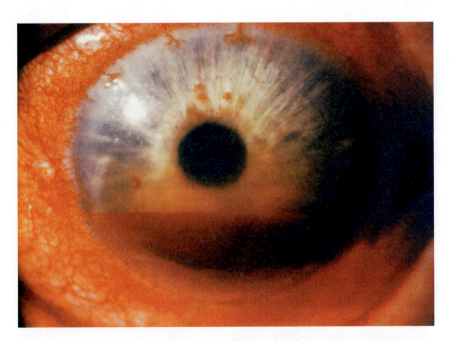

conjunctival hemorrhage or hyphema may be present. Careful inspection of the eye is of the utmost importance when attempting to identify globe rupture. (See Figure 17-23 ■.)

OCULAR AVULSION

In severe maxillofacial trauma **enucleation** (removal) of the globe from the orbit may occur. Despite the often dramatic presentation of these injuries, loss of vision can be avoided and depends on the extent of injury as well as the quality of care. Of course, the tearing and shearing forces associated with an ocular avulsion often result in significant damage to the major blood vessels and optic nerve, which decreases the likelihood that normal vision can be restored. Care must be taken in such circumstances to control active hemorrhaging and rule out additional, potential life-threatening injuries.

enucleation *traumatic removal of the globe from the orbit.*

TRAUMATIC RETINAL DETACHMENT

Traumatic retinal detachment occurs most often as a result of blunt trauma and is considered a surgical emergency. In retinal detachment, the outer, pigmented layer of the retina separates from the inner, neural layer. There are three mechanisms by which this can happen. First, increased intraocular pressure from blunt force trauma can tear the retina and force vitreous humor from the posterior chamber into the defect, resulting in a dissection-like injury between the layers. Second, tractional retinal detachment can occur when adhesions form between the vitreous humor and the retina and mechanical forces within the globe secondary to blunt or penetrating trauma separate the layers of the retina (with or without tearing it). Third, blood can escape from damaged vessels, separating and filling the retinal layers. Retinal detachments may have no outward signs, and diagnosis by the critical care paramedic is often made after considering the mechanism of injury and symptoms. Symptoms include seeing flashes of light, curtain-like shadows in the peripheral vision, dimmed vision, and black spots.

PATHOPHYSIOLOGY OF NECK INJURIES

Proper care of the patient with blunt or penetrating neck trauma can prove to be extremely challenging for the critical care paramedic. Seemingly benign injuries can quickly turn life threatening, and delayed or inappropriate treatment can easily result in disability or death.

Seemingly benign injuries can quickly turn life threatening, and delayed or inappropriate treatment can easily result in disability or death.

Horner's syndrome *caused by injury to the sympathetic nerves of the face, it causes a triad of constricted pupil, ptosis, and facial dryness (anhidrosis).*

The critical care paramedic will find it useful to classify neck injuries according to the anatomical zones affected. This will not only aid in providing a clear, comprehensible verbal and written report to the receiving facility, but can also help the critical care paramedic anticipate injuries based on known anatomy within the zones.

Injuries to Zone I are associated with high mortality because they can involve the great vascular structures of the chest, the inferior larynx and trachea, as well as intrathoracic structures such as the lungs. Don't forget, the apex of the lung can extend to just below Zone I, immediately below the level of the clavicle. A high index of suspicion is needed to be alert for developing pneumothorax after a stab wound to Zone I. Injuries to Zone II commonly involve the carotid arteries and airway structures, and are readily identifiable owing to the exposed nature of this area of the neck. Zone III injuries often involve the internal and external carotid arteries, the vertebral artery, and the cranial nerves.

Finally, any wound that obviously penetrates the platysma should immediately increase the index of suspicion for underlying injury to the deeper structures of the neck. This is an injury that will most likely be explored surgically.

VASCULAR NECK INJURIES

The vascular structures of the neck are commonly injured in penetrating neck trauma, and laceration of the carotid arteries or internal jugular veins can result in rapid loss of significant amounts of blood and development of hemorrhagic shock. In addition, insult to the carotid arteries can decrease cerebral perfusion and cause cerebral hypoxia and ischemia, and an expanding hematoma can occlude blood vessels and compromise the airway. Injury to the common carotid artery occurs in 11% to 13% of all penetrating neck trauma. Laceration of the jugular vein can also result in the development of an air embolism as venous pressure drops below atmospheric pressure during deep exhalation.

While not as common as penetrating trauma, blunt trauma can also be associated with significant arterial injury. Mechanisms of injury that result in hyperextension, hyperflexion, hyperrotation, and direct blows to the neck should alert the critical care paramedic to the possibility of vascular injury. Specific carotid artery injuries include pseudoaneurysm and dissection, resulting in hematoma formation, neurologic deficits, carotid bruits, ipsilateral **Horner's syndrome** (which is clinical findings of ptosis, pupillary miosis, and facial anhidrosis), and pulse deficits. Because 25% to 50% of patients with carotid injury secondary to blunt trauma initially present with no external signs of trauma, an appreciation for the mechanism of injury is essential in such cases. Similar injury to the vertebral arteries presents clinically with hemiparesis, diplopia, nystagmus, vertigo, and dysarthria.

LARYNGOTRACHEAL INJURIES

Laryngotracheal injuries include edema and swelling of the soft tissue, thyroid and cricoid cartilage fracture, hyoid bone fracture, and laryngotracheal disruption. Clinical findings include dysphonia (hoarseness), dysphagia, dyspnea, pain, and hemoptysis. "Clothesline" injuries can occur as a result of striking stationary ropes, cords, or wires while operating vehicles such as bicycles, ATVs, or motorcycles. In addition, strangulation or hanging can cause a similar type of insult. These injuries can be overlooked due to their unimpressive initial presentation, but they are at high risk for developing total airway occlusion secondary to swelling and edema of the surrounding tissues. Developing hoarseness is an ominous sign of impending airway occlusion.

Conversely, penetrating trauma injuries to Zones I and II resulting in laryngotracheal injury are seldom occult. Clinical exam findings include obvious airway defect, dyspnea, hemoptysis, air bubbling from the wound, and subcutaneous emphysema.

In cases of both blunt and penetrating trauma, deformity of the normal anatomical landmarks can make oral intubation difficult even for the most experienced provider, and these situations often require the use of a surgical airway. Tracheostomy rather than cricothyrotomy may be the airway of choice, because a cricothyrotomy attempt may worsen existing trauma in that area.

NEUROLOGIC INJURIES

Direct injury to nerves located outside of the spinal cord is the most common etiology of neurologic deficits secondary to neck trauma. Of particular concern are two injuries that are potentially life threatening: injuries to the phrenic nerves, and injuries to the recurrent laryngeal nerves. The paired phrenic nerves provide all of the innervation to the diaphragm, and insult to one can cause a marked insult to normal respiration. Insult to both phrenic nerves, however unlikely, would result in paralysis of the diaphragm. The paired recurrent laryngeal nerves provide innervation allowing for opening of the vocal cords. Insult results in vocal cord paralysis and airway obstruction secondary to a closed glottic opening. In addition, injuries to the deep cervical and brachial plexus can occur.

THYROID INJURIES

Of all the structures in the neck, the thyroid gland is one of the most exposed and is very susceptible to injury. Of primary concern would be the potential for significant hemorrhage secondary to laceration of the superior and inferior thyroid arteries. Although rare, thyrotoxicosis secondary to thyroid trauma can occur and should be considered in any patient with injury to the thyroid or surrounding tissues and presenting with the clinical manifestations associated with thyrotoxicosis.

PHARYNX AND ESOPHAGUS INJURIES

Due to their deep, protected location in the neck, pharyngeal and esophageal injuries are fairly uncommon, and are most often the result of penetrating neck trauma. Esophageal injuries are often difficult to identify clinically, and are often overlooked during the initial assessment. However, due to the close to 100% mortality if treatment is delayed 24 hours, it is imperative that these injuries be identified quickly.

ASSESSMENT FINDINGS AND INTERPRETATION

PRIMARY ASSESSMENT

Assessment of airway, breathing, and circulation are of extreme importance in the patient with maxillofacial or neck trauma, because injuries to these systems can easily become life threatening. Continual reassessment is also required, because airway, breathing, and circulation parameters can change rapidly with facial trauma. What was once a patent airway may become partially or fully occluded in just minutes due to bleeding or swelling. As such, airway control and ventilation decisions should be made early, promptly, and carried out with precision. The maintenance of the airway is equally important because failure to do so will doom all other interventions to failure.

Assessment of circulation in the primary exam revolves around the identification and treatment of life-threatening hemorrhage. Gross hemorrhage from a vascular neck injury is usually obvious. The presence of shock in a patient with maxillofacial injuries is more likely than not due to blood loss at an additional location such as the thorax, abdomen, pelvis, long bones, or externally. Bleeding from these locations should be controlled with direct pressure prior to assessing and addressing any maxillofacial or neck injuries.

Because neck trauma often results in compromise of arterial vascular structures, a rapid neurologic exam to rule out cerebral hypoxia secondary to shock, arterial impingement, or arterial occlusion should be performed in the primary assessment.

Assessment of airway, breathing, and circulation are of extreme importance in the patient with maxillofacial or neck trauma, because injuries to these systems can easily become life threatening.

MAXILLOFACIAL ASSESSMENT

The ears, nose, and mouth should be assessed for the presence of blood or fluid. The mouth should be inspected for teeth, secretions, or blood in the oropharynx and suctioning provided as necessary. The oral cavity should be inspected for malocclusion, lacerations, avulsions, penetrating injury, bone fragments, foreign bodies, and compound fractures.

A systematic inspection and palpation of the bony structures of the midface should reveal the majority of facial fractures. The entire face should be palpated for loss of integrity, crepitus, subcutaneous air, and pain.

Orbital fractures can be identified by loss of integrity of the infraorbital rim, loss of symmetry between the orbits, and periorbital anesthesia. In addition, enophthalmos, restriction of extraocular movement, or diplopia may be present. Radiographic findings consistent with orbital fracture include the "hanging teardrop" and "open bomb-bay door" signs resulting from the herniation of orbital fat and displacement of orbital bone into the maxillary sinus. Air/fluid levels may also be appreciated in the maxillary sinus on the X-ray.

Zygoma fractures can be identified by the presence of a flattened cheek, lateral subconjunctival hemorrhage on the ipsilateral side, and infraorbital anesthesia. If the displaced zygoma impinges the masseter muscle or coronoid process, trismus or limited range of motion can occur. X-ray is adequate for the interpretation of arch injuries, while tripod injuries are best evaluated with CT scanning.

Nasal fractures to the bony or cartilaginous structures can be readily identified by asymmetry, deformity, and pain. The need for nasal films can be described as controversial.

Mandibular fractures can be identified clinically by the presence of malocclusion, instability, crepitation, and immobility of the mandible. The tongue-blade test can be a useful technique for detecting mandibular fractures that are not readily apparent on initial inspection. The examiner instructs the patient to bite down forcefully on a tongue blade inserted between the teeth. The examiner then twists the blade, attempting to break it. The patient with a fractured mandible will experience pain and reflexively open his mouth. A positive tongue blade test is an extremely simple, but very sensitive clinical test for a mandibular fracture.

OCULAR ASSESSMENT

The periorbital area should be inspected for ptosis, lacerations, swelling, deformity, ecchymosis, or any dysfunction. Palpation of the orbital rims should be performed to evaluate for crepitus, loss of integrity, or periorbital anesthesia.

The external eye and anterior chamber should be inspected for penetrating objects, foreign bodies, signs of infection, flattening, protrusion, lacerations, hemorrhage, hyphema, and any other sign of trauma. Pupil assessment is best performed in a slightly underlit or dim environment. Pupils should be assessed for symmetry, shape, accommodation, and reaction to light.

Visual acuity in both eyes should be evaluated in all nonacute patients who are conscious and alert.

Visual acuity in both eyes should be evaluated in all nonacute patients who are conscious and alert. Near or distance charts should be utilized when practical, assessing for the smallest line readable for each eye while the other is covered. Uncorrected vision should be tested first, followed by corrected vision.

OCULAR MOTILITY

Evaluation of the six extraocular muscles and the cranial nerves that innervate them can be performed by having the patient move his eyes through all six positions of gaze. Disconjugate gaze, diplopia, or limitation in motility should be recorded.

FUNDOSCOPIC EXAMINATION

An ophthalmoscope can be utilized to magnify and visualize the anterior and posterior cavities of the eye, allowing for evaluation of the retina, optic nerve, and macula. Dilation of the pupils makes the visualization of these structures easier. This can be useful since many types of traumatic insults to the head can result in clinical findings discernible with an ophthalmoscope. (See Figure 17-24 ■.)

EXAMINATION OF THE NECK

Inspect and palpate the neck and note any lacerations, asymmetry, swelling, pulsating masses, subcutaneous emphysema, and tracheal deviation. Pay particular attention to the area of Zone III under the mandible, the posterior triangle, and the inferior aspect of Zone I—these areas are often passed over and injuries overlooked with devastating consequences. Remember that penetrating in-

Pay particular attention to the area of Zone III under the mandible, the posterior triangle, and the inferior aspect of Zone I—these areas are often passed over and injuries overlooked with devastating consequences.

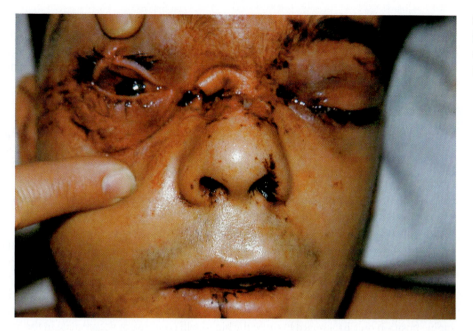

■ **Figure 17-24** Blunt eye injury necessitates opthalmoscopic examination. *(Ben Ho, MD)*

juries to Zone I can result in thoracic injury, and a chest film can be useful to rule out pneumothorax, hemothorax, and pneumomediastinum. Cervical spine films must be evaluated in all patients with neck injury. When looking at a lateral neck X-ray, note the presence of all seven cervical vertebrae. The anterior vertebral bodies should follow the same line, and the spinal processes should be even and symmetrical as well. In general, thoroughly assess the neck film for penetrated foreign bodies, bony fractures, subcutaneous air, soft-tissue injury, hematoma, tracheal disruption or deviation, and retropharyngeal thickening. (See Figure 17-25 ■ and Table 17–2.)

MANAGEMENT

The most urgent complications of maxillofacial and neck trauma are airway compromise and uncontrolled hemorrhage. The extreme and disheartening nature of these injuries must not distract

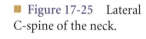

The most urgent complications of maxillofacial and neck trauma are airway compromise and uncontrolled hemorrhage.

■ **Figure 17-25** Lateral C-spine of the neck.

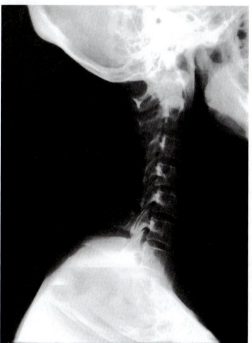

the critical care paramedic from performing an adequate assessment, promptly correcting life-threatening conditions, and continuously reassessing the ABCs. Because a large percentage of patients with maxillofacial and/or neck injury present with multisystem trauma, it is imperative that a thorough initial exam and detailed physical exam of the head and neck be completed and repeated.

AIRWAY

The most common cause of death from maxillofacial trauma is obstruction of the upper airway secondary to posterior displacement of the tongue into the hypopharynx.

The most common cause of death from maxillofacial trauma is obstruction of the upper airway secondary to posterior displacement of the tongue into the hypopharynx (from atonia of the submandibular muscles in the obtunded patient). It is also arguably the most preventable. Manual BLS airway maneuvers should always precede the initiation of ALS mechanical procedures. The modified jaw thrust and suctioning of the oropharyngeal cavity are often sufficient to open up the airway and keep it clear for initial oxygenation. And obviously, care must be exercised so as to not manipulate the cervical spine if cervical injury is suspected.

If however, manual airway maneuvers are not sufficient to open the airway, a simple mechanical adjunct, the oropharyngeal airway, can be inserted. Use of a nasopharyngeal airway is generally contraindicated in cases of suspected fracture of the cribriform plate, because the airway may pass through the fracture and into the cranial vault. Frequent suctioning of the airway is often required in maxillofacial trauma, and particular care should be paid to patients who are immobilized in a supine position on a backboard because the blood will continue to accumulate in the hypopharynx of the supine, nonintubated patient.

Distortion of the soft tissue and bony structures of the face can make achieving a proper mask seal difficult at best, and impossible at worst. A flail mandible not only makes the mask seal difficult to maintain, but may allow the tongue to fall into the posterior hypopharynx, thereby obstructing the airway as well. In neck injuries, air dissecting into the surrounding tissue and facial compartments can quickly distort airway anatomy and make ventilation as well as recognition of laryngeal structures difficult if not impossible. Again, diligent airway assessment and maintenance cannot be stressed enough.

Developing airway compromise should be suspected if worsening dyspnea, tachypnea, cyanosis, agitation, altered mental status, loss of consciousness, accessory muscle use, nasal flaring, subcutaneous emphysema, or hoarseness is noted. In such cases, endotracheal intubation should be considered. The use of endotracheal intubation is frequently required to ensure adequate oxygenation and ventilation, and the decision to perform intubation is a critical one that should be made decisively.

Developing airway compromise should be suspected if worsening dyspnea, tachypnea, cyanosis, agitation, altered mental status, loss of consciousness, accessory muscle use, nasal flaring, subcutaneous emphysema, or hoarseness is noted.

When attempting intubation with these patients, ensure the equipment is properly prepared and set up so your first attempt at intubation is your best attempt. Orotracheal intubation is preferred over nasotracheal intubation in most cases because of the risk of basilar skull fracture in this population of patients. In-line cervical spine stabilization should be held in those patients identified to be at risk for cervical spine injury. Numerous tools, such as the Viewmax, fiber-optic stylettes, and the gum elastic bougie, can facilitate intubation of the difficult airway, and are discussed in greater depth in Chapter 7. In addition, advanced techniques such as retrograde intubation can be utilized in situations where routine endotracheal intubation is difficult or impossible.

Rapid-sequence intubation (RSI) in patients with severe maxillofacial or neck injury is not without significant risk. Failure to intubate a paralyzed patient can be further complicated by failure to adequately ventilate with a bag-value mask (BVM) due to distortion of normal facial anatomy. These patients are prime candidates for facilitated intubation, in which sedation with benzodiazepines, barbiturates, droperidol, or other induction agent is administered to increase the likelihood of successful intubation without rendering the patient paralyzed and apneic. Whether RSI or sedation is used, a backup method of securing the airway in case of failed intubation must be prepared. Options for backup include alternative airways such as the CombiTube, the Intubating LMA device, or a surgical airway technique. If a surgical airway is to be considered, it is necessary to properly and completely prepare both the patient and your equipment. Preparation means that a surgical airway tray is opened and ready for use, the patient's neck is prepared per protocol, and an endotracheal or tracheostomy tube is selected and opened.

Surgical airway options for the patient with maxillofacial trauma include needle cricothyroidotomy, surgical cricothyroidotomy, and tracheostomy. Severe neck trauma that includes the larynx may result in the deformation of landmarks, effectively excluding cricothyroidotomy as an option. In such cases, tracheostomy is the airway of choice. It is important to remember that the gold standard surgical airway in cases of neck trauma is surgical tracheostomy by an experienced surgical team.

Ideally, the decision to perform advanced airway procedures should be made earlier rather than later. Attempt to arrive at a definitive airway prior to transport, because performing advanced procedures in the back of a ground ambulance or helicopter can prove challenging due to cramped conditions and limited help. It is always better to secure the airway prior to leaving a scene or facility, in a more stable environment, with additional personnel to assist if needed.

HEMORRHAGE CONTROL

Although patients rarely develop shock secondary to facial hemorrhage, care should be taken to control any bleeding with a pressure dressing. Clamping of wounds with hemostats should be avoided, because inadvertent damage to facial nerves or salivary ducts may occur. Pinching the upper nasal cartilage together often easily controls nasal hemorrhage. In rare cases, packing of the anterior or posterior nasal cavity may be necessary for severe bleeds, but care must be taken not to pack the cranium as well. A Foley catheter inserted through the nasal cavity, filled with saline, and then pulled back out until the balloon lodges is often used in such circumstances. Patients should be encouraged, if possible, not to swallow any blood because that can lead to gastric irritation and vomiting (again further complicating the airway status). Very often, conscious and alert patients are able to suction their airway themselves if given a rigid tip suction device and instructions on its use.

Bleeding from neck injuries is controlled in the same manner—direct pressure with a sterile dressing, avoiding the practice of blind clamping of vessels. Avoid placing an IV in any location that would flow toward a vascular injury site. Any fluid administered through such an IV would potentially extravasate through the vascular insult. A general rule of thumb is to place IVs on the opposite side of Zone I injuries, or consider cannulation of other peripheral sites. Consider also the use of an occlusive dressing on large open neck wounds to eliminate the potential of air being entrained into the wound site.

IMPALED OBJECTS

Unless it interferes with airway control, any impaled object in the face, neck, or eye should be immobilized in place. This can be accomplished in any number of ways, and creativity is sometimes required when patients are impaled with unusually shaped objects. More often than not, penetrating objects can be stabilized with bulky dressings placed and secured around the object. Often, an additional support such as a cup with a hole punched out is placed over the object and dressings to provide additional support. When stabilizing objects that have penetrated the eye, it is advisable to also cover the unaffected eye to prevent the patient from looking about his surroundings, which encourages conjugate movement of the affected eye and could result in increased damage.

FACIAL FRACTURES

In and of themselves, facial fractures are not treated by the critical care paramedic, but complications arising from facial fractures are. As discussed previously, mandibular fractures can result in posterior displacement of the tongue into the posterior hypopharynx, complicating the airway. Le Fort fractures that are hemorrhaging significantly can also be reduced with gentle inferior traction in an attempt to control bleeding.

OCULAR INJURIES

Corneal abrasions and foreign bodies can be treated initially with application of an eye shield and soft packing to prevent blinking; then hold the lid in place. Care should be taken not to put any pressure on the globe. Corneal foreign bodies that have penetrated the cornea should be removed under magnification, by an ophthalmologist. (See Figure 17-26 ■.) Foreign bodies not penetrating the cornea can be removed with irrigation, a cotton-tipped applicator or the corner of a 2×2 gauze. Inversion of the eyelid can help in locating and removing foreign bodies in this situation.

It is always better to secure the airway prior to leaving a scene or facility, in a more stable environment, with additional personnel to assist if needed.

A general rule of thumb is to place IVs on the opposite side of Zone I injuries, or consider cannulation of other peripheral sites. Consider also the use of an occlusive dressing on large open neck wounds to eliminate the potential of air being entrained into the wound site.

Unless it interferes with airway control, any impaled object in the face, neck, or eye should be immobilized in place.

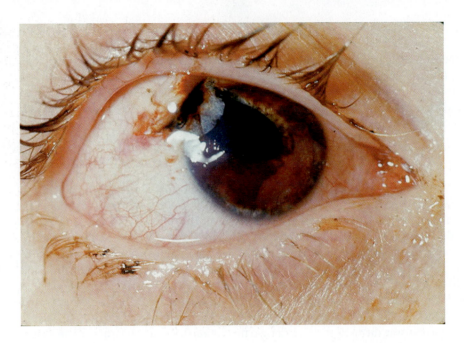

The enucleated or avulsed eyeball should be treated with care, and never be pushed back into the orbit. Rather, it should be shielded from further trauma by placement beneath a rigid patch or similar device.

CONTACT LENS REMOVAL

Contact lenses must be removed in all patients with chemical burns to the eye, and strongly considered in all unconscious patients. A ruptured globe is a contraindication to contact lens removal in the field. Removal of contact lenses can be achieved by several methods. Soft lenses can be removed in the normal fashion by "pinching" the lens with the thumb and forefinger, or sliding the lens off the cornea and onto the sclera where it can be "pushed" off. Rigid contact lenses need to be pushed down (gently), on one side to break the seal created by the moist corneal surface. The lens can then be lifted off the eye. Irrigation with saline can also remove contact lenses, but they are often lost in the irrigation runoff.

AUDITORY INJURIES

The critical care paramedic cannot effectively treat auditory injuries to the middle and inner ear, which often require thorough evaluation and treatment by an otolaryngologist. In cases where injury results in otorrhea or hemorrhage, external application of sterile gauze dressing is warranted, but packing of the external ear canal is not suggested. Care should also be taken to ensure that water or other fluids are not allowed to enter the ear canal.

MANDIBULAR DISLOCATION

In cases where isolated temporomandibular joint dislocation without fracture has been confirmed with radiographic study, mandibular reduction can be performed and is a relatively minor procedure. After sedation with IV benzodiazepines, the reducer wraps his thumbs in gauze and assumes a position behind the patient. Reaching around the patient and grabbing the anterior jaw with gauzed thumbs placed in the mouth on the mandibular ridge, downward and forward traction is applied to rearticulate the joint. The patient should be discouraged from "testing" his jaw after the procedure, because redislocation may occur due to the stretched or torn ligaments. Application of a Barton bandage immediately after relocation will help prevent repeat dislocation.

DENTAL ALVULSIONS

Although not a priority in a trauma patient, avulsed, intact teeth can be reinserted within 20 minutes of removal into their sockets as long as there are no serious injuries that would demand the critical care paramedic's attention. Tooth reinsertion should never be performed in an unconscious patient due to the risk of aspiration. Care should be taken to handle the tooth by the crown and avoid injuring the root or periodontal fibers. The tooth and socket should both be rinsed clean of dirt and debris with normal saline (or Hank's solution if available). If the tooth has been dry for greater than 20 minutes but less than 1 hour, the tooth should be soaked in Hank's solution for 30 minutes prior to reintroduction into the socket. If rinsing the avulsed tooth is warranted, rinsing of the socket to remove dirt and clots should be performed gently, with as little manipulation as possible. The tooth should be properly aligned after reinsertion, comparing it to the surrounding dentition. If able, the patient should be instructed to bite down on a roll of gauze for a minimum of 20 minutes.

Summary

The critical care paramedic will encounter few situations that are as potentially gruesome, disturbing, and clinically challenging as a patient with severe maxillofacial and neck trauma. A sound understanding and appreciation of anatomy, physiology, pertinent medical equipment, and treatment modalities will ensure that your patients will enjoy the best chance at reduced morbidity and mortality. Most maxillofacial and neck trauma is not life threatening, but it is commonly intimidating to the conscious patient. Fear of long-term disability and disfigurement is justified, because maxillofacial trauma has high potential for physical and psychological impairment. More than 25% of individuals who suffer maxillofacial injury experience post-traumatic stress disorder. This should not be lost on the critical care paramedic, who is likely to be in a position to provide emotional support and reassurance as well as advanced procedures.

Review Questions

1. Decide whether each of the following statements is true or false with regard to the anatomical neck zones used in trauma evaluation.
   a. Zone I injuries can include insult to the larynx, trachea, and thyroid gland.
   b. Zone II injuries are often the most obvious because of location and structures involved.
   c. Zone III injuries may involve the subclavian and pulmonary pleura.
   d. Zone III injuries may involve larynx, recurrent laryngeal nerve, internal carotid artery, and external carotid artery.

2. What is the largest concern the critical care paramedic should have regarding neck and facial trauma?

3. What is the proper management for an avulsed tooth?

4. Identify whether each of the following statements is true or false with regard to Le Fort fractures.
   - A Le Fort I fracture involves the maxilla, orbits, and nasal bones.
   - Manipulation of a Le Fort III fracture results in movement of the maxilla, infraorbital rim, and nose but not the eyes.
   - Manipulation of a Le Fort II fracture results in movement of the maxilla, infraorbital rim, and the eyes.
   - A Le Fort II fracture involves the maxilla, zygomatic arches, frontozygomatic suture, sphenoid bone, and nasal bone.

5. In a patient with penetrating neck trauma, paralysis of the diaphragm would indicate an insult to what nerve?

6. When should an impaled object to the neck be removed?

7. Why would an occlusive dressing be utilized during the management of a patient who suffered a penetration injury to the neck?

8. Paralysis of the vocal cords can occur secondary to what cranial nerve dysfunction?

9. Why is the use of nasopharyngeal airways or nasogastric tubes relatively contraindicated on a patient with severe facial trauma?

See Answers to Review Questions at the back of this book.

Further Reading

Bledsoe BE, Porter RS, Cherry RA. *Paramedic Care: Principles & Practice,* 2nd ed. Upper Saddle River, NJ: Pearson Prentice Hall, 2005.

Bisson JI, Shepherd JP. "Psychological Sequelae of Facial Trauma." *Journal of Trauma: Injury, Infection, and Critical Care,* Vol. 43, No. 3 (September 1997): 496–500.

Hubble MW, Hubble JP. *Principles of Advanced Trauma Care,* 1st ed. Albany, NY: Thompson Delmar Learning, 2002.

Hudak CM, Gallo BM, Morton PG. *Critical Care Nursing: A Holistic Approach,* 7th ed. Philadelphia: Lippincott-Raven Publishers, 1998.

Martini FH, Timmons MJ, McKinley, MP. *Human Anatomy,* 3rd ed. Upper Saddle River, NJ: Pearson Prentice Hall, 2000.

Netter, FH. *Atlas of Human Anatomy.* Summit, NJ: Ciba-Geigy Corporation, 1989.

Revis Jr. DR. *Human Bite Infections.* http://www.emedicine.com/med/topic1033.htm (last updated October 27, 2004).

Sole ML, Lamborn ML, Hartshorn JC. *Introduction to Critical Care Nursing,* 4th ed. Philadelphia: W. B. Saunders Company, 2005.

Tung T-C, Chen Y-R, Chen C-T, Lin C-J. "Full Intrusion of a Tooth after Facial Trauma." *Journal of Trauma: Injury, Infection, and Critical Care,* Vol. 43, No. 2 (August 1997): 357–359.

Wilkins RB, Havins WE. "Current Treatment of Blow-Out Fractures." *Ophthalmology,* Vol. 89, No. 5 (1982): 464–466.

Burns and Electrical Injuries

Lee Richardson, NREMT-P, CCEMT-P, FP-C

Objectives

Upon completion of this chapter, the student should be able to:

1. Describe the epidemiology, including incidence, mortality/morbidity, and risk factors for thermal burn injuries. (p. 490)
2. Describe the effects of heat according to Jackson's theory of thermal wounds, particularly:
   A. Zone of coagulation (p. 490)
   B. Zone of stasis (p. 491)
   C. Zone of hyperemia (p. 491)
3. Describe techniques used to identify and establish priorities for treatment of the burn patient. (p. 493)
4. Identify the techniques used for airway management and ventilation support of the burn patient. (p. 493)
5. Calculate the total percentage of body surface area involved using one or more of the following methods:
   A. "Rule of nines" (adult and pediatric) (p. 497)
   B. "Rule of palms" (p. 497)
   C. Lund and Browder chart (p. 498)
6. Identify and describe the depth classifications of burn injuries:
   A. Superficial burns (first degree) (p. 499)
   B. Partial-thickness burns (second degree) (p. 500)
   C. Full-thickness burns (third degree) (p. 500)
   D. Fourth-degree burns (p. 501)
7. Describe the various formulas used for burn resuscitation and the techniques required to initiate and monitor fluid resuscitation. (p. 503)

8. Discuss the use of pharmacological agents for the management of pain associated with burn trauma. (p. 505)

9. Describe the three types of airway injuries:
   A. Carbon monoxide poisoning (p. 507)
   B. Inhalation injury above the glottis (p. 508)
   C. Inhalation injury below the glottis (p. 508)

10. Understand why pediatric patients with circumferential burns to the thorax require special ventilatory considerations. (p. 509)

11. Discuss the basic assessment and management findings for the following inhalation injuries:
    A. Carbon monoxide (p. 507)
    B. Supraglottic inhalation injury (p. 508)
    C. Subglottic inhalation injury (p. 508)

12. Describe the anticipated signs and symptoms as well as management for the following burns:
    A. Eyes (p. 509)
    B. Ears (p. 509)
    C. Hands (p. 509)
    D. Feet (p. 510)
    E. Genitalia and perineum (p. 510)

13. Describe the specific assessment, management, and prognosis of burn patients with the following mechanisms of injury:
    A. Thermal burns (p. 490)
    B. Chemical burns to the eyes (p. 509)
    C. Electrical burns (p. 510)
    D. Lightning strikes (p. 511)
    E. Chemical burns (p. 513)
    F. Radiation exposure (p. 516)

14. Discuss the importance for assessing the concurrent signs of trauma in the burn patient. (p. 517)

15. Define the American Burn Association criteria/guidelines for patients requiring transport/treatment at a designated burn center. (p. 518)

16. Decide the proper mode of transportation for a burn patient to a designated burn center. (p. 519)

17. Discuss potential complications that the critical care paramedic should be cognizant of while transporting the burn patient. (p. 519)

Key Terms

Case Study

Cyclone Volunteer Fire Department has just responded to its second grass fire of the day. This time of year the grass is so dry, some say it does not ignite—it detonates! Two firefighters are in a brush truck in a rolling and pumping mode with one person driving and the other on back putting water on the fire. The fire has already consumed nearly 100 acres and the wind is picking up making things worse. Suddenly, the wind changes directions and the fire starts to move toward the brush truck. Instinctively, the driver starts to move away. However, he does not see an old water well and drops the truck's wheel into the well. After several attempts to move the truck, it appears hopeless without a winch. Meanwhile, both aggressively fight the fire and try to protect the truck. The fire moves quickly and, within a few seconds, the truck is surrounded by a wall of fire and the truck catches fire. The firefighters suffer burns yet are able to jump clear of the truck. Additional units notice the emergency and call for help and an ambulance.

Other vehicles arrive and begin to administer emergency care. The driver of the truck has only some first- and second-degree burns of the face and arms. His clothing is removed. His airway is patent and he appears well. The other firefighter, a 19-year-old male, is much more seriously injured. His clothing caught fire and had to be extinguished before rescuers could approach.

The patient is in intense pain. He is covered in sterile sheets while first responders administer 100% oxygen. The ambulance arrives and the patient is emergently transferred to the local community hospital emergency department (ED). There, the emergency physician calls the local general surgeon to assist. The patient has first- and second-degree burns to the face and neck. He has second-degree burns across the chest and back with several areas of third-degree burns. There are first- and second-degree burns on the arms. The lower extremities and pelvic region are unaffected.

Two wide-bore IVs of lactated Ringer's are established. The emergency physician orders titrated doses of fentanyl and promethazine (Phenergan) IV. The patient is very anxious and a 2.0-mg dose of midazolam (Versed) is administered IV. The patient's burns are estimated at 35% TBSA. The patient is very anxious and his airway is swelling as evidenced by increasing stridor. The emergency physician performs rapid-sequence intubation with additional midazolam, fentanyl, and succinylcholine. A 7.5-mm endotracheal tube is placed. Oxygen saturation improves and end-tidal CO_2 monitoring ensures proper tube placement. The initial vent settings are a V_t of 500 mL, rate of 14, and FiO_2 of 1.0. A blood gas 15 minutes later reveals a pH of 7.30, PO_2 of 200 mmHg, and PCO_2 of 35 mmHg. Following this, the rate is increased to 16 and the FiO_2 decreased to 0.65. The patient will require burn center care and the surgeon begins the transfer process. Additional lab and X-ray studies are ordered while the ED staff await the critical care transport team. Because he is now stable, the patient will be transferred by ground ambulance.

The critical care team arrives, and assesses the patient, and processes the paperwork. The patient remains stable. Vecuronium (Norcuron) has been administered for continued paralysis. The resultant lab studies are as expected. Additional fentanyl has been administered. The patient is packaged for transport.

Once in the ambulance, care continues. The estimated transport time is approximately 70 minutes. About 25 minutes into the trip, the patient's oxygen saturation starts to fall and $ETCO_2$ starts to rise. First, the attending critical care paramedic ensures that the ET tube is properly placed and the ventilator is working properly. He increases the FiO_2 to 1.0. No improvement is noted. He then increases the rate to 20. Again, no change noted and the SpO_2 continues to fall. He reassesses the patient and finds the skin of the chest has tightened significantly with fluid resuscitation. He takes a #10 scalpel and performs a bilateral chest escharotomy. The tissue spreads wide open behind the blade exposing the subcutaneous fat. Immediately the patient's SpO_2 increases to 100% and the $ETCO_2$ falls to 35 mmHg.

The patient is safely delivered to the burn center. He is admitted and has a stormy and prolonged course. He is discharged to a burn rehab facility closer to home some 55 days post-injury. He still faces years of skin grafts and surgery—but vows to return to firefighting.

INTRODUCTION

The quality of care during the first hours after a burn injury can have a major impact on long-term outcome. Yet most initial burn care is provided outside of the burn center environment. Burns are usually associated with a very dramatic clinical presentation. While the obvious cutaneous manifestations of burns are frequently quite impressive, the critical care paramedic cannot lose sight of the fact that these patients may have associated pathology that is of greater risk to life and limb than the burn is initially. Only after performance of a comprehensive trauma assessment should the critical care paramedic focus attention on the burn injury itself. It is a fact that initial management at the scene and during transport are both prime determinants of survival. Inappropriately assessed patients, inadequate fluid resuscitation, and a delay in aggressive airway management for patients with inhalation injury all significantly contribute to the increase in mortality. In addition, the critical care paramedic also must be aware of the unique metabolic and cardiovascular problems that accompany burn injuries. These associated factors will have important implications especially with respect to transport.

Therefore, it is important that the burn patient receive proper management in the early hours after injury. This chapter will prepare the critical care paramedic for the unique challenges he will face when caring for and transporting the critically burned patient.

EPIDEMIOLOGY

Despite the fact that burn injuries in the United States and other developed countries have been steadily declining for several decades, it still ranks as the fourth leading cause of trauma deaths overall (all age groups) and the second leading cause of death in children under the age of 12 years. Burn deaths are preceded only by incidents involving motor vehicles, penetrating trauma, and falls. Each year, in the United States, an estimated 1.25 to 2 million Americans are treated for burns and 50,000 are hospitalized. Approximately 3% to 5% of these burns are considered life threatening. The types of burns usually follow a predictable pattern usually associated with the age of the group involved (adults, 12 deaths per 1 million population; children, 39 deaths per 1 million population). For instance, scalds from hot liquids are more often found in toddlers, whereas flame burns are most frequently seen in the older child. Industrial burns from liquids or caustic agents are most common in adults. Most (approximately 68%) significant burns occur in the home; most of the remainder (approximately 24%) occur in industry. People at greatest risk for serious burns include the very young, the elderly, and the infirm. These groups make up the majority of the injured, and members of these groups are approximately five times more likely to die from burns than other groups. Also, those who are exposed to occupational sources of combustion and chemicals are at higher risk of burn injury than the general population. Some examples of high-risk occupations include firefighters, metal smelter workers, and chemical workers.

Much of the national decline in burn injuries/mortality can be attributed to improved building codes, safer construction techniques/materials, and the use of early warning devices such as smoke and heat detectors. A smaller, but still important aspect in this reduction is the growing emphasis on injury prevention and public education campaigns aimed primarily at school-aged children. Several relatively inexpensive "canned" injury prevention programs are currently available through organizations such as the **National Fire Protection Association (NFPA) "Risk Watch" program,** which targets kindergartners through eighth graders.

Burn prevention does not have to be expensive or labor intensive, it is primarily common sense and generally carried out or taught by role models such as parents, grandparents, older siblings, or professionals such as firefighters. Examples of simple and inexpensive measures that have helped prevent burns include teaching good fire safety behaviors, keeping cigarette lighters and matches out of reach of children, and reducing household hot-water temperatures to below scalding levels. Half of all tap-water burns occur in children under the age of 5 years old. Merely adjusting the hot-water temperature to below 130° F (54.4° C) can prevent most scalding burns.

Associated injuries account for a significant part of the mortality and morbidity of thermal injuries. Inhalation injuries are present in 20% to 50% of the patients admitted to burn centers and 60% to 70% of the patients who die in burn centers. Chemical injury to the lung tissue and toxic by-products of combustion are both prime contributors to the pulmonary pathology of burn injuries.

The prehospital care of a burn injury has a significant impact on subsequent morbidity and mortality.

The extremes of age (over 50 years and under 2 years) also contribute to the morbidity and mortality rates. This patient population cannot combat the effects of critical burns because of factors such as underlying medical problems, reduced vital organ function, decreased resistance to infection, and the age and condition of their integumentary system. To give you an idea of the impact age plays on mortality in this age group, you can use this simple formula:

$$\text{Patient's age (in years)} + \text{TBSA\% burned} = \text{Probability of mortality}$$

where TBSA stands for *total body surface area.*

TYPES AND EFFECTS OF BURNS

Always look for associated trauma when evaluating a burn patient.

Burn injuries can subject a patient to a variety of complications including severe fluid loss, infection, hypothermia, and organ failure. Burns can be caused by several mechanisms of injury (MOI) including thermal, electrical, chemical, and radiation energies. The critical care paramedic must have the ability to understand the pathophysiology of the various MOIs that cause burns to the skin. By having this understanding, the critical care paramedic will be able to determine the degree and area of burn which will help them in assessing the seriousness of the burn and guide care.

Burns result from disruption of proteins in the cell membrane (usually in the skin). The skin has at least four functions crucial to survival:

★ Protection from infection and injury
★ Prevention of loss of body fluid
★ Regulation of body temperature
★ Sensory contact with the environment

Soft-tissue burns have four common MOIs. While the local and systemic responses to burns are generally similar, the damage process differs with the various mechanisms. The degree of tissue destruction, and thus the depth of burn, correlates with both the temperature and the duration of exposure to the heat source and is influenced by three factors:

1. The intensity of the energy source
2. The duration of exposure to the energy source
3. The conductance of the tissue exposed

The physiological impact of the burn varies with both the extent of the burn (TBSA of second- and third-degree burns involved) and its depth. We will look at each mechanism of burn injury in more detail in the next sections.

THERMAL BURNS

From a pure physics standpoint, heat is the energy of molecules in motion. The greater the heat, the greater the molecular motion. All objects not at absolute zero ($-273°$ C) generate heat. Thus, the greater the movement of molecules within an object, the greater the temperature. As the temperature increases, objects can change their physical form. Objects can change from a solid, to a liquid, to a gas at various temperatures (depending on the nature of the chemical involved). These changes can result in expansion of an object (as seen in steel), combining with other substances (as seen with gasoline and oxygen), or the actual nature of matter may change (as seen when water turns into ice or steam or an egg changes its nature as the proteins break down, called denaturing, because of heat, which is why cooked eggs have a rubbery consistency).

Similar changes also take place in burned tissue. As the molecular speed increases, the cell components, especially membranes and proteins, begin to break down just like the egg in a frying pan. The result of exposure to extreme heat is progressive injury and ultimately cell death. The extent of burn injury relates to the amount of heat that is actually transferred to the patient's skin. The amount of that heat energy in turn depends on three components of the burning agent:

1. Its temperature
2. The concentration of the heat energy it possesses
3. The length of time it's in contact with the patient's skin

Obviously, the greater the temperature of an agent, the greater the potential for damage. However, it is also important to consider the amount of heat energy possessed by the object or substance. Receiving a blast of heated air from an oven at 350° F is much less damaging than contact with hot cooking oil at the same temperature. In general, water, oils, and other liquids have fairly high heat energy content. This content is roughly related to the density of the material. In a similar fashion, solids also usually have high heat content. Gases, on the other hand, usually have less capacity to hold heat owing to their less dense nature.

Duration of exposure to the heat source is also obviously important in determining the severity of a burn. A patient's momentary contact with hot oil would result in less damage than if the oil were poured into his or her shoe.

A burn is a progressive process, similar to a "bull's-eye" with each ring representing a different zone of intensity. The greater the heat energy transmitted to the body, the deeper (more intense) the wound. Initially, the burn damages the epidermis by the increase in temperature. As contact with the substance continues, heat energy penetrates further and deeper into the body tissue. Thus, a burn may involve the epidermis, dermis, and subcutaneous tissue as well as muscles, bone, and other internal tissue.

At the level of local tissues, thermal burns cause a number of effects that are collectively referred to as **Jackson's theory of thermal wounds.** This theory helps us understand the physical effects of high heat and helps explain a number of clinical effects. When a burn occurs, the central area of the burn wound, that is, the skin nearest the heat source, typically suffers the most profound effect or changes. The cell membranes rupture and are destroyed, blood coagulates, and structural proteins denature (coagulation necrosis). This most damaged area is called the **zone of coagulation.**

Jackson's theory of thermal wounds *a zone theory that reflects the effects of high heat on human tissue (zone of coagulation, stasis, and hyperemia).*

zone of coagulation *area of burn where cell membranes rupture and are destroyed, blood coagulates, and structural proteins denature (coagulation necrosis).*

Zone of hyperemia

Zone of stasis

Zone of coagulation

Epidermis

Dermis

Subcutaneous tissue

If the zone of coagulation penetrates the dermis, the resulting injury is termed a full-thickness or third-degree burn.

Extending peripherally from the zone of coagulation is a labile area of injured cells with decreased blood flow, which under ideal circumstances may survive, but which more often than not undergo necrosis in the ensuing 24 to 48 hours post-burn. This zone is called the **zone of stasis.**

Lying farther peripherally is an area where inflammation and changes in blood flow are limited. This area will typically recover in 7 to 10 days post-burn. This area is called the **zone of hyperemia** and accounts for the redness (called erythema) that is associated with some burns. (See Figure 18-1 ■.)

The larger the burn, the more profound the pathologic effects on the body as a whole. In general, these effects are important in any burn that covers more than approximately 20% to 25% TBSA of the patient. To be able to understand these effects and the resulting burn shock, we must look at the progression of burns beyond the zones described earlier.

The body's response to burns occurs over time and can be classified into four stages. The first stage occurs immediately following the burn and is called the **emergent phase.** This is the body's initial reaction to the burn. This phase includes a pain response as well as the systemic effects of the body dumping massive amounts of catecholamines into the blood in response to not only the pain but also to the physical and emotional stresses associated with being burned. It is during this stage that the patient will likely present with tachycardia, tachypnea, mild hypertension, and anxiety.

The next phase is called the **fluid shift phase** and follows the initial phase. The fluid shift phase can last for up to 18 to 24 hours. The fluid shift phase begins shortly after the burn and reaches its peak in 6 to 8 hours. Because of this the critical care paramedic is very likely to see this phase in the prehospital setting as well as in the ED or during interfacility transports. This is the phase in which the damaged cells begin to release agents that initiate the acute inflammatory response in the body. The basic mechanics are always the same with regard to the inflammatory response: (1) Blood flow to the injured site increases due to the contraction and dilation of the vessels; (2) an increase in vascular, specifically capillary, permeability occurs so that (3) white blood cells and plasma proteins can move from the capillaries into the tissues by crossing the permeable capillary walls to begin destroying the invaders and begin the healing process. The chief activator of the inflammatory process is the mast cells.

Mast cells resemble bags of granules. They are not blood cells but live in the connective tissues just outside the blood vessels. The inflammatory process is activated by the mast cells in two ways or functions: degranulation and synthesis. Degranulation is what the mast cells do when activated. The cells empty granules from their interior into the extracellular environment. Degranulation can occur as a result of physical injury, such as a burn; chemical agents, such as toxins; or through immunological and direct processes such as allergic reactions that release IgE antibodies or actual activation of the complement components.

zone of stasis *labile area of injured cells with decreased blood flow where tissue can undergo necrosis in the 24–48 hours post-burn.*

zone of hyperemia *area of burn where inflammation and changes in blood flow are limited.*

emergent phase *the initial phase immediately following the burn; includes pain response and the systemic effects of massive catecholamine release, as well as the physical and emotional stresses associated with being burned.*

fluid shift phase *phase in which fluid movement occurs; begins shortly after the burn, reaches a peak in 6–8 hours, and can last for up to 18–24 hours.*

During degranulation the various biochemical agents in the mast cell granules are released. These include the vasoactive amines and certain chemotactic factors. Vasoactive amines cause the constriction of the smooth muscle of large vessel walls and the dilation of the post-capillary sphincter, which results in increased blood flow to the injury site. The primary amine is histamine. In addition, basophils, which are a type of white blood cell (very similar to mast cells), also release histamine, with the same effects as previously described. Also at the same time, serotonin is released by the platelets. Serotonin can have an effect on both vasoconstriction and vasodilation, which may effect blood flow to the site of injury.

Chemotactic factors are another consequence realized by mast cell degranulation. Chemotactic factors are chemicals that attract white blood cells to the site of inflammation. This attraction is called *chemotaxis*. Once stimulated, mast cells also synthesize two substances that have very important roles in the inflammatory process: leukotrienes and prostaglandins. Leukotrienes, also known as slow-reacting substances of anaphylaxis (SRS-A), act very similar to histamine, that is, they vasoconstrict, increasing capillary permeability and chemotaxis. They are also important in later stages of inflammation because they promote slower and longer lasting effects than histamines. Prostaglandins, like leukotrienes, cause increased vasoconstriction and capillary permeability and chemotaxis. Prostaglandins are also the substances that cause pain and help control the inflammation by suppressing the release of histamine and lysosomal enzymes for some white cells.

Other responses are also seen such as systemic responses, chronic inflammatory responses, and local inflammatory responses. So how does this affect the burn patient? When you put it all together, this is what it looks like: The inflammatory mechanisms increase blood flow to the capillaries that surround the injured area, thus increasing the permeability of the capillaries to fluid. This increased capillary permeability results in the loss of proteins (hypoproteinemia), which aggravates edema in the nonburned tissues due to a large fluid shift away from the *intravascular space* into the *extravascular space* (massive tissue edema). This insensible fluid loss from the burn wound increases the basal metabolic rate and, along with the fluid shift, leads to hypovolemia. Note that the capillaries leak fluids such as water, electrolytes, and dissolved proteins, but not blood cells. Blood loss from burns not associated with other trauma is typically minimal and very rarely requires that blood be administered to the burn patient. The exception would be if the patient had some underlying condition which caused them to be anemic requiring blood replacement in conjunction with treatment of the burn injury.

The next phase is called the **hypermetabolic phase.** This phase may last from days to weeks depending on the severity of the burn injury. In this phase the body has a large increase in demands for nutrients as it begins the long process of healing. After time this phase evolves into the **resolution phase,** in which scar tissue is laid down and remodeled, and the burn patient begins the long road to rehabilitation. Nutrition is extremely important in burn rehabilitation. During the healing phase, burn patients can require a tremendous number of calories. While nutrition is usually not a major concern during interhospital transport, it is important. In many instances, burn patients will be receiving their nutrition intravenously (total parenteral nutrition). With long transports critical care paramedics may need to assure that such therapy be maintained. (See Figure 18-2 ■.)

The critical care paramedic should also realize that improper wound care and resuscitation may lead to extensive injury, permanent disability, and increased mortality and morbidity rates. By simply following the standard of care, potential complications can be kept to a minimum. Remember, the likelihood of survival depends on optimizing resuscitation; improper fluid management (either underhydration or overhydration) and hypothermia can actually worsen the burn injury by extending the zone of stasis and causing conversion into the zone of coagulation.

In addition to the complications mentioned, the burn patient may experience a variety of other physiological responses to burn injuries that can compromise patient outcome. With the decrease in circulating plasma comes an increase in hematocrit. This increased hematocrit level can lead to hemoglobinuria, when the hemoglobin is filtered through the kidneys, and can contribute to renal failure. In addition, increased peripheral vascular resistance leads to a decrease in venous return to the heart, decreased cardiac output, impaired tissue perfusion, and a decrease in renal perfusion, which can also contribute to renal failure.

A decrease in splanchnic blood flow occurs, which increases the occurrence of mucosal hemorrhages in the stomach and duodenum. There may also be an increased risk for sepsis from bacterial translocation owing to diminished mucosal barrier function in the intestine. Patients with burns of greater than 20% TBSA can also experience a dynamic ileus, which can be of special concern when transporting by air at high altitudes.

hypermetabolic phase *the healing phase of a burn; may last from days to weeks depending on the severity of the injury.*

resolution phase *scar tissue is laid down and remodeled, allowing rehabilitation to begin.*

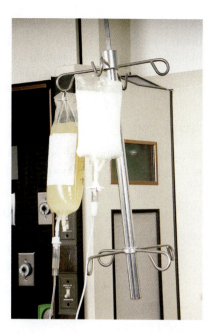

Burn patients also have decreased immune responses, which greatly increases the risk of infection. This requires the critical care paramedic to take some extra precautions to prevent further injury to the burn victim through exposure to contaminated environments. Some of these precautions include the use of dry sterile sheets (one under the patient and one covering the patient) and blankets added over the sterile sheets as needed. Avoid the use of wet dressings (remove if already in place) because they provide a direct pathway for bacteria. An additional measure that may also help decrease the contamination of the burn injury is reverse isolation by wearing gowns, gloves, and masks while caring for the patient.

INITIAL ASSESSMENT AND MANAGEMENT

The initial assessment of the burn patient is no different than with any other trauma patient. Once you have determined that the scene is safe for you to enter, you should follow a systematic approach giving particular attention to life-threatening and potentially life-threatening conditions first.

The ABCDE method is an easy-to-use approach:

★ **A**irway maintenance with cervical spine protection
★ **B**reathing and ventilation
★ **C**irculation with bleeding control
★ **D**isability (assess neurologic deficits)
★ **E**xpose/Examine (completely undress the patient, but protect from hypothermia)

AIRWAY

The airway should be your first priority and assessed immediately. A compromised airway may be controlled by:

★ Chin lift
★ Jaw thrust
★ Insertion of an oropharygeal or nasopharyngeal airway in patients with a decreased level of consciousness (LOC)
★ Assessment of the need for endotracheal intubation

Have a low threshold for intubating the burn patient with possible airway burns.

As with any other trauma patient it is important to protect the integrity of the cervical spine before doing anything that will cause flexion or extension of the neck. In-line manual cervical immobilization is performed during the initial assessment, in general, and during endotracheal intubation, in particular, for those patients in whom cervical spine injury is suspected by the mechanism of injury or for those with altered mental states.

BREATHING AND VENTILATION

Adequate ventilation requires adequate functioning of the lungs, chest wall, and diaphragm. Each of these must be evaluated as part of the initial assessment:

★ Verify breath sounds (bilaterally) by auscultation of the chest.

★ Assess adequacy (rate and depth) of respirations.

★ Administer high concentrations (100%) of oxygen via appropriate device (this not only treats hypoxia but helps to wash out CO_2).

★ Monitor closely any circumferential full-thickness burns of the trunk because such burns may impair ventilation.

CIRCULATION

Assessment of the adequacy of circulation includes evaluation of blood pressure, pulse rate, and skin color (of unburned skin). Intravenous cannulation is performed by inserting two large-bore catheters (in unburned skin, if possible) to begin fluid administration. It may be necessary to use a Doppler to determine whether there is a circulation deficit in a circumferentially burned extremity. Physical indicators of a circulation deficit include decreased sensation, diminished distal pulses, and decreased capillary refill time. The circulation in a limb with full-thickness circumferential burns may be impaired as a result of subeschar edema formation.

DISABILITY AND NEUROLOGIC DEFICIT

Typically, most burn patients present initially awake, alert, and oriented. If they don't, the critical care paramedic should consider associated injuries [i.e., motor vehicle collisions (MVCs), jumped from a building on fire to save themselves], carbon monoxide (CO) poisoning, substance abuse (i.e., ETOH), hypoxia, or preexisting medical conditions, particularly acute myocardial infarction (AMI) or patients at risk for AMI. Use the Glasgow Coma Score (GCS) to assess the patient's LOC:

★ Eye opening

★ Verbal response

★ Motor response

The GCS is the most reliable universally accepted method of documenting trends in a patient's level of consciousness. Each category should be documented based on the patient's best response for each of the criteria (for example, E3, V4, M5). The critical care paramedic should be very familiar with the individual scoring components of the GCS and should assess and document the GCS with each reassessment of the patient.

EXAMINE/EXPOSURE

All clothing should be removed to facilitate a complete patient assessment. In addition, all jewelry should be removed to prevent potential complications (impaired circulation due to swelling). Evaporative heat loss mechanisms and hypermetabolic states of burn patients leave them at high risk of hypothermia, therefore, maintaining the patient's temperature is a priority. Once you have completed your examination, the patient should be covered with dry sterile sheets and blankets to prevent hypothermia. Another means that will assist you with the prevention of hypothermia is to increase the temperature of the environment (i.e., ED room,

MICU). You can use the same rule that is used for neonates: "If you aren't sweating, it ain't warm enough."

In addition, intravenous fluids should be warmed (37°–40° C) for use during resuscitation.

DETAILED EXAM

As with any critically injured trauma patient, addressing the ABCDEs and managing any life threats found should be the first priority in the care of the burn patient. Once this is complete and proper resuscitative efforts are well established, more detailed exam and patient history can be addressed.

Typically this detailed exam consists of reevaluation of the initial assessment and then a detailed head-to-toe examination of the patient. The burn is often the most obvious injury, but other serious and even life-threatening injuries may be present. A complete detailed exam is necessary to ensure that all injuries and preexisting diseases are identified and appropriately managed to minimize any potential complications. A complete neurologic exam should be performed, and any radiologic and laboratory studies obtained, if time allows. (Do not delay treatment/transportation to obtain these.)

PATIENT HISTORY

Every effort should be made to obtain as much information as possible regarding the circumstances surrounding the incident. Initial management as well as definitive care is dictated by things such as MOI, duration, and severity of the injury. The following information about the MOI must be obtained:

Injuries Caused by Flames

★ How did the burn occur?

★ Did the burn occur inside or outside?

★ Did the clothes catch on fire?

★ How long did it take to extinguish the flames?

★ How were the flames extinguished?

★ Was gasoline or another fuel involved?

★ Was there an explosion?

★ Did the patient get thrown?

★ Was there a house fire?

★ Was the patient found inside a smoke-filled room?

★ How did the patient escape?

★ If the patient jumped out of a window, from what floor?

★ Were others killed at the incident?

★ Was the patient unconscious at the scene?

★ Was there a motor vehicle crash?

★ How badly was the patient's vehicle damaged?

★ Was there a vehicle fire?

★ Is there any associated trauma?

★ Are the reported circumstances of the injury consistent with the burn characteristics (i.e., is abuse a possibility)?

Scald

★ How did the burn occur?

★ What was the temperature of the liquid?

★ What was the liquid? (Oil has more heat content than H_2O.)

★ How much liquid was involved?

★ What was the water heater set at?

★ Was the patient wearing clothes?

★ How quickly were the patient's clothes removed? (the longer it takes to remove the clothes, the greater the burning)

★ Was the burned area cooled?

★ Who was with the patient when the burn took place?

★ How quickly was care sought?

★ Where did the burn occur (e.g., bathtub, sink)?

★ Are the reported circumstances of the injury consistent with the burn characteristics (i.e., is abuse a possibility)?

Chemical

★ What was the agent?

★ How did the exposure occur?

★ What was the duration of contact?

★ What decontamination occurred? (Do not use bathtub full of H_2O; it will spread the agent and the burn.)

★ Is there a Material Safety Data Sheet (MSDS)? (Check to see if there is a vapor potential.)

★ Was there an explosion?

Electrical

★ What kind of electricity was involved? (AC vs. DC, high vs. low voltage)

★ What was the duration of contact?

★ Was the patient thrown or did he/she fall (possible associated trauma, especially spinal)?

★ What was the estimated voltage (higher voltage = increased risk of other injury)?

★ Was there loss of consciousness?

★ Was CPR or defibrillation administered at the scene?

MEDICAL HISTORY TAKING

Things to Consider

★ The patient's age, because extremes of ages have different responses, needs, and considerations

★ Are there any preexisting diseases or associated illnesses (e.g., diabetes, HTN, cardiac or renal disease, seizure disorders)?

★ Medications/alcohol/illegal drugs (these may mask signs and symptoms, is there a possibility of ETOH withdrawal?)

★ Allergies

★ Tetanus immunization history (Burns are the leading cause of tetanus in the United States.)

An Easy-to-Remember Mnemonic for obtaining a SAMPLE history

★ **S** Signs and symptoms

★ **A** Allergies

★ **M** Medications

★ **P** Pertinent past history

★ **L** Last oral intake

★ **E** Events/environment related to the injury

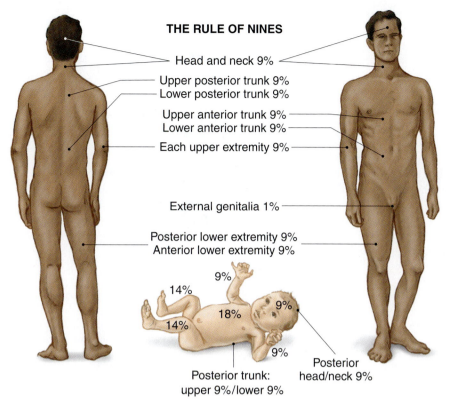

THE RULE OF NINES

Head and neck 9%

Upper posterior trunk 9%
Lower posterior trunk 9%

Upper anterior trunk 9%
Lower anterior trunk 9%

Each upper extremity 9%

External genitalia 1%

Posterior lower extremity 9%
Anterior lower extremity 9%

9%

14%

18%

14%

9%

9%

Posterior head/neck 9%

Posterior trunk:
upper 9%/lower 9%

■ Figure 18-3   The rule of nines.

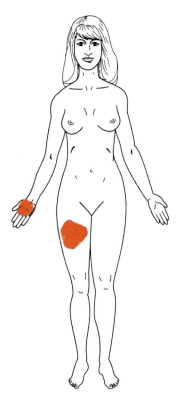

■ **Figure 18-4**   Using the rule of palms, the surface of the patient's palm represents approximately 1 percent of TBSA and is helpful in estimating the area of small burns.

Performing the Detailed "Head-to-Toe" Exam

★ Head/face (maxillofacial)

★ Neck/cervical spine

★ Chest

★ Abdomen

★ Perineum/genitalia

★ Back/spine (including the buttocks)

★ Extremities (musculoskeletal)

★ Vascular

★ Neurologic

As a general rule, the severity of a burn injury is usually determined based on the extent of **total body surface area (TBSA)** involved and the depth of the burn. However, other factors such as extremes of age, preexisting medical conditions, associated trauma, and complications associated with critical areas of the body such as the hands, face, and genitalia must also be considered when determining the burn severity. Remember only partial-thickness (second-degree) and full-thickness (third-degree) burns are used when calculating TBSA.

When determining the severity of a burn, the critical care paramedic must calculate the percentage of TBSA involved. This can be accomplished by using one of several methods. The first and most widely used is the "rule of nines." The **rule of nines** is based on the fact that in the adult body each anatomical region represents approximately 9%, or a multiple thereof, of the TBSA. (See Figure 18-3 ■.) Another method that works particularly well with scattered burns is called the **rule of palms (palmar method)** or "walking out the burn." (See Figure 18-4 ■.) This method is based on the fact that the size of a patient's palm represents approximately 1% of the patient's TBSA. The last

total body surface area (TBSA)   *the total extent of body surface area by the burn. TBSA, specific locations, and depth combine to determine severity of the injury.*

rule of nines   *anatomic regions of the body are assigned percentage designations that represent approximately 9 percent (or multiples thereof); the sum is TBSA.*

rule of palms (palmar method)   *method of measuring the area of a burn based upon the size of a patient's own palm (approximately 1 percent of TBSA).*

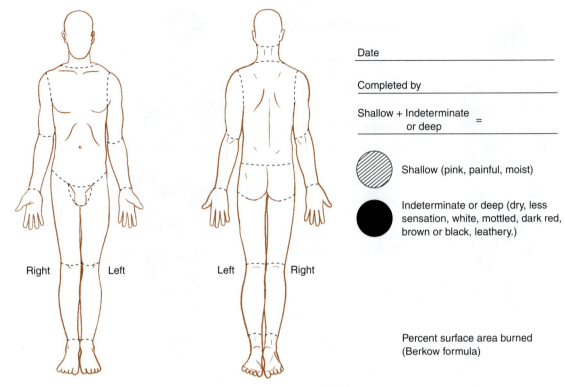

Date _____

Completed by _____

Shallow + Indeterminate
      or deep = _____

⬚ Shallow (pink, painful, moist)

⬤ Indeterminate or deep (dry, less
sensation, white, mottled, dark red,
brown or black, leathery.)

Percent surface area burned
(Berkow formula)

Area	1 year	1-4 years	5-9 years	10-14 years	Y>15 years	Adult	Shallow	Indeterminate or deep
Head	19	17	13	11	9	7		
Neck	2	2	2	2	2	2		
Ant. trunk	13	13	13	13	13	13		
Post. trunk	13	13	13	13	13	13		
R. buttock	2.5	2.5	2.5	2.5	2.5	2.5		
L. Buttock	2.5	2.5	2.5	2.5	2.5	2.5		
Genitalia	1	1	1	1	1	1		
R.U. arm	4	4	4	4	4	4		
L.U. arm	4	4	4	4	4	4		
R.L. arm	3	3	3	3	3	3		
L.L. arm	3	3	3	3	3	3		
R. hand	2.5	2.5	2.5	2.5	2.5	2.5		
L. hand	2.5	2.5	2.5	2.5	2.5	2.5		
R. thigh	5.5	6.5	8	8.5	9	9.5		
L. thigh	5.5	6.5	8	8.5	9	9.5		
R. leg	5	5	5.5	6	6.5	7		
L. leg	5	5	3.5	6	6.5	7		
R. foot	3.5	3.5	3.5	3.5	3.5	3.5		
L. foot	3.5	3.5	3.5	3.5	3.5	3.5		
Total								

■ **Figure 18-5** Lund and Browder chart.

Lund and Browder method *accurate method of determining the area of a burn; calculates TBSA while accounting for developmental (age) changes in percentage.*

method, which is the **Lund and Browder method,** is more commonly used in the hospital. (See Figure 18-5 ■.) This method is difficult to use in the prehospital environment because it takes more time to calculate but this method is the most accurate, especially in infants and children, because it allows for developmental changes in percentage of TBSA.

Determining the depth of burns is directly related to the amount of tissue that is damaged. Tissue damage due to burn injury is largely dependent on four major factors (see Figure 18-6 ■):

★ Temperature (of the burning agent)

★ Duration of contact (exposure)

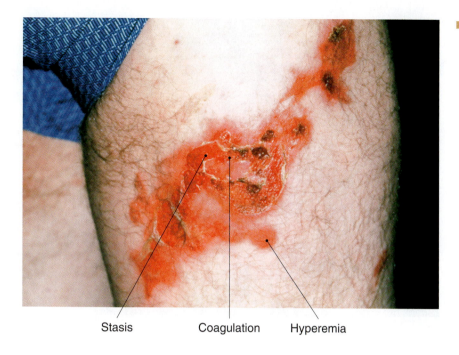

Stasis   Coagulation   Hyperemia

★ Thickness of the dermis (conductance of involved tissue)

★ Blood supply (typically, the better the supply, the less the depth of the burn)

The evaluation of burn injuries merely provides estimates because the full extent of the injury may not be apparent for several days. Burn injuries are typically classified into four categories:

Superficial Burns (First-Degree Burns) (See Figure 18-7 ■).

★ Injury involving only the epidermis

★ Characterized by red, inflamed skin that is painful to touch

★ Generally does not require prehospital interventions

★ Healing time is usually 5 days with no scarring

★ Typical cause is sun

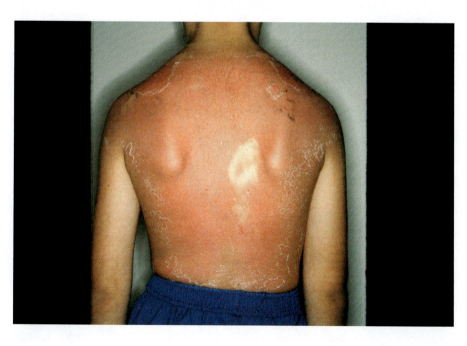

■ Figure 18-7   A superficial burn on the back of a male patient. *(Charles Stewart and Associates)*

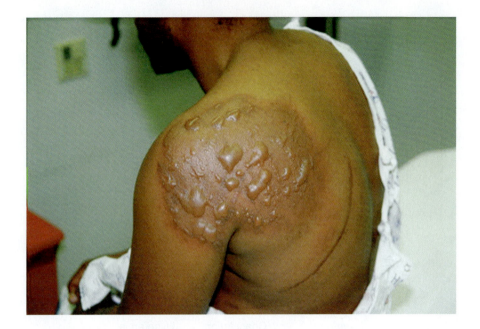

Figure 18-8 Partial-thickness burn. *(Edward T. Dickinson, MD)*

Partial-Thickness Burns (Second-Degree Burns) (See Figure 18-8 ■.)

★ Injury involving both the epidermis and dermis

★ Characterized by reddened areas, blisters, or open weeping wounds

★ Causes significant pain to the patient

★ Significant fluid loss occurs with subsequent hypovolemic shock

★ Healing time is usually 30 days with late hypertropic scarring and possibly contracture formation

Full-Thickness Burns (Third-Degree Burns) (See Figure 18-9 ■.)

★ Injury involving the epidermis, dermis, and the subcutaneous tissue (and possibly deeper)

★ Characterized by charred or leathery appearance

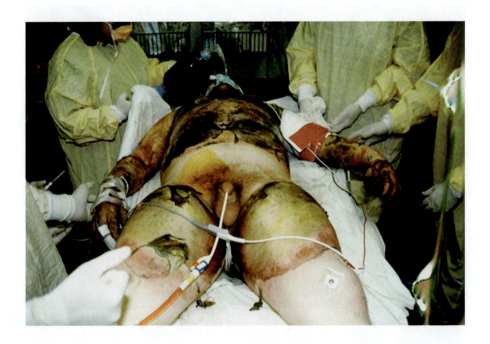

Figure 18-9 Full-thickness burn. *(Edward T. Dickinson, MD)*

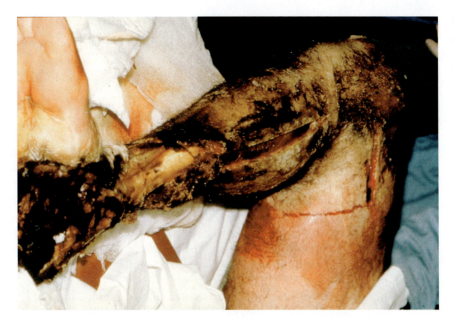

■ **Figure 18-10** Fourth-degree burn. A charring electrical burn covers the lacerated leg of an emergency room hospital patient. *(Roy Alson, MD, FACEP)*

★ Not painful (nerve endings are destroyed), but may have pain if associated with second-degree burns

★ No capillary refill to the burned area

★ Healing time is extensive because the area cannot regenerate and will require skin grafting to heal; scarring will be significant

Fourth-Degree Burns (See Figure 18-10 ■.)

★ Injury (full-thickness burn) that also penetrates the subcutaneous tissue, muscles, fascia, periosteum, or bone

★ Usually caused by incineration-type exposure and electrical burns in which the heat is sufficient to destroy tissues below the skin

MANAGEMENT AND FURTHER EVALUATION OF THE BURN PATIENT

As discussed earlier, with the exception of stopping the burning process, the management of the burn patient is essentially the same as any other trauma patient, that is, use the ABCDE method, addressing any life threats (i.e., other trauma, or abnormalities with the ABCs) first.

Once life-threatening and potentially life-threatening injuries have been addressed, specific treatments can be started based on the patient's needs. Some general guidelines that should be used on all burn patients include:

★ Don't become a victim, make sure the scene is secure.

★ Stop the burning process.

★ Remove all clothing and jewelry.

★ Estimate the extent of surface burns.

★ Identify points of contact on electrical burns paying special attention to areas such as hands, feet, and scalp (look carefully; hair can hide wounds).

★ Perform a detailed neurologic examination and document any trends.

★ Assess for any occult injuries, fractured or dislocated extremities, and any evidence that compartment syndrome is developing.

★ Start fluid resuscitation using the 4 mL/kg/%TBSA formula and constantly evaluate the patient's clinical response for the possible need to increase the fluid rates.

★ Insert a Foley catheter as soon as possible (in severe burns).

★ Perform 12-lead ECG and cardiac monitoring on any critical burn patient or patients who have experienced an electrical injury.

★ Protect the patient from hypothermia.

GENERAL TREATMENT CONSIDERATIONS

As with any critically ill or injured patient, airway management and ventilation are the priority. Assessing the airway of a burn patient is of particular concern, and management decisions may prove difficult for the critical care paramedic. A high index of suspicion should be used with burn patients who are thought to have a compromised airway (i.e., signs or symptoms of inhalation injury), and aggressive airway management should be started early to avoid the need for more invasive techniques such as a tracheostomy, which leads to a higher mortality/morbidity rate due to the inherent complications associated with the procedure. A good rule of thumb is "It is better to perform prophylactic intubation (early) than waiting until it becomes an emergency intubation (late)."

In critical patients the airway should be secured with an appropriate sized endotracheal tube (ETT). The decision to intubate or not should be based on the critical care paramedic's experience and the patient's clinical assessment. Although most schools of thought say "when in doubt intubate," there are basic guidelines to assist the critical care paramedic with determining whether to intubate a burn patient. (See Table 18–1.)

Table 18–1	Indications for Endotracheal Intubation

Findings to indicate the possible need for endotracheal intubation include:

Physical Findings

Obvious inhalation injury on physical exam

Airway obstruction imminent (progressive hoarseness and/or stridor)

Decreased LOC which impairs protective mechanisms (despite the cause)

Signs of carbonaceous sputum

Obvious facial burns

Singed facial or nasal hairs

Agitation (hypoxia)

Tachypnea, intercostal retractions

History

Unconsciousness

Exposure to noxious chemicals

Fire in an enclosed space

Hoarseness

Rales, rhonchi, diminished breath sounds

Naso- or oropharynx erythema

Inability to swallow

Other Considerations

Underlying medical conditions

Associated trauma

Extensive TBSA involvement

Extended transport time

Also, when evaluating the history of the event, be particularly cognizant of facts such as history of unconsciousness, noxious chemicals involvement, and injuries that occur in a closed space.

Intubating the burn patient may require the critical care paramedic to use various pharmacologic agents such as amnestics, sedatives, paralytics, and analgesics (rapid-sequence induction) to facilitate ETT placement. The provider must be thoroughly familiar with each agent's pharmacodynamics, particularly with paralytic agents such as succinylcholine, so the patient's condition is not further compromised by his actions.

Once the burn patient's airway has been secured with an ETT the tube's placement must be not only confirmed initially but monitored throughout transport to ensure tube vigilance. In addition to the standard methods of confirming tube placement that the critical care paramedic learned during initial training, there are several newer methods to confirm the placement of the ETT such as end-tidal CO_2 (ETCO$_2$) monitoring (capnography), which is rapidly becoming the "gold standard" and the esophageal detector device (EDD). Once placement is confirmed, continuous monitoring by means of capnography is the preferred method of avoiding potentially lethal consequences associated with inadvertent and unrecognized tube displacement.

In addition to ETT placement, the patient must be ventilated at an appropriate rate and administered 100% oxygen. Some burn patients will require the use of higher airway pressure (due to the effects of the inhalation injury) to provide adequate ventilatory support. The critical care paramedic must be familiar with making adjustment to advanced airway adjuncts such as PEEP valves, CPAP/BIPAP, and the advanced mechanisms and settings on mechanical ventilators such as peek airway pressures, I/E ratios, rates and volumes so that patient care can be optimized based on the clinical responses of the patient. (See Figure 18-11 ■.)

FLUID RESUSCITATION

Proper fluid management is critical to the survival of patients with extensive burn injuries, who will need aggressive fluid replacement to maintain some form of homeostasis. The goal of fluid resuscitation is to maintain an adequate amount of perfusion to the vital organs by ensuring adequate circulating volume while avoiding the complications associated with inadequate or excessive fluid therapy. Fluid resuscitation is monitored not by the amount of fluid that is administered but by maintaining an adequate amount of urine output (normal adult: 0.5–1.0 mL/kg/hr; normal child: 1.0 mL/kg/hr). The best method to monitor urine output is early placement of a Foley catheter. There are, however, general guidelines to fluid resuscitation in the critical burn patient. The standard for fluid administration rate most widely used is the **Parkland formula.** The Parkland formula

Fluid resuscitation is an important aspect of emergency burn care.

Parkland formula *widely used standard for fluid resuscitation (partial- and full-thickness burns); utilizes patient's weight, and percentage of TBSA involved. Represented in formula as: 4 mL × kg of body wt × TBSA%.*

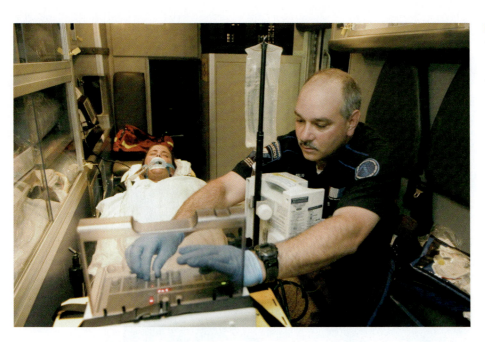

■ **Figure 18-11** Patient on transport ventilator. *(© Craig Jackson/In the Dark Photography)*

utilizes the patient's weight, percentage of TBSA involved (partial- and full-thickness burns only), and a standard fluid replacement amount. The actual formula is

$$4 \text{ mL} \times \text{kg of body wt} \times \text{TBSA\%}$$

The fluid should be a crystalloid solution such as the preferred Ringer's lactate (RL) or normal saline (NS). Half of this fluid is given to the patient during the first 8 hours post-burn injury (not from the time you transport the patient). This fluid is not given as a bolus but in an hourly rate, ideally via an infusion pump. Then the rate is reduced to achieve the administration of the rest of the calculated fluid during the next 16 hours. Again, this is only a guideline and should be adjusted based on patient's clinical responses.

RL should be started in burn patients of all age groups. Every effort should be made to administer warmed fluids to burn patients. Warmed fluids (38° C) are essential to avoid the complications of hypothermia. (See Figure 18-12 ■.) Glucose-containing solutions are not typically given to adult patients in the first 24 hours post-burn; early use of glucose may induce an unwanted, and dangerous, osmotic diuresis. However, in the pediatric patient, hypoglycemia may develop due to limited glycogen reserves; therefore, blood glucose levels must be monitored and maintenance rate infusions of RL with 5% dextrose should be included in resuscitation fluids.

Because pediatric patients have a greater surface area to body mass they typically require the administration of greater amounts of resuscitation fluids than adults do. In addition, pediatric patients have higher metabolic demands, especially with burns, which require the administration of solutions that contain glucose. Maintenance fluid requirements for the pediatric patient can be calculated as follows:

For the first 10 kg of body weight:	100 mL/kg over 24 hours
For the second 10 kg of body weight:	50 mL/kg over 24 hours
For each kilogram of weight above 20 kg:	20 mL/kg over 24 hours

Example: Initial fluid requirements for a child who weighs 33 kg and has sustained burns over 30% TBSA would be calculated as follows:

Resuscitation fluids:	$4 \text{ mL} \times 33 \text{ kg} \times 30\% = 3{,}960 \text{ mL of RL}$
Maintenance fluids:	$100 \text{ mL} \times 10 \text{ kg} = 1{,}000 \text{ mL}$
	$50 \text{ mL} \times 10 \text{ kg} = 500 \text{ mL}$
	$20 \text{ mL} \times 13 \text{ kg} = \underline{260 \text{ mL}}$
	Total 1,760 mL of D₅RL

■ **Figure 18-12** Thermal Angel IV warmer. *(Courtesy of Estill Medical Technologies, Inc.)*

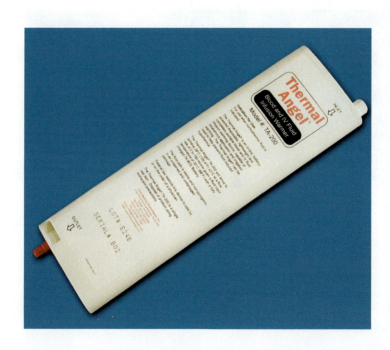

Total fluid requirements for 24 hours = 3,960 (resuscitative)
$$\underline{+\ 1{,}760}\ \text{(maintenance)}$$
5,720 mL (238.3 mL/hr)

There are several types of burn patients who will have a special fluid need beyond the standard requirements. Some of these patients are:

★ Patients with associated injuries

★ Patients with electrical injuries

★ Patients who sustain inhalation injuries

★ Patients in whom resuscitation is delayed

★ Patients with preexisting dehydration

★ Patients with very deep burns (i.e., fourth degree)

In addition, for some patients, the critical care paramedic must be cautious with fluid administration. Some of these patients are:

★ Pediatric patients

★ Elderly patients

★ Patients with preexisting cardiac disease

In addition to proper fluid administration, the critical care paramedic must be cognizant of the potential complications associated with transporting the critically burned patient. It should be noted that ALL fluid resuscitation should be managed via an infusion pump. As stated before, the amount of fluid administered is centered around the actual time of injury and not the time of transport. Therefore, the critical care paramedic must anticipate clinical situations that may dictate the need for additional treatment modalities prior to initiating transport. One example is the patient who is 3 hours post-burn injury and is behind 2 liters of fluid on your arrival. The anticipated transport time (ED to burn center) is approximately 1 hour. The critical care paramedic must "catch the patient up" on fluids by arrival at the burn center. By administering 2,000 mL of fluid in addition to the calculated resuscitation fluid rate, the patient's condition has a high probability of deterioration because of the complications that are associated with "catching up" on fluid during transport. One of the most critical situations the critical care paramedic must evaluate in a situation such as this is the potential for airway compromise (airway swelling and loss of landmarks), and she must also recognize the need for aggressive airway management (i.e., ETT placement) prior to transport.

PAIN MANAGEMENT

Pain management in the burn patient is probably one of the most challenging issues that the critical care paramedic will face. Proper doses of narcotic agents, such as morphine and fentanyl, are usually the medication of choice for analgesia. Several recent studies have shown that burn patients in the United States receive inadequate doses of analgesia in the prehospital and emergency department setting. In addition to analgesics, sedatives, such as benzodiazepines, are needed for procedural and background pain in patients who have experienced a significant burn injury. Combinations of drugs such as narcotics and benzodiazepines need to be used in high doses in patients undergoing special procedures such as wound debridement. The critical care paramedic must be cognizant of the potential side effects of these particular types of medications and dosages and be prepared to manage any complications that may arise.

Pain from the burn injury itself is related to the severity of the injury. Several methods of pain management are available to the critical care paramedic. The preferred analgesic agents for the management of acute burn injuries are the opiates fentanyl or morphine. Nitrous oxide can be useful—especially during procedures such as debridement. All medications, other than nitrous oxide, are best given by IV ONLY.

Burn patients need aggressive analgesia therapy—usually with intravenous opiates such as fentanyl or morphine.

WOUND CARE

The general approach to wound care is to prevent further contamination of the wound and its associated complications and to protect the patient from hypothermia. In burn injuries that are less than 10%

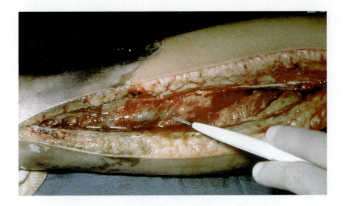

■ **Figure 18-13** Fasciotomy is required when tissue constriction caused by the burn injury adversely affects pulses or neurological function.

TBSA, it is acceptable to use wet sterile dressings on the injuries. Any burn injury greater than 10% should be covered with DRY STERILE dressings only. Do not use gels, ointments, shaving cream, and so on. Using these products will only complicate wound care at the burn center and cause the patient additional pain when they are removed. Wound debridement is not indicated in the first 24 hours post-burn injury and should not be done prior to transfer to the burn center. The use of antimicrobial agents is also not indicated. The use of wet dressings on large burns can cause evaporative heat loss leading to hypothermia and extension of the burn severity and therefore should be avoided. Note that many surgeons are advocating the use of white petroleum in the dressing of facial burns and CCPs may see this during interfacility transports. Consult with the burn center PRIOR to applying any substance to a burn.

Escharotomies (surgically incising into the eschar and surrounding tissues to relieve pressure) and fasciotomies (incising the fascia to to relieve pressures) are rarely indicated prior to transfer of a burn patient to a burn center. However, certain patients may require these procedures to allow for normal ventilation and peripheral perfusion (see Figure 18-13 ■):

★ Circumferential burns
★ Very deep burns
★ Delayed resuscitations
★ Cyanosis refractory to airway management
★ Deep tissue pain
★ Progressive decrease or absence of pulses (compartment syndrome)
★ Progressive paresthesias

These procedures are life/limb saving interventions and should be treated as such. As a general rule they should only be performed after consultation with the burn center and should be performed by the most qualified medical professional available at the time of transfer. In addition, the use of electric cautery is encouraged to minimize blood loss. (See Figure 18-14 ■.)

TETANUS IMMUNIZATION

Always determine a burn patient's tetanus immunization status.

The patient's tetanus status must be evaluated and prophylactic administration should follow the recommendations from the American College of Surgeons.

MANAGEMENT OF SPECIFIC INJURIES

After general treatment has begun, the critical care paramedic can focus on specific injuries and their treatment. The critical care paramedic must be vigilant in his assessment of these specific burn injuries so early, aggressive treatment can be started. In addition to the general management discussed earlier, we will now address some specific injuries and their treatments.

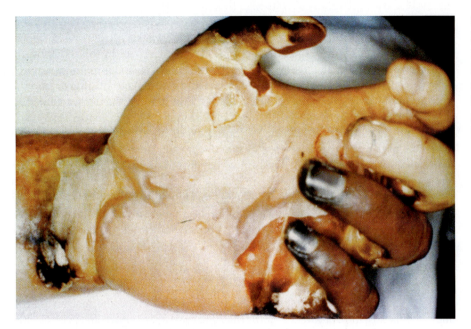

■ Figure 18-14 A person's hand covered with painful marks from an electrical burn. The skill of escharotomy and cautery may be needed in the management of this critical hand injury.

INHALATION INJURIES

By definition, an inhalation injury is an injury that is manifested by the pathology and dysfunction in the airways, lungs, and respiratory system that occurs during and up to 5 days after the burn injury (i.e., inhaling smoke and other products of incomplete combustion or toxic chemicals). According to the American Burn Association, inhalation injury is an important factor in determining the mortality of burn patients. Inhalation injuries are present in anywhere from 20% to 50% of patients who are admitted to burn centers and 60% to 70% of patients who die in burn centers. It cannot be emphasized enough that the critical care paramedic needs to use a high index of suspicion when assessing the burn patient who may have sustained an inhalation injury, and prophylactic intubation should be given a great deal of thought.

The ABA breaks down inhalation injuries into three categories:

★ Carbon monoxide poisoning
★ Inhalation injury above the glottis
★ Inhalation injury below the glottis

Carbon Monoxide Poisoning

As you already know, most fire deaths are caused by asphyxiation and/or carbon monoxide poisoning. It is not uncommon to find carboxyhemoglobin levels of 50% to 70% or more. Among patients who survive the fire itself, carbon monoxide poisoning may be the most immediate threat to life.

In addition to administering 100% oxygen, the carboxyhemoglobin level should be checked, whenever possible, especially in those patients who present with respiratory complaints and those with altered mental status. Dysfunction of hypoxia-sensitive organs, such as the brain, can occur with levels as low as 15% to 40%. Levels of 40% to 60% can cause obtundation and coma. Carboxyhemoglobin levels must be correlated with the clinical presentation of your patient. For example, levels as high as 5% to 10% have been found in patients who have no clinical signs and symptoms such as smokers and those exposed to heavy traffic. Administration of 100% oxygen should continue until the carboxyhemoglobin levels return to normal values.

When assessing the patient with CO poisoning, critical care paramedics must remember that the typical assessment findings taught in their initial training program may steer them down the wrong clinical pathway due to the false sense of security they may get from the lack of typical signs and symptoms present. For instance, a finding such as cherry red skin is actually an uncommon finding, occurring in less than 50% of patients with severe carbon monoxide hypoxemia. In fact, patients who have severe carbon monoxide hypoxemia may not exhibit any of the abnormal signs and symptoms one typically might expect in this situation. Typical signs such as cyanosis and tachypnea are not usually present because CO_2 removal is not affected. Another area that may give the critical care paramedic a false sense of security about his patient's clinical condition is arterial blood gases (ABGs). Even though the oxygen content of the blood is reduced, the amount of oxygen dissolved in the blood (PaO_2) is unaffected by carbon monoxide poisoning, making the ABG analysis normal with the exception of the carboxyhemoglobin level. Due to the variety and severity of symptoms associated with CO poisoning it is essential to measure carboxyhemoglobin levels in all patients suspected of having been exposed to carbon monoxide.

The critical care paramedic must not forget that the use of pulse oximetry is of little or no value when assessing the patient with potential CO poisoning or smoke inhalation and may give you a false sense of security (falsely high saturation) because of the affinity to hemoglobin that CO has versus oxygen (200 times greater).

Carbon monoxide poisoning can complicate any closed space burn injury.

Inhalation Injury above the Glottis

Because of the heat exchange abilities of the respiratory tract, most thermal burns to the airway are limited to the structures above the glottis (nasopharynx, oropharynx, and larynx), although chemical burns can also cause injury above the glottis. The heat exchange capabilities of the respiratory tract are so efficient that most of the heat is absorbed above the true vocal cords and this is where the majority of the damage will occur. In addition, any damage to the pharynx caused by heat can be severe enough to cause upper airway obstruction at any time during the resuscitation.

As mentioned earlier, unresuscitated or underresuscitated patients are of particular concern in this situation because the potential for airway swelling (supraglottic) may not present until fluid resuscitation has been under way for a while (i.e., during a long transport). This is one of those situations where aggressive airway management (i.e., prophylactic intubation) may be lifesaving.

Inhalation Injury below the Glottis

In contrast to injuries above the glottis, which can be thermal (most common) or chemical in nature, inhalation injuries occurring below the glottis are almost always chemical. Some exceptions to this rule are steam inhalation, aspiration of scalding liquids, and explosions occurring while a patient is breathing very high concentrations of oxygen or flammable gases under pressure. Smoke contains several chemicals that cause direct damage to the epithelium of the larger airways. Once the patient has been exposed to these chemicals (smoke) for a prolonged amount of time, especially if he has lost his protective airway reflexes (i.e., unconscious), the smaller airways and bronchi can be affected.

Some of the pathophysiological changes that are usually associated with lower airway injuries (i.e., injuries below the glottis) are:

★ Increased blood flow (promotes edema formation)
★ Edema
★ Hypersecretion
★ Bronchospasms
★ Impaired immune defenses
★ Airway mucosal ulcerations
★ Impaired ciliary activity

The critical care paramedic must be aware that, although typical signs and symptoms such as severe bronchospasms (tracheobronchitis) may occur in the first minutes to hours post-burn injury, the severity of the inhalation injury and the amount of damage done to the underlying respiratory structures are clinically unpredictable in the first few hours post-burn (i.e., initial history and physical including chest X-ray). Thus, the patient who presents with possible inhalation injury, especially below the glottis, should be closely observed for signs and symptoms of complications for at least 24 hours.

INHALATION INJURY AND THE PEDIATRIC PATIENT

The critical care paramedic must be keenly aware of the anatomical differences between the adult and pediatric airways that serve to make the pediatric airway much more susceptible to obstruction (i.e., relatively smaller). Once successful ET intubation has been accomplished in the pediatric patient, with an appropriately sized uncuffed tube, extra care must be given to securing the ETT to prevent dislodgement.

Another concern with pediatric burn patients is that due to their rib cage and sternum not yet being ossified they are more pliable than the adults. Clinically significant signs of respiratory distress, such as retractions of the sternum, can be used to guide treatment. Patients who sustain significant circumferential burns to the chest and abdomen may be at higher risk for respiratory failure due to the extra effort to overcome the decrease in compliance of their chest wall and their limited glycogen stores. In these cases an escharotomy should be performed at the first onset of ventilatory impairment.

FACIAL BURNS

Burns to the face are usually considered serious and almost always require hospitalization. Any patient who has sustained burns to the face must be evaluated with a high index of suspicion for inhalation injury.

Facial burns tend to be associated with extensive swelling, this is due to the fact that the face has a very rich blood supply and loose areolar tissue. Edema can be minimized by elevating the patient's head and trunk 30 degrees if not contraindicated (i.e., hypotensive).

Another common complication seen in patients with facial burns is chemical conjunctivitis. To avoid this complication, as much as possible, clean the face with only water or saline (no soap) and protect the eyes during the procedure.

BURNS TO THE EYES

Due to the possibility of rapid swelling of the eyelids, a thorough ocular examination should be performed as quickly as possible. Once the swelling starts, this exam will prove difficult at best. Corneal injury should be evaluated with the use of fluorescein, and ophthalmic antibiotic ointments or drops may be instilled after consultation with the burn center. Also, during times of maximal eyelid edema, the patient should have a mild ophthalmic solution instilled. Solutions that contain steroids should be avoided.

As with any chemical burn, chemical burns to the eyes should be flushed with copious amounts of saline or sterile water as soon as possible.

Do not apply any substance to a burn (except sterile saline or dressings) without contacting the burn center.

BURNS TO THE EARS

Evaluation of the ears should be performed as quickly as possible before swelling occurs. Both the canal and the drum should be evaluated to determine whether external otitis or otitis media is present, especially in pediatric patients. Also, in patients who are injured in an explosion (or other blast-type environment) or who have sustained a lightning strike, the tympanic membrane should be evaluated for possible perforation.

All trauma and excessive pressure should be avoided when dealing with burns to the ear to help minimize potential complications (i.e., no occlusive dressings, no pillow under the head).

BURNS TO THE HANDS

Burns to the hands may range from temporary disability and inconvenience to permanent loss of function depending on the severity of the burn.

Without a doubt, the most important aspect of evaluating burns to the hands is to evaluate the vascular status (both digital and palmar pulses) and the possible need for escharotomy. Evaluation of vascular status is usually best accomplished with the use of an ultrasonic flowmeter such as a

Doppler. This method is also the most accurate for trending (the plotting of results over time) and should be done at least hourly. In addition to monitoring perfusion to the burned hand, movement and sensory functions in the hand (radial, median, and ulnar nerves) should also be evaluated frequently if possible.

Burns to the hands should be elevated above the level of the heart (i.e., on pillows) to decrease potential swelling. Dressings should be avoided because of the potential to impede the ability to assess perfusion as well as perfusion itself. Digital escharotomies are usually not indicated prior to transfer to the burn center.

BURNS TO THE FEET

Evaluating burns to the feet should follow the same guidelines as burns to the hands with emphasis again being on assessing perfusion and minimizing swelling.

BURNS TO THE GENITALIA AND PERINEUM

Burns involving the penis require immediate insertion of a Foley catheter to maintain the patency of the urethra. Consulting with the burn center is highly advised in these situations.

Swelling to the scrotum, despite its significant presentation, does not typically require specific treatment, and diverting colostomies are not indicated for perineum burns.

ELECTRICAL BURNS

Electrical burns are the most difficult of all burn injuries to assess and manage because relatively small surface injuries can and typically do cause devastating internal injuries. These burns often cannot be actually examined, thus making it difficult to predict the extent of the burn injury. Because of this characteristic, the electrical burn is called the "grand masquerader" of burn injuries.

Electrical burn injuries account for only about 3% of all burn center admissions, but cause approximately 1,000 deaths per year in the United States. Because most of these injuries are occupational in nature, they have a significant economic as well as public health impact on our country.

Electrical burns can be caused by several mechanisms. The most common are current, arcing, flash, and ignition of the patient's clothing. Understanding the kinematics related to each of these mechanisms my assist the critical care paramedic with assessing the electrical burn-injured patient and predicting potential complications associated with them.

Electrical injuries are typically classified as low-voltage injuries or high-voltage injuries depending on the energy involved. Generally high-voltage energy is considered anything over 1,000 volts.

When a patient is injured by electricity, the extent of the damage is determined by the strength of the electrical current and how long (duration) the patient was exposed. Ohm's law defines this concept:

$$I = V/R$$

where current (I) is directly proportional to the voltage (V) and inversely proportional to the resistance (R).

Electrical burns cause tissue damage because once in the body the energy is converted to heat. Heat production (in joules) is the current times the resistance, multiplied by the time of contact:

$$J = I^2 \times R \times T.$$

The extent of electrical injury depends on several variables such as type of current, the pathway of flow, the local tissue resistance, and the duration of contact. Current flow can also be influenced by the cross-sectional area of the body part that is contacted. The body's most resistant organ is the skin. Once the current overcomes the resistance of the skin, the entire body then becomes a volume conductor with each underlying organ and tissue having a different resistance. Typically electrical current takes the path of least resistance. For example, because of its high density, bone makes a poor conductor of electricity, therefore, when the electrical flow hits a bone it typically will flow down the surface of the bone instead of penetrating it, but during this mechanism the heat generated by the electricity will cause significant damage to underlying tissues such as muscles. The critical care paramedic must realize that a patient who has sustained an electrical injury (particularly high-voltage injuries) may have extensive deep muscle injury and the superficial muscles may appear normal or uninjured initially.

Typical exam findings that should raise the critical care paramedic's index of suspicion that a patient has sustained a significant electrical burn injury include:

★ Loss of consciousness

★ Paralysis or mummified extremity

★ Loss of peripheral pulse

★ Flexor surface burns (especially to antecubital, axillary, inguinal, or popliteal areas)

★ Presence of myoglobinuria

★ Serum creatine kinase (CK) levels above 1,000 IU

★ Superior point of contact injury with very distal exit injuries (i.e., head/feet)

Current is measured in amperes (A) and is divided into two categories: alternating current (AC) or direct current (DC). AC electricity is produced by the reversal of electron flow every half cycle.

Most commercial devices made today, such as home appliances, are operated with alternating current because it is more economical to produce. Direct current injuries are generally from one of two sources: lightning strikes or automobile batteries. Modern hybrid gasoline/electric cars pose a particular risk for high-voltage DC current injuries. In comparison, AC electrical injuries are far more severe than DC injuries. Some of the more life-threatening injuries associated with AC current include cardiac arrest (ventricular fibrillation) and asphyxia from paralysis of the respiratory muscles.

> The severity of an electrical burn can be deceiving.

SPECIFIC MECHANISMS OF ELECTRICAL BURN INJURIES

★ *Current.* AC electricity flows back and forth between the power source and the anatomical point of contact on the patient. There are typically no signs of electrical injury (entrance/exit wounds). DC electricity flows in only one direction (path of least resistance) and therefore will have signs of entrance and exit from the body.

★ *Arcing.* By definition arcing refers to the ionization of air particles between two conductors. The heat generated by arcing can be very high (>4,000° C). That is hot enough to vaporize metal. Because of the intense heat generated by arcing, patients frequently have associated thermal burns caused by ignition of their clothing. Also, excess energy from the arc dissipates in the form of an explosion, which may also cause other blunt trauma injuries to the patient.

★ *Flash.* Flash burns can be caused by the power source itself or by ignition of the patient's clothing or surroundings and may occur without significant injuries to underlying tissues.

★ *Lightning strikes.* Statistically the chance of a person being struck by a lightning bolt is somewhere around 1 in 280,000. Even with these odds, lightning injuries kill somewhere between 80 and 100 people in the United States annually. The mortality rate of lightning injuries is somewhere around 30% but close to 70% of those who survive a lightning strike have severe complications.

Despite the fact that lightning strikes are DC and the median current of a lightning strike is somewhere around 30,000 A (range of 10,000 to 50,000 A) and can be as high as 1,000,000 volts, they are not usually associated with deep tissue burns. The most life-threatening injuries from a lightning strike are cardiac and neurologic in nature.

Although lightning injuries can be from a direct strike, most lightning injuries are created by electricity that is discharged through the air or ground after striking an object or person, called *splash* or *side flash*. Splash or side flashes can kill or injure people standing near the point of contact. This is probably the most common situation that will be seen in the prehospital environment.

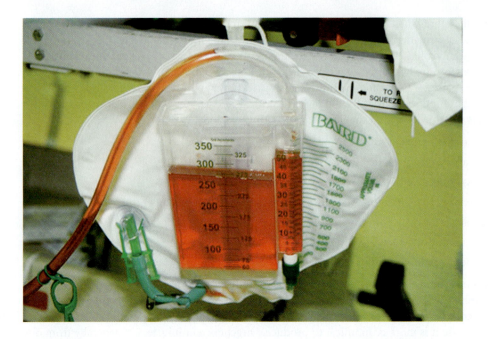

■ **Figure 18-15**
Rhabdomylosis in urine.
(Edward T. Dickinson, MD)

MANAGEMENT OF ELECTRICAL BURN INJURIES

The management of electrical burn injuries should follow the ABCDE format as with any other burn injury. Some special situations unique to electrical burn injuries are cardiac arrest, muscle compartment syndrome, and hemochromogens in the urine. Treatment guidelines for these are as follows:

★ *Cardiac arrest.* Treatment should follow the standard guidelines outlined in advanced cardiac life support courses.

★ *Muscle compartment syndrome.* If signs of muscle compartment syndrome are present, it must be relieved quickly to protect the underlying muscle from necrosis. Compartment syndrome is treated by performing either an escharotomy or fasciotomy. As stated earlier, however, these procedures are not commonly indicated prior to transfer to the burn center but if the patient's condition warrants, it should be done in consultation with the burn center.

hemochromogens *oxygen-carrying compounds (hemoglobin and myoglobin) found in the body; they are released through the process of rhabdomyolysis.*

★ **Hemochromogens.** The presence of rhabdomyolysis (port wine-colored pigments) in the urine is an indication of significant damage to underlying muscles. (See Figure 18-15 ■.) In these cases the urine output must be maintained between 75 and 100 mL/hr to ensure clearing of the kidneys. Fluid resuscitation should be titrated to facilitate this amount of urine output and will probably require an increase in fluid administration. This urine output should be maintained until the urine becomes grossly clear. Also, sodium bicarbonate (44 mEq in each liter of RL) should be administered until the pH of the urine is >6.0. Mannitol (0.5 g/kg) should be given immediately if hemochromogens are seen in the urine. This will aid in initiating urine output. Consultation with the burn center should be made prior to administration.

ELECTRICAL BURNS IN PEDIATRIC PATIENTS

Most pediatric electrical burn injuries occur in the home and are typically low-voltage injuries. (See Figure 18-16 ■.) Common causes include inserting metal objects into electrical sockets, chewing/biting on electrical cords, and faulty insulation on electrical appliance cords. Most electrical burns in pediatric patients are limited to cutaneous injury and typically do not involve the muscles.

Injuries that involve the oral commissure or other facial areas generally look worse than they are and do not require debridement. Consultation with the burn center is advised before the patient is discharged.

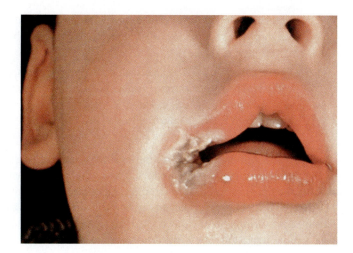

CHEMICAL BURNS

Like electrical burns, the extent of injury sustained by chemical burns may be deceiving. Chemical burns account for somewhere between 2% and 6% of burn center admissions; another 60,000 seek some type of medical treatment for chemical burns each year. That is a relatively small number when you consider that currently in the United States more than 500,000 chemicals are in use of which over 30,000 of them have been designated as hazardous by one or more regulatory agencies.

The extent of injury caused by chemical burns is directly related to the interval of time between the injury and when appropriate treatment began. Several factors influence the severity of a chemical injury:

★ Agent

★ Concentration (influences depth)

★ Volume (influences extent of TBSA involved)

★ Duration of contact (longer contact = deeper burn)

★ Mechanism of action of the agent

Chemicals capable of causing cutaneous burns are typically placed into one of three categories:

★ Alkalis

★ Acids

★ Organic compounds

Alkalis and acids are commonly found in the home or business in the form of cleaning solutions such as oven cleaners, drain cleaners, fertilizers, and heavy industrial cleaning agents. Organic compounds, typically found in petroleum products such as gasoline and creosote, are not only topically irritants but may have significant systemic toxicity. Let's look at each substance closer:

★ *Alkalis*—chemicals which include hydroxides, carbonates or caustic sodas of sodium, potassium, ammonium, lithium, barium, and calcium. The most common application of these chemicals is in oven or drain cleaners. They are also used to form the structural bond in cement and concrete. Severe alkali burns can occur from exposure to wet cement because the pH is approximately 12. Alkalis damage tissue by liquefaction necrosis and protein denaturation. Because of the way alkalis act on the skin they can spread deeper and are typically more severe.

★ *Acids*—chemicals which include muriatic acid, hydrochloric acid, oxalic acid, and hydrofluoric acid. The most common application of these chemicals is in bathroom cleaners, rust removers, and swimming pool chemicals. Acids damage tissue by coagulation necrosis and protein precipitation. Because of the way acids act on the skin they do not generally cause deep tissue damage. The exception to this rule is hydrofluoric acid.

★ *Organic compounds*—chemicals which include phenols, creosote, and petroleum products. The most common application of these chemicals is in disinfectants and petroleum products such as gasoline. Organic compounds cause cutaneous tissue damage from their fat solvent actions (also called cell membrane solvent action). After absorption they can produce severe toxic effects on the renal and hepatic systems.

Treatment for chemical burn injuries differs somewhat from other burns because you must take extra precautions to protect yourself and others from chemical exposure. Although this may prolong the time interval to start patient treatment you can't help anyone if you become a victim.

Prior to initiating treatment, care must be taken to remove as much of the chemical as possible. This means brushing off any powder agents, removing all contaminated clothing, and then beginning copious irrigation. The irrigation should be continued from the prehospital arena through the emergency department. A general guideline to irrigation is to continue it until the patient experiences a decrease in pain or burning sensation in the wound or the patient is evaluated at a burn center.

Universal Precautions, including gloves, gown, eye, and face protection, should be used. The patient should be thoroughly decontaminated prior to transport to minimize the risk of spreading the exposure. Of significant importance is chemicals that put off noxious vapors. Inhaling noxious vapors can prove deadly and most EMS vehicles do not have adequate ventilation in the patient compartment. The use of air evacuation, if appropriate, can be considered as long as the patient can be properly decontaminated prior to flight; otherwise it may be safer to transport the patient by ground vehicle.

Attempts to neutralize the chemical are usually contraindicated due to the potential generation of heat, which could contribute to making the burn more severe. Personnel with specific training in handling hazardous material incidents may neutralize specific chemicals if possible but should only do so after consultation with the burn center.

Certain chemical burns must often be immediately neutralized before patient care can begin.

MANAGEMENT OF SPECIFIC CHEMICAL BURNS

Specific burn injuries often require specific care, as discussed in the following subsections.

Injuries to the Eyes

Chemical injuries to the eyes, especially those involving alkalis, are commonly seen with young adults in the home setting, in industrial accidents, and as a result of aggravated assaults. Alkali burns occur twice as frequently as acid burns. Due to the mechanism of eye injuries, the patient may experience pain, swelling, and/or spasm of the eyelid. In addition, because alkalis bind with tissue proteins, they will require prolonged and copious irrigation to help dilute the chemical and stop the progression of injury. This irrigation should continue from the prehospital environment through to the emergency department.

The use of devices such as the Morgan lens can be used as long as caution is taken to prevent additional injury to the eye globe. Another alternative is to use a nasal cannula placed in the medial sulcus for irrigation with saline or sterile water. Make sure that any excess runoff does not contaminate the other eye. All chemical burn injuries to the eyes should be evaluated by an ophthalmologist in conjunction with the burn center physicians.

Hydrofluoric Acid

Even though hydrofluoric is a weak acid, the fluoride ion that is in it is extremely toxic. Hydrofluoric acid is commonly seen in industry to etch glass, make coatings such as Teflon, and in products designed to clean delicate semiconductors. The clinical presentation of your patient can give you a great deal of information about the concentration of the exposure. Exposure to low concentrations (typically less than 10%) will present with severe pain but this generally does not appear for 6 to 18 hours postexposure. A patient who has been exposed to higher concentrations may appear with severe pain and tissue necrosis. In addition, high concentrations can cause death from hypocalcemia because the fluoride rapidly binds free calcium in the blood.

Specific treatment of hydrofluoric acid burns includes flooding the wounds with water and then applying a topical calcium gel to neutralize the fluoride. This gel is easily made by mixing one ampule of calcium gluconate and 100 g of lubricating jelly. When applying this gel, make sure you protect yourself and the patient's other body parts from contamination by wearing gloves. Patients presenting with severe persistent pain may require intra-arterial or intravenous calcium infusions. This should only be started after consultation with the burn center. Because of the potential cardiovascular effects of high exposure, cardiac monitoring should be started as soon as possible. The burn center may also order excision of the wound early in the initial treatment phase, which could be lifesaving.

Phenol Burns

Disinfectants and chemical solvents typically contain phenol, which is an acidic alcohol that has poor solubility in water. Phenol does its damage by causing coagulation necrosis of the dermal proteins. In addition to copious irrigation of the affected area, cleaning the area with 50% polyethylene glycol (PEG) or ethyl alcohol is useful to increase the solubility of the phenol, which will allow for faster removal of the compound. One negative aspect of this treatment is that once diluted phenol can actually penetrate the skin quicker than when it was in a more concentrated solution, which will typically form a thick eschar due to the coagulation necrosis.

Petroleum Burns (Nonflame)

Because of the process of delipidation (breakdown of lipids) that is produced by prolonged contact with petroleum products such as gasoline and diesel fuel, significant tissue damage may occur. Full-thickness burns can occur but initially have the appearance of partial-thickness burns. Large amounts of hydrocarbon absorption can cause severe complications such as multiple system organ failure and even death. Systemic toxicity generally presents within 6 to 24 hours postexposure and is manifested by respiratory failure or insufficiency and hepatic and renal failure.

The critical care paramedic must evaluate the mechanism of injury and have a high index of suspicion if the patient was in any incident that involved petroleum products (i.e., MVCs), and a thorough exam of the lower extremities, back, and buttocks should be done to identify any possible exposure that could cause burns later. These patients should be evaluated at a burn center as soon as possible.

Tar Burns

Even though tar burns are actually contact in nature they are usually considered to be chemical burns. However, the compound found is tar, called bitumen, is nontoxic. The priority in tar burns is to rapidly cool the molten material (tar) with cold water to stop the burning process. The actual removal of the tar is not considered a priority. Once the tar has been cooled, it should be covered with a petroleum-based ointment, such as white petroleum jelly, and dressed in a manner to promote emulsification of the tar. Consultation with the burn center may also be helpful in managing these patients.

Anhydrous Ammonia Burns

Anhydrous ammonia is a very strong base that has a penetrating odor to it. The critical care paramedic may see burns from anhydrous ammonia in a variety of environments but the most common ones are farms/ranches, where it is used as fertilizer; industry, where it is used as a refrigerant; or in conjunction with an illicit drug manufacturing process, such as methamphetamine production.

Exposure to anhydrous ammonia causes blisters at the point of contact as well as pulmonary injuries if it is inhaled. These burns should be irrigated with copious amounts of water with the end point being removal of the ammonia smell. This may prevent the need for skin grafts down the road. Removal of this smell indicates that most of the ammonia is gone. Eye injuries from this chemical should also be irrigated with copious amounts of water and should be evaluated by an ophthalmologist. If inhaled, anhydrous ammonia can cause severe hypoxemia and copious secretions, which will probably require the patient to be intubated and placed on a ventilator.

Chemical and Biological Warfare Agents (Weapons of Mass Destruction)

Although a comprehensive chapter on chemical, biological, radiological, nuclear and explosives, or CBRNE, follows later in this text (Chapter 33), a brief introduction in this section is warranted.

Chemical warfare has been used by the military for more than 100 years. This form of warfare played a vital role in the mortality/morbidity rates in World War I. In the not so distant past, these agents have been used in terroristic attacks in both the United States and abroad. These agents are generally classified as either vesicants, such as mustard agents and lewisite, or nerve agents, such as sarin. Law enforcement agencies use a form of these agents to subdue and apprehend violent suspects with minimal risk of injury.

The most recent terrorist activity in the United States has been centered around anthrax. Anthrax comes in two distinct forms: inhalation anthrax and cutaneous anthrax. Both forms of the disease are potentially deadly but once diagnosed are easily treated with a common antibiotic called ciprofloxacin (Cipro). This particular strain of anthrax was spread by mail that had been contaminated with the anthrax strain.

When faced with any of these agents the critical care paramedic should follow the same guidelines as any other chemical or hazardous materials exposure: personal protection, isolate the patient(s), remove contaminated clothing, brush off any powder, and use copious irrigation. Any patient with signs or symptoms of respiratory distress/failure should, in most cases, receive prophylactic intubation.

RADIATION INJURY

Nuclear radiation is a natural, daily phenomenon and has affected the earth for centuries. Radiation does not become a danger to people until they are exposed to synthetic sources of radiation. This increased danger is due to the greater intensity of the radiation that is produced synthetically. Radiation is used everyday in both medicine and industry for things such as diagnostic testing and energy production, respectively. Death and serious injury are very rare because of the safety measures commonly used with the handling of nuclear materials. Typically, injuries and death are caused by carelessness, improper handling, or as a result of terroristic activities. Incidents can occur either on site or during transport. The possibility of large-scale incidents with multiple casualties is an ever-increasing risk associated with terrorism.

Ionization is the removal of an electron from a neutral atom. Through this, ionization energy is released, which in turn, can cause damage to human tissues. In the body, for instance, one of three things happens in the cell: It either repairs the damage, dies, or produces damaged cells (cancer). Some cells within the human body are more susceptible to radiation than others. Typically these are the cells that reproduce quickly, such as those responsible for red blood cells (erythrocyte), white blood cells (leukocyte), and platelet production (bone marrow). Also susceptible are cells that line the intestinal tract and those involved in reproduction. These factors explain the prevalence of cancer in these areas (osteosarcoma, colon cancer, and ovarian cancer).

The radiation we come in contact with can be divided into four types, but only three are clinically important:

★ *Alpha radiation.* The nucleus of an atom releases alpha radiation in the form of a small helium nucleus. Alpha radiation is considered the weakest of the four types of energy. Alpha radiation can only travel inches through the air and can be easily stopped with items such as paper or clothing. Alpha radiation cannot penetrate even the epidermis of the human body. Although weak, on a subatomic scale, the alpha particles are massive and can be very destructive over the short distance they can travel. The only significant hazard to humans associated with alpha radiation is through either inhalation or ingestion of contaminated material. The injury occurs as a result of bringing the source too close to areas such as the tissues of the respiratory and digestive tracts.

★ *Beta radiation.* A second type of radiological particles produces beta radiation. Beta energy is greater than that of alpha radiation. A beta particle is lightweight and has the mass of an electron. It can travel up to 10 feet and has the ability to penetrate several layers of clothes. Beta particles can also penetrate the first few millimeters of skin, thus having the potential to cause not only external injury but internal injury as well.

★ *Gamma radiation.* The strongest type of radiation is known as gamma radiation. This type of radiation is primarily used in X-rays. Gamma radiation is so strong it can

With the escalation of terrorism, radiation injuries have become a distinct possibility.

travel through the entire body or ionize any atom within. Because it is pure electromagnetic energy (no mass or charge), it has great penetrating power. This type of radiation poses the greatest risk, is the most dangerous, and, due to it being difficult to protect against, is the most feared. It requires several feet of concrete or several inches of lead to protect against gamma rays. Fortunately, high-energy gamma radiation is usually confined to nuclear reactors, nuclear weapons, and a few other highly radioactive materials. Anyone who has an occupation that exposes them to any of these areas is at a greater risk of exposure than other people. This is why we see specialized construction techniques used in areas of high use of gamma radiation, such as hospital X-ray and emergency departments.

Typically, exposure to ionized radiation occurs by one of two means. The first is unshielded exposure to a strong radioactive source such as uranium. The second is exposure to contaminated dust, debris, or fluids that contain small particles of radioactive materials.

The critical care paramedic should be cognizant of the following when caring for a patient with radiological exposure or if responding to a potential incident such as a MVC involving radioactive materials. There are three factors to consider: duration, distance, and shielding. In general, if you are shielded, are a significant distance away, and limit the duration of exposure, you minimize the potential negative effects of exposure.

Ionizing radiation is measured with the use of a Geiger counter (acute). Long-term exposure, as in people exposed to X-rays on a daily basis (X-ray technicians), is measured with a dosimeter. Both devices measure exposure in either the rad or the Gray (Gy), with 1 Gray being equal to 100 rads.

The critical care paramedic must limit his exposure to radiation and take proper precautions (shielding) to protect himself and his patients from the potential long-term effects of radiation exposure.

In the event the critical care paramedic is faced with a mass or multiple casualty incident (i.e., terrorist attack), great care must be taken to establish a single zone of isolation for evaluating and treating patients to avoid potential provider injury from environmental contamination. Typically, the best means of dealing with large-scale incidents is by following the incident management system in conjunction with departmental standard operating guidelines for hazardous materials responses. Following these established guidelines will not only minimize spread of the hazard, but will facilitate a much smoother operation, which will ultimately lead to better patient care. Because most of the agents used in chemical warfare have both short- and long-term morbidity and toxicity, all patients should be transported to a burn center for definitive care.

MANAGEMENT OF ASSOCIATED NONBURN INJURIES

When evaluating a burn patient, the critical care paramedic must determine if the patient has sustained any associated nonburn injuries. Evaluation of the circumstances surrounding the burn injury may provide valuable information and raise the index of suspicion for associated injuries. Some of these circumstances include MVCs, trauma from jumping/falling from significant heights, electrical burns, and acts of violence such as aggravated assaults and suicide attempts. In general, a patient found to be in shock soon after the event should be treated for hypovolemia and hypoxia as the cause of the shock, not the burn itself. Shock, when caused by the burn injury, appears late not early.

CRITERIA FOR BURN CENTER REFERRAL

According to the American Burn Association, the following burn injuries should be referred to a burn center (Table 18–2):

* ★ Partial thickness (second-degree) burns greater than 10% TBSA
* ★ Any burns involving the face, hands, feet, genitalia, perineum, or major joints
* ★ Full-thickness (third-degree) burns in any age group
* ★ Any electrical burns, including lightning injuries

Table 18-2	Criteria for Burn Center Referral

1. 2nd degree burns > 10 percent TBSA
2. Burns to face, hands, feet, genitalia, perineum, major joints
3. All 3rd degree burns
4. Any electrical burns (lightening included)
5. Any chemical burns
6. Inhalation injuries
7. Burns accompanied by preexisting medical conditions
8. Burns accompanied by trauma, where the burn injury poses the greatest risk of morbidity or mortality
9. Burns to children in hospitals without pediatric services
10. Patients with special social, emotional, or rehabilitative needs
11. Extremes of age (pediatric and geriatric)

Source: American Burn Association

★ Any chemical burns

★ Any inhalation burns

★ Any burn patient who has some preexisting condition that may complicate management, prolong recovery, or affect mortality. This could include diabetes, cardiovascular disease, and so on.

★ Any patient who has sustained concomitant trauma (i.e., fractures) in which the burn injury poses the greatest immediate risk. If trauma poses the greatest risk, then the patient should be evaluated and treated in a trauma center prior to transfer to the burn center. Physician judgment and communication with the burn center is the best course of action in these patients

★ Burned pediatric patients in hospitals without qualified personnel or equipment to care for the child

★ Burn injury in patients who will require special social, emotional, and/or long-term rehabilitative intervention

Consult your local burn center early for burns which may require their care.

Patients at the extremes of age are subject to variable physiological responses to thermal injury. Infants and elderly patients are much less tolerant of thermal, electrical, and chemical injuries. Burn centers use a multidisciplinary approach to managing these patients. The team typically includes physicians, nurses, psychologists, dieticians, social workers, and physical and occupational therapists. This approach has a significant influence on outcome for major burn and electrical injuries.

ADDITIONAL MANAGEMENT (DIAGNOSTIC TESTS)

Because burn injuries can cause dysfunction of any organ system, certain diagnostic evaluations should be performed on every critically burned patient to aid in guiding resuscitation and the treatment of any abnormal values that may be detrimental to the patient's clinical condition. The following are considered the standard initial tests that should be performed:

★ Hematocrit/hemoglobin levels

★ Electrolyte levels

★ Blood urea nitrogen levels (BUN)

★ Urinalysis (UA)

★ Chest X-ray

★ Arterial blood gas analysis

★ Carboxyhemoglobin levels

★ ECG with all electrical burns and preexisting cardiac problems

★ Glucose levels (especially in pediatric patients)

These should be done prior to transport if possible but transport must not be delayed to accomplish them.

PREPARING THE PATIENT FOR TRANSPORT

When the critical care paramedic is called on to transfer the burn-injured patient to the burn center, he must ensure that the patient has been adequately stabilized prior to transport and that the correct mode of transportation has been chosen. (See Figure 18-17 ■.) This has typically been accomplished prior to your arrival, but the critical care paramedic should at least evaluate the following:

★ *Adequate oxygenation/ventilatory support.* Administration of 100% oxygen and prophylactic intubation should both be considered if indicated. All intubated patients must have their ETT placement monitored, ideally by capnography, to avert any catastrophic airway mishap during the transport.

★ *Adequate circulatory support.* This includes establishing at least two large-bore IVs, preferably in nonburned areas or a venous cutdown in lieu of central venous access to avoid the complications associated with the procedures. Ringer's lactate (warm if possible) should be infused based on the Parkland formula and titrated to the appropriate amount of urine output for the patient's injuries. A Foley catheter should be placed as soon as possible after initial life threats have been addressed.

★ *Gastrointestinal management.* This includes keeping the patient NPO until the transfer has been completed. NG/OG tubes should be inserted in all patients with burns greater than 20% TBSA as well as all intubated patients.

★ *The need for dressings.* All wounds should be covered with dry sterile sheets. The addition of blankets over the dressings will assist in preventing hypothermia during the transport.

★ *Pain medication.* Patients should be administered pain medication (narcotics) via IV only. Carefully monitor the patient for any complications associated with the administration of narcotics.

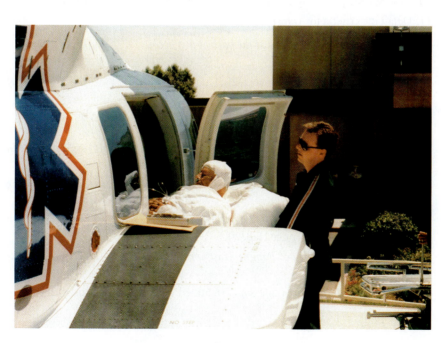

■ **Figure 18-17** A scientist in bandages is placed on a helicopter for airlifting to a hospital after being injured in an explosion at a rocket plant. (*Wendy Lamm/Tribune Media Services TMS Reprints*)

★ *The need for a tetanus injection.* Prophylactic tetanus injections should be administered per the American College of Surgeons' recommendations.

★ *Documentation.* Thorough documentation should accompany the patient to the burn center. This includes memorandum of transfer agreements, consents, prehospital run sheets, resuscitation flowsheets, history and physical exams, radiology reports/X-rays, and any lab results.

Summary

Caring for the critically injured burn patient presents some of the most challenging care situations the critical care paramedic will encounter. By being vigilant in the evaluation and management of these patients, particularly airway management and fluid resuscitation, the critical care paramedic can provide the patient with the best chance of a meaningful recovery and return to a functional lifestyle.

Review Questions

1. Discuss the epidemiology of burn injuries.
2. Detail Jackson's theory of thermal wounds.
3. What component of the initial assessment is most critical to the burn patient?
4. Describe the common burn scoring systems.
5. Calculate the 24-hour fluid requirement using the Parkland formula for a 101-kg patient who has 65% TBSA burns.
6. Discuss the care of suspected inhalational injuries.
7. Detail the effect of carbon monoxide on the burn patient.
8. Describe the management of an electrical burn.
9. Detail the approach to patients with possible chemical burn injuries.
10. Describe the pathophysiology of ionizing radiation-induced burn injuries.
11. Detail the criteria for transport to a burn center.

See Answers to Review Questions at the back of this book.

Further Reading

American Burn Association. *Advanced Burn Life Support Course Providers Manual.* Chicago: Author, 2001.

American College of Surgeons. *Advanced Trauma Life Support Instructors Manual,* 6th ed. Chicago: Author, 1997.

Bledsoe BE, Porter RS, Cherry RA. *Paramedic Care: Principles & Practice,* 2nd ed. Upper Saddle River, NJ: Pearson Prentice Hall, 2005

Holeran RS. *Air and Surface Patient Transport: Principles and Practices,* 3rd ed. St. Louis, MO: Mosby, 2003.

NAEMT. *PreHospital Trauma Life Support,* 5th ed. St. Louis, MO: Mosby, 2004.

Principles of Orthopedic Care

Jeffrey R. Brosius, B.S., NREMTP, FP-C, and Bryan E. Bledsoe, DO, FACEP

Objectives

Upon completion of this chapter, the student should be able to:

1. Describe the skeletal anatomy and physiology, using appropriate medical terminology. (p. 523)
2. Discuss the primary concerns regarding treatment of orthopedic injuries, including the following:
   A. Describe the differences in orthopedic injuries, including fractures, dislocations, and subluxations. (p. 524)
   B. Describe fractures using current and correct medical definitions. (p. 524)
   C. Briefly discuss the pathophysiology of orthopedic injuries. (p. 526)
   D. Describe and demonstrate the proper assessment of the skeletal system. (p. 527)
   E. Discuss the proper treatment of orthopedic injuries. (p. 530)
   F. Identify the orthopedic injuries that are most likely to cause hemodynamic instability, and discuss the specific treatment considerations for each. (p. 532)
3. Identify and discuss various pharmacologic agents utilized as supportive agents for orthopedic injuries, including antibiotics and analgesics. (p. 538)
4. Identify simple orthopedic injuries from radiographic images. (p. 540)

Key Terms

amphiarthrosis, p. 523
arthrodia, p. 523
condyloid, p. 523
deep peroneal reflex, p. 528
Denis system, p. 535
diarthrosis, p. 523
enarthrosis, p. 523
epiphysis, p. 528
external fixation, p. 530

ginglymus, p. 523
Gustilo grading system, p. 525
hangman's fracture, p. 535
internal fixation, p. 531
Jefferson (burst) fracture, p. 535
roentgenogram, p. 540

Salter-Harris system, p. 528
subluxation, p. 524
synarthrosis, p. 523
teardrop fracture, p. 535
trochoid, p. 523
Tscherne method, p. 525

Case Study

You are called to transfer a 61-year-old male patient from a community hospital to a major teaching hospital for definitive care. You are staffing a ground transport unit with another critical care paramedic. While en route, you review the essential information. The patient is a farmer who was plowing a wet field and overturned his tractor, trapping himself underneath it. He lay in the field for about 2 hours before family members noticed he was late for lunch. His wife found him and summoned the local fire department. They were able to free him after approximately 30 minutes, through a combination of digging and use of hydraulic lifts and cribbing. The patient was transported to the local hospital where he was found to be hypothermic and in shock. He had multiple fractures, but no other injuries. He required transfusion of 4 units of packed red blood cells over the first 24 hours of hospital admission. He is being transferred for highly specialized internal fixation of a complex pelvic fracture.

You arrive at the two-bed ICU of a small community hospital and find the patient sleeping. A unit of blood is slowly infusing. Both of the patient's forearms are splinted and his left leg is splinted. He has a Foley catheter in place. You quickly review the chart and find that he has continued to slowly bleed from the pelvic fracture. CT scan of the abdomen and chest were normal. As you flip through the X-rays you see that he has a complex fracture of the distal right radius and ulna. He has an incomplete fracture of the left ulna. His left distal tibia and fibula are shattered. His pelvis has multiple fractures and these are displaced. You ask the ICU nurse about hematuria and she replies that, much to her surprise, there was no blood in the urine.

You apply the monitors and switch the IV and blood to your equipment. As you prepare to move the patient, he moans in pain. The nurse reports that he has had no pain medication in 2 hours. You do a quick check of vitals and administer 100 mcg of fentanyl. After a few minutes, the patient is at ease. You move him to the stretcher and carefully to the ambulance.

The trip to the university hospital is slow to keep from jarring the patient. The blood infusion finishes. You remove the blood bag and place it in a biohazard bag to give to the receiving hospital. The trip is otherwise unremarkable.

The patient is admitted and, the next day, undergoes a 5-hour operation where internal fixation of the pelvis is completed. At the same time, his left tibia is fixed with an internal rod and placed into a cast. The right forearm fracture is opened and reduced by the placement of a plate and screws in the distal radius. Both forearms are casted. The patient does well and is moved to the physical and rehabilitative medicine service. After 4 weeks of hospitalization, he is discharged home and ultimately does well. It is almost a year before he can return to active farming.

INTRODUCTION

During transport of the sick and injured, the critical care paramedic will often find that the patient has some type of orthopedic problem. Most commonly, this will be found in the form of a fracture or multiple fractures in a patient who has suffered multisystem trauma and needs transport to a tertiary facility for definitive care. While isolated orthopedic injuries are rarely fatal, multiple injuries, with the resultant blood loss and potential for infection, can complicate the treatment and recovery of a critical patient. Although it is infrequent that the critical care paramedic will need to perform any significant intervention for an orthopedic injury, knowledge of orthopedic injuries and the proper care for such injuries will allow greater patient comfort, promote recovery, and help to limit long-term disability.

INCIDENCE

Orthopedic injuries and illness are quite prevalent in today's society. As the human life expectancy increases, the predisposition to injury or illness is manifested by higher occurrence of orthopedic injury or disease. Some statistics regarding injuries quickly reveal the prevalence of the problem:

★ In 2000, 1.6 million seniors were treated in emergency departments for fall-related injuries and 353,000 were hospitalized. The chance that a fall will cause a severe injury requiring hospitalization greatly increases with age.

★ Of those who fall, 20% to 30% suffer moderate to severe injuries such as hip fractures or head traumas that reduce mobility and independence and increase the risk of premature death.

★ Among older adults, the majority of fractures are caused by falls.

★ The most common fractures are of the vertebrae, hip, forearm, leg, ankle, pelvis, upper arm, and hand.

★ Approximately 3% to 5% of older adult falls cause fractures. Based on the 2000 census, this translates to 360,000 to 480,000 fall-related fractures each year.

★ In 1999 in the United States, hip fractures resulted in approximately 338,000 hospital admissions.

★ The total cost of all fall injuries for people age 65 or older in 1994 was $20.2 billion. By 2020, the cost of fall injuries is expected to reach $32.4 billion (before adjusting for inflation).

★ Each year in the United States, emergency departments treat more than 200,000 children ages 14 and younger for playground-related injuries. About 45% of playground-related injuries are severe—fractures, internal injuries, concussions, dislocations, and amputations.

Obviously, from the brief statistics shown, orthopedic injuries constitute a major part of medical treatment in the United States. The cost, both in terms of monetary expenditure and loss of functional time, is enormous.

SKELETAL ANATOMY AND PHYSIOLOGY

A solid working knowledge of the skeletal system is vital to proper assessment and care of orthopedic injuries. The critical care paramedic needs to understand the utility of the skeleton, the different types of bones, different types of joints, and how bone growth occurs in order to provide optimal care of orthopedic injuries.

Bones are described with regard to their shape and size, and can be long (femur), short (phalanges), flat (skull bones), or irregular (vertebrae.) Joints, or the connection between two bones, can be classified as either movable (**diarthrosis**), slightly movable (**amphiarthrosis**), or nonmovable (**synarthrosis**). Movable joints can be further subdivided into ball and socket (**enarthrosis**), hinge (**ginglymus**), gliding (**arthrodia**), pivot (**trochoid**), **condyloid**, or saddle.

The skeleton is frequently subdivided into the axial skeleton and the appendicular skeleton. Axial bones include those of the skull, spinal column, torso, and pelvis, while the bones of the arms, legs, hands, and feet comprise the appendicular skeleton. Muscles, attached to the bones by tendons, provide movement, while ligaments that connect bone to bone provide an interconnected structure capable of movement and articulation.

The musculoskeletal system serves several vital life functions, including providing structure and facilitating movement, protection of internal organs, formation of red blood cells, and mineral homeostasis.

diarthrosis *joints, or the connection between two bones, classified as movable.*

amphiarthrosis *joints, or the connection between two bones, classified as slightly movable.*

synarthrosis *joints, or the connection between two bones, classified as nonmovable.*

enarthrosis *ball and socket movable joints.*

ginglymus *hinge movable joints.*

arthrodia *gliding movable joints.*

trochoid *pivot movable joints.*

condyloid *pivot movable joints.*

While structure and movement are the most obvious functions of the skeletal system, protection of internal organs is also of vital importance. The skull provides a protective covering for the brain, the vertebrae protect the spinal cord, and the ribs provide coverage of the heart and lungs. Without such skeletal protection, the rate of injuries to these structures would be greatly increased. Thus, protection is a vital role of the skeleton.

Within the bone marrow of the major bones, red blood cells are produced. Red blood cells typically have a life span of approximately 120 days, and new erythrocytes are produced constantly. Most of the red blood cells are produced in the femur, but the tibia and the pelvis also contribute to erythrocyte formation.

Finally, the bones of the skeleton serve as the primary reservoir for mineral storage, specifically calcium, phosphorus, sodium, magnesium, and carbonate. These minerals serve essential roles in various physiological functions, including the Kreb's cycle, nerve impulse conduction, muscle contraction, and endocrine function.

TYPES OF INJURIES

subluxation *orthopedic injury classified as partial dislocation.*

Most orthopedic injuries can be classified as a fracture, dislocation, **subluxation** (aka "partial dislocation"), or a combination of these. Sprains, strains, and muscle rupture are also orthopedic in nature, but seldom are a concern in the critical care setting because they are limited to the muscles, ligaments, and tendons. Traumatic amputations can require critical care intervention, but this too is rare. Fractures, dislocations, and subluxations are defined as follows:

★ *Fracture (Latin fractura, break)* —a sudden breaking of a bone or a break of a bone

★ *Dislocation (Latin dis, apart, + locare, to place)* —the displacement of any part, especially the temporary displacement of a bone from its normal position in a joint

★ *Subluxation (Latin sub, under, below, + luxatio, dislocation)* —a partial or incomplete dislocation that has spontaneously returned to proper positioning

These definitions are adequate as a general description of the injury, but more precise definitions are commonly used to describe the exact pathology. While dislocations and subluxations are simply defined with anatomical direction (i.e., "lateral patellar dislocation"), fractures are more specifically delineated into one of several types (Figure 19-1 ■):

★ *Open:* The fractured bone is protruding through the skin.

★ *Closed:* The fractured bone does not break the skin.

★ *Complete:* The bone is broken completely through all layers.

★ *Incomplete:* The fracture line does not extend through the entire bone.

★ *Displaced:* The broken ends of the bone are no longer aligned.

★ *Greenstick:* Part of the bone is broken along the length, much as when a green tree branch is broken. Most common in children whose bones have not fully calcified.

★ *Comminuted:* The bone is fragmented into several small parts.

★ *Segmental:* Two complete fractures of the same bone that cause a segment to be free floating.

★ *Butterfly:* A small portion of the bone breaks free, but there is no complete fracture.

★ *Spiral:* The fracture line extends circumferentially around the bone.

★ *Hairline:* A minute fracture, often difficult to see on a radiograph.

★ *Occult:* A fracture not visible on simple radiograph.

★ *Epiphyseal:* A fracture through the growth plate (epiphysis) of a bone.

★ *Oblique:* Breaks in a bone running across it an angle other than 90 degrees. (See Figure 19-2 ■.)

★ *Transverse:* A break that runs across a bone perpendicular to the bone's orientation.

★ *Fatigue:* Breaks in a bone associated with prolonged or repeated stress.

★ *Impacted:* A break in a bone in which the bone is compressed on itself.

Impacted

Oblique

Transverse

Comminuted

Greenstick

Spiral

Further, open and closed injuries are classified with unique descriptive grading systems. Closed fractures are typically graded using the **Tscherne method** (see Table 19–1), while open fractures are classified using the **Gustilo grading system** (see Table 19–2). Of note is that all fractures caused by shotgun wounds, high-velocity gunshot wounds, major crush injury, or agricultural injuries are classified as Gustilo Type III, regardless of size or extent. These injuries all have high levels of wound

Tscherne method *method of grading closed fractures.*

Gustilo grading system *method of grading open fractures.*

■ Figure 19-2   X-ray of displaced fracture of the tibia and fibula. *(Howard Kingsnorth/Getty Images, Inc.)*

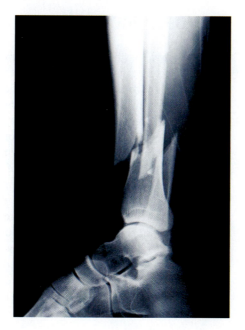

Table 19-1	Tscherne Method for Grading Closed Fractures
Grade 0	Negligible soft-tissue injury
Grade 1	Abrasions or contusions (superficial) over the site of the fracture
Grade 2	Significant muscle contusion; contaminated abrasions
Grade 3	Severe soft-tissue injury, including degloving, crush injury, or vascular damage

contamination and require aggressive management. It should also be mentioned that while these grading systems are acceptable terminology, it is also common practice to simply use nontechnical terms to describe the injury: "Open fracture of left radius and ulna, approximately 4 cm break in skin, minimal soft-tissue damage."

When these descriptors and grading systems are combined with anatomical terminology, an excellent description of the fracture can be obtained. For example, a physician might describe a fracture as follows: "Right-sided Gustilo IIIa midshaft humerus fracture." The knowledgeable critical care paramedic would understand that the fracture is to the right humerus, it is an open fracture, there is contamination of the wound, but the neurovascular structures are not compromised. Specific descriptors of fractures to the pelvis and vertebrae are discussed later in respective sections.

A fracture can be a debilitating injury.

Table 19-2	Gustilo Grading System for Open Fractures
Type I	Small and clean wound (<1 cm); minimal muscle injury; no stripping of periosteum
Type II	Larger open wound (>1 cm); no significant soft-tissue damage; minimal, if any, periosteum damage
Type III	Larger open wounds; extensive muscle and soft-tissue damage; subdivided into three types (a, b, and c)
Type IIIa	Extensive contamination of underlying soft tissue; still enough soft tissue to cover bone and vasculature
Type IIIb	Extensive muscle and soft-tissue damage; will require muscle transfer; major contamination
Type IIIc	Open injury with vascular damage that requires surgical repair

PATHOPHYSIOLOGY

The pathophysiology of a fracture or other orthopedic injury is greatly inferred by the type of injury. The exact mechanism will often point to the injuries suffered. Therefore, an adequate history of the event and a comprehensive knowledge of functional human anatomy are of vital importance. A patient who complains of pain and a sensation of joint slippage while swimming, for example, should be evaluated for shoulder instability. Understanding that most glenohumeral dislocations are caused by extension and external rotation of the shoulder should lead the paramedic to the correct diagnosis. Similarly, leg pain in a new military recruit may be suggestive of a stress fracture, since repetitive impact is the major cause of stress fractures.

Regardless of the exact cause, the common factor in any orthopedic injury is that of impact force. Application of external (or internal, in the case of an avulsion fracture) force in sufficient quantity to the structures of the skeletal system can cause injury. Additionally, external force applied frequently over a period of time can also cause injury. As expected, the amount of force needed will depend on several factors: what bone is involved, any other concurrent force, and any underlying pathology (i.e., osteoporosis.) An extensive discussion about the pathophysiology of orthopedic injury is beyond the scope of this text and is readily available in any number of orthopedic textbooks. (See the Further Reading list at the end of the chapter.)

ASSESSMENT OF THE SKELETAL SYSTEM

Patient assessment should reveal any significant injury. Obviously, assessment of the airway, breathing, and circulation should be the priority. Skeletal assessment is often deferred to the end of the patient assessment. Once the initial assessment is complete, the detailed assessment is performed. After the chest, abdomen, and neurologic status have been evaluated, the skeleton should be assessed. The fundamental aspects of skeletal assessment are little different than that learned in initial paramedic education. Look for obvious signs of orthopedic injury: deformity, contusions, abrasions, pain, lacerations, swelling, tenderness, instability, or crepitus.

Any acute deformity should be assumed to be the result of a fracture unless proven otherwise. Contusions indicate blunt force trauma, and may indicate a fracture. Abrasions are rarely a cause for concern, but large and extensive abrasions may indicate a significant mechanism of injury (MOI). The pain associated with a fracture is often pinpointed, and the patient should be given the "one finger, one place" test. This simple test is accomplished by asking the patient to place one finger on the one place where the pain is greatest. A patient who can accomplish this and point directly to the spot of pain has a positive result. A negative test is found when a patient cannot specify a single area and instead describes a more generalized pain. Lacerations over a deformity should be treated as an open fracture until radiographs can conclusively prove the lack of a fracture. Swelling and tenderness can accompany fractures, sprains, strains, or dislocations, and are therefore poor prognosticators of specific injury, but may help trend the progression of the injury. Instability and crepitus are common with fractures and dislocations, and should therefore be accurately noted.

Various imaging modalities may offer assistance in assessing skeletal integrity. By and far, the most common is the roentgenogram or X-ray. Some basic steps for reading X-rays are provided later in this chapter. Other helpful imaging devices include computed tomography (CT) scans and magnetic resonance imaging (MRI). A short discussion on how to read radiographic images is included later in this chapter, but the skills needed to expertly evaluate CT and MRI images are beyond the scope of this text.

As a general rule, only fractures to the larger bones of the body will cause hemodynamic compromise or significant further injury. Rarely will a radius fracture be cause for great concern. Conversely, a pelvic fracture can be the source of life-threatening hemorrhage. Therefore, your assessment should be focused on those major bones that have the greatest likelihood of causing life threats: pelvis, femur, spine, tibia/fibula, and humerus. Table 19–3 gives a relative indication of hemorrhage from various bones.

Once all life-threatening injures are found, the severity of those injuries should be evaluated. Take time to evaluate distal pulses, and mark the location of the pulse. The risk of vascular injury from a fracture is significant, and the "Six P" approach can aid in evaluating the vascular status. The Six Ps to be assessed are pain, pallor, paralysis, paresthesia, pressure, and pulses. If the cast or splint prevents assessing pulse quality, capillary refill time should be evaluated and recorded. If any abnormalities are found, they should be addressed in the care plan, when possible. In the event an orthopedic injury results in lack of peripheral pulses, reduction of the injury may be required to salvage the limb and prevent amputation.

Check the neurologic function, both sensory and motor function, as well as tendon reflexes. To evaluate sensation, a light tactile stimulus—finger or sharp safety pin—should be applied to the

Anytime you have hypotension in a trauma patient, fractures may be the cause—but first look for more pressing sources (intra-abdominal or intrathoracic hemorrhage).

Table 19–3	Estimated Blood Loss from Select Long-Bone Fractures	
Fractured Bone	**Estimated Blood Loss (mL)**
Humerus	750
Tibia	1,000
Femur	1,500 (per femur)
Pelvis	1,500+

Table 19–4	Deep Tendon Reflexes	
Muscle	**Peripheral Nerve**	**Nerve Root**
Biceps	Musculocutaneous	C5
Brachioradialis	Radial	C6
Triceps	Radial	C7
Quadriceps	Femoral	L4
Posterior tibialis	Deep peroneal	L5
Triceps surae (gastrocnemius/soleus)	Tibial	S1

skin, following the dermatomes. The patient should be able to report the sensation applied. Lack of sensation indicates neurologic compromise, and this increases the urgency of the orthopedic injury. Motor function includes movement of the extremity, and should be evaluated with consideration given to the injury. For example, it would be inappropriate to ask a patient with a fracture of the humerus to flex his elbow, as this would likely exacerbate the injury. However, the patient's motor function can still be assessed in a limited fashion by having him move the fingers of the hand.

In the event the patient is unresponsive, either from injury or sedation, neurologic function is evaluated by testing for the presence or absence of reflexes. While these reflexes can provide valuable information, they are sometimes difficult to evaluate unless one is well practiced at assessment (especially the **deep peroneal reflex,** which is rarely elicited by even the most experienced personnel). (See Table 19–4.) More easily evaluated, and just as valuable, are the superficial reflexes. These are easier to elicit for most health care providers.

deep peroneal reflex *reflex arc involving L_4, L_5, and S_1 spinal segments mediated through deep peroneal nerve.*

Figure 19-3 ■ provides a handy reference for the dermatomes of the spinal nerve roots. A simple evaluation of the ability to sense a pinprick will usually suffice. Evaluate range of motion, and compare to the uninjured side. If any interventions have been made for orthopedic injuries, they need to be evaluated as well. Splints should be checked to ensure they are not overly constrictive and compromising circulation. Traction should be evaluated to ensure it is still effective. External fixation devices, such as pins, need to be checked for tightness, stability, and position. Observe for any signs of infection, such as pus drainage, redness, or necrotic tissue, and note those indicators properly.

SPECIAL PATIENTS: PEDIATRIC FRACTURES

epiphysis *the cartilaginous bone growth plate, also called the physis.*

In children, the bone growth plate is still active. Fractures involving the **epiphysis** can result in various growth abnormalities. The cartilaginous epiphyseal plate, also called the physis, is readily injured in that it is weaker than ossified bone or ligaments. (See Figure 19-4 ■.) Damage to the epiphyseal plate during a child's growth may destroy all or part of the bone's ability to produce new bone. The potential for a growth disturbance from a growth-plate injury is related to the number of years the child has to grow. Thus, the older the child, the less time remains for a deformity to develop. The **Salter-Harris system** is often used to classify growth-plate injuries. The potential for growth disturbances increases as the classification number increases. The prognosis is best for Salter-Harris Type I fractures and worst for Salter-Harris Type V fractures. The Salter-Harris classifications for growth-plate injuries are as follows (Figure 19-5 ■):

Salter-Harris system *method of classifying growth plate injuries.*

★ *Salter-Harris Type I.* The fracture line runs through the physis. There is usually little, if any, separation of the epiphysis from the rest of the bone. It is often difficult to see the fracture line on X-ray, because the line is often hidden within the growth plate. A Type I injury is the least severe epiphyseal fracture type.

★ *Salter-Harris Type II.* The entire epiphysis and a portion of the metaphysis are broken off. The fracture line runs through the physis into the metaphysis.

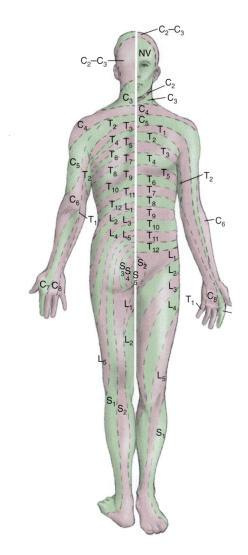

★ *Salter-Harris Type III.* A portion of the epiphysis is broken off. The fracture line runs through the physis, the epiphysis, and into the joint.

★ *Salter-Harris Type IV.* A portion of the epiphysis and a portion of the metaphysis are broken off. The fracture line runs through the metaphysis, the physis, the epiphysis, and into the joint.

★ *Salter-Harris Type V.* The epiphyseal plate is compressed, usually through an axial loading type force. These injuries are difficult to diagnose and are sometimes only evident retrospectively.

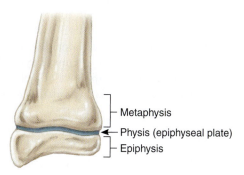

Metaphysis
Physis (epiphyseal plate)
Epiphysis

■ Figure 19-4　Growth plate in a child's long bone. The growth plate is also called the physis or epiphyseal plate. The portion of bone proximal to the physis is the metaphysis; the segment distal to the physis is the epiphysis.

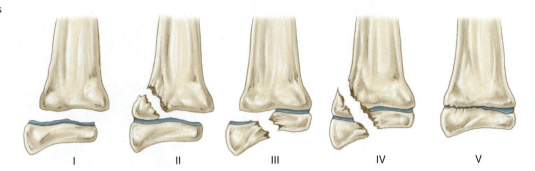

■ **Figure 19-5** Salter-Harris system of classifying growth-plate injuries. The likelihood of a permanent growth-plate deformity increases as the classification number increases.

I   II   III   IV   V

TREATMENT

Treatment of orthopedic injuries is, at the fundamental level, very straightforward: Place the bone into proper alignment, keep it in place, and let it heal. The manner in which the orthopedic surgeon elects to accomplish this goal will vary greatly, depending on the nature of the injury and the capability of the hospital. With the exception of pelvic fractures, which will be discussed later, most orthopedic injuries can be stabilized with one of several methods: splint, cast, reduction/realignment, external fixation, internal fixation, or amputation.

SPLINT

The most basic level of orthopedic injury treatment is the simple splint. The bone is returned to normal alignment (or as close to normal as possible) and secured with a rigid splint. One of the most commonly used materials is called OrthoGlass®, a fiberglass material that is soft and pliable, but becomes rigid once soaked with water and allowed to dry. Splints are temporizing measures until a more permanent solution can be placed and most splints are in place for no more than 72 hours. This allows the swelling that often accompanies an orthopedic injury to abate somewhat, before any restrictive casting material is applied.

CASTING

A rigid material is applied over the extremity once proper alignment is established. Plaster was once the most commonly used material, but it is rapidly becoming obsolete and replaced by lightweight fiberglass casting material. Casts are more permanent than splints, and are commonly left in place for several weeks. Typically, casting is used for closed, simple fractures without complicating infections or soft-tissue injury. Casts are rarely applied in the first 24 to 36 hours after an injury, because swelling within a rigid cast may exacerbate tissue damage and prolong healing.

REDUCTION/REALIGNMENT

In certain cases, the orthopedic injury can be easily treated by reducing the injury back to normal (or near-normal) position. This is most applicable to dislocations where the patient suffers pain, neurovascular deficit, or functional loss. Reduction of a dislocation is typically a simple task, but there is risk of increasing the damage to underlying structures if done improperly. All reductions should be done with the approval of a physician, under controlled circumstances, and with adequate amounts of analgesia and sedation to provide comfort.

external fixation
application of external metal or composite framework applied with pins, screws, and rods to the bone, keeping proper alignment, while fracture is visualized under fluoroscopy.

EXTERNAL FIXATION

External fixation refers to a procedure where the fracture is visualized under fluoroscopy, and then a metal or composite framework is applied with pins, screws, and rods to the bone, keeping proper

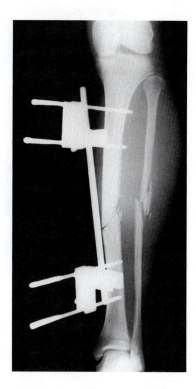

■ **Figure 19-6** X-ray of a pinned fracture of both the tibia and fibula. The tibia has been immobilized by metal pins (lower and upper center). The pins are held in place by an external metal frame. *(SPL/Photo Researchers, Inc.)*

alignment. (See Figure 19-6 ■.) An external fixator is placed in the operating room and is an invasive technique. External fixation is indicated for open fractures, closed fractures with extensive soft-tissue trauma, and infected fractures. Several different external fixation devices exist, but the general principle behind all is the same. External fixation is commonly referred to as "ExFix."

INTERNAL FIXATION

During **internal fixation,** the skin is opened surgically, the fracture is reduced into proper alignment, and the placement of rods, plates, screws, and nails is performed. This technique is commonly called open reduction with internal fixation (ORIF) and may be done under fluoroscopy. ORIF is employed when the fracture is displaced, segmented, comminuted, or otherwise complicated and simple reduction is ineffective. (See Figure 19-7 ■.)

internal fixation *the internal placement of rods, plates, screws, and nails is performed through a surgical opening in the skin to stabilize a fractured bone.*

AMPUTATION

The critical care paramedic should bear in mind that repair of orthopedic injuries is often delayed several hours, and even days. While there has been much debate in the past about the appropriate time frame in which to address orthopedic injuries in the multisystem trauma patient, this issue has been addressed by the Eastern Association of Surgery for Trauma (EAST) in their Trauma Practice Guidelines. The available literature shows little benefit to early repair of fractures, and concerns about potential complications [emboli, acute respiratory distress syndrome (ARDS), and so on] are unsupported by current research. Therefore, do not be surprised if an open tibia fracture is left unrepaired for several hours. If vascular integrity is maintained and tissue perfusion is adequate, simple splinting will suffice while you treat other, more significant injuries.

When a fracture and the resultant soft-tissue injury are so extensive and complicated that repair is not feasible, the orthopedic surgeon or trauma surgeon may elect to perform an amputation of the affected limb. Primary emergent amputation results in fewer infectious complications than prolonged wound healing, but obviously creates future challenges for the long-term recovery of the patient.

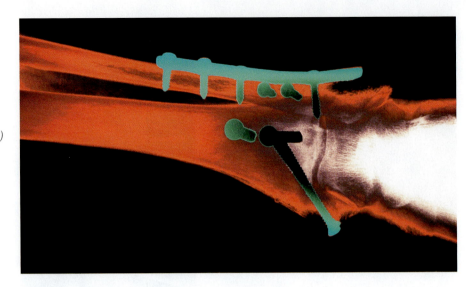

■ **Figure 19-7** X-ray of an ankle fracture complicated by osteoporosis. The bone has been surgically immobilized by the insertion of a long metal plate fixed to the bone with metal screws. *(Airelle-Joubert/Photo Researchers, Inc.)*

CRITICAL FRACTURES AND INJURIES

Compartment syndrome is a limb-threatening emergency.

As mentioned earlier, most fractures are not a major concern for a critical patient. While they do need to be addressed in the course of the treatment plan, definitive care can be delayed, often for 24 hours or more. A few fractures, however, require immediate management to prevent hemodynamic instability. Specifically, pelvic fractures, femur fractures, spinal fractures, humerus fractures, and certain rib fractures can all be critical in nature, because these bones can be the source of life-threatening hemorrhage, permanent neurologic damage, or pulmonary injury. Traumatic amputations are included, since they are a time-sensitive injury and proper early treatment can greatly enhance the chances of successful repair. Also included in this section is the treatment and care of a pulseless extremity, with descriptions of the proper reduction techniques. Further, the pathology of orthopedic injury can lead to a special condition known as compartment syndrome. The frequency and seriousness of compartment syndrome leads to its inclusion as a critical injury. Each of these situations is discussed in the following sections.

PELVIC FRACTURES

One of the five places in the body that can hold enough blood to cause cardiovascular collapse is the pelvic girdle. A pelvic fracture can be the cause of life-threatening hemorrhage (1,500+ mL blood loss), and such bleeding can easily go unnoticed until the patient is well into Stage IV shock. Therefore, any suspected pelvic fracture must be given the utmost attention.

Pelvic fractures are typically classified into one of three major types, according to the Tile Classification System: Type A (stable), Type B (rotationally unstable, vertically stable), or Type C (rotationally and vertically unstable). The classification is dependent on the exact location of the fracture.

Pelvic fractures are typically stabilized with a bed sheet wrap, C-clamp, or external or internal fixation. Some experts promote the use of pneumatic antishock garment (PASG) for emergent stabilization of pelvic fractures, but this approach is not without drawbacks, most notably the limiting of lung expansion and possibility of iatrogenic lower extremity compartment syndrome. (See Figure 19-8 ■.)

FEMUR FRACTURES

The femur, the longest bone in the human body, is not easily fractured. The forces required to cause femoral fracture are tremendous, and femur fractures are commonly associated with other injuries (e.g., multisystem trauma). However, an isolated femur fracture is possible, and these fractures re-

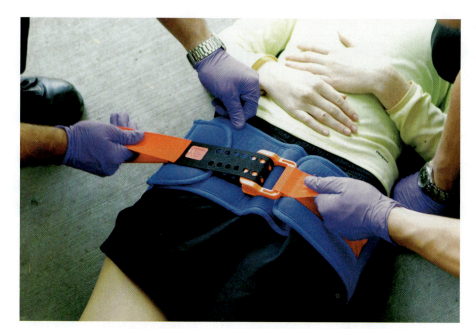

■ **Figure 19-8** SAM Splint for suspected pelvic fracture immobilization. *(SAM Medical Products, Portland, OR)*

quire specialized care to minimize morbidity and mortality. Recall that one fractured femur can be the source of nearly 1,500 mL of blood loss. While this volume alone may not cause cardiovascular collapse, other associated injuries may combine with a femur fracture to create hemodynamic instability. Hence, any femur fracture should be treated as potentially life threatening.

Splinting of a femur fracture is most easily performed with a traction splint, such as the Hare Traction Splint®, Sager Traction Splint®, or Kendrick Traction Device®. Additionally, the MAST/pneumatic anti-shock garment (PASG) might be utilized for initial stabilization of a femur fracture by 911 responders. While this approach can be effective as a splint, it is not without drawbacks, notably the limited assessment that can be done after the MAST are applied. Thus, careful evaluation of the injured leg must be done before application of the MAST. Further, the use of a simple air splint can stabilize many femur fractures, and is easy to apply. If the patient is to be evacuated by aircraft, both MAST/PASG and air splints should be closely monitored, because the pressure gradients associated with aviation can cause expansion of the air inside the splint.

Alternatively, a rod may be nailed through the distal end of the femur and a weight (i.e., sandbag) attached to this rod, and then hung off the edge of the bed, creating a gravity-induced traction. Whatever method is selected, the primary objective is to reduce pain, minimize soft-tissue injury, and maintain neurologic function and peripheral circulation. Later, surgical repair often requires placement of a rod.

The proximal portion of the femur is referred to as the hip and is often fractured, especially in elderly patients. Hip fractures are extremely debilitating. Emergency care includes treatment with immobilization, analgesia, and transport. Most hip fractures require open reduction and internal fixation, usually with metal pins and nails. Following surgery, early ambulation is usually possible.

The hip is a ball-and-socket joint consisting of the acetabulum and the proximal femur, 2 to 3 inches below the lesser trochanter. The incidence of hip fracture increases with age and doubles for every decade past the age of 50. The incidence is two to three times higher in women than men, primarily due to decreased bone density secondary to osteoporosis. Hip fractures are usually classified as extracapsular or intracapsular, depending on their location. With intracapsular fractures, the blood vessels supplying the femoral head are often compromised, which can lead to necrosis of the femoral head. The four types of intracapsular hip fractures are capital, subcapital, transcervical, and basicervical. (See Figure 19-9 ■.) Subcapital fractures are by far the most common type of intracapsular hip fracture. There are three types of extracapsular hip fractures: trochanteric, intertrochanteric, and subtrochanteric. Of these, intertrochanteric fractures are the most common. All hip fractures in ambulatory patients require open reduction and internal fixation in the operating room. Intracapsular fractures usually require replacement of the entire hip joint with a prosthetic hip and acetabulum. Most extracapsular fractures can be stabilized by placement of a surgical

Analgesia is essential to critical care transport of patients with multiple fractures.

An isolated hip fracture in an elderly person is often the first step in a downward spiral leading to loss of mobility, nursing home admission, and ultimately death.

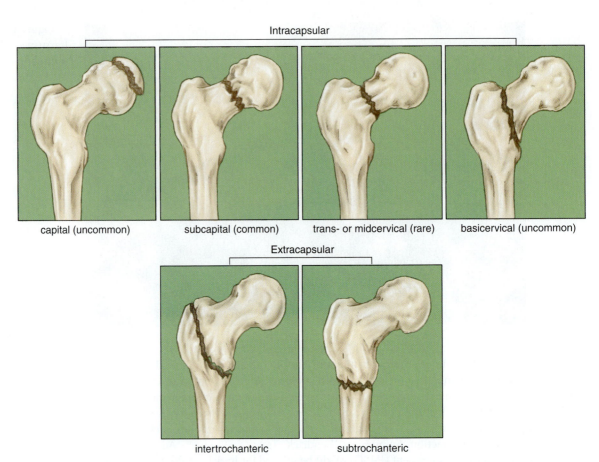

Intracapsular

capital (uncommon) subcapital (common) trans- or midcervical (rare) basicervical (uncommon)

Extracapsular

intertrochanteric subtrochanteric

■ Figure 19-9   Types of hip fractures. Subcapital and intertrochanteric fractures are the most common.

pin or nail to hold the bone segments in place while healing. As a rule, early fixation of hip fractures (<72 hours) in the elderly reduces morbidity and mortality.

VERTEBRAL FRACTURES

Perhaps no injury is as of much concern as a fracture to the vertebrae. These injuries have a very real potential to be catastrophic and, if improperly managed, may cause serious impairment, permanent disability, or death. Those spinal injuries that result in permanent impairment or disability contribute to other, long-term problems. Limb function may be diminished or absent, leading to skin ulcers, muscle atrophy, and infection. Lifestyle changes may need to be made, because the components of normal daily activity are no longer possible. Spinal injuries are also the cause of a large portion of health care expenditures, with the cost of treating an individual spinal injury reaching $1 million or more in a lifetime. Therefore, vertebral injuries warrant very close attention.

Trauma is the leading cause of vertebral injuries. It is estimated that between 15,000 and 20,000 spinal cord injuries occur annually. Most of these (48%) are from motor vehicle collisions, while falls, penetrating injuries, and sports injuries account for 21%, 15%, and 14%, respectively. More than 450 catastrophic injuries were reported in sports between the years of 1982 and 1994. Seventy-five percent of these were cervical spine injuries.

CERVICAL FRACTURES

A fracture to the cervical spine will be classified according to the specific vertebra involved. In 1982, Allen and colleagues introduced a comprehensive classification system of injuries. This classification system includes three common mechanisms: compression-flexion, distraction-flexion, and compression-extension. Vertical compression injury results in the burst-type injury with anterior column failure. C1, or atlas, fractures usually result from axial loading and rarely result in neurologic deficits. They can be described as anterior arch fractures, posterior arch fractures, lateral mass fractures, or a **Jefferson (burst) fracture.** Injuries to C2 also can occur. These fractures may be referred to as a "**hangman's fracture,**" and are easily seen on lateral C-spine radiographs. Neurologic injury usually does not occur unless a C2/C3 facet dislocation is present. There are four types of traumatic spondylolistheses of C2: Type I (nondisplaced or less than 3 mm of C2/C3 translation, no angulation of the fracture fragments), Type II (significant translation of more than 3 mm with angulation), and Type III (severe angulation and translation, often with dislocation of the facets of the vertebral body).

The other cervical vertebrae are equally at risk for injury. Most vertebral fractures fall into one of these categories: avulsion, compression, facet joint, vertebral burst, or teardrop fractures. An avulsion fracture will typically occur at the spinous process, and often requires nothing more than a soft cervical collar to provide comfort. Treatment of a compression fracture will vary depending on the severity of the fracture. Facet joint fractures occur as a result of disruption of the supraspinous ligaments, interspinous ligaments, *ligamentum flavum,* and facet capsule. Treatment of this type of fracture is rather controversial. Some experts advocate early and prompt reduction of the injury, despite the risk of further neurologic injury. Other experts suggest a more conservative approach, using various imaging techniques to evaluate the specifics of the injury, then performing reduction of the fracture if it can be safely done without exacerbating any neurologic deficit. Vertebral burst fractures are simply comminuted fractures of the middle vertebral body. Spinal cord injury is common with these fractures, as bony fragments are propelled into the cord. This type of fracture may require fusion of the bones. Finally, a **teardrop fracture** is identified by the presence of a displaced fracture of the antero-inferior corner of the superior body, segmental disk disruption, posterior ligament injury, and retropulsion of the proximal body into the neural canal. They are approached in much the same manner as a burst fracture.

THORACIC FRACTURES

Less common than cervical fractures, injuries of the thoracic vertebrae comprise a significant portion of spinal injuries. These injuries still have great potential for long-term neurologic deficits, and the primary goals of treatment for thoracic spine fractures include protecting the neural elements and preventing deformity and instability. The choice of surgical or nonsurgical treatment depends on several factors, including extent of injury, neurologic defects, resultant kyphosis ("hunchback"), and comorbid factors (multisystem injuries, age, general health, and so on). Thoracic vertebrae fractures are classified much the same way as cervical fractures, with the Denis system most commonly used: (1) primarily axial load injuries including compression and burst fractures, (2) flexion-distraction injuries, and (3) fracture subluxation and/or dislocation. The majority of thoracic vertebrae injuries can be seen on either plain radiographs or CT scan film.

LUMBAR SPINE FRACTURES

The lumbar vertebrae are the largest of all the vertebrae, and this size gives them great strength. In the absence of bone disease, a fractured lumbar vertebra indicates a significant impact force. Falls from heights, motor vehicle collisions, and auto-pedestrian impacts are the most common causes of lumbar injury, and associated injuries are common, especially pelvic fractures and thoracic spine injuries. Rarely, a fall where the patient lands on the buttocks can transfer the impact force up the entire length of the spine and cause a concussion.

Similar to cervical and thoracic fractures, lumbar vertebral fractures are classified to provide a standard descriptor system. Since lumbar fractures are almost exclusively of a compression nature, the **Denis system** is extrapolated and applied to the lumbar vertebrae:

Type A—involvement of both endplates

Type B—involvement of the superior endplate

Type C—involvement of the inferior endplate

Type D—buckling of the anterior cortex with both endplates intact

Jefferson (burst) fracture *vertebral fractures normally associated with spinal compression injury, as in anterior arch, posterior arch, and lateral mass fractures.*

hangman's fracture *injury and fracture of the C2 vertebral body; usually without obvious neurological deficit, unless a C2–C3 facet dislocation is present.*

teardrop fracture *displaced fracture of the antero-inferior corner of the superior vertebral body, with segmental disc disruption, posterior ligament injury, and retropulsion of the proximal body into the neural canal.*

Denis system *method most commonly used to describe lumbar vertebral fractures.*

Further, a burst fracture is possible, and these typically result from an extreme hyperflexion of the spine. Treatment of lumbar fractures depends greatly on the extent and degree of the fracture. Compromise of the spinal canal greater than 40%, kyphosis greater than 25 degrees, or neurologic compromise will typically require surgical intervention to fuse the vertebrae. For additional information on spinal injuries see Chapter 14.

HUMERUS FRACTURES

The humerus is classified as a long bone, and may be a source of significant hemorrhage when fractured. Much like the femur, 750 mL of blood loss may not seem significant until combined with other sources of bleeding; taken in total, this may be enough to cause hemorrhagic shock. The prudent paramedic will address a fractured humerus promptly, thus preventing or mitigating this possible complication.

Humerus fractures are classified using the simple method of location and type of fracture (i.e., complete midshaft oblique fracture). There is a growing trend toward further subclassification, depending on the general location. Proximal humerus and distal humerus can be further subdivided. Proximal humerus fractures have been classified as early as 1970 by Neer, and are described as nondisplaced, two-part, three-part, or four-part fractures. Distal humerus fractures, while quite rare in adults, can be described as single-column or bicolumn fractures. The most common distal humerus fracture seen in children is the supracondylar fracture. (See Figure 19-10 ■.) These fractures often require immediate care because of possible vascular and neurologic compromise. In children, supracondylar fractures can involve the growth plate resulting in a growth deformity.

The treatment in the emergent setting primarily focuses on splinting and application of traction. For humerus fractures, overhead traction is typically the best option. Later, definitive treatment will consist of either rigid casting or surgical repair. For humeral shaft fractures, closed treatment with a cast will nearly always result in 90% to 100% union of the fracture. ORIF may be required for more extensive fractures, such as a comminuted or severely displaced fracture.

RIB FRACTURES

The rib cage performs remarkably well in its function of protecting the organs within the thoracic cavity, but these bones are just as susceptible to injury and fracture as any other. One of the primary concerns with rib fractures is that of pulmonary injury and ventilatory compromise. The pain associated with a rib fracture may preclude the patient from full volume inhalation, leading to decreased ventilation and gas exchange. Further, a fractured rib may displace and cause direct pulmonary injury, such as a pneumothorax. Lower rib fractures can also cause liver or spleen injury,

■ Figure 19-10
Supracondylar fracture. These have a high incidence of associated nervous and vascular tissue injury. In children, some supracondylar fractures can involve the growth plate, possibly leading to permanent deformity or disability.

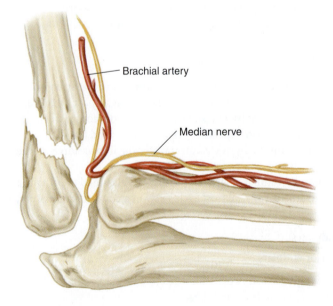

Brachial artery

Median nerve

with the potential for serious hemorrhage. Finally, a fracture of the first rib carries a 30% association of aortic injury.

Rare is the rib fracture that requires intervention beyond adequate analgesia for pain. Plating of rib fractures has fallen out of favor, and rib belts or other devices once used to restrict movement of the thoracic cage have been shown to have deleterious effects on the pulmonary system, and are associated with a higher incidence of atelectasis, pneumonia, and ARDS, a poorly understood and frequently fatal complication of trauma.

Since rib fractures may cause pneumothorax, hemothorax, or tension pneumothorax, careful assessment of the chest and thorax is of vital importance. Significant pulmonary injury should be evident on physical examination, and the health care provider should not delay treatment to obtain a chest X-ray. Treatment of a pneumothorax, hemothorax, or tension pneumothorax is straightforward, and well covered in the chapter on thoracic injuries.

As discussed in Chapter 15, the appropriate and effective administration of analgesia for a noncomplicated rib fracture will promote normal inhalation, reducing the potential for further complications.

AMPUTATIONS

Amputation of an extremity, from a foot or finger, to a hand, arm, or leg, can be an eye-catching injury. It is easy, even for experienced providers, to focus on the amputated part and fail to treat other, more urgent injuries. In the event of an amputated body part, the paramedic should remember that life takes precedence over limb, and that close attention should be paid to the ABCs before any treatment of arms and legs begins. Once the ABCs are stable, the amputation can be given due attention.

The treatment of a traumatic amputated extremity is straightforward in the prehospital setting. The stump of the injury should be bandaged with a clean, sterile, moist dressing, and if there is significant bleeding, it should be managed with direct pressure, elevation if possible, and the use of a pressure point. The amputated part should be gently cleansed with Ringer's lactate, then wrapped in sterile gauze moistened with Ringer's lactate. Place the amputated part in a plastic bag, and transport it in a box or container filled with ice. The body part should not be placed directly on the ice, nor placed on dry ice. Transport the amputated body part along with the patient to the hospital. In the event that the amputated part is not immediately found, do not delay transport of the patient to look for the amputated part. Instead, the local law enforcement agency, fire department, or other emergency responders can stay behind and look for the body part while EMS transports the patient.

PULSELESS EXTREMITY

A fracture to an arm or leg has a high chance of causing vascular damage. If the fracture causes enough vascular compromise, distal circulation may be impaired, resulting in the loss of peripheral pulses. For a pulseless extremity, it may be possible to reduce the fracture or realign the extremity in an attempt to restore adequate circulation. The decision to reduce or not to reduce requires good judgment, a complete physical exam, careful consideration of all other factors involved, and sufficient skill in the technique of reduction and realignment. In the event that transport time is short, and the circulation is compromised but still intact, it may be best to splint, transport, and leave the reduction for the more skilled physician. Conversely, if transport time is long, and the distal circulation is absent, then realignment or reduction may be warranted.

In many cases, simple repositioning of the injured extremity may be enough to restore adequate circulation. If this is successful, a splint should then be applied to prevent further movement, pulse location and quality recorded, and frequent reassessment performed. Adequate analgesia, along with possible diazepam to facilitate muscle relaxation, can be helpful and will make the treatment less painful for the patient.

If the orthopedic injury is a dislocation that has caused vascular compromise, the treatment will depend on the exact injury. Easily reduced dislocations include the ankle, patella, elbow, and fingers. More difficult to reduce are the knee and elbow, while a hip dislocation is often possible only under deep sedation or general anesthesia. Local protocol and experience will dictate which of these dislocations can be done by the paramedic, and which should be left for physician intervention.

COMPARTMENT SYNDROME

A potential complication of orthopedic injuries, compartment syndrome is a critical finding, requiring prompt intervention for the best outcome. First described by Volkman in the 1880s, compartment syndrome is ischemia of soft tissues in the compartments of extremities. While this is usually found as a result of a single traumatic incident, it can also result from prolonged and repetitive injury. The exact pathophysiology behind compartment syndrome is still a matter of some controversy and debate, but the most commonly accepted theory is that the buildup of fluid in a compartment is a result of vascular permeability changes due to the inflammatory response. This change in vascular permeability allows shifting of fluid from the intravascular space to the interstitial space, or compartment. Compartment syndrome can result from isolated fracture, crush injury, internal bleeding of an extremity, or from repeated stress (i.e., frequent long-distance running).

The clinical picture is, unfortunately, rather vague and nonspecific for compartment syndrome. The most common reported symptom is a feeling of fullness or tightness in the leg (or arm). The Six Ps discussed under Assessment (pain, pallor, paralysis, pulselessness, pressure, and paresthesia) may be present, but these are typically late findings, and the lack of these clinical signs should not be used to rule out compartment syndrome. Once the Six Ps are found, the compartment syndrome has been present for some time, and the chances of full recovery are reduced. Muscle necrosis has been reported after only 4 hours of compartment pressures of 50 mmHg, or in as little as 6 hours with pressures of 40 mmHg. Obviously, early recognition is the key to treatment of compartment syndrome. Internal compartment pressures can be measured via any number of commercial devices, but a transducer connected to a catheter is the easiest and most common method.

Frequently, chronic compartment syndrome (and, to a lesser extent, mild cases of acute compartment syndrome) can be treated conservatively with rest, ice, elevation, nonsteroidal anti-inflammatory drugs, and physical therapy. In more serious cases, however, surgical intervention—a fasciotomy—is needed to release the buildup of pressure within the inured extremity. For such cases, an orthopedic surgery specialist should be consulted.

PHARMACOLOGY

During the course of treating an orthopedic injury or disease, various pharmacologic agents are used for the treatment of pain, inflammation, infection, and thrombus. The critical care paramedic should have a working knowledge of the properties of these medications, including indications, contraindications, pharmacokinetics, pharmacodynamics, side effects, and dosing. Generally, the medications used will fall into one of several categories: nonsteroidal anti-inflammatory drugs (NSAIDs), opiate analgesics, antibiotics, muscle relaxants, or anticoagulants.

NSAIDS

Nonsteroidal anti-inflammatory drugs play a fundamental role in the treatment of orthopedic injuries. The role of NSAIDs is to decrease inflammation, thereby reducing the cause of pain felt by the patient. While narcotics are often used to treat "breakthrough" pain, NSAIDs work on the fundamental cause of the pain. Hence, patients are commonly given a combination of an NSAID and a narcotic analgesic.

NSAIDs promote healing by mitigating the inflammatory response that accompanies acute injury, though the exact action of each NSAID is different. Ibuprofen, for example, inhibits prostaglandin synthesis, while ketorolac's primary mechanism of action is inhibition of cyclooxygenase activity. The specifics of each NSAID can be obtained from a variety of reference materials, including a *Physicians' Desk Reference* (PDR) or other medical drug reference.

NSAIDs are generally safe for most patients, but select groups will need special considerations. Patients who have aspirin sensitivity should be given NSAIDs with caution, due to the potential for cross-reactivity, increased risk of bronchospasm, and higher incidence of anaphylaxis. NSAIDs should also be used with caution in any patient who has a history of peptic ulcer disease, renal failure or insufficiency, coagulopathies, congestive heart failure, or uncontrolled hypertension. Patients who take ACE (angiotensin-converting enzyme) inhibitors should not be given NSAIDs, because the combination may precipitate renal failure and acute hypercalcemia in patients with congestive heart failure or renal disease.

Some of the NSAIDs used for orthopedic injury include ibuprofen, naproxen, ketoprofen, ketorolac, and aspirin. Acetaminophen, while not technically an NSAID, is included in this category, because it has indications and actions more similar to NSAIDs than any other category.

OPIATE ANALGESICS

Opiate analgesics, or narcotic analgesics, form the second pillar of the treatment of pain in the orthopedic patient. As mentioned in the previous section, NSAIDs work on the cause of the pain, while narcotics treat pain levels that exceed that controlled by the NSAIDs.

All opiates have similar properties for pain control. The interaction with the opiate receptor sites—specifically the μ (mu) receptors—in the terminal neurons, hypothalamus, and thalamus provides pain relief. This abundance of opiate receptor sites provides the caregiver a wide variety of options for narcotic pain relief.

Narcotic medications have the potential for serious side effects, including respiratory depression, hypotension, nausea, vomiting, decreased gastrointestinal motility, sedation, euphoria, and physical dependence. The majority of these side effects can be easily controlled with careful and controlled administration of the narcotic.

Common narcotic medications utilized in critical care of orthopedic injuries include morphine sulfate, hydrocodone, fentanyl, oxycodone, and hydromorphone.

ANTIBIOTICS

Infection is a common occurrence in patients with open fractures, extensive soft-tissue trauma, or those who have sustained multisystem trauma. Antimicrobial therapy is indicated to promote healing of tissue, prevent sepsis, and enhance new cell formation. The specific antibiotic agent used depends greatly on the specific bacteria strain causing the infection. There are, however, a few generalities regarding antibiotic therapy.

Cephalosporins comprise the most frequently used class of antibiotics used in orthopedic injuries. Cephalosporins consist of three broad categories, including first generation, second generation, and third generation. The differences between the generations are primarily based on which organisms they inhibit. Other classes of antibiotic medications include penicillin, penicillin derivatives, and sulfonamides. A full discussion of cephalosporins or other antibiotics can be found in numerous texts.

Some of the most common antibiotics used in critical care of orthopedic injuries include amoxicillin, cephalexin, cefazolin, gentamicin, and vancomycin. As with any other medication, a thorough review of current medications and allergies to medications is essential to prevent any allergic reaction from antibiotics.

MUSCLE RELAXANTS

Orthopedic injuries in general, and fractures in particular, often cause spasm of the musculature surrounding the injured site. This spasm can exacerbate the pain of the fracture, and inhibit recovery. Hence, the use of muscle relaxants is frequently indicated as part of a treatment plan.

Muscle relaxants may cause side effects including hypotension, respiratory depression, drowsiness, sedation, or somnolence, especially when used in conjunction with opiates. Benzodiazapines (primarily Valium), cyclobenzaprine (Flexeril), and carisoprodol (Soma) are the most commonly used muscle relaxants.

ANTICOAGULANTS

Deep venous thrombosis (DVT) and pulmonary embolus are potentially life-threatening situations that may occur with orthopedic injury or invasive orthopedic procedures (nailing, internal fixation, and so on). The prevention of DVT requires close monitoring of hemodynamic status, coagulation factors, patient status, and consideration of all contributing factors (including obesity, cigarette smoking, age, prolonged immobilization, and oral contraceptive use).

Prophylactic use of anticoagulants is frequently employed to mitigate the possibility of clot formation or DVT. Choices for anticoagulation include aspirin, warfarin (Coumadin), heparin, and low-molecular-weight heparin (LMWH.) All anticoagulants must be monitored for effectiveness by routine testing of the prothrombin time (PT), partial thromboplastin time (PTT), and International Normalized Ratio (INR).

Aspirin is a mainstay in anticoagulant therapy, inhibiting platelet aggregation by binding and deactivating cyclooxygenase. This, in turn, blocks the production of thromboxane, and without thromboxane, platelets cannot aggregate into a clot. Standard dosing of aspirin is 325 to 1,200 mg orally every day, with close attention to the coagulation lab results.

Warfarin (Coumadin) is one of the most frequently used anticoagulants in orthopedics, specifically for DVT prophylaxis following knee or hip arthroplasty. Warfarin acts on the clotting cascade by limiting the proteins that are dependent on vitamin K. Prothrombin, Factor VII, Factor IX, Factor X, Protein C, and Protein S, all crucial aspects of the clotting cascade, are inhibited, thus reducing the risk of coagulation. Note that due to the various half-lives of these proteins, it is possible to encounter a hypercoagulable stage during the first 72 to 96 hours of warfarin use.

Standard heparin binds to anti-thrombin III, and this bond causes the anti-thrombin III to become more active. Anti-thrombin is an endogenous inhibitor of the coagulation cycle, and when combined with heparin, coagulation Factors II-a and X-a are inhibited to a greater degree, providing anticoagulation. The effects of heparin must be closely monitored, and this is best achieved by following PTT levels. Another risk of standard heparin is heparin-induced thrombocytopenia.

Low-molecular-weight heparin is rapidly gaining popularity in the treatment of orthopedic injury. LMWH is derived from standard heparin, but functions in a vastly different manner. LMWH permits Factor IIa to function, thus allowing localized hemostasis, yet it inhibits Factor Xa, the clotting factor responsible for large thrombosis formation. While this selective inhibition of coagulation is beneficial in many patients, it is not without risk. LMWH is injected via the subcutaneous route, and is not as easily titrated as IV heparin infusions. Conversely, however, LMWH has less chance of causing heparin-induced thrombocytopenia, and does not require the close scrutiny of PT/PTT and INR results.

ROENTGENOGRAM/X-RAY EVALUATION

roentgenogram *X-ray; the primary imaging method for orthopedic injuries.*

The **roentgenogram,** or X-ray, is the primary imaging method for orthopedic injuries. Despite major advances in other imaging technologies, including MRI and CT scan, the "plain film" X-ray still holds the distinction of the most used image in medicine. To properly evaluate an X-ray, a systemic approach must be applied, and careful scrutiny of the film is essential.

It is important to recognize that reading an X-ray is much like any other skill: It takes years of practice and repetition to become proficient. Minute details that appear obvious to an experienced orthopedic surgeon may not even appear to a novice. For this reason, the paramedic is urged to take every opportunity to look at various X-rays, applying the approach taught here. Further, it should be understood that different X-rays require different approaches. A chest film, for example, may be evaluated differently than a pelvic film. The following guidelines are thus general concepts, and much flexibility is allowed the paramedic in the reading of X-ray films.

To "read" an X-ray, the paramedic first needs to know several key components: What body part is being shown? What angle or perspective—anterior, posterior, lateral, and so forth—does the X-ray film show? What are the potential injuries to this body part that will appear on the film? Of those injuries, which are the highest priorities?

The practical application of these questions is obvious: It makes little sense to scrutinize a chest X-ray for a minor rib fracture before looking for a hemothorax or a widened mediastinum. Placing a chest tube on the wrong side of the chest would further complicate this error. A femur X-ray can reveal arthritis of the knee, but this is of little consequence when a comminuted fracture of the shaft is missed.

Once these primary questions are answered, apply a systematic approach to evaluating the X-ray picture. Observe the bones, and look for smoothness of the contours. An irregularity of a bone should raise the suspicion of a fracture. Look at the joints involved, and determine the quality of the articulating area. Check for symmetry, if possible, by comparing both sides of the X-ray. Rib fractures are easily observed in this manner. Irregularities of spacing should be noted as well. A normal X-ray will have smooth contours of the bones, with clear articulation of the joints, and a symmetrical appearance, with regular and equal spacing of bones, compared bilaterally. In a chest X-ray, look closely for evidence of a pneumothorax, hemothorax, or widened mediastinum, and evaluate the upper chest for signs of tracheal damage. Soft-tissue injury is often visible on an X-ray, and any evidence of soft-tissue injury should raise questions about the integrity of the bone below.

The better the prehospital treatment of orthopedic injuries, the better the ultimate outcome.

Summary

Orthopedic injuries are a common aspect of patient care for the critical care paramedic. The ability to provide assessment, treatment, and intervention of serious orthopedic injuries should be within the scope of any individual providing acute critical medical treatment. While most orthopedic injuries are not life threatening, there are several fractures that may create or exacerbate life threats, and these injuries should be addressed promptly in the course of patient care. Having a current and functional knowledge of orthopedics will provide a critical care paramedic with the ability to make the appropriate interventions in a timely fashion, reducing morbidity and mortality from orthopedic injury.

Review Questions

1. Discuss the incidence and costs of orthopedic injuries in medicine.
2. Briefly describe the various classifications of fractures.
3. Describe the Tscherne and Gustilo grading system for open fractures.
4. Discuss the implications of fractures involving the growth plate.
5. Describe the Salter-Harris classification system.
6. Describe treatment modalities for orthopedic injuries.
7. List critical fractures that may be seen during critical care transport.
8. Discuss pharmacologic management of orthopedic injuries.

See Answers to Review Questions at the back of this book.

Further Reading

Alexander BH, Rivara FP, Wolf ME. "The Cost and Frequency of Hospitalization for Fall-Related Injuries in Older Adults." *American Journal of Public Health,* Vol. 82, No. 7 (1992): 1020–1023.

Allen BL, Ferguson RL, Lehmann TR, et al. "A Mechanistic Classification of Closed, Indirect Fractures and Dislocations of the Lower Cervical Spine." *Spine,* Vol. 7 (1982) 7: 1–27.

Aluisio FV, Christensen CP, Urbaniak JR. *Orthopedics,* 2nd ed. Philadelphia: Williams & Wilkins, 1998.

Bell AJ, Talbot-Stern JK, Hennessy A. "Characteristics and Outcomes of Older Patients Presenting to the Emergency Department after a Fall: A Retrospective Analysis." *Medical Journal of Australia,* Vol. 173, No. 4 (2000): 176–177.

Cooper C, Campion G, Melton LJ. "Hip Fractures in the Elderly: A Worldwide Projection." *Osteoporosis International,* Vol. 2, No. 6 (1992): 285–289.

Englander F, Hodson TJ, Terregrossa RA. "Economic Dimensions of Slip and Fall Injuries." *Journal of Forensic Science,* Vol. 41, No. 5 (1996): 733–746.

Holmes JF, Miller PQ, Panacek EA, et al. "Epidemiology of Thoracolumbar Spine Injury in Blunt Trauma." *Academic Emergency Medicine,* Vol. 8, No. 9 (September 2001): 866–872.

Martini FH, Bartholomew EF, Bledsoe BE. *Anatomy and Phsyiology for Emergency Care.* Upper Saddle River, NJ: Pearson Prentice Hall, 2002.

National Center for Injury Prevention and Control, Centers for Disease Control and Prevention. http://www.cdc.gov/ncipc/wisqars (accessed 2001). *Web-Based Injury Statistics Query and Reporting System (WISQARS)* [database].

Pape HC, et al. "Changes in the Management of Femoral Shaft Fractures in Polytrauma Patients: From Early Total Care to Damage Control Orthopedic Surgery." *Journal of Trauma,* Vol. 53, No. 3 (September, 2002): 452–461, discussion 461–462.

Praemer A, Furner S, Rice DP. *Musculoskeletal Conditions in the United States.* Rosemont, IL: American Academy of Orthopaedic Surgeons, 1999.

Scott JC. "Osteoporosis and Hip Fractures." *Rheumatic Diseases Clinics of North America,* Vol. 16, No. 3 (1990): 717–740.

Sterling DA, O'Connor JA, Bonadies J. "Geriatric Falls: Injury Severity Is High and Disproportionate to Mechanism." *Journal of Trauma: Injury, Infection, and Critical Care,* Vol. 50, No. 1 (2001): 116–119.

Tinsworth D, McDonald J. *Special Study: Injuries and Deaths Associated with Children's Playground Equipment.* Washington, DC: U.S. Consumer Product Safety Commission, 2001.

Wilkins K. "Healthcare Consequences of Falls for Seniors." *Health Reports,* Vol. 10, No. 4 (1999): 47–55.

Special Patients: Pediatric, Geriatric, and Obstetrical Trauma

Larry D. Johnson, NREMT-P

Objectives

Upon completion of this chapter, the student should be able to:

1. Discuss and detail the epidemiology of the following:
   A. Pediatric trauma patients (p. 545)
   B. Geriatric trauma patients (p. 565)
   C. Obstetrical trauma patients (p. 572)
2. Examine important aspects of interaction with the critically ill child and family that will enhance interventions. (p. 547)
3. Analyze developmental aspects that necessitate the modification of physical assessment parameters and intervention techniques for the pediatric patient. (p. 549)
4. Identify the components of the initial patient assessment that can be done during a visual examination of the pediatric patient. (p. 552)
5. List the pertinent information that the critical care paramedic should obtain from the sending facility regarding special patients. (p. 552)
6. Identify goals of therapy that maximize oxygen delivery and minimize oxygen demand in the pediatric patient. (p. 554)
7. Discuss the difference between oxygenation and ventilation. (p. 555)
8. Identify normal values pertaining to the pediatric patient for the following:
   A. Vital signs for infants and children (p. 557)
   B. Continuous intracranial pressure (p. 562)

9. Discuss and apply the modified GCS for infants. (p. 558)
10. Identify the three components that influence the rise in intracranial pressure. (p. 562)
11. Identify actions that are recommended to reestablish chest tube patency. (p. 563)
12. Discuss system pathophysiology and organ system decline as it pertains to the geriatric patient in relation to the:
    A. Respiratory system (p. 566)
    B. Cardiovascular system (p. 567)
    C. Renal system (p. 568)
    D. Nervous system (p. 568)
    E. Musculoskeletal system (p. 568)
13. Discuss age-related changes in sensation in the elderly. (p. 567)
14. Discuss considerations in trauma care of the elderly patient. (p. 568)
15. Discuss transport considerations and management of:
    A. Pediatric patients (p. 561)
    B. Geriatric patients (p. 571)
    C. Obstetrical patients (p. 575)
16. Identify and discuss the physiological changes during pregnancy. (p. 573)
17. Identify the most common post-traumatic condition that the critical care paramedic might encounter. (p. 573)
18. Discuss the effects of disruption of normal uterine and fetal physiology during critical care transport. (p. 573)

Key Terms

Case Study

You are dispatched as the safety officer to support a high-risk obstetrical team on an interfacility transport. The weather has been bad and the pilot says a flight is a no-go and the decision is made to retrieve the patient by ground ambulance.

The patient is an 18-year-old female, $G_1P_0Ab_0$, who at 30 weeks' gestation was involved in a motor vehicle collision. She was the restrained driver of a small foreign pickup struck on the driver's side. She was wearing a seat belt, but an air bag was not on the vehicle or not deployed based on the angle of the collision. The patient was transported to the local community hospital where she was evaluated by the obstetrician on call after being cleared of other injuries by the emergency physician. The patient had not had any prior prenatal care although she remembers precisely the date of her last menstrual period.

The travel time to the hospital is approximately 1 hour. Upon arrival, the OB nurse/respiratory therapist team members begin their assessment of the patient. While they are assessing the patient, you review the chart. An ultrasound revealed a small placental abruption. Also, the patient was having some contractions. A Level II sonogram revealed a normal fetus with a gestational age of 30 ±1.5 weeks. The placental abruption was noted and estimated at approximately 10%. The patient is being transferred to a university hospital in case the labor cannot be stopped and neonatal intensive care is required.

The patient is moved to the stretcher and to the ambulance. A fetal monitor is in place. You hear good beat-to-beat variability in the heart rate and there is an occasional uterine contraction. No decelerations are noted. The patient has an infusion of magnesium sulfate running and is taking ritodrine (Yutopar) orally as a tocolytic. She has received a dose of steroid to promote fetal lung maturity. No vaginal bleeding is noted.

The transport is uneventful and you catch up on some reading while the OB team cares for the patient. The patient is admitted to the hospital. The tocolytics are successful in suppressing labor and the fetus remains well. The patient is kept on bed rest at the hospital and gives birth to a healthy baby boy at 36 week's gestation. No neonatal intensive care is required and mother and baby go home together 3 days after delivery.

INTRODUCTION

Because of physiological and anatomical factors, trauma can affect different persons and different patient populations in different ways. In this chapter, we will discuss the effects of trauma on certain frequently encountered patient populations: pediatrics, geriatrics, and obstetrics.

Part 1: Pediatric Trauma

INTRODUCTION

Occasionally, the critical care paramedic will be called on to transfer a critically ill or injured child from one facility to another, frequently from a smaller outlying facility to a larger specialty care facility. Critical care transport of the ill or injured child presents a challenge for the critical care paramedic. The care of an ill or injured child requires an incisive assessment, with excellent patient management skills. It cannot be overemphasized that the margin of error, in both time and intervention, can be extremely narrow with the pediatric patient. A child's cardiovascular, pulmonary, and neurologic systems often operate with little physiological reserve. Decompensation must be anticipated whenever the child is severely ill or injured. Anticipation, assessment, and correction of airway problems are critical.

EPIDEMIOLOGY OF PEDIATRIC TRAUMA

Injuries are the leading cause of death and disabilities in children and adolescents older than 1 year. According to the **National Pediatric Trauma Registry (NPTR),** trauma kills more children than all other diseases combined. Annually in children and adolescents, trauma is responsible for approximately 25,000 deaths, more than 500,000 hospitalizations, and 16 million emergency department visits, at a cost of over $7.5 billion. More than 30,000 children will have permanent disabilities because of injuries to the brain. Blunt trauma accounts for approximately 85% of all injuries.

National Pediatric Trauma Registry (NPTR) *organization that monitors and tracks annual statistical figures related to injuries and deaths in children and adolescents.*

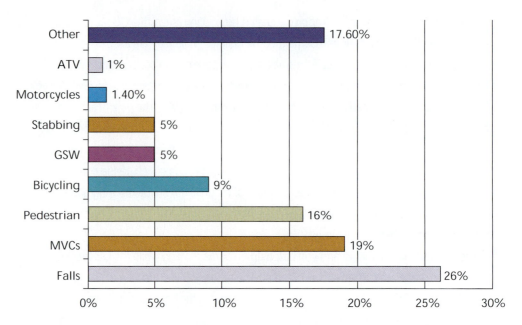

Figure 20-1 Pediatric trauma by type of injury. *(CDC, Atlanta, GA)*

FALLS

According to the NPTR, falls are the single most common cause of injuries in children. A child's gross motor skills and balance are incompletely developed, contributing to falls. Infants and children have little concept of those activities that may be harmful to them, and are unaware of their limitations. Falls among young children are often from furniture such as couches or cribs or they may fall down stairs in walkers. (See Figure 20-1 ■.)

MOTOR VEHICLE COLLISIONS

Another major mechanism and the largest cause of traumatic deaths and permanent brain injuries are motor vehicle-related collisions. Car versus child pedestrian injuries are more common in cities where children play close to the street. Auto-pedestrian injuries are a particularly lethal form of trauma in children, because their short stature tends to push them down under the car. The implementation of children's car seats has decreased the fatality rate associated with motor vehicle collisions (MVCs). Used correctly, child safety seats are 71% effective in reducing infant deaths in passenger cars and 54% effective in reducing toddler deaths. They reduce the need for hospitalization by 69%. However, despite recent advancements in technology and education, the National Highway Traffic Safety Administration (NHTSA) recently reported that 51% of children younger than 5 years ride in vehicles unrestrained, and that 8 out of 10 child seats are misused. Counseling parents about the proper use of child seats and learning to detect and correct misuse will help save lives.

DROWNING AND NEAR-DROWNING

Drowning is the third leading cause of death in children between birth and 4 years of age, with approximately 2,000 deaths occurring in the United States annually. The term *drowning* is used to describe deaths that occur within 24 hours of the accident. Near-drowning refers to injuries where the child did not die or where the death occurred more than 24 hours after the injury. Many children who do not die from drowning suffer severe and irreversible brain injuries because of anoxia. Approximately 20% to 25% of near-drowning survivors exhibit severe neurologic deficits. The outcomes are better when the water is cold. In addition, the body's protective mechanisms protect against brain injury.

PENETRATING INJURIES

Until 20 years ago, penetrating injuries in children were uncommon. Since then, an increase in violent crime (although violent crime rates have both risen and fallen within that period) has resulted in an increasing number of children sustaining penetrating trauma. Stab wounds and firearm injuries account for approximately 10% to 15% of all pediatric trauma admissions. The risk of death increases with age. Children are usually innocent victims of crimes perpetrated against adults. However, children are sometimes the intended victims of gunfire and stabbings, as in the shootings that have taken place in schools. Homicide is the leading cause of death for young black males and the second leading cause of death for young Hispanic males in the United States. Homicide rates for young black and Hispanic males remain substantially higher than for their young non-Hispanic white male counterparts.

BURNS

Burn injuries are the leading cause of accidental death in the home for children under 14 years of age. Children can sustain both burn injuries and smoke inhalation in house fires. Unsupervised children with matches or cigarette lighters are responsible for many fires that result in pediatric injury. Fires kill about 500 children age 14 and under each year and injure approximately 40,000 other children. The majority of fire-related deaths (70%) are caused by smoke inhalation of the toxic gases produced by fires. Actual flames and burns only account for about 30% of fire-related deaths and injuries. The majority of fires that kill or injure children are residential fires. The majority of children ages 4 and younger who are hospitalized for burn-related injuries suffer from scald burns (65%) or contact burns (20%).

PHYSICAL ABUSE

Unfortunately, children are at risk for physical abuse by adults and older children. Factors leading to child abuse are known to include social phenomena such as poverty, domestic disturbances, younger-aged parents, substance abuse, and community violence. According to the American Academy of Pediatrics, each week, child protective services (CPS) agencies throughout the United States receive more than 50,000 reports of suspected child abuse or neglect. For example, in 2002 there were 2.6 million reports made concerning the welfare of approximately 4.5 million children. Of these, the information provided in the report was sufficient to prompt an assessment or investigation in approximately two-thirds of these cases. As a result of these investigations, approximately 896,000 children were found to have been victims of abuse or neglect—an average of more than 2,450 children per day. More than half (60%) of these victims experienced some form of neglect, meaning a caretaker failed to provide for the child's basic needs. Fewer victims experienced physical abuse (nearly 20%) or sexual abuse (10%), although these cases are more likely to be publicized. The smallest number (7%) was found to be victims of emotional abuse, which includes criticizing, rejecting, or refusing to nurture a child. In the United States, an average of nearly four children die every day as a result of child abuse or neglect.

GENERAL APPROACH TO PEDIATRIC TRAUMA

Children are not small adults.

The approach to the pediatric patient varies with the age of the patient and with the problem being treated. Foremost in approaching any pediatric emergency is consideration of the patient's emotional and physiological development. Care also involves the family members or caregivers responsible for the child. They will demand information, express fears, and, ultimately, give or refuse consent for treatment and/or transport.

COMMUNICATION AND PSYCHOLOGICAL SUPPORT

Children have small physiological reserves.

The signs and symptoms of physiological deterioration in a child can be subtle.

Treatment of an infant, child, or teenager begins with communication and psychological support. Interaction with pediatric patients and related adults continues throughout assessment, management, and transport. The parents are often the primary source of information, especially in the case of infants and young children. However, as children become older, they can also be a good source of information. Older children, for example, can often give accurate descriptions of symptoms or other details. Treat all pediatric patients with respect, allowing them to express opinions and ask questions. Your listening skills will play an important role in alleviating the fears of pediatric patients. You can even communicate a calm and caring attitude to infants, who respond to touch and voice just like any other human being.

RESPONDING TO PATIENT NEEDS

As previously mentioned, a child's response to an emergency will vary, depending on the age and emotional maturity of the child. The child's most common response to illness or injury is fear. Common fears of children include:

★ Fear of being separated from the parents or caregivers

★ Fear of being removed from a family place, such as home, and never returning

★ Fear of being hurt

★ Fear of being mutilated or disfigured

★ Fear of the unknown

These fears may be intensified if the child detects fear or anxiety from the parents or caregivers. The general chaos and panic that often surround pediatric emergencies may further distress the child. Remember that children have the right to know what is being done to them. You should be as honest as possible with them. If a procedure such as an IV needle stick will hurt, tell them so. Tell them immediately before performing a procedure. Do not say that a procedure will be painful and then take 5 minutes to prepare the equipment, allowing time for the child's anticipation of pain to build. Always use language that is appropriate for the age of the child. Medical and anatomical terms that we routinely use may be foreign to children. Telling a child that you are going to "apply an ECG electrode" means nothing. Instead, tell the child: "I'm going to put this funny sticky thing on you. Try to hold still." Communication such as this will involve children in their own care and reduce their feelings of helplessness.

RESPONDING TO PARENTS OR CAREGIVERS

As you might expect, the reaction of parents or caregivers to a critical care pediatric patient will vary. Initial reactions might include shock, grief, denial, anger, guilt, fear, or complete loss of control. Their behavior may change during the course of the transport. Communication is the key. Preferably, only one critical care paramedic will speak with the health care provider at the sending facility. This will avoid any chance of conflicting information and allow a second critical care paramedic to focus on the child. If parents or caregivers sense your confidence and professionalism, they will trust your suggestions for care. As with the child, most parents and caregivers feel overwhelmed by fear. They often express their fears in questions such as the following:

"Is my child going to die?"

"Did my child suffer brain damage?"

"Is my child going to be all right?"

"What are you doing to my child?"

"Will my child be able to walk?"

It may be difficult to answer these questions. However, the following actions may help allay parents' fears:

★ Tell them your name and qualifications.

★ Acknowledge their fears and concerns.

★ Reassure them that it is all right to feel the way they do.

★ Redirect their energies toward helping you care for the child.

★ Remain calm and appear in control of the transport.

★ Keep the parents or caregivers informed as to what you are doing.

★ Don't "talk down" to them.

★ Assure parents or caregivers that everything possible is being done for their child.

If conditions permit, you should allow one of the parents or caregivers to remain with the child at all times. Some family members may be extremely emotional in emergent situations. The child will react more positively to a family member who appears calm and reassuring. If a parent or caregiver is "out of control," have another person take him or her away from the immediate area to settle down.

GROWTH AND DEVELOPMENT

Children progress through developmental stages on their way to adulthood. You should tailor your approach to the developmental level of your pediatric patient, as discussed in the following sections.

NEWBORNS (FIRST HOURS AFTER BIRTH)

Although the terms *newborn* and *neonate* are often used interchangeably, *newborn* refers to a baby in the first hours of extrauterine life. The term *neonate* describes infants from birth to 1 month of age. The method most frequently used to assess newborns is the APGAR scoring system. (See Figure 20-2 ■.) Resuscitation of the newborn generally follows the inverted pyramid and the guidelines established in the neonatal advanced life support (NALS) curriculum.

NEONATES (AGES BIRTH TO 1 MONTH)

The neonate, as just noted, is an infant up to 1 month of age. This is a major stage of development. Soon after birth, the neonate typically loses up to 10% of its birth weight as it adjusts to extrauterine life. This lost weight, however, is ordinarily recovered within 10 days. Gestational age affects

APGAR Scoring			
APGAR Sign	2	1	0
Heart Rate (pulse)	Normal (above 100 beats per minute)	Below 100 beats per minute	Absent (no pulse)
Breathing (rate and effort)	Normal rate and effort	Slow or irregular breathing	Absent (no breathing)
Grimace (Responsiveness or "reflex irritability")	Pulls away, sneezes, or coughs with stimulation	Facial movement only (grimace) with stimulation	Absent (no response to stimulation)
Activity (muscle tone)	Active, spontaneous movement	Arms and legs flexed with little movement	No movement, "floppy" tone
Appearance (skin coloration)	Normal color all over (hands and feet are pink)	Normal color (but hands and feet are bluish)	Bluish-gray or pale all over

■ Figure 20-2 APGAR scoring.

early growth. Children born at term (40 weeks) should follow accepted developmental guidelines. Infants born prematurely will not be as developed, either neurologically or physically, as their term counterparts.

The neonatal stage of development centers on reflexes. The neonate's personality also begins to form. The infant is close to the mother and may stare at faces and smile. The mother, and occasionally the father, can comfort and quiet the child. Obviously, the history must be obtained from the parents or caregivers. However, it is also important to observe the child. Common illnesses in this age group include jaundice, vomiting, and respiratory distress. Serious illnesses, such as meningitis, are difficult to distinguish from minor illnesses in neonates. Often, fever is the only sign, although the majority of neonates with fever have minor illnesses (96% to 97%). The few that are seriously ill can be easily missed. For this reason, any fever in a neonate requires extensive evaluation.

The approach to this age group should include several factors. First, the child should always be kept warm. Observe skin color, tone, and respiratory activity. The absence of tears when crying may indicate dehydration. The lungs should be auscultated early during the exam, while the infant is quiet. You might find it helpful to have the child suck on a pacifier during the examination. Allowing the infant to remain in a parent's or caregiver's lap may help calm the child.

INFANTS (AGES 1 TO 5 MONTHS)

Infants should have doubled their birth weight by 5 to 6 months of age. They should be able to follow the movements of others with their eyes. Muscle control develops in a cephalocaudal progression. This means, literally, that development of muscular control begins at the head (cephalo) and moves toward the tail (caudal). Muscular control also spreads from the trunk toward the extremities during this period. The infant's personality at this stage still centers closely on the parents or caregivers. The history must be obtained from these individuals, with close attention to possible illnesses and accidents, including SIDS, vomiting, dehydration, meningitis, child abuse, and household accidents.

Concentrate on keeping these patients warm and comfortable. Allow the infant to remain in a parent's or caregiver's lap. A pacifier or bottle can be used to help keep the baby quiet during the examination.

INFANTS (AGES 6 TO 12 MONTHS)

Infants in this age group may stand or even walk with assistance. They are quite active and enjoy exploring the world with their mouths. In this stage of development, the risk of foreign body airway obstruction (FBAO) becomes a serious concern.

Infants 6 months and older have more fully formed personalities and express themselves more readily. They have considerable anxiety toward strangers. They do not like lying on their backs. Children in this age group tend to cling to the mother, though the father "will do" in many cases. Common illnesses and accidents include febrile seizures, vomiting, diarrhea, dehydration, bronchiolitis, car accidents, croup, child abuse, poisonings, falls, airway obstructions, and meningitis.

These children should be examined while sitting in the lap of the parent or caregiver. The exam should progress in a toe-to-head order, since starting at the face may upset the child. If time and conditions permit, allow the child to become familiar with you before beginning the examination.

TODDLERS (AGES 1 TO 3 YEARS)

Great strides occur in gross motor development during this stage. Children tend to run underneath or stand on almost everything. They seem to always be on the move. As they grow older, toddlers become braver and more curious or stubborn. They begin to stray away from the parents or caregivers more frequently. Yet, these remain the only people who can comfort them quickly, and most children will cling to a parent or caregiver if frightened.

At ages 1 to 3 years, language development begins. Often children can understand better than they can speak. Therefore, the majority of the medical history will still come from the parents or caregivers. Remember, however, that you can ask toddlers simple and specific questions.

Accidents of all types are the leading cause of injury deaths in pediatric patients ages 1 to 15 years. Common accidents in this age group include MVCs, homicides, falls, burn injuries, drowning, and pedestrian accidents. Common illnesses and injuries in the toddler age group include vomiting, diarrhea, febrile seizures, poisonings, child abuse, croup, and meningitis. Keep in mind that FBAO is still a high risk for toddlers.

Be cautious when treating toddlers. Approach toddlers slowly and try to gain their confidence. Conduct the exam in a toe-to-head order. The child may be difficult to examine and may resist being touched. Speak quietly and use only simple words. Avoid asking questions that allow the child to say "no." If the situation permits, allow toddlers to hold transitional objects such as a favorite blanket or toy. Be sure to tell the child if something will hurt. If possible, avoid procedures on the dominant arm and hand, which the child will try to pull away.

PRESCHOOLERS (AGES 3 TO 5 YEARS)

Children in this age group show a tremendous increase in fine and gross motor development. Language skills increase greatly. Children in this age group know how to talk. However, if frightened, they often refuse to speak, especially to strangers. They often have vivid imaginations and may see monsters as part of their world. Preschoolers may have tempers and will express them. During this stage of development, children fear mutilation and may feel threatened by treatment. Avoid frightening or misleading comments.

Preschoolers often run to a particular parent or caregiver, depending on the occasion. They stick up for the people they love and are openly affectionate. They still seek support and comfort from within the home.

When evaluating children in this age group, question the child first, keeping in mind that imagination may interfere with the facts. The child often has a distorted sense of time, and thus you must rely on the parents or caregivers to fill in the gaps. Common illnesses and accidents in this age group include croup, asthma, poisonings, MVC injuries, burns, child abuse, ingestion of foreign bodies, drowning, epiglottitis, febrile seizures, and meningitis.

Treatment of preschoolers requires tact. Avoid baby talk. If time and situation permit, give the child health care choices. Often the use of a doll or stuffed animal will assist in the examination. Allow the child to hold a piece of equipment, such as a stethoscope, and to use it. Let the child sit on your lap. Start the examination with the chest and evaluate the head last. Avoid misleading comments. Do not trick or lie to the child, and always explain what you are going to do.

SCHOOL-AGE CHILDREN (AGES 6 TO 12 YEARS)

Children in this age group are active and carefree. Growth spurts sometimes lead to clumsiness. The personality continues to develop. School-age children are protective and proud of their parents or caregivers and seek their attention. They value peers, but also need home support.

When examining school-age children, give them the responsibility of providing the history, if possible. However, remember that children may be reluctant to provide information if they sustained an injury while doing something forbidden. The parents or caregivers can fill in the pertinent details. When assessing children in this age group, it is important to respect their modesty. Be honest and tell the child what is wrong. A small toy may help to calm the child. Common illnesses and injuries for this age group include drowning, MVC injuries, bicycle accidents, falls, fractures, sports injuries, child abuse, and burns.

ADOLESCENTS (AGES 13 TO 18 YEARS)

Adolescence covers the period from the end of childhood to the start of adulthood (age 18). It begins with puberty, roughly age 13 for male children and age 11 for female children. (For this reason, adolescence is often defined as including ages 11 to 18, rather than 13 to 18.) Puberty is highly child specific and can begin at various ages. A female child, for example, may experience her first menstrual period as early as age 7 or 8.

Adolescents vary significantly in their development. Those over age 15 are physically nearer to adults in terms of their vital signs but emotionally may still be children. Regardless of physical maturity, remember that teenagers as a group are "body conscious." They worry about their physical image more than any other pediatric age group. You should tactfully address their stated concerns about body integrity or disfigurement. The slightest possibility of a lasting scar may be a tremendous issue to the adolescent patient.

Although patients in this age are not yet legally adults, most consider themselves to be grown up. They take offense at the use of the word *child*. They have a strong desire to be liked by their peers and to be included. Relationships with parents and caregivers may at times be strained as the adolescent demands greater independence. They value the opinions of other adolescents, especially members of the opposite sex. Generally, these patients make good historians. Do not be surprised, however, if their perception of events differs from that of their parents or caregivers.

Common illnesses and injuries in this age group include mononucleosis, asthma, MVC injuries, sports injuries, drug and alcohol problems, suicide gestures, and sexual abuse. Remember that pregnancy is also possible in female adolescents. When assessing teenagers, remember that their vital signs are similar to those of adults. In gathering a history, be factual and address the patient's questions. It may be wise to interview the patient away from the parents or caregivers. Listen to what the teenager is saying, as well as what he or she is not saying. If you suspect substance abuse or endangerment of the patient or others, approach the subject with tact and compassion. If you must perform a detailed physical exam, respect the teenager's sense of privacy. If the patient exhibits modesty or bodily shame, have a critical care paramedic of the same sex as the teenager conduct the examination, if possible. Regardless of the situation, provide psychological support and reassurance.

FACILITY ARRIVAL AND INITIAL TRAUMA ASSESSMENT

Once you enter the referring facility, ask to speak with the individual (usually a nurse) in charge of the patient. When obtaining the medical history of the pediatric patient, you should gather information such as:

★ Nurse/physician notes

★ Lab values

★ X-rays

★ Ventilator settings

★ Transfer orders (memorandum of transfer)

★ Nature of the illness/injury

★ Length of time the patient has been sick/injured

★ Presence of fever

★ Effects of the illness/injury on patient behavior

★ Bowel/urine habits

★ Presence of vomiting/diarrhea

★ Frequency of urination

When obtaining your report from the caregiver in charge make certain you understand and document all physician orders accurately.

When entering the patient's room do so without your equipment. This will help alleviate the patient's and parent's anxiety. Introduce yourself in a professional and caring manner. Hold a conversation with the parents and relatives within the child's view. Remember that in the eyes of your pediatric patient, you are an outsider. Win the parents' trust and confidence first before you make contact with the child.

Many components of the initial patient assessment can be done during a visual examination. A child's general appearance is extremely important. In most cases if a child "looks bad," he or she is bad. An excellent tool to refer to is the **pediatric assessment triangle (PAT).** (See Figure 20-3 ■.)

pediatric assessment triangle (PAT) *method assessment that uses appearance, breathing, and circulation status to determine a child's overall condition.*

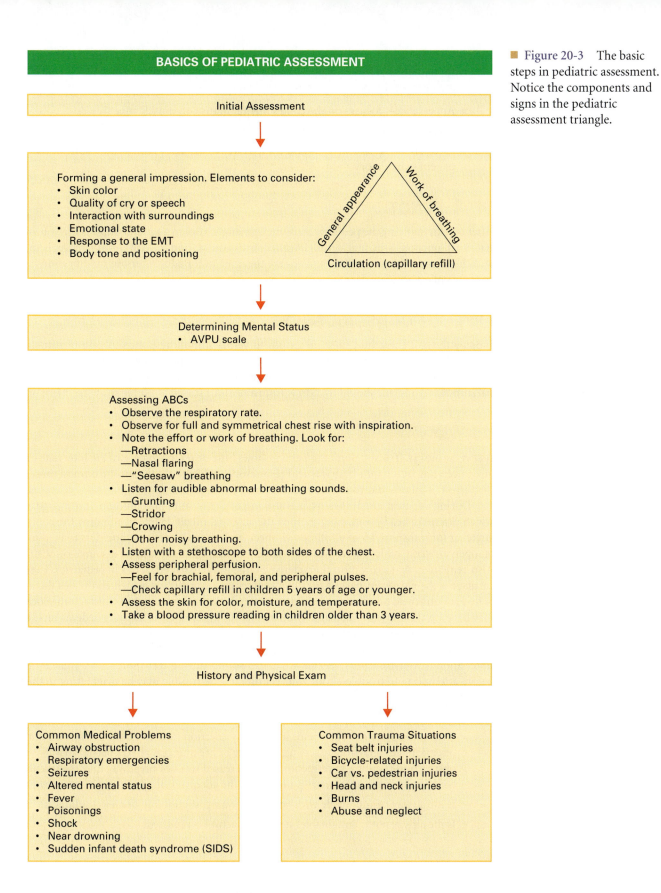

Figure 20-3 The basic steps in pediatric assessment. Notice the components and signs in the pediatric assessment triangle.

BASICS OF PEDIATRIC ASSESSMENT

Initial Assessment

Forming a general impression. Elements to consider:
- Skin color
- Quality of cry or speech
- Interaction with surroundings
- Emotional state
- Response to the EMT
- Body tone and positioning

General appearance

Work of breathing

Circulation (capillary refill)

Determining Mental Status
- AVPU scale

Assessing ABCs
- Observe the respiratory rate.
- Observe for full and symmetrical chest rise with inspiration.
- Note the effort or work of breathing. Look for:
  —Retractions
  —Nasal flaring
  —"Seesaw" breathing
- Listen for audible abnormal breathing sounds.
  —Grunting
  —Stridor
  —Crowing
  —Other noisy breathing.
- Listen with a stethoscope to both sides of the chest.
- Assess peripheral perfusion.
  —Feel for brachial, femoral, and peripheral pulses.
  —Check capillary refill in children 5 years of age or younger.
- Assess the skin for color, moisture, and temperature.
- Take a blood pressure reading in children older than 3 years.

History and Physical Exam

Common Medical Problems
- Airway obstruction
- Respiratory emergencies
- Seizures
- Altered mental status
- Fever
- Poisonings
- Shock
- Near drowning
- Sudden infant death syndrome (SIDS)

Common Trauma Situations
- Seat belt injuries
- Bicycle-related injuries
- Car vs. pedestrian injuries
- Head and neck injuries
- Burns
- Abuse and neglect

By utilizing the pediatric assessment triangle, you can form a rapid general impression of the patient without the use of a stethoscope, blood pressure cuff, pulse oximeter, or other medical devices. The triangle's three components are:

★ Appearance—focuses on the child's mental status and muscle tone

★ Breathing—directs attention to respiratory rate and respiratory effort

★ Circulation—uses skin signs and color as well as capillary refill as indicators of the patient's circulatory status

VITAL FUNCTIONS

After quickly applying the pediatric assessment triangle to form a general impression, you will evaluate vital functions—mental status (level of consciousness) and the ABCs—as they apply to infants and children. Although assessment steps are the same as for adults, certain modifications must be made to collect accurate data.

LEVEL OF CONSCIOUSNESS

Employ the AVPU method (alert, responds to verbal stimuli, responds to painful stimuli, unresponsive) to evaluate the pediatric patient's level of consciousness (LOC). Adjust the techniques for the child's age. With an infant, you may need to shout to elicit a response (perhaps crying) to verbal stimulus. An infant should withdraw from a noxious stimulus. Never shake an infant or child.

AIRWAY

Assess the airway. If at any point the patient shows little or no movement of air, intervene immediately. Keep this fact in mind: Airway and respiratory problems are the most common cause of cardiac arrest in infants and young children.

During a critical care transport, it is also important to note that children have a large occiput, which can make head positioning to open the airway difficult. While positioning the child on the stretcher for transport, place a roll (towel, sheet, and so on) under the shoulders to help maintain an open airway. Children have relatively large tongues; this may also be a source of obstruction. Also, remember that a common characteristic is the funnel-shaped larynx in pediatrics. The cricoid cartilage is the narrowest part of the child's upper airway anatomy, which eliminates the need for cuffed endotracheal tubes in small children. An endotracheal tube that fits through the vocal cords may hang up at the cricoid cartilage. The small radius means greater impact of edema on the cross-sectional area of airway, greater resistance to air flow, so a 1-mm layer of edema that may be well tolerated in an adult-sized airway can cause significant airway obstruction in a child. **Important note:** Should your transport ventilator's alarm sound during transport, *check your patient first* before attempting to trouble-shoot your ventilator. The trouble may be originating in the upper airway.

As you inspect the airway, ask yourself the following questions:

★ Is the airway patent? This seems like an easy question to answer, but this assessment is ofter skipped in favor of assessing adequacy of breathing. A child's partial airway obstruction resulting in retractions and increased work of breathing may mistakenly be judged to have pulmonary pathology if the adequacy of the airway is not assessed.

★ Is the airway maintainable with head positioning, suctioning, or airway adjuncts?

★ Is the airway not maintainable? If so, what action is required?

BREATHING

In assessing the breathing of a pediatric patient, recall the CPR certification courses in which you learned to "Look, Listen, and Feel." *Look* at the patient's chest and abdomen for movement. *Listen* for breath sounds—both normal and abnormal. *Feel* for air movement at the patient's mouth.

Is the breathing adequate? This is often a more important assessment and certainly a more difficult assessment than simply establishing whether a child is breathing. Children frequently require intervention even if a respiratory rate is present, due to inadequacy of breathing or fatigue with risk of respiratory failure.

To simplify discussion, breathing can be thought of as providing two separate functions, oxygenation and ventilation. Both can be judged as to their adequacy in an ill child.

OXYGENATION

Clinical findings can be used to judge adequacy of oxygenation:

★ *Color.* Check nail beds, lips, and tongue for evidence of cyanosis.

★ *Oxygen saturation measurement.* This measurement is much less invasive than an arterial blood gas, but will only give information about oxygenation, not about adequacy of ventilation.

★ *Level of consciousness.* Obviously, LOC may be depressed by a variety of factors; however, a normal LOC is reassuring that adequate levels of oxygen are reaching the brain.

VENTILATION

★ Adequacy of ventilation may be more difficult to assess than oxygenation. An arterial blood gas will give objective information about CO_2 levels, but represents only a single moment in time. Continuous waveform capnography can provide constant and ongoing evaluation of the patient's ventilatory status. As you will recall:

$$\text{Minute ventilation} = \text{Tidal volume} \times \text{Respiratory rate}$$

All of these are used to clinically judge adequacy of ventilation.

★ Air entry is essentially a clinical estimate of tidal volume. If air entry (depth of inspiration) is very good or very poor its assessment is straightforward, but that same assessment can be quite subjective if air entry is somewhere in between.

★ Beware of respiratory rates that are too low. Avoid being lulled into a false sense of security if the breathing rate falls quickly or the child presents with a low respiratory rate and a depressed level of consciousness. This is likely to represent inadequate ventilation.

★ Work of breathing. Even if oxygenation and ventilation are judged adequate, increased work of breathing may eventually lead to fatigue and respiratory failure in a child. Clinical indicators of increased work of breathing include the following:

  – *Respiratory rate.* Be familiar with normal respiratory rates in children, so that an abnormally high rate will be recognized.

  – *Retractions.* Includes retractions of intercostal muscles, suprasternal and substernal areas. May also include retractions of sternum in small children.

  – Use of accessory muscles.

  – Paradoxical abdominal breathing (inward movement of the abdomen with inspiration—the so-called abdominal paradox).

Keep in mind that pediatric patients have small chests. For this reason, place the stethoscope near each axillary region in order to minimize transmitted breath sounds. When considering the respiratory rate, remember that pain or fear can increase a child's respiratory efforts. Tachypnea, an abnormally rapid rate of breathing, may indicate fear, pain, inadequate oxygenation, or, in the case of neonates, exposure to cold. (See Table 20–1.)

In severe chest trauma, check the infant or child's chest tube (if applicable) making sure that the dressing is clean and dry. If the dressing appears to be stained with blood, take a pen and lightly draw a circle to mark the perimeter of the stain. Monitor dressing for evidence of leakage. Check chest tube for kinks and/or obstructions. Observe the Pleurovac's water level and ensure that the air bubbles are moving freely. Keep in mind that even a minor injury to the chest can interfere with a child's breathing efforts. A chest injury can also interfere with your effort to provide adequate oxygenation or ventilation.

A slight increase in the respiratory rate is one of the earliest indicators of a respiratory problem in a child and one that can only be detected by properly measuring the respiratory rate.

Table 20–1	Signs of Increased Respiratory Effort
Retraction	Visible sinking of the skin and soft tissues of the chest around and below the ribs and above the collarbone
Nasal flaring	Widening of the nostrils; seen primarily on inspiration
Head bobbing	Observed when the head lifts and tilts back as the child inhales and then moves forward as the child exhales
Grunting	Sound heard when an infant attempts to keep the alveoli open by building back pressure during expiration
Wheezing	Passage of air over mucous secretions in bronchi; heard more commonly upon expiration; a low- or high-pitched sound
Gurgling	Coarse, abnormal bubbling sound heard in the airway during inspiration or expiration; may indicate an open chest wound
Stridor	Abnormal, musical, high-pitched sound, more commonly heard on inspiration

Your goal is to identify any evidence of compromised breathing. Evaluation of breathing includes assessment of the following conditions:

★ *Respiratory rate.* Tachypnea is often the first manifestation of respiratory distress in infants. Regardless of the cause, an infant breathing at a rapid rate will eventually tire. Keep in mind that a decreasing respiratory rate may be a result of tiring and is not necessarily a sign of improvement. A slow respiratory rate in an acutely ill infant or child is an ominous sign. (Normal respiratory rates are listed in Table 20–2.) In short, be alert for a respiratory rate that is either abnormally fast or abnormally slow.

★ *Respiratory effort.* The quality of air entry can be assessed by observing for chest rise, breath sounds, stridor, or wheezing. An increased respiratory effort in the infant or child is also evidenced by nasal flaring and the use of accessory respiratory muscles. (Signs of respiratory effort are listed in Table 20–1.)

★ *Color.* Cyanosis is a fairly late sign of respiratory failure and is most frequently seen in the mucous membranes of the mouth and the nail beds. Cyanosis of the extremities alone is more likely due to circulatory failure (shock) than to respiratory failure.

CIRCULATION

As mentioned earlier, you should assess a pediatric patient's circulation by first checking the child's color. Keep in mind that the pediatric patient tends to become hypothermic; therefore, you should check the capillary refill time in an area of central circulation, such as the sternum or forehead. (Note that capillary refill time, as discussed later in this chapter, is considered reliable as a sign of perfusion primarily in children less than 6 years of age.) In general, evaluate the following conditions when assessing circulation during the initial assessment:

★ *Heart rate.* As previously mentioned, infants develop sinus tachycardia in response to stress. Thus, any tachycardia in an infant or child requires further evaluation to determine the cause. Bradycardia in a distressed infant or child may indicate hypoxia and is an ominous sign of cardiac arrest. (Normal heart rates are listed in Table 20–2.)

★ *Peripheral circulation.* The presence of peripheral pulses is a good indicator of the adequacy of end-organ perfusion. Loss of central pulses is an ominous sign.

★ *End-organ perfusion.* End-organ perfusion is most evident in the skin, kidneys, and brain. Decreased perfusion of the skin is an early sign of shock. A capillary refill time of greater than 2 seconds is indicative of low cardiac output although an unreliable indicator. Impairment of brain perfusion is usually evidenced by a change in mental

Table 20–2 | Normal Vital Signs: Infants and Children*

Normal Pulse Rates (Beats per Minute, at Rest)

Newborn	100 to 180
Infant (0–5 Months)	100 to 160
Infant (6–12 Months)	100 to 160
Toddler (1–3 Years)	80 to 110
Preschooler (3–5 Years)	70 to 110
School Age (6–10 Years)	65 to 110
Early Adolescence (11–14 Years)	60 to 90

Normal Respiration Rates (Breaths per Minute, at Rest)

Newborn	30 to 60
Infant (0–5 Months)	30 to 60
Infant (6–12 Months)	30 to 60
Toddler (1–3 Years)	24 to 40
Preschooler (3–5 Years)	22 to 34
School Age (6–10 Years)	18 to 30
Early Adolescence (11–14 Years)	12 to 26

Normal Blood Pressure Ranges (mmHg, at Rest)

	Systolic	Diastolic
	Approx. 90 plus 2 × age	Approx. 2/3 systolic
Preschooler (3–5 Years)	Average 98 (78 to 116)	Average 65
School age (6–10 Years)	Average 105 (80 to 122)	Average 69
Early Adolescence (11–14 Years)	Average 114 (88 to 140)	Average 76

* Adolescents ages 15 to 18 approach the vital signs of adults.

Note: Blood pressure is usually not taken in a child under 3 years of age. In cases of blood loss or shock, a child's blood pressure will remain within normal limits until near the end, then fall swiftly.

status. The child may become confused or lethargic. Seizures may occur. Failure of the child to recognize the parents' faces is often an ominous sign. Urine output directly relates to kidney perfusion. Normal urine output is 1 to 2 mL/kg/hr. Urine flow of less than 1 mL/kg/hr is an indicator of poor renal perfusion.

Remember that evaluation of mental status and ABCs during the initial assessment is rapid and not detailed—it is aimed at discovering and correcting immediate life threats. Measurements that are more thorough will be performed during the focused history and physical exam.

PHYSICAL EXAM

When conducting the physical exam use the toe-to-head approach with the younger child (or begin with the chest and examine the head last) and the head-to-toe approach in the older child. If the ill patient is responsive, perform a physical exam that is focused on the affected areas and systems.

SPECIFIC INJURIES

It is not the intent of this chapter to cover in detail all aspects of trauma associated with the pediatric patient. In approximately 90% of all traumatic events one of three if not all body systems (chest, and/or abdomen) are involved. Although management of trauma is the same for children as adults, anatomical and physiological differences cause pediatric patients to have different patterns of injury.

HEAD TRAUMA AND NEUROLOGIC STATUS

The leading cause of death in the pediatric patient is head trauma. The most common head injury in children is a closed head injury, which may not produce any visible signs of injury. Closed head trauma should be suspected in the unconscious trauma victim and should be assumed present if signs of increased intracranial pressure (ICP) are observed. An ongoing evaluation of the patient's mental status is required with the use of a standardized scoring system, as discussed next.

Pediatric Glasgow Coma Scale

In cases of trauma, you may need to apply the Glasgow Coma Scale (GCS), a scoring system for monitoring the neurologic status of patients with possible head injuries. The GCS assigns scores based on verbal responses, motor functions, and eye movements.

In using the Glasgow Coma Scale with pediatric patients, you will have to make certain modifications. The younger the patient, the more adjustments you will need to make. Verbal responses, for example, will not be possible for neonates and infants. However, motor function may be assessed in very young children by observing voluntary movement. Infants under 4 months of age should have a grasp reflex when an object is placed on the palmar surface of their hand. The grasp should be immediate. Children over 3 years of age will follow directions, when encouraged. Sensory function can be observed by the withdrawal reaction from "tickling" the patient. (See Table 20–3 for a modified GCS for infants.)

Table 20–3		Glasgow Coma Scale		
		>1 year	<1 year	
Eyes Opening	4	Spontaneously	Spontaneously	
	3	To verbal command	To shout	
	2	To pain	To pain	
	1	No response	No response	
		>1 year	<1 year	
Best Motor Response	6	Obeys		
	5	Localizes pain	Localizes pain	
	4	Flexion-withdrawal	Flexion-normal	
	3	Flexion-abnormal (decorticate rigidity)	Flexion-abnormal (decorticate rigidity)	
	2	Extension (decerebrate rigidity)	Extension (decerebrate rigidity)	
	1	No response	No response	
		>5 years	2–5 years	0–23 months
Best Verbal Response	5	Oriented and converses	Appropriate words and phrases	Smiles, coos, cries appropriately
	4	Disoriented and converses	Inappropriate words	Cries
	3	Inappropriate words	Cries and/or screams	Inappropriate crying and/or screaming
	2	Incomprehensible sounds	Grunts	Grunts
	1	No response	No response	No response

After you score the **pediatric Glasgow Coma Scale** for the patient, prioritize the patient according to severity. Guidelines are:

- ★ *Mild* —GCS 13 to 15
- ★ *Moderate* —GCS 9 to 12
- ★ *Severe* —GCS less than or equal to 8

pediatric Glasgow Coma Scale *a method of assessing and monitoring neurological status; assigns a numerical value to different levels of verbal response, motor function, and eye movement.*

CHEST

Chest injuries are the second most common cause of pediatric trauma deaths. Because of the compliance of the chest wall, severe intrathoracic injury can be present without signs of external injury. In fact, significant pulmonary contusions occur in children because the absence of a rigid chest wall fails to protect the lungs from blunt trauma. Pulmonary contusions can decrease the gas exchange in the alveoli resulting in hypoxia.

Pneumothorax and hemothorax can occur in the pediatric patient, especially if the mechanism of injury was a motor vehicle collision. Also remember that flail chest is an uncommon injury in children. When noted without a significant mechanism of injury, suspect child abuse. Tension pneumothorax can also occur in children. Tension pneumothorax presents with the following signs and symptoms:

- ★ Respiratory distress
- ★ Worsening hypoxia
- ★ Diminished breath sounds over the affected lung
- ★ A progressive decrease in ventilatory compliance
- ★ Shift of the trachea to the opposite side (a late sign)

The diagnosis of a tension pneumothorax in a child is based on physical exam findings and not chest X-ray. Delaying treatment of a suspected tension pneumothorax for an X-ray may result in the death of the child. In the critical care tranport arena, these patients will have a chest tube in place that will need to be continuously monitored during transport.

ABDOMEN

Significant blunt trauma to the abdomen can result in injury to the spleen or liver. In fact, the spleen is the most commonly injured organ in children. Signs and symptoms of a splenic injury include tenderness in the left upper quadrant of the abdomen, abrasions on the abdomen, and hematoma of the abdominal wall. Symptoms of liver injury include right upper quadrant abdominal pain and/or right lower chest pain. Both splenic and hepatic injuries can cause life-threatening internal hemorrhage.

In treating blunt abdominal trauma, keep in mind the small size of the pediatric abdomen. Be certain to palpate only one quadrant at a time. The pediatric patient with a history of blunt trauma must be monitored continuously, and the critical care paramedic must be able to recognize subtle signs of pain and developing shock.

The treatment of pediatric trauma has changed significantly. The need for surgical intervention post-trauma has decreased significantly. This is primarily a result of much improved medical imaging technologies (i.e., CT scans, ultrasound). Most solid organ injuries were once treated surgically. Now, most are treated conservatively with observation.

SHOCK

Shock is a condition of sustained and progressive circulatory dysfunction that results in inadequate delivery of substrates to meet tissue metabolic demands. It may also be characterized by a compromise in tissue utilization of oxygen. (See Figure 20-4 ■.) Shock is most often the end result of:

- ★ Severe dehydration
- ★ Hemorrhage
- ★ Progressive heart failure
- ★ Sepsis

Patient Assessment Using Priority Plan

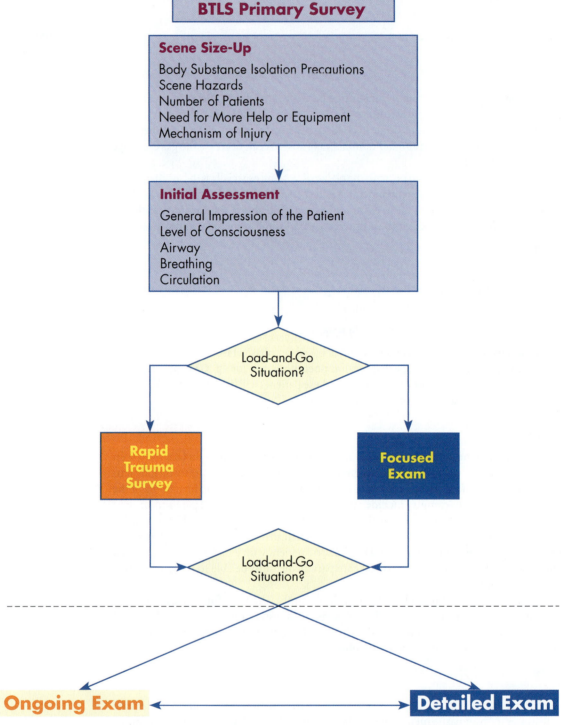

BTLS Primary Survey

Scene Size-Up

Body Substance Isolation Precautions
Scene Hazards
Number of Patients
Need for More Help or Equipment
Mechanism of Injury

Initial Assessment

General Impression of the Patient
Level of Consciousness
Airway
Breathing
Circulation

Load-and-Go
Situation?

**Rapid
Trauma
Survey**

**Focused
Exam**

Load-and-Go
Situation?

Ongoing Exam   **Detailed Exam**

■ Figure 20-4   Steps in the assessment and management of the trauma patient. This is the same for both children and adults.

Ongoing Assessment

Clinical signs of all forms of shock in children include nonspecific signs of distress or deterioration (child "looks bad"), plus signs of inadequate tissue perfusion. These latter signs are usually associated with signs of organ dysfunction. Classic signs of shock include:

★ "Looks bad"—deterioration in color (skin appears mottled, or nail beds are pale), irritability or a decrease in responsiveness, reduced level of activity.

★ Signs of inadequate tissue perfusion and organ function. Lactic acidosis and oliguria (urine output <1 mL/kg/hr despite an adequate fluid intake) both indicate inadequate tissue perfusion.

★ Diminished peripheral pulses and delayed capillary refill despite a warm ambient temperature.

★ Hypotension is typically only a late sign of decompensated shock in children.

Management

Early recognition and therapy are the keys to the successful management of pediatric shock. Therefore, signs of poor systemic perfusion should be identified as soon as they appear, and supportive therapy should be provided to optimize each aspect of cardiovascular and pulmonary function.

The goals of therapy are maximization of oxygen delivery and minimization of oxygen demand. Supporting arterial oxygen content, as well as cardiac output, maximizes oxygen delivery:

★ Optimize arterial oxygen content (support airway, oxygenation, and ventilation).

★ Optimize cardiac output (support heart rate for clinical condition and ensure adequate cardiac preload, maximal contractility, and ideal afterload).

★ Control oxygen demand (treat pain and fever, prevent cold stress, and eliminate needless sources of stress).

An essential aspect of care of the child in shock is reassessment. The child should be reevaluated constantly to determine response to therapy, identify the need for changes in therapy, and detect any signs of further deterioration. When possible, use an objective measure, such as the pediatric trauma score, to monitor the patient for changes. (See Table 20–4.)

TRANSPORT CONSIDERATIONS AND MANAGEMENT

During the critical care transport of a pediatric patient with significant head injuries, the critical care paramedic may need to continually monitor ICP levels and identify trends. ICP is the amount

Table 20–4	Pediatric Trauma Score		
Score	+2	+1	−1
Weight	>44 lb (>20 kg)	22–44 lb (10–20 kg)	<22 lb (<10 kg)
Airway	Normal	Oral or nasal airway	Intubated tracheostomy invasive airway
Blood pressure	Pulse at wrist >90 mmHg	Carotid or femoral pulse palpable 50–90 mmHg	No palpable pulse <50 mmHg
Level of consciousness	Completely awake	Obtunded or any loss of consciousness	Comatose
Open wound	None	Minor	Major or penetrating
Fractures	None	Closed fracture	Open or multiple fractures

of pressure exerted on the cranial vault. Because the cranium is a rigid structure and cannot expand, if any three components of the head increase, the ICP will increase. The three components are:

★ Brain volume

★ Blood volume

★ Cerebrospinal fluid (CSF) volume

ICP monitoring is indicated in trauma patients at risk for cerebral edema, patients with subarachnoid hemorrhage, tumors that obstruct the ventricular system, cerebral aneurysm, and intracranial hemorrhage. The follow is a brief description of ICP monitoring.

continuous intracranial pressure monitoring (ICP)
a continuous, direct intracranial pressure measurement technique using an intracranial sensor, transducer, and recording device.

Continuous intracranial pressure monitoring (ICP) is considered commonplace in most critical care units. ICP monitoring is a continuous, direct measurement technique that uses an intracranial sensor, transducer, and recording device. ICP monitoring allows for the early detection of intracranial hypertension as a complication of head trauma and for aggressive treatment of these patients. ICP monitoring devices also allow for the evaluation of the treatments and care activities being used to prevent or control intracranial hypertension. ICP fluctuates continuously as ventricular fluid patterns change. Normal ICP ranges from 4 to 15 mmHg. However, trends are more important than isolated values. Pressures above 20 mmHg for 30 minutes or more or levels above 40 mmHg for 15 minutes that do not respond to conventional therapy are considered evidence of uncontrolled ICP levels.

During transport, any ICP readings that trend upward or radically decrease should be documented and immediately communicated to the patient's receiving physician. This may identify the need for immediate surgical intervention, and it may indicate potential causes of further clinical deterioration.

An important distinction to remember is that the critical care paramedic will see ICP readings change long before there are clinical signs and symptoms. The critical care transport unit that is equipped with a transport ICP monitor such as a Propaq will have the advantage of treating the patient for increased pressures before any clinical signs appear, thereby preventing any unnecessary damage to the patient's condition. Additional assessments that will contribute to neurologic evaluation include:

★ Vital signs. Note that increased ICP may produce bradycardia, hypertension, and apnea, but these "classic" signs typically appear late in the clinical arena. Watch for any change associated with poor perfusion or neurologic deterioration.

★ Pupil size and response to light.

★ Cranial nerve function, anatomical site of injury, cranial nerve involvement, and spontaneous breathing pattern. Note presence and absence of cough, gag during suctioning.

★ Ability to follow commands. Ask the child to hold up two fingers, wiggle toes, or stick out his or her tongue. Document any deterioration in the child's condition immediately.

Management includes the support of oxygenation and ventilation, since both hypoxemia and hypercarbia can decrease cerebral blood flow, as well as increase intracranial volume and pressure. Treat seizures and fever, since these factors can increase cerebral oxygen demand. If blood pressure and perfusion are adequate and oxygenation and ventilation are optimized, yet ICP remains high, diuresis with mannitol may be needed. Finally, barbiturates may be used if all other methods to control ICP have been tried.

The chest must be reexamined if at any time during the critical care transport any of the following are observed: tachypnea with or without respiratory distress, continuous hemodynamic instability (see Chapter 9), chest pain or tenderness, hypoxemia, hemoptysis, crepitus, or abdominal breath sounds. These signs may be caused by thoracic injury. Common thoracic injuries that may be detected during the assessment include pulmonary contusion, pneumothorax, hemothorax, cardiac contusion, flail chest, rib fractures, and diaphragm rupture.

CHEST TUBES

During the transport of a pediatric chest injury, the critical care paramedic will most likely be faced with the task of monitoring the chest tube of a pediatric patient.

Drainage Monitoring

The critical care paramedic during transport should assess and document the color, consistency, and amount of drainage, remaining alert to sudden changes. A sudden increase in drainage indicates hemorrhage or sudden patency of a previously obstructed tube. A sudden decrease in drainage indicates chest tube obstruction or failure of the chest tube or drainage system.

The following actions are recommended to reestablish chest tube patency:

★ Attempt to alleviate the obstruction by repositioning the patient.

★ If the clot is visible, straighten the tubing between the chest and drainage unit and raise the proximal end of the tube to enhance the effect of gravity.

Water Seal Monitoring

Monitoring the water seal of the chest tube drainage system is as important as observing the drainage. Visual checks are made to ensure water seal chambers are filled to the 2-cm water line. If suction is applied, the critical care paramedic must ensure the water line in the suction chamber is at the ordered level, because water evaporates over time, decreasing the amount of suction being applied.

Respiratory fluctuations are observed in the underwater seal. The absence of fluctuations can indicate that the lung is reexpanded or that there is an obstruction in the system. Continuous vigorous bubbling in the water seal without suction indicates continued pneumothorax or can indicate the tube has been dislodged or disconnected. The entire system has to be checked for disconnections and the chest tube inspected to see if it is displaced outside the chest.

Complications

The most serious complication of a chest tube is tension pneumothorax, which can develop if there is any obstruction in the chest tube drainage system. Clamping chest tubes as a routine practice predisposes patients to this complication. Clamping of chest tubes is recommended in only two situations:

★ To locate the source of an air leak if bubbling occurs in the water seal chamber

★ To replace the chest tube drainage unit (clamping is done only momentarily)

If the tube must be clamped, padded hemostats are used to avoid cutting the vinyl chest tube. Occasionally the chest tube may fall out or be accidentally pulled out. In such a circumstance, the insertion site is quickly sealed off to prevent air from entering the pleural cavity.

Ongoing Monitoring

Physical findings may be minimal despite serious injury, delaying diagnosis and prompt, appropriate intervention. Findings during critical care transport, including hemodynamic instability, an enlarging abdomen with no other site of intravascular volume loss, peritoneal irritation with involuntary guarding, and abdominal wall rigidity, should all be well documented. Children with major trauma often have a head injury that has the potential to mask lethal abdominal trauma. Respiratory rate, pattern, and response to pain are all indicators on which the critical care paramedic relies. It is important to keep in mind that signs and symptoms may be dramatically affected by head injury.

Management includes serial measurements of abdominal girth at the level of the umbilicus as another helpful evaluation tool and one not altered by a decreased level of consciousness. The abdomen may distend due to accumulation of gas (swallowed air or an intestinal obstruction) or liquid (blood, intestinal contents, urine, bile, pancreatic juices), or both. Absent or decreased bowel sounds may be normal or may indicate an obstruction. A bruit may indicate significant arterial injury. Monitor patient closely for signs and symptoms of shock.

NONINVASIVE MONITORING

Modern **noninvasive monitoring devices** all have their application in pediatric critical care. These may include the pulse oximeter, continuous waveform capnography, automated blood pressure devices, self-registering thermometers, and ECGs. To promote the goal of early recognition of cardiopulmonary arrest, every seriously ill or injured child should receive continuous pulse oximetry.

The fluid bolus regimen for children is 20 mL/kg boluses of an isotonic crystalloid solution.

noninvasive monitoring devices *devices used to assist in patient trending and care; they include pulse oximeters, continuous waveform capnography units, automated blood pressure devices, self-registering or digital thermometers, and ECG machines.*

This will provide you with essential information regarding the patient's heart rate and peripheral O$_2$ saturation. It will also help you to monitor the effects of any medications administered. ECGs and an automated blood pressure/pulse monitor should also be considered. However, these devices may frighten the child. Before applying any monitoring device, explain what you are going to do. Demonstrate the display or lights. If the monitoring device makes noise, allow the child to hear the noise before you apply it. Reassure the child that the device will not hurt him.

INVASIVE MONITORING

The direct recording of blood pressure is recommended for critical care patients who require accurate monitoring of arterial pressure. However, direct monitoring of arterial blood pressure is an invasive monitoring procedure that requires sophisticated equipment and frequent calibration and maintenance.

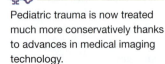
Don't forget the IO route when venous access in a child is difficult or impossible.

For direct arterial monitoring, a catheter is placed into a suitable artery. Most commonly, the radial or femoral artery is used. In neonates, umbilical or temporal arteries may be used. The catheter is usually filled with heparinized saline or dextrose solution that serves as a fluid column between the blood and the diaphragm of the pressure transducer. A transducer is a device that changes energy from one form to another. In this case, the transducer changes the mechanical pressure pulse into an electrical signal. The electrical signal from the transducer is often weak and an amplifier is usually required. Finally, the signal is displayed on an oscilloscope or graph. Most critical care units utilize an electronic monitor that displays the arterial waveform and also provides a numerical value for the systolic, diastolic, and mean arterial pressure (MAP). (Please refer to Chapter 9, "Cardiac and Hemodynamic Monitoring," for more details.)

MECHANICAL VENTILATION

When caring for the pediatric patient receiving mechanical ventilation, the critical care paramedic must continually assess the patient for problems and complications. A combination of data from the patient's physical assessment, the ventilator, and invasive and noninvasive monitoring devices should be evaluated at least every 5 minutes during transport. The following measurements are part of the critical care paramedic's ongoing assessment regarding mechanical ventilation:

- ★ Observe and listen over the artificial airway. Assess for secure taping, proper position, and presence of cuff leak or heavy secretions.
- ★ Auscultate the patient's chest for adventitious breath sounds: crackles (pulmonary edema and atelectasis) and rhonchi (may need suctioning).
- ★ Compare breath sounds bilaterally.
- ★ Observe for asymmetry of chest movement indicating pneumothorax, splinting due to pain, and massive atelectasis. Assess for synchronization of chest movement with ventilator.
- ★ Assess patient for proper positioning for maximum lung expansion.
- ★ Continually monitor ventilator settings.
- ★ Use continuous waveform capnography.

DEFINITIVE MANAGEMENT OF PEDIATRIC TRAUMA

Pediatric trauma is now treated much more conservatively thanks to advances in medical imaging technology.

There has been a significant change in the way pediatric trauma is definitively managed. Formerly, most children who sustained serious trauma received an exploratory operation. Today, however, with the significant advances in diagnostic imaging (CT scanning, ultrasound, magnetic resonance imaging), it is easy to detect internal injuries without an exploratory operation. In addition, we have found that children are amazingly resilient and most injuries will heal without operative intervention. The most commonly injured organ in pediatric blunt trauma is the spleen, followed by the liver, kidney, GI tract, and pancreas in descending order. Solid organ injuries often can be monitored with diagnostic imaging and operated on only if bleeding is excessive and does not slow. The changes in pediatric trauma care during the last decade have been remarkable and pediatric trauma mortality rates continue to improve.

SUMMARY

During critical care transport, your pediatric patient's condition can rapidly change for the better or the worse, making it necessary to repeat relevant portions of the assessment. (For this reason, ongoing assessment is sometimes called *reassessment*.) You should continually monitor the patient's respiratory effort, skin color, mental status, temperature, and pulse oximetry. Retake vital signs and compare them with baseline vitals. In general, reassess stable patients every 15 minutes, critical patients every 5 minutes.

Part 2: Geriatric Trauma

INTRODUCTION

Older patients who sustain moderate to severe injuries are more likely to die than their younger counterparts. Post-injury disability is also more common in the elderly than in the young. It is safe to estimate that a fair number of critical care transports will involve the aging population. As a result, the critical care paramedic must understand normal, age-related physiological changes. All physiological processes alter as a person ages. These alterations are progressive and usually are not apparent or pathologic. Because of these age-related changes, however, the older critically injured patient requires more intense observation.

EPIDEMIOLOGY OF THE GERIATRIC POPULATION

Currently more than 35 million Americans are over the age of 65. This is the age that has been established by the federal government to signify that the individual has reached the age where retirement, in the form of Social Security and Medicare, is available. You may be familiar with the phrase "America is getting older." The number of elderly people has nearly doubled in the last 40 years. There are a number of reasons for the ever-expanding numbers of Americans reaching age 65 in good health:

★ The mean survival rate of old persons is increasing.

★ Medical care, disease control, and nutrition have improved since World War II.

★ There has been an absence of major wars and other catastrophes.

★ The birth rate is declining.

During the next three to four decades, we can expect a very dramatic increase both in the number of elderly persons and in the proportion of elderly persons in the population. Changes in the overall population age 65 and over and in the population 65 to 74 years of age will remain constant until the year 2010. Then, however, the arrival of the large baby boomer cohort at age 65 will trigger large increases in the number and percentage of elderly in the next half century. The record large proportion of elderly persons now in the population, 13%, will rise to perhaps 20% by the year 2030, and the number of elderly is expected to double by that year. These prospective demographic changes have given rise to a general concern about the social, economic, and physical "health" of the U.S. population.

The most rapid increases in the number and share of persons 85 years and over (the so-called "old, old") will occur between 2030 and 2050, when the baby boomer cohort reaches these ages. The cumulative growth of the population 85 years and over from 1995 to 2050 is expected to be more than 400%, and the group should make up nearly 5% of the population in 2050 as compared with 1.4% today. When the post–World War II baby boomers enter their 80s, more than 70 million people will be age 65 or older. By 2040, the elderly will represent roughly 20% of the population. In other words, one in five Americans will be age 65 or older.

Not only will the elderly population increase in size, its members will live longer. Preconceived ideas of what the elderly "look like" is more appropriate for those individuals currently over age 80. The maximum life span is now expected to be 100+ years barring significant disease processes.

As stated, the geriatric population makes up approximately 13% of the population in the United States and 30% of all prehospital calls on an annual basis. When providing health care for the elderly it is important to understand the following:

★ Organ system function declines.

★ The body's effectiveness in dealing with disease is progressively reduced.

★ Total body water decreases.

★ Total body fat is reduced by 15% to 30%.

★ The body's ability to regenerate body cells is reduced.

Let's set some ground rules so that our time discussing the elderly population will truly benefit our patients and not just serve to build a meaningless tally of runs completed during our illustrious and awe-inspiring careers.

We must recognize that the attitudes displayed by elderly patients have formed as a result of their life experiences. For instance, a patient who is 102 years old was born before the first airplane and has lived to see men go to the moon, the International Space Station, and the pictures from Mars rovers.

What does this add up to? In a single word—RESPECT. These individuals deserve and have earned every kindness and respect we can show them for the lives they have lived. Most have fought in major wars that allow us all to have the freedom we Americans so deeply cherish.

SYSTEM PATHOPHYSIOLOGY AND ORGAN SYSTEM DECLINE

Although aging begins at the cellular level, it eventually affects virtually every system in the body. (See Table 20–5.) Age-related changes in the structure and function of organs increase the probability of disease, modify the threshold at which signs and symptoms appear, and affect assessment and treatment of the elderly patient. You should be familiar with normal systematic changes related to aging so that you can more easily identify the abnormal changes that may point to a serious underlying problem.

RESPIRATORY SYSTEM

Changes begin at approximately 30 years of age, marked change after age 60. Pulmonary circulation is reduced 33%, which reduces O_2 and CO_2 exchange in the alveoli. This slowly shifts the body's pH balance toward the acidosis side of the equation. As with any substance subjected to acid, the body tissues will slowly deteriorate and die. Reduced chest wall excursion and loss of muscle flexibility leads to shallow, rapid respirations to compensate for the decreased tidal volume. The tidal volume can decrease by as much as 50%. Maximum respiratory capacity may be reduced by as much as 60%. Maximum oxygen uptake to supply the needs of the cells may be reduced by 70%. These changes and reductions in oxygen capacity should make the critical care paramedic especially attentive to the need for supplemental oxygen administration with all patients. In this patient population, a critical vital sign is the oxygen saturation reading obtained by the pulse oximetry unit. Also, remember that underlying pulmonary disease also will play a large contributing factor in the condition of your patient.

Table 20-5	Common Age-Related Systemic Changes	
Body System	**Changes with Age**	**Clinical Importance**
Respiratory	Loss of strength and coordination in respiratory muscles Cough and gag reflex reduced	Increased likelihood of respiratory failure
Cardiovascular	Loss of elasticity and hardening of arteries Changes in heart rate, rhythm, efficiency	Hypertension common Greater likelihood of strokes, heart attacks Great likelihood of bleeding from minor trauma
Neurological	Brain tissue shrinks Loss of memory Clinical depression common Altered mental status common Impaired balance	Delay in appearance of symptoms with head injury Difficulty in patient assessment Increased likelihood of falls
Endocrine	Lowered estrogen production (women) Decline in insulin sensitivity Increase in insulin resistance	Increased likelihood of fractures (bone loss) and heart disease Diabetes mellitus common with greater possibility of hyperglycemia
Gastrointestinal	Diminished digestive functions	Constipation common Greater likelihood of malnutrition
Thermoregulatory	Reduced sweating Decreased shivering	Environmental emergencies more common
Integumentary (Skin)	Thins and becomes more fragile	More subject to tears and sores Bruising more common Heals more slowly
Musculoskeletal	Loss of bone strength (osteoporosis) Loss of joint flexibility and strength (osteoarthritis)	Greater likelihood of fractures Slower healing Increased likelihood of falls
Renal	Loss of kidney size and function	Increased problems with drug toxicity
Genitourinary	Loss of bladder function	Increased urination/incontinence Increased urinary tract infection
Immune	Diminished immune response	More susceptible to infections Impaired immune response to vaccines
Hematological	Decrease in blood volume and/or RBCs	Slower recuperation from illness/injury Greater risk of trauma-related complications

CARDIOVASCULAR SYSTEM

Cardiac output may be reduced by as much as 50%. Remember, the formula for cardiac output (CO) is:

$$CO = \text{Heart rate} \times \text{Stroke volume}$$

Either part of the equation may be affected by a number of factors—medications, dehydration, previous cardiac events. The decrease in the contractility of cardiac muscle affects the stroke volume due to amount of blood that can be ejected from the heart with each contraction. A conduction problem may be affecting the heart that comes to bear on the rate of contractions, with them being either too slow or too fast to adequately provide for the body's needs. The systemic vascular resistance the heart must overcome to circulate the blood also plays a large part in the ability of the heart to meet the body's needs.

RENAL SYSTEM

Elderly patients experience a 30% to 40% decrease in functioning nephrons. There is as much as a 50% decrease in renal blood flow. Filtration of solutes from the bloodstream may be reduced, leading to electrolyte imbalances. The renal system plays an intimate part in the survival of the organs of the body; when electrolytes are out of normal ranges, the end result—if not corrected—is death. The kidneys also control the reabsorption of fluids in the system to maintain blood pressure and system perfusion.

NERVOUS SYSTEM

Both the central and peripheral nervous systems are degraded through the aging process. In the central nervous system as much as 45% of brain cells may be lost through injury, disease, or previous poor perfusion episodes. The development of plaque within the vessels of the brain leads to further deterioration of the brain tissue; the peripheral nervous system suffers a loss of electrical conductivity along the nerve. This reduction of impulse velocity results in a slowing of reaction time and reduction in the response to pain. In cases of altered mental status, maintain a suspicion of trauma, especially when an accident has been reported.

MUSCULOSKELETAL SYSTEM

Arthritis means pain, swelling, or loss of movement in the joints throughout the body. More than 100 separate diseases can cause arthritis and related disorders of the joints, bones, and muscles. Arthritis can occur in any person at any age.

osteoarthritis
inflammation of a joint resulting from wearing of the articular cartilage.

The specific causes of most forms of arthritis are not known. **Osteoarthritis** causes the breakdown of cartilage and other joint tissue. Cartilage is a firm, slippery material that covers the end of each bone in a joint to act as a cushion or shock absorber between the bones. In osteoarthritis, the cartilage wears away, causing the bones to rub or grind against each other causing pain and loss of movement. That is why the condition is sometimes called degenerative joint disease (DJD). All forms of arthritis are chronic, which means they are diseases that last a lifetime. You cannot prevent or reverse the process of arthritis, but you can slow the progression of the disease and maintain the highest quality of life by getting help early from a health care professional and following your treatment plan.

In aging, the body loses as much as 35% of muscle mass, resulting in injury to both the skin and underlying structures. The skin loses elasticity and the ability to heal is greatly decreased. The process of osteoporosis, which begins in the 30s, is manifest in the late 60s. This process results in numerous fractures and debilitating injuries.

TRAUMA IN THE ELDERLY

The elderly are more at risk from trauma, especially from falls. Contributing factors include slower reflexes, failing eyesight and hearing, and arthritis, and tissue and bones are more fragile. The elderly are also more at risk from criminal assault and abuse.

Head injury is more serious in geriatric patients due to the fact that the brain diminishes in size with age, allowing more potential space within the cranial vault. Due to the larger space it is easier for vessels to lacerate and bleed into the skull. The downside to this is that signs of head injury may take longer to develop with a geriatric patient.

Cervical spine injury can be complicated by osteoporosis and spondylolysis (degeneration of vertebral disks) making the cervical spine more prone to injury. Arthritic changes can compress nerves in the arms and spinal nerve roots. Even sudden neck movement may result in cervical spinal injury.

Considerations in trauma care of the elderly include the following:

★ Past cardiac history may have contributed to the traumatic event.

★ Carefully monitor fluid administration.

★ Hypotension and hypovolemia are both very poorly tolerated.

★ Kidneys cannot compensate for fluid changes.

★ Organs are less tolerant of hypoxia and anoxia.

★ Airway management must be early and aggressive.

★ May need to modify immobilization to accommodate deformities.

FACILITY ARRIVAL AND INITIAL TRAUMA ASSESSMENT

Once you enter the referring facility, ask to speak with the individual (usually a nurse) in charge of the patient. When obtaining the medical history of the geriatric patient, you should gather information such as:

★ Nurse/physician notes

★ Lab values

★ X-rays

★ Ventilator settings

★ Transfer orders (memorandum of transfer)

★ Nature of the illness/injury

★ Length of time the patient has been sick/injured

★ Presence of fever

★ Effects of the illness/injury on patient behavior

★ Bowel/urine habits

★ Presence of vomiting/diarrhea

★ Frequency of urination

Often the chief complaint of the elderly patient may seem trivial, and the patient may fail to relate the important symptoms he is experiencing. It is the responsibility of the critical care paramedic to complete a thorough examination of the patient to include the physical condition, living conditions, and social status of the patient. Any one of these factors may finally point you in the direction that will enable you to determine the patient's problem. The critical care paramedic must be able to differentiate between the chief complaint and the primary problem. A patient may complain of abdominal pain; this is the chief complaint. However, the primary problem may be rectal bleeding.

The geriatric patient frequently suffers from more than one disease process, making assessment more difficult. It is easy to confuse symptoms of chronic illness with symptoms from an acute problem. Remember that trivial complaints often indicate a serious underlying disease.

Common complaints in the elderly include:

★ Fatigue and weakness

★ Depression

★ Dizziness, vertigo, or syncope

★ Falls

★ Headache

★ Insomnia

★ Dysphasia (difficulty swallowing)

★ Loss of appetite

★ Inability to void

★ Constipation or diarrhea

Communications often become difficult; sight and hearing is diminished. Eyesight is diminished due to cataracts and glaucoma. Blindness in the elderly is common, often resulting from diabetes, stroke, or secondary to smoking (macular degeneration). Because the patient cannot control the situation, he may be displaying a high level of anxiety. It is important to speak clearly and calmly to the geriatric patient. Position yourself to be seen clearly by your patient. Diminished hearing or deafness may make it difficult or impossible to obtain a clear history. You may need to speak with friends or family, but maintain contact with the patient.

Often, mental status is decreased in elderly patients. This makes communication more difficult. Noise from radios, equipment, and personnel may add to the patient's confusion. Senility and organic brain syndrome may manifest themselves similarly. Common symptoms include:

★ Delirium

★ Confusion

★ Distractibility

★ Restlessness

★ Excitability

★ Hostility or fear

When dealing with a confused patient, determine if this is a change from the normal. DO NOT ASSUME A CONFUSED GERIATRIC PATIENT IS SENILE! (See Figure 20-5 ■.)

Alcohol abuse is common in the elderly and complicates both your ability to collect a history and perform physical assessment. A review of the literature suggests that lower levels of alcohol consumption (compared to younger adults) can reduce stress, induce pleasant and carefree feelings; and decrease tension, anxiety, and self-consciousness. In the elderly, moderate drinking has been reported to stimulate appetite, promote regular bowel function, and improve mood. However, a review of epidemiological evidence found that moderate alcohol consumption increased the potential risk of hemorrhagic stroke, although it decreased the risk of occlusive strokes. Alcohol may

■ Figure 20-5   *Do not assume that an altered mental status is a normal age-related change. A number of serious underlying problems may be responsible for changes in consciousness.*

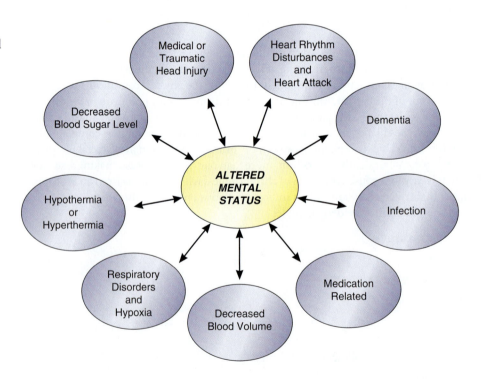

interact harmfully with more than 100 medications, including some sold over the counter. The effects of alcohol are especially augmented by medications that depress the function of the central nervous system, such as sedatives, sleeping pills, anticonvulsants, antidepressants, antianxiety drugs, and certain painkillers. In advanced heart failure, alcohol may not only worsen the disease, but also interfere with the function of medications to treat the disease.

TRANSPORT CONSIDERATIONS AND MANAGEMENT

The priorities of care for the elderly trauma patient are similar to those for any trauma patient. However, you must keep in mind age-related systemic changes and the presence of chronic diseases. This is especially true of the cardiovascular, respiratory, and renal systems.

CARDIOVASCULAR CONSIDERATIONS

Recent or past myocardial infarctions may contribute to the risk of dysrhythmia or congestive heart failure in the trauma patient. In addition, there may be a decreased response of the heart, in adjusting heart rate and stroke volume, to hypovolemia. An elderly trauma patient may require higher than usual arterial pressures for perfusion of vital organs, due to increased peripheral vascular resistance and hypertension. Care must be taken in intravenous fluid administration because of decreased myocardial reserves. Hypotension, hypovolemia, and hypervolemia are poorly tolerated in the elderly patient.

RESPIRATORY CONSIDERATIONS

In managing the airway and ventilation in an elderly trauma patient, you must consider the physical changes that may affect treatment. Check for dentures and determine whether they should be removed. Keep in mind that age-related changes can decrease chest wall movement and vital capacity. Age also reduces the tolerance of all organs for anoxia. Remember, too, that chronic obstructive pulmonary disease is widespread among the elderly.

Make necessary adjustments in treatment to provide adequate oxygenation and appropriate CO_2 removal. It is important to remember that use of 50% nitrous oxide (Nitronox) for elderly patients may result in more respiratory depression than would occur in younger patients. Positive pressure ventilations should also be used cautiously. There is an increased danger of resultant alkalosis and rupture of emphysematous bullae, making the elderly more vulnerable to pneumothorax.

RENAL CONSIDERATIONS

The decreased ability of the kidneys to maintain normal acid–base balance and to compensate for fluid changes can further complicate the management of the elderly trauma patient. Any preexisting renal disease can decrease the kidney's ability to compensate. The decrease in renal function, along with a decrease in cardiac reserve, places the elderly injured patient at risk for fluid overload and pulmonary edema. Remember, too, that renal changes allow toxins and medications to accumulate more readily in the elderly.

TRANSPORT

You may have to modify the positioning, immobilization, and packaging of the elderly trauma patient before transport. Be attentive to physical deformities such as arthritis, spinal abnormalities, or frozen limbs that may cause pain or special care. Recall the frailty of an elderly person's skin and avoid creating skin tears or pressure sores. Keep in mind that trauma places an elderly person at increased risk of hypothermia. Ensure that the patient is kept warm at all times.

HOSPICE

hospice *medical institutions designed to care for and relieve the physical and emotional suffering of the dying.*

Institutions designed to relieve the physical and emotional suffering of the dying are called hospices. The term **hospice** is derived from the same Latin word from which come "hospital" and "hospitality." In the Middle Ages hospices were places of refuge that provided rest and refreshment to travelers, not unlike inns or hotels. Today, hospices offer an alternative form of care for terminally ill patients; they also provide emotional support for the patient's relatives.

Hospice care emerged as an alternative to hospital confinement for several reasons. The primary one is probably the very high cost of keeping terminally ill patients alive indefinitely with respirators and other means. Second, aggressive life-prolonging measures, usually undertaken in intensive care units, frequently do nothing more than add to the discomfort and isolation of dying persons. Hospices, while staffed with physicians, nurses, and other medical personnel, create a home-like and sympathetic environment dedicated to making the last days of the dying as pleasant as possible. Hospice care is also much less expensive than a hospital stay. In the United States, Medicare provides some financial support for hospice care, and in Great Britain, the National Health Service subsidizes hospice care.

More than 90% of hospice patients suffer from cancer. Therefore, the first priority is the alleviation of pain using analgesics, tranquilizers, and a variety of physical therapies. Hospices emphasize the prevention of pain through vigilant monitoring and by the careful dispensing of painkillers. In the United States, there are hospices to care for patients with AIDS (acquired immunodeficiency syndrome), normally a terminal condition, which reached epidemic proportions in the 1980s.

The modern hospice movement began in England with the founding of St. Christopher's Hospice at Sydenham, near London, by Cicely Saunders in 1967. The movement came to the United States in 1975, after Saunders lectured on the subject at Yale University in Connecticut. There were about 1,400 hospices in the United States in the mid-1980s. A useful book on the subject is *Hospice Programs and Public Policy,* edited by Paul Toffens (American Hospital Publishing, Inc., 1985).

SUMMARY

The practice of critical care paramedicine in the 21st century means treating a growing elderly population. The "Graying of America" has resulted in a greater number of people age 65 and older. When treating elderly patients, keep in mind the anatomical, physiological, and emotional changes that occur with age. Weigh normal age-related changes against abnormal changes, that is, those resulting from a medical condition or trauma. Recall that elderly patients are much more susceptible to medication side effects and toxicity than younger patients.

Part 3: Obstetrical Trauma

INTRODUCTION

Although the initial assessment and management priorities for resuscitation of the injured pregnant patient are the same as those for other traumatized patients, the specific anatomical and physiological changes that occur during pregnancy may alter the response to injury and hence necessitate a modified approach to the resuscitation process. The main principle guiding therapy must be that resuscitating the mother will resuscitate the fetus.

EPIDEMIOLOGY OF OBSTETRICAL TRAUMA

Trauma has become the number one cause of morbidity and mortality in pregnant patients. Although maternal mortality due to other causes such as infection, hemorrhage, hypertension, and thromboembolism has declined over the years, the number of maternal deaths due to penetrating trauma, suicide, homicide and motor vehicle collisions has risen steadily. Accidental injuries occur in 6% to 7% of all pregnant patients. Penetrating trauma accounts for as many as 36% of maternal deaths. However, the uterus acts as a short of "shield" resulting in lower than expected maternal intra-abdominal injuries. For example, in the case of gunshot wounds to the pregnant abdomen, overall maternal mortality is low (3.9%). Fetal mortality, on the other hand, is high, ranging between 50% and 70%.

GENERAL APPROACH TO OBSTETRICAL TRAUMA

Because two lives are at risk with the traumatized pregnant patient, assessment and treatment should be oriented to both, but because the primary cause of fetal death is maternal death, attempting to save the mother's life ultimately takes precedence.

The effect of trauma on pregnancy depends on the gestational age of the fetus, the type and severity of the trauma, and the extent of disruption of normal uterine and fetal physiology. The survival of the fetus depends on adequate uterine perfusion and delivery of oxygen. The uterine circulation has no autoregulation, which implies that uterine blood flow is related directly to maternal systemic blood pressure, at least until the mother approaches hypovolemic shock. At that point, peripheral vasoconstriction will further compromise uterine perfusion. Once obvious shock develops in the mother, the chances of saving the fetus are about 20%. When severe injuries such as head trauma, chest trauma, and pelvic fracture are present in the pregnant patient, maternal mortality can be as high as 16%, and fetal demise can be as high as 42%.

If fetal oxygenation or perfusion is compromised by trauma, the response of the fetus may include bradycardia or tachycardia, a decrease in the baseline variability of the heart rate, the absence of normal accelerations in the heart rate, or recurrent decelerations. Note that an abnormal fetal heart rate might be the first indication of an important disruption in fetal homeostasis.

The most common post-traumatic condition the critical care paramedic will have to deal with in OB trauma is placental separation. Placental separation is the second most common cause of fetal death (the most frequent cause is maternal death). Placental separation after trauma occurs in 1% to 5% of minor accidents and in up to 20% to 50% of major injuries. Separation results as the inelastic placenta shears away from the elastic uterus during sudden deformation of the uterus. Abruption can occur with little or no external signs of injury to the abdominal wall. Maternal mortality from abruption is less than 1%, but fetal death ranges from 20% to 35%. Clinical findings that indicate abruption include vaginal bleeding, abdominal cramps, uterine tenderness, amniotic fluid leakage, maternal hypovolemia, a uterus larger than normal for the gestational age, or a change in the fetal heart rate. When present after trauma, vaginal bleeding is an ominous sign often indicative of placental separation.

PHYSIOLOGICAL CHANGES DURING PREGNANCY

During pregnancy, normal physiological changes occur to provide for growth of the fetus and to prepare the mother for birth. Complications as the result of trauma may alter this adaptation and shift an uncomplicated pregnancy into a critical situation. (See Figure 20-6 ▪.)

The pregnant patient will have an increased circulatory volume. Increases in cardiac output and blood volume begin early in the first trimester and are 30% to 50% above the nonpregnant state by 28 weeks. This relative hypervolemic state and hemodilution is protective for the mother because fewer red blood cells are lost during hemorrhage. The hypervolemia prepares the mother for the blood loss that accompanies vaginal delivery (500 mL) or cesarean section (1000 mL). However, almost 40% of maternal blood volume may be lost before the manifestation of signs of maternal shock. As blood volume is lost after injury, blood is shunted away from the uterus first. A much greater degree of blood loss is required to produce compensatory tachycardia.

Cardiac output and heart rate increase in later pregnancy. The heart rate will be about 20 beats per minute above the patient's baseline. Blood pressure usually decreases about 10 mmHg, but rises to normal toward the end of pregnancy. (See Table 20–6.)

Respiratory changes occur to accommodate the enlarged uterus and the increased oxygen demands of the mother and fetus. Mechanical changes include the upward shift of the diaphragm,

Factors Associated with Increased Fetal Mortality after Trauma
Maternal hypotension/hemorrhage
High maternal Injury Severity Score (ISS)
Ejection from a motor vehicle
Maternal pelvic fracture
Auto versus pedestrian accidents
Maternal alcohol usage
Young maternal age (<18 years)
Motorcycle crashes
Maternal smoking history
Uterine rupture

Increasing Frequency

which decreases functional residual capacity, and rib cage volume displacement, which increases tidal volume by 30% to 35%. Respiratory alkalosis can be present because of the increased respiratory rate.

To accommodate both maternal and fetal metabolic and circulatory requirements, renal blood flow increases by 25% to 50% during gestation. Blood urea nitrogen (BUN) and serum creatinine are reduced. In addition, the kidneys enlarge through both hypertrophy and hyperemia as early as the 10th week of gestation secondary to hormonal and mechanical factors.

Hematocrit falls in pregnancy as circulating volume increases—a "dilution anemia." The complete blood count shows an elevated white blood count—usually around 15,000. Although clotting studies remain normal, levels of coagulation factors and fibrinogen increase. This change puts the pregnant trauma victim at increased risk of venous thrombosis or DIC (disseminated intravascular coagulation).

FACILITY ARRIVAL AND INITIAL TRAUMA ASSESSMENT

As previously mentioned in this chapter, once you enter the referring facility, ask to speak with the individual in charge of the patient. When obtaining the medical history of the obstetrical patient, you should gather information such as:

★ Nurse/physician notes

★ Lab values (especially PT, PTT, and fibrinogen studies)

★ X-rays

★ Ventilator settings

Table 20–6	Selected Physiological Changes of Pregnancy
Finding	**Change Observed in Normal Pregnancy**
Systolic blood pressure	Decreased by 5–15 mmHg
Diastolic blood pressure	Decreased by 5–15 mmHg
Heart rate	Increased by 10–15 beats/minute
Blood volume	Increased by 30–50%
Cardiac output	Increased by 1.0–1.5 L/minute
ECG	Flat or inverted T waves in III, V_1 and V_2; Q waves in leads III and aV_F
White blood cell count	Increased to 5–25 K per mm^3
D-Dimer	Often positive
PO_2	Increased to 100–108 mmHg
PCO_2	Decreased to 27–32 mmHg

- ★ Transfer orders (memorandum of transfer)
- ★ Nature of the illness/injury
- ★ Length of time the patient has been sick/injured
- ★ Presence of fever
- ★ Effects of the illness/injury on patient behavior
- ★ Fetal heart tones (FHT)
- ★ Results of electronic fetal heart-rate monitoring (EFM)
- ★ Bowel/urine habits
- ★ Presence of vomiting/diarrhea
- ★ Frequency of urination

When obtaining your report from the caregiver in charge make certain you understand and document all physician orders accurately.

To ensure the best possible chance of maternal and fetal survival, the primary goal in treating a pregnant trauma victim is to stabilize the mother's condition. The pregnant trauma patient should be properly stabilized at the referring facility and transported to the nearest Level I facility capable of treating both mother and fetus. As previously mentioned, the priorities for treatment of an injured pregnant patient remain the same as those for the nonpregnant patient.

The critical care paramedic must obtain a complete history, including an obstetrical history, perform a physical examination, and evaluate and monitor the fetus. The obstetrical history is important because the identification of comorbid factors may alter management decisions. A history of preterm labor or placental abruption puts the patient at increased risk for the recurrence of the condition. The obstetrical history should include the date of the last menstruation, expected date of delivery, and any problems or complications of the current and previous pregnancies. Determination of the uterine size provides an approximation of gestational age (i.e., measurement of fundal height is a rapid method for estimating fetal age). Determination of fetal age and hence of fetal maturity is an important factor in the decision making regarding early delivery. (See Figure 20-7 ■.)

FETAL ASSESSMENT

Fetal evaluation begins with checking fetal heart rate and noting fetal movement. Auscultation or Doppler can detect fetal heart tones. This should be done early after the critical care paramedics' arrival and repeated frequently. The normal range for the fetal heart rate is 120 to 160 beats/minute. Continuous EFM remains the most widely used modality for evaluation of the fetus, and is an adjunct to the monitoring of the maternal condition. The use of EFM permits prompt identification of the fetus at great risk for asphyxia and fetal death. (EFM is discussed in greater detail in Chapter 28, "High-Risk Obstetrical/Gynecological Emergencies.") Any viable fetus of 24 or more weeks' gestation requires monitoring after a trauma event. This includes patients with no obvious signs of abdominal injury because direct impact is not necessary for fetal trauma to be present.

TRANSPORT CONSIDERATIONS AND MANAGEMENT

The pregnant patient needs to be transported in a position of comfort unless she is hypotensive. If so, tilt or rotate the patient 20 to 30 degrees to the left. Manually displace the uterus to the left side during transport, especially in the 7-month or later gestation. Venous return to the maternal heart may be decreased up to 30% because of uterine compression by the fetus.

Hemodynamic monitoring may be indicated to accurately assess cardiac output and fluid volume status. Elevated pulmonary wedge pressure (PAWP) and pulmonary artery pressure (PAP) values may indicate hypervolemia, thus placing the woman at risk for cardiogenic pulmonary edema. Interventions to reduce preload include restricting intravenous fluids, repositioning the patient on her side, and administering diuretics when fluid overload or pulmonary edema is present. Decreased central venous pressure, PAP, and PAWP values indicate hypovolemia, and the patient may need a fluid challenge.

Figure 20-7 Approximate height of the fundus at various weeks of pregnancy.

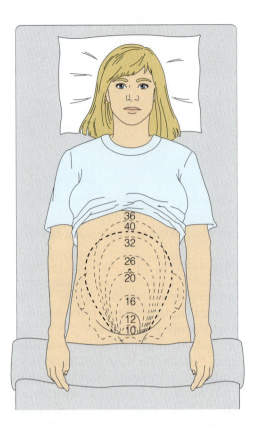

Summary

When a pregnant patient becomes critically injured, it is essential for the critical care paramedic to understand the physiological changes that occur during pregnancy. This knowledge can help the critical care paramedic recognize subtle changes to reduce morbidity and mortality. Collaboration between the referring facility staff and the critical care paramedic will facilitate appropriate management for both mother and her fetus.

Remember that the pregnant patient presents an emotional challenge to any health care provider. Not only do anatomical changes make the patient difficult to transport, but you are also treating two patients simultaneously. Maintaining an air of confidence will calm the patient and aid in your effective assessment and treatment in the prehospital setting.

Review Questions

1. Describe the significance and incidence of pediatric trauma.
2. Discuss the general approach of the Critical Care Paramedic to pediatric trauma.
3. Describe common growth and development of a child from a critical care perspective.
4. Discuss the paradigm shift seen in pediatric trauma care.
5. Describe the pediatric Glasgow Coma Scale.
6. Describe how to use the pediatric trauma score to determine the severity of pediatric injuries.
7. Discuss the critical care and transport of the geriatric patient with altered mental status.
8. Detail the transport considerations of the patient with obstetrical trauma.

See Answers to Review Questions at the back of this book.

Further Reading

Bledsoe BE, Porter RS, Cherry RA. *Paramedic Care: Principles & Practice, Volume 5,* 2nd ed., Upper Saddle River, NJ: Pearson Prentice Hall, 2005.

Eckstein M. "Double Trouble: Managing the Pregnant Trauma Patient." *Journal of Emergency Medical Services,* Vol. 30, No. 5 (2005): 110–131.

Hazinshi MF. *Manual of Pediatric Critical Care.* St. Louis, MO: Mosby, 1999.

Hudak CM, Gallo BM, Morton PG. *Critical Care Nursing: A Holistic Approach,* 7th ed. Philadelphia: J. B. Lippincott, 1998.

Kuhlman RS, Cruikshank DP. "Maternal Trauma during Pregnancy." *Clinical Obstetrics and Gynecology,* Vol. 37 (1994): 274–293.

Lapinsky SE. "Critical Care in the Pregnant Patient." *American Journal of Respiratory and Critical Care Medicine,* Vol. 152 (1995): 427–455.

Lee G. *Flight Nursing: Principles and Practice.* St. Louis, MO: Mosby, 1991.

Pearlman MD. "Blunt Trauma during Pregnancy." *New England Journal of Medicine,* Vol. 323 (1990): 1609–1613.

United States Department of Transportation, National Highway Traffic Safety Administration. *Standardized Child Passenger Safety Training Program, Participant Manual, 2000.* DOT HS 366 R2/00: Module C–5.

United States Department of Transportation, National Highway Traffic Safety Administration, National Center for Statistics and Analysis. *Traffic Safety Facts 1998: Children.* DOT HS 808 951: 1–5.

Pulmonary Emergencies

Scott R. Snyder, B.S., CCEMTP

Objectives

Upon completion of this chapter, the student should be able to:

1. Describe basic pulmonary anatomy and physiology. (p. 580)
2. Define acute respiratory failure. (p. 588)
3. Discuss and differentiate the pathology of common respiratory diseases seen in the critical care environment. (p. 588)
4. Define how the following assessment parameters assist in determining the severity of a pulmonary emergency:
   A. Inspection (p. 591)
   B. Palpation (p. 592)
   C. Percussion (p. 592)
   D. Auscultation (p. 593)
   E. Arterial blood gasses (p. 594)
   F. Pulse oximetry (p. 594)
   G. End tidal capnography (p. 595)
5. Discuss the basic management of the following pulmonary diseases:
   A. Acute respiratory failure (p. 597)
   B. Asthma (p. 601)
   C. Chronic obstructive pulmonary disease (p. 608)
   D. Acute respiratory distress syndrome (p. 610)
   E. Pneumonia (p. 613)
   F. Pneumothorax (p. 616)

Key Terms

acute respiratory failure (ARF), p. 588
egophony, p. 593
capnography, p. 595
hypercapnia, p. 588

noninvasive positive-pressure ventilation (NPPV), p. 603
$PaCO_2$, p. 588
PaO_2, p. 588
perialveolar capillary bed, p. 589

physiological shunt, p. 589
pulmonary surfactant, p. 286
ventilation/perfusion (V/Q) mismatch, p. 589
whispered pectoriloquy, p. 594

Case Study

Your critical care transport team is dispatched to a rural health care facility to transport a 44-year-old female suffering from severe exacerbation of asthma to your tertiary health care facility. Due to lightning storms in the area however, the pilot of your BK-117 helicopter informs you that he is refusing the flight, and you will have to go by ground. You and your partner gather your equipment, load the ambulance, and with the driver begin the 1.5-hour response to the transferring facility.

Upon arrival at the transferring ED, you take a quick glance into the treatment room and see a 44-year-old female who is conscious and in respiratory distress. You note that she is experiencing severe dyspnea, and her responses to questions asked by the hospital staff are given in three- to four-word sentences. The attending physician approaches you and your partner, introduces himself, and starts to give your partner the patient report as you enter the treatment room to perform a physical assessment.

You introduce yourself to the patient, who nods her head quickly and gives you a wave as she is inhaling the mist created by a nebulizer in her hand. As you watch the mist disappear from the end of the nebulizer with each breath you notice, to your dismay, that her tidal volume is quite diminished. "I can tell that you are having a hard time breathing," you tell her, "so I will keep my questions simple, just nod your head yes or no, OK? Is it OK if I examine you?" She nods her head yes and you begin your physical exam.

You note that she is using her accessory muscles, and has slight suprasternal and intercostal retractions with each respiration. The exhalation phase of each breath is noticeably prolonged, and you can hear wheezing despite the fact that your stethoscope is still around your neck. When you auscultate her lung fields, you appreciate diminished breath sounds in all fields with inspiratory and expiratory wheezing. "At least I hear air movement in all fields," you think to yourself as you take your stethoscope out of your ears and place it back around your neck. You palpate a strong, rapid radial pulse as you reach over to activate the automated blood pressure cuff, and note that her skin is cool, slightly diaphoretic, and pale. You glance over at the pulse oximeter and capnography reading as the BP cuff deflates. Her vital signs are HR = 124 sinus tachycardia, BP = 132/78, RR = 28, SpO_2 = 93%, and $PetCO_2$ = 48 mmHg.

Your partner enters the room, and you introduce her to the patient. You and your partner then proceed to exchange the information you have accumulated. She informs you that the patient has a long history of asthma (her only history) treated at home with β-agonist and anticholinergic metered-dose inhalers (MDIs) and theophylline PO. She arrived at the ED 2 hours ago by personal vehicle after experiencing an acute onset of difficulty breathing that was not relieved by her MDIs after 2 hours of home treatment. "So we're now four hours into this attack," you think, "Phase II." Upon her initial arrival at the ED she was placed on continuous albuterol treatment via nebulizer, and 1.5 hours ago was administered 125 mg of Solu-Medrol IV. The staff states that while her condition has not worsened, it has not improved.

"We have some lab data and an X-ray to consider," your partner says as she slides an upright AP chest radiograph on the lightbox. You both note a slightly hyperinflated thorax, characteristic of asthma. ABG analysis reveals PaO_2 = 85 mmHg, $PaCO_2$ = 48 mmHg, pH = 7.32, and HCO_3^- = 26.

You both look at the patient, and your partner asks you "So, do you think we should intubate her before we transport?" "Well," you say, "she's working hard to breathe, but does not appear to be tired yet. And while her lung sounds are diminished, she is at least moving air to all fields, which is good. Her chest X-ray and ABG both indicate that she has some diminished pulmonary function, but she is in no way in extremis."

Your partner looks at you and says "I agree. Considering the clinical and diagnostic information, I'm a little hesitant to intubate, as she may not need it, and it may end up complicating things." You nod your head in agreement. "We will initiate noninvasive positive-pressure ventilation while we prepare to leave, and see if she improves a bit." "I think that would be a wise decision," the attending adds. "Plus, the Solu-Medrol should start having some effect any time now."

"Yeah, but let's see what our med direction thinks also. . . ," you say as you walk over to the nurses' station to call the receiving physician. Your partner and the attending walk over to the patient and explain the noninvasive positive-pressure ventilation therapy to the patient as they set up the required equipment. You give a report to the receiving physician, who agrees with your management decision. You initiate the pressure support ventilation and after a few minutes of coaching the patient gets used to the apparatus and can relax with the mask on. You note an almost immediate SpO_2 increase to 98%, the $PetCO_2$ lowers some, and the patient's respiratory rate soon drops to 22 a minute.

During the course of transport, the patient's vital signs improve slightly, and while you haven't necessarily cured her on the way to your facility, you are able to complete the transport without incident.

INTRODUCTION

This chapter reviews the pathophysiology of acute respiratory failure (ARF) and several of the pulmonary emergencies that can result in ARF. It is worth noting that while the critical care paramedic will often have diagnostic test information available to aid in clinical decision making, it is important to remember that these diagnostic tests are not a "holy grail" that replaces a sound understanding of pulmonary disease processes and good clinical examination. Rather, diagnostics that may be available at the sending facility are designed to augment understanding and clinical judgment.

The critical care paramedic will often have diagnostic test information available to aid in clinical decision making. It is important to remember that these diagnostic tests are not a "holy grail" that replaces a sound understanding of pulmonary disease processes and good clinical examination.

ANATOMY AND PHYSIOLOGY

The cells of the body rely on aerobic metabolism as the preferred method of producing energy. This process requires that O_2 be delivered from the atmosphere to the cellular mitochondria, and that CO_2 be removed from the intracellular environment and transported to the atmosphere. A lack of O_2 or the accumulation of CO_2 in the blood leads to cellular hypoxia, hypercapnia, and eventual hemodynamic derangement. The role of the respiratory system is to facilitate the transfer of these gases between the atmosphere and the circulatory system. Other functions include defense against infection, and the synthesis of chemicals such as surfactant and angiotensin-converting enzyme.

The respiratory system can be divided into the upper and lower airways, with the glottic opening being the transition between the two. In addition, the respiratory system can be considered in terms of function and divided into the conducting zone and respiratory zone. The conducting zone extends from the entrance of the nasal and oral cavities to the terminal bronchioles of the lungs, and the respiratory zone from the respiratory bronchioles to the individual alveoli, the functional unit of the lung and the site of gas exchange. The conducting zone, due to its lack of alveoli and inability to exchange gas, constitutes the anatomical dead space of the airway. (See Figure 21-1 ■.)

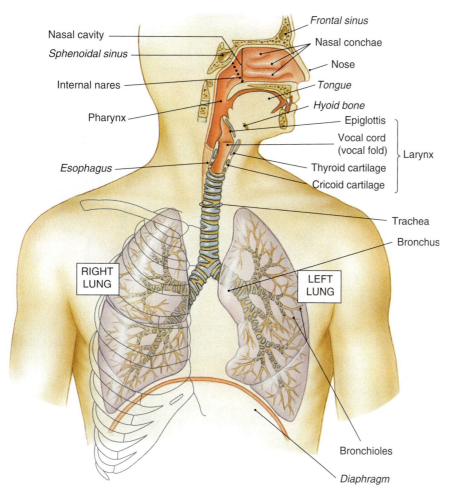

Nasal cavity
Sphenoidal sinus
Internal nares
Pharynx
Esophagus

Frontal sinus
Nasal conchae
Nose
Tongue
Hyoid bone
Epiglottis
Vocal cord (vocal fold)
Thyroid cartilage
Cricoid cartilage
} Larynx

RIGHT LUNG
LEFT LUNG

Trachea
Bronchus
Bronchioles
Diaphragm

■ **Figure 21-1** The components of the respiratory system. *(Fig. 16-1, p. 438, from* Essentials of Anatomy & Physiology, *2nd ed., by Frederic H. Martini, Ph.D. and Edwin F. Bartholomew, M.S. Copyright © 2000 by Frederic H. Martini, Inc. Published by Pearson Education, Inc. Reprinted by permission.)*

THE UPPER AIRWAY

RESPIRATORY EPITHELIUM

Although not a structure specific to the upper airway, the respiratory epithelium is a unique tissue structure that lines most of the respiratory tree, so its structure and function are discussed here first. (See Figure 21-2 ■.) This specialized respiratory epithelium consists of goblet and psuedostratified, ciliated, columnar epithelial cells, which line the respiratory tract in the nasal cavity and extend from the trachea through the alveolar ducts. Goblet cells produce and secrete mucus that covers the exposed respiratory lumen. Cilia in the nasopharynx sweep trapped particulate matter backward to the pharynx, and cilia in the lower respiratory tract sweep particulate material up to the pharynx. This combination of goblet cells and ciliated epithelium form the mucociliary escalator, which effectively traps and removes foreign debris from the respiratory passageways down to the level of the respiratory bronchioles.

NASAL CAVITY

The upper airway's primary function is to filter, warm, and humidify inspired atmospheric air. Filtering is achieved by the coarse hairs that pack the nasal vestibule and extend across the external nares. Warming and humidification are accomplished by the nasal conchae (or turbinates), located in the nasal cavity, whose structure creates turbulent airflow over their warm, moist, mucous-covered surfaces. This creation of turbulent airflow increases the amount of air coming into contact with the conchae surface, increasing heat and moisture transfer and increasing the likelihood that fine, inhaled debris not filtered by the nasal hair will become entrapped in mucus. The nasal hairs and turbinates remove most particles greater than 10 μm in diameter. (See Figure 21-3 ■.)

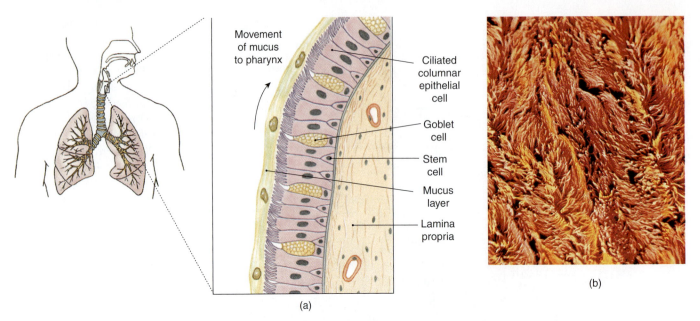

(a)

(b)

■ **Figure 21-2** The respiratory epithelium. (a) A sketch showing the sectional appearance of the respiratory epithelium and its role in mucus transport. (b) A surface view of the epithelium. The cilia of the epithelial cells form a dense layer that resembles a shag carpet. The movement of these cilia propels mucus across the epithelial surface. *(a from Fig. 16-3, p. 440, from* Essentials of Anatomy & Physiology, *2nd ed., by Frederic H. Martini, Ph.D. and Edwin F. Bartholomew, M.S. Copyright © 2000 by Frederic H. Martini, Inc. Published by Pearson Education, Inc. Reprinted by permission. b from Photo Researchers, Inc.)*

PHARYNX

The nose, mouth, and throat are all connected posteriorly by the pharynx, which is divided into the nasopharynx, oropharynx, and laryngopharynx (hypopharynx). Components of both the respiratory and the gastrointestinal tracts share the pharynx. The nasopharynx is the most superior division of the pharynx, located behind the nasal cavity, and is lined with respiratory epithelium. The oropharynx is located posterior to the oral cavity, and extends from the soft palate superiorly to the hyoid bone inferiorly. It is lined not with respiratory epithelium, but with stratified squamous epithelium. The laryngopharynx is the inferior-most division of the pharynx, bordered by the hyoid superiorly and the glottis inferiorly. It too is lined with stratified squamous epithelium that can resist the mechanical abrasion and pathogenic introduction common with the ingestion of food. Occasionally, the term *hypopharynx* is used to describe the inferior portion of the pharynx, corresponding to the height of the epiglottis.

THE LOWER AIRWAY

LARYNX

The larynx protective structure encloses the glottis, and also serves as a filtering device of sorts, with the epiglottis directing food into the esophagus, and inspired air allowed to enter the trachea via the glottic opening, or glottis. It extends between the level of vertebrae C4 and C6. Three cartilagenous structures form the larynx: the thyroid cartilage, cricoid cartilage, and the epiglottis. Additional small cartilages located on the posterior surface of the larynx include two cuneiform cartilages, two corniculate cartilages, and two arytenoid cartilages (to be discussed later).

The thyroid cartilage is the largest of the three. It forms the anterior and lateral walls of the larynx and is open posteriorly. It is commonly referred to as the Adam's apple, and is easily inspected and palpated. The cricoid cartilage is located inferior to the thyroid cartilage, and attaches to the thyroid by means of the cricothyroid (or intrinsic), ligament. Unlike the thyroid cartilage, the cricoid is complete posteriorly, giving it a ring-like appearance; hence, the common moniker "cricoid ring." The inferior cricoid attaches to the first cartilagenous ring of the trachea via the cricotracheal (or extrinsic) ligament. The epiglottis, located posterior to the thyroid and superior

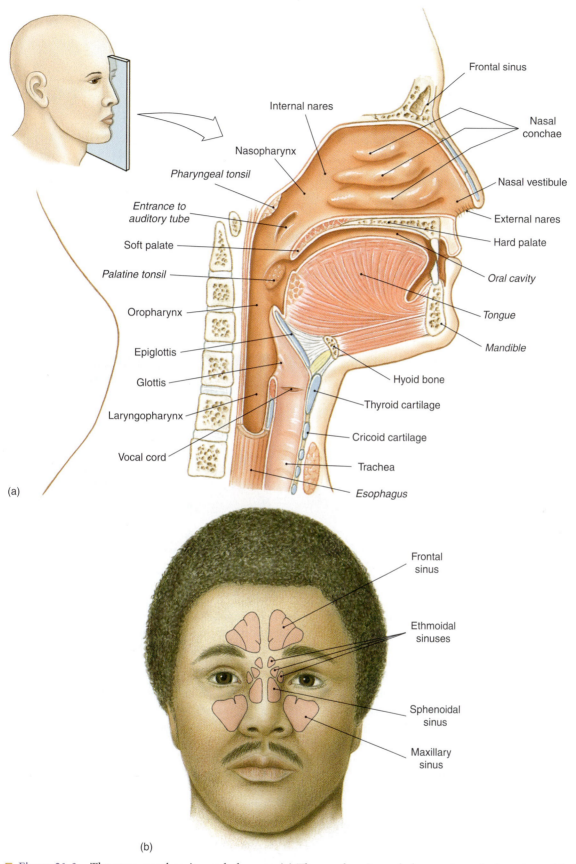

Figure 21-3 The nose, nasal cavity, and pharynx. (a) The nasal cavity and pharynx in sagittal section, with the nasal septum removed. (b) The locations of the paranasal sinuses. *(Fig. 16-2, p. 439, from* Essentials of Anatomy & Physiology, *2nd ed., by Frederic H. Martini, Ph.D. and Edwin F. Bartholomew, M.S. Copyright © 2000 by Frederic H. Martini, Inc. Published by Pearson Education, Inc. Reprinted by permission.)*

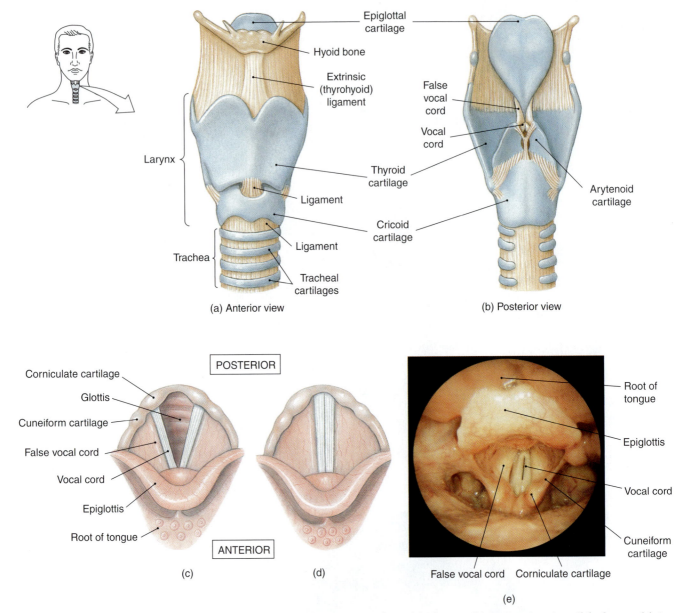

Labels in figure (a) Anterior view:
- Epiglottal cartilage
- Hyoid bone
- Extrinsic (thyrohyoid) ligament
- Larynx
- Thyroid cartilage
- Ligament
- Cricoid cartilage
- Trachea
- Ligament
- Tracheal cartilages

(a) Anterior view

Labels in figure (b) Posterior view:
- False vocal cord
- Vocal cord
- Arytenoid cartilage
- Cricoid cartilage

(b) Posterior view

Labels in figures (c) and (d):
- POSTERIOR
- Corniculate cartilage
- Glottis
- Cuneiform cartilage
- False vocal cord
- Vocal cord
- Epiglottis
- Root of tongue
- ANTERIOR

(c)   (d)

Labels in figure (e):
- Root of tongue
- Epiglottis
- Vocal cord
- Cuneiform cartilage
- False vocal cord
- Corniculate cartilage

(e)

■ **Figure 21-4**   The anatomy of the larynx and vocal cords. (a) An anterior view of the larynx. (b) A posterior view of the larynx. (c) A superior view of the larynx with the glottis open and (d) with the glottis closed. (e) A fiber-optic view of the larynx with the glottis closed. *(a–d from Fig. 16-4, p. 441, from Essentials of Anatomy & Physiology, 2nd ed., by Frederic H. Martini, Ph.D. and Edwin F. Bartholomew, M.S. Copyright © 2000 by Frederic H. Martini, Inc. Published by Pearson Education, Inc. Reprinted by permission. e from Phototake NYC.)*

to the glottis, has ligamentous attachments to the thyroid cartilage inferiorly and the hyoid bone superiorly. It effectively covers the glottis when the larynx is elevated during swallowing.

Additional structures in the larynx include the arytenoid, corniculate and cuneiform cartilages, the vocal cords, and the glottis (the space located between the vocal cords through which all inspired air must pass on its way to the lungs). A point of clinical reference is that if any occlusion exists between the glottic opening and the carina inferiorly, it will result in a fatal airway obstruction if not relieved. (See Figure 21-4 ■.)

TRACHEA AND PRIMARY BRONCHI

The trachea begins at about the level of C5/C6, and extends about 11 cm to its terminus at the carina, where it divides into the right and left main stem bronchi. The trachea has a diameter of about 2.5 cm, and is a moderately flexible tube whose anterior and lateral walls consist of numerous C-shaped cartilaginous rings connected by intercartilagenous (or annular) ligaments. This construction prevents the trachea from collapsing or overexpanding secondary to airway pressure

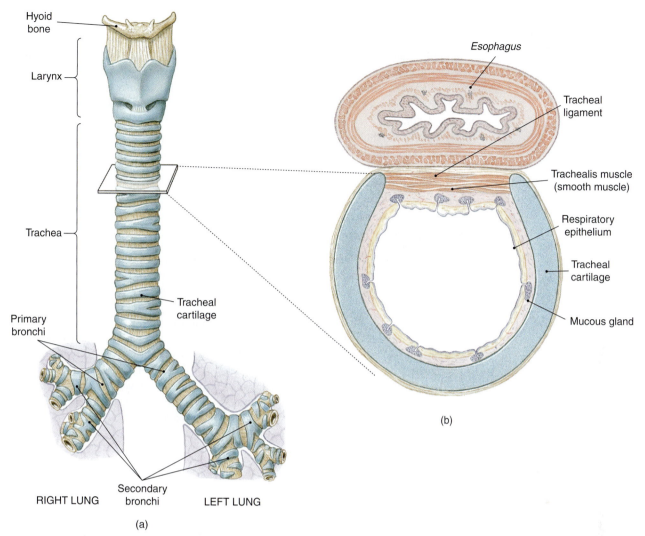

Hyoid bone

Larynx

Trachea

Tracheal cartilage

Primary bronchi

Secondary bronchi

RIGHT LUNG

LEFT LUNG

(a)

Esophagus

Tracheal ligament

Trachealis muscle (smooth muscle)

Respiratory epithelium

Tracheal cartilage

Mucous gland

(b)

■ **Figure 21-5**   The anatomy of the trachea. (a) An anterior view, showing the plane of section. (b) A cross-sectional view of the trachea and esophagus. *(Fig. 16-5, p. 442, from* Essentials of Anatomy & Physiology, *2nd ed., by Frederic H. Martini, Ph.D. and Edwin F. Bartholomew, M.S. Copyright © 2000 by Frederic H. Martini, Inc. Published by Pearson Education, Inc. Reprinted by permission.)*

changes. The posterior wall of the trachea is made up of a layer of smooth muscle termed the trachialis. The lining of the trachea consists of a layer of respiratory epithelium bound to the underlying cartilage and ligaments by a layer of loose connective tissue, the lamina propria. (See Figure 21-5 ■.)

The trachea bifurcates at the carina to form the right and left main stem, or primary, bronchi. The primary bronchi are often termed the extrapulmonary bronchi due to their location outside of the lungs. Each primary bronchus enters the lung, along with the pulmonary vessels, lymph vessels, and nerves, through the hilus. Like the trachea, the primary bronchi are held open by cartilagenous rings. This collection of structures is held in place by a network of dense connective tissue called the root of the lung. The two roots are located at the level of vertebrae T5 on the right, and T6 on the left. The left side is slightly higher owing to the location of the heart in the thoracic mediastinal cavity.

BRONCHIAL TREE

The primary bronchi, after entering the lungs, divide to form the secondary bronchi, and then the tertiary bronchi—all of which have progressively lesser amounts of cartilaginous support. This cartilaginous support ends at the level of the terminal brochi, and the first smooth muscle starts to appear in the walls of the terminal bronchioles. This allows autonomic control of the terminal bronchiole lumen diameter. Terminal bronchioles divide to form respiratory bronchioles, so named for the individual alveoli that start to appear on their outer wall. Respiratory bronchioles give way to alveolar ducts, alveolar sacs, and then individual alveoli, the site of gas exchange in the lung.

ALVEOLI

The lungs contain approximately 300 million individual alveoli, each of which is almost completely enveloped in pulmonary capillaries. It has been estimated that each alveolus has nearly 1,000 pulmonary capillaries associated with it. Gas exchange takes place across the alveolar-capillary membrane, which consists of three layers: the alveolar epithelial cell, the capillary endothelial cell, and the fused basil lamina of each in the interstitial space between them. At this level, the total distance separating the alveolar and capillary lumens is between 0.1 and 0.5 μm, allowing gas exchange to take place rapidly. Factors that will decrease the efficacy of gas exchange between the respiratory and circulatory systems include:

1. Increased width of the interstitial space
2. Lack of perfusion of the pulmonary capillaries
3. Interruption of the alveolar endothelial membrane
4. Filling of alveoli with fluid

Small holes in some of the alveolar walls, called pores of Kohn, allow for limited interalveolar communication. Likewise, the canals of Lambert allow collateral circulation of air between adjacent bronchiole structures. The net effect of these pores and canals is to allow better air distribution to occur without increasing the amount of airway resistance.

Three types of cells are present in the alveoli: Type I pneumocytes, Type II pneumocytes, and alveolar macrophages. The alveolar epithelium is made up primarily of a single layer of Type I alveolar cells and these cells are the ones that allow gas exchange. Interspersed among the Type I cells are Type II surfactant-producing cells. **Pulmonary surfactant** consists of an assortment of phospholipids that serve to decrease the surface tension of water in the alveoli, preventing alveolar collapse and atelectasis. The third type of alveolar cell is phagocytic alveolar macrophages, which roam the alveolar epithelium surface, cleaning up debris such as dust or bacteria that eludes the respiratory defenses. The engulfed material is broken down by the macrophage's lysosomes. (See Figure 21-6 ■.)

pulmonary surfactant *a combination of phospholipids that serve to decrease the surface tension of water in the alveoli, preventing alveolar collapse and atelectasis.*

LUNGS

The lungs are located in the pleural cavity of the thorax, with the base of each resting on the diaphragm and the apex of each extending superior to Zone I of the neck immediately superior to the first rib. The lungs are divided into distinct lobes separated by fissures; the left lung has two lobes, and the right lung three. To the left lung, the oblique fissure separates the lung's superior and inferior lobes. On the right larger lung, the horizontal fissure separates the superior and middle lobes, while the oblique fissure separates the middle and inferior lobes. The connective tissue of the root penetrates each lung into the parenchyma, branching often to divide each lobe into smaller and smaller compartments, called lobules. Each lobule receives a tributary of the bronchial tree, pulmonary artery, and pulmonary vein.

Each lung is covered with visceral pleura, which reflects with the parietal pleura that adheres to the inside surface of the chest wall. The pleurae are serous membranes, and secrete pleural fluid that provides lubrication between the lung and chest wall as the two surfaces move over one another during the respiratory cycle. In addition, the pleural fluid helps to bind the two pleurae together via the hydrostatic attraction of water molecules in the fluid. This attraction, in effect, helps to create a negative pressure between the two pleural layers (along with the normal elasticity of the pulmonary tissue), and subsequently keeps the lung "attached" to the inside surface of the chest wall. An analogy to help understand this action is when a slide plate is placed on a slide for viewing under a microscope. The slide is held firmly together by the surface tension of a drop of water placed between them; separating the two requires some effort.

There is a potential space between the visceral and parietal pleurae, which can create an actual space if the negative pressure between the two is broken, as in the case of pneumothorax.

BLOOD SUPPLY TO THE LUNGS

The pulmonary arteries enter the lungs at the hilus, and branch with the bronchial tree so that each lobule receives its own pulmonary arteriole and vein. The pulmonary vein divides further to form the pulmonary capillaries, which surround and cover the alveolus. Gas exchange takes place across

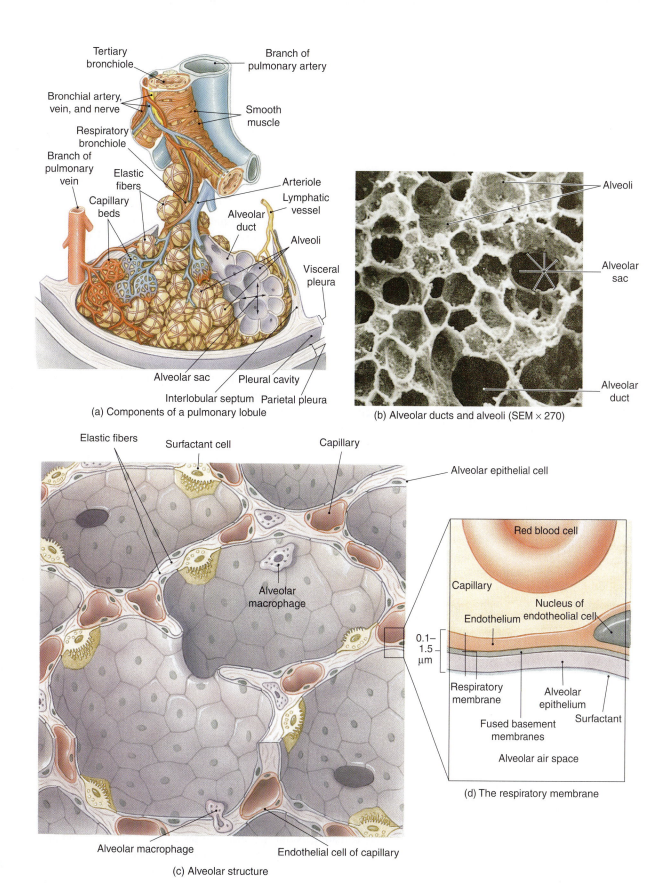

(a) Components of a pulmonary lobule

Tertiary bronchiole

Branch of pulmonary artery

Bronchial artery, vein, and nerve

Smooth muscle

Respiratory bronchiole

Branch of pulmonary vein

Elastic fibers

Arteriole

Lymphatic vessel

Capillary beds

Alveolar duct

Alveoli

Visceral pleura

Alveolar sac

Pleural cavity

Interlobular septum

Parietal pleura

(b) Alveolar ducts and alveoli (SEM × 270)

Alveoli

Alveolar sac

Alveolar duct

Elastic fibers

Surfactant cell

Capillary

Alveolar epithelial cell

Alveolar macrophage

Red blood cell

Capillary

Nucleus of endotheolial cell

Endothelium

0.1– 1.5 μm

Respiratory membrane

Fused basement membranes

Alveolar epithelium

Surfactant

Alveolar air space

(d) The respiratory membrane

Alveolar macrophage

Endothelial cell of capillary

(c) Alveolar structure

■ **Figure 21-6** Alveolar organization. (a) The basic structure of a lobule. A network of capillaries surrounds each alveolus. (b) A scanning electron micrograph of the lung. (c) A diagrammatic view of alveolar structure. (d) The respiratory membrane. *(a, c, and d from Fig. 16-6, p. 444, from* Essentials of Anatomy & Physiology, *2nd ed., by Frederic H. Martini, Ph.D. and Edwin F. Bartholomew, M.S. Copyright © 2000 by Frederic H. Martini, Inc. Published by Pearson Education, Inc. Reprinted by permission. b from Micrograph by P. Gehr, from Bloom & Fawcett,* Textbook of Histology, *W. B. Saunders Co.)*

the alveolar-capillary membrane, and blood returns to the left atrium via the pulmonary venules and vein. In addition to their role in gas exchange, the pulmonary capillaries are the site of production of angiotensin-converting enzyme.

Like all other tissue in the body, the conducting tissue of the lung must receive it's own blood supply to deliver oxygen and nutrients and remove metabolic waste. The bronchial arteries supply arterial blood to the bronchial tree, and venous blood flows into the pulmonary veins, mixing with the oxygen-rich blood leaving the alveoli and returning via the left ventricle.

PATHOPHYSIOLOGY, ASSESSMENT, AND MANAGEMENT

The potential end result of all pulmonary emergencies left unidentified or unmanaged is acute respiratory failure and eventual cardiovascular collapse.

The potential end result of all pulmonary emergencies left unidentified or unmanaged is acute respiratory failure and eventual cardiovascular collapse. It is therefore imperative that all members of the critical care transport team be able to identify the clinical conditions associated with impending respiratory failure, and the management to prevent it. We will first discuss the pathophysiology, assessment, and management of ARF. Afterward, we will review some of the various disease processes that may result in ARF, and discuss the assessment findings and management modalities that are specific to each.

ACUTE RESPIRATORY FAILURE

ARF occurs as a result of many etiologies and may be the patient's primary problem, or a secondary result to an existing disease process. ARF differs from chronic respiratory failure (CRF) in that it develops rapidly, not allowing adequate time for the normal compensatory mechanisms to alleviate the insult. However, ARF and CRF are not mutually exclusive of one another; ARF frequently develops as an exacerbation of a preexisting respiratory condition.

acute respiratory failure (ARF) *defined as a state of inadequate gas exchange resulting from the inability of the respiratory system to absorb O_2 and/or excrete CO_2.*

PaO_2 *oxygen level in arterial blood.*

$PaCO_2$ *carbon dioxide level in arterial blood.*

hypercapnia *high levels of carbon dioxide in arterial blood.*

Acute respiratory failure (ARF) can be defined as a state of inadequate gas exchange, and occurs when the respiratory system is unable to absorb oxygen and/or excrete carbon dioxide. While ARF can be suspected based on purely clinical findings, the best method for diagnosing ARF is an arterial blood gas (ABG) analysis. While no rigid criteria exist, it is generally accepted that ARF exists when the arterial oxygenation level (**PaO_2**) is less than 60 mmHg and the level of arterial carbon dioxide (**$PaCO_2$**) is greater than 50 mmHg, with an arterial pH of less than 7.30 on room air. ARF can be categorized as a failure of oxygenation resulting in hypoxemia, a failure of ventilation resulting in high levels of arterial carbon dioxide (**hypercapnia**), or a combination of both.

OXYGENATION FAILURE

Oxygenation failure resulting in hypoxemia has six generally accepted mechanisms:

1. Hypoventilation
2. Ventilation/perfusion mismatch
3. Intrapulmonary shunting
4. Cardiogenic shock
5. Diffusion defects
6. Low FiO_2

Hypoventilation

Alveolar hypoventilation resulting in hypoxemia can have many different causes.

Alveolar hypoventilation resulting in hypoxemia can have many different causes. To this end, foreign body airway obstruction of the upper airway is perhaps one of the most easily recognizable and rapidly reversible causes of hypoventilation. Numerous other causes, however, also exist and many times are seen by the critical care paramedic. Depression of the respiratory center located in the medulla from drug intoxication, rising intracranial pressure, central nervous system (CNS) sedation, or cerebrovascular accidents can cause the same type of effect. Interruption or impairment of nervous impulses from the CNS to the pulmonary inspiratory musculature may occur in incidences of cervical spinal cord injury, phrenic nerve insult, or disease states that interfere with nervous impulse transmission. Examples of diseases such as these include muscular dystrophy, multiple sclerosis, poliomyelitis, and polyneuritis. Pathology resulting in mechanical abnormalities to the lung or chest wall can also result in alveolar hypoventilation.

Injuries that decrease chest wall or lung compliance such as fractured ribs, a flailed chest, pleural effusion, or pneumothorax can result in decreased lung expansion and precipitate alveolar hypoventilation. Post-traumatic or post-thoracoabdominal surgical pain may result in shallow breathing due to the discomfort of taking deep or normal breaths. All of these causes of alveolar hypoventilation result in the same outcome: decreased minute ventilation and alveolar hypoventilation. The drop in PAO_2 will invariably lead to derangements in the patient's PaO_2, and in addition it is worth noting that alveolar hypoventilation will also result in an increased $PACO_2$ (and eventually an increased $PaCO_2$), as the body continues to produce and transport CO_2 to the lungs. Therefore, all of these mechanisms described as contributing to hypoxemia secondary to inadequate oxygenation can also contribute to hypercapnia secondary to ventilation failure as well.

Ventilation/Perfusion Mismatch

A **ventilation/perfusion (V/Q) mismatch** occurs when either perfusion or ventilation to an area of lung decreases, resulting in diminished gas exchange, hypoxemia, and hypercapnia. In a healthy lung, there should be (theoretically) an equal amount of perfusion for the amount of ventilation that a particular region of the lung receives. What this means is that in the theoretical lung, there is no wasted ventilation (all oxygen and carbon dioxide are exchanged), and there is no wasted perfusion (all RBCs passing through the **perialveolar capillary bed**—the network of capillaries surrounding the alveoli—are fully oxygenated). Realistically, this ideal state never occurs, even in the healthy lung, because of preferential perfusion of the basal pulmonary vascular (due to effects of gravity and other influences), as well as relative hyperventilation to the more compliant apical alveoli. The actual V/Q ratio in the healthy adult is 4/5 (or 0.8).

If, in the diseased or injured lung, ventilation is even more impaired, then there will be a greater amount of wasted perfusion (called *shunting*), and the V/Q ratio will diminish (that is, be <0.8). This may occur in situations of poor lung compliance (from a flail chest) or heightened airway resistance (such as asthma with severe bronchospasm and mucous secretion). Hypoxemia develops because blood directed to the affected region of the lung does not have the opportunity to receive oxygen from the hypoventilated alveoli.

In situations where a section of the lung tissue receives adequate ventilation, but inadequate perfusion, the V/Q ratio will begin to exceed 0.8. Situations where the lung may receive inadequate perfusion could include a pulmonary embolus, severe volume depletion, or a failing right ventricle that can no longer maintain good pulmonary perfusion pressures. The consequences of this type of V/Q mismatch are discussed in greater detail in the ventilation failure section.

Intrapulmonary Shunting

Normal cardiopulmonary anatomy and resultant blood flow results in what is commonly termed the **physiological shunt,** in which a small amount of blood returning to the left side of the heart from the lungs does not participate in alveolar gas exchange. This physiological shunt exists because of the introduction of deoxygenated blood into the pulmonary vein from drainage of the coronary and bronchial veins, and the normal variances of alveolar perfusion and ventilation secondary to gravity (as discussed earlier). The physiological shunt can be calculated using the following equation:

$$\frac{QPS}{QT} = \frac{CiO_2 - CaO_2}{CiO_2 - CvO_2}$$

where QPS is the physiological shunt flow, QT is the cardiac output per minute, CiO_2 is the concentration of oxygen in arterial blood when the V/Q ratio is ideal, CaO_2 is the measured arterial blood oxygen concentration, and CvO_2 is the measured oxygen concentration in mixed-venous blood. If, as in the case of a V/Q ratio of less than 0.8, an area of the lung is not properly ventilated and perfusion remains normal, the PaO_2 will decrease and a "right-to-left" shunt is said to occur. More simply worded, the perfusing RBCs "see no air" in the lung, and return to the left atrium with some degree of underoxygenation. Note that the development of a pathologic right-to-left shunt

ventilation/perfusion (V/Q) mismatch
phenomenon where either perfusion or ventilation to an area of lung decreases; results in diminished gas exchange, hypoxemia, and hypercapnia.

perialveolar capillary bed
the network of capillaries surrounding the alveoli.

A ventilation/perfusion (V/Q) mismatch occurs when either perfusion or ventilation to an area of lung decreases, resulting in diminished gas exchange, hypoxemia, and hypercapnia.

physiologic shunt
introduction of deoxygenated blood into the pulmonary vein from drainage of the coronary and bronchial veins, combined with the normal variances of alveolar perfusion and ventilation secondary to gravity.

occurs as a result of ongoing V/Q mismatching. Although separately described, these two pathologies, in effect, go hand in hand.

Cardiogenic Shock

Normal oxygen transport to the peripheral tissues is 600 to 1,000 mL/min, of which cardiac output (CO) is a major determinant, shown in the formula:

$$O_2 \text{ transport} = CaO_2 \times CO \times 10$$

where CaO_2 is the arterial oxygen content in mL/cc. Cardiogenic shock develops secondary to ventricular heart failure, and is typified by the presence of diminished ventricular ejection and a drop in cardiac output. Thus, the decreased CO associated with cardiogenic shock results in impaired blood flow to (and perfusion of) the peripheral tissues. This includes blood flow through the pulmonary capillaries, resulting in a decrease in gas exchange, and hypoxemia. In this situation, the drop in perfusion to the lungs, which may precipitate hypoxemia and hypercapnia, would be a perfusion deficit to the V/Q ratio.

Diffusion Deficits

Diffusion of CO_2 and O_2 between the pulmonary capillaries and alveoli occurs because (1) a concentration gradient exists and (2) the pulmonary-capillary membrane is between 0.1 and 0.5 µm thick, facilitating rapid and efficient gas exchange. Any disturbance to the delicate alveolar-capillary membrane will result in decreased diffusion of gas across it. Interstitial edema can occur secondary to damaged capillary membranes, pulmonary hypertension, and the leaking of plasma proteins into the interstitial space. The alveolar-capillary membrane may also thicken as a result of fibrotic changes in the lung, thus reducing diffusion. The introduction of plasma into the alveoli, as in the case of heart failure, increases the distance that O_2 and CO_2 must travel during diffusion across the interstitial space and, therefore, hampers diffusion. Important to note clinically regarding this abnormality is that O_2 diffuses less readily than CO_2 and, as such, hypoxemia often results well before hypercapnia in diffusion deficits.

Low FiO$_2$

Low FiO$_2$ can also occur at altitude recreationally, and even during aeromedical transport (to some degree). In addition, it can occur in enclosed and unventilated spaces. For example, the inattentive use of oxygenation adjuncts can result in this if a nonrebreather oxygen mask is used with an inadequate O_2 flow rate. Since the design of a nonrebreather mask relies on the oxygen flow rate to meet the inspiratory needs of the patient, if the flow rate is too low, then the patient's FiO$_2$ will suffer and hypoxemia will result. The same would also occur if an inadequate oxygen flow rate to an intubated and ventilated patient were allowed to exist.

VENTILATION FAILURE

Hypoventilation and V/Q mismatch are the primary mechanisms responsible for hypercapnia.

Ventilation failure resulting in hypercapnia is measured by evaluating the PaCO$_2$ via ABG analysis. Hypoventilation and V/Q mismatch are the primary mechanisms responsible for this hypercapnia. Hypercapnia develops when CO_2 accumulates in the alveoli, thereby eliminating the concentration gradient necessary for CO_2 to diffuse from the blood into the alveoli. Respiratory acidosis develops quickly, and is not attenuated by renal compensation.

Hypoventilation-induced hypercapnia, as discussed earlier, is any situation in which there is inadequate ventilation to the alveoli, a situation that is typically easy for critical care providers to understand. Simply, inadequate minute ventilations that promote poor alveolar ventilation allow carbon dioxide levels to build, and oxygen levels to diminish.

The V/Q mismatch that results in hypercapnia occurs when ventilation to any area of the lung is greater than blood flow to that same area of the lung. This results in a situation where the "air sees no blood" (such as in the case of a pulmonary embolus), and carbon dioxide cannot be offloaded to the alveoli for exhalation. In effect, this condition results in an increase in the amount of physiological dead space that exists in the lung (25% to 30% of inspired volume normally occupies dead space). This increase in dead space cannot be recognized clinically by auscultating breath sounds, nor by noting changes in the patient's minute ventilation. It is suspected based on the patient's history and on clinical and diagnostic evidence of hypercapnia (to be discussed later). In summation, the critical care paramedic should remember that alterations in the amount of dead space directly influence $PaCO_2$; as dead air space increases, $PaCO_2$ increases, and vice versa.

ASSESSMENT OF THE PULMONARY PATIENT

For purposes other than academic, it is almost impossible to separate the discussion of airway assessment from pulmonary assessment due to the inextricably intertwined nature of the airway and breathing components. An occluded airway cannot allow adequate ventilations any more effectively than an open airway would in an apneic patient. As such, components of the following discussion were first introduced in Chapter 7, "Airway Management and Ventilation," but are again mentioned here for completeness.

Every patient's past medical history (PMH) and history of present illness should be obtained. This can prove challenging in a critically ill patient who is experiencing a decreased level of consciousness or altered mental status secondary to his clinical condition. In such cases, efforts should be made to obtain information from family members or friends who may be present. Of particular interest in patients experiencing ARF are their respiratory and cardiac histories. Obtain information of recent illnesses and treatments, and note the dates and outcomes of recent diagnostic studies such as pulmonary function tests and imaging studies.

The physical assessment of the respiratory system begins with inspection and should proceed in a methodic fashion through auscultation, palpation, and percussion. If possible, the physical exam should be performed in a private, well-lit, warm, and quiet room, although the nature of critical care transport may at times exclude all of these desired criteria.

> The physical assessment of the respiratory system begins with inspection and should proceed in a methodic fashion through auscultation, palpation, and percussion.

INSPECTION

Begin the physical examination with a general, global view of the patient. Is the patient conscious and alert? Does she seem aware of her surroundings? Is she agitated or combative? One of the earliest signs of developing hypoxemia may be an altered mental status (hypercapnia typically induces lethargy). Look for obvious signs of respiratory distress. Is the patient assuming a posture, such as the tripod position, to help facilitate breathing? Inspect for accessory muscle use, nasal flaring, pursed lipped breathing, a gaping mouth, and head-bobbing—all of which suggests that a patient is experiencing difficulty breathing. Note the color of the patient's skin as well. Pallor is an early sign and cyanosis a late sign of developing hypoxemia. Evaluate the trachea as well, ensuring that it is midline and is not "tugging" toward one side or the other.

Expose and inspect the chest. Note the presence of accessory muscle use and intercostal, supraclavicular, or suprasternal retractions. Accessory muscles recruited to aid breathing include the scalenes, sternocleidomastoids, trapezius, intercostals, and abdominals. Assess for symmetry of the chest wall, and assess the rate and quality of respirations. Observe the amount of chest expansion. This can be done generally by watching the thorax, or specifically by lying your hands along the bottom costal border with your thumbs at the xyphoid process and noting the separation of your thumbs during inhalation. While normal breathing creates a roughly 1- to 1.5-inch separation of your thumbs, a 3.0-inch separation may be noted with a maximal inhalation. Note the duration of inspiration and expiration. Normal expiration is about 1.5 times as long as inspiration, and a prolonged expiratory phase could indicate air trapping. Abnormal breathing patterns should be identified and corrected (by PPV) if possible, and includes Biot's, Cheyne-Stokes, Kussmaul's, and apneustic respirations.

Assess the contour of the chest wall closely. The normal anteroposterior (AP) diameter of the thorax is half that of the lateral diameter, or a ratio of 1:2. The air trapping common in obstructive pulmonary disease often causes an increased AP diameter, commonly referred to as a "barrel chest." Other chest contour variations include funnel chest, pigeon breast, scoliosis, and kyphosis. Assess the chest for the presence of surgical scars and evidence of recent trauma. Surgical scarring can suggest PMH and provide clues as to the etiology of a patient's respiratory distress. Observe closely for new or healing stab or gunshot wounds, abrasions, contusions, lacerations, hematomas, burns, or any other indicator of traumatic insult to the chest wall.

Some patients with critical pulmonary disorders or traumatic thoracic injuries may have a chest tube placed prior to transport. Chest tubes are inserted primarily to serve as a drainage system for the thoracic cavity. The chest tubes can remove air, fluid, or blood from the pleural space, promote the normal reexpansion of a collapsed lung, prevent the reflux of drainage back into the chest, and allow the return of the negative intrapleural pressure needed for normal lung function.

The transport of a patient with a chest tube also comes with special considerations the critical care paramedic needs to be cognizant of. First and foremost is careful handling of the patient to prevent accidental removal of the chest tube; removal could result in the development of a pneumothorax. Additionally, maintain the chest drainage system that is attached to the chest tube by positioning the drainage system below the level of the chest. Secure the drainage system and arrange the tubing so that it does not become crushed or kinked. Some drainage systems for chest tubes require the application of suction to ensure adequate chest evacuation (both wet and dry drainage systems exist). Frequent assessment of the patient and drainage system should be performed by the critical care paramedic to include assessment for proper tube placement (not outward displaced allowing the chest tube eyelets to exit the thorax); also check for an absence of any air leaks, dressing integrity around the chest tube insertion site, water seal integrity to include water level, and drainage. Finally, the chest tube may be attached to a Heimlich valve and not a more complex drainage system that uses suctioning. The Heimlich valve is a one-way valve encased in plastic that attaches to the end of the chest tube and prevents the accidental entrainment of air into the pleural cavity. Heimlich valves are used for pneumothoraces, and are not used when the chest tube system needs to evacuate fluid from the chest.

Also assess the insertion sites of the chest tube, or any central lines for that matter, for infection. Signs of an infection can be seen if the skin surrounding the insertion site displays swelling, redness, weeping, or purulent discharge from the insertion site. Note the presence of blood or fluid in a chest tube drainage chamber. Be sure to inquire if the system has been emptied, and ensure that you are aware of the total amount of fluid drained.

PALPATION

Palpation often occurs simultaneously with inspection, and both should include the anterior, lateral, and posterior chest walls. Palpation should proceed in a systematic, methodical progression that ensures that no area of the chest is unexamined. Attempt to identify pain, tenderness, masses, or the presence of subcutaneous emphysema. Palpate for chest wall symmetry with deep inspiration. Asymmetry can indicate the presence of trauma or unilateral ventilation issues. The trachea should be palpated from its origin inferior to the larynx to the suprasternal notch for deviation from the midline. Conditions such as tension pneumothorax, pleural effusion, and hemothorax may result in deviation away from the affected side, whereas atelectasis, fibrosis, and phrenic nerve paralysis may result in deviation toward the affected side. Tracheal tugging, if it is observed, may be due to obstruction of a bronchi.

Assess for tactile fremitus by placing the palmar or ulnar surface of one hand on the patient's chest wall. Palpable vibrations are transmitted from the bronchial tree through the chest wall when the patient speaks. Fremitus is best appreciated in thin, healthy males, and is more pronounced over the larger bronchi, dissipating toward the distal bronchial tree. The patient is asked to repeat the word *ninety-nine* as the examiner moves her hand over the patient's chest wall, palpating for disparity between bilateral regions. Tactile fremitus is increased over areas of lung consolidation, such as in pneumonia, and decreased over areas where the bronchi are obstructed, the lung is hyperinflated, or where the pleural space is occupied by air.

PERCUSSION

Percussion can be a valuable tool if performed by an examiner familiar with its execution and interpretation of findings. If percussion is performed in a systematic fashion, results can be used to determine if underlying tissues are air filled, fluid filled, or solid. The five types of sounds produced by percussion are resonant, hyperresonant, tympanic, dull, and flat, and should be described in terms of their pitch, intensity, and duration.

Resonant sounds are the normal sounds associated with the lungs, and are of low pitch, low intensity, long duration, and often described as "hollow" sounding. Hyperresonant sounds are abnormal sounds percussed over the lungs, and are suggestive of air building up in the thoracic cavity, as in emphysema. Hyperresonant sounds are of low pitch, low intensity, and long duration, and often described as a "booming" sound when compared to the "hollow" sound of resonant. Tympanic sounds occur secondary to significant free air buildup in the thoracic cavity, as in cases of pneumothorax, and are normally heard over hollow organs such as the empty stomach and bowel. They are of high pitch, loud intensity, and long duration. Dull sounds appear in the chest exam when air is removed from the lung field, as in atelectasis or consolidation. Dull sounds are of high pitch, low intensity, and short duration. Flat sounds are normally percussed over solid organs such as the liver, and appear in the chest exam when the thorax is filled with blood, fluid, or a solid mass. Flat sounds are of higher pitch than dull sounds and of low intensity and very short duration.

AUSCULTATION

Auscultation of the lung fields should take place in a systematic, methodical manner that allows comparison of bilateral lung areas. It is important to take your time with your assessment, ensuring that the patient is taking a deep breath with his mouth open, or a critical care transport team member is giving an adequate tidal volume when squeezing the bag-valve mask (BVM) so as to best appreciate the underlying pathology. Auscultation can prove difficult in many transport environments, so it is important to perform a good exam when pretransport conditions allow it.

It is important to be familiar not only with adventitious lung sounds, but with normal lung sounds as well. Normal lung sounds are described as tracheal, bronchial, bronchovesicular, and vesicular. Tracheal breath sounds are loud, harsh sounds with an equal inspiratory and expiratory duration appreciated over the trachea. Bronchial are loud, high-pitched sounds with a longer expiratory phase normally heard over the manubrium. Bronchovesicular sounds are of medium pitch, have an almost equal inspiratory and expiratory phase, and are heard over the main stem bronchi and larger divisions of the bronchial tree. Vesicular lung sounds are auscultated over the majority of the lung fields, and are the result of air being ventilated into and out of the bronchi and alveoli. They are described as soft, low-pitched sounds with a long inspiratory phase and a short expiratory phase.

Adventitious lung sounds include crackles (rales), ronchi, wheezes, and friction rub. Crackles, also referred to as rales, can be described as fine, coarse, and audible. Fine crackles are often described as small "pops" or akin to the sound hair makes when rolled and rubbed together between one's fingers next to the ear. This sound is the result of deflated, slightly edematous alveoli reinflating during inspiration, and is often appreciated at the end of inspiration. Coarse crackles are produced when the alveoli are more filled with fluid, pus, or blood, and are heard earlier in the inspiratory phase. They are present in pathologies such as pneumonia or pulmonary edema. They commonly have a more moist, wet sound then do fine crackles. Audible crackles are appreciated when edema buildup is significant enough to include the larger bronchial airways, and are often associated with fulminating pulmonary edema.

Ronchi are produced when mucus or secretions are present in the larger divisions of the bronchial tree. The sound is often described as a wet, sticky, deep, and low-pitched noise akin to the sound of sucking a thick liquid out of the bottom of a cup through a straw. Because of the mucus in the larger airways, often asking the patient to cough forcibly will cause the mucus to shift and produce a change in the characteristics of the sound.

Wheezes are the result of airflow through a constricted or partially obstructed airway such as occurs in asthma, emphysema, chronic bronchitis, pneumonia, and allergic reactions. Bronchoconstriction can occur secondary to bronchial smooth muscle contraction, and increased edema and mucous production. Wheezes are often described as a musical, high-pitched sound that can occur late in the expiratory phase with slight constriction and obstruction, and progress over the whole respiratory cycle in cases of severe constriction and obstruction.

Friction rub is a cracking, grating sound appreciated during both inspiration and expiration, caused by the rubbing together of inflamed visceral and parietal pleurae. The presence of infection, pus, or fluid in the pleural space can also create the sound. Etiologies include pneumothorax, pleural effusion, and pleurisy.

While the critical care paramedic is utilizing the stethoscope for assessment of breath sounds, additional assessment findings can also be easily ascertained to help understand the patient's underlying pulmonary pathology. One such assessment technique is called egophony. **Egophony** is the

Auscultation can prove difficult in many transport environments, so it is important to perform a good exam when pretransport conditions allow it.

egophony   describes the distortion of voice transmission, as heard through the stethoscope, when a patient is instructed to speak during auscultation of the lungs.

While the critical care paramedic is utilizing the stethoscope for assessment of breath sounds, additional assessment findings can also be easily ascertained to help understand the patient's underlying pulmonary pathology.

term used to describe the distortion of voice as heard through the stethoscope when the patient is instructed to speak during auscultation. With this assessment technique, the patient is instructed to verbalize a long "E" (i.e., "eeeeeeeeeeeeeee") while the stethoscope is on the thorax. If the long "E" sound that is spoken sounds like a flat "A" sound, then "E to A" egophony is said to be present. What this assessment finding infers is that there is consolidation of lung tissue beneath the stethoscope (e.g. pneumothorax, tumor, pulmonary edema, pleural effusion, hemothorax). The denser tissue from the consolidation creates the "E to A" change. With the absence of egophony, no discernible "flat A" sound should be auscultated.

whispered pectoriloquy
assessment tool used to determine areas of consolidation in the lung tissues.

Another auscultated assessment finding along the same lines is known as **whispered pectoriloquy.** This is the presence of loud and clear sound heard while auscultating and instructing the patient to speak in a whispered voice. Again, the finding indicates lung consolidation, and the finding exists because sound vibration travels better through dense lung tissue rather than normally aerated lung tissue.

ARTERIAL BLOOD GAS

An ABG analysis provides information regarding a patient's ventilation and perfusion status, as well as data concerning the overall acid–base balance status. Information provided by an ABG includes the SaO_2, PaO_2, $PaCO_2$, pH, and bicarbonate (HCO_3^-) level. Acid–base balance is discussed in greater detail in Chapter 25. In an ABG blood draw, arterial blood is drawn from a direct arterial puncture, most often at the radial artery, or from an existing arterial catheter. Blood is then sent to a lab for analysis, or a portable ABG unit can be utilized at the bedside. Normal values for an ABG are as follows:

★ SaO_2: 94%–99%

★ PaO_2: 80–100 mmHg

★ $PaCO_2$: 35–45 mmHg

★ pH: 7.35–7.45

★ HCO_3^- : 22–26 mEq/L

ABG analysis can indicate the presence of hypercapnia, hypoxemia, acidosis, alkalosis, and the body's attempt at correcting acid–base disturbances with compensatory measures.

ABGs are useful in both the evaluation of respiratory function in a patient as well as the need for and efficacy of therapeutic interventions. ABG analysis can indicate the presence of hypercapnia, hypoxemia, acidosis, alkalosis, and the body's attempt at correcting acid–base disturbances with compensatory measures.

PULSE OXIMETRY

Pulse oximetry works by the determining the percentage of saturated hemoglobin in arterial blood. Oxygen binding to hemoglobin has a predictable relationship as described and demonstrated by the oxygen-hemoglobin dissociation curve. According to this relationship, the affinity for oxygen on the iron sites of the hemoglobin increases as more iron sites are occupied by oxygen molecules. The release of oxygen according to the curve depends on factors such as blood pH, temperature, and blood levels of 2,3-DPG.

The abbreviation SaO_2 is used to represent the oxygen saturation determined by arterial blood gas measurement while SpO_2 is used for oxygen saturation readings determined by pulse oximetry.

Beyond this, it is known that given the saturation patterns, when arterial oxygen saturations are above 70%, the oxygen saturation recorded by pulse oximetry varies from actual arterial saturation by only about 3%. This makes it an ideal tool for continuous monitoring and evaluation of therapeutic interventions. In addition, it is a valuable tool for identifying and recording hypoxemic episodes. Compared to ABG determination of arterial oxygenation, pulse oximetry is as accurate, is faster, is less invasive, has fewer complications, and is less expensive. In addition, pulse oximetry allows for continuous monitoring of arterial blood oxygenation, making it ideal for transport situations, especially in intubated patients. The following chart is a rough estimate that can be used when estimating PaO_2 from SpO_2:

Monitored SpO_2	Estimated PaO_2
90%	60 mmHg
80%	50 mmHg
70%	40 mmHg

Given this relationship, it is easy to understand why a pulse oximeter reading of less than 90% is considered to be an "objective" sign of severe hypoxemia (as would a PaO_2 level of 60 mmHg or less). Normal SpO_2 is 98% to 99%, with an acceptable SpO_2 value being >95%. SpO_2 readings between 90% and 95% are in that "gray" zone of not being too low, but not being "normal." As such, a thorough pulmonary assessment is still warranted in order for the critical care paramedic to make the best care decisions possible.

A critical limitation of pulse oximetry is that while it does offer valuable data regarding a patient's oxygenation status, it does not offer data concerning a patient's ventilation status. Thus, a patient can be oxygenated adequately and demonstrate an acceptable SpO_2 reading, but still have issues with pulmonary gas exchange resulting in hypercapnia.

END-TIDAL CAPNOGRAPHY

End-tidal **capnography** is the monitoring of exhaled carbon dioxide by way of a sampling device that assesses the concentration of carbon dioxide in the exhaled gas. The end-tidal carbon dioxide (abbreviated $ETCO_2$) level is an approximation of $PaCO_2$ since both are a reflection of alveolar ventilation. Whereas a normal disparity between $PaCO_2$ and $ETCO_2$ may exist (end tidal is usually 1 to 2 mmHg lower than arterial carbon dioxide), the monitoring of exhaled carbon dioxide still allows gross interpretation as to the quality of alveolar ventilation in the spontaneously breathing or mechanically ventilated patient.

The exhaled carbon dioxide levels can be displayed via a waveform on the monitor. Thus, the capnogram is a continuous and graphic reading of exhaled carbon dioxide with each breath. As mentioned previously, exhaled carbon dioxide equates roughly with arterial carbon dioxide, and as such any elevations or depressions in the $ETCO_2$ value can reflect a change in the patient's physiological status, mechanical change in ventilations, or both.

A normal capnogram is represented by four phases described here (and can be seen later in Figure 21-7 ■, the upper tracing):

1. The first phase is a flat line that stays at a base of 0 mmHg (in the healthy adult). This phase corresponds to the patient as he is either completing the inhalatory phase or just beginning an exhalation phase (i.e., sampled gas is devoid of all but traces of carbon dioxide).

2. The second phase is a rapid upstroke, and represents the exhalation of carbon dioxide from the lungs.

3. The third phase in the capnogram waveform is a plateau phase that corresponds to the exhalation of carbon dioxide from the terminal airways and alveolar spaces. The plateau phase should trace up slightly higher at the end as compared to the beginning of the plateau. The end of the plateau phase is where the CO_2 level is the highest, and corresponds to the end of the tidal volume (hence the name *end-tidal carbon dioxide*).

4. The final phase occurs when the patient starts the next inhalatory phase and the capnogram rapidly returns to the baseline of zero (due to an absence of carbon dioxide).

Indications for continuous $ETCO_2$ monitoring include, but are not limited to:

★ Augment placement of an endotracheal tube

A critical limitation of pulse oximetry is that while it does offer valuable data regarding a patient's oxygenation status, it does not offer data concerning a patient's ventilation status.

capnography *a monitoring device that samples and reports the concentration of carbon dioxide (CO_2) in exhaled gases.*

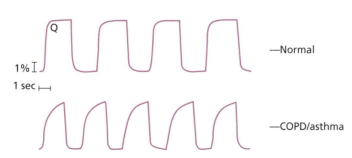

■ Figure 21-7
Capnography waveforms Normal (top) COPD/Asthma (bottom). Note "shark fin" appearance of waveform with obstructive pulmonary disease.

★ Continuous monitoring of a critical patient when repeated arterial blood gas analysis is not available, or practical

★ When desiring to maintain a specific carbon dioxide level due to a concurrent medical condition (such as a traumatic or nontraumatic brain injury)

Should the $ETCO_2$ level present as elevated (or continuously rising), the critical care paramedic should consider:

★ Conditions resulting in increased CO_2 production (fever, bicarbonate administration, seizures, and so forth)

★ Decreased alveolar ventilation (CNS depression, diminishing minute ventilation, muscular disorder, and so forth)

★ Equipment malfunction (bad sensor, rebreathing carbon dioxide in the circuit, high levels of PEEP in the ventilated patient, and so forth)

Should the $ETCO_2$ level present as lowered (or continuously diminishing), the critical care paramedic should consider:

★ Decreased CO_2 production (hypothermia, cardiac arrest, pulmonary embolus, and so forth)

★ Increased alveolar ventilation (tachypnea and/or hyperpnea in the breathing patient, increased minute ventilation in the mechanically ventilated patient, and so forth)

★ Equipment malfunction (obstruction of ventilation tubing, bad sampling head, displacement of endotracheal tube into esophagus, and so forth)

As a warning, the critical care paramedic needs to be cognizant of the limitations of end-tidal carbon dioxide monitoring:

★ It does not detect main stem intubations.

★ It may be affected by high concentrations of oxygen (false low readings).

★ It can be influenced by excessive water vapor (false high readings).

The use of medical technology in the assessment of pulmonary patients is simply an adjunct available to incorporate into your clinical assessment of pulmonary function and treatment efficacy.

The use of $ETCO_2$ monitoring (or even the use of pulse oximetry for that matter) was never intended to be a sole diagnostic device. Rather the use of medical technology in the assessment of pulmonary patients is simply an adjunct available to incorporate into your clinical assessment of pulmonary function and treatment efficacy.

The basic goals of management in acute respiratory failure are to ensure adequate ventilation, oxygenation, and CO_2 elimination.

MANAGEMENT

The basic goals of management in acute respiratory failure are to ensure adequate ventilation, oxygenation, and CO_2 elimination. Airway control is, of course, of paramount importance, and the critical care transport team should be aggressive in this respect. All patients in respiratory distress should receive high-concentration oxygen, and ventilations can be assisted or provided to those patients who have a labored or absent respiratory drive. BLS airway maneuvers, including proper positioning, use of the jaw thrust, and BLS airway adjuncts should be utilized prior to intubation. The familiar adage "BLS before ALS" applies even when the critical care transport team has numerous advanced airway adjuncts and procedures available to them.

The decision to intubate, when possible, should be made prior to the initiation of transport, in the transporting facility or on scene. This allows the critical care transport team the luxury of additional personnel to assist is any procedure, better access to the patient, and often provides a better lit, more stable environment than does the patient compartment of a moving ambulance or aircraft.

While no set criteria exist for the indication of intubation, it is generally accepted that intubation is required when the PaO_2 is less than 60 mmHg, the $PaCO_2$ is greater than 50 mmHg, and the arterial pH is less than 7.30 on room air. Various methods for endotracheal intubation are available to the transport team and are detailed in Chapter 7.

Airway control aside, specific treatment of ARF is directed at the underlying disease process, the more frequent of which are discussed next.

CAPNOGRAPHY

As discussed earlier, end-tidal carbon dioxide monitoring is a noninvasive method of measuring the levels of carbon dioxide in the exhaled breath. CO_2 is a normal end product of metabolism and is transported by the venous system to the right side of the heart. It is then pumped from the right ventricle to the pulmonary artery and eventually enters the pulmonary capillaries. There it diffuses into the alveoli and is removed from the body through exhalation. When circulation is normal, $ETCO_2$ levels change with ventilation and are a reliable estimate of the partial pressure of carbon dioxide in the arterial system ($PaCO_2$). Normal $ETCO_2$ is 1 to 2 mm less than the $PaCO_2$, or approximately 5%. A normal $ETCO_2$ is approximately 38 mmHg (0.05×760 mmHg = 38 mmHg). When perfusion decreases, as occurs in shock or cardiac arrest, $ETCO_2$ levels reflect pulmonary blood flow and cardiac output, not ventilation.

Capnometry provides a noninvasive measure of $ETCO_2$ levels, thus providing medical personnel with information about the status of systemic metabolism, circulation, and ventilation. The use of capnography has become commonplace in the operating room, in the emergency department, and in the prehospital setting.

ASTHMA

EPIDEMIOLOGY

Asthma affects about 4% to 5% of the total population in the United States. The disease can afflict patients of any age, but children younger than 10 years old account for about 50% of all patients, with males outnumbering females about 2:1. About 33% of all cases of asthma occur in individuals between the ages of 10 and 40 years old, with the disparity between the sexes evening out in this age group. The elderly are particularly susceptible to disease, and asthma affects about 7% to 10% of the elderly population in the United States. It is believed that patients at risk for fatal or near-fatal asthma exacerbations include those with a high degree of bronchial reactivity, a high occurrence of poor compliance with therapy and follow-up, and a history of frequent admissions or previous intubations.

PATHOPHYSIOLOGY

Asthma is a chronic inflammatory disorder of the lower airways characterized by hyperresponsiveness of the airways to various stimuli, inflammation and edema of the airways, and increased mucous production. Although this disorder is commonly reversible with proper medications, during the asthmatic episode, these three pathophysiological changes serve to decrease the bronchiole lumen diameter, making it difficult for ventilation of the alveoli and gas exchange to take place. It is important for the critical care paramedic to appreciate that asthma is not simply a matter of bronchoconstriction; while bronchoconstriction plays a role in asthma, by arguably one-third, it is not the only pathology present in the disease state, and failure to consider or recognize such can lead to disastrous consequences for your patient.

The airway inflammation accompanying asthma may be acute or chronic, and an acute episode usually follows a two-phased response. When an antigen is inhaled and presents in the lower airway, sensitized IgE antibodies trigger mast-cell degranulation in the airway submucosa resulting in the release of histamine, prostaglandins, thromboxanes, leukotrienes, cytokines, interleukins, and eosinophil chemotaxic factors. The release of these chemicals results in an inflammatory response that includes immediate bronchoconstriction and developing submucosal edema, vascular congestion, mucous production, and impaired mucociliary clearance. This first phase of an asthma attack typically occurs within the first 90 minutes of the introduction of an antigen. The second phase occurs about 3 to 4 hours later, and occurs secondary to invasion of the submucosa by esinophils, platelets, lymphocytes, and leukocytes. These immune cells contribute further chemical factors that promote additional, sustained inflammation, mucous production, and edema. Chronic inflammation results in persistent submucosal cell damage and repair, resulting in microscopic airway changes including basement membrane thickening, hypertrophied airway smooth muscle, microvascular leakage, epithelial disruption, and increased numbers of goblet cells. Gross changes include the formation of mucous plugs in the large and small airways containing mucus, cellular debris, and immune cells.

SIGNS AND SYMPTOMS

An asthma attack may begin suddenly and severely, with a rapid onset of signs and symptoms, or may progress more insidiously, with a gradual onset of difficulty breathing.

An asthma attack may begin suddenly and severely, with a rapid onset of signs and symptoms, or may progress more insidiously, with a gradual onset of difficulty breathing. Regardless of the onset, the classic early signs of asthma include end-expiratory wheezing, dyspnea, tachycardia, cough, and chest tightness. As the exacerbation continues, increasing bronchonstriction and developing edema will result is a progression of wheezing from late in the expiratory phase to early in the expiratory phase, and eventually into the inspiratory phase. This progression of wheezing through the respiratory cycle occurs as the airways become increasingly constricted and edematous. In addition, increased mucous production may result in the production of thick, viscous mucus. As airway resistance increases, accessory muscles are recruited to assist in ventilation, wheezing may become audible without a stethoscope, and the expiratory phase becomes noticeably longer.

Severe cases of asthma may result in a "silent chest" as a result of severe airflow obstruction, and air trapping may result in hyperinflation of the chest and an exaggerated anteroposterior chest diameter.

Physical exam will further reveal hyperresonance to percussion and pulsus paradoxus. Pulsus paradoxus greater than 20 mmHg is considered indicative of serious asthma exacerbation. In addition, severe cases of asthma may result in a "silent chest" as a result of severe airflow obstruction, and air trapping may result in hyperinflation of the chest and an exaggerated anteroposterior chest diameter. Head-bobbing, paradoxical breathing, combativeness, and altered mental status should be considered ominous signs, indicating that respiratory failure is imminent. Asthma can be generally defined based on the clinical findings as mild, moderate, severe, and impending respiratory failure. (See Figure 21-8 ■.)

Continuous waveform capnography can aid in diagnosing airflow obstruction as seen in asthma or chronic obstructive pulmonary disease. With asthma, the waveform begins to assume a "shark fin" appearance—namely a loss of vertical E_2, opening and blunting of angle Q, and tilting of E_3.

In severe or prolonged cases there may be noticeable changes to the ECG findings as well when looking at a 12-lead ECG. Beyond the expected sinus tachycardia from hypoxemia, hypercapnia, and sympathetic discharge, there may be additional findings of right ventricular strain, right axis deviation, or early R-wave progression.

With the hyperinflation of the lungs from air trapping, there is increased pulmonary resistance that the right ventricle has to overcome from forcing blood through the perialveolar capillary beds of overly inflated alveoli. This heightened pulmonary resistance is an atypical strain that the right ventricle typically encounters so evidence of a laboring right ventricle may be present on the 12-lead ECG. Finally, although sinus tachycardia is an extremely common finding with any type of respiratory distress, if a supraventricular tachycardic rhythm is present, do not exclude the possibility of theophylline toxicity in the patient receiving any type of methyl xanthine.

DIAGNOSIS

Spirometry provides a rapid, reproducible, objective, and cheap modality for the assessment, diagnosis, and evaluation of therapy in the asthma patient. Both the peak expiratory flow rate (PEFR) and the forced expiratory volume over 1 second (FEV 1) reveal the degree of large airway obstruction. Often, changes in PEFR and FEV1 precede the clinical manifestations of physiological alterations in the airway, providing warning of a worsening condition, or confirmation that therapy is working. (See Figure 21-9 A-C ■.)

Chest radiography may show hyperinflation of the lung fields, focal atelectasis, or be normal, depending on the severity of the exacerbation. A chest X-ray is indicated in any patient suspected of having complications such as pneumothorax or pneumomediastinum, especially if subcutaneous emphysema is present, and an X-ray can be useful to rule out other respiratory disease states. Other indications of hyperinflation include an increased anteroposterior chest diameter, enlarged

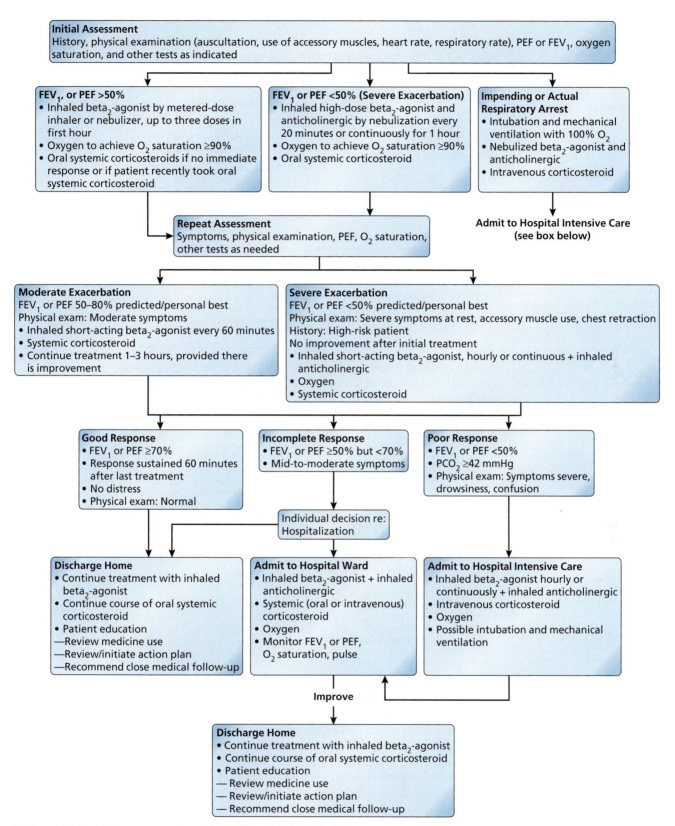

Initial Assessment
History, physical examination (auscultation, use of accessory muscles, heart rate, respiratory rate), PEF or FEV_1, oxygen saturation, and other tests as indicated

FEV_1, or PEF >50%
- Inhaled beta$_2$-agonist by metered-dose inhaler or nebulizer, up to three doses in first hour
- Oxygen to achieve O_2 saturation ≥90%
- Oral systemic corticosteroids if no immediate response or if patient recently took oral systemic corticosteroid

FEV_1 or PEF <50% (Severe Exacerbation)
- Inhaled high-dose beta$_2$-agonist and anticholinergic by nebulization every 20 minutes or continuously for 1 hour
- Oxygen to achieve O_2 saturation ≥90%
- Oral systemic corticosteroid

Impending or Actual Respiratory Arrest
- Intubation and mechanical ventilation with 100% O_2
- Nebulized beta$_2$-agonist and anticholinergic
- Intravenous corticosteroid

Admit to Hospital Intensive Care
(see box below)

Repeat Assessment
Symptoms, physical examination, PEF, O_2 saturation, other tests as needed

Moderate Exacerbation
FEV_1 or PEF 50–80% predicted/personal best
Physical exam: Moderate symptoms
- Inhaled short-acting beta$_2$-agonist every 60 minutes
- Systemic corticosteroid
- Continue treatment 1–3 hours, provided there is improvement

Severe Exacerbation
FEV_1 or PEF <50% predicted/personal best
Physical exam: Severe symptoms at rest, accessory muscle use, chest retraction
History: High-risk patient
No improvement after initial treatment
- Inhaled short-acting beta$_2$-agonist, hourly or continuous + inhaled anticholinergic
- Oxygen
- Systemic corticosteroid

Good Response
- FEV_1 or PEF ≥70%
- Response sustained 60 minutes after last treatment
- No distress
- Physical exam: Normal

Incomplete Response
- FEV_1 or PEF ≥50% but <70%
- Mid-to-moderate symptoms

Poor Response
- FEV_1 or PEF <50%
- PCO_2 ≥42 mmHg
- Physical exam: Symptoms severe, drowsiness, confusion

Individual decision re: Hospitalization

Discharge Home
- Continue treatment with inhaled beta$_2$-agonist
- Continue course of oral systemic corticosteroid
- Patient education
—Review medicine use
—Review/initiate action plan
—Recommend close medical follow-up

Admit to Hospital Ward
- Inhaled beta$_2$-agonist + inhaled anticholinergic
- Systemic (oral or intravenous) corticosteroid
- Oxygen
- Monitor FEV_1 or PEF, O_2 saturation, pulse

Admit to Hospital Intensive Care
- Inhaled beta$_2$-agonist hourly or continuously + inhaled anticholinergic
- Intravenous corticosteroid
- Oxygen
- Possible intubation and mechanical ventilation

Improve

Discharge Home
- Continue treatment with inhaled beta$_2$-agonist
- Continue course of oral systemic corticosteroid
- Patient education
— Review medicine use
— Review/initiate action plan
— Recommend close medical follow-up

Figure 21-8 Asthma treatment. *(National Institutes of Health).*

Figure 21-9A

Spirometry. Forced vital capacity (top) and forced expiratory volume in 1 second (bottom) *(National Institutes of Health)*

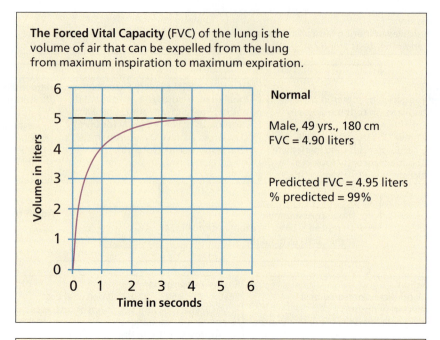

The Forced Vital Capacity (FVC) of the lung is the volume of air that can be expelled from the lung from maximum inspiration to maximum expiration.

Normal

Male, 49 yrs., 180 cm
FVC = 4.90 liters

Predicted FVC = 4.95 liters
% predicted = 99%

Volume in liters

Time in seconds

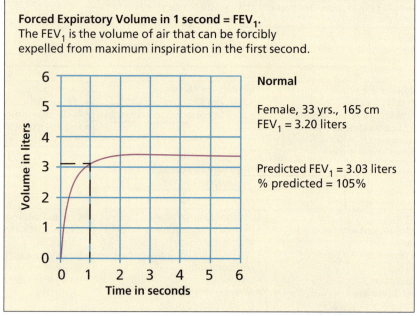

Forced Expiratory Volume in 1 second = FEV_1.
The FEV_1 is the volume of air that can be forcibly expelled from maximum inspiration in the first second.

Normal

Female, 33 yrs., 165 cm
FEV_1 = 3.20 liters

Predicted FEV_1 = 3.03 liters
% predicted = 105%

Volume in liters

Time in seconds

thoracic cage, increased width of the intercostal spaces, flattened diaphragm, increased pulmonary shadowing, and increased pulmonary parenchymal lucency.

While performing an ABG on an asthma patient is never contraindicated, ABG analysis is indicated only in those patients with severe asthma exacerbation resulting in air trapping, hypoventilation, hypercapnia, and respiratory acidosis. These patients can usually be identified based on their clinical exam findings or spirometry results indicating less than 25% of normal predicted or actual values. In acute asthma, the resultant tachypnea results in a blowing off of CO_2 and therefore a slightly lowered $PaCO_2$. A $PaCO_2$ that is normal or slightly elevated is suggestive of severe exacerbation. PaO_2 in severe asthma is less than 60 mmHg. Pulse oximetry is a valuable tool for the continuous monitoring of the asthma patient, both to identify progression of the exacerbation, efficacy of therapy, and trends.

A complete blood count with differential (CBC) is usually not necessary but can be expected to show an increased eosinophil count. In addition, leukocytosis may be present, especially if the patient has received β-agonist or corticosteroid therapy. A serum theophylline level should be determined on all patients who use it at home, or have received it prior to your arrival.

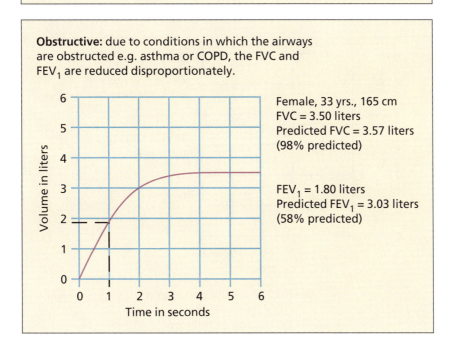

Restrictive: due to conditions in which the lung volume is reduced, e.g. fibrosing alveolitis, scoliosis. The FVC and FEV_1 are reduced proportionately.

Male, 49 yrs., 180 cm
FVC = 2.00 liters
Predicted FVC = 4.90 liters
(40% predicted)

FEV_1 = 1.80 liters
Predicted FEV_1 = 4.02 liters
(45% predicted)

Obstructive: due to conditions in which the airways are obstructed e.g. asthma or COPD, the FVC and FEV_1 are reduced disproportionately.

Female, 33 yrs., 165 cm
FVC = 3.50 liters
Predicted FVC = 3.57 liters
(98% predicted)

FEV_1 = 1.80 liters
Predicted FEV_1 = 3.03 liters
(58% predicted)

■ **Figure 21-9B**
Spirometry. Abnormal pattern due to restrictive lung disease (top) and obstructive lung disease (bottom). *(National Institutes of Health)*

MANAGEMENT

The goal of the treatment of asthma by the critical care team is simple: Reverse bronchoconstriction and airway inflammation and edema to increase ventilation, oxygenation, and CO_2 elimination. The medications utilized to achieve this goal include oxygen, β-agonists, anticholinergics, corticosteroids, theophylline, and magnesium. Patients who do not respond to pharmacologic therapy and are in impending respiratory arrest are candidates for intubation and mechanical ventilation.

β-Agonists and anticholinergics are considered first-line medications in an asthma attack. While dramatic improvement can be expected in the early phase of an asthma exacerbation, these medications tend to result in limited improvement in patients experiencing late-phase asthma exacerbations. This can be explained by the fact that early-phase asthma is characterized primarily by bronchoconstriction, which responds to β-agonists and anticholinergics; late phase asthma is characterized by bronchoconstriction as well as airway inflammation and edema, which do not respond to these medications.

Figure 21-9C
Spirometry. Restrictive
pattern (top) and obstructive
pattern (bottom). *(National
Institutes of Health)*

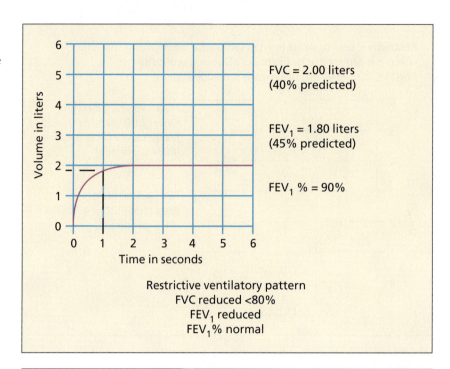

FVC = 2.00 liters
(40% predicted)

FEV$_1$ = 1.80 liters
(45% predicted)

FEV$_1$ % = 90%

Restrictive ventilatory pattern
FVC reduced <80%
FEV$_1$ reduced
FEV$_1$% normal

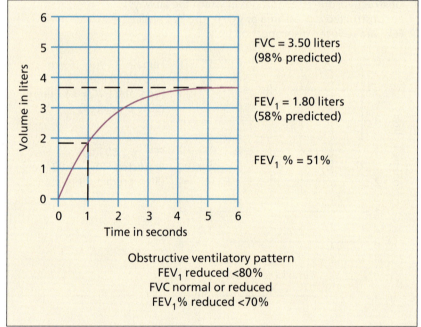

FVC = 3.50 liters
(98% predicted)

FEV$_1$ = 1.80 liters
(58% predicted)

FEV$_1$ % = 51%

Obstructive ventilatory pattern
FEV$_1$ reduced <80%
FVC normal or reduced
FEV$_1$% reduced <70%

β-Agonists, preferably β$_2$-specific agonists, are beneficial in asthma for three reasons: They result in bronchial smooth muscle relaxation of the smaller airways, they inhibit mediator release, and they promote mucociliary clearance. Inhaled forms of β-agonists are preferred over the oral, intravenous, or subcutaneous routes. This method results in topical administration of a small dose of medication and local effects, rather than the systemic distribution and potentially serious side effects typical of parenteral administration. Aerosolization can be achieved via a nebulizer or metered-dose inhaler (MDI), providing that a properly fitted spacing device and proper technique are utilized. Parenteral routes can be considered in patients who are too dyspneic to take adequate tidal volumes needed to deposit the medication on the bronchiole smooth muscle, and may be considered at this point. Another consideration for the extremely dyspneic patient in extremis is elective endotracheal intubation, with this intervention, aerosolized β-agonists can be administered via the endotracheal tube. Aerosolized treatments can be administered every 15 to 20 minutes in cases of mild exacerbation, or continuously if the patient's clinical condition warrants it. Side effects of β-agonist medications include tremors, palpitations, headache, hyperglycemia, tachycardia, and hypertension. The often talked about concerns over cardiac complications have not proven to be supported in the literature, but the critical care paramedic should be aware of and be alert for the potential of cardiac affects. Examples of β-agonists frequently used are listed at the top of Table 21–1.

Anticholinergic drugs act as a competitive antagonist to acetylcholine at the acetylcholine receptor located on the postsynaptic membrane of the postganglionic nerve fiber and the effector cell. This action blocks vagal tone to the larger central airways, resulting in bronchodilation. Used in conjunction with a β-agonist, bronchoconstriction is thus addressed from both the sympathetic and parasympathetic influences, and recent studies have shown that FEV1 and PEFR both increase by 10% when ipratropium bromide is added to standard β-agonist regimens. Aerosolized ipratropium bromide, a synthetic derivitive of atropine sulfate, is the most often used anticholinergic, and is administered in doses of 0.5 mg via a nebulizer every 15 to 20 minutes or continuously if needed. MDI preparations are also available. Common side effects include thirst, dry mouth, and difficulty swallowing.

Corticosteroids are highly effective at reducing the airway inflammation and edema characteristic of asthma, and are used in the management of both acute and chronic asthma. Because the onset of action can be 4 to 8 hours by both the intravenous and oral routes, the goal of the critical care paramedic should be to get corticosteroids administered as soon as possible. Common treatment regimes are oral prednisone, 40 to 60 mg; or intravenous Solu-Medrol, 60 to 125 mg every 6 hours for the first 24 hours. Solu-Medrol administration is continued until clinical findings and spirometry results normalize, and is then tapered over days or weeks.

While oral theophylline seems to be enjoying a bit of resurgence in the treatment of chronic asthma, the use of theophylline or IV aminophylline as a first-line treatment for asthma remains controversial. The use of oral theophylline in combination with inhaled β-agonists appears to increase the toxicity of treatment, but not the efficacy. Whether intravenous aminophylline results in any benefit when used in conjunction with normal treatment modalities for asthma remains unknown. What is known is that when used to manage chronic asthma, oral theophylline contributes to a decrease in airway inflammation and swelling, but its overall bronchodilatory effects are limited. Common side effects of theophylline include nausea, vomiting, headache, and anxiety. Theophylline toxicity occurs at plasma levels greater than 30 mcg/mL, with cardiac dysrhythmia and seizures a serious risk. The arguably meager benefits of theophylline or aminophylline must be weighed against the potentially undesirable side effects.

Intravenous magnesium sulfate relaxes bronchial smooth muscle via the blocking of calcium channels in muscle cells. In addition, it may inhibit mast-cell degranulation, resulting in decreased airway inflammation and edema, and can improve respiratory muscle function in cases of serum magnesium deficiency. While magnesium's role in the management of mild and moderate asthma has not been established, it seems to benefit those patients with severe exacerbations (FEV1 < 25% predicted). The medication is usually administered 1 to 2 g in 50 mL of normal saline over 20 to 30 minutes.

Patients with severe asthma and hypercapnia who are unresponsive to pharmacologic and supplemental oxygen therapy, are hemodynamically stable, and still possess an adequate respiratory drive may benefit from **noninvasive positive-pressure ventilation (NPPV).**

NPPV is an intervention strategy for spontaneously breathing patients who are having trouble keeping smaller bronchiole airways open, or would benefit from the displacement of excessive fluid accumulation in the alveoli back into interstitial spaces and the perialveolar capillary network. This intervention works by providing a constant "back pressure" of air against which the patient must exhale. The back pressure helps to keep the alveoli open, diminishes alveolar fluid accumulation, assists in keeping smaller bronchioles open that in turn allow a more effective exhalation and removal of carbon dioxide from the lungs, and finally decreases the work of breathing necessary during inhalation due to the positive pressure of air entering into the mask. Two forms of NPPV exist, continuous positive airway pressure (CPAP), and bilevel positive airway pressure (BiPAP). Whereas CPAP delivers constant pressure through a mask that is positioned securely on the face during inhalation and exhalation, BiPAP alternates the positive pressure from a higher level during inhalation (to decrease work of breathing) to a lower level during exhalation (to allow effective exhalation while promoting bronchiole patency and decreasing atelectasis). Either form of NPPV can be delivered via a nasal mask, full face mask, or mouthpiece. One key with this intervention is the

noninvasive positive-pressure ventilation (NPPV) *ventilatory therapy that provides constant positive gas pressure via mask. Also known as CPAP (continuous positive airway pressure) and BiPap (bilevel positive airway pressure).*

Table 21–1 | Quick-Relief Medications

Name/Products	Indications/Mechanisms	Potential Adverse Effects	Therapeutic Issues
Short-acting inhaled beta$_2$-agonists Albuterol Bitolterol Pirbuterol Terbutaline Levalbuterol	**Indications** • Relief of acute symptoms; quick-relief medication. • Preventive treatment prior to exercise for exercise-induced bronchospasm. **Mechanisms** • Bronchodilation. Smooth muscle relaxation following adenylate cyclase activation and increase in cyclic AMP producing functional antagonism of bronchoconstriction.	Tachycardia, skeletal muscle tremor, hypokalemia, increased lactic acid, headache, hyperglycemia. Inhaled route, in general, causes few systemic adverse effects. Patients with preexisting cardiovascular disease, especially the elderly, may have adverse cardiovascular reactions with inhaled therapy.	• Drugs of choice for acute bronchospasm. Inhaled route has faster onset, fewer adverse effects, and is more effective than systemic routes. The less beta$_2$-selective agents (isoproterenol, metaproterenol, isoetharine, and epinephrine) are not recommended due to their potential for excessive cardiac stimulation, especially in high doses. Albuterol liquid is not recommended. • For patients with mild intermittent asthma, regularly scheduled daily use neither harms nor benefits asthma control. Regularly scheduled daily use is not generally recommended. • Increasing use or lack of expected effect indicates inadequate asthma control. >1 canister a month (e.g., albuterol-200 puffs per canister) may indicate overreliance on this drug; ≥2 canisters in 1 month poses additional adverse risks. • For patients frequently using beta$_2$-agonist, anti-inflammatory medication should be initiated or intensified.
Anticholinergics Ipratropium bromide	**Indications** • Relief of acute bronchospasm (see Therapeutic Issues column). **Mechanisms** • Bronchodilation. Competitive inhibition of muscarinic cholinergic receptors. • Reduces intrinsic vagal tone to the airways. May block reflex bronchoconstriction secondary to irritants or to reflux esophagitis. • May decrease mucous gland secretion.	Drying of mouth and respiratory secretions, increased wheezing in some individuals, blurred vision if sprayed in eyes.	• Reverses only cholinergically mediated bronchospasm; does not modify reaction to antigen. Does not block exercise-induced bronchospasm. • May provide additive effects to beta$_2$-agonist but has slower onset of action. • Is an alternative for patients with intolerance to beta$_2$-agonists. • Treatment of choice for bronchospasm due to beta-blocker medication.

Table 21-1	Quick-Relief Medications (continued)		
Name/Products	**Indications/Mechanisms**	**Potential Adverse Effects**	**Therapeutic Issues**
Corticosteroids *Systemic:* Methylprednisolone Prednisolone Prednisone	*Indications* • For moderate-to-severe exacerbations to prevent progression of exacerbation, reverse inflammation, speed recovery, and reduce rate of relapse. *Mechanisms* • Anti-inflammatory. See Figure 3-1.	• Short-term use: reversible abnormalities in glucose metabolism, increased appetite, fluid retention, weight gain, mood alteration, hypertension, peptic ulcer, and rarely aseptic necrosis of femur. • Consideration should be given to coexisting conditions that could be worsened by systemic corticosteroids, such as herpes virus infections, varicella, tuberculosis, hypertension, peptic ulcer, and *Strongyloides*.	• Short-term therapy should continue until patient achieves 80% PEF personal best or symptoms resolve. This usually requires 3 to 10 days but may require longer. • There is no evidence that tapering the dose following improvement prevents relapse.

adequate preparation and coaching of the patient who has never received this intervention to not "fight" the system. If the patient remains calm and learns how to breathe with the assistance of this device, he often will start to feel more comfortable.

Any patient who experiences progressive lethargy, near exhaustion, somnolence, or apnea will require intubation. Nasotracheal intubation may be better tolerated in a conscious patient, but the orotracheal route permits the use of a larger diameter endotracheal tube (ETT), allowing for deep suctioning of the airway and the use of a bronchoscope if necessary. In addition, a larger diameter ETT will lower the resistance in the airway circuit, because the resistance of airflow through a tube is inversely proportional to its internal radius to the fourth power. Thus, the resistance of an 8-mm ETT is less than one-third that of a 6-mm tube. Sedation may be necessary in a conscious patient, but the use of neuromuscular blocking agents should be avoided if at all possible. In addition, the use of opioids or barbiturates should be avoided, because they both encourage histamine release and can worsen bronchoconstriction.

There is significant potential for barotrauma in a patient who is receiving mechanical ventilation. Severe airflow obstruction can lead to air trapping and the "stacking" of respirations. This occurs when tidal volume is greater than returned volume; with each tidal volume delivered, some portion is not exhaled, and each successive breath leads to greater residual volume and the eventual "stacking" of breaths in the lung. Pneumothorax and pneumomediastinum are potential complications, and can be avoided by administering ventilations at a rapid inspiratory flow rate with a frequency of 12 to 14 breaths per minute, then allowing for a prolonged respiratory phase. While this "relative hypoventilation" may not resolve an elevated $PaCO_2$, it is adequate for maintaining a PaO_2 above 90 mmHg. This methodology has been termed *permissive hypoventilation*.

> Any patient who experiences progressive lethargy, near exhaustion, somnolence, or apnea will require intubation.

CHRONIC OBSTRUCTIVE PULMONARY DISEASE

EPIDEMIOLOGY

As the sixth leading cause of death in the world, chronic obstructive pulmonary disease (COPD) is a worldwide health issue, and represents the fourth-leading cause of death in the United States. In 2000, 119,000 deaths, 726,000 hospitalizations, and 1.5 million hospital emergency department visits were caused by COPD. In the United States, COPD is rare in adults under 40 years of age, appears in about 10% of the population age 55 to 85 years old, and is more common in males than females. In recent years, however, the prevalence of females diagnosed with COPD has more than doubled, reflecting the increased incidence of smoking of females. In 2000, the number of COPD deaths among women surpassed the number among men.

For patients hospitalized with exacerbation of COPD, mortality is about 5% to 14%, and rises to 24% in those admitted to an intensive care unit. For those patients over 65 years old and who are discharged from an ICU after exacerbation of COPD, the 1-year mortality is an astounding 59%, considering that the expected mortality is about 30%.

PATHOPHYSIOLOGY

The Global Initiative for Chronic Obstructive Lung Disease (GOLD), published in 2001, describes COPD as a disease state characterized by airflow limitation that is not fully reversible. COPD is an umbrella term, covering the disease states of emphysema and chronic bronchitis. Traditionally, asthma was considered a disease state of COPD, but many authorities argue that its reversible nature excludes it from this classification. About 85% of patients with COPD suffer from chronic bronchitis, and 15% suffer from emphysema. The condition is usually progressive, and is associated with an abnormal inflammatory response in the lungs secondary to noxious gases and particles. Although tobacco smoking is the most critical risk factor for both development and progression of COPD, asthma, exposure to ambient air pollution in the home and workplace, and respiratory infections are also key risk factors. The only proven genetic risk factor is α_1-antitrypsin deficiency (<1% of all cases). As an interesting aside, despite the fact that cigarette smoking is responsible for 80% to 90% of all cases of COPD, only about 15% of individuals who smoke develop COPD.

Repeated exposure to noxious stimuli results in pathologic changes to the large and small airways. In the trachea, bronchi, and larger bronchioles, immune cells infiltrate the surface epithelium, resulting in edema. In addition, mucous-secreting glands and goblet cells become hypertrophic and secrete copious amounts of mucus, which cannot be removed due to destruction of the mucocilicary escalator. In the smaller bronchioles, repeated injury and repair of the airway walls results in weakening and subsequent loss of recoil and collapse. In the alveoli, destruction of the walls between individual alveoli leads to the creation of enlarged terminal air spaces, called *blebs,* that contain far less surface area for gas exchange to take place across. In addition, pulmonary capillaries experience a thickening of their endothelial walls, further impeding gas exchange across the alveolar-capillary membrane.

These pathologic changes lead to the characteristic physiological changes associated with the disease state. Early COPD is characterized by increased mucous secretion and decreased mucous elimination secondary to mucociliary escalator dysfunction. Late in the disease state, pulmonary hypertension develops secondary to the impedance of pulmonary blood flow through damaged pulmonary capillaries. The increased pulmonary pressures can lead to cor pulmonale. In addition, the increased pulmonary capillary impedence leads to a diminished output state from the pulmonary circulation, which subsequently results in a low-output state from the left ventricle. Increased airway resistance, secondary to decreased mucous elimination and bronchiole collapse, leads to decreased alveolar ventilation and air trapping; hypoxemia and hypercapnia result. The likelihood of hypoxemia is further increased with the destruction of the alveolar membrane and thickening of the pulmonary capillary walls; a V/Q mismatch is created, and a right-to-left shunt results. As a result of chronic hypercapnia, COPD patients can develop a hypoxic drive.

SIGNS AND SYMPTOMS

An exacerbation of COPD may develop slowly and insidiously, or can be impressive in its rapid development and severity.

Like asthma, an exacerbation of COPD may develop slowly and insidiously, or can be impressive in its rapid development and severity. In addition, the patient with pure emphysema will present slightly differently than the patient with pure chronic bronchitis, so we will first consider the signs and symptoms of each separately. The critical care paramedic must remember, however, that a patient can have pathophysiologic changes consistent with both diseases, and the clinical findings of both may be present to some degree.

The patient suffering from chronic bronchitis presents with the morphologic appearance typically labeled the "blue bloater." An exacerbation of chronic bronchitis will be typified by a history of increased sputum production and expectoration, dyspnea, weakness, and the development of a productive cough. If sputum production exceeds elimination, common because of decreased ciliary clearance, heavy rhonchi will be audible upon auscultation. Wheezing might also be appreciated secondary to local airway irritation and subsequent bronchoconstriction. In severe cases, mucous plugs can form, resulting in diminished or absent lung sounds to the areas distal. Tachypnea results in the drying of mucus and formation of plugs, and can also lead to dehydration in an individual too dyspneic to ingest fluids.

The patient suffering from emphysema will present as the archetypical "pink puffer." An exacerbation of chronic emphysema will typically present with decreased lung sounds in all fields and diffuse wheezing. Like asthma, a "silent chest" with evidence of hypoxemia is an ominous finding. Increased mucous production is not an issue to the extent that it is in chronic bronchitis, and a productive cough is not typical. Rather, destruction of the airways distal to the terminal bronchiole is the primary insult. Significant air trapping can occur, resulting in an increased anteroposterior chest diameter, in which case percussion will reveal tympany. Patients will often breathe through pursed lips in order to create a physiological positive end-expiratory pressure (PEEP) to keep collapsed bronchioles open and permit exhalation, which is often prolonged. Accessory muscles, usually prominent in emphysema patients, may be utilized.

Many factors can result in an exacerbation of COPD, including noncompliance with medications, underlying respiratory infection (a factor in 70% to 75% of all exacerbations), increased bronchospasm, smoking, cardiovascular deterioration, or ingestion of drugs or medications that reduce respiratory drive. Despite their slightly different pathologies, acute, severe exacerbations of chronic bronchitis and emphysema both result in a worsening obstruction to airflow, decreased alveolar ventilation, and eventual hypoxemia and hypercapnia. As such, diagnosis and management of the two diseases are similar.

DIAGNOSIS

The GOLD criteria allow clinicians to diagnose and classify COPD on the basis of pulmonary function testing via spirometry. These criteria recognize that the disease state may be subclinical, even among persons with substantial degrees of impairment. The GOLD methodology uses observed diminishment in the forced vital capacity (FVC) and the percentage of predicted FEV1 to determine disease severity. (See Table 21–2.) In addition, decreased pulmonary function secondary to COPD can include a decreased forced expiratory volume, prolonged expiration, decreased maximum voluntary ventilation, increased total lung capacity, and increased residual volume. In severe, acute exacerbation of COPD, spirometry may be impossible due to the severity of difficulty breathing. In those patients able to perform the exam, a FEV1 of less than 1.00 L or a peak expiratory flow rate of less that 100 L/min in a patient without severe chronic obstruction is considered severe exacerbation. Serial spirometry is also a useful tool to monitor a patient's response to therapy.

While chest radiographs can be valuable in diagnosing complications such as pneumothorax, pneumomediastinum, and concomitant respiratory illness, results can be misleading in cases of mild COPD. Initial diagnosis and determination of severity should never be made on radiographic evidence alone. In acute exacerbations of COPD, findings may include evidence of hyperinflation, including increased anteroposterior chest diameter, enlarged thoracic cage, increased width of the intercostal spaces, flattened diaphragm, increased pulmonary shadowing, and increased pulmonary parenchymal lucency.

Table 21–2	GOLD Methodology for Diagnosing and Classifying COPD			
Stage 0: At Risk	**Stage I: Mild COPD**	**Stage II: Moderate COPD**	**Stage III: Severe COPD**	**Stage IV: Very Severe COPD**
• Normal spirometry	• FEV_1/FVC <70%	• FEV_1/FVC <70%	• FEV_1/FVC <70%	• FEV_1/FVC <70%
• Chronic symptoms (cough sputum production)	• FEV_1 >80% predicted	• 50% FEV_1 <80% predicted	• 30% FEV_1 <50% predicted	• FEV_1 <30% predicted or FEV_1 <50% predicted plus chronic respiratory failure
	• With or without chronic symptoms (cough, sputum production)	• With or without chronic symptoms (cough, sputum production)	• With or without chronic symptoms (cough, sputum production)	

ABG analysis is an essential tool in determining the oxygenation, CO_2 elimination, and pH status of the patient in acute exacerbation of COPD. A PaO_2 of less than 60 mmHg or an SaO_2 of less than 90% on room air is suggestive for respiratory failure. Ventilatory failure is suggested in those patients who present with a pH of less than 7.30 or $PaCO_2$ greater than 70 mmHg. While pulse oximetry is useful for identifying hypoxemia and monitoring a patient's oxygenation status during transport, it cannot identify hypercapnia or acid–base disturbances. Short of ABGs the only other method available to assess $PaCO_2$ and draw correlations is end-tidal capnography.

MANAGEMENT

The goal for the critical care transport team in treatment of acute exacerbation of COPD is to improve oxygenation and CO_2 elimination, correct reversible bronchospasm, and begin (or continue) treatment of the underlying etiology of the exacerbation. The methods utilized to achieve this goal are similar to those used in the management of asthma, and include oxygen, β-agonists, anticholinergics, corticosteroids, and theophylline. Patients who do not respond to pharmacologic therapy and are in impending respiratory arrest are candidates for intubation and mechanical ventilation.

The first and easiest intervention to initiate is oxygen therapy. The patient should be provided high-flow, high-concentration oxygen via the oxygenation adjunct most appropriate for the patient's minute ventilation. While pulse oximetry may be artificially lower in the COPD patient due to the polycythemia commonly present, SpO_2 values above 95% are still desired in the acute setting. Although there was a concern once that the administration of high-flow, high-concentration oxygen to a COPD patient would wipe out her hypoxic drive and promote depression of spontaneous breathing, numerous studies in more current literature have shown that this is not the case in the acute setting. Simply put, using high-flow, high-concentration oxygen in a severely dyspneic patient is not nearly as detrimental as denying them oxygen for the fear of depressing their respiratory drive. Never withhold oxygen in the critical care environment.

The uses of aerosolized β-agonist and anticholinergic medications are considered first-line therapies in the management of acute exacerbation of COPD, and both produce similar improvements in FEV1 and PEFR. Further information on these medications is presented in the asthma section.

While the use of corticosteroids in the treatment of acute exacerbation of COPD is fairly widespread, controversy remains as to whether they are truly beneficial. What is fairly certain is that they are not harmful if administered for a few days. The general consensus is that while there may be a benefit in mild exacerbation of COPD, its efficacy in moderate and severe exacerbation is unknown.

Likewise, the use of theophylline in acute exacerbation of COPD is also controversial. The current trend calls for its use when other pharmacologic management has failed, or when plasma theophylline levels in a chronic user are subtherapeutic. As stated earlier, the risk of serious side effects from theophylline is significant. Furthermore, its therapeutic index narrow and its bronchodilatory effects are limited.

Antibiotics should be administered in acute exacerbation of COPD when the clinical condition suggests infection. The most common pathogens associated with COPD exacerbations include *Streptococcus pneumoniae, Haemophilus influenzae* and *Moraxella catarrhalis,* accounting for up to 60% of all exacerbations resulting from bacterial infection. Mild to moderate exacerbations are usually treated with older broad-spectrum antibiotics such as doxycycline, trimethoprim-sulfamethoxazole, and amoxicillin. Treatment with penicillins, fluoroquinolones, and third-generation cephalosporins or aminoglycosides are often used in patients with severe exacerbations. While the critical care paramedic will most likely not initiate antibiotics during the course of transport, the critical care paramedic may continue an administration that was started at the sending facility.

The indications for NPPV and endotrachial intubation in the management of acute exacerbation of COPD mirror that of asthma. Despite hypercapnia, hyperventilation is to be avoided in the intubated COPD patient who is chronically hypercapnic and has developed renal compensation to maintain normal acid–base balance. Hyperventilation will result in the excess elimination of CO_2, leaving the compensatory metabolic alkalosis that is present unchecked. Side effects would include decreased cardiac output, impaired cerebral blood flow, decreased respiratory drive, and cardiac dysrhythmia. In addition, as in asthma, hyperventilation can result in "air stacking," hyperinflation, and subsequent barotrauma.

ACUTE RESPIRATORY DISTRESS SYNDROME

EPIDEMIOLOGY

Since first being described in 12 patients in 1967, acute respiratory distress syndrome (ARDS) has become the leading cause of respiratory failure in the United States, with a mortality that has ranged from 60% in those first 12 patients to 40% in the past decade. High-risk conditions for developing ARDS include sepsis syndrome, multiple blood transfusions, and pulmonary contusion, of which 41%, 36%, and 22% of patients in one study developed ARDS, respectively. ARDS develops quickly, with 80% of patients developing the syndrome within 24 hours of the onset of a high-risk condition, and 95% developing the syndrome within 72 hours. Of those patients who develop ARDS, only 10% to 40% suffer mortality secondary to respiratory failure. The majority of deaths that occur within the first 72 hours are secondary to the original insult or organ failure, and after 72 hours mortality is often secondary to infection.

Since first being described in 12 patients in 1967, acute respiratory distress syndrome has become the leading cause of respiratory failure in the United States.

PATHOPHYSIOLOGY

Clinically, ARDS is characterized by impaired oxygenation, rapidly progressive hypoxemia, the presence of diffuse bilateral infiltrates on chest radiograph, and decreased lung compliance following a known predisposing insult. Simply put, ARDS is the presence of pulmonary edema in the absence of depressed left ventricular function or volume overload in the presence of a known insult.

It is important to remember that ARDS is not a primary disease; rather, it is a complication that occurs when a disease or traumatic insult produces a severe and progressive systemic inflammatory response that ultimately involves the lungs. A wide and varying range of conditions is associated with ARDS. (See Table 21–3.) Direct injuries, such as thoracic trauma, aspiration of gastric contents, or toxic gas inhalation, result in direct damage to the lung epithelium. Indirect injuries include sepsis, pancreatitis, and major nonthoracic trauma.

What direct and indirect injuries have in common is that they all result in a release of systemic activation of circulating neutrophils and macrophages. These activated cells become sticky and adhere to the pulmonary capillary endothelium, where they release proteases, oxygen metabolites, and leukotrines. These chemicals increase capillary permeability, allowing neutrophilic invasion of the lung parenchyma and causing the inflammatory process to continue. The developing inflammation and capillary permeability result in the accumulation of interstitial and alveolar edema.

This initial accumulation of interstitial and alveolar edema causes a decrease in lung compliance; that is, the lung stiffens, and blood flow to the lung is reduced. As a result of this diminished blood flow, platelets aggregate in the pulmonary capillaries, which may give rise to microthrombi that can obstruct the pulmonary capillaries and produce ischemic injury. In addition, the platelets are also a source of additional inflammatory mediators, which further damage the capillary membrane, increasing capillary permeability to plasma proteins. The movement of proteins into the interstitial space increases the interstitial osmotic pressure, drawing more fluid from the vascular

Table 21–3	Factors Associated with Acute Respiratory Distress Syndrome	
Direct Injury		**Indirect Injury**
Near-drowning		Burns
Pulmonary contusion		Multiple trauma
Pneumonia		Sepsis
Chemical exposure		Multiple blood transfusions
Gastric aspiration		Drug overdose
Fat emboli		Acute pancreatitis
Reperfusion pulmonary edema		

space and causing pulmonary edema. As CO_2 dissolves more readily in water than does O_2, PaO_2 starts to diminish, and $PaCO_2$ remains normal or can decrease as respiratory rate increases and excess CO_2 is eliminated. As fluid accumulates in the alveolar space, pulmonary surfactant is washed from the alveoli epithelium surface, and pulmonary Type II surfactant-producing cells are damaged, resulting in atelectasis. As alveolar edema and atelectasis worsen, a V/Q mismatch occurs and a right-to-left shunt develops. Further injury to the lung results in fibrosis, and CO_2 elimination is affected, resulting in hypercapnia. This late stage of ARDS is known as the fibroproliferative phase.

The end result of ARDS is naturally, respiratory failure, yet only 10% to 40% of patients who develop ARDS subsequently die from respiratory failure. Many patients suffer mortality secondary to the original insult that resulted in ARDS. Recall that ARDS was a result of a systematic inflammatory response that resulted in pulmonary inflammation; the same process can occur, and often does, in any capillary network in any organ in the body, resulting in multisystem organ dysfunction syndrome (MODS).

SIGNS AND SYMPTOMS

Early ARDS may be subclinical, with only tachypnea suggestive of the condition developing secondary to the original insult. Progressive hypoxemia and severe respiratory distress typically develop within 24 hours. Crackles may be appreciated upon auscultation, but can often be surprisingly insignificant or absent compared to the edema present on chest radiograph. Pertinent negatives in ARDS include the absence of jugular venous distention (JVD) an S3 heart sound, or other signs of left ventricular failure or volume overload.

DIAGNOSIS

Clinical diagnosis of ARDS is made when bilateral infiltrates on chest radiograph are present, $PaO_2/FiO_2 < 100$, no evidence of left atrial hypertension is present in a patient with a defined risk factor for ARDS, and finally when there is no severe chronic pulmonary disease.

ABG analysis is usually significant for hypoxia, and respiratory alkalosis may be present early in the disease from the initial tachypnea. Hypercarbia and respiratory alkalosis may develop late in the disease as blood gases become more deranged. In addition to the bilateral diffuse infiltrates evident in the early stage of ARDS, chest radiograph findings will progress to complete bilateral whiteout of the lung fields late in the disease state.

MANAGEMENT

The primary goal of management for the critical care transport team will be to ensure oxygenation to an SpO_2 of greater than 90%. Early in the disease process, this may be accomplished with a nonrebreather mask, while late phases of the disease will require endotracheal intubation and the use of significant PEEP.

Whatever the delivery modality, the FiO_2 should be kept low, 50% or lower, in an effort to minimize the risk of oxygen toxicity. Recall that one of the classes of destructive chemicals released by neutrophils during the progression of ARDS is oxygen metabolites, which result in alveolar epithelial damage. The same destruction can occur with the long-term administration of high concentrations of oxygen, a powerful oxidant. Endogenous pulmonary antioxidants in the lung usually protect against the destructive nature of oxygen, but are overwhelmed by the development of ARDS. Thus, the very oxygen that is needed to maintain adequate tissue perfusion in ARDS can further damage the lung parenchyma if administered in high concentrations. If an FiO_2 of 50% is insufficient to achieve an SpO_2 of 90%, external PEEP should be provided incrementally to increase oxygenation at nontoxic levels.

The growing consensus is that intubated patients with ARDS should be ventilated at low tidal volumes to prevent overpressure injuries to the lung. The damage to the lung in ARDS is not equally distributed, with some areas experiencing significant insult and others seemingly none.

These unaffected regions receive the majority of delivered tidal volume and experience high peak inspiratory pressures (PIP), resulting in hyperinflation and barotrauma including disruption of the alveolar-capillary membrane and surfactant depletion. To prevent overinflation injury, an effort should be made to limit PIP to 35 cm H_2O by utilizing tidal volumes of 7 to 10 mL/kg. A suggested strategy is to initiate mechanical ventilation at 10 mL/kg. If the PIP is greater than 35 cm H_2O, the tidal volume is reduced in increments of 2 mL/kg until PIP is 35 cm H_2O or lower. If inflation pressures of less than 6 cm H_2O result, PEEP should be utilized to prevent distal airway and alveolar collapse. PEEP should be added in increments of 2 cm H_2O until adequate ventilation is achieved. Late in ARDS, especially when there is significant interstitial edema and fibrosis, significant PEEP (>20 cm H_2O) may be needed to ensure airway patency and adequate ventilation.

One emerging trend with the mechanical ventilation of the ARDS patient is to decrease the delivered tidal volume in order to keep airway pressures low and avoid barotraumas. Doing this, though, has a tendency to allow the arterial levels of carbon dioxide to rise. This "permissive hypercapnia" is felt by some to be a reasonable trade-off in the attempt to avoid excessive lung stretch and barotraumas from mechanical ventilation. Because this is still a newer concept to ARDS management in the mechanically ventilated patient, the critical care paramedic should check with medical direction prior to considering it a viable option.

Along with permissive hypercapnia, some pulmonary physicians will reverse the inspiratory/expiratory (I/E ratio) times on the ventilator so that the inhalation phase is longer than the exhalation phase. A longer inhalation time will typically lower peak airway pressures, promote a less turbulent gas flow, and provide more time for good tidal volume distribution through the damaged lung tissue. Surfactant therapy to replicate the lost or damaged layer of surfactant in the alveoli is also gaining popularity, as is the use of inhaled nitric oxide (NO). Early studies have shown that nitric oxide can modulate pulmonary blood flow and and improve gas exchange in the lungs, and a growing body of literature suggests that it might alter several events in the pathogenesis of acute lung injury and ARDS.

In intubated patients who are resisting mechanical ventilation, sedation or neuromuscular blockade should be considered. "Fighting the vent" can result in poor oxygenation, high airway pressures and barotraumas, and episodes of hypotension secondary to the high intrathoracic pressures generated during combativeness.

Some treatment options available to the critical care transport team that may seem intuitive in the treatment of ARDS are the use of corticosteroids to attenuate the inflammatory response, the use of diuretics or PEEP to relieve pulmonary edema, and the use of dopamine to improve impaired cardiac output. Unfortunately, these treatment modalities are of little use in ARDS. The literature has failed to show a decrease in the development of ARDS when corticosteroids are used as prophylaxis in high-risk patients, or a reduction in mortality when used in the early stages of ARDS. In addition, secondary infection seems to be more common in ARDS patients who receive corticosteroids, making their use potentially harmful. The use of diuretics, such as furosemide, does not result in the reduction of pulmonary edema characteristic of ARDS, for the simple reason that pulmonary edema in ARDS is secondary to inflammation, and diuretics have no effect on inflammation. PEEP is a useful tool for reducing the alveolar edema typical of heart failure, but like furosemide, has no such role in the treatment of ARDS. In fact, it has been shown that high levels of PEEP actually result in an increase of alveolar edema, for reasons that are not fully understood. It must be understood that PEEP use in ARDS is not a therapy strategy, but an adjunct that allows the use of decreased tidal volumes in an effort to prevent iatrogenic lung injury.

Reduced pulmonary capillary perfusion (if present) results in decreased blood return to the left ventricle, decreased left ventricle end-diastolic pressure, decreased stroke volume, and decreased cardiac output. In cases of decreased cardiac output, the use of dobutamine is recommended when fluid volume is not warranted. The use of dopamine to correct decreased cardiac output is to be avoided, because dopamine will constrict the pulmonary veins, reducing an already limited blood flow to the pulmonary vasculature. Dobutamine, however, increases the cardiac output, but does not promote pulmonary vasoconstriction.

PNEUMONIA

EPIDEMIOLOGY

Pneumonia is the seventh leading cause of death in the United States. Estimates of the incidence of community-acquired pneumonia (CAP) range from 4 to 5 million cases per year, resulting in 1 million hospitalizations. Nosocomial pneumonia has an occurrence of about 250,000 to 300,000 cases per year. Left untreated, pneumonia may have a mortality of more than 30%, but that drops to 3% to 5% with treatment. Males have a higher incidence of infection than females, and the geriatric population is at particular risk and has an increased mortality (up to 40%) when compared to those younger than age 65. As such, pneumonia is the fifth leading cause of death in the elderly population.

PATHOPHYSIOLOGY

Pneumonia is an infection of the alveoli and gas-exchanging units of the lungs, including the respiratory bronchioles, alveolar ducts, and alveolar sacs. Infectious agents causing pneumonia include bacteria, viruses, fungi, protozoa, or rickettsia. Common bacterial pathogens include *Streptococcus pneumoniae* (up to 70% of all cases of bacterial pneumonia), *Staphylococcus aureus*, *Pneumococcus*, *Haemophilus influenzae*, and *Pseudomonas*. Common viral causes include influenza virus types A and B, RSV, adenovirus, parainfluenza virus, rhinovirus, Hantavirus, and cytomegalovirus. Very often, coinfection with bacterial and viral agents identified occurs, and no etiologic pathogen is identified in 40% to 60% of pneumonias. Atypical agents such as *Mycoplasma*, *Legionella*, *Chlamydia*, and SARS may also produce infection.

Normal defense mechanisms that protect against pneumonia include the filtration and humidification of inspired air as it passes through the upper airway, mucous secretion and mucociliary clearance, the cough reflex, cellular immunity, humoral immunity, and circulating neutrophils. Numerous routes of infection exist, and include the inhalation of infectious pathogens, the aspiration of oral or gastric contents, reactivation of a previous infection (common in immunocompromised individuals), and hematogenous seeding. Considering both the natural defenses and routes of infection, patients most at risk are those who have impaired mucocilicary clearance, are at increased risk of aspiration, are immunocompromised, or have a risk of bacteremia.

Introduction of a pathogen into the airways distal to the respiratory bronchioles results in colonization and infection of the affected portion. The infection can spread throughout the lung utilizing the bronchial tree and the pores of Kohn between adjacent alveoli. Some forms of pneumonia can elicit a severe inflammatory response resulting in the accumulation of immune cells, pathogenic material, cellular debris, pus, and fluid in the airway, while others will result in a less severe response and a much more subtle pathophysiology.

NOSOCOMIAL PNEUMONIA

Nosocomial pneumonia is pneumonia acquired in a hospital, and represents the second most common nosocomial infection in the United States. Mortality for nosocomial pneumonia (20% to 50%) is significantly higher than that of other types. Most bacterial nosocomial pneumonias occur by aspiration of bacteria colonizing the oropharynx or upper gastrointestinal tract of the patient. Contributing to the rate of this infection is the use of mechanical ventilation through an endotracheal tube (intubation bypasses the normal filtration of the upper airway), and bacteria tends to pool just above the endotracheal cuff in a location hard to access with traditional suctioning techniques. The pH of the stomach has also been shown to be a contributing factor for nosocomial pneumonia in that incidence rates for infection increase as the gastric pH increases above >4.0 (In fact, research has shown that the use of antacids and/or H blockers is associated with increased rate of nosocomial pneumonia in mechanically ventilated patients.) This is a special concern for the critical care paramedic who cares for patients who have been intubated and patients who have been admitted to an ICU.

Pneumonia is an infection of the alveoli and gas-exchanging units of the lungs, including the respiratory bronchioles, alveolar ducts, and alveolar sacs.

Endotracheal intubation, as stated earlier, bypasses the normal defenses of the upper airway, thus providing a more direct access to the lung; as many as 20% of intubated patients in the ICU develop pneumonia. In addition, the wide use of antibiotics in the ICU setting has led to the selection of antibiotic-resistant strains of microbes and more severe courses of illness.

SIGNS AND SYMPTOMS

The clinical manifestations of pneumonia are as varied as the causes themselves, ranging from the inflammation and productive cough typical of bacterial pneumonia to the nonproductive cough secondary to an atypical infection. The classic clinical picture is one of fever, sputum production, productive cough, dyspnea, tachycardia, fever, and pleuritic chest pain. Additional findings may include hemoptysis, blood-tinged sputum, and a history of upper respiratory infection. Weakness, general malaise, anorexia, and recent weight loss may also be present.

Ausculation of lung fields may reveal crackles from fluid accumulation, decreased sounds secondary to consolidation, or ronchi and wheezing from accumulation of pus and debris. In cases of consolidation, dullness to percussion and increased tactile fremitus may be appreciated.

Severe tachycardia, tachypnea, fever, and hypotension associated with pneumonia are ominous signs, and could herald respiratory failure or be suggestive of septicemia. Most patients with CAP will not require ICU admission, but high-risk patients include those with pneumonia and preexisting lung disease, pneumonia resulting in septicemia or coexisting with ARDS, patients with a history of alcoholism or diabetes, and the elderly.

DIAGNOSIS

The individualized nature of pneumonia and the wide range of clinical presentations make it challenging to establish clear criteria for the diagnosis of pneumonia. Commonly accepted clinical criteria for the identification of serious pneumonia include tachypnea greater than 30 breaths per minute, temperature greater than 101° F, hypotension, and altered mental status. The following laboratory exams may aid the critical care transport team in the identification of pneumonia.

Leukopenia in the patient with pneumonia is considered an ominous sign and is suggestive for sepsis. Leukocytosis with a left shift indicates bacterial infection, but not necessarily pneumonia; it can also be present in cases of viral pneumonia. The absence of leukocytosis, especially in the elderly, does not rule out the possibility of pneumonia.

Blood cultures, sputum cultures, and Gram stains may be helpful in identifying the etiology of the pneumonia, but are frequently useless. Rapid antigen detection kits can detect influenza, RSV, parainfluenza, and other viruses rapidly enough for critical care transport or ED use.

Chest radiograph may reveal consolidation, pleural effusion, patchy interstitial or alveolar infiltrates, or peribronchial thickening. Depending on the pathogen and extent of the disease, findings may be lobular, multilobular, unilateral, or bilateral.

ABG analysis may reveal hypoxemia in severe cases of pneumonia, but are arguably not necessary in mild or moderate cases in which oxygenation determination via pulse oximetry is sufficient.

A summary of the laboratory results that influence the decision for hospitalization of a patient with pneumonia include leukopenia less than 4,000 to 5,000 cells/mm^3, leukocytosis greater than 30,000 cells/mm^3, a PaO_2 of less than 50 mmHg, and involvement of more than 50% of the lung.

MANAGEMENT

The management of a patient with pneumonia will be mostly supportive, consisting primarily of oxygenation and ventilatory support. In cases of severe pneumonia, endotracheal intubation may be necessary.

Treatment with antibiotic therapy should be initiated within the first 8 hours, if possible, because the early administration of antibiotics has been shown to improve morbidity and mortality for those patients who are going to require hospitalization for their pneumonia. Typical treatment for unidentified etiologies includes a second- or third-generation cephalosporin or penicillin plus a beta-lactamase inhibitor. Patients may also receive a macrolide to address atypical agents. If the etiology has been determined, more specific antibiotic treatment can be initiated.

For those patients with wheezing that is audible on auscultation, an inhaled agonist may be considered, but its benefit should be weighed against the potential for cardiac involvement of the drug.

SPONTANEOUS AND IATROGENIC PNEUMOTHORAX

EPIDEMIOLOGY

It has been estimated that up to 20,000 cases of spontaneous pneumothorax occur in the United States each year, with about 9,000 being primary pneumothoraces and the remaining secondary pneumothoraces. The description of the tall, thin male who has exerted himself and suffered a spontaneous pneumothorax has reached urban legend status among prehospital care providers, and the critical care paramedic will be pleased to know that this categorization has basis in reality, according to the literature. Males have a 6:1 relative risk of pneumothorax compared to females, and a tall, thin stature contributes to that risk. Physical exertion has not proved to be a significant risk factor (about 10% to 20% of all cases), but smoking has. Smokers have a 20:1 relative risk compared to nonsmokers, and may very well be the cause of the increase of spontaneous pneumothoraces in the female population in the past decades, mirroring the increasing number of women smokers.

A primary risk factor in the occurrence of secondary spontaneous pneumothorax is COPD, which is present in up to 67% of cases. These patients experience a 3.5-fold increase in relative mortality when compared to those COPD patients without spontaneous pneumothoracies. Mortality percentages in patients with COPD and pneumothorax have ranged from 1% to 17%. The *Patient Safety in American Hospitals, Health Grades 2004,* report determined that 33,571 iatrogenic pneumothoraces occurred in U.S. hospitals between 2000 and 2002. Transthoracic needle aspiration (biopsy), needle thoracentesis, and subclavicular catheterization attempts account for about 75% of all iatrogenic pneumothoraces, and it has been reported that pneumothorax occurs in 2% to 6 % of all subclavian catheterization attempts.

PATHOPHYSIOLOGY

A pneumothorax occurs when a hole in the lung, the chest wall, or both penetrates the visceral or parietal pleura and transforms the intrapleural region from a potential space into an actual one. Without the subatmospheric (negative) pressure within the pleural cavity to hold the lung up to the inner chest wall, the lung's tendency to collapse is unopposed.

Spontaneous pneumothoraces are those that occur without a prior event or any other apparent cause. A spontaneous pneumothorax that occurs in an individual without any underlying lung disease is termed a primary spontaneous pneumothorax, and one that occurs in the presence of underlying disease is termed a secondary spontaneous pneumothorax. Traumatic pneumothorax results from direct or indirect trauma to the thorax and can be further delineated as iatrogenic or noniatrogenic.

Primary spontaneous pneumothorax results from the rupture of a subpleural emphysematous bleb, most often in the upper lobe. Exact mechanisms of bleb formation are unknown, but it is suspected that cigarette smoking and subsequent airway inflammation are a cause, as is local ischemia secondary to decreased upper lobe blood flow, and increased upper lobe pulmonary airflow pressure.

Secondary spontaneous pneumothorax occurs as a complication of lung disease, most often COPD (67% of cases). Additional lung diseases associated with spontaneous pneumothorax include asthma, cystic fibrosis, *P. carinii* pneumonia secondary to AIDS, interstitial lung diseases, and granulomatous lung diseases.

Iatrogenic pneumothorax occurs secondary to transthoracic needle aspiration, needle thoracentesis, subclavicular catheterization attempts, broncoscopy, pericardiocentesis, nasogastric tube placement into the bronchial tree, mechanical ventilation, and CPR. Use of the low tidal volume, minimal PEEP method of ventilation detailed in the ARDS section may prove helpful in preventing iatrogenic pneumothorax in patients with underlying lung disease.

SIGNS AND SYMPTOMS

As the pleura is innervated, greater than 95% of patients will experience pleuritic chest pain secondary to primary spontaneous pneumothorax, which is localized to the side of the pneumothorax about 90% of the time. Pleuritic chest pain and dyspnea are the most common clinical findings in primary spontaneous pneumothorax. Tachycardia secondary to catecholamine release from pain will be present to some degree, and increases with the size of the pneumothorax and resulting oxygenation deficits. Auscultation of lung fields may reveal decreased or absent lung sounds, depending on the degree of collapse; it has been estimated that 30% of the lung must be involved before a decrease in lung sounds is detectable. In cases of significant percentage of lung involvement, ipsilateral hyperresonance and decreased chest wall motion may be appreciated.

Signs and symptoms in cases of secondary spontaneous pneumothorax mirror those of primary pneumothorax, but are commonly much more severe due to decreased pulmonary reserve secondary to underlying lung disease. Severe dyspnea, hypotension, and hypoxemia are more common in this population.

Developing pneumothorax and tension pneumothorax in a mechanically ventilated patient may be difficult for the critical care paramedic to detect. In addition, sedation or neuromuscular blockade and the ground and especially aeromedical transport environments may make recognition even more difficult. A patient may not be able to communicate the onset of pleuritic chest pain and developing shortness of breath typical of pneumothorax to the caregiver because of being intubated, sedated, or pharmacologically paralyzed. A noisy environment or helmet will impede the critical care paramedic's ability to auscultate lung sounds as well. A pneumothorax in a ventilated patient can quickly develop into a tension pneumothorax if unidentified. The acute onset of decreased SaO_2, hypotension, tachycardia, increases in airway pressure, and pulseless electrical activity (PEA) should alert the critical care paramedic to developing tension pneumothorax in the paralyzed, intubated patient. For those patients not under the influence of neuromuscular blockade, combativeness, restlessness, and "fighting the vent" are additional indications of developing pneumothorax and tension pneumothorax.

Many times care providers will look for changes in capnography or end-tidal carbon dioxide levels for evidence of a pneumothorax, but this may not be much help. The interpretation of the capnogram depends on the size of the pneumothorax, the evolutionary stage of the pneumothorax, and whether or not the patient is being ventilated. If the pneumothorax is small, then changes to the $PetCO_2$ will be minimal or nonexistent and capnography is nondiagnostic. If the pneumothorax is larger, then the $PetCO_2$ may become elevated due to poor alveolar ventilation, but if the pneumothorax progresses to a tension status, then the diminishment in cardiac output as a consequence of mechanical pressure on the heart will inhibit cardiac output and may actually cause the exhaled carbon dioxide level to decrease from poor pulmonary perfusion. Or conversely, if the patient's tidal volume is diminishing due to a collapsed lung (poor alveolar ventilation), then the exhaled gas sampled by the machine will initially increase until the point at which the tidal volume is only ventilating pulmonary dead space, and the $PetCO_2$ could then decrease. In conclusion, the critical care paramedic is again cautioned to use the $PetCO_2$ waveform and reading as a supportive diagnostic adjunct only.

DIAGNOSIS

First and foremost, the diagnosis and treatment of tension pneumothorax are achieved based on clinical observations, not diagnostic studies. Tension pneumothorax is a life-threatening and easily reversible pathology that must be corrected immediately.

Chest radiograph, specifically a 6-foot upright posteroanterior view, is considered the "gold standard" for the diagnosis of pneumothorax. A thin pleural line and the absence of lung marking between the pleural line and the chest wall are suggestive of pneumothorax, and may be hard to identify in patients with underlying pulmonary disease. For patients who are unable to sit upright and must be evaluated supine, the presence of a wide and deep costophrenic angle, often called the deep sulcus sign, is suggestive of a pneumothorax. In addition, an enlarged ipsilateral hemithorax secondary to contralateral shift of the mediastinum may be appreciated. A chest CT can be utilized if a radiograph proves nondiagnostic for suspected pneumothorax, because a CT scan would be expected to be more sensitive.

ABG analysis is not necessary for the diagnosis of pneumothorax, and will not reveal anything that the clinical picture cannot yield. Hypoxemia would be expected as a pneumothorax progresses, as well as possible hypocapnia secondary to an elevated respiratory rate and excess CO_2 elimination early on. In severe cases of pneumothorax, hypoxia and hypercapnia may be seen, as well as a respiratory acidosis.

Although not commonly used in the United States, ultrasound is widely used in Europe to identify both traumatic and nontraumatic pneumothorax with a sensitivity approaching 100%. One study in the United States showed that a wide range of emergency medicine providers, including attending and resident physicians, nurse practitioners, medical students, and physician assistants, could successfully identify pneumothorax greater than 90% of the time after attending an ultrasound educational session. This, along with the fact that portable ultrasound units are readily available and in use in many critical care programs already, suggests that this diagnostic modality might be of benefit to, and within the scope of learning of the critical care transport team.

MANAGEMENT

The management goals for the critical care transport team regarding pneumothorax include removing intrapleural air, ensuring proper oxygenation, and preventing recurrences.

Many small, primary pneumothoraces do not require treatment other than the administration of oxygen at 3 to 4 lpm and a serial chest radiograph to ensure that the injury is not expanding. Intrapleural air is reabsorbed at a rate of 1.25% per day, and the lung will frequently readhere to the chest wall without complication. However, 20% to 40% of patients who are initially treated with observation ultimately require chest thoracostomy. Needle aspiration is also an option in a small, primary pneumothorax.

Chest tube thoracostomy is the standard of care for almost all cases of secondary spontaneous pneumothorax, and is always required if mechanical ventilation is going to be utilized. Other indications for tube thoracostomy include a pneumothorax greater than 40%, a pneumothorax that does not respond to aspiration, and ABG abnormalities.

The development of tension pneumothorax necessitates the need for immediate needle decompression of the affected side of the chest. A chest thoracostomy tube should not be used to treat a tension pneumothorax unless it can be performed more rapidly than needle decompression.

Summary

The intent of this chapter was to introduce the critical care paramedic to the types of pulmonary emergencies that are commonly seen in the critical care environment. Unlike prehospital care, where many of the causes of respiratory distress are of a minor cause, the transport of a patient with persistent respiratory distress should raise alarm. Common sense would dictate that if the etiology of the pulmonary dysfunction could have been managed at the original facility, then transport of the patient would be unnecessary. The simple fact that the critical care paramedic is responding to a patient with respiratory distress speaks to the fact it is most likely a significantly ill patient.

The critical care paramedic should, regardless of the etiology of respiratory distress, develop a process approach to the management of pulmonary emergencies. Almost without exception, the overarching goals in the management of these patients is to ensure airway adequacy, restore or promote ventilatory sufficiency, monitor and maintain acceptable arterial blood gases, and prevent continued deterioration. The information provided in this chapter was designed to allow the critical care paramedic to do this.

Review Questions

1. Briefly describe acute respiratory failure.

2. Name the common precipitating events of acute respiratory failure.

3. Discuss some of the factors regarding oxygenation failure as it pertains to acute respiratory failure.

4. Describe the effects of ventilatory failure in acute respiratory failure.

5. What are the pharmacologic and nonpharmacologic management principles for a patient with acute respiratory failure?

6. Why is the use of a mechanical ventilator cautioned when a patient has end-stage ARDS?

7. What would be some of the clinical indications of impending respiratory failure that would cause the critical care paramedic to provide rapid-sequence intubation to a patient?

8. What diagnostic studies are beneficial to the critical care paramedic in deciding what treatment modalities to employ while transporting a patient with ARDS?

9. What clinical indications would need to be present for a critical care paramedic to decide to decompress a suspected tension pneumothorax?

See Answers to Review Questions at the back of this book.

Further Reading

Allen G, Kaminsky DA. "Asthma." In *Critical Care Secrets,* 3rd ed. Parsons PE, Wiener-Kronish JP, editors. Philadelphia: Hanley & Belfus, 2003.

Ashbaugh DG, Bigelow DB, Petty TL, Levine BE. "Acute Respiratory Distress in Adults." *Lancet,* Vol. 2, No. 7511 (August 12, 1967): 319–323.

Bledsoe BE, Porter RS, Cherry RA. *Paramedic Care: Principles & Practice,* 2nd ed. Upper Saddle River, NJ: Pearson Prentice Hall, 2005.

Butler TJ, Monahan FD. "Knowledge Basic to the Nursing Care of Adults with Respiratory Disfunction." In *Nursing Care of Adults,* Monahan FD, Drake T, Neighbors M, editors. Philadelphia: W. B. Saunders, 1994.

CDC MMWR Survalence Summary. *Surveillance for Asthma—United States, 1960–1995.* http://www.cdc.gov/mmwr/preview/mmwrhtml/00052262.htm.

Chang AK, Barton ED. "Pneumothorax, Iatrogenic, Spontaneous, and Pneumomediastinum." http://www.emedicine.com/EMERG/topic469.htm (accessed 2002).

Cydulka RK. "Acute Asthma in Adults." In *Emergency Medicine: A Comprehensive Study Guide,* 6th ed. Tintinelli JE, Kelen JD, Stapczynski JS, editors. New York: McGraw-Hill, 2004.

Cydulka RK, Dave M. "Chronic Obstructive Pulmonary Disease." In *Emergency Medicine: A Comprehensive Study Guide,* 6th ed. Tintinelli JE, Kelen JD, Stapczynski JS, editors. New York: McGraw-Hill, 2004.

Cydulka RK, McFadden ER, Emerman CL, et al. "Patterns of Hospitalization in Elderly Patients with Asthma and Chronic Obstructive Pulmonary Disease." *American Journal of Respiratory and Critical Care Medicine,* Vol. 156 (1997): 1807.

Fernandez E. "Chronic Obstructive Pulmonary Disease." In *Critical Care Secrets,* 3rd ed. Parsons PE, Wiener-Kronish JP, editors. Philadelphia: Hanley & Belfus, 2003.

Halm EA, Teirstein AS. "Management of Community Acquired Pneumonia." *New England Journal of Medicine,* Vol. 347 (2002): 2039.

Hasegawa N, Husari AW, Hart WT, et al. "Role of the Coagulation System in ARDS." *Chest,* Vol. 105 (1994): 268–277.

Hix CD, Tamburri LM. "Acute Respiratory Failure." In *Introduction to Critical Care Nursing*, 3rd ed. Sole ML, Lamborn ML, Hartshorn JC, editors. Philadelphia: W. B. Saunders, 2000.

Hubble MW, Hubble JP. *Principles of Advanced Trauma Care*, 1st ed. Albany, NY: Thompson Delmar Learning, 2002.

Hudac CM. "Common Respiratory Disorders." In *Critical Care Nursing: A Holistic Approach*, 7th ed. Hudak CM, Gallo BM, Morton PG, editors. Philadelphia: Lippincott-Raven Publishers, 1998.

Hudson LD, Milberg JA, Anardi D, Maunder RJ. "Clinical Risks for Development of the Acute Respiratory Distress Syndrome." *American Journal of Respiratory and Critical Care Medicine*, Vol. 151, No. 2, Pt. 1 (February 1995): 293–301.

Hunter MH, King DA. "COPD: Management of Acute Exacerbations and Chronic Stable Disease." *American Family Physician*, Vol. 64 (2001): 603–612, 621–622.

Irish C, Owens W, Gibbs M. "Bedside Ultrasound for the Diagnosis of Pneumothorax: A Teaching Module for Emergency Medicine Providers." *Academic Emergency Medicine*, Vol. 11, No. 5 (2004): 579–580.

Lichtenstein DA. "Lung Ultrasound in the Intensive Care Unit." *Recent Research Developments in Respiratory and Critical Care Medicine*, Vol. 1 (2001): 83.

Mannino DM, Homa DM, Akinbami LJ, et al. "Chronic Obstructive Pulmonary Disease Surveillance—United States, 1971–2000." *MMWR Surveillance Summary*, Vol. 51 (2002): 1.

Mannino DM, Homa DM, Akinbami LJ, et al. "Surveillance for Asthma—United States." *MMWR Surveillance Summary*, Vol. 51 (2002): 1.

Marino, PL. *The ICU Book*, 2nd ed. Baltimore, MD: Williams & Williams, 1998.

Martini FH, Timmons MJ, McKinley MP. *Human Anatomy*, 3rd ed. Upper Saddle River, NJ: Pearson Prentice Hall, 2000.

Melton LJ, Hepper NGG, Offord KP. "Incidence of Spontaneous Pneumothorax in Olmsted County, Minnesota: 1950–1974." *American Review of Respiratory Disease*, Vol. 120 (1979): 1379.

Minino AM, Smith BL. "Deaths: Preliminary Data for 2000." *National Vital Statistics Reports*, Vol. 49 (2001): 1–40.

Moffa DA, Emerman CL. "Bronchitis, Pneumonia, and Pleural Emphysema." In *Emergency Medicine: A Comprehensive Study Guide*, 6th ed. Tintinelli JE, Kelen JD, Stapczynski JS, editors. New York: McGraw-Hill, 2004.

Monahan FD, White MA, Rinne CW. "Respiratory Care of Adults with Lower Respiratory Disorders." In *Nursing Care of Adults*. Monahan FD, Drake T, Neighbors M, editors. Philadelphia: W. B. Saunders, 1994.

Morton PG. "Patient Assessment: Respiratory System." In *Critical Care Nursing: A Holistic Approach*, 7th ed. Hudak CM, Gallo BM, Morton PG, editors. Philadelphia: Lippincott-Raven Publishers, 1998.

Netter, FH. *Atlas of Human Anatomy*. Summit, NJ: Ciba-Geigy Corporation, 1989.

Pauwels RA, Buist AS, Calverley PM, Jenkins CR, Hurd SS. "Global Strategy for the Diagnosis, Management, and Prevention of Chronic Obstructive Pulmonary Disease. NHLBI/WHO Global Initiative for Chronic Obstructive Lung Disease (GOLD) Workshop Summary." *American Journal of Respiratory and Critical Care Medicine*, Vol. 163 (2001): 1256–1276.

Rothenhaus, T. *Acute Respiratory Distress Syndrome*. http://www.emedicine.com/emerg/topic15.htm (accessed 2004).

Scalera TM, Boswell SA. "Abdominal Injuries." In *Emergency Medicine: A Comprehensive Study Guide*, 6th ed. Tintinelli JE, Kelen JD, Stapczynski JS, editors. New York: McGraw-Hill, 2004.

Schwartz MI. "Acute Pneumonia." In *Critical Care Secrets*, 3rd ed. Parsons PE, Wiener-Kronish JP, editors. Philadelphia: Hanley & Belfus, 2003.

Skobeloff EM, Spivey WH, St Clair SS, Schoffstall JM. "The Influence of Age and Sex on Asthma Admissions." *Journal of the American Medical Association*, Vol. 268, No. 24 (December 23–30, 1992): 3437–3440.

Soler N, Torres A, Ewing S, Gonzalez J, Celis R, El-Ebiary M, et al. "Bronchial Microbial Patterns in Severe Exacerbations of Chronic Obstructive Pulmonary Disease (COPD) Requiring Mechanical Ventilation." *American Journal of Respiratory and Critical Care Medicine,* Vol. 157 (1998): 1498–1505.

Turki M, Parsons PE. "Acute Respiratory Distress Syndrome." In *Critical Care Secrets,* 3rd ed. Parsons PE, Wiener-Kronish JP, editors. Philadelphia: Hanley & Belfus, 2003.

Young Jr WF, Humphries RL. "Spontaneous and Iatrogenic Pneumothorax." In *Emergency Medicine: A Comprehensive Study Guide,* 6th ed. Tintinelli JE, Kelen JD, Stapczynski JS, editors. New York: McGraw-Hill, 2004.

Zamora MR, Burkhardt D. "Acute Respiratory Failure." In *Critical Care Secrets,* 3rd ed. Parsons PE, Wiener-Kronish JP. Philadelphia: Hanley & Belfus, 2003.

Cardiovascular Emergencies

Arthur Kanowitz, MD, FACEP

Objectives

Upon completion of this chapter, the student should be able to:

1. Understand and discuss the anatomy and physiology of the heart as it pertains to the critical care paramedic. (p. 623)
2. Understand the pathophysiology, clinical manifestation, diagnostics, and management guidelines of patients with the following disorders:
   A. Acute coronary syndrome (p. 631)
   B. Aortic aneurysm (p. 639)
   C. Aortic dissection (p. 641)
   D. Cardiogenic shock (p. 643)
   E. Adult cardiomyopathies (p. 647)
   F. Cardiopulmonary arrest (p. 649)
   G. Congestive heart failure (p. 651)
   H. Hypertensive emergencies (p. 652)
   I. Pericarditis, pericardial effusion, and cardiac tamponade (p. 656)
   J. Valvular dysfunction (p. 658)
   K. Disorders of the aortic valve (p. 659)
   L. Disorders of the mitral valve (p. 660)
3. Be familiar with those procedures with which competency is expected in the critical care transport environment including:
   A. Ventricular assist device (p. 645)
   B. Arterial line placement (p. 662)
   C. Central venous access (p. 669)
   D. Intra-aortic balloon pump (p. 671)
   E. Pericardiocentesis (p. 672)
4. Understand the general considerations for interfacility critical care transport. (p. 673)

5. Understand the special considerations related to air critical care transport:
  A. Preparation for flight (p. 674)
  B. Alterations in cardiovascular physiology at altitude (p. 674)
  C. Handling of in-flight cardiopulmonary arrest (p. 674)

Key Terms

Case Study

You and your flight crew are just getting settled down in your quarters after a long day of missions when you are again alerted for a mission coming out of a very rural hospital near the border of the county. The pilot checks the coordinates and weather conditions as you get further information on your patient, and before long you are in the air in your EC 135 helicopter flying at 145 knots towards the hospital. You remark on how the weather couldn't possibly be better for flying today, and you land 25 minutes later at the hospital.

As you enter the emergency department, the staff seems unusually concerned about the patient as they give you a report. Your patient, Frank, is a 58-year-old male who was brought in by the local volunteer EMS squads with crushing substernal chest pain radiating down his left arm and into his jaw. Paramedics stated that upon their arrival his pain was at 10/10. They followed their chest pain protocol, which included chewable aspirin, nitroglycerin 0.4 mg × 2 sublingual, IV therapy, and O_2 at 15 liters per minute. The paramedics stated that following this therapy the pain reduced to 7/10. At the emergency department, the physician ordered the administration of another nitroglycerin sublingual and morphine 2 mg × 2 in 10-minute intervals. This promoted further reduction in pain to 4/10. A 12-lead ECG was obtained showing ST elevation in leads V1–V4, and the cardiac enzyme markers troponin and myoglobin are markedly elevated upon blood analysis. The physician tells you that the patient is being transferred to your facility for PTCA since he has a recent history of GI ulcerations with hemorrhage and is not a fibrinolytic candidate. Currently the patient seems to be resting comfortably and states he is pain free.

You quickly perform a bedside physical assessment of the patient, and start attaching the patient to your portable equipment. Following the movement of the patient to your cot, you obtain the transfer documents, X-rays, and blood work from the staff in the ED. The patient's family says their good-byes to the patient, and you whisk the patient back to your EC 135 running hot on the helipad, and prepare for liftoff. Before you lift off however, Frank begins to complain of his pain worsening (now at a 4/10), and he starts to become very nauseous. You also notice his anxiety level rising.

You quickly scan the 12-lead and see the V-leads starting to elevate, so you continue on with your chest pain management protocol for an active myocardial infarction. Your partner begins to set up the syringe pump with a nitroglycerin infusion as you administer an additional 2 mg of morphine for pain relief and then Phenergan 12.5 mg for nausea. The patient states no relief from the morphine and the nitroglycerin infusion is initiated at 10 mcg/min. After a brief reassessment of the patient's hemodynamics, you find no change in the patient's clinical condition. You increase the drip rate to 20 mcg/min with still no relief, and only after the infusion is raised to 30 mcg/min is the pain resolved. You decide to hold on any additional medication as the pilot announces the final approach to the helipad. You lean over and tell the patient you'll be on the ground in about 2 minutes. He smiles, and thanks you for your care.

INTRODUCTION

Patients with cardiovascular emergencies are not only among the most common patient scenarios encountered in critical care transport, but they are also among the most challenging cases.

Patients with cardiovascular emergencies are not only among the most common patient scenarios encountered in critical care transport, but they are also among the most challenging cases. These patients frequently require the critical care paramedic to have an in-depth understanding of cardiovascular pathophysiology as well as the ability to handle invasive cardiac monitoring and sophisticated cardiovascular support equipment.

Critical care transport may be accomplished via ground or air. The critical care paramedic frequently must be able to care for a critically ill patient while simultaneously managing an extensive amount of equipment. This may include multiple IV pumps, mechanical ventilation, and an intra-aortic balloon pump or ventricular assist device. Appropriately managing the patient dependent on this sophisticated medical equipment requires preparation prior to transport and diligent monitoring while en route to the final destination.

The decision to utilize a critical care transport team rather than an advanced life support (ALS) unit for a patient with a cardiovascular emergency is usually based on criteria set by local protocol. Typical criteria might include the following:

1. Any patient who is being admitted to an intensive care unit
2. Any patient who is being admitted directly to a cardiac cath lab
3. Any patient who will require medications, equipment, or procedures during transport that may be outside the street-level paramedic's scope of practice
4. Specific request by the sending physician for a critical care transport team

The critical care transport of patients with cardiovascular emergencies typically involves the following types of interfacility transfers:

1. Emergency department to emergency department
2. Emergency department to intensive care unit
3. Emergency department to cardiac cath lab
4. Intensive care unit to intensive care unit

Considerations regarding the preparation and safe transfer of patients by both air and ground transport will be covered in this chapter.

ANATOMY AND PHYSIOLOGY OF THE HEART

LOCATION

The heart, a hollow muscular organ, is located in the mediastinal cavity just to the left of the sternum. The superior border of the heart rests approximately at the second intercostal space, with the inferior border at the sixth rib. The heart is rotated slightly to the left, with allows the right ventricle to be the anterior surface.

PHYSIOLOGY

The purpose of the heart is to pump blood throughout the circulatory system, a task it cannot fail in—even for a moment—without disastrous effects. It is comprised of four chambers, divided into receiving upper chambers (**atria**) and bottom pumping chambers (**ventricles**). The right atrium receives deoxygenated blood from the venous system and delivers it to the left ventricle for pumping through the pulmonary circuit so as to allow oxygenation to take place. After passing through the lungs, the blood is received by the left atrium, which provides it to the left ventricle so that it may be pumped through the systemic circulation, which allows respiration of the tissue cells of the body.

The left and right sides of the heart can also be divided into (and discussed as) two completely separate hemispheres. The left side of the heart is a high-pressure system that circulates oxygenated blood throughout the body's arteries, while the right side is a low-pressure system circulating deoxygenated blood through the pulmonary vasculature for the lungs where it can be reoxygenated and again circulated throughout the body on return to the left side. The flow of blood is maintained through the heart by way of sequential contraction of the atria prior to the ventricles, and the flow of blood from the ventricles is controlled by way of the valves. Following the contraction of the atria, blood from the right atrium passes through the tricuspid valve, and blood from the left atrium passes through the bicuspid valve. These atrioventricular valves prevent the backflow of blood as the ventricular pressure rises during systole. The papillary muscles and *chordae tendonae* are tethered from the ventricle to the inferior surface of the atrioventricular valves in order to prevent them from prolapsing into the atria when the ventricles contract. In summation then, it takes both the sequential pumping of the chambers of the heart and the opening and closing of the atrioventricular valves to keep blood flowing in a proper direction through the heart.

Following this, the blood vessels that carry the blood from the heart, the pulmonary arteries beyond the right ventricle and the aorta beyond the left ventricle, also have blood flow to them controlled by a set of valves. The pulmonic valve is positioned between the right ventricle and the pulmonary artery, and the aortic valve is positioned between the left ventricle and the aorta. These semilunar valves open during ventricular systole due to the rising intraventricular pressure and allow blood to pass into either the pulmonary artery from the right ventricle or the aorta from the left ventricle. Once the pressure in the aortic root or pulmonary artery exceeds the pressure of its respective ventricle following contraction, the semilunar valves shut, and retrograde blood flow is prevented.

atria *thin-walled, upper chambers of the heart that receive venous blood from the pulmonary or systemic circulation.*

ventricles *thick-walled, lower chambers of the heart that discharge blood into the pulmonary or systemic circulation.*

The purpose of the heart is to pump blood throughout the circulatory system, a task it cannot fail in—even for a moment—without disastrous effects.

CARDIAC CONDUCTION

As mentioned previously, the heart has to operate in a rhythmic fashion in order for there to be forward propulsion of blood. This is achieved universally by cells of the heart that have differing action. First, there are cells of the heart that comprise the conduction system. These cells do not participate in contraction, because they do not have contractile properties. The conduction cells of the heart simply transmit impulses from the sinoatrial node throughout the rest of the myocardium in an organized fashion so that cellular contraction is uniform. A special subset of the conduction cells comprises the pacemaker sites, and the cells of this subset have the capability of automaticity. Automaticity is the property of pacemaker cells that allows them to initiate their own impulse, which is then transmitted to the working cells of the myocardium by way of the conduction system. Pacemaker cells are located at specific points along the conduction system, to include the sinoatrial node, the atrioventricular junction, and the Purkinje network.

The conduction system starts with the primary pacemaker site, the **sinoatrial (SA) node.** The SA node has an intrinsic discharge rate of 60–100 impulses per minute. The impulse is then spread through the atria by way of intra-atrial pathways, allowing for uniform atrial contraction. The impulse travels down the internodal pathway to the **atrioventricular (AV) node,** where it is delayed so that the ventricles have a chance to be filled by blood leaving the atria. Once the impulse emerges from the AV node, it passes through the bundle of His where it then divides into the right and left bundle branch within the interventricular septum. Each bundle branch is responsible for transmitting the impulse through the ventricles in a uniform fashion, progressing to the **Purkinje fibers,** which then stimulate the myocardial working cells so that uniform contraction of the ventricles can occur. The AV node has an intrinsic discharge rate of 40–60 impulses per minute and the Purkinje fibers have an intrinsic rate of 20–40 per minute. This decreasing intrinsic rate is designed to allow the SA node to remain as the primary pacemaker for the heart. But should the SA node fail, the AV node will reach threshold next and establish a junctional escape rhythm. If, however, the SA and AV nodes fail to initiate an impulse, or if the impulse generated does not reach the ventricles, the Purkinje network can initiate an escape rhythm. The escape rhythm from the ventricles, however, is slow, unreliable, and prone to failing rapidly.

The contractile force of the myocardium is generated from the second type of cardiac cell, the contractile cell. The contractile cell is where the actual work of pumping the blood is done. As the electrical current generated from the conductive cells passes through a contractile cell, the contractile cell shortens in length, and blood is ejected from the heart as the chamber size decreases in response to this contraction. (See Figure 22-1 ■.)

CORONARY PERFUSION

The heart is justifiably the most important muscle of the body, and it ensures the adequacy of its own blood supply by taking its arterial blood flow directly off the aorta, prior to the generation of any other blood vessel. The heart is perfused during diastole, through two major coronary arteries that branch directly off from the aorta. The right coronary artery perfuses the SA node, AV node, right atrium, and ventricle as it circles around the back side of the heart to perfuse the posterior wall and ultimately the inferior wall of the left ventricle. The left common coronary artery branches into two smaller arteries called the left anterior descending artery and the left circumflex artery. The left anterior descending artery perfuses the septal and anterior walls of the left ventricle. The left circumflex artery continues beyond the generation of the left anterior descending artery to wrap around the lateral side of the ventricle. It ultimately terminates at the apex of the heart. As such, the circumflex perfuses the lateral and posterior wall of the left ventricle. Numerous other smaller arteries originate off left and right coronary arteries as mentioned, and they complete the arterial supply to the heart. (See Figure 22-2 ■.)

CARDIAC AUSCULTATION

Due to the potential complications with cardiac patients, a good assessment of your patient's cardiac status cannot be emphasized enough. Along with obtaining a good history and interpreting the ECG, cardiac auscultation will yield the best clue to your patient's cardiac function without additional invasive hemodynamic monitoring. The key to good auscultation lies in both proper use of the stethoscope and a quiet environment. Stethoscope tubing should be no longer than 12 inches to prevent distortion of sound. Ear pieces should point toward and fit snugly into the external ear canal. A stethoscope with both a diaphragm, for listening to high-pitched sounds, and a bell, for low-pitched sounds, is recommended.

Another component of auscultating heart tones is understanding where to auscultate in order to hear the best sounds for the normal valve action or valve dysfunction, whatever you're listening for. Table 22–1 identifies these common auscultation areas by name and location.

HEART SOUNDS

Starting with the basic heart sounds, S_1 and S_2 should be the first identifiable heart tones heard. S_1 precedes S_2 and they can be described as the basic "lub-dub" sounds. When the atria contract and

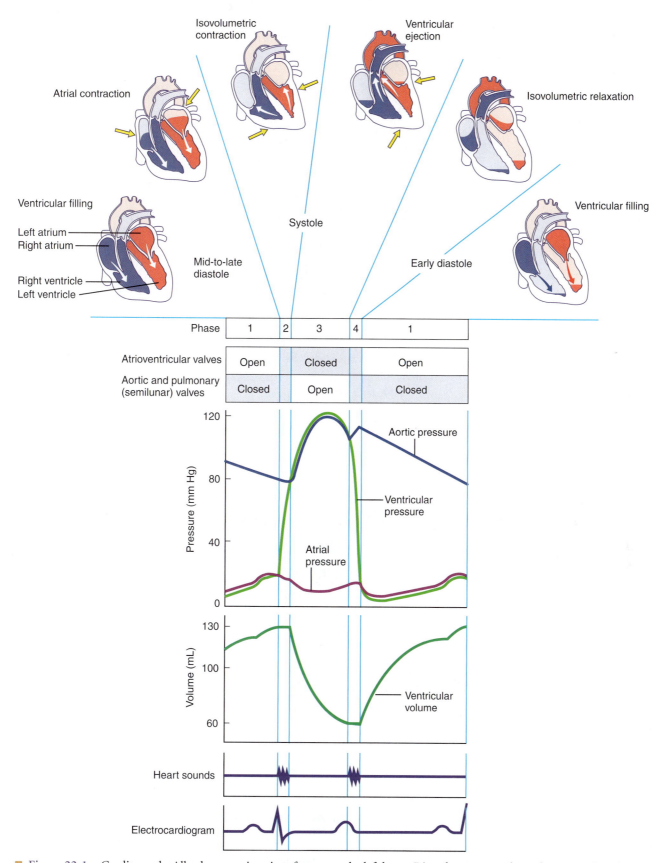

■ **Figure 22-1**   Cardiac cycle. All values are given in reference to the left heart. Diastole corresponds to phases 4 and 1, whereas systole corresponds to phases 2 and 3. Note the correlations between changes in pressure gradients across valves and the open/closed state of the valve and the changes in ventricular volume. Heart sounds are correlated with the closing of the valves. ECG waves correlate to the mechanical events of the heart; the P wave precedes atrial contraction (evident as an increase in atrial pressure), the QRS complex precedes ventricular contraction (evident as the rapid increase in ventricular pressure), and the T wave precedes ventricular relaxation (evident as the rapid decrease in ventricular pressure). *(Fig. 14-17, p. 434, from* Principles of Human Physiology, *2nd ed., by William J. Germann and Cindy L. Stanfield. Copyright © 2005 by Pearson Education, Inc. Reprinted by permission.)*

Figure 22-2 The coronary circulation. Coronary vessels supplying the (a) anterior and (b) posterior surfaces of the heart. *(Fig. 13-7, p. 363, from Essentials of Anatomy & Physiology, 2nd ed., by Frederic H. Martini, Ph.D. and Edwin F. Bartholomew, M.S. Copyright © 2000 by Frederic H. Martini, Inc. Published by Pearson Education, Inc. Reprinted by permission.)*

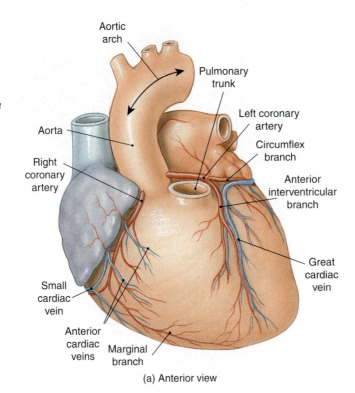

(a) Anterior view

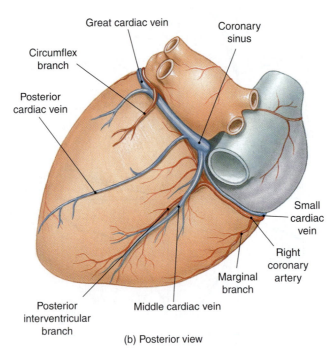

(b) Posterior view

Table 22–1	Common Auscultation by Name and Location		
Aortic Area	**Pulmonic Area**	**Tricuspid Area**	**Mitral or Apical Area**
Second intercostal space (ICS) to the right of the sternum	Second ICS to the left of the sternum	Fifth ICS to the left of the sternum	Fifth ICS on the midclavicular line

eject the remaining atrial blood into the ventricles, in the ventricular filling pressure rises. This rise in ventricular pressure causes the atrioventricular valves to snap shut, thus producing the S_1 (or first) heart sound.

During ventricular systole, the ventricles contract and cause the pressure in the ventricles to exceed the pressure in the aorta and pulmonary artery; the semilunar valves are forced open and blood is ejected into the corresponding blood vessel. Eventually at the end of systole, the pressure within the ventricles starts to fall as the ventricles eject blood. As the intraventricular pressure drops below the pressure in the aorta and pulmonary artery, the aortic and pulmonic valves snap shut, eliciting the S_2 (or second) heart sound, as shown in Figure 22-3 ■.

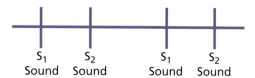

■ **Figure 22-3** Normal heart sounds displayed graphically (S_1 and S_2).

With this explained, we will now consider how closure of certain valves manifests as certain heart sounds. The first thing to mention are split heart sounds. When S_2 occurs, it is essentially the closure of the louder aortic valve first followed by the pulmonic valve closing a split second later. This is referred to as physiological splitting and normally occurs on inspiration when there is an increased venous return and negative intrathoracic pressure, which delays the emptying of the right ventricle and thus delays the closure of the pulmonic valve. It basically sounds like "lub/dubdub." The two sounds should normally be fused on expiration. This is referred to as a normal or physiologic split. If at any time the split does not present itself in this manner, further investigation is called for. When assessing, the S_2 sound can best be auscultated with the diaphragm at the second intercostal spaces on the right for the aortic closure and on the left for the pulmonic closure.

The S_1 sound may also split into a louder mitral sound, which precedes a softer tricuspid sound. As should make sense, sounds originating from the left side of the heart tend to be louder since the pressure tends to be higher on the left. S_1 sound is best heard at the apex of the heart. Since mitral closure is louder and may mask tricuspid closure, you may not be able to hear the S_1 split as easily as the S_2 split.

In addition, other sounds may be auscultated in correlation to specific events in the cardiac cycle. Although not considered normal, the opening of the aortic valve may be accompanied by a high-pitched "ejection sound" best heard over the aortic auscultatory point. This sound, when heard, follows S_1 and may suggest aortic valve stenosis, systemic hypertension, or dilated aorta. Another valvular sound, the "opening snap," may be auscultated at the apex as a high-pitched sound. This is the opening snap of the mitral valve. Not normally audible, this sound may clue you into the existence of mitral stenosis. It usually closely follows S_2.

As the ventricles fill following opening of the AV valves, a third heart sound may be auscultated, called S_3. This sound is due to the rapid filling of noncompliant or diseased ventricles and is also occasionally referred to as a ventricular gallop. Since the ventricle cannot distend to accept the rapid inflow of blood, turbulent blood flow results in the vibration of the AV valvular structures or the ventricles. It follows S_2 in the cardiac cycle and may be confused with an S_2 split. However, remember that an S_2 split should normally split on inspiration, whereas an S_3 will not. It is a lower-pitched sound than the S_2 and can best be heard with the bell with the patient turned slightly to the left side. S_3 sound is considered by most sources to be normal in children and young adults, but suggests ventricular dysfunction or left ventricular hypertrophy in adults older than 35 years of age (Figure 22-4 ■).

The S_3 sound is due to the rapid filling of noncompliant or diseased ventricles and is also occasionally referred to as a ventricular gallop.

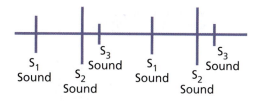

■ **Figure 22-4** Graphic display of the S_3 or third heart sound—an abnormal finding.

The S$_4$ sound or atrial gallop is a low-frequency sound that is audible late in the diastolic phase, just before S$_1$. S$_4$ occurs as a result of vigorous atrial contraction as it tries to eject blood into a noncompliant ventricle that is resistant to filling. It occurs in patients with systemic hypertension, aortic stenosis, acute myocardial infarction, or cardiomyopathy. The sound could be created as well by the right side of the heart if the patient has pulmonary hypertension or pulmonary stenosis (Figure 22-5 ■).

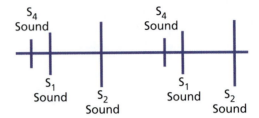

■ **Figure 22-5** Graphical display of the S$_4$ or atrial gallop.

The occurrence of both S$_3$ and S$_4$ is a summation gallop and is described as sounding similar to a horse's gallop. This occurs due to a shortening ventricular diastolic phase from tachycardic rates and the S$_3$ and S$_4$ sounds become fused together (Figure 22-6 ■).

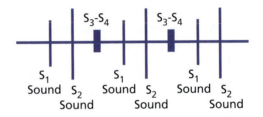

■ **Figure 22-6** Graphical display of both S$_3$ and S$_4$ or summation gallop.

To summarize the auscultatory findings mentioned thus far, refer to Table 22–2.

Table 22–2	Auscultatory Findings				
				Ejection Sound (ES)	**Opening Snap (OS)**
S₁ Sound	**S₂ Sound**	**S₃ Sound**	**S₄ Sound**		
Mitral and tricuspid valve closure	Aortic and pulmonic valve closure	Abnormal ventricular filling due to noncompliant ventricle	Atrial contraction into diseased ventricle	Ventricular ejection through aortic valve stenosis or dilated aorta	Opening of mitral valve during ventricular diastole
S₁ sound is heard when?	*S₂ sound is heard when?*	*S₃ sound is heard when?*	*S₄ sound is heard when?*	*Ejection sound is heard when?*	*Opening snap is heard when?*
First "normal" heart tone	Second "normal" heart tone	Early diastole, following S₂	Late diastole, just prior to S₁	Late after S₁, just prior to S₂	Closely follows S₂ sound
Where is S₁ best heard?	*Where is S₂ best heard?*	*Where is S₃ best heard?*	*Where is S₄ best heard?*	*Where is ES best heard?*	*Where is OS best heard?*
Apex auscultatory point	Aortic auscultatory point	Lower left sternal border with patient turned to left	Lower left sternal border, increases with inspiration	Aortic auscultatory point	Apex auscultatory point

HEART MURMURS

With an initial discussion of heart sounds complete, the second concern with cardiac auscultation is the appreciation of murmurs. The sound that creates the murmurs is either from a stenosed valve or an abnormally functioning valve that allows for regurgitation. If the critical care paramedic keeps in mind that a stenosed valve is open (but the opening is narrowed) and a regurgitating valve is closed (but allowing blood to regurgitate), he will make determining the source of the murmur easier. They are distinguished from basic heart sounds by their longer duration and are classified by their timing within the cardiac cycle, their location of maximum intensity, their patterns of radiation, their pitch or tonal quality, their configuration, and their intensity.

Perhaps the most diagnostic classification of murmurs lies in their timing, that is, where they fall with the cardiac cycle. For example, one must determine whether the murmur is systolic or diastolic. This is important because "innocent" murmurs may occur in systole, whereas diastolic murmurs are never innocent.

Systolic Murmur

A systolic murmur occurs between S_1 (AV valve closure) and S_2 (semilunar valve closure). As such, the systolic murmur occurs during ventricular systole and results from abnormalities from blood passing through the stenotic or narrowed semilunar valves. Because the AV valves are already closed prior to the ejection of the blood through the aortic and pulmonic valves, there is a delay between S_1 and the beginning of the murmur. Additionally, the murmur created is described as crescendo–decrescendo (or diamond shaped). This means that the sound rises to a peak and then falls in intensity (Figure 22-7 ■).

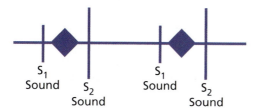

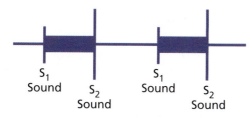

Systolic regurgitation murmurs result from faulty AV valves. The sound is created as blood regurgitates from higher pressure in the ventricles to lower pressure in the atria. The sound is usually more harsh, with a blowing quality, and is described as holosystolic, which means that the sound begins immediately after S_1 and continues until S_2 (Figure 22-8 ■).

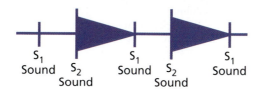

Diastolic Murmur

Diastolic murmurs occur during ventricular diastole. This means that they fall after S_2, but precede the next S_1. (During this phase the atrioventricular valves are opening and blood is filling the ventricles.) If either the aortic or the pulmonic valve is faulty and allowing regurgitation, there will be a blowing sound that begins immediately after S_2 and decreases in intensity due to the drop in the blood pressure of the aortic and pulmonary arteries. Formally, these diastolic murmurs are described as early diastolic decrescendo murmur (Figure 22-9 ■).

If the critical care paramedic keeps in mind that a stenosed valve is open (but the opening is narrowed) and a regurgitating valve is closed (but allowing blood to regurgitate), he will make determining the source of the murmur easier.

Perhaps the most diagnostic classification of murmurs lies in their timing, that is, where they fall with the cardiac cycle.

■ Figure 22-7 Graphical display of systolic murmur.

■ Figure 22-8 Graphical display of systolic regurgitation murmur.

Diastolic murmurs occur during ventricular diastole. This means that they fall after S_2, but precede the next S_1. (During this phase the atrioventricular valves are opening and blood is filling the ventricles.)

■ Figure 22-9 Graphical display of diastolic murmur.

There can also be a narrowing and stenosis to the mitral and tricuspid valve as well. This will also produce a sound that is heard during the diastolic phase. The difference with this is the timing and characteristics of the sound heard. An AV valve murmur from stenosis will be a low-frequency sound that occurs a short time after the S_1 sound (due to the AV valves not opening until mid-diastole). Furthermore, the characteristics will be decrescendo–crescendo. The initial phase is decrescendo as the ventricles fill passively, but then as the atria contract, the intensity increases and the sound becomes crescendo again (Figure 22-10 ■).

 Figure 22-10 Graphical display of AV valve murmur from stenosis.

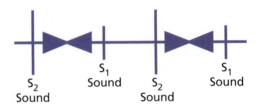

S_2 Sound S_1 Sound S_2 Sound S_1 Sound

Table 22–3 summarizes systolic and diastolic murmurs.

The classification of murmurs by intensity is probably the most subjective category of classification. Intensity is, to a degree, related to the volume of blood flow. In the United States, the Levin scale of Grades I through VI is used. Unfortunately, what one person may hear as a Grade II may be a Grade III to a more experienced care provider. Regarding the descriptions, however, a Grade I murmur is considered very faint, barely audible in a quiet room with a stethoscope. A Grade II is also quiet, but definitely audible. Subsequently then with each grade, the sound becomes louder and louder with the highest category being a Grade VI. Grade VI can be heard audibly with the stethoscope off the chest.

⚷ ───────────

Like any other skill the critical care paramedic will learn about, auscultation and interpretation of cardiac sounds will take patience and practice.

Like any other skill the critical care paramedic will learn about, auscultation and interpretation of cardiac sounds will take patience and practice. Once the skill becomes better entrenched into the critical care paramedic's repertoire of assessment tools, a more complete assessment and appreciation of the patient's status can be done. In conclusion, aside from history, auscultation is one of the most diagnostic tools when assessing cardiac status. A good history and physical exam should alert you to the development of new cardiac symptomatology or the worsening of a previous cardiac disorder.

Table 22–3	Summary of Systolic and Diastolic Murmurs		
Systolic Semilunar Murmur	**Systolic Regurgitant Murmur**	**Diastolic Semilunar Murmur**	**Diastolic Atrioventricular Valve Murmur**
Forward blood flow through a stenotic aortic or pulmonic valve	Regurgitation of blood flow from ventricles to atria due to incompetent AV valve	Regurgitation of blood flow back into ventricles due to faulty semilunar valve	Forward blood flow through a stenotic bicuspid or tricuspid valve
When is this sound heard?	*When is this sound heard?*	*When is this sound heard?*	*When is this sound heard?*
Between S_1 and S_2, crescendo–decrescendo, midsystolic ejection	Between S_1 and S_2 throughout systole, holosystolic murmur	Between S_2 and next S_1, early diastolic decrescendo murmur	Between S_2 and next S_1, decrescendo–crescendo murmur
Where is this sound best heard?	*Where is this sound best heard?*	*Where is this sound best heard?*	*Where is this sound best heard?*
Aortic valve stenosis is heard in aortic area. Pulmonic valve stenosis can be heard over pulmonic area.	Bicuspid valve insufficiency heard in apical area. Tricuspid valve insufficiency can be heard over left sternal border.	Aortic valve insufficiency heard over aortic area. Pulmonic valve insufficiency can be heard in pulmonic area.	Bicuspid valve stenosis heard best at apex with patient turned to left side. Tricuspid valve stenosis can be heard at 5th ICS, left sternal border.

ACUTE CORONARY SYNDROME

Acute coronary syndrome (ACS) includes a spectrum of coronary artery disease (CAD) processes from myocardial ischemia and myocardial injury to myocardial infarction. The progressive narrowing of the lumen of the coronary arteries causes this spectrum of diseases and the severity of clinical symptoms is dependent on the location and extent of narrowing. Acute coronary syndrome includes the clinical entities of stable angina, unstable angina, and acute myocardial infarction.

Stable angina is defined as transient, episodic chest discomfort resulting from myocardial ischemia. The discomfort is typically predictable and reproducible with the frequency of attacks constant over time. The discomfort is frequently provoked by physical exertion or intense emotional stress. These episodes usually resolve with the use of palliative maneuvers, such as rest or medications, to open the coronary arteries and relieve the symptoms.

Unstable angina is defined as angina that meets any one of the following three presentations:

1. Angina at rest that lasts longer than 20 minutes

2. New onset angina

3. Crescendo (increasing) angina or preinfarction angina

Acute myocardial infarction is defined as irreversible injury (necrosis) of the myocardium. Diagnosis typically relies on the combined presentation of three specific findings. These findings include a clinical history suggestive of CAD, evidence of ischemic changes on the electrocardiogram, and elevated myocardial enzymes in the blood. (See Figure 22-11 ■.)

PATHOPHYSIOLOGY

Coronary artery disease involves progressive narrowing of the lumen of the coronary arteries (atherosclerosis) caused by the development of thick, hard plaques (atheromas). As the narrowing of the coronary arteries progresses, it leads to the clinical spectrum of myocardial ischemia, injury, and infarction. This spectrum of coronary occlusive disease is known as acute coronary syndrome.

Myocardial **ischemia** is caused by an imbalance of oxygen supply and demand: either a decreased oxygen supply or increased oxygen demand. The net result of this process is injury to myocardial cells followed by cellular death (infarction) if the process is not reversed. Impairment of oxygen delivery is the primary contributor to decreased oxygen supply. Impaired oxygen delivery is caused by occlusion of the coronary arteries either by spasm, stenosis, thrombus, or a combination of these. Other factors that might contribute to the decreased oxygen supply to the coronary arteries

acute coronary syndrome (ACS) *a spectrum of coronary artery disease (CAD) processes including myocardial ischemia, myocardial injury, and myocardial infarction.*

Acute coronary syndrome includes the clinical entities of stable angina, unstable angina, and acute myocardial infarction.

ischemia *injury to an area of myocardial cells that may be followed by cellular death (infarction) if perfusion of oxygenated blood is not restored.*

■ **Figure 22-11** Acute coronary syndrome.

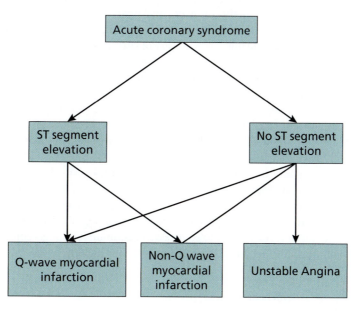

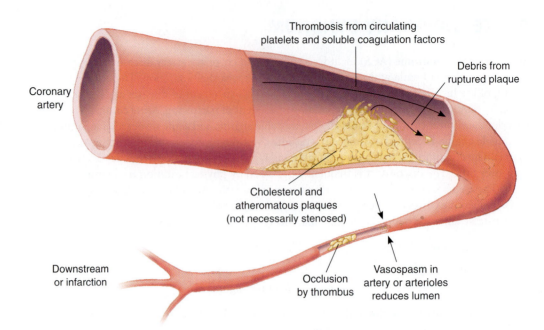

■ **Figure 22-12** Acute coronary syndrome pathophysiology.

Thrombosis from circulating platelets and soluble coagulation factors

Debris from ruptured plaque

Coronary artery

Cholesterol and atheromatous plaques (not necessarily stenosed)

Downstream or infarction

Occlusion by thrombus

Vasospasm in artery or arterioles reduces lumen

Impairment of oxygen delivery is the primary contributor to decreased oxygen supply. Impaired oxygen delivery is caused by occlusion of the coronary arteries either by spasm, stenosis, thrombus, or a combination of these.

are any factors that produce low blood pressure, such as volume loss, drug effects, and infection. Physical exertion and emotional stress are factors that increase myocardial oxygen demand.

Thrombus formation is considered an integral factor in coronary artery disease. The process is usually initiated by endothelial damage, usually from disruption of an atherosclerotic plaque, which leads to platelet aggregation and thrombus formation. The resulting thrombus can occlude the vessel lumen, leading to myocardial ischemia, injury, and infarction. The consequences of coronary artery occlusion depend on the preexisting atherosclerotic plaque, the extent of occlusion by the thrombus formation, and the rate of development of the occlusion. Occlusions that occur more slowly give the body time to develop collateral circulation in an attempt to compensate for the decrease in blood flow to the area involved. (See Figure 22-12 ■.)

CLINICAL MANIFESTATIONS

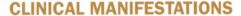

The history is the foundation of the assessment of patients with suspected ACS.

The history is the foundation of the assessment of patients with suspected ACS. The classic features of myocardial ischemia are chest discomfort or pressure with radiation to the left arm or jaw, dyspnea, and diaphoresis. Presence of these symptoms significantly increases the likelihood of the diagnosis of unstable angina or myocardial infarction. The presence of risk factors for coronary artery disease also increases the likelihood of the symptoms being related to acute coronary syndrome. Such risk factors include a past history of coronary or vascular disease, a family history of coronary or vascular disease, smoking, hypertension, hypercholesterolemia, and diabetes mellitus. Artificial or early menopause and the use of contraceptives also increase the likelihood of ischemic heart disease in women.

Patients with classic angina will have a history of substernal chest pain or discomfort. The pain is usually described as a pressure or heaviness on the center of the chest and usually occurs with activity and is relieved by rest. It may radiate to the left arm or jaw. The pain is frequently associated with dyspnea, nausea and vomiting, and diaphoresis.

Symptoms from an ACS may present as just described; however, there is one population of patients who may have slightly different presentation patterns—women. Current literature from the past several years reveals that female heart attacks have a tendency to present slightly differently than do those of their male counterparts. Although all of the aforementioned symptoms may be present in men or women to some extent, additional findings commonly reported in the literature about female heart attack clinical presentations include:

★ Indigestion or gas-like pain

★ Dizziness or nausea

Symptoms from an ACS may present as just described; however, there is one population of patients who may have slightly different presentation patterns—women.

- ★ Unexplained weakness or fatigue
- ★ Discomfort or pain between the shoulder blades
- ★ Recurring chest discomfort
- ★ Sense of impending doom
- ★ Atypical presentations

Patients may present with atypical presentations, with chest pain being absent from their complaints. Atypical presentations include dyspnea alone, syncope, fatigue or generalized weakness, nausea and vomiting, sharp or pleuritic chest pain, or confusion and stroke-like symptoms. In fact, only about 50% of all acute coronary events present with the stereotypical presentation of chest pain as described earlier. Of the remaining 50%, roughly 25% do not have any chest pain, and the other 25% have many of the findings described as "atypical."

The findings on physical exam are generally nonspecific and frequently the exam is normal, unless significant cardiac dysfunction is present. When significant cardiac dysfunction is present, the following physical findings may be present: altered mental status, hypotension, diaphoresis, rales, elevated jugular venous distention, and S_3 and S_4 heart sounds. Otherwise, the dysfunction may reveal a pale or dusky-appearing individual with cool, clammy skin and labored breathing.

DIAGNOSTICS

The electrocardiogram (ECG) can be used to support the diagnosis of ischemia, injury, and infarction. It may also be used to screen patients with atypical presentations for unsuspected myocardial infarction. The ECG is often nondiagnostic (>50%). However, despite the frequency of nondiagnostic findings, when it is positive it is one of the main diagnostic tools for cardiac ischemia or infarction and frequently is used as the main criterion for initiating fibrinolytic therapy and other pharmacologic interventions as well as activating the cardiac cath lab. The ECG can also be used to screen for nonischemic, but potentially life-threatening causes of chest pain such as pulmonary embolism or pericarditis.

ST segment and/or J-point elevation greater than 1 mm off of baseline may be a manifestation of myocardial injury. But remember that ST and J-point elevation can also occur in the absence of ischemia from numerous causes such as bundle branch blocks, left ventricular hypertrophy, ventricular pacemakers, pericarditis, or early repolarization. Q waves indicate the presence of a myocardial infarction (MI) but they do not indicate the age or acuteness of the infarct. The ECG finding most indicative of acute myocardial infarction (AMI) is ST segment elevation of >0.1 mV (>1 mm) in at least two consecutive leads corresponding to the involved coronary artery. Reciprocal ST segment depression may be evident in the reciprocal leads, but the absence of reciprocal changes does not rule out the presence of an evolving MI. The location of MI and the associated changes on ECG are summarized in Table 22–4.

Acute myocardial infarction is now classified based on ECG findings:

- ★ Non–ST elevation myocardial infarction (Non-STEMI)
- ★ ST elevation myocardial infarction (STEMI)

Table 22–4	Localization of Infarction by ECG Changes	
Location of Infarct	**Leads**	**ST Segment**
Inferior wall of left ventricle	II, III, AVF	Elevation
Septal wall	V1, V2	Elevation
Anterior wall of left ventricle	V3, V4	Elevation
Lateral wall of left ventricle	I, AVL, V5, and V6	Elevation
Posterior wall	V1–V3	Depression
Right ventricle	V4R	Elevation

Elevated serum cardiac enzymes, measured over several days of hospitalization, have been the standard for diagnosing acute myocardial infarction.

Elevated serum cardiac enzymes, measured over several days of hospitalization, have been the standard for diagnosing acute myocardial infarction. The creatine kinase (CK) MB marker is used by most clinical laboratories to detect AMI. In the past, it was sufficient to measure serial cardiac enzymes over a period of 48 to 72 hours. However, with the advent of therapeutics such as fibrinolytic therapy and percutaneous transluminal coronary angioplasty (PTCA), and the ability of those interventions to quickly reverse the obstructions that lead to cardiac ischemia and infarction, there is now significant pressure to diagnose AMI as early as possible. Therefore, an immunochemical test for CK-MB has been developed that allows for quick automated tests. The diagnosis of a patient with a nondiagnostic ECG is now possible within several hours after symptom onset. Serial CK-MB testing has a sensitivity and specificity greater than 90% within 3 hours, using immunochemical assays. The sensitivity approaches 100% within 10–12 hours after symptom onset. If the value of CK-MB is elevated and the ratio of CK-MB to total CK (relative index) is more than 2.5 to 3, it is likely that the heart was damaged. A high CK with a relative index below this value suggests that skeletal muscles were damaged.

Another serum marker that is frequently used is troponin. Troponin is a family of proteins found in skeletal and heart muscle fibers where it helps muscles contract. There are two forms (troponin I and troponin T) found in the heart and in other muscles. The tests for these forms of troponin measure only the type found in heart muscle. When a person experiences a myocardial infarction, troponin T is released into the blood. Troponin levels remain high longer than some other substances (such as CK-MB) that are measured if an ACS is suspected. Troponin T appears in the serum within 3–4 hours after symptom onset and remains elevated for up to 14 days. Diagnostic accuracy, which is correctly identifying AMI patients with positive levels and non-AMI patients with negative levels, is 98% for troponin T and 97% for CK-MB.

GENERAL MANAGEMENT

Current interventions, including fibrinolytic therapy, PTCA, and bypass surgery, are all aimed at reperfusing the ischemic myocardium in time to preserve left ventricular function and thereby decreasing morbidity and mortality.

Current interventions, including fibrinolytic therapy, PTCA, and bypass surgery, are all aimed at reperfusing the ischemic myocardium in time to preserve left ventricular function and thereby decreasing morbidity and mortality.

The approach to the treatment of ACS includes the following:

1. *Increase myocardial oxygen supply.* This is accomplished by administering supplemental oxygen via nasal cannula or mask. Improving coronary blood flow further increases myocardial oxygen supply. Nitrates and calcium channel blockers improve coronary blood flow via direct smooth muscle relaxation. Fibrinolytic therapy improves coronary blood flow by dissolving intracoronary thrombi. PTCA and bypass surgery are invasive procedures used to increase myocardial oxygen supply when medical treatment is unsuccessful.

2. *Decrease myocardial oxygen demand.* Nitrates, beta-blockers, and calcium channel blockers decrease myocardial oxygen demand. Nitrates accomplish this by reducing preload and afterload. Beta-blockers inhibit beta-adrenergic receptors, thus decreasing heart rate and contractility. Calcium channel blockers decrease myocardial contractility. They also vasodilate peripheral arteries, thus reducing afterload and thereby decreasing myocardial oxygen demand.

3. *Correct disturbances to the heart rate and rhythm.* During the management of an AMI, cardiac rate and rhythm disturbances may present and must be corrected immediately. Generally speaking, if the patient is experiencing a severe MI complicated by dysrhythmias, the critical care paramedic should first normalize the heart rate, then administer medications to correct rhythm disorders.

4. *Prevent reocclusion of coronary arteries.* Aspirin, the standard antiplatelet medication, inhibits platelet formation during the thrombotic response to the rupture of coronary artery plaque, thereby preventing reocclusion of the coronary arteries.

5. *Reduce pain and relieve stress.* Both of these interventions will contribute to the lessening workload placed on the heart by heightened sympathetic tone from the stress response. The goal for pain reduction is "0." That means the goal is to continue to relieve pain until the patient states their pain is a "0" on a scale of "1 to 10." This is

achieved with the use of oxygen, nitroglycerin, nitrous oxide, morphine sulfate, and so on. The relief of stress should be done by constant verbal reassurance by health care providers, keeping the patient in a comfortable position, and completing similar tasks that will ease the mind of the patient.

Several classes of pharmacologic agents and interventions are used in the treatment of acute coronary syndromes. They include analgesics, antiplatelets and anticoagulants, nitrates, beta-blockers, calcium channel blockers, antidysrhythmics, cardiac pacing interventions, and fibrinolytics. The analgesics treat pain. The antiplatelet/anticoagulants prevent further thrombus formation or platelet aggregation. The nitrates, beta-blockers, and calcium channel blockers alter the supply-demand equation by either improving oxygen supply to the heart muscle or by decreasing oxygen demand. The antidysrhythmics correct underlying rate or rhythm disturbances. And finally, the **fibrinolytics** are used to lyse coronary thrombi, thus improving oxygen supply to the myocardium.

RIGHT VENTRICULAR MYOCARDIAL INFARCTIONS

Prior to a full discussion on the pharmacology for AMI management, one important point needs to be considered by the critical care paramedic who is deciding to initiate care for a suspected MI patient. The issue concerns the presence of a right ventricular infarction (RVI).

The right ventricle is perfused by the right coronary artery, so if it becomes occluded during an ACS, the patient may experience an MI. Because the coronary artery is occluded, the patient will initially display an inferior wall MI on the 12-lead ECG (leads II, III, AVF) assuming the electrodes are placed in their traditional locations. Should this be the case, the critical care paramedic should take the precordial leads and place them in a mirror location on the right thoracic wall. This will give a picture of the right ventricular wall. Although V3 through V6 are most commonly used to assess for right ventricular involvement it has been shown that moving V4 to its mirror location on the right thorax (V4R) will provide 90% specific and sensitive data regarding the presence of right ventricular ischemia or infarction.

Should ST segment and/or J-point elevation be identified with the right precordial lead(s), the critical care paramedic should conclude that the right coronary artery occlusion that spawned the inferior wall MI seen initially is a proximal occlusion and is also resulting in a right ventricular infarction. The reason this is clinically important is because the preload to the right side of the heart is dependent on central venous pressure (CVP). If the patient is administered nitrates and opioids for the chest pain, this will reduce CVP and right heart preload. The right ventricular cardiac output will diminish and deliver less pulmonary perfusion to the lungs and less preload to the left side of the heart. Since the left side of the heart can only pump what it receives, if preload drops then so will left ventricular cardiac output. This in turn lowers systolic perfusion pressure and there will be reflexive tachycardia. The tachycardia will only worsen the situation as it results in a shortened diastolic phase, which means coronary artery perfusion will decrease (recall that the coronary arteries are perfused during ventricular diastole). The end result can be an enlargement of the ischemic zone with further myocardial wall depression and failing cardiac output.

For the patient with an inferior wall MI *and* evidence of a right ventricular involvement as seen on the right precordial leads, the critical care paramedic may wish to consider the early administration of fluids. The administration of an IV bolus will help to elevate CVP prior to it being diminished by the nitrates and opioids. Essentially the critical care paramedic will be "filling up the tank" prior to making the "tank" larger with the use of vasodilators. With this special treatment consideration, the drop in left ventricular afterload (a desired result of the medication) will be offset by a relative maintenance of CVP. Prior to the initiation of a fluid bolus for the MI patient, however, the critical care paramedic may wish to consult medical direction to confirm this treatment path or to discuss an alternative.

ANALGESICS

One of the goals in the treatment of ACS or AMI is to reduce the myocardial oxygen demand. Analgesics, such as morphine sulfate, do this in several ways. First, reduction of pain results in a diminished sympathetic discharge in response to pain with resultant reduced heart rate and force of contraction, and thus reduced oxygen demand. Morphine also reduces preload and afterload, which

fibrinolytics
chemicals/drugs used to lyse coronary thrombi, thus improving oxygen supply to the myocardium. Also known as thrombolytics.

Although V3 through V6 are most commonly used to assess for right ventricular infarction, it has been shown that moving V4 to its mirror location on the right thorax (V4R) will provide 90% specific and sensitive data regarding the presence of right ventricular involvement.

For the patient with an inferior wall MI *and* evidence of a right ventricular MI as seen on the right precordial leads, the critical care paramedic may wish to consider the early administration of fluids.

then requires decreased cardiac contractility and heart rate and therefore decreased oxygen demand. Morphine is usually given 2–4 mg at 5- to 15-minute intervals. The major side effects include hypotension, decreased respirations, and decreased mentation.

ANTIPLATELETS/ANTICOAGULANTS

Aspirin is the standard antiplatelet drug used in ACS. It is also the most cost-effective treatment for ACS. Clinical studies have shown a clear benefit from the use of aspirin alone: a 23% reduction in mortality. Aspirin, when used in combination with fibrinolytic therapy attains a 42% reduction in mortality. Aspirin works by inhibiting platelet formation during the thrombotic response to ruptured coronary artery plaque. Standard doses range from 160 to 324 mg given orally. Contraindications include life-threatening hemorrhage or a history of significant allergy to aspirin.

Heparin accelerates the action of antithrombin III and activated Factors IX, X, and XI. This indirectly inhibits clot propagation. Heparin has a significant synergistic effect with aspirin in reducing AMI and death. The initial dose is 80 U/kg by IV bolus followed by a maintenance infusion of 18 U/kg/hr. The maintenance dose is then adjusted based on maintaining the partial thromboplastin time (PTT) of 1.5 to 2.5 times control. Contraindications to heparin include life-threatening hemorrhage or a history of significant allergy to heparin.

NITRATES

Nitrates are widely accepted as the first-line treatment for angina and AMI. They work by direct smooth muscle relaxation of the coronary arteries, improving coronary blood flow and thus increasing myocardial oxygen supply. They also decrease myocardial oxygen demand by reducing preload and afterload. Long-acting nitrates can be used to prevent angina. Short-acting nitrates are used sublingually or intravenously to treat angina. Patients with ACS and a blood pressure greater than 90 mmHg should receive sublingual (SL) nitroglycerin (0.4 mg) on presentation and then every 5 minutes until pain is relieved. If the pain is not relieved after 3 SL tablets, then the patient should be started on IV nitroglycerin. The nitroglycerin infusion is started at 5 mcg/min and is increase by 5 mcg/min every 3–5 minutes. The infusion is titrated to relieve pain. If the pain is not relieved by 20 mcg/min then the infusion is increased by 10 mcg/min every 3–5 minutes until pain is relieved or up to 200 mcg/min. Care must be taken when administering nitrates to patients with a right ventricular infarct because nitrates may cause a sudden, precipitous fall in blood pressure. If that occurs discontinue the nitroglycerin and resuscitate with IV fluids.

HEART RATE AND RHYTHM CONTROL

The need to correct fatal dysrhythmias cannot be overstated (whether or not they exist in the presence of an MI). To do this, the critical care paramedic should first normalize the heart rate. If the patient is symptomatic from a tachydysrhythmic rate, consideration of vagal maneuvers, adenosine, calcium channel blockers, beta-blockers, and amiodarone can be entertained (according to NATIONAL standards). If the patient is symptomatic from a bradydysrhythmia, consider the use of transcutaneous cardiac pacing for stabilization of the heart rate. Beyond the use of transcutaneous pacing common to prehospital use, the critical care paramedic may encounter the CCU/ICU patient who has a temporary cardiac pacemaker system already placed, utilizing one of the following designs:

★ Epicardial wires that are attached to the heart and exit the thorax through a subxiphoid incision. These are often used as a temporary adjunct during (and after) open heart surgery.

★ Temporary transvenous pacing in which a catheter is introduced via a large vein and the pacing catheter is threaded through a sheath and into the right ventricle where it is placed in contact with the endocardial surface of the right ventricular apex.

★ Pulmonary artery balloon flotation catheters that have both atrial and ventricular pacing ports for dual-chamber pacing.

Table 22–5	NBG* Pacemaker Code			
I—Chamber(s) Paced	**II—Chamber(s) Sensed**	**III—Response to Setting**	**IV—Rate Modulation**	**V—Multisite Pacing**
O = None	O = None	O = None	O = None	O = None
A = Atrium	A = Atrium	T = Triggered	R = Rate modulation	A = Atrium
V = Ventricle	V = Ventricle			V = Ventricle
D = Dual (A + V)	D = Dual (A + V)	D = Dual (A + I)		D = Dual (A + V)
S = Single (A or V)	S = Single (A or V)			

*NBG = North American Society of Pacing and Electrophysiology (N), British Pacing and Electrophysiology Group (B) and generic (G) code.

The pulse generator for a temporary transvenous or epicardial pacing system is an external device, often called a *temporary pacemaker,* that is operated by a 9-V alkaline or lithium battery. The generator contains several controls that regulate the current output, heart rate, sensitivity, and mode of pacing (synchronous or asynchronous). The dual-chamber pulse generators also have separate terminals for the atrial and ventricular inputs. Due to the complexity and diversity of cardiac pacemakers, a universal coding system has been designed for uniformity. Understanding this five-letter pacemaker code will assist the critical care paramedic in determining the type of pacing used, the intended mode of operation, and the actual mode of operation. Table 22–5 illustrates this generic pacemaker code.

Following (or in tandem with) emergency cardiac pacing for bradycardiac rate control, the critical care paramedic can also consider the use of parasympatholytics (i.e., atropine sulfate) for noninfranodal bradydysrhythmias. Sympathomimetic infusions of dopamine, epinephrine, or iso-proterenol can also be considered in refractory bradycardias according to current American Heart Association/Emergency Cardiac Care (AHA/ECC) guidelines.

After rate control is achieved, the critical care paramedic should then turn attention to any rhythm and/or blood pressure disturbances. Rhythm disturbances should be treated according to current AHA/ECC standards, in concert with medical direction guidelines. If after rate and rhythm control are achieved, the blood pressure is still not at a desired level, specific management for this can be initiated. (Refer to Chapter 11 for a full discussion of antidysrhythmic and blood pressure control pharmacology.) One word of caution: The critical care paramedic needs to remain aware that with every drug given, there is increasing opportunity for prodysrhythmic side effects to occur.

BETA-BLOCKERS

Beta-blockers inhibit beta-adrenergic receptors, decreasing heart rate and contractility and thereby reducing myocardial oxygen demand. The use of beta-blockers for unstable angina reduces the risk of subsequent AMI by 13%. IV metoprolol can be given in 5-mg increments by slow IV infusion with repeated doses at 5-minute intervals up to 15 mg.

CALCIUM CHANNEL BLOCKERS

Calcium channel blockers inhibit the movement of Ca^{2+} ions across myocardial and vascular smooth muscle. This leads to decreased myocardial contractility and thus decreased myocardial oxygen demand. Calcium channel blockers also improve coronary blood flow via direct smooth muscle relaxation. However, they also can cause peripheral vasodilation, which may lead to hypotension. IV diltiazem is probably the best choice for AMI. Diltiazem is generally administered as follows: an initial bolus of 0.25 mg/kg IV (typically 20 mg) over 2 minutes followed by a maintenance infusion of 10 mg/hr. Calcium cannel blockers should be used with caution if used in combination with beta-blockers.

FIBRINOLYTICS

Acute coronary thrombosis is primary to the pathogenesis of acute MI. Fibrinolytics are used to lyse coronary thrombi, thus improving oxygen supply to the myocardium. The common pathway for all fibrinolytics is via activation of plasminogen. Plasminogen is converted to plasmin, which has potent fibrinolytic activity.

Once fissuring of an atherosclerotic plaque has occurred, whether the coronary vessel becomes totally occluded, develops a severe flow-limiting stenosis, or heals without incident depends largely on the degree to which thrombus propagates in the vessel lumen. The balance between activation and inhibition of platelet aggregation as well as of the coagulation cascade are critical in this process.

The therapeutic goal is to lyse clots and prevent further propagation of clot to improve coronary patency while minimizing the risk of intracerebral hemorrhage (ICH). This is accomplished by combination therapy using a fibrinolytic drug (streptokinase, alteplase, reteplase, anistreplase), an antiplatelet drug (aspirin, tirofiban), and an anticoagulant (heparin). Several studies suggest that accelerated dosing regimens of alteplase and reteplase with intravenous heparin are currently the most effective therapies for achieving early coronary reperfusion, but both are substantially more expensive and carry a slightly greater risk of ICH than streptokinase. The cost-to-benefit ratio must be weighed in deciding which thrombolytic to use. Factors include the time interval elapsed since onset of symptoms, the size and location of the infarct, and the patient's risk for ICH.

The emergency physician or cardiologist makes the decision on which drug or combination of drugs to use based on the aforementioned criteria and taking into consideration the patient's history and clinical presentation. The critical care paramedic must be familiar with all of the available fibrinolytic agents, methods of dosing, and the care of patients receiving fibrinolytic therapy if he is to properly care for those patients receiving fibrinolytics during transport. Clearly being able to anticipate and recognize early complications such as intracerebral hemorrhage is necessary. A patient receiving fibrinolytic therapy is also at high risk for other bleeding complications. Therefore, to minimize potential complications, all invasive procedures and venipunctures should be avoided, if at all possible. If bleeding does occur from venipuncture sites, compression dressings should be applied to decrease the amount of oozing. All sites should be monitored closely. If pacing is required, external pacing is recommended.

MECHANICAL REPERFUSION

percutaneous transluminal coronary angioplasty (PTCA) *mechanical method used to restore perfusion in coronary arteries blocked or constricted by atherosclerotic disease.*

Although the critical care paramedic will not be directly involved in these mechanical reperfusion techniques, he will certainly be involved in the transport of patients who must be taken to regional tertiary care facilities to receive one of these procedures.

An alternative to fibrinolytic therapy to attain coronary reperfusion is **percutaneous transluminal coronary angioplasty (PTCA).** It is a mechanical method used for obtaining reperfusion of the coronary arteries. PTCA is the most commonly used type of mechanical reperfusion technique. Percutaneous coronary interventions (PCIs) make up a group of mechanical reperfusion techniques that include PTCA as well as other new techniques capable of relieving coronary narrowing. Components of PCI include rotational atherectomy, directional atherectomy, extraction atherectomy, laser angioplasty, and implantation of intracoronary stents and other catheter devices for treating coronary atherosclerosis.

Although the critical care paramedic will not be directly involved in these mechanical reperfusion techniques, he will certainly be involved in the transport of patients who must be taken to regional tertiary care facilities to receive one of these procedures. Patients with the following criteria may be candidates for mechanical reperfusion rather than fibrinolytics:

1. Contraindication to fibrinolytic therapy
2. Persistent hemodynamic instability
3. Post-infarct or post-reperfusion ischemia

The benefits of PTCA include improvement in coronary perfusion with improvement in global and regional left ventricular function. Complications of PTCA include coronary artery dissection, reocclusion, coronary spasm, dysrhythmias, hemorrhage, and impairment of circulation in the extremity in which the catheter is placed. Some of these complications may require emergent surgical intervention to correct.

SURGICAL REPERFUSION

Coronary artery bypass graft (CABG), a surgical reperfusion technique, is performed to improve the myocardial blood supply for patients with significant coronary artery occlusion, and more recently has been used as an intervention for AMI. It is also used to treat complications of PTCA such as coronary artery dissection. The indications for emergency CABG include unstable angina unresponsive to medical therapy and evolving AMI when fibrinolytic therapy and/or PTCA are unsuccessful.

AORTIC ANEURYSM

An **aortic aneurysm** is a localized dilatation of the aorta caused by weakening of its wall. It involves all three layers of the aorta (intima, media, and adventitia). Aneurysms can develop in any portion of the aorta, but most involve the aorta below the renal arteries. Although there is no universally accepted definition of an abdominal aortic aneurysm, an infrarenal aortic diameter of 3 cm or greater can be defined as an abdominal aortic aneurysm (AAA).

Aortic aneurysms are commonly confused with aortic dissections. In aortic dissections, blood enters the tunica media of the aorta and splits (dissects) the aortic wall. Unlike aneurysms they seldom originate in the abdominal aorta. They commonly originate in the thoracic aorta but they may extend throughout the entire aorta. There is a distinct difference in the etiology, signs and symptoms, and progression of the two disease processes that must be recognized by the critical care paramedic. (See Table 22–6.)

PATHOPHYSIOLOGY

As mentioned, an abdominal aortic aneurysm is a weakening of all three layers of the aortic wall. The weakening of the aortic wall is believed to be due to the loss of collagen and connective tissue components of the aorta.

coronary artery bypass graft (CABG) *surgical reperfusion technique used to improve the myocardial blood supply for patients with significant coronary artery occlusion, complications of PTCA (such as coronary artery dissection), or AMI.*

aortic aneurysm *a localized dilatation of the aorta caused by weakening of the aortic wall; can involve all three layers of the aorta (intima, media, and adventitia).*

Aneurysms can develop in any portion of the aorta, but most involve the aorta below the renal arteries.

Table 22–6	Comparison of Aortic Aneurysm versus Aortic Dissection	
	Aortic Aneurysm	**Aortic Dissection**
Etiology	Primarily arteriosclerotic	Arterial hypertension
Pathophysiology	Weakening of arterial wall All three layers involved	Initiated by an intimal tear Dissection into media Develops false lumen
Location	Abdominal (90%)	Thoracic aorta
Prevalence	Men > women 6:1	Men > 60 yrs old Marfan's disease Syphylis
Signs	Enlarged aorta on exam or X-ray Hypotension if ruptured	Hypertension Loss of pulse in neck, arms AR (diastolic) murmur Focal neurologic deficits
Symptoms	Clincally silent initially Abdominal fullness Abdominal pulsations Back pain, throbbing or colicky	Sharp "tearing"-type chest pain
Management	Asymptomatic: referral for surgical evaluation Symptomatic, intact: besides US or CT Symptomatic, ruptured: Rapid transport Notify surgery at receiving hospital Multiple large-bore IVs, fluid resuscitation Type and cross-match 10 units blood Immediate surgical intervention	Nitroprusside, propranolol Maintain systolic presure between 100 and 120 Surgical correction of intimal tear

The etiology of an AAA is highly associated with age and coronary artery disease, specifically atherosclerosis. Risk factors include increasing age, gender (men > women), peripheral vascular disease, extremity arterial aneurysms, and history of a first degree relative with AAA. In these populations, AAA can be expected in up to 30% to 40% of patients as compared to the general incidence of 2% to 4% in the elderly population over age 50. Abdominal aortic aneurysms become clinically significant when they reach a certain size or rate of expansion. Any AAA with the following criteria should be considered for surgical intervention:

★ Greater than 5 cm in diameter
★ Greater than 1 cm growth in 12 months
★ Symptomatic pain or hypotension

Individuals meeting these criteria are at increased risk for rupture, with incidence approaching 60% for those aneurysms reaching up to 10 cm. (See Figure 22-13 ■.)

CLINICAL MANIFESTATION

Most abdominal aortic aneurysms are clinically silent until they rupture. However, clinical manifestations may include abdominal pulsations, back pain, throbbing or colicky pain, oliguria, or a sensation of abdominal "fullness." It is important to note that pain often indicates rupture and is a late symptom of the progressing AAA. Physical exam may reveal an expanding aorta, abdominal bruits, and decreased femoral pulses. The clinical finding of hypotension is the hallmark of a ruptured AAA.

DIAGNOSTICS

Signs of AAA are seen on plain radiographs in two-thirds to three-fourths of cases. Either ultrasound or abdominal CT best determines the diagnosis of an abdominal aortic aneurysm. Since AAAs are commonly misdiagnosed, all providers should have a high index of suspicion with any patient presenting with abdominal pain.

MANAGEMENT

The management of an intact, asymptomatic aneurysm involves referral for further evaluation and surgical repair. The surgeon will evaluate the patient and, depending on the size of the aneurysm,

■ Figure 22-13 Abdominal aortic aneurysm.

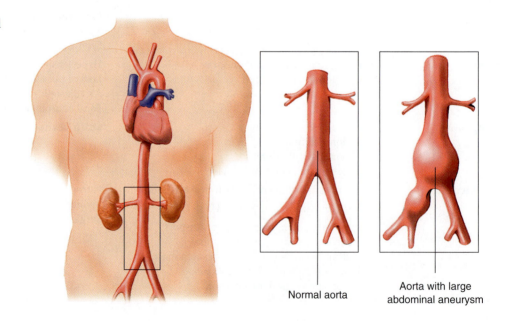

Normal aorta

Aorta with large abdominal aneurysm

patient age, underlying health, and other factors, will either follow the patient with serial scans or consider early elective surgery.

The management of a symptomatic aortic aneurysm is dependent on the patient's hemodynamic stability. In patients with acute abdominal or back pain without hypotension, time can be taken to confirm the presence of an AAA either by bedside ultrasound or CT scan.

If a patient with a known history of AAA presents with hypotension and therefore a ruptured AAA is highly suspected, the patient should be taken to the operating room as early as possible. A ruptured aneurysm is a true emergency. Once the aneurysm ruptures, the prognosis is grim. Few patients survive ruptured aneurysms unless they are in the emergency department or the operating suite at the time.

Sudden onset hypotension with or without new onset of pain is suggestive of rupture and should be treated aggressively. The patient should be transported to the nearest appropriate emergency department in a facility that has immediate surgical capabilities. Multiple large-bore IVs with packed red cells and blood pumps should be started. Crystalloid infusion is the most immediate supportive measure; however, avoid overaggressive fluid resuscitation to limit blood loss. Infusion of blood products may be necessary and therefore the patient should be immediately type and cross-matched for 10 units of blood. The definitive treatment of a ruptured abdominal aortic aneurysm is aimed at immediate surgical intervention.

AORTIC DISSECTION

Aortic dissection involves dissection of the layers of the aorta initiated by an intimal tear. Blood, under the force of arterial pressure, goes through the intimal tear and enters the media of the aorta and splits (dissects) the aortic wall. Dissection of the layers results in a false lumen.

Aortic dissections are commonly confused with aortic aneurysms, and the management of a true aneurysm with the pharmacology used for a dissection can be disastrous to the patient. Aortic dissections are also sometimes referred to as a "dissecting aortic aneurysm," but this is also inappropriate (an aneurysm does not have a "false passage," nor does a dissection result from a weakening and ballooning out of a vascular wall). Pathophysiologically, the dissection results in altered blood flow through the aorta (typically the ascending aorta and aortic arch), and the aneurysm results in the hemorrhaging of blood into the abdominal cavity due to a breech in all three vascular layers of the aorta.

The patient's medical history can also be contributory in alerting the clinician about the possibility of an aortic dissection. Unlike the aortic aneurysm, an aortic dissection is not usually caused by atherosclerosis, but by arterial hypertension. Other risk factors for aortic dissection include **Marfan's disease** (a genetic connective tissue disorder that causes a weakening of vascular tissue, among other problems), inflammatory disorders of the aorta (syphilis), smoking, and pregnancy.

Aortic dissections most commonly originate in the thoracic aorta but they may extend throughout the entire aorta, whereas aortic aneurysms most commonly involve the abdominal region of the aorta. There is a distinct difference in the etiology, signs and symptoms, and progression of the two disease processes that must be recognized by the critical care paramedic.

PATHOPHYSIOLOGY

An aortic dissection begins as a tear in the tunica intima, usually in the ascending thoracic portion of the aorta. Over time the systolic pressure associated with systemic arterial hypertension allows for a dissection between the intima and media layers of the aortic wall. Collagenous deterioration can accelerate the process, as is hypothesized in syndromes such as Marfan's. Inflammatory processes of the aorta also can initiate the intimal tear. As a result of this pathology, the dissection may extend both distally and proximally. If the dissection extends proximally, it may involve the aortic valve rendering it incompetent. As the dissection progresses forward, it may result in disruption of the arteries that originate off the arch and proximal descending aorta.

For purposes of categorization and identification, there are three types of aortic dissections. With DeBakey Type I, the intimal tear is in the ascending aorta and extends to involve the ascending

aortic dissection *a potentially lethal dissection of the intimal layers of the aorta. Blood, under the force of arterial pressure, goes through an intimal tear and enters the media of the aorta and splits (dissects) the aortic wall.*

Aortic dissections are commonly confused with aortic aneurysms, and the management of a true aneurysm with the pharmacology used for a dissection can be disastrous to the patient.

Marfan's disease *a genetic connective tissue disorder that causes a weakening of vascular tissue, among other problems.*

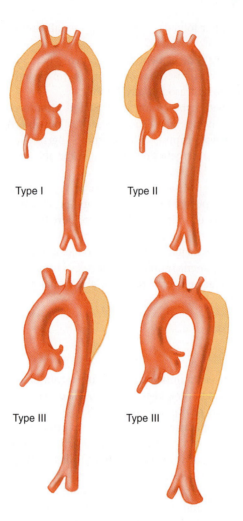

■ **Figure 22-14** DeBakey classification system of thoracic aortic aneurysm.

Type I   Type II

Type III   Type III

aorta, the aortic arch, and the descending aorta. With DeBakey Type II, the intimal tear is in the ascending aorta and is confined to the ascending aorta. With DeBakey Type III, the intimal tear is in the descending aorta and is confined to the descending aorta, distal to the left subclavian artery (Figure 22-14 ■).

CLINICAL MANIFESTATIONS

Clinical presentation can vary with the type of dissection that occurs, but management in the acute phase is almost always similar. Dissection of the aorta typically presents with a severe, sharp "tearing"-type chest pain radiating to the upper back or scapula. Depending on the structures involved, neck or arm pain may also be present. Hypertension is another associated finding seen in 60% to 70% of patients. Given the location of the dissection for both DeBakey Type I and Type II classes, they both may exhibit varied pulse pressures between the left and right sides of the body (if the dissection progresses though the aortic arch and involves the arterial originations of the vessels located there). As well, decreased carotid pulses may also be present on one or both sides of the neck. Further or prolonged dissection may result in altered mental status or neurologic compromise from the vascular disruption. Additional signs or symptoms include any of the following:

– Loss of speech	– Dyspnea
– Paraplegia	– Pleural effusion
– Myocardial infarction	– Abdominal pain (mesenteric infarction)
– Extremity paresthesias	– Diastolic murmur
– Hematuria	– Decreased bowel sounds

DIAGNOSTICS

ECG changes consistent with AMI are seen in 10% to 20% of patients with aortic dissection. Therefore, an ECG positive for AMI on a patient presenting with chest pain does not rule out aortic dissection. Further workup and clinical correlations need to be made in order to rule out the presence (or absence) of dissection. The ECG in this situation may show evidence of LVH and left axis deviation that reflects longstanding hypertension. Routine laboratory tests are of little value for this patient and should not precede more appropriate therapy designed to limit the progression of the dissection. Aortography, contrast-enhanced computed tomography, magnetic resonance imagery, and echocardiography have been shown useful in establishing a definitive diagnosis. For those who are misdiagnosed, the prognosis is extremely poor. Roughly 90% of untreated dissections will rupture within 3 months.

MANAGEMENT

All patients suspected of having an aortic dissection should have ongoing monitoring of the cardiac rhythm, blood pressure, and urine output. Therapy is geared at decreasing the forces that favor progression of the dissection. This is accomplished by maintaining systolic blood pressure between 100 and 120 mmHg and by reduction of cardiac contractility. For patients who present with hypertension, prompt reduction of the blood pressure can be accomplished in a controlled manner with sodium nitroprusside by mixing 50 mg in 250 mL of D_5W and infusing it at a rate of 0.5 to 3.0 mcg/kg/min. The rate is adjusted to maintain the blood pressure between 100 and 120 mmHg. A beta-adrenergic blocker should be used in conjunction with nitroprusside to decrease cardiac contractility and heart rate. Propranolol may be administered with a starting dose of 1 mg IV every 5 minutes with a target reduction of heart rate to 60 to 80 beats/min. Esmolol, a short-acting beta-blocker administered by continuous infusion at 50 to 200 mcg/kg/min, may be preferable. Caution should be used though to not accidentally drop the heart rate too low with beta-blocking therapy, nor should a beta-blocker be used if the patient's heart rate is already too slow. Definitive therapy for an aortic dissection is oftentimes operative. Unlike AAA, nearly all aortic dissections must undergo surgical intervention.

All patients suspected of having an aortic dissection should have ongoing monitoring of the cardiac rhythm, blood pressure, and urine output. Therapy is geared at decreasing the forces that favor progression of the dissection.

POSTOPERATIVE TRANSPORT

In some instances, critical care transport may be utilized to transport postoperative patients recovering from aortic dissection. Care should be taken to maintain antihypertensive and anticoagulation medications as ordered by the physician. In addition, utilization of a "cough pillow" helps the patient minimize the increased thoracic pressure associated with coughing. This in turn decreases the likelihood of damaging the repaired structures. The critical care paramedic provider should be on the lookout for any signs or symptoms suggestive of a leaking or ruptured repair.

CARDIOGENIC SHOCK

Cardiogenic shock is the clinical entity of circulatory failure seen when the heart has suffered its most extreme form of pump failure. The severe left ventricular dysfunction manifested by a weak ventricular contraction leads to diminished ejection fraction (this refers to the percentage of blood that is pumped out of a filled ventricle with each heartbeat), decreased cardiac output, and inadequate perfusion of vital organs.

Cardiogenic shock can be caused by dysfunction of ventricular filling (preload), myocardial contractility (stroke volume), or ventricular emptying (excessive afterload). The most common cause of cardiogenic shock is myocardial infarction, usually involving greater than 40% of the left ventricle, leading to significant dysfunction of left ventricular myocardial contractility. Other causes of dysfunction of myocardial contractility include diffuse myocardial ischemia, cardiomyopathy, myocarditis, and myocardial contusion. Tension pneumothorax, pericardial tamponade, and valvular dysfunctions such as mitral stenosis and tricuspid stenosis also diminish ventricular

cardiogenic shock *the clinical state of circulatory failure occurs when the heart suffers its most extreme form of pump failure, manifested by severe left ventricular dysfunction.*

Cardiogenic shock can be caused by dysfunction of ventricular filling (preload), myocardial contractility (stroke volume), or ventricular emptying (excessive afterload).

filling and can lead to cardiogenic shock. Pulmonary embolism, ventricular septal defect, and valvular dysfunctions such as aortic stenosis, pulmonic stenosis, and mitral insufficiency produce ventricular emptying deficits that may lead to cardiogenic shock.

PATHOPHYSIOLOGY

All causes of cardiogenic shock lead to decreased cardiac output and hypoperfusion of vital organs. Initially, as the baroreceptors in the aortic arch and carotid bodies sense a fall in cardiac output and blood pressure, the cardiovascular system attempts to compensate by increasing heart rate and peripheral vascular resistance. These compensatory mechanisms manifest in tachycardia, pallor, cool skin and diaphoresis, and a narrowing pulse pressure. As cardiac output and blood pressure fall due to the body's inability to compensate, the hypoperfusion of the brain manifests in restlessness, anxiety, altered mental status (confusion), and eventually unconsciousness.

CLINICAL MANIFESTATIONS

The history may help the critical care practitioner narrow the cause of cardiogenic shock. For instance, if a patient who presents with clinical findings consistent with cardiogenic shock has a history of coronary artery disease and currently has severe chest pain, ECG findings consistent with AMI, and elevated cardiac enzymes, then myocardial infarction with dysfunction of myocardial contractility would most likely be the cause. However, if a patient who presents with clinical findings consistent with cardiogenic shock presents with severe chest pain, but has a history of recent trauma to the chest and now presents with a clinical picture consistent with a tension pneumothorax, then dysfunction of ventricular filling caused by tension pneumothorax is likely the cause of the cardiogenic shock.

Patients in cardiogenic shock appear acutely ill. They manifest varying levels of altered mental status, from restlessness and anxiety to varying levels of confusion and ultimately unconsciousness. On physical examination they are frequently very diaphoretic and their skin is pale and cool. Their vital signs exhibit tachycardia and hypotension. They also exhibit oliguria secondary to tissue hypoperfusion of the kidneys.

In cases of acute myocardial infarction or other clinical entities that lead to dysfunction of myocardial contractility, the damaged heart muscle prevents the heart from pumping efficiently. There is a decrease in stroke volume that leads to a backup of blood into the pulmonary circulation. Due to this backpressure into the pulmonary circulation, patients may manifest with signs of congestive heart failure including pulmonary edema (rales), tachypnea, distended neck veins, and elevated pulmonary capillary wedge pressures as noted with hemodynamic monitoring. Similar clinical manifestations are found in cases caused by dysfunction of ventricular emptying caused by valvular dysfunction.

Patients with dysfunction of ventricular filling that leads to cardiogenic shock, similar to those patients with dysfunction of myocardial contractility, manifest with the general findings of shock including altered mental status; pale, cool, diaphoretic skin; tachycardia; hypotension; and oliguria. However, they do not manifest with signs of left ventricular failure and pulmonary edema.

The management of patients in cardiogenic shock includes treating the underlying cause (AMI), monitoring the hemodynamic status (invasively and noninvasively), and providing pharmacologic treatment and alternative devices such as an intra-aortic balloon pump or left ventricular assist device to enhance cardiac output, stabilize blood pressure, and improve tissue perfusion.

DIAGNOSTICS

Laboratory findings include hypoxemia and acidosis. There may be laboratory and ECG evidence of acute myocardial infarction. Right-sided leads should be obtained to rule out right ventricular infarct. Chest X-ray often reveals pulmonary congestion, and the urinary output is significantly reduced or absent. Blood gases and hemoglobin/hematocrit levels are often assessed to determine oxygen-carrying capacity. A Swan-Ganz catheter is frequently used to measure pulmonary capillary wedge pressures.

MANAGEMENT

The management of patients in cardiogenic shock includes treating the underlying cause (AMI), monitoring the hemodynamic status (invasively and noninvasively), and providing pharmacologic treatment and alternative devices such as an intra-aortic balloon pump or left ventricular assist device (both discussed later) to enhance cardiac output, stabilize blood pressure, and improve tissue perfusion.

The primary key to managing patients in cardiogenic shock is to closely monitor their hemodynamic status. Heart rate, blood pressure, pulse oximetry, and pulmonary artery pressures (if a Swan-Ganz line is present) should be frequently assessed.

The patient should be placed in the supine position to improve cerebral and coronary blood flow. Intravenous access must be obtained and the patient should be continuously monitored. Oxygen should be administered at 100% via a nonrebreather mask. Endotracheal intubation with positive end-expiratory pressure (PEEP) ventilation may be necessary to maintain adequate oxygenation.

Pharmacologic management is used to improve cardiac output. Inotropic agents such as dopamine, dobutamine, and Inocor increase cardiac output by increasing myocardial contractility. Vasodilators such as nitroprusside and nitroglycerin are used to decrease afterload in an attempt to improve output from the heart. Diuretics can be considered for fluid overload, but must be used with caution and appropriate central venous pressure monitoring to avoid worsening hypotension. If profound hypotension develops, vasoconstrictive agents such as norepinephrine (Levophed) may be necessary.

If the cardiogenic shock is due to a right ventricular infarct, the patient will need volume resuscitation. Avoid diuretics and nitroglycerin, which reduce preload and can worsen the hypotension. Dobutamine can be considered if fluids do not lead to improvement, or if an inotropic and vasopressor agent is needed that does not simultaneously vasoconstrict pulmonary vasculature. Dopamine should also be avoided in right ventricular infarct since it increases pulmonary vascular resistance and can worsen hypotension.

When standard management including pharmacologic therapies fails to improve the patient's condition, then specialized equipment such as the intra-aortic balloon pump and left ventricular assist device are frequently employed.

INTRA-AORTIC BALLOON PUMP

The **intra-aortic balloon pump (IABP)** is used to increase cardiac output. Balloon pump counterpulsation can augment cardiac output by as much as 10% to 20%. Raising the intra-aortic pressure during diastole and lowering the intra-aortic pressure during systole accomplish this augmentation in cardiac output. Insertion of the intra-aortic balloon involves percutaneously placing a balloon device into the femoral artery and advancing the balloon until it lies in the thoracic aorta 2 cm distal to the aortic arch. The balloon is inflated and deflated synchronously with the cardiac cycle. During diastole, the balloon is inflated, thereby displacing blood both proximally and distally to the balloon. Proximal displacement of blood enhances both coronary artery and cerebral perfusion; distal displacement of blood enhances systemic perfusion. The deflation of the cuff at the onset of ventricular systole causes a rapid drop in afterload pressure in the aorta, and the ejection fraction of the patient improves. (See Figure 22-15 ■.)

Managing patients who require IABP support during transport should include three primary goals:

1. Evaluation of patient response to counterpulsation in terms of hemodynamic status, control of dysrhythmias, systemic perfusion, and relief of symptoms of cardiac ischemia

2. Observation of early signs of complications from IABP therapy such as limb ischemia, bleeding, infection, thrombus formation, malpositioning of the balloon catheter, and arterial damage

3. Ensuring proper functioning of the IABP including correct timing, consistent triggering, appropriate troubleshooting of all alarm situations, and safe operation

LEFT VENTRICULAR ASSIST DEVICES

The left ventricular assist device (LVAD) allows an injured myocardium to rest by diverting blood from the natural ventricle to an artificial pump that maintains the circulation. LVADs are indicated

intra-aortic balloon pump (IABP) *a balloon inserted into the aortic arch controlled by an external pulsating pump; used to augment cardiac output when other therapies available for cardiogenic shock have failed or cannot be used.*

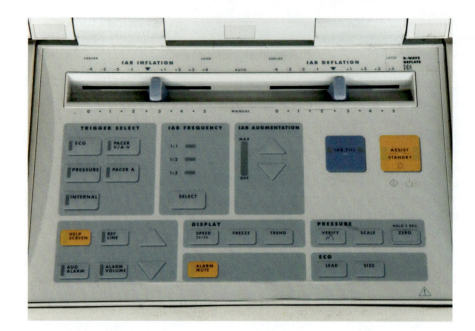

when profound cardiogenic shock develops despite maximal conventional therapy. There are typically three groups of patients that can benefit from the use of a ventricular assist device: (1) patients in cardiogenic shock secondary to acute myocardial infarction, (2) patients with postcardiotomy left ventricular failure who cannot be weaned from cardiopulmonary bypass, and (3) candidates for cardiac transplantation whose condition deteriorates before a donor can be found. (See Figure 22-16 ■.)

Transport of patients in cardiogenic shock requiring the use of either the IABP or LVAD requires organizing a smooth and safe transition from the critical care area to the receiving facility. This requires a team effort to ensure that the hemodynamic stability of the patient is not adversely affected. All equipment must be properly secured prior to transport. During transport, whether by

■ **Figure 22-16** Ventricular assist device.

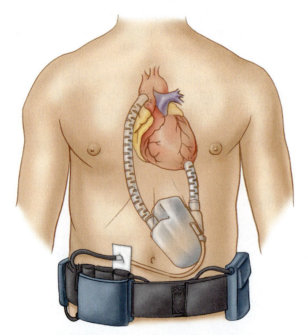

A ventricular assist device is a device that is used to help a heart that can no longer pump blood effectively due to heart failure. This illustration shows a left ventricular assist device (LVAD).

ground or air, the transport team must be able to adequately visualize the patient, monitors, and medication pumps. Adequate supplies of oxygen, medical air if needed to power devices, and electrical power must be readily available to complete the transport safely.

AIR MEDICAL TRANSPORT SPECIAL CONSIDERATIONS

The hypobaric environment experienced during transport of a patient by air can adversely affect the functioning of the intra-aortic balloon pump. As the patient descends in altitude, the barometric pressure increases, thus volume within the intra-aortic balloon will decrease, thereby resulting in incomplete inflation of the balloon and less than optimal augmentation of cardiac output. The opposite occurs during ascent. Therefore, the IABP may need to be reprimed during ascent, at cruising altitude, and during descent.

CARDIOMYOPATHY

The **cardiomyopathies** are a group of cardiac disorders in which the dominant feature is involvement of the heart muscle itself. Cardiomyopathies are characterized as primary or secondary. Primary cardiomyopathies are those in which no cause can be identified. Secondary cardiomyopathies are those in which there is a demonstrable underlying cause. The cardiomyopathies are also classified into three major categories: dilated cardiomyopathies, hypertrophic cardiomyopathies, and restrictive cardiomyopathies.

DILATED CARDIOMYOPATHY

Dilated cardiomyopathy is a disorder that involves a dilated failing heart. In most cases no cause can be identified (idiopathic). However, a number of toxic, metabolic, and infectious factors may be involved. These factors include myocarditis, coronary artery disease, HIV, alcohol, hypertension, pregnancy, hyperthyroidism, and connective tissue diseases. Cardiac enlargement is a prominent feature with all four chambers involved.

Pathophysiology

A decrease in stroke volume and decrease in ejection fraction lead to an increase in end systolic volume. This increased end systolic residual volume leads to dilated chambers as well as a predisposition to clot formation. It is the increased end-systolic volume, and subsequent increased end-systolic ventricular pressure, that leads to a backup of pressure into the pulmonary circulation. This backup of pressure leads to the progressive symptoms of CHF.

Clinical Manifestations

General symptoms include fatigue and weakness. The patient may also present with chest pain. The typical picture is progressive symptoms of CHF, including dyspnea on exertion, orthopnea, paroxysmal nocturnal dyspnea, and dyspnea at rest.

On physical examination the patient's skin may be pale, cool, or cyanotic. Signs of right-sided failure can be seen including elevated jugular venous distention, hepatomegaly, splenomegaly, ascites, and peripheral edema. Presence of S_3 and S_4 heart sounds may be heard as a summation gallop. Mitral or tricuspid regurgitation murmurs may also be heard.

Diagnostics

Chest X-ray reveals cardiomegaly and may reveal evidence of pulmonary edema or pleural effusions. The electrocardiogram is usually nonspecific but may show evidence of an intraventricular conduction delay or bundle branch block. The echocardiogram is most diagnostic with evidence of a dilated left ventricle and ejection fraction of less than 45%. A cardiac catheterization may be done if ischemia is suspected as the cause.

cardiomyopathies *a group of cardiac disorders in which the dominant feature is dysfunctional involvement of the heart muscle itself.*

The cardiomyopathies are classified into three major categories: dilated cardiomyopathies, hypertrophic cardiomyopathies, and restrictive cardiomyopathies.

Management

Treatment is generally supportive and symptomatic treatment of heart failure. The goal is reduction in both preload and afterload by vasodilators such as the nitrates. Diuretics are used to decrease blood volume. Anticoagulants are used to prevent clots from forming and thereby prevent pulmonary emboli. Although positive inotropic agents such as amrinone and dobutamine have been used, their results have been mixed.

HYPERTROPHIC CARDIOMYOPATHY

Hypertrophic cardiomyopathy (HCM) involves a nondilated, hypertrophic left ventricle and no cardiac or systemic disease process found that could produce the left ventricular hypertrophy. Although the cause is unknown, it is thought to have an autosomal dominant inheritance trait. The disease has previously been known as idiopathic hypertrophic subaortic stenosis (IHSS) or hypertrophic obstructive cardiomyopathy.

Pathophysiology

The abnormalities of hypertrophic cardiomyopathy involve an asymmetric thickening of predominantly the septum but also involving the ventricular free wall. There is thickening of the anterior and posterior leaflets of the mitral valve, and the asymmetric hypertrophy produces asymmetric pull on the papillary muscles leading to mitral regurgitation. There is decreased ventricular compliance, a decrease in left ventricular end-diastolic volume, and an increased pressure gradient across the outflow tract.

Clinical Manifestations

Typically hypertrophic cardiomyopathy involves young athletic males in their second or third decade. Most commonly patients are asymptomatic. They may present for an unrelated problem and demonstrate a systolic murmur on examination. The murmur is best appreciated at the left sternal border with radiation to the apex and into the axilla. This systolic flow murmur increases with standing and decreases with squatting.

Dominant clinical features include dyspnea, chest pain, fatigue, palpitations, syncope, angina, paroxysmal nocturnal dyspnea, and vertigo, all of which are worsened with exertion. Atrial fibrillation may be present.

Diagnostics

Chest X-ray reveals left ventricular hypertrophy. The electrocardiogram is usually nonspecific but may show evidence of a nonspecific intraventricular conduction delay or bundle branch block. The echocardiogram is most diagnostic with evidence of depressed left ventricle ejection fraction. A cardiac catheterization may be utilized to assess hemodynamic abnormalities.

Management

Treatment is essentially symptomatic relief. Propranolol, a beta-blocker, is the mainstay for treatment of hypertrophic cardiomyopathy. It has the ability to decrease dysrhythmias seen with HCM. It also reduces the pressure gradient across the outflow tract. It is a negative inotropic and negative chronotropic agent and lengthens diastolic filling time. Verapamil, a calcium channel blocker, may also be considered. Prophylactic antibiotics are given for procedures to prevent infective endocarditis.

RESTRICTIVE CARDIOMYOPATHY

Pathophysiology

Restrictive cardiomyopathy is a disorder that resembles constrictive pericarditis. Abnormal ventricular stiffness leads to abnormal diastolic function. There is a gradual but progressive limitation of ventricular filling due to endocardial and myocardial lesions. The ventricular walls are thick and noncompliant. The stiffness of the heart also reduces the ability to increase cardiac output.

CONGESTIVE HEART FAILURE

Congestive heart failure (CHF) is a pathophysiological state in which the heart is unable to pump enough blood to meet the metabolic needs of the body. This inability of the heart to pump adequately leads to a clinical picture of shortness of breath and fluid overload. The causes of congestive heart failure are many and include coronary artery disease, valvular disease, and myocardial disease. Other factors that may contribute to CHF include excessive salt or water intake, hypertension, thyrotoxicosis, pulmonary embolism, alcohol/drug abuse, and anemia.

congestive heart failure (CHF) *a pathophysiologic state in which the heart is unable to maintain sufficient cardiac output to meet the metabolic needs of the body, leading to increased dyspnea and pulmonary or systemic edema.*

PATHOPHYSIOLOGY

Heart failure is generally divided into left ventricular failure and right ventricular failure. Left ventricular failure occurs when the left ventricle is unable to pump adequately, and there can be multiple reasons why the heart pumps inadequately. Dysfunction of the heart muscle itself, as is seen with a myocardial infarction, is one of the main causes of left ventricular pump failure. Dysrhythmias also inhibit the heart's ability to pump normally. Obstruction of outflow from the heart, such as is seen in valvular disease or chronic hypertension, causes an undue burden on the heart muscle and leads to left ventricular failure. All of the above disorders lead to a backup of blood into the pulmonary circulation and then to pulmonary congestion/edema.

In right heart failure the right side of the heart fails to function as an adequate pump, which leads to back pressure of blood into the venous circulation. This most commonly is caused by left heart failure, which subsequently progresses to right heart failure. Similar to left ventricular failure, disorders that can cause the right side to fail include dysfunction of the heart muscle itself and things that diminish the outflow from the pump. Right ventricular MI is less common than left ventricular MI but is seen. Pulmonary hypertension and valvular disease can cause right heart failure.

Heart failure results in the reduction of cardiac output and may be due to a decrease in stroke volume or a decrease in heart rate. **Cardiac output** by definition, is the amount of blood pumped by the heart over 1 minute of time. The relationship of cardiac output (CO), stroke volume (SV), and heart rate (HR) is found in the following equation:

cardiac output *the amount of blood pumped by the heart in one minute.*

$$CO = SV \times HR$$

A reduction in cardiac output leads to compensatory mechanisms that act to restore cardiac output. For instance, when a patient sustains a myocardial infarction, the dead heart muscle prevents the heart from pumping normally, thus leading to a decreased cardiac output. The body senses the decrease in cardiac output and tries to compensate. Since it cannot increase stroke volume, due to the damaged pump, it must compensate by increasing the heart rate. If a patient has a dysrhythmia that affects only the heart rate (i.e., bradycardia), the decreased heart rate leads to a decreased cardiac output. In that case the body tries to compensate by increasing the stroke volume.

The body has several other mechanisms it can use to compensate for decreased cardiac output. These include vasoconstriction of peripheral vessels and activation of the renin-angiotensin-aldosterone system. Unfortunately, all of the compensatory mechanisms actually increase myocardial oxygen demand and thus are potentially detrimental to myocardial function.

CLINICAL MANIFESTATIONS

The patient history will usually point the practitioner in the direction of the diagnosis of congestive heart failure. The typical clinical history for CHF includes shortness of breath, orthopnea, paroxysmal nocturnal dyspnea, and peripheral edema. The shortness of breath is usually exertional at the onset and may progress to dyspnea at rest. The history may also point to the cause of the heart failure. For example, you would suspect an acute MI as the cause for heart failure if the patient had a history of recent chest pain. If the patient had a history of valvular disease that had been steadily worsening, then valvular disease may be considered to be the cause of heart failure.

On physical examination the following may be noted: pulmonary crackles, distended jugular veins, peripheral pitting edema, tachypnea, and oxygen desaturation on pulse oximetry. If central venous monitoring is available, the patient may also exhibit an elevated CVP. In left ventricular failure, the apical pulse is usually displaced laterally and downward. There may be a paradoxically split S_2 and an S_3 gallop present as well. A systolic murmur, if heard, is suggestive of mitral regurgitation. In right ventricular failure, S_3 is often heard as well as a holosystolic murmur of tricuspid regurgitation.

DIAGNOSTICS

The chest radiograph is essential in confirming the diagnosis of CHF and in assessing the severity. Chest X-ray may reveal cardiomegaly and pulmonary congestion or frank pulmonary edema. The ECG may assist in determining the cause of CHF. A finding on ECG such as ischemia would suggest myocardial infarction as the cause. A finding of left ventricular hypertrophy might suggest hypertension as the cause.

Laboratory data are generally nonspecific, other than elevated cardiac enzymes, which may be helpful in confirming an AMI as the source of the CHF. Invasive monitoring reveals an elevated pulmonary capillary wedge pressure, elevated systemic vascular resistance, and low cardiac output.

MANAGEMENT

The general management of patients with congestive heart failure involves decreasing cardiac workload by reducing both preload and afterload. Traditional treatment for preload reduction is accomplished by use of morphine sulfate, nitrates, and lasix. Afterload reduction is accomplished with an angiotensin-converting enzyme inhibitor (ACE inhibitor). Alternatively, a beta-agonist such as dobutamine can be used to improve stroke volume and unload the heart, thus reducing pulmonary edema. In addition, controlling excessive retention of salt and water will improve congestive heart failure.

Some additional therapies, however, are being used with increasing frequency in hospital intensive care units that the critical care paramedic may encounter. These include the use of fluids to increase pressure during the period of isovolemic contraction in cases of diastolic dysfunction. This increases the ventricular ejection fraction and helps to decrease left atrial and PCWP pressures. Even the use of beta-blockers is gaining acceptance for patients who fit the criteria for Grade II to IV of the New York Heart Association (NYHA) functional classification of heart failure. Although these latter two treatments are not universal for the critical care paramedic, it is important for the critical care paramedic to be aware of these modalities, especially since it is counter to what most paramedics are initially taught.

Although the critical care paramedic will consult with his or her medical director prior to transport in most instances, the current mainstay treatment for acute CHF includes sitting the patient upright, administering high-flow, high-concentration oxygen, and administering morphine, nitrates, and lasix to reduce afterload. This will often provide prompt relief. Although oxygen frequently works to relieve hypoxemia, some patients require more aggressive noninvasive therapies. CPAP (continuous positive airway pressure) can be applied with a tight-fitting face mask and a ventilator that provides continuous positive airway pressures. BiPAP utilizes biphasic airway pressures. Both modalities improve oxygenation, decrease the work of breathing, and decrease left ventricular preload by increasing intrathoracic pressure. The goal of these respiratory therapies is to improve oxygenation noninvasively in an attempt to improve the patient's condition without using more invasive treatment such as endotracheal intubation.

HYPERTENSIVE EMERGENCIES

hypertensive emergency
severe, accelerated hypertension, with a diastolic blood pressure greater than 140 mmHg, leading to a constellation of systemic findings that can include end-organ damage or "shut down."

A **hypertensive emergency** is defined as severe, accelerated hypertension, with a diastolic blood pressure greater than 140 mmHg and a constellation of findings representing end-organ damage. This constellation of findings includes papilledema (edema of optic nerve), acute left ventricular failure (CHF), myocardial ischemia or infarction, acute renal failure, hypertensive encephalopathy, cerebrovascular accident, eclampsia, aortic dissection, postoperative bleeding, head trauma, extensive burns, and microangiopathic hemolytic anemia.

Since hypertensive emergencies result from a variety of etiologies they require a thorough assessment and efficient diagnosis in order to determine the appropriate type of therapy. A hand guide or drug chart for hypertensive emergencies provides a useful tool for the critical care paramedic provider in rapid selection and administration of the appropriate antihypertensive agents. The provider must be prepared for recurrent, acute episodes of hypertensive emergencies while transporting patients recently treated for medical conditions associated with hypertension.

PATHOPHYSIOLOGY

The most common category of hypertension is primary or essential hypertension. Essential hypertension is a hypertensive state in which no specific cause has been identified. Essential hypertension is chronic in nature and seldom do patients with essential hypertension progress to hypertensive emergencies.

Several theories exist with respect to the acute onset of hypertensive emergencies. One popular theory stems from the belief that chronic hypertensive disease eventually causes permanent changes in arterial wall smooth muscle, resulting in overreactive vasoconstriction. Other theories suggest that these emergencies stem from a loss of autoregulatory mechanisms in the central nervous system.

CLINICAL MANIFESTATIONS

Myocardial Infarction

Hypertension in the face of an acute MI is likely to manifest with signs of left ventricular heart failure. Symptoms progress nearly identical to that of any acute MI, but with a greater likelihood of pulmonary edema. Shortness of breath, dyspnea on exertion (DOE), and chest pain are common presenting symptoms. Physical signs include cyanosis, clubbing, crackles on auscultation of lung sounds, and production of pink, frothy sputum, and hemoptysis. Jugular venous pressures may be elevated, with an S_3 or S_4 gallop heard on auscultation of heart sounds.

Intracranial Hemorrhage and Hypertensive Encephalopathy

Patients may present initially with severe headaches, accompanied by nausea, vomiting, drowsiness, confusion, and decreased level of consciousness. Left unchecked, seizures, blindness, various neurologic deficits, coma, and death can result. Key presenting signs reside in the neurologic changes found on exam. Partial paralysis, and focal neurologic findings differentiate a hypertensive origin from that of an intracranial lesion.

Aortic Dissection

Aortic dissections associated with hypertension present with severe onset of "tearing" back or chest pain. Patients may have partial or full paralysis when dissections interrupt spinal blood supply. Syncope, cardiac tamponade, and shortness of breath may also be present. Additional physical signs can include varying blood pressures on the left side as compared to the right, unequal jugular vein distention, physical manifestations of cardiac tamponade, and loss of unilateral pulses. Myocardial infarction must be ruled out before proceeding to interventional therapy.

Pregnancy

Hypertensive emergencies during pregnancy are considered to be an impending sign of eclampsia, and require rapid intervention. The hypertensive disorders of pregnancy are among the most common complications of pregnancy, and present with slightly elevated blood pressure (130/70 in pregnant females), or a progressive rise in blood pressure. Increase of greater than 30 mmHg systolic or 15 mmHg diastolic is clinically significant for hypertension in gravid females. A blood pressure of 160/110 is considered representative of severe preeclampsia and impending seizures. Physical manifestations include swelling and edema of the face and distal extremities, visual changes, headache with nausea and vomiting, and epigastric pain. Laboratory assessment of urine samples should be done to assess for proteinuria. Seizures may be precipitated by prolonged incidence of hypertension. Note that the incidence of seizures is associated with increased mortality with evidence of cerebral hemorrhage as the cause.

Malignant Hypertension

Malignant hypertension results from end-organ damage secondary to both acute and chronic episodes of hypertension. Therefore, clinical signs and symptoms can vary with the organs involved. Changes in vision are significant indicators of changes within the retinal arteries. On funduscopic exam by a physician, exudates, cotton wool spots, or punctate hemorrhages may be present. Hematuria and oliguria are present with renal damage. Systemic signs and symptoms include headache with blurred vision, dyspnea, chest pain, and neurologic changes. It is extremely difficult to differentiate malignant hypertension from other etiologies by exam alone.

DIAGNOSIS

Myocardial Infarction

Hypertensive patients with characteristic findings on 12-lead ECG, elevated cardiac enzymes, and pulmonary congestion on chest X-ray are diagnostic for an AMI with pulmonary edema (CHF). Increased pulmonary wedge pressures and decreased cardiac output are indicative of left ventricular failure, while ECGs may reveal left ventricular hypertrophy from chronic hypertension.

Intracranial Hemorrhage and Hypertensive Encephalopathy

Hypertensive patients with altered mental status must be evaluated for hypertensive encephalopathy or intracranial hemorrhage. Serum chemistries should be obtained to rule out any metabolic causes of altered mental status. Head CT is often normal in encephalopathy but will be diagnostic for intracranial hemorrhage. Electroencephalogram yields little in encephalopathy, as does analysis of cerebrospinal fluid. Diagnosis is often made based on recent onset of an abnormal neurologic exam in the presence of acute hypertension.

Aortic Dissection

The critical care paramedic must have a high index of suspicion for aortic dissection in hypertensive patients with chest pain. Bedside ultrasonography may rapidly reveal a clinically significant aortic dissection. Additional tests that are useful include transesophageal ultrasound, CT or MRI, and aortography. These additional tests will make a more definitive case where the providers are uncertain of the diagnosis.

Pregnancy

The American College of Obstetricians and Gynecologists define the following hypertensive categories:

★ *Pregnancy-induced hypertension*—systolic BP > 140 or diastolic > 90 on more than one occasion

★ *Mild preeclampsia*—systolic BP > 140 or diastolic BP > 90 on more than one occasion and proteinuria

★ *Severe preeclampsia*—systolic BP > 160 or diastolic BP > 110 on two occasions more than 6 hours apart with patient resting, OR 24-hour urine output < 400 mL OR proteinuria greater than 5 g/24 hr, OR visual disturbances, pulmonary edema, or cyanosis

★ *Eclampsia*—seizures without underlying CNS lesion in a patient with preeclampsia

Malignant Hypertension

To make the diagnosis of malignant hypertension, patients must demonstrate evidence of end-organ damage in addition to elevated blood pressures. Elevated kidney function tests (BUN and creatinine), along with hematuria and proteinuria, suggest kidney damage. Left ventricular hypertrophy with strain pattern on ECG and cardiomegaly and pulmonary congestion on chest X-ray suggest end-organ damage to the heart. Red blood cell fragments and fibrin degradation products on the blood smear suggest microangiopathic hemolytic anemia.

MANAGEMENT

The overall goal of treatment is to judiciously lower the mean arterial blood pressure. The target reduction in blood pressure is modest, preferably resulting in a 20% to 25% decrease in mean arterial pressure or a resulting diastolic blood pressure between 100 and 110 mmHg. Care should be taken to hold the BP at a moderately high level for up to 12 to 24 hours and then to begin slower, more methodical blood pressure control in order to avoid hypotensive or vasoconstrictive side effects. The management of specific disease processes related to hypertensive emergencies is described next.

Myocardial Infarction

Initial stabilization and treatment of a new-onset MI should follow guidelines for acute coronary syndromes. Nitroglycerin infusions will assist in the lowering of blood pressure. Other medications may be appropriate in addition to nitroglycerin. In the presence of pulmonary edema, furosemide 40 to 80 mg IV bolus will assist in lowering the blood pressure via diuresis of fluid. Labetalol IV can provide additional decrease in blood pressure by decreasing heart rate and stroke volume. Nitroprusside is avoided in the AMI setting due to the decrease in preload resulting from venous dilatation.

Intracranial Hemorrhage and Hypertensive Encephalopathy

In this instance, nitroprusside is the preferred drug of choice to decrease hypertension resulting from an increase in intracranial pressure. An IV infusion of 0.5 to 3.0 mcg/kg/min is titrated to maintain a diastolic BP less than 110 mmHg. Labetalol IV and calcium channel blockers have also been shown to have some positive effect in treating ICP-related hypertension.

Aortic Dissection

It is imperative, when treating an aortic dissection, to reduce the BP much further than in other conditions. A systolic range of 100 to 120 should be the target in rapid medical management of aortic dissection. Ultimately, dissection is managed surgically, but in the interim, nitroprusside infusion of 0.5 to 3.0 mcg/kg/min can be initiated. Adjust the rate of infusion to maintain a systolic blood pressure between 100 and 120. The use of beta-blockers can also be considered for BP regulation in the aortic dissection patient. Propranolol can be administered at 1 mg IV every 5 minutes until a target heart rate of 60–80 bpm is obtained. Or, esmolol can be administered via infusion at 50 to 200 mcg/kg/min and titrate to maintain a target heart rate of 60–80 bpm.

Pregnancy

Rapid consultation with an obstetrician should be initiated while providing stabilization to the pregnant patient with an acute hypertensive emergency. Magnesium sulfate remains the mainstay of treatment in pregnancy-induced hypertension. Dilute 6 grams of magnesium sulfate in 50 mL of 0.9% normal saline (NS) and administer over 20 minutes. This initial bolus can be followed with a maintenance infusion of 2 g/hr. This dose may be increased up to a dose of 3 g but should be done in consultation with a physician. For rapid reduction of blood pressure in a hypertensive emergency, administer a 5-mg bolus of hydralazine. Repeat doses of 1 mg every 20 minutes may be utilized to achieve a diastolic below 100 mmHg. Labetalol is an effective alternative, while nitroprusside is usually withheld due to the potential for cyanide poisoning of the fetus.

Malignant Hypertension

Intravenous nitroprusside or labetalol must be instituted immediately to lower systemic blood pressure when a diagnosis of malignant hypertension is made. Nifedipine in particular must be avoided because of its tendency to cause a rapid crash in BP. Furosemide 40 mg IV bolus may also be added when organ damage results in water retention. ACE inhibitors are often utilized post-emergency for their salvage effect on the kidneys.

PERICARDITIS, PERICARDIAL EFFUSION, AND CARDIAC TAMPONADE

Pericardial diseases, including pericarditis, pericardial effusion, and cardiac (pericardial) tamponade, make up a large group of inflammatory, infectious, and infiltrative disorders of the pericardium. The causes of acute and chronic pericardial disease include trauma, viral infections, bacterial infections, fungal infections, parasitic infections, myocardial infarction, drugs, radiation, neoplasms, autoimmune disease, and other miscellaneous causes. The pericarditis can be seen with or without a pericardial effusion and may progress to one of the restrictive pericardial complications, pericardial tamponade, or restrictive pericarditis.

The pericardium is a smooth sac containing the heart. This sac is made up of visceral and parietal layers, with a small potential space between the pericardial wall and the heart. This space may contain from 15 to 60 mL of fluid in the normal adult. Though its true function is not well established, it is widely held that the pericardium serves to provide a lubricated container for the heart, and possibly to augment the normal pressures that exist between each of the heart chambers. The pericardial diseases discussed in this chapter include pericarditis, pericardial effusion, and cardiac tamponade.

PERICARDITIS

Pathophysiology

Pericarditis involves inflammation, infection, or infiltration of the pericardium. These processes maybe complicated by the accumulation of pericardial fluid (pericardial effusion), which subsequently may lead to pericardial tamponade.

Clinical Manifestations

Clinically, pericarditis presents with substernal chest pain. The pain is usually retrosternal or precordial. It is usually a sharp, pleuritic pain that may radiate to the shoulder. It is worsened by inspiration or cough. The pain can also be worsened by lying down in the recumbent position. It is improved by leaning forward.

While the initial presentation can mimic an acute myocardial infarction, there are several characteristic signs and symptoms that may assist the provider in distinguishing pericarditis from acute coronary syndrome. However, myocardial infarction should be ruled out prior to making the diagnosis of pericarditis.

The history is very valuable. The critical care paramedic should ask the following questions when considering pericarditis:

★ Does sitting up or leaning forward relieve the chest pain?
★ Does lying down worsen the chest pain?
★ Was there a prodrome of fever or muscle aches?
★ Is there any history of recent illnesses or infection?
★ Is there any history of malignancy or trauma of the chest?

Affirmative answers to these questions should encourage the provider to keep pericarditis in the differential diagnosis.

Physical exam reveals the characteristic pericardial friction rub, usually best auscultated at the left lower sternal border. The friction rub is intermittent and is increased when leaning forward. Heart sounds may be muffled. Arterial pressure may be decreased and venous pressure may be increased with distended jugular veins.

Diagnostics

Laboratory evaluation may reveal the cause of pericarditis but there are no diagnostic laboratory tests. An elevated white cell count may be indicative of an infectious origin. An elevated erythrocyte sedimentation rate (ESR) may be indicative of an inflammatory process as the cause. While true diagnosis depends on echocardiography of the pericardium, the ECG can assist the provider in early recognition of pericarditis. The typical findings of pericarditis on ECG are diffuse ST segment changes, specifically initial ST segment elevation in all leads except for reciprocal depression in AVR and VI. Most of these patients will have PR segment depression as well. As pericarditis progresses, the ST and PR segments normalize, providing almost a "lucid interval" of the ECG. The tracing then may develop deeply inverted T waves, and finally resolve without any obvious ST or PR segment or T wave changes.

Management

Treatment consists of nonsteroidal anti-inflammatory drugs (NSAIDs) and oral steroids. In some cases certain anti-uremic or antibiotic therapies may be indicated. The critical care transport provider will rarely be called on to initiate any such treatment, but care should be taken to ensure familiarity with the class and type of medications associated with the transport of a newly diagnosed pericarditis.

PERICARDIAL EFFUSION
Pathophysiology

An abnormal buildup of fluid in the pericardial sac is known as a pericardial effusion. The effusion is usually a complication of one of the many inflammatory, infectious, or infiltrative processes that cause pericarditis or as a response to traumatic injury of the pericardium. The major problem with this process is the exudates that collect in the pericardial sac and may provide mechanical pressure on the heart, which limits diastolic filling pressures.

Clinical Manifestation and Diagnostics

Pericardial effusion is often asymptomatic and is usually found in conjunction with the workup for other associated diseases. Pericardial effusion should be suspected when an enlarged silhouette is noted on chest X-ray, in the presence of an appropriate clinical history. Echocardiogram or CT scan may easily distinguish a forming effusion.

Management

Pericardiocentesis is an intervention in which fluid is removed from the pericardial space so that the heart can better accommodate preload and allow improved cardiac output. Pericardiocentesis is used as both a diagnostic and a treatment modality. In the event pericardiocentesis has been performed prior to transport, it is imperative that the provider be prepared for subsequent emergency pericardiocentesis if the patient's pericardial effusion increases significantly enough to produce hemodynamic instability. Further treatment on the part of the transport provider revolves around supportive therapy.

pericardiocentesis *an invasive technique using a needle and syringe to aspirate fluid from the pericardial space.*

CARDIAC TAMPONADE
Pathophysiology

Cardiac tamponade occurs when the accumulation of fluid in the pericardial sac (pericardial effusion) occurs to such an extent that cardiac output is significantly compromised. Cardiac tamponade should be considered by the critical care transport provider to be a true emergency. The causes of cardiac tamponade are varied, and can include both traumatic (penetrating and blunt trauma) etiologies, as well as medical etiologies (viral and bacterial infections, certain drug therapy, and so on).

Reduced ventricular filling, decreased cardiac output, and increased end-diastolic pressures characterize cardiac tamponade. The hemodynamic effects of cardiac tamponade are related to the speed of accumulation. A rapid accumulation of 150 to 200 mL of fluid in the pericardium may produce a cardiac tamponade. On the other hand, a slow accumulation of 1,000 mL of pericardial fluid may be tolerated. The presence of additional fluid above the usual 15 to 50 mL normally found in the pericardial sac causes the intrapericardial pressure to increase. Increased intrapericardial pressure results in decreased right ventricular filling and thus decreased cardiac output. As the pressure increases to a critical level, a precipitous drop in arterial pressure occurs.

Clinical Manifestations

The clinical presentation of tamponade can be insidious or may be immediate. Dr. Claude Beck first described the typical clinical presentation of cardiac tamponade in the early 1930s. **Beck's triad,** as it would come to be known, presents as hypotension (often with narrowing pulse pressures), jugular venous distention, and muffled heart tones. While this is pathognomonic for cardiac tamponade, other presentations do exist. Symptoms may include fever, fatigue, malaise, pleuritic chest pain, dyspnea, orthopnea, a sensation of fullness in the chest, and oliguria. In addition, the physical exam may reveal any of the following: increased jugular venous pulses, jugular venous distention, narrowing pulse pressures (rising diastolic in the face of sustained or decreasing systolic pressure), a friction rub, or pulsus paradoxus. The patient may present with signs of right heart failure or shock.

Pulsus paradoxus exists when systolic arterial pulse pressures drop during inspiration. On exam, direct palpation may reveal either a detectable decreased pulse or an absent arterial pulse when the patient inspires. To quantify this, the provider should utilize a BP cuff and assess the point at which the auscultated pulse disappears on inspiration. As the cuff is deflated, the *paradoxus* measurement is the difference between this point and the point at which pulsing is heard during both inspiration and expiration.

MANAGEMENT

Treatment of cardiac tamponade involves three components. The first is aggressive fluid resuscitation in the early phase of tamponade. This is supported by the theory behind Starling's law, which states that the energy liberated by the heart when it contracts is a function of the length of its muscle fibers at the end of diastole. This can be achieved with the use of a fluid bolus that enhances myocardial preload filling, which in turn causes a more vigorous contraction and enhanced cardiac output. Thus, as the patient begins to exhibit signs of decreased cardiac output, intravenous crystalloid fluids may prolong the perfusion of vital organs.

The second component involves removing some of the pericardial fluid to relieve the buildup of pressure. The critical care paramedic may be called on to perform this procedure known as pericardiocentesis (see procedure at end of chapter). Therefore, the critical care provider must be well trained and experienced at performing this procedure. In most emergent situations, a small amount of fluid (less than 20 mL) may be sufficient to relieve the immediate harmful effects of external pressure on the ventricular chambers. These patients must be monitored with routine 12-lead ECGs to rule out any inadvertent complications such as a lacerated coronary artery. Such complications may manifest as a new-onset myocardial infarction of the anterior, anteroseptal, or inferior myocardium.

The third component involves treating the cause of the fluid buildup. Antibiotic therapy will be used if the cause is bacterial. Anti-inflammatory drugs will be used if the cause is an inflammatory process such as post-infarction or post-radiation pericardial effusions. If the pericardial effusion that caused the tamponade is uremic, then dialysis should be considered.

VALVULAR DYSFUNCTION

Valvular dysfunction can be categorized by its two basic presentations: valvular **stenosis** (abnormal narrowing of the structure which inhibits normal blood flow) and valvular insufficiency. They result from a myriad of congenital and acquired causes and are further exacerbated by continuous

Beck's triad *the clinical presentation of cardiac tamponade, first described by Dr. Claude Beck in the early 1930s, it includes hypotension (often with narrowing pulse pressures), jugular venous distension, and muffled heart tones.*

pulsus paradoxus *a physical manifestation felt on palpation of arterial pulses; may reveal either a decreased or absent arterial pulse wave during inspiratory phase.*

stenosis *abnormal narrowing of a structure, inhibiting normal blood flow.*

immunologic or hemodynamic stressors. Each of the four valves of the heart may become involved in either category, though some are more serious than others. The following valvular heart diseases involving the aortic and mitral valves are among the more significant with respect to hemodynamic compromise. This is primarily due to the location of the aortic and mitral valves on the left side of the heart, thus significantly affecting cardiac output.

DISORDERS OF THE AORTIC VALVE

AORTIC STENOSIS

Pathophysiology

Aortic stenosis (AS) is the most common isolated valvular lesion. In individuals under 65 years of age, aortic stenosis is caused by a congenitally acquired bicuspid aortic valve. In patients over 65 years of age, aortic stenosis is caused by calcific degeneration of the aortic valve cusp. Other etiologies include rheumatic disease, infection, and idiopathic calcification. As the valve becomes stenotic, pressures in the left ventricle begin to increase due to increased outflow resistance. To compensate for the outflow obstruction, the left ventricle attempts to maintain stroke volume and cardiac output. As a result, aortic stenosis leads to left ventricular hypertrophy.

A critical level of obstruction of the outflow tract from AS is thought to occur when the valve orifice becomes less than 1.0 cm or the pressure gradient across the valve is greater than 50 mmHg. The aortic valve is able to maintain cardiac output until the valve reaches this critical level of stenosis. Because symptoms are only seen after the stenosis reaches this critical level, symptoms are usually seen late in the disease process.

Clinical Presentation

AS typically presents with the triad of angina, exertional syncope, and dyspnea on exertion. Angina is the result of the increased demand placed on the heart from the outflow obstruction. Dyspnea on exertion is usually secondary to the left ventricular failure. Syncope is usually the result of inadequate perfusion of the brain.

Physical exam will reveal a crescendo–decrescendo systolic murmur best auscultated at the second intercostal space, right sternal border with radiation to the carotid arteries. Another physical finding is pulsus parvus et tardus, which is a delay in the carotid pulse after auscultated systole, usually with a decreased amplitude of the pulse wave. Narrowing pulse pressures, a fixed A2-P2 split, and an ejection click are also specific findings suggestive of AS. A late sign is that of a left ventricular lift or heave. These occur when the left ventricle is enlarged enough to visibly determine the cardiac lift by observing the chest.

Diagnostics

Chest X-ray reveals evidence of left ventricular hypertrophy and pulmonary congestion. Aortic calcification may be seen. The ECG most commonly reveals a pattern consistent with left ventricular hypertrophy along with an idioventricular conduction delay and left axis deviation. Left atrial enlargement may be noted as well. A definitive diagnosis is made by echocardiography, which is able to define the valvular anatomy, aortic root size, left ventricular size and function, and aortic size.

Management

Left untreated, symptomatic AS has a 10-year mortality rate of 100%. Once symptomatic, surgery is the only definitive option. Asymptomatic patients or symptomatic patients considered to be poor surgical candidates may receive medical therapy consisting of digitalis, diuretics, nitrates, and inotropic agents. Gentle diuresis is used if patients have CHF. Mild hydration may be considered if they are hypotensive and not in failure. If the patient is hemodynamically unstable an intra-aortic balloon pump may be required until the patient is prepared for surgery. Any of these treatments may be encountered when transporting an individual with symptomatic AS.

AORTIC REGURGITATION

Pathophysiology

Aortic regurgitation (AR) arises from a variety of different causes. Marfan's disease, rheumatic fever, endocarditis, aortic dissection, and calcification are all possible causes of AR. Due to acute aortic regurgitation, left ventricular diastolic pressures rise rapidly resulting in left ventricular failure and pulmonary edema. AR typically results in left ventricular dilation, sometimes accompanied with hypertrophy, as a result of volume overload. Decreased cardiac output can occur with time, and chronic retention of fluid becomes a consideration.

Clinical Manifestations

The typical presentation of aortic regurgitation is that of fulminant congestive heart failure including fatigue, dyspnea, orthopnea, paroxysmal nocturnal dyspnea, and peripheral edema. They may present with angina as well.

Physical exam reveals crackles, cyanosis, and hypotension. A blowing, decrescendo diastolic murmur may be auscultated along the left sternal border on cardiac exam. Widened pulse pressures, and a rapidly rising and falling carotid pulse wave known as Corrigan's pulse (or water hammer pulse), may also be present.

Diagnostics

With acute aortic regurgitation, chest X-ray reveals pulmonary edema with a normal heart. With chronic aortic regurgitation the chest X-ray reveals an enlarged left ventricle and dilated aorta. ECG findings will exhibit left ventricular hypertrophy with a strain pattern.

Diagnosis is made by echocardiogram, multiple gated acquisition scan (MUGA for short), or ventriculogram. Serial studies of ECGs and echocardiogram are used to identify slower, chronic cases. Because physical exam may sometimes mimic the presentation of other valvular dysfunctions, diagnosis of AR by physical exam alone is not sufficient.

Management

As with AS, AR is definitively treated by surgical valve replacement. While the 10-year mortality rate of untreated AR is less than 40%, most cases are considered for valve replacement once they become symptomatic. Treatment of acute onset AR is identical to the treatment of congestive heart failure and includes the use of preload and afterload reducers and diuresis.

DISORDERS OF THE MITRAL VALVE

MITRAL STENOSIS

Rheumatic fever is the most common cause of mitral stenosis (MS). Several decades may pass from the time of infection to the time of symptomatic presentation. Other causes include cardiac tumors, rheumatologic disorders (lupus, rheumatoid arthritis), congential defects, and calcification.

Pathophysiology

Stenosis of the mitral valve impedes the flow of blood from the left atrium into the left ventricle leading to elevated left atrial pressures. This further backs up into the pulmonary circulation manifesting with pulmonary edema. With further backup, pulmonary hypertension and subsequent right ventricular failure result.

Clinical Presentation

Patients with mitral stenosis manifest with exertional dyspnea, orthopnea, paroxysmal nocturnal dyspnea, and fatigue. Often hemoptysis may develop as a result of pulmonary damage secondary to pulmonary hypertension.

Physical exam reveals a palpable diastolic thrill over the apex, a loud S_1 snap, and an opening snap of the mitral valve in early diastole follow by a low-pitched rumbling diastolic murmur best auscultated at the apex.

Diagnostics

Chest roentgenogram may reveal increased vascular markings or frank pulmonary edema. Left atrial enlargement is seen on chest X-ray as a straightening of the left heart border. The most common findings on ECG include atrial fibrillation and left atrial enlargement. In more advanced stages right ventricular hypertrophy may be noted. As with prior valvular dysfunctions, MS is diagnosed by echocardiogram.

Management

Management of MS is directed at treating the symptoms of congestive heart failure and controlling the ventricular rate if atrial fibrillation is present. Acute presentations of congestive heart failure should be treated symptomatically with diuresis and salt restriction as the primary considerations. Digitalis is used to control the rate in atrial fibrillation. Anticoagulation may be considered with new-onset atrial fibrillation. Surgical intervention is an option when MS reaches a critical degree.

MITRAL REGURGITATION

Pathophysiology

Rheumatic fever is the cause of mitral regurgitation (MR) in 40% to 45% of cases. Other causes include mitral valve prolapse, infection, trauma, cardiomyopathies, and myocardial ischemia.

The amount of regurgitant blood flow in acute mitral regurgitation can be three to four times the amount of forward flow resulting in acute pulmonary edema. In chronic mitral regurgitation, the left ventricle compensates by increasing stroke volume and cardiac output. CHF is uncommon. MR may result in left ventricular hypertrophy due to increased left ventricular preload. Left atrial enlargement and atrial fibrillation may develop.

Clinical Manifestations

Presentation of MR is often insidious. Patients may remain asymptomatic throughout their lifetime. Primary chief complaints are fatigue, dyspnea, and palpitations. In acute mitral regurgitation secondary to acute myocardial infarction, fulminant pulmonary edema is seen.

In acute mitral regurgitation, physical findings consistent with acute pulmonary edema are notable. Physical exam will reveal a loud harsh crescendo–decrescendo murmur, loudest at the apex and sometimes radiating to the axilla. There is a palpable thrill at the apex and S_3 and S_4 heart sounds are notable.

In chronic mitral regurgitation a left ventricular heave and thrill is frequently palpable at the apex. The murmur is holosystolic and is best heard at the apex radiating to the axilla. The S_1 heart sound is decreased or obscured and the S_2 heart sound is widely split.

Diagnostics

ECG may be helpful in diagnosing an AMI as the cause for acute mitral regurgitation. Atrial fibrillation is frequently noted, as is left atrial hypertrophy on the ECG. The left atrial enlargement may be confirmed on the chest X-ray. Diagnosis is made by echocardiography. MUGA scan may add some value, but echocardiography remains the primary diagnostic tool for MR.

Management

Treatment of mitral regurgitation is similar to that of mitral stenosis and is directed at treating the symptoms of congestive heart failure and controlling the ventricular rate if atrial fibrillation is present. Acute presentations of congestive heart failure should be treated symptomatically with diuresis and salt restriction as the primary considerations. Digitalis is used to control the rate in atrial fibrillation. Anticoagulation may be considered with new-onset atrial fibrillation. Surgical intervention is an option when MR reaches a critical degree, and an intra-aortic balloon pump may be necessary to support the patient in acute mitral regurgitation until surgical intervention is available.

DISORDERS OF THE TRICUSPID AND PULMONARY VALVES

While the tricuspid and pulmonary valves will present with various abnormalities, the aortic and mitral valves typically cause the emergent or critical problems requiring rapid intervention. Table 22–7 summarizes the etiology, clinical findings, and treatment of the four cardiac valves, and highlights the important findings associated with the tricuspid and pulmonic valves. The critical care transport provider should always be aware of the various valvular disease presentations, but preparation remains focused on those that severely limit cardiac output or induce congestive heart failure.

CRITICAL CARE PROCEDURES FOR CARDIOVASCULAR EMERGENCIES

ARTERIAL LINE

Arterial lines are often in place for critical care patients prior to transport. The presence of an arterial line allows for hemodynamic monitoring and for the sampling of arterial blood gases without repeating the arterial stick. In the event that the critical care paramedic is called on to catheterize an artery, the preferred location is the radial artery due to its location. The superficial location of the radial artery makes it easy to localize the artery and maintain a sterile field during the procedure. The following protocol should be utilized for radial arterial line placement:

Indications

- ★ Hemodynamic monitoring for
  - – Hypotension
  - – Arterial hypertension requiring vasodilator therapy
- ★ Unstable ischemic heart disease
- ★ Post-cardiac surgery
- ★ Inotropic therapy
- ★ Frequent blood gas sampling
- ★ Intra-aortic balloon pump use

Precautions

A modified Allen test should be performed as a screening test prior to radial artery cannulation. The Allen test ensures good collateral flow of blood to the hand. The test is performed by first extending the patient's arm and wrist out in a 45-degree angle, with the anterior forearm presenting and the hand in a position of dorsiflexion. Then occlude both the radial and ulnar arteries digitally with your hands. After noting the pallor that will start to become evident to the hand due to arterial occlusion, release your pressure on the radial artery. Perfusion should return to the hand almost spontaneously as evidenced by the hand "pinking up." Then repeat the procedure, but this time release pressure to only the ulnar artery and observe for the same finding. If there is evidence of good collateral circulation, then this site is considered acceptable for performing the arterial stick. As a general rule though, use the patient's nondominant arm whenever possible.

Technique

The technique for arterial line placement described here utilizes the radial artery site, which is the site where it is most commonly performed. Although the critical care paramedic should consider

Table 22-7 | Valvular Disorders and their Presentations

Valvular Disorders and their Presentations

	Etiology	Physiology	Symptoms	Exam	Lab Studies	Treatment
Aortic regurgitation	Infectious, congenital, hypertension	LV volume overload	Edema, dyspnea, fatigue	Diastolic rumble, SEM	Echocardiogram	Surgical, diuretics
Aortic stenosis	Congenital, degenerative, rheumatic	LV pressure overload	Chest pain, syncope, heart failure	Delay pulse wave, aortic thrill	Echocardiogram, cath lab	Surgery
Mitral regurgitation	Degenerative, CAD, connective d/o	LV volume overload	Dyspnea, fatigue	Apical holosystolic murmur	ECG, echocardiogram	Digitalis, surgical
Mitral stenosis	Rheumatic, lesion, congenital, calcific	LA pressure overload	Dyspnea, syncope, palpitations	Loud S1, diastolic rumble	Echocardiogram, ECG	Coumadin, surgical
Tricuspid regurgitation	RV dilation, infectious, trauma	RV dilation	Peripheral edema	Atrial fibrillation	CXR, ECG, echocardiogram	Limited to RV failure
Tricuspid stenosis	Rheumatic, lesion	RA hypertension	Dyspnea, fatigue	Increased JVP	ECG, echocardiogram	Antibiotics
Pulmonic regurgitation	Pulmonary hypertension, infectious	Pulmonary hypertension	Mimics pulmonary hypertension	High-pitched diastolic blow	CXR, echocardiogram	Treat pulmonary HTN
Pulmonic stenosis	Congenital	RV pressure overload	Edema	Slight increased JVP	CXR, echocardiogram	Treat RV failure

the radial artery as the primary site, the femoral, brachial, or dorsalis pedis arteries may be utilized for arterial line placement.

- ★ Equipment
  - – 20-gauge, nontapered, 1.5- or 2-inch over-the-needle catheter
  - – Fluid-filled noncompliant tubing with stopcocks
  - – A constant flush device
  - – 4-0 suture material
  - – 1% lidocaine in a syringe attached to a 25-gauge needle
- ★ Perform a modified Allen's test and/or Doppler examination of the wrists to demonstrate that the blood supply to the hand would not be eliminated by a catheter-induced thrombus. Place the hand in 45 degrees of dorsiflexion with the aid of a roll of gauze and armband. Utilize appropriate body substance isolation (BSI) precautions. Prepare and drape the volar (palm side) aspect of the wrist.
- ★ Infiltrate 0.5 mL of lidocaine on both sides of the artery using a 25-gauge needle.
- ★ Puncture the skin approximately 5 cm proximal to the wrist crease at an angle of 30 to 60 degrees. Advance until blood is noted in the hub. Holding the needle steady, advance the catheter over it and into the lumen of the artery. If the catheter does not advance smoothly, it may be necessary to advance the needle and catheter together, 1–2 mm. Attach the catheter to the Luer-Lok three-way stopcock, which in turn is attached to a pressure-infused heparin solution, an intraflow device, and an arterial pressure monitor. One to two units of heparin per milliliter of saline should be concentrated in the intravenous solution. A continuous infusion of 1–3 mL/hr should be maintained. Suture the catheter in place, and apply antibiotic ointment and sterile dressing. Extension of the wrist may now be reduced and the tubing taped to the arm. Zero the transducer and observe the waveform. Correlate the invasive blood pressure with the noninvasive reading.

Complications

No technique is devoid of any complications, and arterial cannulation is no exception. Although some complications may potentially be severe, the critical care paramedic's attention to these will limit their effect.

- ★ As with any type of venipuncture, the patient may complain of pain.
- ★ The catheter must be firmly attached to the three-way stopcock via a Luer-Lok fitting. Use of a non–Luer-Lok fitting, which can become disconnected, can result in exsanguinating hemorrhage.
- ★ Inattention to the heparin infusion may result in thrombosis of the line.
- ★ Arterial spasm may be induced by performance of the procedure. This may be reduced by administration of peri-arterial local anesthetic.
- ★ Hematoma formation may occur if the posterior wall of the vessel is inadvertently perforated. If this occurs, firm pressure over the hematoma of 5–10 minutes duration is indicated.
- ★ Limb ischemia
- ★ Infection
- ★ Air embolism

SUBCLAVIAN VEIN

Gaining access to the central circulation via subclavian vein allows for the provision of multiple interventions by the critical care team. First, the administration of medications by the central line affords predictable absorption patterns since its delivery is so close to the heart. Secondly, it allows for the placement of sensors needed for hemodynamic monitoring, and also affords the ability for emergency transvenous pacing.

Indications

★ Emergency intravenous route in seriously ill or injured patients

★ Central venous pressure monitoring

★ Insertion of transvenous pacemaker

★ Intravenous access in patients without peripheral veins

★ Infusion of hypertonic or irritant solutions

Precautions

The critical care paramedic should ensure that the patient has airway control established, is being oxygenated and ventilated as appropriate, and any emergent cardiac dysrhythmias are being managed.

★ This procedure has a significant increase in serious complications when performed on uncooperative or agitated patients.

★ The most experienced provider should attempt insertion because rates of complication are directly influenced by operator experience.

★ When using a Seldinger technique for subclavian vein access, you must maintain control of the J-wire at all times.

★ This procedure is contraindicated for patients with deformity of the chest wall, previous surgery or trauma in this area, fibrotic changes, radiation therapy, or any other situations that would distort the landmarks and anatomy of the region.

Technique

Like arterial line placement, the critical care paramedic will uncommonly have opportunities to perform the skill. This is because the skill is usually already performed by the hospital staff prior to the establishment of patient transfer. This does not, however remove the responsibility on the part of the critical care paramedic to be familiar with the indications and techniques for insertion.

★ Equipment

   – Double- or triple-lumen, J-wire-guided, subclavian kit

   – Normal saline or heparin flush

★ Utilize appropriate BSI procedures.

★ Prepare your equipment. If using a triple-lumen catheter, flush the two accessory ports with heparin.

★ Place the patient in 10–20 degrees of Trendelenburg.

★ Prep and drape the area appropriately.

★ Locate the appropriate landmarks. The subclavian vein is entered infraclavicularly at the junction of the medial and middle thirds of the clavicle. The target landmark will be just above the sternoclavicular notch.

★ If the patient is conscious and his condition warrants anesthesia, a skin wheal of 1% lidocaine is raised at the proposed vena puncture site, approximately 2 cm lateral to the medial and middle thirds of the clavicle.

★ Attach the 18-gauge introducer needle to a syringe. Line up the bevel of the needle with the markings on the syringe. Insert the needle through the skin at the vena puncture site described above and advance the needle into the side of the clavicle. Place the index finger of your left hand in the sternoclavicular notch. Apply a downward pressure on the needle with the thumb of your left hand until the needle goes under the clavicle. Keeping the angle of the needle shallow, advance the needle forward, directed toward the target landmark, just above the sternoclavicular notch.

Too deep an angle increases the likelihood of puncturing the lung and causing a pneumothorax. Continue to advance the catheter, maintaining negative pressure on the syringe, until blood is noted to flow freely into the syringe. Rotate the syringe 90 degrees so that the markings on the syringe are pointed toward the patient's feet. Place the J-wire through the side port and advance the wire, then remove the catheter over the wire. Make sure to always maintain control of the wire. Make a small incision through the skin at the site of the wire, large enough to easily advance the dilator catheter through the skin. Place the dilator over the wire. Advance the dilator to the hub. Again maintaining stability of the wire, remove the dilator. Next place the triple-lumen catheter over the wire and advance so that the catheter is in the proximal aspect of the superior vena cava. Remove the wire and check to ensure that blood is still flowing freely into the syringe.

★ Attach intravenous tubing to the catheter and ensure that the line is flowing properly.

★ Apply antibiotic ointment and suture the catheter in place. Then apply a sterile gauze dressing.

★ An X-ray should be obtained as early as possible after the placement of a subclavian line. If the line is placed in the field, monitor the patient's respiratory status and breath sounds and obtain an X-ray after arrival at the hospital.

Complications

Subclavian complications are similar to those found with other types of peripheral cannulation. Additionally, there may be risks to other organs or structures as discussed later.

★ Pneumothorax
★ Venous thrombosis
★ Thrombophlebitis
★ Hematoma formation
★ Infections

FEMORAL VEIN

The femoral vein is cannulated as an alternative site for access to the central circulation, when needed. It is also used when performing PTCA in patients not eligible for fibrinolytic therapy.

Indications

★ Emergency intravenous route when unable to find access elsewhere
★ When rapid placement of a large-bore central venous catheter is necessary
★ A central line for hemodynamic monitoring or medications that require administration through a central venous catheter

Precautions

★ Operator inexperience may increase the number of attempts required and rate of complications.
★ As with all central venous catheterizations, caution must be exercised to prevent air embolization.
★ A common error is to direct the needle tip medially, toward the umbilicus.
★ All central lines should be flushed prior to insertion.
★ Application of a knee immobilizer will limit movement of the cannulated extremity. This site should not be used if there is infection or lesions at the desired site or if there is known thrombosis of the desired vessel.

Technique

- ★ Equipment
  - – Double- or triple-lumen, J-wire-guided, subclavian kit
  - – Central venous access kit
  - – Normal saline/heparin flush
  - – IV fluids
  - – Skin prep and sterile dressing supplies
  - – Local anesthetic (1% lidocaine) with 25-gauge 3 mL syringe
- ★ Utilize appropriate BSI procedures.
- ★ Locate the vein by first palpating the femoral artery pulse. The vein is located 1 cm medial to the artery. In the patient with vascular collapse or cardiac arrest in whom the arterial pulse cannot be palpated, one can find the vein by extending an imaginary line between the symphysis pubis and the anterior superior iliac spine. The vein is located midway between these two structures.
- ★ Anesthetize the area with 1% lidocaine if the patient is conscious.
- ★ Position the catheter approximately 2 cm distal to the inguinal ligament and medial to the artery. Direct the needle cephalad at a 45-degree angle with the skin. Advance the catheter, maintaining negative pressure on the syringe, until a flash of blood is noted in the hub. Then advance the catheter while removing the needle.
- ★ If arterial blood is encountered, remove the needle and place continuous pressure on the site for 10 minutes.
- ★ Attach intravenous tubing to the catheter and ensure that the line is flowing properly.
- ★ Apply antibiotic ointment and secure the catheter and tubing in place. Then apply a sterile gauze dressing.

Complications

- ★ Venous thrombosis
- ★ Thrombophlebitis
- ★ Hematoma formation
- ★ Infections
- ★ Septic arthritis of the hip
- ★ Femoral nerve damage

Special Notes

A Seldinger wire technique may be used in place of the above procedure.

INTERNAL JUGULAR VEIN

Internal jugular cannulation is yet another method for gaining access to the core circulation when previous attempts at alternative locations fail or when the patient's condition precludes the use of alternative sites. The following outlines this procedure.

Indications

- ★ Emergency intravenous route in seriously ill or injured patients
- ★ Central venous pressure monitoring
- ★ Insertion of transvenous pacemaker
- ★ Intravenous access in patients without peripheral veins
- ★ Infusion of hypertonic or irritant solutions

Precautions

★ This procedure has a significant increase in serious complications when performed on uncooperative or agitated patients.

★ Central venous catheters should be used with caution in patients with known coagulopathies.

Technique

★ Equipment:

– Double- or triple-lumen, J-wire-guided, subclavian kit

★ Utilize appropriate BSI procedures.

★ Prepare your equipment. If using a double- or triple-lumen catheter, flush the accessory ports with heparin.

★ Place the patient in 10–20 degrees of Trendelenburg.

★ Turn the patient's head to the contralateral side.

★ Prep and drape the area appropriately.

★ Locate the appropriate landmarks.

★ *Anterior approach:* Locate the triangle formed by the sternal and clavicular heads of the sternocleidomastoid muscle and the clavicle inferiorly. The point of insertion is at the apex of the triangle. Direct the needle inferiorly and laterally toward the ipsilateral nipple.

★ *Posterior approach:* The site of insertion is along the posterior border of the sternocleidomastoid muscle just cephalad to where the external jugular vein crosses that border. Advance the needle under the sternocleidomastoid, aiming at the midpoint of the suprasternal notch.

★ If the patient is conscious and his condition warrants anesthesia, a skin wheal of 1% lidocaine is raised at the proposed vena puncture site.

★ Attach the 18-gauge introducer needle to a syringe. Line up the bevel of the needle with the markings on the syringe. Insert the needle through the skin at the vena puncture site described above.

★ Continue to advance the catheter, maintaining negative pressure on the syringe, until blood is noted to flow freely into the syringe. Rotate the syringe 90 degrees so that the markings on the syringe are pointed toward the patient's feet. Place the J-wire through the side port and advance the wire, then remove the catheter over the wire. Make sure to always maintain control of the wire. Make a small incision through the skin at the site of the wire, large enough to easily advance the dilator catheter through the skin. Place the dilator over the wire. Advance the dilator to the hub. Again maintaining stability of the wire, remove the dilator. Next place the triple-lumen catheter over the wire and advance so that the catheter is in the proximal aspect of the superior vena cava. Remove the wire and check to ensure that blood is still flowing freely into the syringe.

★ Attach intravenous tubing to the catheter and ensure that the line is flowing properly.

★ Apply antibiotic ointment and suture the catheter in place. Then apply a sterile gauze dressing.

★ An X-ray should be obtained as early as possible after the placement of an internal jugular line. If the line is placed in the field, monitor the patient's respiratory status and breath sounds and obtain an X-ray after arrival at the hospital to confirm proper placement.

Complications

- ★ Pneumothorax
- ★ Venous thrombosis
- ★ Thrombophlebitis
- ★ Hematoma formation
- ★ Infections
- ★ Arterial catheterization

VASCULAR ACCESS DEVICE

When attempts at peripheral or central line access fails, and the patient's hemodynamic status warrants immediate fluid resuscitation or pharmacologic intervention, the critical care provider may need to utilize existing vascular access devices (VADs). The following protocol should be utilized when accessing VADs.

Indications

To obtain rapid venous access for the critical patient when peripheral access cannot be otherwise obtained and the patient already has a vascular access device in place

Precautions

- ★ Obtain information and assistance from family members or home health professionals who are familiar with the device.
- ★ Discontinue any intermittent or continuous infusion pumps.
- ★ Ensure placement and patency of the VAD prior to infusing any fluids or medications.
- ★ Flush the catheter completely with sterile normal saline.
- ★ Use aseptic technique.

Central Venous Catheters or PICC Lines

- ★ Attempt peripheral external jugular or intraosseous access before utilizing a peripherally-inserted central catheter (PICC) line, unless the patient or patient's family insists on direct usage of the VAD.
- ★ Identify the location and type of VAD (i.e., central venous catheter, peripheral inserted central catheter).
- ★ Utilize knowledgeable family members, significant others, or home visiting nurses, if available.
- ★ If the patient has fluids or medications already infusing into the device, consult with the base physician to determine compatibility and/or need to continue/discontinue that medication or fluid.
- ★ Use appropriate BSI precaution.
- ★ Clamp the VAD closed to prevent air embolus.
- ★ If multiple lumens are present, identify the lumen to be used.
- ★ Utilize aseptic technique.
- ★ Briskly wipe the injection cap with an alcohol and/or povidone-iodine pad.
- ★ Insert the needle (attached to syringe) into the cap.
- ★ Aspirate slowly for a blood return. Obtain blood samples, if necessary. Then flush the line with solution.

★ Insert the needle (attached to a medication syringe or IV tubing) and infuse medications or fluids.

★ Secure the IV tubing.

★ Reassess the infusion site.

★ Reassess patient condition.

Technique: Implanted Ports

★ Attempt peripheral, external jugular, or intraosseous access before utilizing an implanted port, unless the patient or patient's family insists on direct usage of the VAD.

★ Identify the location and type of VAD (e.g., implanted port).

★ Utilize knowledgeable family members, significant others, or the home visiting nurse, if available.

★ If the patient has fluids or medications already infusing into the device, consult with the base physician to determine compatibility and/or need to continue/discontinue that medication or fluid.

★ Carefully palpate the location of the implanted port.

★ If multiple ports are available, identify the port to be used.

★ Using sterile technique, prep the site with alcohol and/or povidone-iodine. Wipe from the center outward three times in a circular motion.

★ Using a sterile gloved hand, press the skin firmly around the edges of the port.

★ Using a syringe filled with solution, insert the needle perpendicular to the skin.

★ Aspirate slowly for blood return, and then flush the port prior to infusion.

★ Secure the IV tubing.

★ Reassess the infusion site.

★ Reassess the patient.

Complications

★ Patients with vascular access devices are very susceptible to site infections or sepsis. Use sterile techniques at all times.

★ Sluggish flow or no flow may indicate a thrombosis. If a thrombosis is suspected, do not utilize the lumen.

★ Rarely, a catheter will migrate. The symptoms may include the following:
  – Burning with infusion
  – Site bleeding
  – Shortness of breath
  – Chest pain
  – Tachycardia and/or hypotension
  – If a catheter migration is suspected, do not use the VAD and treat the patient according to symptoms.

★ Catheters are durable but may leak or tear. Extravasation of fluids or medications may occur and may cause burning and tissue damage. Clamp the catheter and do not use.

★ Air embolism may occur if the VAD is not clamped in between infusions. Avoid this by properly clamping the catheter and preventing air from entering the system.

INTRA-AORTIC BALLOON PUMP MANAGEMENT

Indications

- ★ Cardiogenic/septic shock
- ★ Unstable angina/myocardial infarction
- ★ Weaning from cardiopulmonary bypass
- ★ Preoperative and postoperative myocardial dysfunction
- ★ Bridge to transplantation
- ★ Percutaneous coronary angioplasty

Precautions

- ★ Critical care team members will not be responsible for the insertion of intra-aortic balloon pumps but will responsible for maintaining both triggering and timing during interfacility transfers.
- ★ Keep a 60-cc syringe present in order to exercise the balloon in the event of pump failure.
- ★ Consider placing the patient's leg (with the IABP insertion site) in a knee immobilizer to prevent movement.
- ★ Do not allow the patient to sit up greater than 30 degrees.
- ★ Maintain access to cannulation site and monitor leads.
- ★ Determine the patient's ability to tolerate brief periods without counterpulsation prior to departing the sending facility.
- ★ Most triggering problems are due to an ECG with an R wave of low amplitude.
- ★ Timing should be rechecked every 1 to 2 hours and whenever there is a >20% change in heart rate, change in cardiac output, development of an dysrhythmia, or change in triggering mode.
- ★ Do not use the central lumen of the intra-aortic balloon catheter for blood sampling.
- ★ Ensure that the patient does not have a history of AAA or AV insufficiency.

Technique: Transporting a Patient with an IABP

- ★ Equipment
  - Intra-aortic balloon pump
  - IABP equipment kit:
    - 60-cc slip-tip syringe
    - Appropriate IAB/IABP adapters
    - Scissors
    - Kelly clamp
    - ECG patches
    - Extra helium tank
    - ECG cable and arterial pressure cable
    - IABP flowsheet
    - IABP operator's manual
- ★ Confirm that a bed at the accepting facility is ready and confirm the name of the accepting physician.
- ★ Review the patient condition and current triggering and timing of the IABP with the referring physician.

- ★ Review the post-insertion X-ray to confirm proper placement (second to third intercostal space, below left subclavian).
- ★ Verify clean ECG and arterial pulse (AP) transducer signals on the monitor.
- ★ Check the IABP battery for sufficient charge.
- ★ Verify that an adequate amount of helium is available to complete transport safely.
- ★ If the patient can tolerate the reduction in counterpulsation (i.e., <20% change in HR, BP, CO), set the assist ratio to 1:2 and confirm timing. Return to a 1:1 ratio after confirming proper timing.
- ★ Timing is set and changed using two separate controls that move the timing markers to the left and right. The inflate control is moved to the left to adjust the inflate time to occur earlier and to the right to occur later. The deflate control operates in a similar manner: moved to the left for earlier deflation, to the right for later deflation.
- ★ Properly secure the IABP in the ambulance.
- ★ During transport the operator must constantly monitor the console and make adjustments for timing errors as needed.
- ★ Timing is evaluated by utilizing timing markers on an arterial pressure waveform to ensure inflation and deflation correspond with appropriate stages of diastole.
- ★ Blood in the connecting tubing is a hallmark of balloon rupture and requires immediate cessation of counterpulsation to prevent cerebral gas embolization.
- ★ Alarms indicated on the console are accompanied by an indicated corrective action.

Complications

- ★ Aortic wall dissection, rupture, or local vascular injury
- ★ Balloon rupture with helium embolus or catheter entrapment
- ★ Limb ischemia or compartment syndrome
- ★ Infection
- ★ Thrombocytopenia
- ★ Hemorrhage
- ★ Obstruction of the left subclavian artery, carotid arteries, renal arteries, or mesenteric arteries

PERICARDIOCENTESIS

Indications

As discussed earlier in the chapter, this technique is used for the management of suspected cardiac tamponade causing hemodynamic compromise.

Precautions

Pericadiocentesis must be viewed as a temporary measure only. It must not be viewed as a definitive therapeutic procedure. The patient must be observed closely for the recurrence of tamponade and readied for surgery if this is indicated.

Technique

1. Prepare equipment
   - Iodinated prep solution
   - Sterile towels
   - 10- and 50-cc syringes
   - 3-inch 18-gauge spinal needle
   - Use proper BSI techniques

2. Prep the skin in the substernal area with Betadine solution and drape the area. Sterile technique should be scrupulously adhered to.

3. Attach the limb leads of the ECG to the patient.

4. Place the patient with the upper torso elevated at 30 degrees.

5. Attach an 18-guage spinal needle to a syringe via a three-way stopcock. Attach one end of an alligator clip to the base of the spinal needle and the other end to the chest lead of an electrocardiograph. The four limb leads should be attached normally to the extremities.

6. Introduce the spinal needle into the left costal arch and direct the tip toward the right shoulder or directly cephalad. The needle may be aimed at the tip of the left shoulder. It is gently passed through the diaphragm, and as the pericardium is entered a "pop" is often felt. Maintain negative pressure on the syringe during advancement of the needle. During the time the procedure is being performed, the V lead of the ECG should be carefully monitored for the appearance of a myocardial injury pattern. If an injury pattern is noted, the needle is in contact with the epicardium and should be withdrawn 1–2 mm until the normal electrocardiographic complex returns.

7. With the needle tip in the pericardial sac, aspiration can be performed.

8. Withdraw the catheter and apply a sterile dressing and adhesive tape.

9. Repeated aspirations may be necessary as the patient's condition warrants.

Complications

★ Myocardial injury

★ Coronary artery injury

★ Dysrhythmias

★ Pneumothorax

GROUND AND AIR TRANSPORT CONSIDERATIONS FOR THE CARDIAC PATIENT

SPECIAL CONSIDERATIONS FOR INTERFACILITY TRANSPORT

An independent evaluation by the critical care paramedic is warranted. While the sending physician has already made a diagnosis for you to follow through with, do not hesitate to evaluate the patient yourself. Sometimes a new diagnosis may result from missed signs or symptoms, or developing complications of the initial diagnosis (such as a tamponade resulting from purulent pericarditis). Look at the radiology results, interpret the laboratory values, and develop your own differential diagnosis list. Failure to do so may result in further delay in appropriate care for new or developing medical complications.

Inform the receiving facility of your arrival. An early call to the receiving facility will alert them to any necessary preparations such as ventilators, IV pumps, or surgeon notification and operating room preparation. Base the time allowed for notification on the patient's status and anticipated needs.

Ensure that the receiving facility has the necessary verbal and written reports sufficient to carry out all needed interventions for the patient. If time allows during transport, attempt to obtain any information necessary to fill in gaps of information not obtained by the sending facility.

Know the level of interventions your critical care transportation unit is capable of and trained to perform, and obtain any necessary written medication orders prior to receiving the patient. Consider recommending other types of transport in the event your transport unit will not facilitate the needs of the patient (i.e., sending a neonatal transport unit with a pediatric isolette for a 1-week-old premature infant).

Be aware of the types of medication being administered during transport and their compatibility with any medications you may potentially administer. Carrying an ICU medication handbook may be useful in such circumstances.

Ensure vascular access. Cardiac patients decompensate quickly under extreme circumstances. Vascular access is a necessity prior to initiating transport. Do not allow the sending facility to speed transportation without appropriate vascular access. Failure to do so could result in delayed medication administration vital to the treatment of cardiac complications.

Secure all devices prior to transport. Large equipment such as intra-aortic balloon pumps and ventilators can be dangerous if left unsecured to slip and slide in the back of the transport unit. These devices must be placed and preferably tied down to ensure minimal movement during transport.

In the event the critical care ground ambulance is involved in an accident, the provider must first ensure safety to themselves and the patient. In a safe environment void of immediate fire hazard, the provider should reassess the patient and any invasive tubes or catheters for any change or dislodgement. If necessary, intubated patients may need the application of the bag-valve-mask unit until they can be safely reattached to a ventilator.

SPECIAL CONSIDERATIONS FOR AIR TRANSPORT

PREPARATION FOR TRANSPORT AND FLIGHT

The patient is prepared for transport on the basis of information obtained from the history, patient assessment, type of aircraft the patient will be transported in, the expected amount of time to complete the transfer, the type of equipment and monitoring required, and the anticipated problems that may develop based on the patient's illness.

The critical care paramedic must determine both the in-flight and ground times required to complete the transfer so he can determine the oxygen requirements needed to meet the patient's needs. The flight team must then ensure that sufficient oxygen is available to safely complete the transport. Similarly, if medical air is needed to power a mechanical ventilator, sufficient amounts must be available to safely complete the transport.

Any medical equipment that requires batteries should also have auxiliary power capabilities that can use the aircraft's inverter power source. Ventilators, intra-aortic balloon pumps, ventricular assist devices, and IV pumps may all require an alternate source of power. The aircraft must be stocked with sufficient supplies and medications to provide quality patient care as a continuation of what is being provided at the hospital.

ALTERATIONS IN CARDIOVASCULAR PHYSIOLOGY AT ALTITUDE

Physiological changes occur as barometric pressure at altitude decreases, causing a reduction in the alveolar pressure of oxygen. A reduction in alveolar pressure leads to a reduction in the amount of oxygen that gets into the blood, which in turn decreases the amount of oxygen available to the tissues. The body attempts to compensate for the decreased oxygen supply by increasing the respiratory rate, heart rate, and cardiac output. Patients with cardiovascular disease may not be able to support a response to compensate for the decreased oxygen supply. Patients with CAD who are unable to compensate for the increased workload imposed on the heart by decreased oxygen tension of high altitude may experience chest pain, congestive heart failure, pulmonary edema, cardiac dysrhythmias, or cardiac arrest. Therefore, all patients with cardiovascular disease should receive supplemental oxygen while in flight. The American College of Chest Physicians has recommended altitude limits for patients with known cardiovascular disease when supplemental oxygen is not available. Limiting the cabin altitude pressure to a maximum of 6,000 feet has been shown to eliminate problems for people with cardiovascular disease.

CARDIOVASCULAR EMERGENCIES AT ALTITUDE

FLIGHT CARDIOPULMONARY ARREST

The flight team must be aware of the patient's Do Not Resuscitate order or code status prior to leaving the referring facility. In addition, before transport, the patient and family members accompanying the patient on flight should be made aware of the risks of air medical transport and the potential for diversions should the patient's condition deteriorate.

The flight critical care paramedic must address the issues of a full cardiopulmonary arrest during transport. The flight medic must consider:

1. Code status of the patient
2. Company policies and procedures for in-flight arrests
3. The decision to return, divert, or proceed to the destination
4. Availability of resuscitation equipment
5. Time frames and endurance of the air medical personnel

If a patient's code status is "full resuscitation or full code" and the patient suffers a cardiopulmonary arrest, then the company's policies and procedures must be followed and must take into consideration the legal aspects of interstate transport and state laws. The program's policies and procedures should clearly delineate what should be done if a patient arrests in flight. The flight team must weigh both state and interstate laws. The team may need to weigh distance and time factors to decide the appropriate destination. This may require returning to the sending facility, diverting to the closest facility, or continuing to the receiving facility. The flight team may need to consider terminating resuscitative efforts based on the amount of resuscitative medications available, the time anticipated to get the patient to an appropriate facility, and the endurance capabilities of the medical personnel onboard. Usually consultation with medical direction to determine cessation of resuscitation is recommended.

Preparation for in-flight cardiac arrest includes ensuring that resuscitative equipment is easily accessible. Oxygen should be readily available and ACLS drugs must be labeled and within easy reach. The flight team must establish well-defined roles and responsibilities in order to effectively respond in the event of a cardiac arrest. There must be access to the patient's head so that endotracheal intubation can be performed. A cardiac defibrillator must be readily available. Studies have shown that defibrillation with current equipment can be safely administered. Standard defibrillation precautions should be followed. If the patient is at high risk for cardiopulmonary arrest, defibrillation pads should be placed on the patient's chest and equipment readied prior to transport.

Summary

Patients with cardiovascular emergencies are a common source of interhospital transports for the critical care paramedic. Due to the critical nature of such patient's needs, the transport team may find itself dealing with the transport and maintenance of multiple IV pumps, mechanical ventilation, an intra-aortic balloon pump, or even a ventricular assist device. Appropriately managing the patient is often dependent on this sophisticated medical equipment, and it requires the critical care paramedic to be properly prepared prior to transport and to maintain diligent monitoring while en route to the final destination. These types of patients may be most demanding on the critical care paramedic due to the needed in-depth understanding of cardiovascular pathophysiology as well as the ability to handle invasive cardiac monitoring and sophisticated cardiovascular support equipment.

Review Questions

1. What are the intrinsic discharge rates of each of the heart's three pacemaker sites?
2. Explain the pathophysiological difference between angina and infarction.
3. A patient with an occlusion to the left anterior descending artery would infarct what walls of the heart?

4. What are the major categories of medications used on the patient with an actively occurring myocardial infarction?

5. How does an aortic aneurysm differ from an aortic dissection?

6. What are the treatment goals for a patient with an aortic dissection?

7. What are the three types of cardiac myopathies, and how do they present?

8. Why would a patient with CHF benefit from dobutamine rather than dopamine?

9. A faulty aortic valve would present how clinically?

10. What aspects of normal blood flow does the IABP help compensate? How does this device achieve this?

See Answers to Review Questions at the back of this book.

Further Reading

Bickley LS. *Bates' Guide to Physical Examination and History Taking,* 8th ed. Philadelphia: Lippincott Williams & Wilkins, 2003.

Crawford MH, DiMarco JP, et al. *Cardiology.* London, England: Mosby, 2001.

Czarnecki M, Stone R, Seaman K. *UMBC Critical Care Transport Field Guide.* Sudbury, MA: Jones and Bartlett, 2001.

Hamilton GC. *Emergency Medicine: An Approach to Clinical Problem-Solving,* 2nd ed. Philadelphia: W. B. Saunders, 2003.

Martini FH, Bartholmoew EF, Bledsoe BE. *Anatomy and Physiology for Emergency Care.* Upper Saddle River, NJ: Pearson Prentice Hall, 2002.

Morton PG, et al. *Critical Care Nursing: A Holistic Approach,* 8th ed. Philadelphia: Lippincott Williams & Wilkins, 2005.

Rosen P, Barkin R, Danzl DF, Hockberger RS, Ling LJ, Markovchick V, Marx JA, Newton E, Walls RM. *Emergency Medicine: Concepts and Clinical Practice,* 4th ed. St. Louis, MO: Mosby, 1998.

Rosen P, Chan TC, Vilke GM, Sternbach G. *Atlas of Emergency Procedures.* St. Louis, MO: Mosby, 2001.

Tintinalli JE, Kelen GD, Stapczynski JS. *Emergency Medicine: A Comprehensive Study Guide,* 5th ed. New York: McGraw-Hill, 1999.

Chapter 23

Neurologic Emergencies

Donald J. Perreault, Jr., RN, BSN, CCRN, EMT

Objectives

Upon completion of this chapter, the student should be able to:

1. Develop and enhance neurologic assessment skills. (p. 688)
2. Identify common neurologic emergencies that may result in the need for critical care intervention. (p. 688)
3. Recognize the potential for secondary injury and understand treatment options to minimize its effects. (p. 690)
4. Become familiar with the pathophysiology of thromboembolic and hemorrhagic cerebrovascular accidents, as well as the treatment of both. (p. 691)
5. Identify patients who are candidates for fibrinolytic therapy. (p. 695)
6. Identify infectious processes found in the central nervous system and their effects. (p. 701)

Key Terms

Case Study

Your ambulance is dispatched to a small clinic in a nearby rural town for a 25-year-old man named Mr. Sample with an altered mental status. The patient has a medical history that is remarkable for generalized anxiety and genital herpes. The only medication that Mr. Sample takes is acyclovir as needed to help treat herpes outbreaks. He is allergic to penicillin.

The patient's girlfriend claims that he had been complaining of a progressively worsening headache for the last 3 days. He had developed a fever that morning, and she was able to convince him to come to the doctor's office for evaluation. While en route, she noticed that the patient seemed uncharacteristically irritable.

In the 45 minutes that have passed since Mr. Sample arrived at the office, he has grown confused and somewhat lethargic. The physician called 911 to have him transported to the emergency department for a more detailed neurologic evaluation. After a brief assessment, you move Mr. Sample to the ambulance to begin the transport and reassess him.

Mr. Sample opens his eyes spontaneously, but does not seem able to focus on you well. His pupils are reactive bilaterally, and he will not follow your commands to assess his extraocular movement. His face is symmetric bilaterally, and his tongue is midline. His speech is somewhat slurred, and he is oriented only to his own name. He becomes agitated with repeated questioning. Mr. Sample will not follow your commands to move his extremities, but localizes all of them with equal strength, and has no apparent sensory deficit. He complains of a headache and neck pain.

Mr. Sample's vital signs are as follows:

HR 90 and NSR

RR 18

BP 158/84

Temp. 102.4

The remainder of his physical examination yields no findings of consequence, except for hot, diaphoretic skin.

You establish IV access with an 18-gauge angiocath in Mr. Sample's left antecubital vein and begin a normal saline drip at a rate of 125 mL/hr. You attempt to cool him passively by removing his heavy clothing. The total transport time is approximately 25 minutes from the clinic to the hospital. You notice that Mr. Sample is no longer keeping his eyes open spontaneously, and he has stopped answering your questions entirely.

When you are about 10 minutes away from the ED, Mr. Sample suddenly goes unresponsive and begins to have a tonic-clonic seizure. You administer 5 mg of IV midazolam to stop the seizure and elect to intubate him to protect his airway. Your partner pulls the vehicle over to assist. He administers 100 mg of IV lidocaine because you are concerned about the possibility of intracranial pathology, and do not wish to elevate his intracranial pressure during the intubation. He administers 100 mg of IV succinylcholine and an additional 5 mg of midazolam and you successfully intubate Mr. Sample with a 7.5 ETT. Your partner resumes transport as you ventilate Mr. Sample with a bag-valve-mask unit and alert the receiving ED.

Upon arrival, Mr. Sample is quickly stabilized in the trauma room. He receives additional IV access and has blood cultures and other lab work drawn. He is given an acetaminophen suppository and is loaded with 1000 mg of IV phenytoin (Dilantin). His sedation is maintained with periodic doses of midazolam. A CT scan is unremarkable for acute pathology. A lumbar puncture is performed and yields clear CSF that is sampled and cultured. The opening pressure is 28 mmHg. The patient is started on broad-spectrum antibiotics, as well as intravenous acyclovir with a presumptive diagnosis of herpes simplex encephalitis. CSF cultures indicate the presence of herpes simplex virus type 1 (HSV-1) and antibiotic therapy is discontinued.

Serial CT scans reveal progressive encephalitis. A fiber-optic ICP bolt is inserted, and Mr. Sample receives periodic doses of IV mannitol over the next few days to maintain his ICP at less than

20 mmHg. The acyclovir therapy continues, and Mr. Sample remains intubated and sedated with a propofol infusion that is lifted every 2 hours for a bedside neurologic exam. On post-admission day 5, Mr. Sample begins following motor commands with all four extremities, is weaned from the sedation and ventilatory support, and extubated. He has not had any substantial elevation in his ICP for 2 days, and the bolt is also discontinued. After an additional 3 days in the ICU, Mr. Sample is deemed stable for the floor, and is transferred to continue on IV acyclovir until his discharge. He remains impulsive, forgetful, and confused at times, but his neurologic exam returns to baseline by the time he is discharged 8 days later.

INTRODUCTION

Critical care medicine has evolved tremendously in the treatment of neurologic disorders during the past few decades. The same risks for secondary injury are present within the neuromedical critical care population as in victims of central nervous system (CNS) trauma. However, the damage caused by many primary neurologic emergencies can also be attenuated by prompt recognition and intervention. The critical care paramedic must learn how to recognize neurologic emergencies early in their development and initiate timely treatment and preventive care.

NEUROANATOMY AND PHYSIOLOGY

The anatomy and physiology of the human central nervous system is an extremely complex subject to which entire textbooks have been dedicated. However, a basic understanding of neurologic anatomy and physiology is essential for understanding the neuro patient in the critical care setting. Because of the complexity of these structures, basic gross anatomy and physiology will be reviewed here with an emphasis on functional structures and systems, and specifically how they relate to critical care pathology.

THE BRAIN

The brain is the major organ of the central nervous system and the principal control organ in the body. Situated in the cranial vault, it consists of several readily identifiable features.

CEREBRUM

The cerebral hemispheres are comprised of both white matter, containing neuronal axons, and gray matter. This gray matter, also known as the **cortex,** is a thin layer that is comprised of neuronal cell bodies and supporting structures, and is therefore the epicenter of higher forms of consciousness, thought, and control. The axons and fiber tracts of the white matter serve as connective wiring between the cortex and other brain and body structures. Interspersed within the white matter are functionally significant areas of neuronal cell bodies known as *nuclei.*

The cerebrum is divided laterally into left and right hemispheres in the midline by the *longitudinal fissure.* The surface area of the cerebrum is increased by *sulci* and *gyri.* A sulcus is a furrow or valley that invaginates into the surface of the brain. Those with greater depth are known as *fissures.* A gyrus, by contrast, is a ridge of nervous tissue that projects outward from the surface of the cortex. Deeper sulci help to separate the cerebrum into functionally distinct areas known as *lobes,* which should be familiar to all critical care paramedics: the *frontal, temporal, parietal,* and *occipital* lobes. The specific effects of damage to each of these, as well as their functional significance, will be discussed later.

cortex *a thin layer in the brain comprised of neuronal cell bodies and supporting structures; the epicenter of higher forms of consciousness, thought, and control.*

The cerebral cortex is the seat of consciousness.

CEREBELLUM

cerebellum *area of the brain responsible for coordination and stabilization of fine and complex movements; helps determine body's external spatial relationships.*

The cerebellum is the second largest distinct structure in the brain, and sits in the posterior fossa. The **cerebellum** is responsible for the coordination and stabilization of fine and complex movements, as well as a subconscious understanding of how the body is positioned in space, known as *proprioception*. It connects to the brainstem via the *cerebellar peduncles*, which are fiber tracts.

DIENCEPHALON

Diencephalon is a term used to describe a structure deep to the cerebrum that is composed of the thalamus, hypothalamus, and epithalamus. The diencephalon encases the third ventricle, and the epithalamus is home to the *choroid plexus*, which is responsible for the production of cerebrospinal fluid (CSF), as well as the *pineal gland*.

Thalamus

The thalamus is known as the "gateway to the cortex." It is comprised of several functionally significant nuclei, which essentially all serve to filter almost every piece of information passing between the cerebral cortex and elsewhere in the body.

Hypothalamus

The hypothalamus is a vital neurohormonal structure, closely associated with the adjacent *pituitary gland*, that controls much of the body's endocrine system. In addition, the hypothalamus is ultimately responsible for the autonomic nervous system, helps to regulate sleep–wake cycles, and regulates satiety with regard to food and water intake, as well as body temperature regulation. The hypothalamus also interacts with other structures in the brain to define physiological responses to emotion and behavior.

BRAINSTEM

The brainstem is the deepest and most protected structure in the brain, and also represents some of the most physiologically primitive functions. It is composed of the *midbrain, pons*, and *medulla*, and is home to the nuclei of the majority of the cranial nerves. Pathology in the brainstem can prove to be rapidly fatal, and the close association of the cranial nerves with it underscores the need for accurate cranial nerve assessment.

Midbrain

The midbrain is where the *cerebral peduncles* that form the pyramidal motor tracts are found. It encases the cerebral aqueduct that connects the third and fourth ventricles. It is also the site of physiologically significant nuclei.

Pons

The pons is essentially a relay station for information within the brainstem, and also houses a respiratory control center known as the pneumotaxic center.

Medulla

The medulla is the most inferior structure in the brainstem, and merges with the spinal cord at the *foramen magnum*, a large hole in the base of the skull. The medulla is responsible for the maintenance of the most fundamental functions in the body, specifically regulation of the respiratory and cardiovascular systems. It is also part of the pyramidal motor tract, and is the site of physiologically significant nuclei.

VENTRICULAR SYSTEM

Cerebrospinal fluid circulates around the brain, and through hollow spaces within its interior known as ventricles. There are two *lateral ventricles* located deep to the cerebrum, which drain into *intraventricular foramina*, drainage points whereby CSF passes into the *third ventricle* located inferiorly, and abutting the midbrain. The third ventricle drains into the *fourth ventricle*, which lies at the level of the brainstem, via the *aqueduct of Sylvius*. The fourth ventricle has three openings that allow CSF to exit the ventricular system and enter the subarachnoid space: the *foramen of Magendie* and the paired *foramina of Luschka*. CSF is eventually reabsorbed into the sagittal sinus via finger-like projections known as *arachnoid villi*. Some CSF will enter the central canal of the spine to help cushion the structures there as well.

THE MENINGES

Three layers of coverings protect the brain and spinal cord. The first of these, the pia mater, clings to their surface. Overlying this is a spiderweb-like layer known appropriately as the arachnoid layer. Between the pia and arachnoid mater is the subarachnoid space, wherein most of the arterial structures, as well as CSF, can be found. Above the arachnoid layer is the dura mater, a tough, fibrous, bilevel structure that occasionally dips into areas of the brain and spinal cord to form anatomical barriers. The dura is contiguous with the periosteum, and penetrating it are venous structures that feed both bone and nervous tissue.

THE SPINE

The spinal cord, whose cephalad end is contiguous with the medulla oblongata, is composed of white and gray matter, just as the brain is. A transverse cross section of the spinal cord looks vaguely like an oval of white matter with a butterfly-shaped mass of gray matter located in the center. The central canal runs through the middle of this gray matter. Two anatomical structures serve to divide the spinal cord nearly into two lateral halves, the *anterior median fissure* and the *posterior median sulcus*.

Each half of the white matter is divided physiologically into columns of axons that run cephalocaudally through the cord. These are known as the *posterior, anterior,* and *lateral funiculus* (plural: funiculi).

The cell bodies comprising the gray matter in each conceptual half are also divided into three lobes, the *dorsal (posterior), ventral (anterior),* and *lateral horns*. The two halves are joined by a thin strip of gray matter known as the *gray commissure*, through which the central canal runs longitudinally in the midline.

The spinal cord's vascular supply runs cephalocaudally along the anterior and posterior aspects of the cord. The lateral aspects of the cord give rise to the peripheral nervous system. A *ventral* spinal nerve root projects laterally from the anterior portion of the cord in either direction, and merges with a *dorsal root* which projects from the posterior to form a *spinal nerve*. These then branch into the peripheral nervous system.

The ventral root carries efferent motor impulses from the cell bodies in the anterior horns of the gray matter to skeletal muscles.

The dorsal root carries afferent sensory information from the body's periphery to a specialized structure comprised of neuronal bodies within the root itself, known as the *dorsal root ganglion*. The axons progressing into the spinal cord from these ganglia may then synapse either in the cord directly or run up the white matter to the brain. The dorsal horn of the gray matter contains *interneurons* which are responsible for facilitating the relay of sensory input to other areas of the CNS.

The lateral horns of the gray matter are responsible for autonomic control of the sensory organs, sending their axons through the ventral root along with those from the anterior horn.

The white matter of the spinal cord is comprised of several tracts that carry both afferent and efferent impulses. Certain tracts are responsible for the conveyance of certain types of information. Ascending tracts carry sensory information such as sensations of pressure, light touch, and proprioception. Descending tracts carry motor information from the brain to the body.

These tracts do not end when they enter the brain. Certain tracts synapse with different nuclei before they reach the final destination that controls their coordinated purpose. Some systems will be discussed in greater detail to emphasize the effects on the critical care patient when these areas are compromised by pathology.

CEREBRAL VASCULATURE

Blood supply to the brain is through a network of arteries that arise from the carotid and vertebral arteries (Figure 23-1 ■). Venous drainage is through the jugular veins.

ARTERIAL SYSTEM

Remember that the arteries perfusing the brain do not behave in quite the same fashion as those which perfuse the rest of the body. The driving phenomenon behind the behavior of the cerebral vasculature is the autoregulation of cerebral blood flow. The maintenance of consistent perfusion to the neurons is the most important task with which the cerebral vasculature is charged. Cerebral perfusion pressure remains the bottom line of autoregulation.

$$\text{Cerebral perfusion pressure (CPP)} = \text{Mean arterial pressure (MAP)} - \text{Intracranial pressure (ICP)}$$

Thus, if CPP is decreased by relative systemic hypotension or intracranial hypertension, cerebral vasodilation occurs to increase cerebral blood flow. If CPP increases due to systemic hypertension, the cerebral vasculature vasoconstricts to reduce cerebral blood flow.

Diagrams of the cerebral arteries are helpful in understanding their complexity. In essence, the aorta branches into the two large brachiocephalic arteries, which then give rise to both the common carotid arteries and the right subclavian artery. The left subclavian arises directly from the aorta. The common carotids bifurcate into the external and internal carotids, which form part of the foundation of the cerebral arterial system. The other part of that foundation is formed by the vertebral arteries, which arise from the subclavians.

It is helpful to imagine the brain as being divided into two distinct areas with regard to circulation: the anterior and posterior circulation. The anterior circulation is perfused by offshoots of the internal carotids, while the posterior circulation, also known as the vertebrobasilar circulation, is perfused by the vertebral arteries and their tributaries.

At the level of, and wrapped around the inferior surface of, the brainstem, both internal carotids and vertebral arteries merge to form a specialized structure known as the **circle of Willis** (Figure 23-2 ■). The physiological circle formed by these arteries and the smaller arteries that connect them provides some degree of collateral circulation and becomes the jumping-off point for all of the major tributary cerebral arteries.

Starting from the posterior circulation, the vertebral arteries merge to form a single, large *basilar artery*. The right and left *posterior cerebral arteries (PCAs)*, diverge from this. The posterior portion of the circle of Willis is formed by these two PCAs, which then connect to the internal carotid arteries via the *posterior communicating arteries*. At the approximate point of this nexus, the two internal carotids bifurcate into the right and left *middle cerebral arteries (MCAs)* and the *anterior cerebral arteries (ACAs)*, which form most of the rest of the circle of Willis. These follow a somewhat angular course and track up the midline of the anterior portion of the brain. They are connected by the *anterior communicating artery*, which is a tiny artery that completes the circle of Willis.

Just before the merger of the two vertebral arteries into the basilar artery, each vertebral artery gives rise to the *posterior inferior cerebellar artery (PICA)*, as well as two additional small tributaries that merge caudally to form the *anterior spinal artery (ASA)*. At the point of the union of the vertebral arteries into the single vertebral artery, two additional offshoots form the *anterior inferior cerebellar arteries (AICAs)*. This union is mirrored at the caudal end of the basilar artery by the formation of the two *superior cerebellar arteries (SCAs)*, which form at the same junction as the PCAs. For the sake of clarification, the PICAs and PCAs are at opposite poles of the pons.

With regard to perfusion, the MCAs perfuse the bulk of each cerebral hemisphere, occupying the lateral aspect of each. The ACAs perfuse the midline portion of each, and the PCAs perfuse only the most inferior layer.

These are not the only arteries that arise from the circle of Willis or its major tributaries, but they comprise the bulk of the brain's primary circulation and are sufficient to formulate an adequate understanding.

circle of Willis *a series of constituent cerebral arteries located at the midline, anterior portion of the brain that form a circle around the brainstem; the foundation of the arterial system that perfuses the brain, and other collateral areas.*

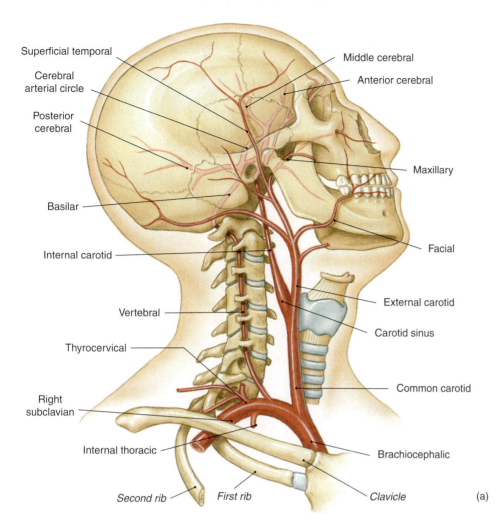

Superficial temporal

Cerebral
arterial circle

Posterior
cerebral

Basilar

Internal carotid

Vertebral

Thyrocervical

Right
subclavian

Internal thoracic

Second rib

First rib

Middle cerebral

Anterior cerebral

Maxillary

Facial

External carotid

Carotid sinus

Common carotid

Brachiocephalic

Clavicle

(a)

■ **Figure 23-1** Arteries of the neck, head, and brain. (a) The general circulation pattern of arteries supplying the neck and superficial structures of the head. (b) The arterial supply to the brain. *(Fig. 14-15, p. 395, from Essentials of Anatomy & Physiology, 2nd ed., by Frederic H. Martini, Ph.D. and Edwin F. Bartholomew, M.S. Copyright © 2000 by Frederic H. Martini, Inc. Published by Pearson Education, Inc. Reprinted by permission.)*

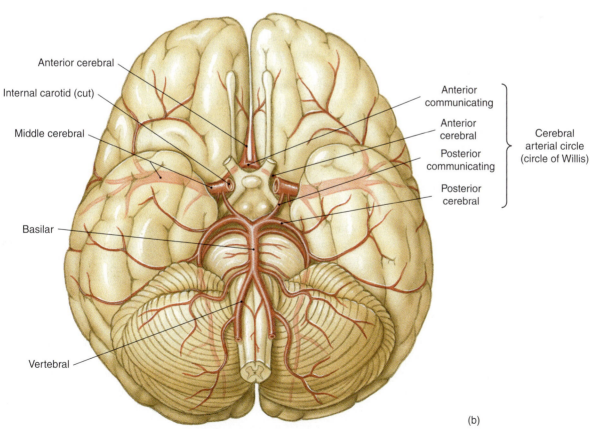

Anterior cerebral

Internal carotid (cut)

Middle cerebral

Basilar

Vertebral

Anterior
communicating

Anterior
cerebral

Posterior
communicating

Posterior
cerebral

Cerebral
arterial circle
(circle of Willis)

(b)

Cerebral Vasculature **683**

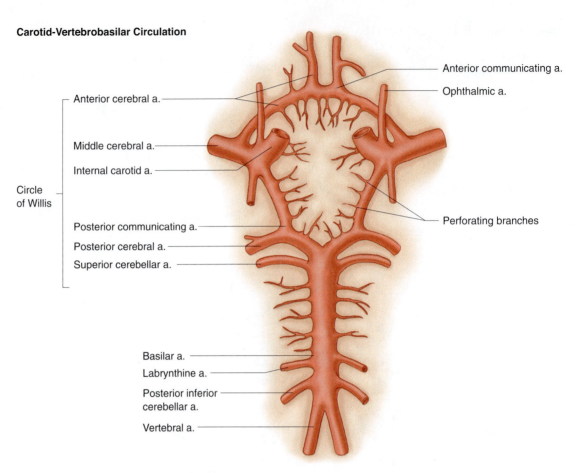

Anterior communicating a.

Ophthalmic a.

Anterior cerebral a.

Middle cerebral a.

Internal carotid a.

Circle
of Willis

Posterior communicating a.

Posterior cerebral a.

Superior cerebellar a.

Perforating branches

Basilar a.

Labrynthine a.

Posterior inferior
cerebellar a.

Vertebral a.

■ Figure 23-2   Circle of Willis.

VENOUS SYSTEM

The venous system of the brain can almost be visualized similar to the collecting system of the kidneys. Small veins merge to form collecting veins known as *sinuses*, all of which eventually merge into the internal jugular vein. Two exceptions are the occipital vein, which flows into the external jugular, and the vertebral vein, which flows directly into the brachiocephalic. Among the more significant of the venous sinuses are the *cavernous sinus*, which lies near the sphenoid, the *sagittal sinus*, which courses along the superior aspect of the cerebrum, and the *transverse sinuses*, which lie in the occiput. Thrombosis of the venous sinuses does occur, but tends to cause far less overt damage than arterial thrombosis.

FUNCTIONAL SYSTEMS OF THE CNS

Although very little occurs within the CNS in isolation, it is helpful to understand neurological pathophysiology by viewing the functional areas of the CNS, to the exclusion of detail with regard to some specific individual structures. However, the complexity of the CNS means that all of its pieces are interconnected to some degree or another.

VOLUNTARY MOTOR CONTROL

Motor control in the nervous system can be either voluntary or involuntary (automatic). Voluntary motor control includes the *pyramidal*, or *corticospinal* motor system. The terms *pyramidal* and *extrapyramidal* are frequently used in neurology and can be somewhat confusing to students, particularly when emphasis is placed on the crossing-over point of the pyramidal tracts within the medulla. It is helpful to break down the compound word describing the tract itself—*corticospinal*. *Cortico* refers to the cerebral cortex, while *spinal* is fairly self-explanatory. Thus, *corticospinal* means from the top of the brain, down the spine, to the periphery. Thus, the pyramidal motor system is the primary voluntary motor control system in the human body.

The highest control center within the CNS over motor function is found in the cortex, specifically within the frontal lobe. The frontal lobe is separated from the parietal lobe by a deep sulcus known as the *central sulcus*. The last gyrus before the central sulcus is known as the *precentral gyrus*. This ridge of brain tissue contains *pyramidal* cells. The axons issuing forth from the cell bodies of these pyramidal cells are the only motor cells that don't synapse elsewhere on the way down through the body. They go directly through to the spine, down to the peripheral nervous system (PNS).

Certain areas of the precentral gyrus exert specific control over certain areas of the body. The homunculus is a conceptual humanoid diagram drawn over a picture of the precentral gyrus to help students to understand the functional regions of the gyrus itself. It is quite simplistic, but gives a reasonably accurate representation of what portion of the gyrus controls which portion of the body. Certain areas of the homunculus are almost comically stretched out to reflect large portions of the gyrus which are dedicated to specific areas of the body, particularly in the face and mouth.

Anterior to the precentral gyrus is the section of the cortex known as the *premotor cortex*. This region has greater control over the intent and higher thought surrounding voluntary movement, as well as learned patterns of complex voluntary motor repetition. Closer to the temporal lobe, but still within the frontal lobe, is Broca's area, a piece of frontal cortex that is responsible for the initiation of and physical formation of speech. Patients with damage to Broca's area are said to have an *expressive aphasia*, meaning that they can receptively understand speech, but may have difficulty forming it on their own. Voluntary eye movement is also controlled by the cortex of the frontal lobe.

The axons of the pyramidal neurons depart from the cortex and travel down through the cerebrum until they come together in an area known as the *internal capsule*. They then enter the *cerebral peduncles*, and move down the brainstem to the lower portion of the medulla. At this point, most of the fibers cross over to where they will enter the anterior horn of the spinal cord on the side contralateral to that from whence they originated in the cortex. This crossing over, or decussation, occurs at the pyramids of the medulla, which give the tract its name. It is because of this decussation that motor control of the body is controlled by the contralateral side of the brain.

Not all of the axons decussate here; some wait instead to cross over at the spinal cord. They are not significant to this text. At this point, it is valuable to mention upper and lower motor neurons. The axons extending from the pyramidal cells of the cortex end when they synapse with another neuron lower down the line whose axon will carry a nerve impulse to the PNS. The *upper motor neuron* describes the neuron in the cortex, as well as its axon all the way down to where it meets the synapsing neuron. The *lower motor neuron* describes the cell body that synapses with the cortical axon, and then sends its own axon out to the periphery.

The terms *upper* and *lower* are relative, and describe sequence, not position. There are upper motor neurons that terminate deep in the spinal cord, and lower motor neurons, such as those of the *corticobulbar tract* that innervates the face, which are found in the head. This can be of significant diagnostic consequence. Upper motor neuron lesions affect the *contralateral* side of the body, whereas lower motor neuron lesions affect the ipsilateral side of the body. A stroke is a perfect example of the difference here. Infarct of the motor cortex on the left side of the brain will cause paralysis on the right side of the body. This is an upper motor neuron lesion. Since the cranial nerves affected by this come after the point of decussation, there will be facial weakness on the opposite side of the body, the right side.

However, infarct that occurs in some areas of the posterior circulation can affect the lower motor neuron directly; thus, there will be weakness on the ipsilateral side of the face. Upper motor neuron lesions only tend to affect the lower half of the face as well, since the upper part and portions of the oropharynx are innervated by both sides of the brain. Lower motor neuron lesions, however, will wipe out an entire half of the face.

With regard to the periphery, upper motor neurons will not affect nerves that directly innervate skeletal muscle. Thus, there is no muscle wasting. A spastic paralysis will result in affected muscles with a great deal of tone. Conversely, flaccid paralysis with early muscle wasting occurs in muscles affected by lower motor neuron lesions.

EXTRAPYRAMIDAL MOTOR SYSTEM

The extrapyramidal motor system is the motor control system that describes everything but the voluntary process of the pyramidal system. It provides involuntary control of musculature for such purposes as maintaining muscle tone and muscular group stability. The extrapyramidal motor system is regulated by the cerebellum indirectly, through a multitude of nuclei buried deep within the white matter of the cortex. These nuclei play a role in stability, coordination, involuntary elimination of aberrant movement, and reflex coordination.

Many neurologic diseases affect these deep nuclei, and the symptoms that they cause are the result of disorderly movement or the loss of control and coordination of movement. A discussion of the specific anatomy and physiology of each of these nuclei and their tracts is unnecessary here. These *basal nuclei*, or *basal ganglia*, include the *caudate, putamen*, and *globus pallidus, red nucleus* and *substantia nigra* of the midbrain, the *subthalamic nucleus*, and to some extent, the *thalamus*. The putamen and globus pallidus are known collectively as the *lentiform nucleus*, and the caudate nucleus and putamen, when taken together, are often referred to as the *striatum*. The basal ganglia is a common site for intracerebral hemorrhage, particularly hypertensive bleeds.

Most critical care paramedics are already familiar with the "extrapyramidal effects" of certain medications, particularly antipsychotic medications such as thorazine derivatives. These may include athetosis, tardive dyskinesia, tremor, or other abnormal disorders of movement. Insults to these nuclei and the axonal tracts that extend from them are the origin of those side effects.

SENSATION

Working backward to the CNS in the other direction, sensory nerves that fill the dermis, muscle, and visceral structures of the body receive information concerning light touch, pain, pressure, stretching, and temperature. This information is passed along to the spinal nerve, and processed through the dorsal root ganglion. Proprioceptive information is also delivered in the same manner. A total of six tracts in the white matter of the spinal cord convey the information to the brain, and again a decussation occurs before the ultimate destination is reached, either in the spinal cord or at the medulla.

Interestingly, only four of these tracts result in higher awareness of specific or generalized sensation. There are two *spinocerebellar tracts* that end in the cerebellum and convey information about unconscious proprioception directly to it. Like the motor tracts, the spinocerebellar tracts have an upper and lower neuron component, called *first-* and *second-order neurons*. The remaining pathways, which contribute to conscious sensation, actually terminate in the thalamus, where a *third-order neuron* sends the information through an axon ultimately to the cortex. Remember that the thalamus serves as the ultimate filter and relay for all information ascending toward the cortex.

Just as the precentral gyrus of the frontal lobe controls motor responses, the *postcentral gyrus* of the parietal lobe, which abuts the central sulcus on the other side, is in control of sensation. There is a homunculus to correspond with the sensory strip of the brain, similar to that which belongs to the motor cortex.

The sensory strip of the postcentral gyrus conveys a rough idea of what is being perceived to the adjacent *somatosensory association area*, which occupies much of the parietal lobe. This area is then responsible for analysis of the information and extrapolation of important pieces of data that can help to define the sensation, much of which is taken from memory.

VISION

The second cranial nerves, the optic nerves, are comprised of axons coming from the retina at the rear of the eye. The optic nerves travel back to the *optic chiasma* where partial decussation occurs. The chiasma is located very near the circle of Willis. After decussation, the optic nerve synapses in the thalamus, which in turn relays the information to the occipital lobe, which is the portion of the brain primarily responsible for vision. As with the primary motor and somatosensory areas, the visual cortex of the occipital lobe is associated with a larger association area that helps to interpret rough images that the eye perceives.

HEARING

The eighth cranial nerve, the vestibulocochlear nerve, conducts auditory information via nuclei within the brainstem back to the auditory cortex, which is located in the temporal lobe, just beneath where the lateral sulcus divides the temporal from the parietal lobe. Interpretation of sound is accomplished by the adjacent auditory association area.

SMELL AND TASTE

The cortical areas involved with the processes of smell and taste are also located in the temporal lobe, which explains why olfactory and gustatory auras often precede seizures in susceptible persons, since seizure activity often originates in the temporal lobes.

AUTONOMIC REGULATION

The primary control of the autonomic nervous system is held by the hypothalamus. The hypothalamus regulates body temperature, thirst, sleep–wake cycles, blood pressure, heart rate, certain emotions, and endocrine activity. Other structures within the brain exert their own influence on the hypothalamus, such as regions of the cortex that deal with emotion and memory. The hypothalamus in turn regulates the reticular formation in the brainstem, which controls the oculomotor nerve (CN III), as well as basic physiological drives such as the heart rate, vascular tone, and respiratory rate.

The hypothalamus also transmits regulatory information to the spinal cord for more direct action on specific organ systems. Both sympathetic and parasympathetic nerves consist of two orders of neurons, and both issue forth from different regions of the spinal cord toward their target organs.

The sympathetic division of nerve fibers can be found in the thoracolumbar spine, arising from the lateral horns of the gray matter between T1 and L2. Fibers synapse *postganglionic* sympathetic nerve fibers in the *paravertebral ganglion*, located near the spinal cord. These fibers may travel to a different ganglion before synapsing and extending a longer postsynaptic fiber toward their target organ. The *preganglionic* fibers are mediated by the neurotransmitter *acetylcholine*, while the postganglionic fibers secrete the neurotransmitter *norepinephrine*. This neurotransmitter can have an inhibitory or excitatory response depending on the receptor type stimulated within the target organ. Receptors for the sympathetic autonomic nervous system (SANS) are known as *adrenergic* receptors and are separated into alpha and beta classes, depending on their action.

The parasympathetic autonomic nervous system's preganglionic fibers tend to be much longer than those of the SANS. The majority originate from the brainstem, while preganglionic parasympathetic fibers controlling the genitourinary system emerge from the sacral region of the spine, from S2 through S4. Second-order synapsing occurs very near the target organ. The vagus nerve alone is responsible for a tremendous amount of the parasympathetic control over the body, and divides into several nerve plexuses for control of specific organ systems. Both the presynaptic and postsynaptic ganglia secrete *acetylcholine*. The acetylcholine secreted by postsynaptic fibers will then have either an excitatory or inhibitory effect on affected organs by stimulation of one of two types of cholinergic receptors, known as the muscarinic and nicotinic receptors.

THOUGHT, EMOTION, AND MEMORY

Thought, emotion, and memory are among the highest and most complex of cortical functions, and are the processes that define us as human beings. It should be obvious by now that functional physiology within the brain is heavily interconnected. In other words, the autonomic nervous system, mediated by the hypothalamus, can be stimulated from fear caused by a cortical response to a memory held within the cortex. Cognitive function that occurs in the frontal lobe may be heavily influenced by visual images processed in the occipital lobe.

The anterior frontal lobes, known as the *prefrontal cortex*, are responsible for the majority of the intellectual processes that occur within the brain. However, a large portion of the cortex within the rest of the brain is also responsible for the analysis of sensory input, the integration of language, and the connection of emotion and memory.

The *limbic system* can be found deep to the cortex, encircling the diencephalon. Also known as the "emotional brain," this series of interconnected structures responds to a variety of physiological and sensory input to define the brain's response to emotion, and contributes heavily to the formation and integration of memory. The limbic system exerts control both intellectually, via the cortex, and physiologically, via such structures as the hypothalamus.

DIAGNOSIS OF NEUROLOGIC EMERGENCIES

As with the victim of CNS trauma, the neurologic examination remains the most important diagnostic tool that a clinician has for the assessment of neurologic emergencies. It is imperative that critical care paramedics practice and develop their clinical neurologic exam so that they can detect what are often subtle changes in presentation that have tremendous implications from a pathological standpoint.

DETAILED NEUROLOGIC ASSESSMENT

The approach to a patient with a possible neurologic problem should be systematic and comprehensive.

THE CONSCIOUS PATIENT

★ Determine if the patient can open his eyes. Does he acknowledge the examiner and track her movement?

★ Assess extraocular movement in all extremes of the visual field, noting abnormal findings including nystagmus or gaze restriction.

★ Cover each eye and assess for visual field deficit by asking the patient to look at your nose. Move your wiggling fingers into each of his four visual quadrants and ask him to identify when he can see them in his peripheral vision. Actual deficits in the visual fields are an important finding.

★ Ask the patient about the presence of visual changes. These can include numerous subjective complaints, such as blurred vision, diplopia (double vision), the perception of "floaters" (spots of light floating across the visual field), and loss of vision, either transient or ongoing, in any aspect of his visual field.

★ Assess facial symmetry.

★ Ask the patient to stick out his tongue and say "ah." Look for tongue deviation to one side or the other, as well as bilateral rise of the soft palate.

★ Ask the patient the standard questions of orientation. Be aware, however, that patients may be able to successfully answer these questions but can still be confused. Be alert to strange behavior, affect, repetitive questioning, or other indications of confusion.

★ Assess speech for clarity.

★ Aphasia may take several forms depending on the structures affected. Aphasia may be expressive (patient is unable to speak or formulate words clearly), receptive (patient is unable to understand speech), global (both receptive and expressive), or conductive (speech is fluent but dysphasic with inappropriate words, yet good comprehension).

★ Ask the patient to hold out his arms at shoulder height with his palms facing upward, and to close his eyes. This simultaneously assesses for motor weakness and a pronator drift. If unilateral weakness is detected, it can be further evaluated by other motor strength assessments. Pronator drift is specific to the cerebellum, and occurs when there is a loss of visual input to help maintain proprioception. One of the hands will invert, and will sink downward.

★ Further assess cerebellar ataxia in a nonambulatory patient by asking him to point his finger to his own nose, and then to reach out and touch your extended index finger in sequence. As you move your finger about to different positions, assess the patient for the inability to accurately localize your finger in space.

★ Assess the patient's hand grasp. Note, however, that hand grasps are a subjective indicator of motor strength and are not the most sensitive indicator of weakness. Be aware also of other limiting factors when assessing motor strength, such as pain, injury, or old deficit. Also, the grasp reflex is an infantile reflex that may reemerge in patients with substantial neurologic compromise and must not be mistaken for purposeful movement or the ability to follow commands.

★ Assess motor strength in the legs by asking the patient to lift them against resistance.

★ Ask the patient about parasthesias or other sensory abnormalities.

THE UNRESPONSIVE PATIENT

★ If the patient is not responsive, determine if he has been chemically paralyzed. If so, this greatly reduces the efficacy of your neurologic exam, since even cranial nerves are affected.

★ If the patient does not open his eyes, determine if there is a gaze preference, a disconjugate gaze, or strange eye movement noted. Repetitive or "roving" eye movements may be indicative of seizure activity.

★ Flick your hand toward the patient's face to elicit a reflexive blink. Does he "blink to threat"?

★ Watch for overt seizure activity. Any repetitive behavior or focal movement is suspicious for seizure activity.

★ Attempt to elicit a motor response with a brisk sternal rub. Patients who do not give a clear response to this should also be assessed by applying nail bed pressure to each extremity.

★ Assess the Babinski reflex by stroking the plantar surface of the foot with a rigid object. Toes that splay outward are a positive, and therefore abnormal, finding, except in very young children.

★ Assess for clonus by holding the plantar surface of the foot and rapidly dorsiflexing the ankle (assuming other injuries do not contraindicate this). If rhythmic jerking occurs, clonus is present and may indicate a seizure state or other abnormal tone.

★ If the patient is not sedated or chemically paralyzed, determine if he has spontaneous respirations.

★ Touch the surface of each eyeball with a sterile wisp of gauze and assess for a blink. This tests the presence or absence of a corneal reflex, and should be done bilaterally.

★ Insert a rigid tonsil tip suction catheter into the patient's oropharynx and assess both sides for the presence of a gag reflex.

★ Determine if the patient coughs on his endotracheal tube, or if he has a cough reflex in response to deep tracheal suctioning.

★ Determine if there is CSF drainage from the ears, nose, or from a surgically placed drain. This holds a potentially severe potential for infection.

DIAGNOSTIC IMAGING

The diagnostic tests and imaging studies performed in the assessment of neurologic emergencies are essentially identical to those performed on the trauma patient. However, certain exams are utilized more frequently or in different ways than in the trauma population, so a quick review is in order.

Advances in diagnostic imaging have significantly changed and improved care of neurologic patients.

COMPUTED TOMOGRAPHY (CT) SCAN

As in the trauma patient, the CT scan is the most fundamental imaging study utilized, allowing a fast but detailed assessment of the brain tissue and bony structures. The CT scan can be augmented by injecting a dye that allows imaging of the cerebral vasculature. This combination CT-angiogram is highly sensitive for detecting the presence of aneurysms, arteriovenous malformations, and occluded vessels when read by an experienced radiologist.

MAGNETIC RESONANCE IMAGING (MRI)

MRI is a lengthier and more involved exam than the CT scan, but is far more effective at assessing the characteristics of brain tissue. Like the CT scan, the use of different types of contrast medium can allow for sophisticated histologic assessment and the visualization of cerebral vasculature. Changes in brain tissue pathology that are too acute to be seen in a CT, such as in the case of a very fresh infarction, can be seen with an MRI.

CEREBRAL ANGIOGRAPHY

Specialized physicians can view cerebral vasculature directly with the use of cerebral angiography. This procedure is similar to performing an angiogram of the heart. Facilities with advanced neuroradiological teams can manipulate the cerebral vasculature by injecting drugs directly into them, or by inserting devices to close off aneurysms.

TRANSCRANIAL DOPPLER ULTRASOUND

This technique utilizes an ultrasonic probe that is placed on the outside of the patient's skull. The ultrasound records the velocity of blood flow through the cerebral arteries, and can be a sensitive indicator for cerebral vasospasm.

ELECTROENCEPHALOGRAM (EEG)

An EEG device measures brain wave activity, and is often used to detect seizure activity in patients.

LUMBAR PUNCTURE

A lumbar puncture involves the insertion of a needle into the subarachnoid space of the patient's spine to collect CSF for analysis and to assess for elevated ICP.

OTHER STUDIES

Numerous other diagnostic tools are available such as the PET scan, which measures the metabolism of certain nutrients by the brain tissue, evoked electrical potential, myelography, and others.

SECONDARY INJURY IN THE NEUROLOGIC PATIENT

The central nervous system reacts to hypoperfusion and hypoxia the same way in the neuromedical patient as it does in the trauma patient. As such, regardless of the mechanism, the patterns of histopathologic secondary brain injury are the same. Infarcted tissue will become edematous and swell just as contused tissue will. Bleeds that are atraumatic in origin, such as from a ruptured aneurysm, are just as dangerous and have the same sequelae as bleeds that are caused by trauma; in some cases, bleeds of an atraumatic origin can be more dangerous.

The trauma principles of the prevention of secondary injury, ICP monitoring and treatment, and maintenance of cerebral perfusion pressure (CPP) apply to the neuromedical patient. Some neurologic emergencies have greater predisposition to certain types of secondary injuries than others, and some have other complications of their own above and beyond those seen in the trauma population. Above all else, the critical care paramedic must be vigilant for change and further injury regardless of the original etiology.

CEREBROVASCULAR DISORDERS

ACUTE ISCHEMIC STROKE

Until quite recently, the victim of an acute stroke had few options available for treatment. Care was primarily preventive and supportive in nature, and little could be done to reverse the neurologic deficits caused by infarction. The development of clot-busting drugs, however, has brought new hope for many stroke patients whose deficits can be greatly reduced or even eliminated if they are treated with alacrity. In addition, new research is being performed to explore the efficacy of alternative treatments, such as therapeutic hypothermia and high-pressure, high-oxygen hyperbaric therapy.

The risk factors for ischemic stroke are the same as those for cardiovascular disease, as is the mechanism of infarction. Hypertension, hyperlipidemia, diabetes mellitus, smoking, obesity, and genetic predisposition may contribute to atherosclerotic changes in the cerebral vasculature just as they do elsewhere in the body. This causes narrowing of the vascular lumen and the formation of blood clots. Other risk factors for infarction include an elevated hematocrit, which may occur in polycythemia vera, or hypercoagulable states, as may occur in systemic inflammation. The use of oral contraceptives, prolonged airplane or car trips, and valvular dysfunction of the heart also elevate the risk for thromboembolic stroke. Patients with chronic atrial fibrillation, particularly those who are improperly anticoagulated, as well as younger patients with a persistent patent foramen ovale, are also at risk for embolic stroke (Figure 23-3 ■).

On a cellular level, ischemia causes a transition to anaerobic metabolism, which produces damaging by-products such as lactate (Figure 23-4 ■). Anaerobic glycolysis does not generate sufficient adenosine triphosphate (ATP) to provide energy for the active transport of the sodium-potassium pump across the cell membrane, and hence intracellular accumulation of sodium occurs. Extracellular water moves into the cell to maintain the osmotic gradient, and cellular edema and death occur (Figure 23-5 ■).

The long-term neurologic effects of acute ischemic stroke may be reduced by aggressive treatment (Figure 23-6 ■). In a given area of infarction, there are two clinically significant regions, the zone of infarction and penumbra. The **zone of infarction** is essentially the locus of the infarction, and is comprised of brain tissue that will become necrotic in the absence of perfusion. Surrounding the infarction is a larger area known as the **penumbra,** (Figure 23-7 ■) which consists of brain tissue that is threatened with cellular death from hypoperfusion, but that may be spared with timely treatment. The new mantra with regard to care of the acute stroke patient is that "Time Is Brain." This slogan emphasizes the importance of seeking early, definitive care for the ischemic stroke

zone of infarction   *a component of ischemic stroke, describes the area of brain tissue distal to an occluded vessel, and without collateral circulation.*

penumbra   *describes a region of tissue that will become necrotic after an infarct occurs if perfusion is not restored.*

■ Figure 23-3   Causes of stroke.

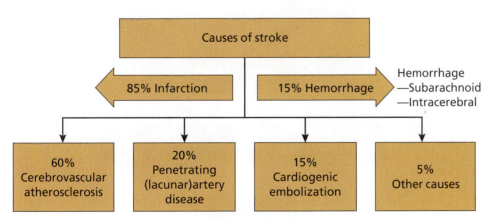

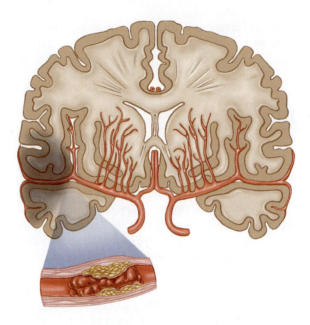

Figure 23-4 Ischemic stroke resulting from thrombosis or embolization of middle cerebral artery.

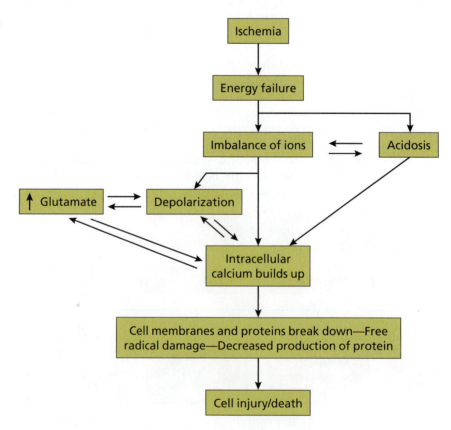

patient to reduce damage to the penumbra, preserve neurologic function, and attempt to restore perfusion quickly if fibrinolytic therapy is indicated.

As with all neurologic disorders, the signs and symptoms, as well as the prognostic outlook, depend on the area of brain tissue affected by hypoperfusion and secondary changes. Of particular importance in the majority of the population is the region of the brain perfused by the left middle cerebral artery (left MCA). The MCAs on both sides of the circle of Willis are responsible for perfusing the majority of the lateral aspects of the frontal, temporal, and parietal lobes. The speech centers of the brain are contained in the left MCA distribution of the temporal lobe in all patients who

Fibrinolytic therapy for stroke remains controversial.

Figure 23-5 Pathogenesis of stroke.

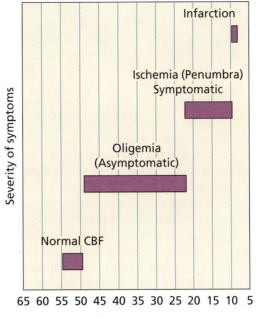

■ **Figure 23-6** Cerebral blood flow thresholds.

Severity of symptoms

Infarction

Ischemia (Penumbra)
Symptomatic

Oligemia
(Asymptomatic)

Normal CBF

65 60 55 50 45 40 35 30 25 20 15 10 5

CBF in mL/100 g/min

are left hemisphere dominant. Damage to the speech centers of the brain may result in the inability to express or understand speech. This can have devastating implications for patients after the acute phase of illness has passed. The majority of the population has left hemisphere dominance, including those who consider themselves to be "right-brained" by virtue of their habits or preferences. All persons with right-handed dominance and roughly 75% to 85% of people with left-handed dominance are left cerebral hemisphere dominant. With a thorough understanding of the

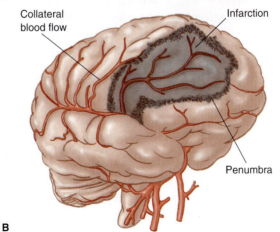

■ **Figure 23-7** Penumbra. A) At orgin of arterial blockage. B) Global effect.

Collateral flow

Penumbra

Infarction

Thrombus

A

Collateral blood flow

Infarction

Penumbra

B

anatomy and physiology of the brain, as well as its vasculature, a knowledgeable critical care provider can predict, with a reasonable degree of accuracy, the region of vascular involvement based solely on the clinical exam. This will allow for early anticipation of a patient's specific treatment needs and prognosis. The following sections review some of the common clinical findings with specific stroke syndromes with regard to specific vessels affected.

MIDDLE CEREBRAL ARTERY (MCA)

The MCA is a large vessel, the primary tributary of the internal carotid. It perfuses much of the frontal lobe, as well as the lateral aspects of the temporal and parietal lobes. As mentioned earlier, MCA occlusion in the dominant hemisphere of the brain, statistically the left MCA, can cause infarction of the speech centers. Proximal, or total, MCA occlusion will cause contralateral hemiplegia and hemisensory loss, global aphasia (if on the dominant side), and a contralateral upper motor neuron facial weakness, and can also cause an ipsilateral gaze preference (eyes look toward the lesion), as well as a homonymous hemianopia in the visual fields contralateral to the side of the lesion. Damage to the speech centers also tends to correlate with damage to the motor function governing a patient's oral motor mechanics. These patients can remain at a high risk for aspiration from loss of control over their oropharynx, and may require enteral feeding on a permanent basis.

MCA infarction can result in significant edema and secondary injury. The degree of deficit resulting from infarct depends on the amount of tissue involved, which directly correlates to the proximity of the lesion to the circle of Willis. As the MCA travels superiorly, it branches into separate vessels. Infarction of more distal aspects of the vessel will result in similar but less severe or incomplete deficits.

ANTERIOR CEREBRAL ARTERY (ACA)

The ACA perfuses the medial aspects of the temporal and parietal lobes of the brain, near the midline, as well as much of the frontal lobes. Occlusion of the ACA can cause contralateral lower extremity weakness, as well as intellectual and behavioral changes from frontal lobe involvement.

POSTERIOR CEREBRAL ARTERY (PCA)

A number of stroke syndromes are based on the loss of the posterior circulation. Involvement of the occipital lobe can contribute to visual or visual accessory loss, including the loss of ability to see in all quadrants of the visual field or to understand written language. There is a bizarre phenomenon known as "cortical blindness" that occurs as the result of either bilateral PCA occlusion or occlusion of the basilar tip, whereby a patient's visual processing cortex is wiped out. However, the patient will actually be unaware of the fact that he cannot see, and his pupils will react normally to changing light. The patient is completely blind, but is in denial of or completely unaware of the fact.

Deeper structural involvement in PCA occlusion affecting the thalamus can cause contralateral hemisensory loss, and the involvement of pyramidal motor tracts can cause contralateral hemiplegia.

VERTEBRAL AND BASILAR ARTERIES

Involvement of these large vessels can be catastrophic. A wide variety of clinical syndromes are associated with vertebrobasilar arterial occlusion, reflective of these arteries' involvement with the brainstem. Varying degrees of motor and sensory loss can occur. Infarction of the entire pons can result in a phenomenon known as "locked-in syndrome." This syndrome refers to the fact that the subcortical pyramidal motor tract is essentially wiped out, as well as many of the cranial nerves. However, there is "cortical sparing," as well as sparing of the structures controlling the reticular activating system. The result is complete, total-body loss of motor control with the exception of minimal extraocular movement and aphasia. However, the patient remains completely awake, aware, and intellectually intact. Moreover, he experiences no sensory loss. Thus, he becomes a thinking, feeling brain trapped inside of, or "locked in," a nonfunctioning body.

CEREBELLAR ARTERIES

Infarction of the cerebellar arteries can also result in a constellation of symptoms depending on the precise structures involved. In general, these tend to include both contralateral and ipsilateral patterns of ataxia, motor weakness, sensory deficit, and vertigo. Because the cerebellum resides in the relatively small posterior fossa of the skull, and in proximity to the brainstem, edema subsequent to infarct can rapidly cause herniation and death.

Critical care paramedics may encounter patients who demonstrate evidence of *lacunar infarction syndromes*. These are syndromes caused by patterns of small infarctions and areas of neuronal necrosis within the deep white matter structures of the brain. Lacunar infarcts tend not to be as severe as infarcts of larger vessels, but will present with similar symptoms, and can often be heralded by transient ischemic attacks (TIAs). Motor, sensory, and movement disorders may be seen, such as the "dysarthria/clumsy hand" syndrome, whereby patients suffering from lacunar infarct can have facial muscle paresis, and unilateral ataxia, particularly with regard to fine motor dexterity in the hand.

Watershed infarction is another term that critical care paramedics may encounter in the critical care environment. This describes numerous small areas of infarcted tissue at the periphery of the smallest extensions of the cerebral arteries. The "watershed" of the cerebrum may be visualized as tissue that is most vulnerable to hypoperfusion because of its peripheral distribution and lack of collateral circulation. Generalized hypoperfusion of this distal tissue, such as in diffuse vasospasm, may cause a syndrome of watershed infarction.

Thromboembolic strokes cannot be differentiated from hemorrhagic strokes without a CT scan. The signs and symptoms of each are far too similar to allow for clinical differentiation without the benefit of imaging studies. However, in the case of any and all apparent cerebrovascular accidents or TIAs, the patients should be considered potential candidates for fibrinolytic therapy until proven otherwise. As such, each patient should be screened for risk factors and contraindications for fibrinolytic therapy, and transported to an appropriate facility as quickly as possible. Special emphasis should be placed on attempting to pinpoint the timing of the onset of symptoms, because this information can be crucial to determining the eligibility of a thromboembolic stroke patient for fibrinolysis.

The degree of deficit caused by stroke should be assessed according to the National Institute of Health Stroke Scale (NIHSS). This tool was developed to allow an objective evaluation of the severity of stroke symptoms based on the patient's level of consciousness, motor and sensory function, and degree of cognitive impairment. The NIHSS provides an extremely detailed assessment and should be familiar to critical care paramedics, since many treatment decisions are often based heavily on it. The Cincinnati Stroke Scale is another effective means of determining the presence of neurologic deficit. The Cincinnati Stroke Scale evaluates for the presence or absence of a facial droop, arm weakness, and the clarity of speech. Any abnormal finding is considered to be evidence of intracerebral pathology.

Fibrinolytic Therapy

The primary purpose of fibrinolytic therapy is the dissolution of thromboembolic clots that have caused infarction of tissue perfused by the vessel that they have occluded. The intent of this therapy is to minimize or eliminate the necrosis of hypoperfused tissue, thereby preserving the function of that tissue. In the case of the acute stroke patient, successful fibrinolysis translates into the preservation of neurons and improvement in functional outcome. Because neuronal necrolysis occurs quickly in event of infarction, it is imperative that fibrinolytic therapy be initiated within a very narrow time frame after the onset of symptoms.

Successful fibrinolysis in the acute stroke patient within an appropriate time frame has been proven to contribute to a dramatic reduction in neurologic morbidity. However, the therapeutic properties of such fibrinolytic drugs as tissue plasminogen activator (tPA) also make them extremely dangerous, and inappropriate administration can have disastrous consequences. The decision to pursue fibrinolytic therapy must be carefully weighed, because the potential for adverse effects is significant. The potential for catastrophic and even fatal bleeding is very real, and the potential benefit of successful therapy must be considered with regard to the risk involved on a case-by-case basis. Patients and their families should form the foundation of the decision-making team to go forward with fibrinolytic therapy whenever possible.

Because the time frame for fibrinolysis in the acute stroke patient is so short, the need for critical care providers to understand its use and administration is extremely high. Furthermore, it is vital that eligible recipients be identified in a timely fashion. The following lists detail inclusion and exclusion criteria found in many fibrinolytic protocols. The guidelines are general and are based on an assessment of several institutional protocols, but are not representative of any official recommendation.

The patient MUST:

★ Be between 18 and 75 years of age

★ Have a clinical diagnosis of stroke with significant neurologic compromise to warrant the risk of fibrinolytic therapy

★ Have symptoms with a definite onset of less than 3 hours prior to the initiation of fibrinolytic therapy

★ Have a CT scan that demonstrates the absence of any sort of intracranial hemorrhage (ICH)

The patient MUST NOT:

★ Have deficits that are improving without treatment

★ Have a CT that demonstrates any suggestion of ICH

★ Have a history of ICH or known aneurysm

★ Have had a seizure when symptoms began

★ Have had a stroke or serious head injury within the prior **3 months**

★ Have a history of IV drug abuse

★ Be under the influence of cocaine

★ Have undergone major surgery or sustained major trauma within the prior **2 weeks**

★ Have suffered gastrointestinal or genitourinary hemorrhage within the prior **3 weeks**

★ Require ongoing aggressive treatment to lower blood pressure

★ Have sustained an arterial puncture at a noncompressible site or lumbar puncture within **1 week**

★ Have undergone heparin therapy **within 48 hours**

★ Have evidence of pericarditis

★ Have a known bleeding diathesis

★ Be pregnant or breast-feeding

The following vital signs are recommended exclusion criteria:

★ Systolic BP > 185 mmHg

★ Diastolic BP > 110 mmHg

The following laboratory values are also recommended as exclusion criteria:

★ Serum glucose < 50 mg/dL or > 400 mg/dL

★ Platelet count < 100,000 /uL

★ Patients currently on anticoagulant therapy with prothrombin time (PT) > 15 seconds or International Normalized Ratio (INR) > 1.7

Tissue plasminogen activator is generally administered at a dose of 0.9 mg/kg, with a maximum dose of 90 mg. Ten percent of the total dose should be administered as a bolus loading dose, with the rest of the total dose infused during the following 60 minutes.

Systemic blood pressure should be tightly controlled after the administration of tPA to minimize the risk of hemorrhage. These patients do not receive additional antithrombotic infusions such as heparin while under the effects of tPA.

Studies have been done to explore the administration of other agents beyond the 3-hour window, up to 6 hours after the onset and beyond. However, generally only intra-arterial tPA will be employed after 3 hours have passed. Clinical evidence of a large ischemic stroke on CT is also cited as a reason NOT to administer fibrinolytic therapy, since extensive changes on CT take time to arise, and are therefore reflective of an event that occurred longer than 3 hours prior.

Patients who do not receive fibrinolysis should receive antiplatelet therapy in the form of aspirin, clopidogrel (Plavix), or similar agents.

Some patients at advanced centers may benefit from the administration of intra-arterial fibrinolysis if major arteries such as the MCA or basilar artery are occluded. This must occur within 6 hours from the onset of symptoms, and must be performed by specially trained physicians utilizing angiography. This is a very experimental therapy, however, with significant risks.

Critical care paramedics who may be responsible for administering and monitoring tPA infusions should review their governing protocols exhaustively. Invasive procedures including the insertion of IV catheters and urinary catheters should be avoided if at all possible after fibrinolytic therapy is begun, and careful physiological monitoring is essential.

HEMORRHAGIC STROKE

Cerebral aneurysm (Figure 23-8 ■) and arteriovenous malformation rupture can cause injury to brain tissue in three primary ways. The first of these is the mass effect of the blood itself, depending on the size and location of the bleed. The second is hypoperfusion in the region of the brain that the compromised vascular structure had supplied. The third mechanism of injury is through cerebral vasospasm.

The major arteries of the brain are contained within the subarachnoid space. Thus, arterial bleeding within the brain from aneurismal or **arteriovenous malformation** (AVM) rupture causes a subarachnoid hemorrhage (SAH) (Figure 23-9 ■). The ventricles of the brain are contiguous with the subarachnoid space, and thus the term *intraventricular hemorrhage (IVH)* may also be used, depending on CT findings. The duration of the active bleeding itself tends to be quite short—often only a few seconds of bleeding actually occurs postrupture. The severity of SAH can be graded with a variety of grading scales. Two of the most common, the Fisher and the Hunt and Hess scales, are

arteriovenous malformation (AVM) *a vascular abnormality caused by the abnormal anastomosis of veins and arteries; a tortuous collection of structurally weak veins and arteries that are vulnerable to rupture.*

■ Figure 23-8 Examples of various types of aneurysms affecting the circle of Willis and adjoining vessels.

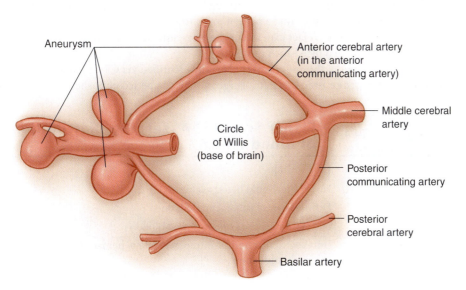

Aneurysm

Anterior cerebral artery (in the anterior communicating artery)

Middle cerebral artery

Circle of Willis (base of brain)

Posterior communicating artery

Posterior cerebral artery

Basilar artery

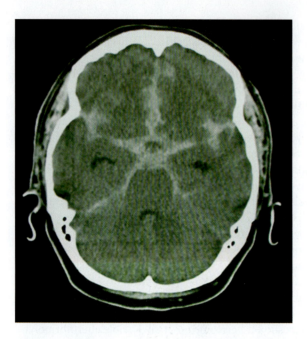

Figure 23-9 CT of subarachnoid hemorrhage. Note blood around circle of Willis and associated vessels.

shown in Tables 23–1 and 23–2, respectively. The Fisher scale describes blood pattern distribution, whereas the Hunt and Hess scale has more direct prognostic implications. The higher the grade on the Hunt and Hess scale, the worse the prognosis.

When blood spills into the subarachnoid space it mixes with the CSF, and can quickly overwhelm the capacity of the arachnoid villi to reabsorb CSF into the venous sinuses. This occurs both as the result of volume increase and mechanical obstruction from clotting. The result is an often rapidly developing hydrocephalus that requires rapid correction via the insertion of an extraventricular drain (EVD). The EVD is covered extensively in Chapter 14, "Neurologic Trauma."

The classic presentation of patients suffering a subarachnoid hemorrhage is that of an individual complaining of "the worst headache of my life" or a "thunderclap" headache. The use of either of these terms should be a red flag to the clinician. Some patients with subarachnoid hemorrhage will present with seizures, unconsciousness, or a decreased level of consciousness, or may in fact die before reaching a hospital. Localizing symptoms such as focal motor weakness are possible, depending on the vascular territory affected. Patients who are awake enough to provide subjective symptoms may also complain of neck pain and stiffness (subsequent to meningeal irritation), photophobia, and nausea.

Unsecured bleeds are inclined to bleed again, particularly if the systemic blood pressure is raised. Thus, it may be possible that a patient presenting with an SAH with a recent prior history of unevaluated symptoms is in fact experiencing a worsening of an existing bleed, or even complications from an undetected bleed such as vasospasm.

In aneurysmal SAH, the aneurysm is generally identified via CT-angiography or similar diagnostic tool and is then secured by a neurosurgeon. This can be accomplished either by the direct ap-

Great strides have been made in the care of certain types of acute stroke.

Table 23–1	Fisher Scale for Assessing Distribution of Blood on CT
Fisher Grade	**CT Findings**
I	No subarachnoid blood visible on CT
II	Diffuse layer of subarachnoid blood
III	Localized region of subarachnoid blood
IV	Intraventricular and/or intraparenchymal hematoma and subarachnoid blood

Table 23-2	Hunt and Hess Scale for Assessing Prognosis Based on Clinical Presentation

Hunt and Hess Grade	Clinical Presentation at Onset
I	Minimal headache and/or nuchal rigidity
II	Moderate headache and/or nuchal rigidity and cranial nerve involvement
III	Lethargy, confusion, and focal motor deficit
IV	Stupor, hemiparesis, extension rigidity
V	Deep coma

plication of a surgical clip or myelin wrapping at the base of the aneurysm, or through interventional angiography via the insertion of coils or a gluelike substance that fills the aneurysm and causes it to clot off.

It has been well documented that aneurysmal rupture can cause indirect damage to the myocardium, ranging from benign ECG changes to myocardial infarction and the development of lethal dysrhythmias. The mechanism for this is believed to be the sudden rush of catecholamines that accompanies aneurysmal rupture. Young, otherwise healthy patients may present with severe left ventricular wall dysfunction, elevated troponin levels, and markedly decreased cardiac output. Patients may present with cardiovascular collapse, including hypotension and florid pulmonary edema. Vasopressors and invasive hemodynamic monitoring may become necessary until the patient stabilizes. If the patient can survive this episode of myocardial "stunning," there is generally a dramatic improvement within days or weeks.

Patients who experience a subarachnoid hemorrhage are at further risk for the development of vasospasm, which holds the potential for devastating secondary injury. *Vasospasm* occurs when blood comes into contact with the outside walls of the brain's arterial blood supply. The blood acts as an irritant, which causes a reflexive spasm of the smooth muscle in the vessel wall, causing a marked decrease in the diameter of the vessel lumen. This process may continue throughout the length of the cerebral arterial system in severe cases. Vasospasm can cause severe hypoperfusion to all distal tissue fed by the affected arterial structures, which can lead to infarction. Large areas of infarction can cause cytoxic cerebral edema, which causes an increase in ICP with a subsequent decrease in CPP, resulting in less perfusion and even wider zones of infarction. Thus, severe cases can perpetuate themselves in an unfortunate cascade that ultimately leads to the functional loss of perfusion to the brain and diffuse neuronal destruction.

Vasospasm does not occur in all cases of subarachnoid hemorrhage, and its severity is equally unpredictable. Interestingly, it does not tend to occur in cases of traumatic SAH.

Transcranial Doppler studies can help to gauge the severity of vasospasm at the bedside. Isolated elevations in the velocity of blood flow through cerebral arteries represent potentially spastic arteries. However, abnormally high values can occur in the absence of vasospasm. Thus, the ratio of the velocity of blood traveling through the MCA to that traveling through the vertebral artery is compared, resulting in the Lindegaard ratio, a determinant of vasospasm severity.

Lindegaard Ratio	Severity of Vasospasm
<3	Normal
3–6	Mild vasospasm
>6	Severe vasospasm

The typical range of onset varies from 3 to 21 days, although cases may persist even beyond this point. It tends to peak between days 8 and 12. Calcium channel blockers such as nimodipine, which is more pharmadynamically specific for cerebral vasculature, are currently being utilized in an effort to decrease the incidence and severity of vasospasm in patients with SAH who are deemed at risk for it. These patients are also regularly monitored with transcranial Doppler ultrasound (TCD), because an increase in the velocity of blood through the narrowed arteries may be one of the first signs of impending vasospasm. Vasospasm is also frequently heralded by deterioration of the patient's neurologic exam, and often presents as increasingly erratic or impulsive behavior in the otherwise cognitively intact patient. Cerebral angiography is considered to be the gold standard of assessment for vasospasm, because it allows for direct visualization of the vasculature itself.

Treatment for vasospasm is primarily intended to ensure adequate perfusion in spite of compromised vasculature. Although controversial and disputed in some research, one strategy for therapy is intended to *h*ypertense, *h*ypervolumize, and *h*emodilute. This so-called "Triple-H" or "HHH" therapy helps to force blood into areas that are being hypoperfused. Patients undergoing HHH therapy should ideally have invasive ICP, arterial line, and central venous pressure monitoring. They receive large volumes of isotonic fluid, often in the form of colloids such as albumin, to maintain a hyperdynamic fluid balance state. This therapy is often titrated to a target central venous pressure to ensure that adequate fluid volume is being maintained. In addition, patients are often placed on vasopressor agents to artificially elevate their systolic and mean arterial pressures. These patients may have perfusion-dependent neurologic function that warrants systolic blood pressure goals as high as 200 mmHg. ICP monitoring and management are essential to observe the patient's CPP; however, hypoperfusion can still occur in the presence of normal CPP values when patients are severely compromised by vasospasm.

Triple-H therapy can be extremely dangerous, particularly in patients who have poor cardiovascular health, either as the result of preexisting comorbidities or from the stunned myocardium that can occur with SAH. Patients may require pulmonary arterial line insertion to monitor fluid balance and cardiac output. High doses of vasopressor agents may be required, many of which have significant side effects. The forced increase in cerebral blood flow may also precipitate an increase in ICP in patients with poor compliance subsequent to space-occupying lesions such as cerebral edema.

Patients with advanced vasospasm may be candidates for direct intra-arterial injection of calcium channel blocking medication similar to nimodipine in specialized facilities. This is most effective for the opening of focal areas of severe spasm, and its effects generally last for about 48 hours. Focal infarction that results in substantial cerebral edema may necessitate surgical decompression via hemicraniectomy with bone flap removal, as detailed in the neurologic trauma chapter. Medical treatment such as the administration of mannitol or hypertonic saline may also be indicated. Ultimately, patients with SAH complicated by vasospasm are critically ill, and their recovery depends on the amount of damage that occurs as the result of secondary injury.

INTRACEREBRAL HEMORRHAGE

Intracerebral hemorrhage occurs when blood vessels running through the brain tissue itself bleed, causing hematoma formation that can occasionally extend into the subarachnoid space or ventricles. The hemorrhage may result from a previously unknown arteriovenous malformation or other vascular defect (Figure 23-10 ■). Generally, in the neuromedical patient, these injuries occur as the result of hypertension and hypertensive crises. Most patients with ICH of a hypertensive origin will have the bleed occur deep in the white matter, near the basal ganglion. Unfortunately, these patients are not candidates for surgical correction. If an ICH occurs focally in a more superficial area of the brain, a neurosurgeon may be able to evacuate it.

Patients with an ICH who do not have a clear history of hypertension may suffer from amyloid angiopathy, a vascular disorder whereby amyloid is deposited in the vessel walls of the cerebral vasculature. This process weakens patients and can form "microaneurysms," leaving them susceptible to hemorrhage. Cerebral amyloid angiopathy may also lead to dementia. Bleeds caused by amyloid angiopathy tend to be more superficial than those caused by hypertension, and there is a high incidence of recurrence.

Patients who sustain an intracerebral hemorrhage are at risk for a variety of secondary injuries, depending on the location of the lesion. Local mass effect can cause herniation and hydrocephalus, and supportive treatment is dictated by the patient's clinical presentation. Care should be taken to

Time is brain tissue!

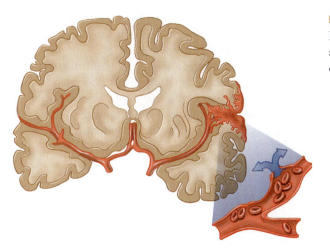

keep the mean arterial pressure at a safe limit to prevent rebleeding and extension, although the fundamental tenets of CPP maintenance take precedent.

INFECTIOUS PROCESSES

MENINGITIS

The meninges covering the brain and spinal cord may become inflamed if exposed to infectious agents, including a variety of bacteria and viruses. The overall mortality and morbidity of patients with meningitis depends heavily on the etiology, as well as secondary complications, speed of onset, and alacrity of treatment.

The homeostatic balance present within the CNS depends on the integrity of the protection offered by the intact bone and meningeal structures, as well as the blood–brain barrier. If these defenses are breached, however, the CNS has a poor capacity to respond to infection. Any patient with an open avenue for infection is at high risk for meningitis or ventriculitis, which is an inflammation of the ventricles of the brain. These patients include those with skull fractures, CSF leaks, and extraventricular drains. In addition, certain patients with predisposing illnesses or conditions are at higher risk. Patients who have a recent history of mild bacterial or viral illness, or those with chronic illness such as HIV or tuberculosis, and who present with meningitic symptoms should be held with a high index of suspicion for meningitis by care providers.

The hallmark signs of meningitis are a high fever and headache, neck, or back pain. There is a high incidence of changes in the level of consciousness, as well as nausea, vomiting, photophobia, and seizure activity. Any febrile patient who complains of a headache or neck pain should be regarded as having a high potential for meningitis.

Meningococcal meningitis may present with a purpuric or petechial rash, particularly over the lower extremities. Although certain bacteria such as *Neisseria meningitidis, Streptococcus pneumoniae, Haemophilus influenzae*, and *Klebsiella pneumoniae* are most commonly implicated, meningitis may be caused by any number of bacterial agents. Immunocompromised patients are highly susceptible to opportunistic infections. Patients with tuberculosis may suffer meningitic infection when the disease spreads to different areas of the CNS in the form of metastatic foci that may lie subclinically dormant for long periods of time.

Spirochettal agents such as syphilis, Lyme disease, and the zoonose *Leptospira interrogans*, as well as protozoan agents such as toxoplasmosis and malaria, may also cause meningitis. Viral etiological agents include mumps, herpes, and the Epstein-Barr virus, among others. Viral infections are the most frequent cause of meningitis, and the offending agent may not be identifiable from CSF culture.

Meningeal inflammation may cause mechanical obstruction of CSF flow, which can be exacerbated by the presence of purulent material in the CSF. This may lead to hydrocephalus. Meningitis may also cause vascular inflammation that can predispose patients to infarction, as well as secondary infection in the form of cerebral abscess or septicemia. Direct involvement of the cranial nerves may lead to permanent damage, including blindness.

Anyone with a suspicion of meningitis will require a CT scan to rule out other differential diagnoses, as well as a lumbar puncture for CSF analysis. Blood cultures should also be obtained, and the administration of antibiotics should be an early and emergent priority where bacterial meningitis is considered. Respiratory precautions should be instituted at the earliest suspicion of meningitis, because some forms can be highly contagious.

Some forms of meningitis are highly contagious.

ENCEPHALITIS

The term *encephalitis* describes inflammation of the brain parenchyma as the result of viral exposure. Viral encephalitis presents clinically with high fever, changes in mental status, and possible nausea, vomiting, and seizures. The most common source in the United States is herpes simplex virus. Cytomegalovirus is also relatively common in severely immunocompromised patients, as is toxoplasmosis, an obligate intracellular protozoan infection that can lead to the development of focal lesions. Other viral origins of encephalitis include mumps and the Epstein-Barr virus. The threat of mosquito-borne encephalitis is growing in the forms of the Eastern Equine and West Nile viruses, which are become increasingly endemic in certain areas of the country.

Parenchymal inflammation can cause elevated ICP and diffuse cerebral edema, as well as hydrocephalus. Care is supportive, although azithromycin can be administered to patients with herpes encephalitis by way of antiviral treatment. The mortality and morbidity of these diseases is dependent on the causative agent and the overall health of the patient prior to illness.

BACTERIAL INFECTION OF THE BRAIN

Bacterial infections within the brain do not cause diffuse encephalitis, but instead tend to occur as localized abscesses. These may occur singly or multiply anywhere inside the skull, including the epidural and subdural spaces. They can be the result of local infection, such as in an open skull fracture or surgical incision, or they may spread from other areas of the body through the blood. Cerebral abscesses may give rise to other abscesses, or may cause meningeal involvement. In addition, they are space-occupying lesions that can cause elevated ICP, mass effect, and herniation. They are generally treated with antibiotics, as well as surgical evacuation or removal.

CNS INFECTION IN IMMUNOCOMPROMISED PATIENTS

A disproportionately high number of dangerous CNS infections occurs in immunocompromised patients and are worthy of mention here. Toxoplasmosis is an infection resulting in single or multiple cerebral abscesses that is caused by exposure in immune-deficient persons to an intracellular protozoon. It may also be associated with meningitis and encephalitis, and is treated with antimicrobial agents.

Cytomegalovirus is a herpes-related virus that is a common cause of encephalitis in AIDS patients. Cryptococcal encephalitis is caused by a fungal pathogen. Antiviral and antimicrobial medication, respectively, can be used to treat these infections, in addition to supportive care. Signs and symptoms depend on the location and extent of CNS involvement. Other structures may be affected as well, including the peripheral nervous system, GI tract, and other organ systems. Mental status changes in immunocompromised patients may be the result of any number of opportunistic infections or neoplasms, and require an extensive workup.

CNS TUMORS

Tumors of the central nervous system are not uncommon and can vary from being highly malignant to totally benign.

BRAIN TUMORS

Brain tumors may be primary lesions or metastatic lesions originating from a primary cancer at another site. Tumors may be benign or malignant, depending on their histological origin, the speed of growth and infiltration, and the degree of cellular differentiation. This holds true for tumors in any part of the body; however, tumors that can be histologically classified as "benign" may in fact be fatal or cause severe neurologic impairment to a patient by virtue of their location, as well as from the secondary complications that can arise from them. All tumors within the brain are pathologic space-occupying lesions and, as such, are capable of causing mass effect, vasogenic edema, hydrocephalus, and increased intracranial pressure. Certain well-differentiated tumors may actually cause hormonal hypersecretion, the physiological effects of which may be among the first diagnostic indicators. Benign tumors can also be life threatening if they arise in locations that are surgically inaccessible or physiologically critical.

Overall, the Brain Tumor Society estimates that 200,000 new intracranial tumors are diagnosed a year.

Brain tumors often present somewhat insidiously. Tumors may arise anywhere within the brain, or within its supporting structures, and symptoms may depend greatly on the location of the tumor and nearby structures. The patient may complain of visual and sensory changes, persistent headaches that are often worse in the morning after awakening, and other less specific symptoms such as nausea and lack of appetite. The patient may present with seizures and behavioral changes as well. Tumors of the brain parenchyma may be vulnerable to hemorrhage within the lesion itself. This type of bleed may in fact be the presenting complaint that brings the patient in for treatment in the first place.

Diagnosis is typically accomplished through CT scan, lumbar puncture, and MRI. The latter is the most sensitive and definitive tool, allowing for more sophisticated viewing of the tumor, particularly when certain types of contrast medium are utilized. The degree of mass effect that is apparent in the initial imaging studies of some patients with relatively slow-growing tumors can be astonishing; similar pathologic changes that occur from acute injury or expanding hemorrhage would have a far more drastic clinical presentation. The fact that the brain is able to compensate over time for the lesion can allow for significant progression with surprisingly benign symptoms.

Tumors are diagnosed, graded, and treated based on their type and location. Some tumors are surgically resected with little complication. Others require more radical surgical intervention or may be completely inoperable. Radiation and chemotherapy remain options for certain types of tumors (Figure 23-11 ■).

Metastatic lesions are also highly variable in nature, and their location and histological characteristics depend greatly on the primary source. As a rule, patients with metastatic disease involving the CNS tend to have a poorer prognosis than those with primary lesions, but this is not always the case.

Higher grades of brain tumors, as determined by grading scales such as that produced by the World Health Organization, translate into more destructive and invasive lesions. With regard to cell characteristics, tumor cells with more advanced differentiation are less malignant than tumor cells that are poorly differentiated. *Differentiation of cells* is a phrase that is used to determine how specialized the structure of an aberrant cell is. New cells begin their lives as precursor cells that have no specialized structures to determine their function. Specific cell types become more specialized as they age to serve a specific functional purpose within the body. Thus, they are said to "differentiate." More primitive cells that lack differentiation tend to be faster growing and, therefore, more malignant when cancerous. Thus, poorly differentiated cells found within a tumor biopsy are indicative of greater malignancy. Primary tumors that are comprised of neuronal tissue also tend to be less malignant than those comprised of the structurally supportive cells within the brain.

Gliomas

The term *glioma* refers to a group of tumors that are formed of the various types of structurally supportive cells within the brain, which are known collectively as the **neuroglia.** These include astrocytomas, which are the most common types of primary lesions, oligodendrogliomas, and ependymomas. Their degree of malignancy is highly variable. High-grade gliomas have a poor

neuroglia *various cells within the brain that comprise the supportive structures surrounding neurons.*

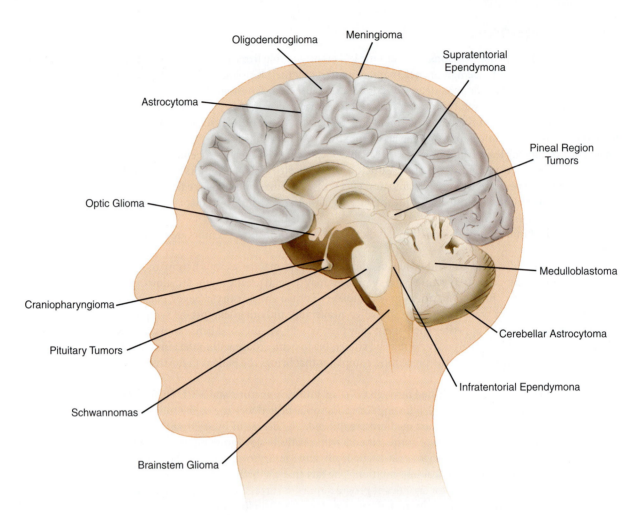

■ **Figure 23-11**   Brain tumor types.

prognosis, and low-grade lesions may develop to become high-grade ones. Perhaps the most common and most malignant of these is glioblastoma multiformes, which often claim victims within 1 year of the presentation of symptoms. The treatment for most gliomas generally consists of surgical debulking and resection, followed by radiation. Oligodendrogliomas tend to be slower growing, more focal, and more susceptible to chemotherapy than astrocytomas. Total resections are associated with better prognoses. In general, gliomas tend to favor the cerebral hemispheres, and can be highly invasive and difficult to eradicate.

Meningiomas

Meningiomas are tumors of the meningeal cells lining the surface of the brain, and are not composed of brain parenchyma. They are the second most common type of intracranial tumor. They are generally benign, although a small percentage may have malignant qualities. The signs and symptoms they produce vary depending on their location, which is also the primary determinant of how life threatening the meningioma is to the patient. Meningiomas may occur alone or may be associated with other lesions. Some may be asymptomatic, and are found only coincidentally or during an autopsy. When possible, surgical excision is the most effective intervention, although rates of recurrence are significant.

Other Types of Intracranial Tumors

There are numerous other primary intracranial tumors that affect different age groups and patient populations, and with varying degrees of malignancy. Tumors may originate from neurons themselves, vascular structures, nerve sheaths, and epithelial cells. Those that are in contact with the CSF may spread or "seed" by releasing tumor cells into the CSF circulation, which then create secondary lesions elsewhere in the CNS. Metastasis of a primary brain lesion cannot occur by lymphatic spread, as do many other types of tumors in the body, because there are no lymphatic structures within CNS tissue. Tumors of the pineal or pituitary glands may have significant systemic effects as a result of hormone secretion.

SPINAL TUMORS

Primary and metastatic tumors can also form in the spinal cord and osseous spinal column. Generally, spinal tumors first become symptomatic when the patient complains of localized back pain. As the tumor progresses, signs and symptoms of cord and nerve root compression may occur, including pain, parasthesias, incontinence, and autonomic dysfunction. The types of tumors found within the spinal cord and its supporting structures are etiologically and histopathologically identical to those found inside the cranium. Some spinal tumors such as the chordoma, a slow-growing osseous tumor that develops from remnants of fetal structures, are unique to the spine, but may metastasize to other areas of the CNS.

The treatment of most spinal tumors is the same as that for most intracranial tumors. Surgical decompression and laminectomy are performed while ensuring adequate stability of the spinal column. As with intracranial tumors, the location of the lesion is of the utmost importance in determining the degree to which surgical intervention can be utilized. Radiotherapy and chemotherapy may follow, depending on the type of tumor found.

From a critical care perspective, the actual histological origin of a CNS neoplasm is of lesser importance. The most significant piece for critical care providers to consider is the physiological effect that the tumor has on the patient. In addition, providers should be sensitive to the psychosocial health of patients with neoplastic lesions in the critical care setting who are awake and oriented.

ENCEPHALOPATHY

The term *encephalopathy* refers to progressive neuronal degeneration and dysfunction that results from pathologic changes that begin outside of the CNS, or from an exogenous source such as ingested or inhaled toxins. Hypoxia, hypercapnia, hypoperfusion, extremes in blood sugar, and numerous metabolic disorders can cause encephalopathy. It is a prominent end-stage feature in patients with severe liver disease, renal dysfunction, or certain nutritional deficiencies, and is also seen in AIDS. Chronic alcoholism is one of the most common causes, but it may also be seen more acutely when certain toxins, medications, or drugs are introduced into the body.

The progression of organic encephalopathies is variable, and depends on the causative agent. When encephalopathy presents with a gradual onset, there are usually subtle changes in behavior, memory, and movement. These are followed by worsening disorders of thought and movement, transitioning to frank dementia, and then degenerating into varying degrees of coma until death occurs. Certain stages of degenerative change may be reversible, again depending on the underlying cause.

Treatment in the critical care setting is supportive, and is determined by the extent of disease progression. Causative disorders must be treated, particularly in the case of metabolic encephalopathies that may be reversible.

AIDS ENCEPHALOPATHY

The degenerative process of AIDS encephalopathy occurs in the brain tissue of patients with HIV, although the exact mechanism is not entirely clear. It is believed that HIV-infected macrophages travel to the brain tissue where the virus is spread to other neuronal and glial cells, causing progressive degenerative destruction. Generally, the white matter and deeper gray matter are more readily affected. Superimposed on AIDS encephalopathy may be other neurologic infections and malignancies associated with immunodeficiency, including tuberculosis or cryptococcal meningitis, cytomegaloviral encephalitis, CNS lymphoma, and toxoplasmosis. The treatment of AIDS encephalopathy is limited, and is based primarily on supportive care and antiretroviral therapy. However, this serves only to slow disease progression, and cannot reverse neuronal degeneration.

WERNICKE'S ENCEPHALOPATHY

Wernicke's encephalopathy is a common encephalopathy caused by vitamin B_1 (thiamine) deficiency. It is most commonly seen in chronic alcoholism, and arises both from poor nutrition and impaired absorption and storage of thiamine. The primary feature of Wernicke's encephalopathy is known as Korsakoff's psychosis, which is a pattern of progressive retrograde and anterograde amnesia with flattening of the affect and intellectual slowing.

One feature of this population is confabulation, which is the invention of fictional accounts to explain for gaps of time lost in the memory from the amnestic progression of the encephalopathy. In addition, the patient may exhibit nystagmus, impaired extraocular movement, and cerebellar ataxia with gait disturbance. The disease is treated in the critical care setting by the provision of thiamine supplementation. This will not reverse memory and cognitive deficits, unfortunately. Patients with advanced Wernicke's encephalopathy may have numerous coexisting metabolic derangements as a result of poor nutrition. Furthermore, many of these patients will present with comorbidities related to chronic alcohol abuse, including hepatic disease, pancreatitis, and acute and chronic traumatic injuries.

HEPATIC ENCEPHALOPATHY

Hepatic encephalopathy is caused by the buildup of toxic by-products of metabolism in the presence of advanced liver disease, as in cirrhosis. Protein metabolism in the gut creates ammonia (NH_3), which is then converted to urea in the liver and excreted by the kidneys. Hepatic impairment can cause a buildup of unmetabolized ammonia, which is believed to have an intoxicating effect on the brain. Cortical function and levels of consciousness are impaired, and cerebellar ataxia may occur. Patients with elevated ammonia levels may demonstrate asterixis, which is a flapping tremor of the hands that occurs when the patient extends his supinated arms in front of himself.

Hepatic encephalopathy may progress to coma and death, and can be a hallmark of end-stage liver disease in the chronic patient. Acute encephalopathic changes may be triggered by stressors such as infection, GI bleeding, or metabolic derangement. Treatment is focused on reversal of the precipitating cause, supportive care, and elimination of ammonia from the body. This is generally accomplished by the administration of Lactulose, a laxative that pulls ammonia into the gut and hastens excretion. The patient should be maintained on a low-protein diet in the critical care setting to ensure minimal ammonia production. Research continues to explore the implications of the accumulation of other metabolic by-products and their contribution to encephalopathic changes in the hepatically compromised patient.

TOXIN-INDUCED ENCEPHALOPATHY

Acute and chronic encephalopathic syndromes may be caused by exposure to numerous drugs and chemicals. Patients at risk for toxin-induced encephalopathy include abusers of volatile solvents (i.e., butane "huffing" and glue sniffing), IV drug abusers, and people in contact with industrial chemicals, heavy metals, and organophosphates. Toxic exposure should always be included in the differential diagnosis of any patient with acute neurologic change, and a careful history should always be taken.

SEIZURE DISORDERS

Seizures are defined as a paroxysmal and abnormal electrical discharge from the brain. They are a common feature of many neurologic complaints, and may also be seen in patients with hypoxia, hypoglycemia, metabolic derangement, or any number of other medical problems. More often than not in the general population, the etiology of seizures is unclear. Seizure disorders are commonly encountered in the prehospital arena, and are perhaps most commonly encountered by providers who deal with chronic seizure disorder patients. Often, paramedics are called on to administer benzodiazepine agents to stop generalized, tonic-clonic seizure activity, or to evaluate and transport patients in the postictal state that follows.

Critical care providers must increase their awareness of seizure activity and its significance, however, and learn to recognize seizures that are not as readily apparent as the tonic-clonic seizure.

Aberrant electrical activity can cause focal signs and symptoms of a wide variety, depending on where and why the seizure began. As a rule, seizures that begin from an epileptic focus in the cerebral cortex will begin with focal symptoms. The electrical discharge may then progress to a generalized seizure, particularly when deeper structures such as the thalamus are involved. Seizures that originate from deeper foci tend to present as generalized activity.

In the conscious patient, be alert for behavioral changes and inattentiveness, as well as sensory complaints including tinnitus, parasthesias, and gustatory, auditory, or visual abnormalities. Patients who are not readily able to communicate such abnormalities may present with abnormal and repetitive actions such as lip smacking or even with more complex motor activities that would seem to require higher cortical input. An example of this would be the removal of a nasal cannula and the repetitive winding of it around the fingers. Seizure activity should be considered in any display of abnormal or seemingly automatic behavior.

Complex partial seizures may present as the repetitive twitching or jerking of one limb or side of the body, or even as a facial tic. Unconscious patients should be evaluated for "roving" or other abnormal eye movements. Focal seizures may hold the potential to progress to generalized seizures at any time.

Seizure activity may also be entirely subclinical, and only recognizable on an EEG. It must be remembered, however, that all seizure activity is clinically significant, even if it is not necessarily clinically evident. Patients who are chemically paralyzed still hold the capacity for electrographic seizures, but will not present with any motor symptoms. Other physiological responses are often present in the paralyzed patient that may be indicative of seizure activity, including apnea, tachycardia, and elevated ICP.

There is a phenomenon known as Todd's paralysis that can present a confusing clinical picture to critical care providers in patients who have sustained a seizure. This may be particularly true for patients with acute mental status changes who have had an unwitnessed seizure, and who present with no apparent radiological evidence of intracranial pathology. In Todd's paralysis, patients in the postictal phase of a seizure can present with hemiparesis, facial droop, and other focal symptoms suggestive of ischemia. These symptoms present on the side of the body contralateral to the side of the brain where the epileptic focus lies. Eye deviation may occur toward the ipsilateral side of the seizure's focus. Clinically, these patients resemble an acute stroke, except for the fact that no focal lesion can be found. The focal deficits imposed by Todd's paralysis will begin to resolve after a short period of time as the postictal state progresses.

STATUS EPILEPTICUS

Patients are considered to be in status epilepticus when they experience seizure activity with little or no recovery between episodes. It can occur in any type of clinical seizure disorder, but is most dangerous in the case of generalized seizures. Generalized status epilepticus is acutely life threatening to patients in a number of ways. Tonic-clonic seizures are typically associated with periods of apnea that may be sustained long enough to cause life-threatening hypoxia, and can cause fatal dysrhythmias. In addition, violent muscle contractions demand high amounts of energy, which must take the form of anaerobic metabolism, particularly in the hypoxic patient. The result is a rapid accumulation of lactic acid that can cause a dangerous metabolic acidosis in a short period of time, an acidotic state that is superimposed on a preexisting respiratory acidosis caused by hypoxia.

Skeletal muscle breakdown caused by unrelenting generalized seizures results in the release of large amounts of creatine kinase into the blood, a phenomenon known as *rhabdomyolysis*, which can lead to renal compromise. Malignant hyperthermia with body core temperatures in excess of 105° F may also result. Hypertension and elevated ICP are also common features of generalized status epilepticus, and leave the patient at risk for aneurysmal or vascular malformation rupture, acute ICH or rebleed, pulmonary edema, and any number of other complications, particularly in the presence of comorbidity or preexisting neurologic compromise. Neuronal destruction is the final result of status epilepticus, and can occur from prolonged electrical hyperstimulation even in the absence of clinical seizure activity, as in the chemically paralyzed patient.

Treatment of status epilepticus must be prompt and aggressive. As always, airway control and hemodynamic stabilization take the highest priority. Benzodiazepenes may be insufficient to stop seizures, particularly in status epilepticus caused by drug or alcohol withdrawal, or from metabolic causes. Anti-epileptics must also be administered as quickly as is safely possible. If any underlying cause can be identified, it must also be reversed. In spite of this, patients in status epilepticus may continue to seize, and may require more aggressive management. This may necessitate the induction of a barbiturate coma to protect the brain from further damage, as well as to break the abnormal electrical cycle and allow status epilepticus to cease.

Seizure activity of any kind does not always begin as a full, generalized seizure. Often, subtle signs may be indicative of a more drastic, possibly imminent worsening of an otherwise benign presentation. The presence of tremors, clonus, or muscle fasciculation, as well as focal motor activity, should be addressed promptly before seizures have an opportunity to become generalized.

In addition, systemic and intracranial hypertension, hyperthermia, and cardiopulmonary compromise must be treated expeditiously. Adequate intravenous hydration should be provided as can be tolerated to prevent renal damage from rhabdomyolysis. All patients with the potential for seizures must be physically protected from secondary trauma caused by convulsions as much as possible, such as by padding siderails on stretchers.

With regard to patients with a poor neurologic exam after status epilepticus has resolved, it must be remembered that even subclinical seizures have a draining effect on the brain. The postictal state imposed by status seizures may remain for days after the seizure activity ceases. Also, deficits imposed by metabolic changes must be considered and reversed. The pharmacologic agents employed to stop status seizures can have a cumulative sedating effect, and may take some time to metabolize completely from the patient's body. Thus, it is difficult to know what a patient's neurologic outcome will be after status epilepticus until all contributing factors can be excluded.

NEUROLOGIC DISORDERS WITH SYSTEMIC MANIFESTATIONS

A wide variety of acute and chronic neurologic disorders can present with generalized or systemic signs and symptoms. These may include neuromuscular disorders, demyelinating diseases, or exposure to neurotoxins. The etiologies of these disorders can be congenital, infectious, autoimmune, hormonal, or subsequent to environmental exposure. Typically, these disorders become significant in the critical care population when they cause respiratory or cardiovascular compromise, or when they develop acutely in the critical care setting in response to the stress of another disease process. In the case of many congenital or progressive degenerative disorders, critical care intervention coincides with end-stage progression and end-of-life care. Critical care paramedics should familiarize themselves with the basic pathophysiology, presentation, and treatment of these disorders.

It is important to note the difference between dementia and delirium, because either or both can be found within this patient population. Dementia is a process of cognitive decline with the loss of higher intellectual abilities, as well as memory. As a rule it tends to occur on a more gradual basis, and is the result of progressive pathology. Delirium is the product of a more acute process, and is characterized by an alteration in the level of consciousness or changes in behavior that cannot be attributed to chronic pathology. Delirium will degrade more quickly than dementia, but is also more reversible, and can also be superimposed on dementia within a given patient. Chronic sleep deprivation and loss of normal circadian rhythms can contribute to a state of delirium known as "ICU psychosis" in critical care patients who are hospitalized for a prolonged period of time. There is also a phenomenon known as "sundown syndrome" which is characterized by delirium that worsens at night.

ALZHEIMER'S DISEASE

Alzheimer's disease is a primary dementia caused by cortical and hippocampal degeneration, as well as the formation of neurofibrillary tangles and senile plaques (Figure 23-12 ■). These are intracellular and extracellular conglomerates of protein, respectively, that contribute to neuronal loss. The primary mechanisms appear to involve the deficiency of numerous neurotransmitters, particularly acetylcholine, and possibly exposure to viruses. Although primarily a disease of the elderly, it may strike younger patients at times. Generally, a younger age of onset and rapid progression are poor prognostic indicators.

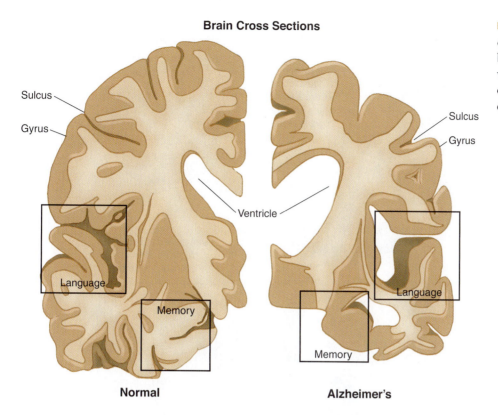

Brain Cross Sections

Sulcus

Gyrus

Sulcus

Gyrus

Ventricle

Language

Language

Memory

Memory

Normal

Alzheimer's

■ **Figure 23-12** Alzheimer's disease. Note decrease in brain mass and expansion in ventricular size. Note effect on memory and language centers.

Signs and symptoms are insidious at onset, and generally involve short-term memory loss and forgetfulness, as well as difficulty in retaining newly learned information. As memory and cognitive impairment progress, motor function is affected and behavioral changes become apparent. Eventually, patients may succumb to near-total mental and physical debilitation and progress to total dependence. Patients with Alzheimer's are vulnerable to infection, accidental injury, exposure after wandering, and violence. Because of its prevalence in the elderly population, critical care paramedics will frequently be exposed to it. Alzheimer's may augment or mask more acute neurologic changes in this patient population, and often contributes to the overall failure of a patient to thrive.

Several therapeutic agents are available on the market now that slow the progression of Alzheimer's through a variety of mechanisms. Some of these medications can precipitate dramatic orthostatic hypotension or increase vagal tone in elderly persons, which the critical care paramedic may encounter. Unfortunately, there is no cure for the disease, and degeneration is ultimately inevitable.

PARKINSON'S DISEASE

Parkinson's disease is another common degenerative brain disorder, and is a major cause of disability in the United States (Figure 23-13 ■). It appears to occur from the loss of dopamine-secreting neurons and dopamine deficiency in the extrapyramidal nuclei of the brain, particularly the substantia nigra, and to a lesser extent the globus pallidus and corpus striatum. This syndrome can be reproduced after exposure to certain drugs and toxins, or after encephalitis.

The primary feature of Parkinson's disease is a coarse, persistent tremor of 3 to 5 hertz while at rest that often begins in the upper extremities and spreads to the lower extremities with disease progression. A "pill-rolling" motion may be seen with the hands and fingers. Muscular rigidity with changes in posture and bradykinesia or slowing of muscular movement will also occur. These changes become more debilitating as the disease advances. Depression from loss of functional ability and dementia, often as a side effect from treatment, may also contribute to decompensation. This disorder is commonly encountered in the critical care setting and may contribute to abnormal neurologic findings in a patient. As with any patient with chronic neurologic disease or past insult, it is important to ascertain the neurologic baseline so that abnormalities in the exam can be assessed.

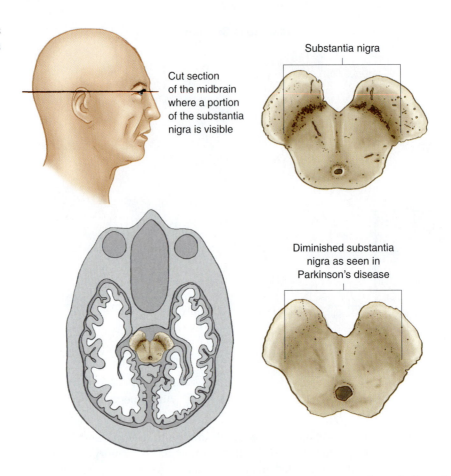

Cut section of the midbrain where a portion of the substantia nigra is visible

Substantia nigra

Diminished substantia nigra as seen in Parkinson's disease

Treatment for Parkinson's disease includes the administration of anticholinergic agents, as well as exogenous dopamine precursors. Other pharmacologic and even surgical options may exist for patients with advanced cases.

MULTIPLE SCLEROSIS (MS)

Multiple sclerosis is an autoimmune disease that results from the demyelination of white matter in the brain and spinal cord, and generally occurs in proximity to the venous system (Figure 23-14 ■). This demyelination occurs in a patchy distribution, known as plaques, and can be associated with axonal destruction. This disease is characterized by remissions and relapses, although rapid progression may occur.

The most common symptoms of relapse are vague sensory alterations, fatigue, and visual disturbance. Cerebellar ataxia, loss of sphincter control, and motor disturbances including spasticity, weakness, and frank paraplegia may also occur. As many as half of those who suffer from MS may demonstrate cognitive dysfunction or behavioral changes as well. Critical illness tends to occur secondary to debilitation that leads to complications from immobility.

Multiple sclerosis manifests differently during periods of relapse depending on the location of axonal demyelination, which can occur anywhere in the white matter of the CNS. Treatment is dictated by the presenting symptoms. In addition, corticosteroids are often given in the acute setting to help reduce inflammatory changes.

AMYOTROPHIC LATERAL SCLEROSIS

Amyotrophic lateral sclerosis (ALS), or Lou Gehrig's disease, is a degenerative disease of the upper and lower motor neurons that tends to begin after the fourth decade of life (Figure 23-15 ■). The etiology is uncertain, although some familial tendency does exist. Motor neuron degeneration results

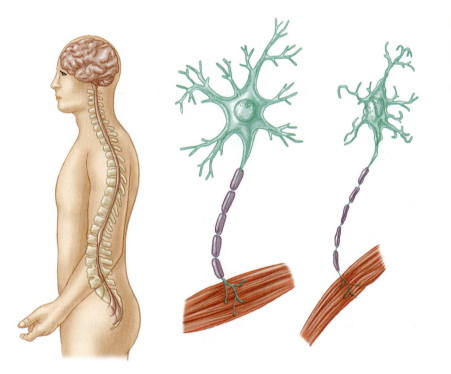

Normal nerve

Myelin

Central nervous system
(Brain and spinal cord)

Immune attack

Nerve
signals

Myelin sheath
of healthy nerve

Axon

In multiple sclerosis the myelin
sheath, which is a single cell
whose membrane wraps
around the axon, is destroyed
with inflammation and scarring.

■ **Figure 23-15**
Amyotrophic lateral sclerosis.
Note degeneration of both
upper and lower motor
neurons.

Pathophysiology of Guillain-
Barré Syndrome (GBS).

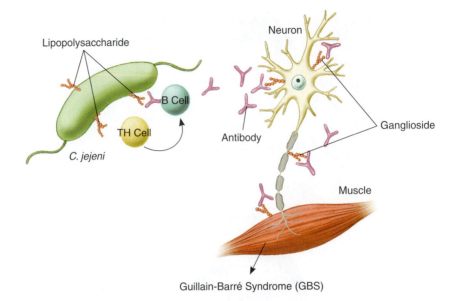

Guillain-Barré Syndrome (GBS)

in atrophic changes in innervated musculature. The cranial nerves and corticospinal pathways may also be affected.

These patients enter the critical care setting when respiratory muscle involvement occurs, or when cranial nerve involvement causes poor airway protection such that aspiration pneumonia results. Treatment is limited to supportive care, because the disease is not reversible and is invariably fatal.

GUILLAIN-BARRÉ SYNDROME

Guillain-Barré syndrome is an autoimmune disorder that results from the inflammatory destruction of the myelin sheaths surrounding spinal cord nerve roots (Figure 23-16 ■). Demyelination causes nerve conduction impairment, and inflammatory changes can cause damage to underlying nerve structures, including extension into the anterior horn of the spinal cord, as well as the motor nuclei of cranial nerves. It is believed that Guillain-Barré syndrome may be triggered by exposure to viral illness, or may occur in response to the stress of a similar acute infection or surgery.

The disease presents with a symmetrical motor weakness that begins distally and inferiorly, and ascends. Sensory changes are usually simultaneous. The disease may be self-limiting, or may progress far enough to impose a functional tetraplegia, mimicking the locked-in syndrome seen in certain pontine lesions. Patients in the critical care setting must be monitored diligently for respiratory compromise as thoracic and diaphragmatic involvement occurs. Autonomic instability with hemodynamic implications may occur in a significant number of these patients. If deeper structures are not permanently damaged by inflammation, recovery is usually virtually complete, although it may not occur for several weeks or even months.

In addition to providing supportive care for patients with Guillain-Barré syndrome, an improvement in symptoms may occur after the timely administration of IV immunoglobulin, as well as plasmapheresis. The latter involves a process of exchanging the plasma in the patient's blood. Hemodynamic compromise from autonomic instability may be treated symptomatically, or preventively with beta-blockers.

MYASTHENIA GRAVIS

Myasthenia gravis is an autoimmune disorder that involves the destruction of acetylcholine receptors in the synaptic cleft at the neuromuscular junction of skeletal muscles (Figure 23-17 ■). In a normal impulse transmission of skeletal muscle, electrical impulses mediated by calcium ions reach the synaptic bouton and cause a release of acetylcholine. The acetylcholine then enters the synaptic cleft, where it binds with acetylcholine receptors. This causes a sodium ion shift in the muscle fiber on the other end of the synaptic cleft, which results in muscle fiber depolarization, assuming the sodium shift is sufficient to reach the action potential. Acetylcholine within the synaptic cleft is quickly degraded by the enzyme acetylcholinesterase (ACE) so that impulse transmission will stop and the synapse can return to its normal electrochemical state.

When acetylcholine receptors are destroyed, as occurs in myasthenia gravis, the repeated transmission of nerve impulses into the skeletal muscles is impaired. Thus, the hallmark symptom of myasthenia gravis is muscular weakness that worsens with repeated muscle stimulation. Patients will fatigue easily as the day continues. This muscular weakness can involve skeletal muscles anywhere in the body, and often affects the facial and extraocular muscles. Involvement of the diaphragm and intercostal muscles can lead to acute respiratory distress, which is termed a "myasthenic" or "gravid" crisis.

Treatment for these patients is primarily supportive. ACE inhibitors will reduce the metabolism of acetylcholine within the synaptic cleft, thus allowing for more acetylcholine to be available for a longer period of time to allow for continued muscle transmission. Diagnosis is achieved through nerve stimulation and action potential investigation. There is a prevalence of thymic disease in these patients, suggesting that the autoimmunologic origin may be in the thymus gland, and therefore related to T lymphocytes. Thymectomy may be beneficial to these patients, particularly those who suffer from a tumor in the thymus gland. Plasmapheresis can also confer a temporary relief of symptoms.

NEUROLEPTIC MALIGNANT SYNDROME (NMS)

Neuroleptic malignant syndrome is a potentially fatal response to neuroleptic medications or similar agents after they have been reintroduced, or after a sudden dosage change. Neuroleptic agents include haloperidol, prochlorperazine, promethazine, risperidone, and metoclopramide. There is an idiopathic blockade of dopamine-2 receptors, which can cause severe hyperthermia and muscular rigidity. A cascade response of the sympathetic autonomic nervous system also occurs, with life-threatening tachycardia and hypertension. Prolonged muscular contraction can lead to acid–base disturbances, as well as elevated creatine kinase (CK) levels and a risk for rhabdomyolysis.

Patients with suspected NMS are generally treated with a muscle relaxant such as Dantrolene, and may also receive dopamine-2 agonists such as bromocriptine and amantadine. Other interventions, including sedation and body core temperature cooling, are further indicated. Obviously, the offending agent must also be removed.

MALIGNANT HYPERTENSION SYNDROME (MHS)

Malignant hypertension syndrome is very similar to NMS, but generally occurs in response to anesthesia. It may, however, occur in individuals after the administration of a depolarizing neuromuscular blockade agent, such as succinylcholine. The etiology differs from NMS in that dopaminergic pathways are not implicated. Instead, patients with malignant hyperthermia, who must be genetically predisposed toward the same, suffer a pathologic excess of calcium ion release from the sarcoplasmic reticulum of muscle fibers, causing abnormal and sustained muscular contractions. Noted that the incidence of this complication is exceedingly rare.

The signs and symptoms of MHS are similar to those of NMS. Dantrolene is the only therapy indicated, in addition to supportive and symptomatic care.

CREUTZFELDT-JAKOB DISEASE (CJD) AND BOVINE SPONGIFORM ENCEPHALOPATHY (BSE)

There are several transmissible degenerative diseases caused by proteins with an abnormal structure known as "prions" that cause widespread glial and neuronal destruction with eventual and inevitable death. The transmission of these disorders depends on their etiology. Creutzfeldt-Jakob disease can follow a familial pattern of genetic transmission. Other variants of this disease are zoonoses, meaning that they are diseases of animals that can be transmitted to humans. Of these, bovine spongiform encephalopathy is the most widely recognized. Also known as "mad cow disease," this prion disorder has received widespread media attention in the past decade because of deaths that have occurred from the ingestion of affected beef products. A similar phenomenon known as *scrapie* has been recognized in sheep for hundreds of years. All prion disorders are fatal, often within a period of several months. The mechanism whereby they cause CNS tissue destruction is not readily apparent; however, patients will present with progressive encephalopathic changes until coma ensues and death occurs.

NEUROTOXIC POISONING

The specific syndromes, symptoms, and treatment of patents suffering from neurotoxic pathology extends well beyond the scope of this text. However, critical care paramedics should be aware that neurotoxicology may play a significant role in acute neuropathology syndromes that develop in patients with no known cause. Many poisonous snakes, snails, arachnids, and plants can cause neurologic symptoms varying in severity worldwide, either through envenomation or ingestion. Organophosphates, organic solvents, certain chemical warfare agents, and some heavy metals are among the myriad numbers of chemical agents that can cause neurologic compromise as well.

Above all, providers must maintain a high index of suspicion for and be prepared to deal with neurotoxic agents and the syndromes they cause, particularly in the setting of potential exposure to weapons of mass destruction. Personal safety and appropriate equipment, resources, and training must be ensured at all times when exposure to toxic entities is possible.

SPINAL CORD DISORDERS

The spinal cord is susceptible to many of the same pathophysiological insults that occur in the brain. Infarction, inflammation, neoplastic growth, and hemorrhagic vascular malformations within the spine do occur, although they are less common than intracranial pathology. Deficits caused by insult to the spinal cord depend on the location of the insult and the degree of secondary injury that occurs subsequently. Structural disorders of the spine may also be encountered by the critical care paramedic.

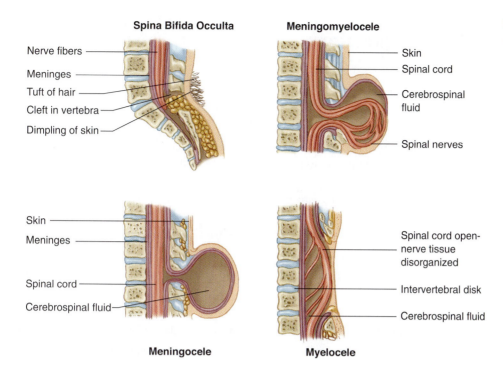

Figure 23-18 Common types of myeloceles.

Spina Bifida Occulta

- Nerve fibers
- Meninges
- Tuft of hair
- Cleft in vertebra
- Dimpling of skin

Meningomyelocele

- Skin
- Spinal cord
- Cerebrospinal fluid
- Spinal nerves

- Skin
- Meninges
- Spinal cord
- Cerebrospinal fluid

Meningocele

- Spinal cord open-nerve tissue disorganized
- Intervertebral disk
- Cerebrospinal fluid

Myelocele

MYELOMENINGOCELE (SPINA BIFIDA)

Myelomeningocele is a congenital disorder that deserves special mention, because it may be encountered by the critical care paramedic who deals commonly with chronic care populations. It is caused by the improper formation of the neural tube, which is the primitive structural precursor to the CNS that forms during fetal development. A defect results, such that incomplete formation of the spinal column leaves meningeal and nervous tissue exposed to potential damage or infection. The disorder has different stages, including an occult form wherein no nervous tissue compromise occurs. In the most advanced form, a sac formed by the meninges and containing nervous tissue protrudes from the patient's back into the open air, generally in the region of the lumbar spine (Figure 23-18 ■). Although surgical correction is possible, myelomeningocele formation is associated with varying degrees of paralysis and neurologic deficit. Prenatal maternal folate deficiency is among the causes implicated in the development of this disorder. Spina bifida can be detected prenatally by the presence of elevated levels of alpha fetoprotein via amniocentesis, as well as by ultrasonography. Because of the extensive supportive care required in infancy by patients with advanced cases and subsequent repeated exposure, there is a high incidence of latex hypersensitivity in this population.

Summary

There are numerous neurologic conditions, both acute and chronic, that may require critical care support and intervention at some point during the natural history of disease progression. Prompt recognition of acute changes and the aggressive prevention of secondary injury are essential if optimal quality of life is to be maintained after the acute phase of neurologic illness. Critical care paramedics must maintain a high index of suspicion in undiagnosed patients who present with acute mental status or other neurologic change. Time is often the most critical factor of all, particularly in acute neurologic emergencies such as ischemic infarct. Thus, it is essential that critical care paramedics maintain their assessment skills and continue to learn about the wide variety of neurologic disorders that they may face.

Review Questions

1. What are the major arteries perfusing the brain that feed the circle of Willis?

2. Which is the dominant hemisphere in the majority of the population and how is hemispherical dominance determined?

3. What is the accepted maximum time frame from the onset of symptoms for the administration of intravenous tissue plasminogen activator (tPA) in patients suffering from acute ischemic stroke?

4. What is the presumptive mechanism for the development of cardiac dysrhythmias and left ventricular wall dysfunction in acute atraumatic subarachnoid hemorrhage (SAH)?

5. What is the typical window after SAH occurs when vasospasm is most likely to occur?

6. What does HHH therapy stand for?

7. What is the most common etiology of atraumatic intracerebral hemorrhage in deep white matter structures?

8. What is Todd's paralysis?

9. What precautions should be taken with any patient complaining of fever and a headache?

10. What is the most sensitive noninvasive tool for brain tumor diagnosis?

See Answers to Review Questions at the back of this book.

Further Reading

American Association of Critical Care Nurses. *Core Curriculum for Critical Care Nursing*, 5th ed. Philadelphia: W. B. Brace, 1998.

Bledsoe BE, Porter RS, Cherry RA. *Paramedic Care: Principles & Practice: Medical Emergencies*, 2nd ed. Upper Saddle River, NJ: Pearson Prentice Hall, 2005.

Cuthbertson BH, Dickson R, Mackenzie A. "Intracranial Pressure Measurement, Induced Hypothermia and Barbiturate Come in Meningitis Associated with Intractable Raised Intracranial Pressure." *Anaesthesia*, Vol. 59 (2004): 908–911.

Devinsky O, Feldmann E, Weinreb HJ, Wilterdink JL. *The Resident's Neurology Book*. Philadelphia: F. A. Davis, 1997.

Hanley DF. "Review of Critical Care and Emergency Approaches to Stroke." *Stroke*, Vol. 34 (2003): 362–364.

Lindsay KW, Bone I, Callander R. *Neurology and Neurosurgery Illustrated*, 3rd ed. Edinburgh, Scotland: Churchill-Livingstone, 1997.

Merino JG, et al. "Extending Tissue Plasminogen Activator Use to Community and Rural Stroke Patients." *Stroke*, Vol. 33 (2002): 141–146.

Schwab S, Spranger M, Schwarz S, Hacke W. "Barbiturate Coma in Severe Hemispheric Stroke: Useful, or Obsolete?" *Neurology*, Vol. 48 (June 1997): 1608–1613.

Seventh ACCP Conference on Antithrombotic and Thrombolytic Therapy. "Antithrombotic and Thrombolytic Therapy for Ischemic Stroke." *Chest*, Vol. 126, No. 3, suppl. (2004): 483S–512S.

Gastrointestinal Emergencies

Scott R. Snyder, B.S., CCEMTP

Objectives

Upon completion of this chapter, the student should be able to:

1. Describe basic gastrointestinal anatomy and physiology. (p. 720)
2. Discuss and differentiate the pathology of common gastrointestinal diseases and complications. (p. 728)
3. Discuss diagnostic studies available to aid in the diagnosis of gastrointestinal disease and complications. (p. 734)
4. Discuss the management of specific gastrointestinal diseases and complications. (p. 735)
5. Understand how to manage various types of gastric management tubes that may be encountered during transport. (p. 739)

Key Terms

Case Study

Your critical care transport team is asked to respond to a rural community ED located approximately 100 miles from the tertiary care facility where your team is based. The dispatch information indicates that you are to transport a 46-year-old male with an active GI bleed to your facility for immediate surgery. With the pilot and critical care nurse, you take the elevator from the dispatch center to the rooftop helipad. During the trip, the pilot reports that a quick check of the radar revealed no weather hazards along the planned route, and a full moon should provide plenty of light for visual navigation.

After the preflight check, the three of you secure yourselves in your seats and begin the 35-minute flight to the transporting facility. While en route, you contact the attending at the transporting facility, let him know that you anticipate arriving in about half an hour, and ask for a quick update. The attending reports that your patient has a suspected upper GI bleed that is actively hemorrhaging, is in compensated shock, and will be transported to your facility for evaluation in the ED.

After touchdown at the helipad of the transporting facility, the pilot shuts down the engines while you and your partner load the stretcher with your equipment and offload from the helicopter. You are greeted at the ED nurses' station by the attending physician and the charge nurse, who begin to give your partner a report while you go into the examination room to assess the patient.

You enter the examination room and are presented with an alert and oriented 46-year-old male lying supine on a stretcher and looking around nervously. You introduce yourself to the patient, and while chatting with him to put him at ease, you start your physical exam. While shaking his hand, you note that his skin is slightly diaphoretic, cool, and pale. His lung sounds upon auscultation are clear and equal bilaterally, and you note that there is no peripheral or sacral edema. His abdomen is unremarkable, and there is no pain with palpation. He is receiving oxygen via a nonrebreather mask at 15 lpm, has large-bore peripheral and central IV lines in place, and is on a cardiac monitor. His vital signs are:

HR: 118 and regular
BP: 96/52
RR: 20 and regular
SpO_2: 96%

During your conversation with the patient, you learn that he has been experiencing abdominal pain for the past 3 weeks, which became acutely worse 3 days ago. Two days ago, he developed dark, tarry, foul-smelling feces. He also reports that he has been experiencing a worsening of general weakness and dizziness when he stands or ambulates. He has a history of CAD, is a social drinker, and smokes a pack of cigarettes a day. Your partner returns from the nurses' station with the patient's chart and reports the following lab values:

Hematocrit: 19%
Hemoglobin: 6
WBC: 22,000
Platelets: 45,000
Na: 138

K: 3.9

Cl: 110

Bicarb: 19

BUN: 42

Creatinine: 1.0

While preparing the patient for transport back to the helicopter and lifting, you and your partner initiate the administration of 2 units of O⁻ whole blood, and request two additional units to bring with you for administration during transport, if necessary. Additionally, you initiate IV pantoprazole sodium (Protonix) administration. You and your partner both agree that he is not in need of sedation and intubation at this time, and feel that he will be able to complete the transfer without respiratory complications; oxygen administration will continue via nonrebreather mask at 15 lpm. You place the patient on your transport monitor, and transfer him to your stretcher. You ensure that he and your equipment are properly secured, brief him on what to expect during the flight, and make your way to the helipad. After a routine load, you are on your way to the receiving facility. Once in the air, your partner calls the surgery department at the receiving facility and gives an update to a member of the surgical team.

Twenty minutes into the transport, you note that the two units of blood have been infused. Evaluation of vital signs reveals:

HR: 88 and regular

BP: 106/78

RR: 16 and regular

SpO₂: 100%

While your team has not identified the source of the GI bleed or controlled it, you have successfully stabilized you patient during transport. Upon arrival at the receiving facility, you deliver the patient to the ED, where a bleeding duodenal ulcer is found on endoscopy. Attempts at controlling the bleed are unsuccessful, and the patient is taken to surgery where a segmental bowel recession is performed to control the bleeding. Your patient spends 3 days in the ICU post-surgery before being transferred to the step-down unit for 2 days. On the sixth day after transport, the patient goes home after an uncomplicated recovery.

INTRODUCTION

The purpose of the gastrointestinal (GI) tract is digestion of food and absorption of water and nutrients. The GI tract breaks down ingested food so that the ingested nutrients in the diet can be converted to simpler forms that can be circulated in the body and used for the numerous metabolic processes of the body. The GI system also assists in the roles of detoxification and elimination of bacteria, viruses, chemical toxins, and drugs. To fulfill these roles, there is a complex system of mechanical, hormonal, and neural influences that allows normal homeostasis to be maintained within this body system. Any disturbance of the GI system as a result of traumatic or medical problems or any disturbance in the GI regulatory influences can result in not only nutritional deficits, but grave disturbances in the body's overall homeostasis. As such, it is important for the critical care paramedic to have a functional understanding of the GI tract so proper assessment, field diagnosis, and intervention strategies can be implemented.

The purpose of the gastrointestinal tract is digestion of food and absorption of water and nutrients.

ANATOMY AND PHYSIOLOGY

The digestive tract is an approximately 9 meter muscular tube consisting of the oral cavity, pharynx, esophagus, stomach, small intestine (duodenum, jejunum, and ileum), large intestine (colon), and rectum. Accessory organs to the digestive tract include the salivary glands, the liver, and the pancreas. These structures secrete various enzymes, buffers, and other digestive aids to increase the effectiveness of the breakdown and absorption of nutrients.

HISTOLOGICAL ANATOMY

The wall of the digestive tract can be divided into four distinct layers: the mucosa, submucosa, muscularis externa, and the serosa. (See Figure 24-1 ■.) Regional variations of these layers occur along the digestive tract and are related to the differences in function along its length.

The inner lumen of the digestive tract is made up of a mucous membrane, the mucosa, and is anchored by an underlying layer of loose connective tissue, the lamina propria. The **mucosa** is made up of a layer of simple or stratified epithelium, depending on the location, and is moistened by the secretions of mucous glands. The mucosa is often organized into longitudinal and horizontal folds, called plicae. These folds significantly increase the surface area available for absorption of nutrients. Two thin layers of smooth muscle, the circular layer and the longitudinal layer, lie on the outside surface of the mucosa between it and the lamina propria. Contraction of these muscle layers, termed the muscularis mucosae, results in changes in the shape of the intestinal lumen and plicae. The loose connective tissue of the lamina propria contains small blood vessels, smooth muscle, lymphatic tissue, and lymphatic vessels. In addition to its role as part of the immune system, the lymphatic vessels absorb long-chain fatty acids from the intestinal lumen as cholimicrons, depositing them in the venous blood via the thoracic duct.

The **submucosa** consists of a layer of dense connective tissue surrounding the mucosal and muscularis layers and contains exocrine glands, larger blood vessels, lymphatic tissue, and collections of nerve fibers called Meissner's plexus. Meissner's plexus contains the sensory nerves, sympathetic postganglionic fibers, and parasympathetic ganglionic neurons that innervate the digestive tract.

mucosa *a layer of simple or stratified epithelium (depending upon the location), moistened by the secretions of mucous glands.*

submucosa *a layer of dense connective tissue surrounding the mucosal and muscularis layers; contains exocrine glands, larger blood vessels, lymphatic tissue, and collections of nerve fibers called Meissner's plexus.*

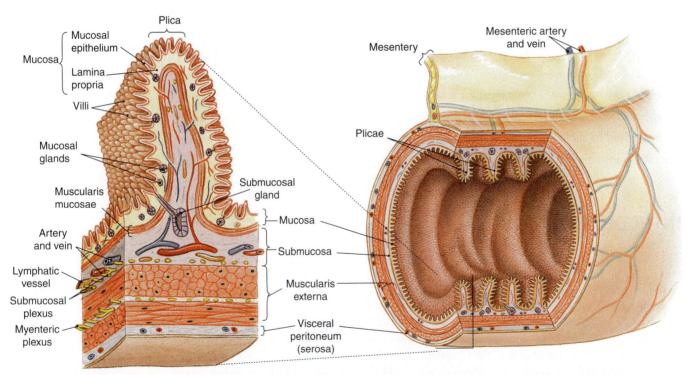

■ **Figure 24-1** Layers and structures of the digestive tract. A representative portion of the digestive tract—the small intestine. *(Fig. 17-2, p. 465, from* Essentials of Anatomy & Physiology, *2nd ed., by Frederic H. Martini, Ph.D. and Edwin F. Bartholomew, M.S. Copyright © 2000 by Frederic H. Martini, Inc. Published by Pearson Education, Inc. Reprinted by permission.)*

The smooth muscle layers that form the **muscularis externa** are arranged in an inner, circular layer covered by an outer, longitudinal layer, as in the muscularis mucosae. Contraction of these muscles results in the peristaltic movement of material along the digestive tract. Stimulation of the parasympathetic nervous system stimulates peristaltic motion, while sympathetic stimulation attenuates peristaltic motion.

The **serosa** consists of a serous membrane that is continuous with the mesentery, and covers the muscularis externa of all parts of the intestinal tract located in the peritoneal cavity. The muscularis externa of the rectum, esophagus, pharynx, and oral cavity is bound to adjacent structures by a support network of collagen fibers.

GROSS ANATOMY

A gross exploration of the digestive tract can follow the passage of a bolus of food as it travels from the mouth to the anus. Lubrication of ingested food and digestion first take place in the oral cavity. Mechanical digestion occurs secondary to the chewing of food, and chemical digestion of carbohydrate begins with the release of the enzyme amylase in saliva. Lingual lipase, secreted by the tongue, also adds to saliva in the oral cavity and initiates the digestion of triglycerides. Saliva also serves to lubricate ingested material, facilitating passage through the esophagus. Saliva is produced and secreted from the parotid, sublingual, and submandibular salivary glands. This process of mechanical digestion, chemical digestion, and lubrication is termed *mastication*.

The tongue helps form the masticated food debris into a bolus, which is then directed to first the oropharynx and then the laryngopharynx. Pharyngeal muscles contract to push the bolus further along into the esophagus, the superior portion of which is located at the level of C6. Involuntary muscle contractions of the esophagus then produce the peristaltic esophageal wall motion that delivers the bolus the length of the esophagus to the stomach. The esophagus receives a rich arterial blood supply, with the superior portion located in the neck supplied by the external carotid and thyrocervical arteries, the mediastinal portion supplied by branches of the bronchial and the esophageal arteries, and the inferior portion supplied by the gastric artery. Venous blood from the esophagus drains into the esophageal, azygos, and gastric veins. Veins draining the inferior esophagus, as well as the cardia of the stomach, communicate with the hepatic portal vein. (See Figure 24-2 ■.)

muscularis externa *smooth muscle layers arranged in an inner, circular layer covered by an outer, longitudinal layer, as in the muscularis mucosae.*

serosa *serous membrane that is continuous with the mesentery, and covers the muscularis externa of all parts of the intestinal tract located in the peritoneal cavity.*

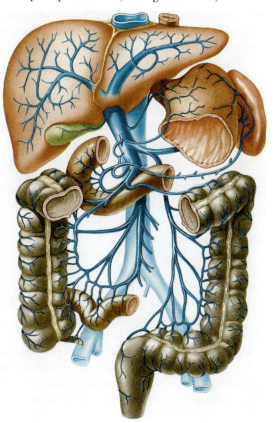

■ Figure 24-2 Blood circulation through the internal organs of the human digestive tract, with cut-away depictions of the stomach, liver, spleen, small, and large intestinal tracts. The inferior vena cava and hepatic portal vein are displayed through and around the organs. Anterior view. (*Dorling Kindersley Media Library*)

The majority of the stomach lies in the upper left quadrant of the abdomen, immediately inferior to the diaphragm, between the level of vertebrae T7 and L3. The exact size and extension can be variable between individuals and meals. The stomach receives food from the upper GI tract via the esophagus and cardiac sphincter, and empties through the pyloric sphincter into the duodenum. The stomach is divided into four regions: the cardia, fundus, body, and pylorus. (See Figure 24-3 ■.) The esophagus enters the stomach at the cardia, so named due to its proximity to the heart located just across the diaphragm. The fundus lies superior to the gastroesophageal junction, and comes into contact with the abdominal surface of the diaphragm. The largest of the four regions is the body, which extends from the fundus to the pylorus, the region that connects to the duodenum via the pyloric sphincter. The stomach has a rich vascular supply consisting of the left gastric artery and branches of the splenic and common hepatic arteries. These arteries together comprise the three branches of the celiac artery, which itself branches off the abdominal aorta.

The digestive functions of the stomach are carried out by chemical and mechanical means. Compared to the rest of the digestive tract, the stomach has an extra, oblique layer of muscle covering the mucosa to aid in mechanical digestion. The longitudinal, circular, and oblique muscle layers of the stomach contract to mechanically break down ingested material and mix it with gastric juice to produce chyme. Gastric juice consists of the secretions of chief cells and parietal cells, which are located in the gastric glands of the stomach walls. Parietal cells secrete hydrochloric acid, and chief cells secrete pepsinogen.

Chyme exits the stomach through the pyloric sphincter and enters the small intestine, where further digestion and up to 90% of nutrient absorption will take place. The small intestine ranges in length from 4 to 6 meters, with a diameter of 3 to 4 centimeters. It is located in every abdominal quadrant and takes up the majority of space in the peritoneal cavity. As such, it is frequently injured when the abdomen is subjected to traumatic insult. The small intestine is suspended in place by the mesentery and protected by the greater omentum.

The duodenum is the shortest segment of the small intestine, approximately 10 inches long and C-shaped, the majority of which is located in the retroperitoneal cavity. In addition to chyme from the stomach, it receives digestive secretions from the pancreas and gallbladder to both aid in digestion and lower the pH of the chyme. The duodenum reenters the peritoneal cavity just before its transition with the jejunum. The jejunum is approximately 8 feet long, and is the site of the bulk of digestion and absorption within the small intestine. The most distal segment of the small intestine is the ileum, which is about 8 feet in length. The ileocecal valve at its terminus regulates the flow of material into the first segment of the large intestine, the cecum. (See Figure 24-4 ■.)

The large intestine, from its beginning at the ileocecal valve, runs a horseshoe-shaped route around the small intestine to its terminus at the anus. It is responsible for the resorption of water, electrolytes, and some vitamins from the intestinal contents. The large intestine has an overall length of about 5 feet, and is divided into the cecum, colon, and rectum. The colon is further divided into the ascending, transverse, and descending colon.

The cecum is a small, expandable pouch that receives material from the ileum and begins the process of fecal impaction. The vermiform appendix is attached to the posteromedial aspect of the cecum. The ascending colon, while covered on its anterior surface by the parietal peritoneum, is considered a retroperitoneal structure. It ascends the right posterolateral wall of the abdominal cavity, and then makes a sharp right-hand turn at the hepatic flexure below the liver and transitions into the transverse colon. The transverse colon curves anteriorly to reenter the peritoneal cavity, where it is suspended in place by the mesentery. Turning posterior and reentering the retroperitoneal space at the splenic flexure, the transverse colon transitions into the descending colon, which travels inferiorly along the left posterolateral wall of the abdominal cavity. Transition to the sigmoid colon takes place at the level of the iliac fossa with the sigmoid flexure before ending at the rectum. The rectum forms the lasts 6 inches of the digestive tract, and is a storage area for fecal material prior to defecation.

The abdominal cavity, in terms of structure, can be divided into three spaces: the peritoneal space, the retroperitoneal space, and the pelvic space. Organs and structures located within the peritoneal space include the stomach, the proximal duodenum, ascending colon, transverse colon, sigmoid colon, liver, gallbladder, and the spleen. Retroperitoneal organs include the kidneys, ureters, distal duodenum, the posterior wall of the ascending and descending colon, and the pancreas. The

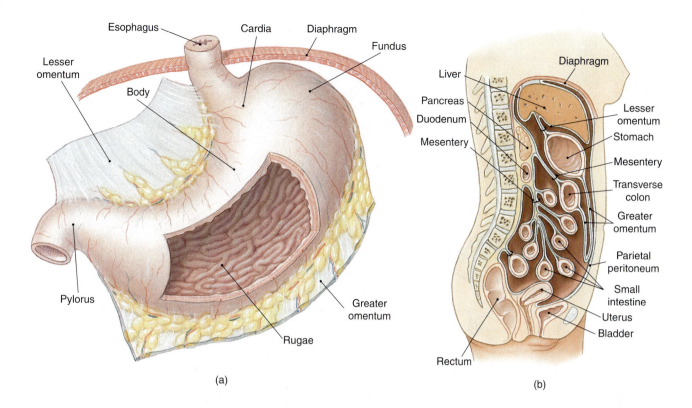

(a)

(b)

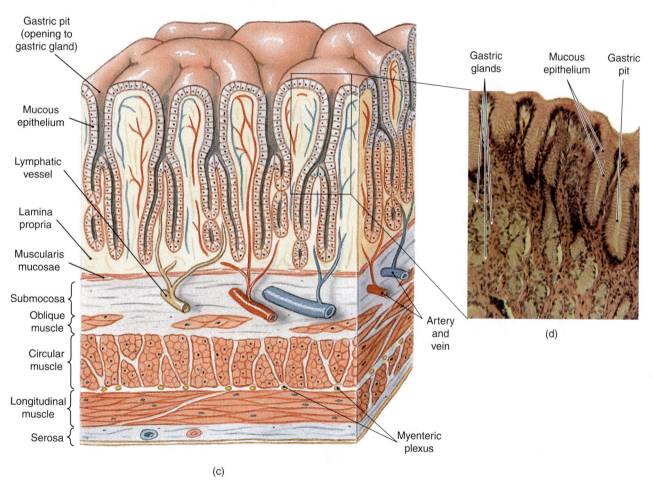

(c)

(d)

■ **Figure 24-3** The gross anatomy of the stomach. (a) An anterior view of the stomach, showing superficial landmarks. (b) The stomach's position in the peritoneal cavity. (c) The organization of the stomach wall. (d) Light micrograph of the lining of the stomach. (*a–c from Fig. 17-8, p. 472, from* Essentials of Anatomy & Physiology, *2nd ed., by Frederic H. Martini, Ph.D. and Edwin F. Bartholomew, M.S. Copyright © 2000 by Frederic H. Martini, Inc. Published by Pearson Education, Inc. Reprinted by permission. d from Ward's Natural Science Establishment, Inc.*)

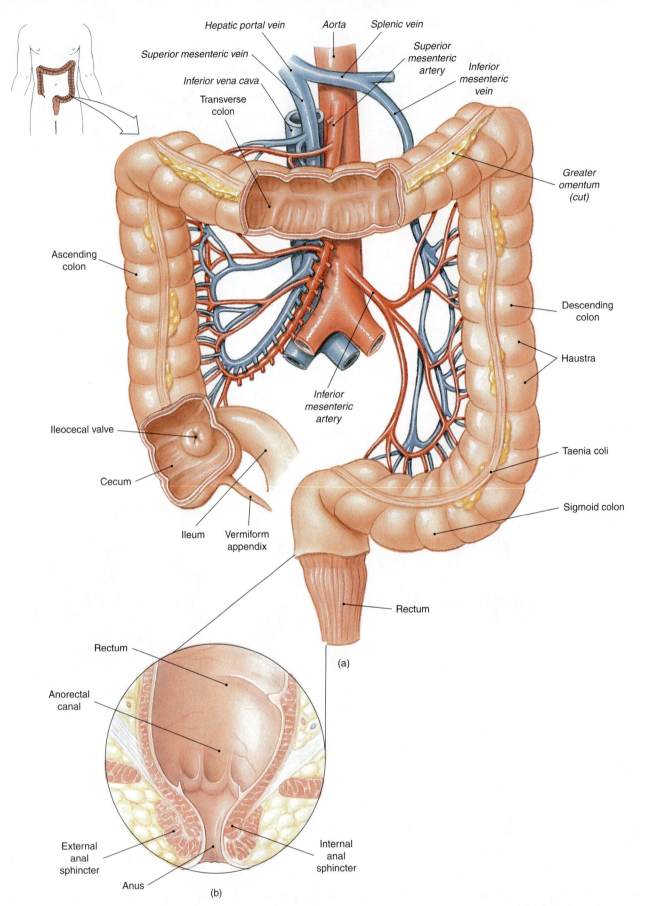

Hepatic portal vein

Aorta

Splenic vein

Superior mesenteric vein

Superior mesenteric artery

Inferior mesenteric vein

Inferior vena cava

Transverse colon

Greater omentum (cut)

Ascending colon

Descending colon

Haustra

Inferior mesenteric artery

Ileocecal valve

Cecum

Taenia coli

Sigmoid colon

Ileum

Vermiform appendix

Rectum

(a)

Rectum

Anorectal canal

External anal sphincter

Anus

(b)

Internal anal sphincter

■ **Figure 24-4** The large intestine. (a) Gross anatomy and regions of the large intestine. (b) Detailed anatomy of the rectum and anus. *(Fig. 17-17, p. 483, from* Essentials of Anatomy & Physiology, *2nd ed., by Frederic H. Martini, Ph.D. and Edwin F. Bartholomew, M.S. Copyright © 2000 by Frederic H. Martini, Inc. Published by Pearson Education, Inc. Reprinted by permission.)*

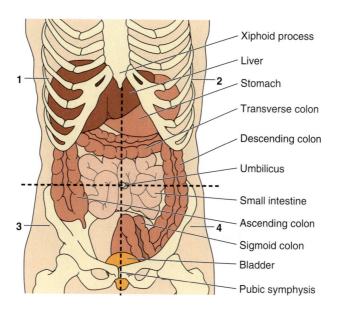

Labels in figure: Xiphoid process, Liver, Stomach, Transverse colon, Descending colon, Umbilicus, Small intestine, Ascending colon, Sigmoid colon, Bladder, Pubic symphysis

urinary bladder, rectum, and urethra are located in the pelvic space. In the female, the ovaries, fallopian tubes, and uterus are also located in the pelvic cavity. Superficially, the abdomen is divided by horizontal and vertical lines, which cross at the umbilicus to form the four quadrants. The critical care paramedic should already be familiar with all organs, including those of the digestive tract, located in the four abdominal quadrants. (See Figure 24-5 ■.)

The peritoneal space is lined with a serous membrane, the parietal peritoneum, which is continuous with the visceral peritoneum covering the abdominal organs. The portions of the digestive tract located within the peritoneal space are suspended by the mesentery, which is continuous with both the visceral and parietal membranes. Thus, the visceral peritoneum, parietal peritoneum, and mesentery form a large, continuous sheet of serous membrane that lines the peritoneal space, suspends the peritoneal organs, and covers the peritoneal organs. Peritoneal fluid is continuously secreted by the serous membrane, which serves to lubricate the peritoneal surfaces. Approximately 7 liters of serous fluid is secreted and reabsorbed every day, and the amount of fluid present can range from little to none in a healthy male and up to 20 mL in a healthy female, depending on the phase of her menstrual cycle.

The mesentery is a double layer of serous membrane connected by loose connective tissue that extends inferiorly from the posterior wall of the abdominal cavity. This space between the double layer serves as a conduit for the vast vascular network, nerves, and lymphatic structures to and from the large and small intestines. In addition, the mesentery acts as a supportive structure for the digestive tract, preventing the movement and entanglement of the intestines.

The greater and lesser omentum are similar double-layer membranes hanging from the greater and lesser curvatures of the stomach, respectively. The greater omentum in effect lies over and conforms to the abdominal viscera, and its rich supply of adipose tissue provides padding, protection, and insulation to the underlying structures. The lesser omentum lies in the space between the liver and stomach, providing an access route for blood vessels entering the liver and support for the stomach.

ACCESSORY ORGANS

The accessory organs of the digestive tract include the salivary glands, liver, gallbladder, and pancreas. The salivary glands are located within the parenchyma of the maxillofacial region. Specific glands include the parotid, sublingual, and submandibular glands. Salivary secretion is controlled by the autonomic nervous system. Parasympathetic stimulation results in increased secretion and copious saliva production, while sympathetic stimulation results in the secretion of smaller volumes of highly concentrated saliva. This smaller volume is the cause of the "dry mouth" associated with sympathetic nervous system activation in a stressful situation.

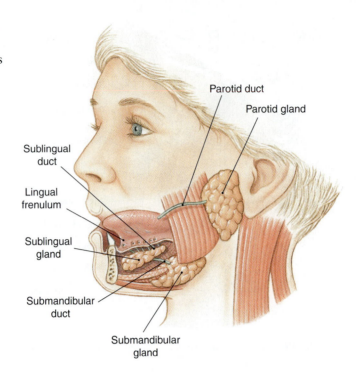

■ **Figure 24-6** The salivary glands. A lateral view, showing the relative positions of the salivary glands and ducts on the left side of the head. *(Fig. 17-5, p. 468, from* Essentials of Anatomy & Physiology, *2nd ed., by Frederic H. Martini, Ph.D. and Edwin F. Bartholomew, M.S. Copyright © 2000 by Frederic H. Martini, Inc. Published by Pearson Education, Inc. Reprinted by permission.)*

Parotid duct

Parotid gland

Sublingual duct

Lingual frenulum

Sublingual gland

Submandibular duct

Submandibular gland

The liver's functions can be divided into three categories: metabolic regulation, hematologic regulation, and bile synthesis and secretion.

The parotid gland lies over the ramis of the mandible, just superior to the angle of the mandible, anterior to the auditory canal, and inferior to the zygomatic arch. The parotid duct exits the gland, then passes over the masseter muscle before draining into the oral cavity by the second upper molar. Parotid secretions contain salivary amylase. Another paired gland, the sublingual gland, is located on the floor of the oral cavity at the base of the tongue. It empties into the oral cavity via numerous sublingual ducts located lateral to the lingual frenulum. The submandibular gland, also paired, lies inferior to the angle of the mandible. Numerous submandibular ducts open into the oral cavity posterior to the front teeth on both sides of the distal lingual frenulum. (See Figure 24-6 ■.)

The liver lies in the upper right quadrant of the abdomen within the peritoneal cavity and is the largest organ in the abdominal compartment. As such, it is frequently the recipient of traumatic forces. The inferior rib cage provides some bony protection to the liver. The falciform ligament bisects the liver, dividing it into the left and right lobes, and anchors the liver to the posterior and anterior abdominal walls. The inferior margin of the falciform ligament thickens to form the ligamentum teres, which is actually the remnant of the fetal umbilical vein. The liver is encapsulated in a tough, fibrous layer that is itself covered with a layer of visceral peritoneum. The hepatic artery provides the liver's enormous blood supply, which is about 25% of cardiac output. Venous return is via the hepatic vein, which deposits blood into the inferior vena cava. In addition to a rich arterial supply, the liver receives all venous blood exiting the digestive system through the hepatic portal vein. The hepatic portal vein, hepatic artery, nerves, lymphatic structures, and the hepatic bile ducts pass through the hilus. (See Figure 24-7 ■.)

The liver's functions can be divided into three categories: metabolic regulation, hematologic regulation, and bile synthesis and secretion. With regard to metabolic regulation, the liver is the primary organ regulating the metabolic composition of the blood. All blood leaving from the absorptive surfaces of the digestive tract is directed to the liver via the hepatic portal system. This allows the liver hepatocytes the opportunity to extract both absorbed nutrients as well as toxins from the blood prior to its entering the systemic circulation. Excess circulating nutrients are stored, and any deficiencies corrected by the mobilization of stored nutrients or the initiation of synthesizing processes.

In addition to monitoring circulating levels of carbohydrates, fats, and amino acids, the liver removes old or damaged red blood cells from circulation and synthesizes plasma proteins. Bile, produced to aid in the digestion of fats, is produced in the liver, travels through the common hepatic duct, is stored in the gallbladder, and is excreted into the duodenum when needed.

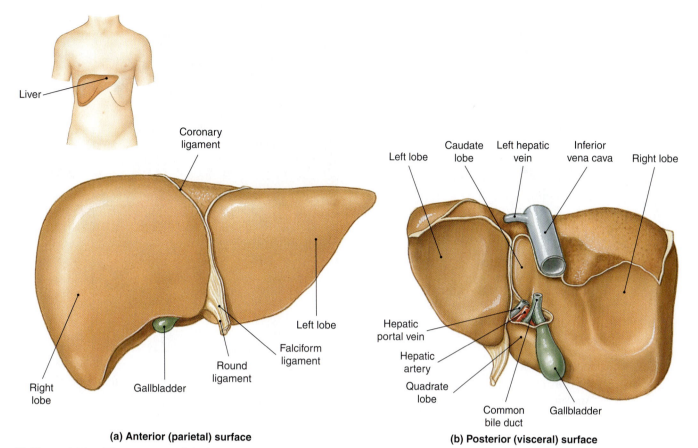

(a) Anterior (parietal) surface

(b) Posterior (visceral) surface

■ **Figure 24-7**   The anatomy of the liver. *(Fig. 17-14, p. 479, from* Essentials of Anatomy & Physiology, *2nd ed., by Frederic H. Martini, Ph.D. and Edwin F. Bartholomew, M.S. Copyright © 2000 by Frederic H. Martini, Inc. Published by Pearson Education, Inc. Reprinted by permission.)*

The gallbladder is located on the posterior surface of the liver, and it stores and concentrates bile produced in the liver prior to secretion into the duodenum. The liver produces approximately 1 liter of bile each day, which is stored in the gallbladder until needed. The typical adult gallbladder can store 50–70 mL of bile. While bile production is continuous, secretion into the duodenum only occurs when acidic chyme in the duodenum increases serum cholecystokinin (CCK) levels. In response to a rising CCK level, muscular contractions of the gallbladder wall propel bile into the small intestine via the cystic duct, which joins the common hepatic duct from the liver to form the common bile duct that terminates at the duodenum. The pancreatic duct shares this terminus, and the hepatopancreatic sphincter controls the secretion of bile and pancreatic juice into the duodenal ampulla, which empties into the duodenum via the duodenal papilla. Rising CCK levels result in the relaxation of the pancreohepatic sphincter, allowing the secretion of bile. Chyme rich in lipids results in a greater release of bile. (See Figure 24-8 ■.)

The pancreas is a retroperitoneal structure that is about 6 inches in length, and located posterior to the stomach. The head of the pancreas is tucked into the C-shaped fold of the duodenum, and its body and tail extend back into the abdominal cavity toward the spleen, coming to a point at, and adhering to, the posterior abdominal wall. The pancreatic duct carries the digestive juice secreted by the pancreas to the duodenum, joining with the common bile duct at the duodenal ampulla. The pancreas receives its arterial blood supply via the pancreatic and pancreaticoduodenal arteries, and venus blood is drained via the splenic vein.

The pancreas has both endocrine and exocrine functions. The functional unit of the exocrine pancreas, accounting for about 99% of the cellular population of the pancreas, is the pancreatic acini. The pancreatic acini secrete pancreatic juice, a mixture of water, sodium bicarbonate, and digestive enzymes including lipase and amylase. The sodium bicarbonate acts as a buffer to neutralize the acidic chyme just released from the stomach, and the digestive enzymes perform the majority of the chemical digestion that takes place in the small intestine. Digestive enzymes released include

The gallbladder is located on the posterior surface of the liver, and it stores and concentrates bile produced in the liver prior to secretion into the duodenum.

The pancreas has both endocrine and exocrine functions.

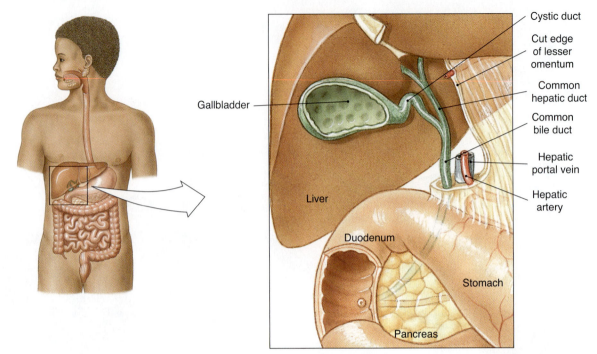

Gallbladder

Cystic duct

Cut edge
of lesser
omentum

Common
hepatic duct

Common
bile duct

Hepatic
portal vein

Hepatic
artery

Liver

Duodenum

Stomach

Pancreas

■ **Figure 24-8** The gallbladder. The inferior surface of the liver, showing the position of the gallbladder and ducts that transport bile from the liver to the gallbladder and duodenum. *(Fig. 17-16, p. 482, from* Essentials of Anatomy & Physiology, *2nd ed., by Frederic H. Martini, Ph.D. and Edwin F. Bartholomew, M.S. Copyright © 2000 by Frederic H. Martini, Inc. Published by Pearson Education, Inc. Reprinted by permission.)*

carbohydrases to digest sugars and starches, lipases to digest lipids, proteinases to break down large protein chains, peptidases to break down smaller peptide chains into individual amino acids, and nucleases, which break down nucleic acids.

The functional unit of the endocrine pancreas is the islets of Langerhans, which account for about 1% of all pancreatic cells, and whose alpha cells secrete glucagon, beta cells secrete insulin, and delta cells secrete somatostatin. In addition, F-cells within the pancreatic islets secrete pancreatic polypeptide, which inhibits gallbladder contraction and increases the rate of nutrient absorption in the small intestine. F-cell secretion is stimulated by the introduction of protein-rich chyme into the duodenum. The endocrine pancreas, by definition, secretes all of its hormones directly into the bloodstream. (See Figure 24-9 ■.)

PATHOPHYSIOLOGY, ASSESSMENT, AND MANAGEMENT OF GASTROINTESTINAL BLEEDING

GI bleeding may occur anywhere along the digestive tract from the mouth to the anus, and may be obvious or occult. GI bleeding is a symptom of a disease rather than a disease itself.

Gastrointestinal bleeding is a common, potentially life-threatening problem both in the emergency department as well as the intensive care unit (ICU), though many cases in the ICU may remain subclinical. GI bleeding may occur anywhere along the digestive tract from the mouth to the anus, and may be obvious or occult. GI bleeding is a symptom of a disease rather than a disease itself, and the different etiologies of GI bleeding will be discussed in this segment.

Upper GI bleeding (UGIB) in adults has an incidence of about 100 per 100,000 population per year, and occurs approximately four times as often as lower GI bleeding (LGIB). Approximately 100,000 patients are admitted every year to U.S. hospitals for UGIB management, and 3% to 15% of patients who develop UGIB will require operative management. Mortality rates for UGIB have remained largely unchanged during the past 30 years, at about 6% to 10% overall, and the rate rises with age. UGIB is more common in the elderly population and in males. Ulcers in the stomach and duodenum (as high as 50% of cases) are the most common causes of UGIB. Gastric erosions (23%), esophageal and gastric varicies (10%), Mallory-Weiss tears (7%), and esophagitis (6%) are responsible for the majority of remaining cases.

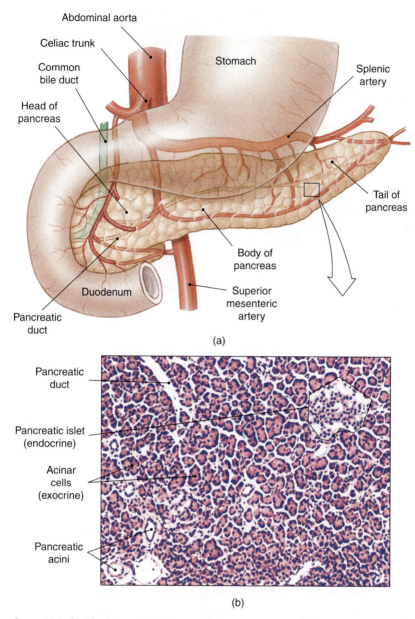

Abdominal aorta
Celiac trunk
Common bile duct
Head of pancreas
Stomach
Splenic artery
Tail of pancreas
Body of pancreas
Duodenum
Superior mesenteric artery
Pancreatic duct

(a)

Pancreatic duct
Pancreatic islet (endocrine)
Acinar cells (exocrine)
Pancreatic acini

(b)

■ **Figure 24-9** The pancreas. (a) Gross anatomy. The head of the pancreas is tucked into a curve of the duodenum than begins at the pylorus of the stomach. (b) Light micrograph of the pancreatic duct and exocrine and endocrine tissues. *(Fig. 17-13, p. 478, from Essentials of Anatomy & Physiology, 2nd ed., by Frederic H. Martini, Ph.D. and Edwin F. Bartholomew, M.S. Copyright © 2000 by Frederic H. Martini, Inc. Published by Pearson Education, Inc. Reprinted by permission.)*

LGIB occurs in about 20 individuals per 100,000 population per year, and also occurs more often in the elderly population and males. Mortality rates are between 10% and 20%. The most common cause of LGIB is diverticular disease (43% of cases), with angiodysplasia (20%), undetermined etiologies (12%), neoplasia (9%), and colitis (9%) accounting for the majority of remaining cases. Diverticular disease, in addition to being the most common cause of LGIB, is also the etiology most likely to require ICU admission.

CAUSES OF UPPER GASTROINTESTINAL BLEEDING

Upper GI bleeds are those hemorrhages that occur proximal to the ligament of Treitz, which supports the duodenojejunal junction and as such include insults to the esophagus, stomach, and duodenum. Etiologies, in order of decreasing frequency of occurrence, include peptic ulcer disease, gastritis and esophagitis, esophageal and gastric varices, and Mallory-Weiss tears.

PEPTIC ULCER DISEASE

An ulcer results secondary to the destruction and sloughing off of the mucosa of the digestive tract, allowing the hydrochloric acid and pepsin present in gastric juice to destroy underlying tissue. Ulcers

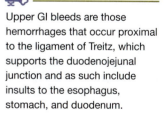

Upper GI bleeds are those hemorrhages that occur proximal to the ligament of Treitz, which supports the duodenojejunal junction and as such include insults to the esophagus, stomach, and duodenum.

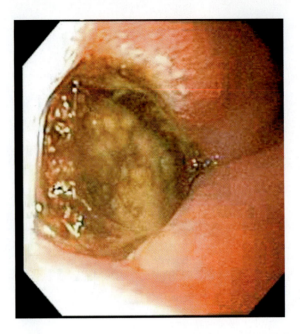

■ **Figure 24-10** Duodenal ulcer.

are most often caused by the action of acidic gastric contents, and tend to appear in areas of the digestive tract that are exposed to these contents. **Peptic ulcer disease (PUD)** involving the stomach and duodenum accounts for up to 50% of all upper GI bleeds. Other possible sites of ulcer formation include the pylorus and esophagus. Duodenal ulcers (about 29% of all ulcers) are more common than gastric ulcers (about 16% of all ulcers), but both have identical instances of bleeding. (See Figure 24-10 ■.) Most often, bleeding results secondary to arterial erosion within the ulcer, and hemorrhage from vessels greater than 1.5 mm in diameter is associated with an increased mortality rate. Large vessels capable of resulting in exsanguinating hemorrhage are usually located deep in the duodenal and gastric submucosa and serosa, and as such require significant ulcer progression for inclusion and subsequent rupture. Bleeding secondary to a peptic ulcer will resolve spontaneously in about 80% of cases, and re-bleeding is associated with a higher mortality. Gastric ulcers are more likely to rebleed than are duodenal ulcers. Increased mortality secondary to upper GI bleeds is associated with a rise with age (especially above 60 years), coexistent organ disease, blood transfusions in excess of 5 units, persistent hypotension, need for surgery, and stress including surgery, sepsis, ventilatory support, and trauma.

Risk factors for PUD include a history of nonsteroidal anti-inflammatory drug (NSAID) use, alcohol abuse, stress, and chronic renal failure. In recent years, appreciation for *Helicobacter pylori* infection as an etiology of PUD has grown, and it is now recognized as the leading etiology of PUD. *H. pylori* infection of the gastric and duodenal mucosa disrupts the mucous barrier, allowing erosion of the underlying tissue by gastric acids. Treatment for, and eradication of, *H. pylori* has been proven to reduce the risk of PUD.

NSAID and salicylate drugs are the second most common etiology of peptic ulcers. Their attenuating effect on cyclooxygenase-1 (COX-1) results in diminished prostaglandin production in the mucosa, thereby decreasing mucous and bicarbonate production and mucosal blood flow, allowing ulcer formation. It has been shown that the combination of *H. pylori* infection and NSAID use increases the risk of peptic ulcer hemorrhage.

Stress ulcers can occur in the stomach and duodenum of critically ill patients secondary to stress from trauma, burns (Curling's ulcer), sepsis, hypotension, cranial or CNS disease (Cushing's ulcer), or long-term ventilatory support. This condition is termed **stress-related erosive syndrome (SRES)**. Long-term ventilatory support and coagulopathy have been identified as the two main risk factors for SRES. Occult bleeding secondary to SRES occurs in more than 25% of critically ill patients, and about 10% experience overt hemorrhage. It is postulated that a breakdown of the GI tract's normal defensive mechanisms allows the acidic gastric juice to erode the mucosal lining. Normal defensive mechanisms include an intact mucosal lining, secretion of alkaline buffers, gastric epithelial migration to areas of mucosal disruption, and the production of mucosal prostaglandin. These factors are significantly impaired in critically ill patients.

GASTRITIS

Gastritis is a superficial erosion and chronic inflammation of the gastric mucosa, and can be thought of as a precursor to an ulcer. Cells of the immune system infiltrate the gastric tissue, resulting in edema irritation. Chronic episodes of gastritis commonly lead to peptic ulcers, perforation, and hemorrhage.

H. pylori infection occurs in 30% to 50% of cases. In response to *H. pylori* infection, the submucosa is initially infiltrated by B and T lymphocytes, followed by infiltration of the lamina propria and gastric epithelium by leukocytes that phagocytize the bacteria. The infection results in localized edema, irritation, and disruption of the mucosal barrier, allowing further irritation and erosion by stomach acids.

Autoimmune gastritis occurs when circulating antibodies mistake the cells of the gastric mucosa for foreign antigens, resulting in destruction of the gastric mucosa layer. The resulting chronic inflammation can result in pernicious anemia secondary to decreased vitamin B_{12} absorption, due to the lack of a key digestive factor destroyed by the chronic inflammation.

Chemical gastritis occurs secondary to the reflux of pancreatic enzymes and bile into the stomach, and to the chronic use of NSAIDs, salicylates, alcohol, and coffee. Compared to other gastritis etiologies, the inflammation associated with chemical gastritis is minimal.

Radiation gastritis can occur at relatively small doses of radiation (<1,500 rad), in which case the mucosal damage is reversible and isolated to the epithelial cells and lamina propria. Higher doses of radiation can result in irreversible changes including mucosal erosion, blood vessel compromise, and mucosal ischemia.

Collectively, gastritis, esophagitis, and duodenitis are responsible for about 15% of all cases of upper GI bleeds.

> **gastritis** *a superficial erosion and chronic inflammation of the gastric mucosa; can be a precursor to peptic ulcers.*

Collectively, gastritis, esophagitis, and duodenitis are responsible for about 15% of all cases of upper GI bleeds.

ESOPHAGEAL AND GASTRIC VARICES

In the United States, esophageal and gastric varices are most often the result of alcoholic and viral cirrhosis of the liver. In chronic cirrhotic liver failure, hepatocyte destruction and resultant fibrosis result in increased resistance to blood flow. The portal vein supplies approximately 1,500 mL/min of blood to the liver from the bowel, spleen, and stomach, and any resistance to blood flow will result in an increase of portal venous pressure. As a result, blood in the splenic system is diverted to the superior and inferior vena cava via collateral circulation through veins in the submucosa of the esophagus, stomach, and anterior abdominal wall. The absence of valves in the portal vasculature aids in the retrograde flow of blood. Normal venous pressure in the portal system is 5 to 10 mmHg, and pressures in excess of 10 mmHg will result in variceal formation.

Around 60% of patients with chronic liver disease will develop varices, and 25% to 30% of those who develop varices will experience hemorrhaging. (See Figure 24-11 ■.) While varices account for only 10% of all upper GI bleeds, the mortality rate is high (20% to 65%), with increased mortality associated with cardiovascular, pulmonary, renal, and immune system compromise. Approximately 70% of patients who have experienced variceal hemorrhage will rebleed, with one-third of those cases proving fatal.

In the United States, esophageal and gastric varices are most often the result of alcoholic and viral cirrhosis of the liver.

MALLORY-WEISS SYNDROME

Mallory-Weiss syndrome is a UGIB secondary to a longitudinal tear in the cardioesophageal region. A Mallory-Weiss tear occurs secondary to a rise in intragastric pressure such as by retching, vomiting, or forceful coughing; it is also associated with long-term NSAID, salicylate, or alcohol use. Bleeding stops spontaneously in 80% to 90% of patients, and about 10% of patients who suffer a Mallory-Weiss tear will experience hemodynamic instability and shock.

> **Mallory-Weiss syndrome** *upper GI bleed secondary to a longitudinal tear in the cardio-esophageal region; can be caused by retching, vomiting, forceful coughing, long-term use of NSAIDs, salicylates, and/or alcohol use.*

CAUSES OF LOWER GASTROINTESTINAL BLEEDING

LGI bleeds are those hemorrhages that occur distal to the ligament of Trietz, and include insults to the jejunum, ileum, large intestine, rectum, and anus. The most common cause of lower GI bleeding is diverticular disease.

The most common cause of lower GI bleeding is diverticular disease.

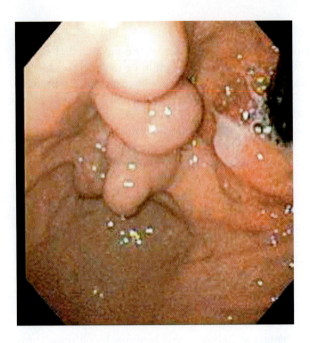

■ **Figure 24-11** Gastric varices.

DIVERTICULAR DISEASE

Diverticula are outpouchings of the colonic mucosa. (See Figure 24-12 ■.) The exact mechanism of diverticular formation in not well understood, but it is thought that areas of increased intraluminal pressure within the colon cause defects in the colon wall. It is also thought that colonic muscle abnormalities or connective tissue disorders weaken the colon wall and contribute to diverticula formation. The acute complications of diverticular disease include inflammation (covered later in this chapter) and bleeding. Bleeding (diverticulosis) can occur secondary to perforation of a blood vessel by a developing diverticula. (See Figure 24-13 ■.) The pain of diverticular disease is sometimes characterized as "left-sided appendicitis."

ASSESSMENT

Patients with a gastrointestinal hemorrhage will often present with a history of weakness, dizziness, near syncope, or syncope, particularly with exertion. Hypotension, tachycardia, and angina are also

Patients with a gastrointestinal hemorrhage will often present with a history of weakness, dizziness, near syncope, or syncope, particularly with exertion.

■ **Figure 24-12** Colon diverticulum.

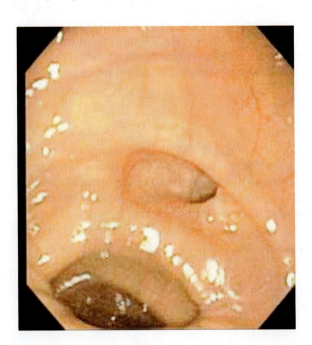

common symptoms. A more dramatic sign of a GI bleed is "coffee-grounds" emesis and hematemesis. Because blood is a gastric irritant, even small amounts in the stomach, secondary to a UGIB, will result in vomiting. A history of retching and vomiting followed by hematemesis is suggestive for a Mallory-Weiss tear. Hematochezia and melena are generally suggestive of a LGIB, but can also occur secondary to UGIB. A bleed producing at least 200 mL of blood is generally needed for the formation of melena, but a tarry stool may be passed with as little as 60 mL of blood in the GI tract.

The physical exam findings of a GI bleed can be extremely subtle. In cases of less than 800 mL of blood loss, tachycardia, weakness, anxiety, and diaphoresis can occur—the classic signs and symptoms of compensated shock. In more severe cases of GI bleeding, physical signs and symptoms will include significant tachycardia, hypotension, and signs and symptoms associated with shock secondary to increased sympathethic nervous system tone.

LABORATORY DATA

Hemoglobin and hematocrit values remain unchanged from baseline immediately after acute blood loss from any type of hemorrhage (GI or otherwise). During the course of resuscitation, the hematocrit may fall secondary to crystalloid infusion and re-equilibration of extracellular fluid into the intravascular space. In less acute hemorrhagic situations, the hematocrit and hemoglobin values provided by a complete blood count are probably still the most useful lab values in a GI bleed because it would be expected that both would be lowered. Even so, due to compensatory mechanisms, it may still take up to 3 to 4 hours for these values to drop. Additionally, in response to the stress associated with a GI bleed, serum glucose and the white blood cell (WBC) count may be elevated.

Electrolyte studies usually are not helpful in the acute setting either. After massive resuscitation, certain abnormalities can occur. Sodium and chloride may increase significantly with administration of large amounts of isotonic sodium chloride. Hyperchloremia may cause a non–ion gap acidosis and significantly worsen an existing acidosis. Calcium levels may fall with large-volume, rapid blood transfusions. (This is secondary to chelation of the calcium by the ethylenediaminetetraacetic acid [EDTA] preservative in stored blood.) Likewise, potassium levels may rise with large-volume blood transfusions. Creatinine is usually within normal limits unless preexisting renal disease is present. Caution should be used when administering iodinated contrast in patients with elevated creatinine because the dye load could initiate a contrast-induced nephropathy in addition to chronic renal impairment.

Coagulation studies are useful to determine liver function, especially in those patients with hepatic disease and those on anticoagulant therapy. In such patients, prolonged prothrombin (PT)

Hemoglobin and hematocrit values remain unchanged from baseline immediately after acute blood loss from any type of hemorrhage (GI or otherwise).

Coagulation studies are useful to determine liver function, especially in those patients with hepatic disease and those on anticoagulant therapy.

and partial thromboplastin (PTT) times are not necessarily suggestive for GI hemorrhage, but do suggest that the patient is at high risk for one. In a patient with normal liver function, a prolonged bleed can result in consumption of coagulation factors, resulting in prolonged times. In addition, it is not abnormal for a healthy individual to have a normal PT and PTT with a GI bleed, especially early in its course. Electrolyte abnormalities, should they occur, can include hypokalemia, hypocalcemia, and, in cases of severe bleeding from any source, elevated lactate.

The BUN can increase secondary to decreased hepatic perfusion and the digestion of blood and subsequent absorption of hemoglobin. In patients with a suspected GI bleed, a BUN greater than 40 with a normal creatinine is suggestive of a substantial hemorrhage. A BUN can be expected to return to normal about 12 hours after the cessation of bleeding. Ammonia can be expected to rise as blood in the GI tract is digested and its metabolites absorbed.

IMAGING STUDIES

Three imaging methods are recognized as procedures of choice for the diagnosis of GI bleeding: endoscopy/colonoscopy, scintigraphy, and angiography. Critical care transport team members will neither perform nor be expected to interpret these studies, but should be familiar with them if presented with results.

Endoscopy and colonoscopy are useful diagnostic as well as therapeutic modalities. **Endoscopy** is utilized to identify and treat UGIBs, while **colonoscopy** is utilized to treat LGIBs. Endoscopy is a more proven intervention than colonoscopy, because defects in the colon, primarily diverticula, tend to be dispersed and difficult to locate in the voluminous colon. (See Figure 24-14 ■.) Specific treatments for particular insults are detailed below.

Scintigraphy, also known as technetium-labeled red blood cell scan, is an effective diagnostic test in cases of brisk bleeding, generally 1 to 2.0 mL/min or greater. In this study, red blood cells absorb radiolabeled potassium that is injected in the bloodstream. The extravasation of blood is then readily identified on X-ray by the presence of the radiolabeled blood found in the GI tract.

Angiography, like scintigraphy, also requires a relatively brisk bleeding rate of 0.5–2.0 mL/min or greater, and is particularly useful in the identification of LGIBs. In this study, radio-opaque dye is injected into the gut vasculature, which is then inspected under a fluoroscope. Subsequent identification of dye in the GI tract is diagnostic for hemorrhage.

Routine abdominal radiographs are of little diagnostic value in the diagnosis of GI bleeding. Barium contrast studies are not very much more useful in the acute setting, but may have more use in the chronic patient. In addition, barium has the disadvantage of contaminating and obscuring the GI tract wall, making the subsequent use of colonoscopy or endoscopy less effective.

endoscopy *diagnostic examination of the insides of organs or body cavities by use of a remote camera on the end of a scope; can be utilized to identify and treat UGIBs.*

colonoscopy *diagnostic examination of the insides of the colon by use of a remote camera on the end of a scope; can be utilized to treat LGIBs.*

scintigraphy *diagnostic test to detect bleeding in the GI tract.*

angiography *diagnostic study of the inside of vasculature by injection of radio-opaque dye, then inspection under a fluoroscope.*

■ Figure 24-14   Colonic mass (cancer).

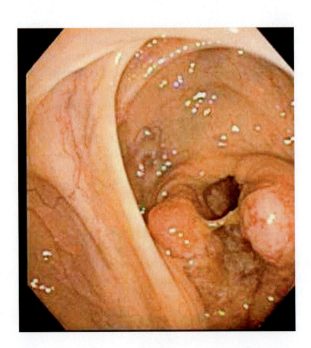

MANAGEMENT

As with all emergencies, priority is placed on ensuring that your patient has an adequate airway, is breathing appropriately, and has a pulse. Patients with UGIBs and hematemesis may require aggressive suctioning and an advanced airway to prevent the aspiration of blood. Oxygen should be administered to all patients suffering from GI bleeding, the delivery method determined by the degree of hypoxia present. In addition, significant blood loss may lead to shock and inadequate breathing, necessitating artificial ventilation.

Signs and symptoms consistent with shock require the aggressive administration of volume-expanding agents. Initial volume replacement can be accomplished with crystalloid solutions; blood products should be administered based on clinical findings suggestive of severe volume depletion (greater than 2 L of crystalloid used). Because hematocrit levels are not always reliable indicators in cases of acute bleeds or after significant volume replacement with nonblood products, they should not be used to determine their need in such cases.

Despite concerns to the contrary, NG tube placement will not result in bleeding in patients with varices, and all patients with significant GI bleeding should have an NG tube placed and the stomach evacuated of any contents. In cases of bright red blood return in a NG tube, gentle gastric lavage can be considered to rid the stomach of blood in an effort to reduce the chances of vomiting and aspiration.

Despite concerns to the contrary, NG tube placement will not result in bleeding in patients with varices, and all patients with significant GI bleeding should have an NG tube placed and the stomach evacuated of any contents.

Esophageal and gastric varices identified by endoscopy can be treated with band ligation or sclerotherapy with a chemical or thermal agent. Treatment modalities that can be initiated by the typical critical care transport team include the administration of vasopressin or somatostatin, and balloon tamponade with a Sengstaken-Blakemore tube. Vasopressin and somatostatin are agents that lower portal hypertension, slowing the rate of variceal bleeding (by vasoconstricting the splanchnic bed). Octreotide is a longer-acting analogue of somatostatin that has been used with success and has fewer side effects than vasopressin.

Variceal bleeding in the esophagus and the gastric cardia can be controlled by direct pressure with the use of a Sengstaken-Blakemore tube. The tip of this device is placed in the stomach, utilizing the nare for entry into the GI tract. A gastric balloon is then inflated with no more than 50 mL of air and positioned so that it rests in the gastric cardia. External traction is supplied to keep the balloon in place against the gastric wall and apply direct pressure to the bleeding varices. If needed, an esophageal balloon can be inflated to a pressure of no more than 25 to 45 mmHg to tamponade esophageal varicies. Use of this device is ideal for critical care transport, but not for longer than 24 to 48 hours, because pressure necrosis can develop secondary to decreased tissue perfusion under the balloon. If all other methods of managing esophageal varices fail, the patient may have a procedure done that is referred to as **transjugular intrahepatic portosystemic shunt** (TIPS) placement. During this radiologic procedure, an intrahepatic shunt is placed in an attempt to decrease portal pressure and slow the hemorrhage of the varices.

Treatment of peptic ulcers is directed at reducing the secretion of gastric acid, attenuating the effects of secreted acid on the gastric mucosa, and eliminating *H. pylori*. Acid-reducing therapy includes the administration of proton pump inhibitors, histamine receptor antagonists (H$_2$RAs), sucralfate, and antacids. An IV proton pump inhibitor (PPI) is considered standard of care. PPIs are extremely effective at decreasing acid secretion by irreversibly binding with the proton pump on gastric parietal cells responsible for pumping hydrogen ions across the gastric lumen. H$_2$RAs inhibit the action of histamine at the H$_2$ receptors of the gastric parietal cells, reducing the secretion of gastric acid. Sucralfate encourages the formation of thick mucus over an ulcer, preventing further erosion via gastric acid and allowing for healing. Antacids buffer gastric acids, allowing for the healing of ulcerations to occur.

transjugular intrahepatic portosystemic shunt (TIPS) *a radiologic procedure that creates an intrahepatic shunt in an attempt to decrease portal pressure and slow the hemorrhage of esophageal varices when other methods have failed.*

PANCREATITIS

Although there are a myriad of known etiologies for acute pancreatitis, the exact physiological mechanism of the disease remains unidentified. Under normal circumstances, pancreatic enzymes are secreted in an inactive form, and then activated upon entering the duodenum. It is postulated that premature activation of pancreatic enzymes that are still within the acinar cells of the pancreas results in the autodigestion of pancreatic tissue. Trypsin, phospholipase A, compliment, kinin, and

Although there are a myriad of known etiologies for acute pancreatitis, the exact physiological mechanism of the disease remains unidentified.

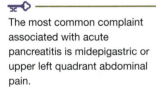

The etiologies of acute pancreatitis can be categorized as obstructive, traumatic, toxin induced, metabolic, infectious, vascular, and idiopathic.

lipase are the primary enzymes responsible for the local necrosis, swelling, and systemic complications. Activation of these digestive enzymes results in edema, vascular damage, interparenchymal hemorrhage, coagulation, and tissue necrosis. This damage results in a local inflammatory reaction that further increases vascular permeability and edema, with the end result being **pancreatitis.**

The etiologies of acute pancreatitis can be categorized as obstructive, traumatic, toxin induced, metabolic, infectious, vascular, and idiopathic. Common causes of obstructive pancreatitis include gallstones (about 45% of all cases), ampullary or pancreatic neoplasms, a hypertensive sphincter of Oddi, and foreign bodies. Blunt or penetrating trauma that insults the pancreohepatic ductal system can result in pancreatitis, as can trauma from iatrogenic sources. Toxic etiologies include methyl and ethyl alcohol and organophosphate insecticides. More than 80 different drugs have been associated with pancreatitis. Bacterial etiologies include *Legionella, Mycobacterium tuberculosis, M. avium,* and *Mycoplasmas.* Parasites such as ascariasis and viral infections including mumps, rubella, HIV, Epstein-Barr, and hepatitis have been shown to contribute to pancreatitis. Vascular occlusion can result in pancreatic tissue necrosis and progression of pancreatitis. About 10% of cases of pancreatitis are idiopathic.

The clinical course of pancreatitis can range from mild to severe and include multiple organ failure, sepsis, and death. The severity of disease can be categorized by the type of lesions present. Edematous pancreatitis is a mild form characterized by the presence of mild pancreatic interstitial edema and the presence of mild peripancreatic fat necrosis. This mild form can be self-limiting or may progress to the more severe necrotizing pancreatitis, characterized by significant parenchymal necrosis, intrapancreatic hemorrhage, and extensive intrapancreatic and peripancreatic fat necrosis. While severe pancreatitis can affect every organ system in the body, 80% to 90% of cases of pancreatitis are self-limiting and will resolve spontaneously within 5–7 days.

Important also during the course of pancreatitis is the release of enzymes (e.g., phospholipase), which is believed to cause the numerous pulmonary complications associated with pancreatitis. The patient with pancreatitis may experience significant changes in pulmonary function such as arterial hypozemia, atelectasis, pleural effusions, ARF, and ARDS. Vigorous pulmonary care with careful fluid administration is necessary to minimize the pulmonary complications of pancreatitis.

Cardiovascular complications include hemodynamically significant fluid sequestration during fulminant pancreatitis. Enzymes released also cause peripheral vasodilation, hypoperfusion, hypotension, and shock. Poor blood flow can also cause the ischemic pancreas to release myocardial depressant factor (MDF). MDF decreases heart contractility and cardiac output leading to multiple-organ dysfunction.

SIGNS AND SYMPTOMS

The most common complaint associated with acute pancreatitis is midepigastric or upper left quadrant abdominal pain. The pain is often described as constant, boring pain that radiates to the back and flanks. The pain often starts suddenly after the ingestion of a meal, and is commonly severe in nature and exacerbated by lying supine; a knee-chest position will often provide some relief. Abdominal guarding and rigidity are often present, and swelling or distention is sometimes appreciated. Palpation of the abdomen will often elicit severe pain.

Nausea and vomiting are common, as is a low-grade fever and tachycardia. Auscultation of bowel sounds may reveal hyperactive or absent sounds in the case of paralytic ileus. In the more severe cases of pancreatitis, bruising of the flanks (Grey Turner's sign) or around the umbilicus (Cullen's sign) may occur, and indicates severe pancreatic insult and hemorrhage; shock and multisystem organ failure are possibilities in such cases.

LABORATORY DATA

Due to the lack of a specific, identifiable clinical syndrome, a diagnosis of pancreatitis cannot be obtained by clinical evaluation alone. Laboratory and imaging studies are helpful for ruling out alternative diagnoses of abdominal pain, and can be helpful to an extent in determining the severity of pancreatitis. For example, radiographs of the chest and abdomen are useful in determining the presence of other pain-provoking etiologies such as intestinal perforation, paralytic ileus, pericardial effusion, and various pulmonary disease processes. Abdominal ultrasound is not extremely useful because of difficulty in visualizing the pancreas due to adipose tissue and/or intestinal gas. CT scanning is helpful in determining the severity of acute pancreatitis due to the ability to visualize the size of the pancreas and to identify the presence of pancreatic fluid, pseudocysts, and abcesses. The only "gold standard" diagnostic study is pathologic examination of the pancreas.

While serum amylase and lipase are the two most commonly utilized serum markers for pancreatitis, both lack the sensitivity and specificity to be used as the sole indicators of disease and should be used in conjunction with the entire clinical picture.

Amylase, a digestive enzyme secreted by the salivary glands and the pancreas, is used to digest starch into smaller carbohydrates. Unfortunately, it is a nonspecific marker for pancreatitis because it is also found in other tissues such as the small intestine, lungs, thyroid, fallopian tubes, ovaries, testes, adipose tissue, and skeletal muscle. In cases of pancreatitis, amylase is released into the bloodstream, causing a rapid rise above the normal levels of 110–300 IU/L. Due to a half-life of about 2 hours, amylase levels will return to normal within 3 to 4 days, even in instances of continued inflammation. As such, amylase has a sensitivity of 81% to 84% within the first 24 hours, and drops to about 33% after 36 hours. With regard to specificity, a level of three times the normal upper level, or 900 IU/L, has a specificity of about 75%. An upper limit five times the normal raises the specificity to about 90%. Amylase is eliminated by the kidney, and may be elevated in patients with renal failure.

Lipase is a digestive enzyme secreted by the pancreas to aid in the digestion of triglycerides. As lipase is also found in the gastric and intestinal mucosa, serum lipase can rise in cases of intestinal disease as well as pancreatitis. As such, it is about 90% specific for pancreatitis, arguably making it a better marker for pancreatitis; sensitivity is about 90% at an upper limit of two times normal. Lipase has a half-life of about 7 hours, and will remain elevated for several days after serum amylase has returned to baseline.

Additional lab studies that may be helpful in determining the extent of cases other than mild pancreatitis include serum calcium, hematocrit, base deficit, BUN, WBC count, glucose, lactate dehydrogenase, and asparate aminotransferase. Serial ABGs are useful in tracking the progression of severe pancreatitis, because pulmonary involvement is a common extrapancreatic sequela in such cases. ABG trends can be useful in determining the need for endotracheal intubation prior to transport in moderate to severe cases of pancreatitis.

IMAGING STUDIES

Imaging studies are extremely helpful in grading the severity of pancreatitis and the ruling out of other etiologies in a differential diagnosis. Modalities include CT, MRI, ultrasound, and radiograph. CT is the imaging study of choice because it provides unsurpassed anatomical detail and allows for not only the diagnosis of pancreatitis, but also the grading of the severity of the disease. CT is not, however, useful in ruling out pancreatitis, because it is insensitive to a mild and early disease process. MRI, as an alternative, has been found to be as effective as CT in identifying and grading pancreatitis. Ultrasound is useful in the evaluation of pancreatitis secondary to biliary obstruction or dilation (67% sensitivity, 100% specificity). It has limited value in the evaluation of nonbiliary etiologies, and practically no value in determining the extent of pancreatic injury. Abdominal radiographs have no use in the evaluation of the pancreas, but are useful to exclude conditions that may mimic pancreatitis, such as bowel infarction.

Determining the severity of pancreatitis can be aided by the use of one or more of the clinical criteria systems that have been developed. These include the commonly used CT severity index and Ranson's criteria for acute pancreatitis. Use of such grading systems can aid the critical care transport team in the appreciation of the severity of disease and aid in management and transport decisions.

MANAGEMENT

After addressing the airway, breathing, and circulation needs of your patient, considerations for transport can be considered. The general principle is to "rest the pancreas," which can be achieved by keeping the patient NPO. Traditionally, insertion of an NG tube has been recommended to decrease pancreatic release of secretin, which is released by the duodenum when acidic gastric content

Imaging studies are extremely helpful in grading the severity of pancreatitis and the ruling out of other etiologies in a differential diagnosis.

enters it. Secretin release results in the secretion of pancreatic juice; thus, an NG tube clears the stomach of acidic content, which decreases secretin secretion, which decreases the release of pancreatic enzymes, alleviating the severity of pancreatitis. While this treatment is often initiated, recent studies have not proven NG tube insertion to be effective. NG tubes can, however, decompress the stomach during air transport and in cases of distention, and is recommended in those patients who are vomiting. Inhibition of pancreatic secretions by the use of anticholinergics or somatostatin can be considered, though their therapeutic benefit is questionable.

In all but severe cases of pancreatitis, small amounts of clear fluids can be administered orally, but hydration needs should be met via IV administration of a balanced electrolyte solution such as 0.9% normal saline. A urinary output of 100 mL per hour is considered ideal. In mild cases, some degree of dehydration will likely be present. In moderate to severe cases, the possibility of significant fluid shifting necessitates the need for central vein catheterization, hemodynamic monitoring, and aggressive fluid replacement with a crystalloid solution or blood products, if needed. In all cases of pancreatitis, a Foley catheter should be inserted prior to transport and urine output recorded.

Because 40% to 60% of all patients with necrotic pancreatic tissue will develop a secondary bacterial infection, antibiotic therapy should be considered in all cases of severe pancreatitis. IV imipenem or a quinolone should be utilized in combination with metronidazole, because these medications are able to successfully penetrate pancreatic tissue. Traditional antibiotics such as penicillins, aminoglycosides, and first- and second-generation cephalosporins should be avoided, because they penetrate pancreatic tissue poorly.

Because pancreatitis frequently results in anything from mild discomfort to significant pain, use of analgesics is encouraged to provide a pain-free transport for your patient. Every effort should be made to alleviate your patient's pain.

Numerous systemic complications can arise secondary to severe pancreatitis. Hypokalemia, hypocalcemia, and hypomagnesemia are common and will require replacement therapy. Patients will commonly require nutritional support in the form of total parenteral nutrition (TPN), requiring caregivers to be familiar with its administration. It is not uncommon for a jejunal feeding tube to be surgically inserted for prolonged TPN.

LIVER FAILURE

Liver failure can be precipitated by either chronic or acute etiologies. Chronic liver failure was the 12th leading cause of death and the 10th leading cause of death in men in the United States in 2000. Liver cirrhosis secondary to alcohol abuse accounts for the vast majority of chronic liver disease in these cases. The most common cause of acute liver is viral hepatitis, and it along with cirrhosis will make up the vast majority of cases of liver failure. Other etiologies of hepatitis and liver failure include drug toxicity, chemical toxicity, and autoimmune reactions.

PATHOPHYSIOLOGY

hepatitis *an inflammation of the liver parenchyma including the Kupffer's cells, bile ducts, and blood vessels.*

Hepatitis is an inflammation of the liver parenchyma including the Kupffer cells, bile ducts, and blood vessels. Inflammation leads to disruption of the hepatic structures, leading to an interrupted blood supply, ischemia, and eventual necrosis. Dead liver cells are removed via the immune system, and some regeneration takes place, allowing for the recovery of some degree of liver function in most cases.

Chronic active hepatitis, along with alcoholic liver disease and diseases causing biliary obstruction, can lead to cirrhosis of the liver. Cirrhosis causes severe changes in the structure and function of hepatic cells. As in hepatitis, an initial inflammation leads to decreased perfusion and necrosis, and fatty deposits also tend to be present. Instead of normal liver cells being regenerated, fibrotic tissue is generated that does not share the physiological characteristics of normal liver cells. This fibrotic tissue distorts the normal anatomy of the liver, leading to further liver dysfunction. In addition to causing a loss of normal metabolic and synthetic function, fibrotic tissue results in increased resistance to blood flow and an increase in portal pressure. These morphological and physiological changes to the liver are irreversible, and will eventually lead to liver failure.

The diagnosis of liver failure is made by the clinical presentation and the evaluation of liver function, determined by laboratory testing. Liver function tests determine the presence of the

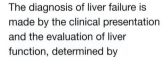

The diagnosis of liver failure is made by the clinical presentation and the evaluation of liver function, determined by laboratory testing.

markers of acute hepatocyte injury and death, the level of hepatocyte catabolic activity, and measure hepatocyte synthetic function.

Fulminant hepatic failure (FHF) is a medical emergency that is described as acute liver failure associated with hepatic encephalopathy. It has a very high mortality rate, and is found most commonly in patients who do not have any preexisting liver disease. Its cause is similar to those that precipitate chronic liver failure, but in this situation, the precipitating cause causes the liver to fail in 1 to 3 weeks. The development of hepatic encephalopathy then develops within 8 weeks. Hepatic encephalopahy is thought to result from failure of the liver to detoxify various substances in the bloodstream, ultimately resulting in metabolic and electrolyte imbalances.

SIGNS AND SYMPTOMS

The signs and symptoms associated with liver disease can be vague, despite the seriousness of the disease state. Nausea, vomiting, abdominal discomfort, and anorexia are also common. GI/GU symptoms include the production of dark urine and clay-colored stools. The liver may be found to be tender to palpation and moderately enlarged, and jaundice may be present. A cirrhotic liver is likely to be enlarged or firm on palpation. In addition ascites secondary to portal hypertension may develop, as can esophageal and gastric bleeding secondary to varices.

In cases of severe liver failure, an altered mental status, decreased level of consciousness, and even coma can result secondary to hepatic encephalopathy. Cardiovascular alterations include a decreased peripheral vascular resistance and an increased cardiac output. This may seem counterintuitive, but results from the opening of myocutaneous shunts.

Critical care paramedics will most likely see liver dysfunction patients during interfacility transports when they are moving patients to hospitals with liver transplant capabilities. The patient with hepatic failure (whether or not it is from FHF) is usually diagnosed prior to transferring the patient.

LABORATORY DATA

In cases of liver dysfunction, several markers of hepatic cellular damage are evaluated. Alanine transferase (ALT or AGOT), aspartate aminotransferase (AST or SGPT), and alkaline phosphatase are all elevated in instances of cellular injury. A prolonged PT and decreased albumin suggest decreased or diminishing hepatic function. In addition, hypoalbuminemia, hypokalemia, and hyponatremia may be present. Increased hepatic catabolic activity also results in elevated bilirubin and serum ammonia. Note, however, that in liver failure the liver enzymes (ALT/AST) may be normal due to profound liver dysfunction and scarring/fibrosis.

MANAGEMENT

No cure for liver failure exists, and the definitive treatment is liver transplant. Thus, the management of liver failure is mostly supportive, with particular attention to the airway, breathing, and circulation deserving obvious attention from the critical care transport team. A patient with hepatic encephalopathy can lose the ability to control his airway and may develop breathing irregularities; as such, he will require an advanced airway and ventilatory support. Hypoalbuminemia can result in changes in oncotic pressure and subsequent fluid shift out of the vascular space, requiring volume support. Alteration in coagulation may require the administration of coagulation factors.

GASTROINTESTINAL MANAGEMENT DEVICES

Both the short- and long-term management of gastrointestinal complications will often require the need for gastrointestinal devices such as drainage tubes, feeding tubes, peritoneal dialysis catheters, and ostomy collection bags. While the critical care paramedic will normally not be responsible for the placement of such devices, an understanding of their role, function, and potential complications is required to ensure adequate continuation of care.

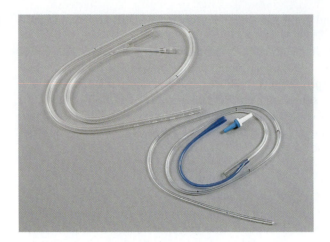

NASOGASTRIC TUBES

A large-bore (14- to 16-French) NG tube may be inserted for a number of reasons, including the decompression of gastric air during artificial ventilation, the removal of gastric contents in cases of obstruction, ileus, or drug overdose, for the removal of gastric acids in cases of ulcerative disease, and to control bleeding in cases of variceal bleeding (addressed later). In addition, an NG tube may be placed for diagnostic purposes such as the evaluation of gastric pH or to determine the presence of blood in the stomach. (See Figure 24-15 ■.)

Large-bore NG tubes commonly used for decompression or drainage include the Salem sump and Levine tubes. The Salem sump tube is a double-lumen device with a small-diameter vent tube housed within a larger-diameter suction tube. (See Figure 24-16 ■.) The suction tube is commonly attached to low continuous suction, but greater suction pressure can be applied when needed. The inner vent tube maintains a suction of less than 25 mmHg through the eyes located at the distal end of the tube, preventing damage to the gastric mucosa. The single-lumen Levine tube is also used to decompress and evacuate the stomach, but the absence of a vent tube necessitates the use of low-pressure intermittent suction to prevent damage to the gastric mucosa should the distal end of the tube come into contact with the gastric wall.

Insertion of an NG tube is a straightforward process within the scope of practice for members of the critical care transport team; however, the procedure is not without potential complications. Improper tube placement is the primary cause of complications, and every serious effort must be

■ Figure 24-16 Salem sump nasogastric tube. (*Craig Jackson/In the Dark Photography*)

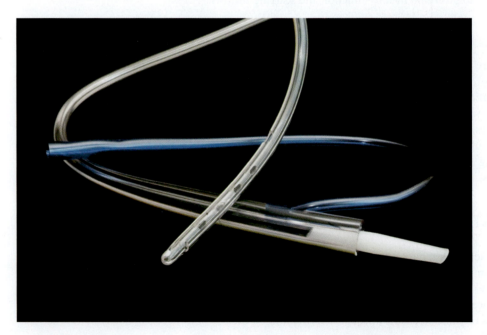

made to ensure that the distal end of the tube is properly placed. Misplacement of NG tubes into the lung is a common occurrence, and placement of NG tubes into the cranial vault has been reported in the literature numerous times. Placement of an NG tube into the respiratory tract can result in pneumothorax and pneumomediastinum, and introduction of material such as charcoal into the lung can prove fatal. Methods to ensure proper NG tube placement include the auscultation of insufflated air into the stomach, aspiration and pH measurement of gastric content, chest radiograph, and capnometry. It is worth noting that endotracheal intubation with an NG tube is often asymptomatic, and the most often used method in the emergent situation, auscultation of the upper abdomen while insufflating the stomach, is a notoriously unreliable method of tube placement confirmation. Therefore, the critical care paramedic should make every effort to utilize pH measurement, chest radiograph, or capnometry to rule out improper tube placement. No confirmation method is foolproof, and common sense must prevail; when in doubt, pull it out and reattempt. As with endotracheal tubes, the critical care paramedic should always reevaluate the placement of NG tubes inserted prior to their arrival.

Prior to transport, the critical care paramedic should confirm proper placement and evaluate the NG tube drainage. Normal drainage color ranges from yellow to green, and will occasionally contain streaks of blood, secondary to the distal end coming into contact with the gastric wall. Frank blood or "coffee-grounds" drainage is not normal and should be noted and the cause of bleeding explored. To prevent accidental extubation of the NG tube, it should be anchored to the nare with tape, and the level of entry marked on the tube with an indelible marker. Because an NG tube is likely to irritate a patient's nasal mucosa and throat, lozenges or other forms of topical anesthetic may be utilized to ensure comfort.

NASOINTESTINAL TUBES

Nasointestinal tubes, commonly referred to as feeding tubes, are small-bore (8- to 10-French) tubes inserted into the small intestine to support nutrition. The most commonly used feeding tube is the Dobhoff tube, a single-lumen tube that is not attached to suction. The smaller diameter of feeding tubes alleviates some of the mucosal irritation that occurs with larger-diameter NG tubes, and can be kept in place for 2 to 3 weeks.

Nasointestinal tubes are placed in the same manner as NG tubes, but are advanced farther along the digestive tract past the pyloric sphincter and into the duodenum, jujenum, or ileum. (See Figure 24-17 ■.) Complications of these tubes mirror those of NG tubes, and feeding tubes, because of their smaller diameter, are more easily dislodged and clogged. Nasointestinal tubes should be securely anchored to the nare, and the insertion level identified with an indelible marker. Clogged feeding tubes can be instilled with saline, left for 30 minutes, and an attempt made to flush the accumulated sediment forward. If this proves unsuccessful, the feeding tube should be replaced.

Prior to transport, a nasointestinal feeding tube should be evaluated to ensure that it is properly placed, patent, and secure. If the tube has been in use without complications, the critical care transport team can be assured that it is properly placed and patent, and the tube should be adequately secured in place. Consideration should be given to slowing the flow rate or stopping feeding altogether during transport to decrease the possibility of gastric regurgitation or vomiting, both of which increase the risk of aspiration and airway compromise. If a new feeding tube is placed immediately prior to transport, tube placement must be confirmed by radiograph prior to use, because introduction of nutritional solutions into the respiratory tract can result in pneumonia, sepsis, and death. In cases where a patient will require enteral feeding for more than 30 days, a more permanent transabdominal feeding tube will be surgically or endoscopically placed.

TRANSABDOMINAL FEEDING TUBES

Although the insertion of a **transabdominal feeding tube** is beyond the scope of practice for critical care transport team members, all should be familiar with their function and the complications associated with these devices. The three types of transabdominal feeding tube procedures often utilized are gastrostomy, jejunostomy, and gastrojejunostomy. Feeding tube placement can be via open surgical technique by a surgeon, under endoscopy by a gastroenterologist, or percutaneously by an interventional radiologist. Catheters often used for gastrostomy include balloon catheters and mushroom

nasointestinal tubes *small-bore (8-to-10 French) tubes inserted via a nare into the small intestine to support nutrition: commonly referred to as feeding tubes.*

transabdominal feeding tube *tube used to support nutrition, and placed via open surgical technique, under endoscopy, or percutaneously. The three types often utilized are gastrostomy, jejunostomy, and gastrojejunostomy.*

Figure 24-17 Naso-jejunal tube. *(Craig Jackson/In the Dark Photography)*

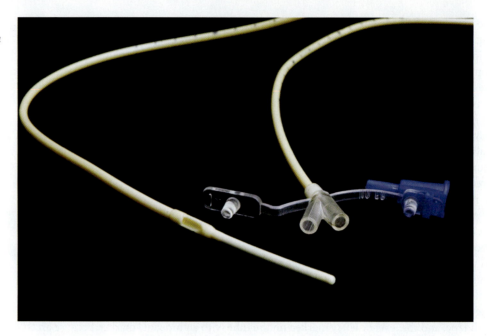

(bumper) catheters, and they often have a double lumen to allow for feeding as well as suctioning bowel contents.

In a gastrostomy, a feeding tube is introduced into the stomach through the abdominal wall. A surgical gastrostomy is usually performed while a patient is already undergoing laparotomy for abdominal complications. A permanent stoma is created by suturing the gastric and abdominal walls to one another, and a feeding tube is inserted into the gastric lumen and held in place with internal and external rubber bumpers and/or bolster.

A percutaneous endoscopic gastrostomy (PEG) is performed by a gastroenterologist with the patient under conscious sedation. An endoscope is passed into the patient's stomach, allowing the gastroenterologist to identify the tube placement site. A guidewire is passed through the abdominal wall, and forceps are used to grab the wire and bring it up through the endoscope into the patient's mouth. The PEG tube is secured to the wire, and then pulled through the mouth, into the stomach, and through the abdominal wall. As with a surgically placed gastrostomy tube, a PEG tube is often held in place with rubber bumpers and/or bolster, or an internal balloon and external disk may be used to secure it in place. (See Figure 24-18 ■.)

An interventional radiologist can also place a gastrostomy tube with the patient under local anesthesia, utilizing fluoroscopic visualization techniques to identify the stomach and avoid other abdominal structures, such as the liver. Gastric distention is performed by introducing gas into the stomach via an NG tube, which facilitates gastric puncture and dilation of the tube tract. A balloon-tipped feeding tube is then introduced into the gastric lumen, the balloon inflated, and an external disk used to further secure the tube in place.

Figure 24-18
Percutaneous endoscopic gastrostomy (PEG) tube.

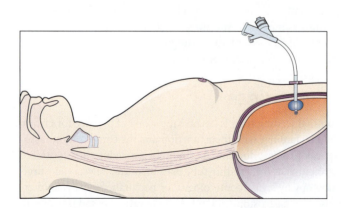

In a jejunostomy, a feeding tube is placed into the jejunal lumen through the abdominal wall. As in gastrostomy, a surgical or percutaneous approach may be used. Due to the high risk associated with direct jejunostomy, a gastrojejunostomy (often called transgastric jejunostomy) is often performed. A percutaneous endoscopic jejunostomy (PEJ) can be considered an extension of a PEG tube. In PEJ, a PEG tube is placed, and a smaller-diameter feeding tube is introduced through the PEG tube into the stomach, and directed into the duodenum. Peristaltic motion of the duodenum then propels the PEJ tube into the jejunum.

Prior to transport, the critical care paramedic should ensure that a previously placed transabdominal feeding tube is adequately secure and patent. As with nasogastric feeding tubes, the critical care team should consider stopping feeding for the duration of the transport, if possible, to help decrease the likelihood of gastric regurgitation, airway compromise, and aspiration. If a transabdominal feeding tube has been placed just prior to transport, ensure that tube placement has been verified prior to the initiation of feeding. In addition, complications such as perforated stomach and bowel, hepatic injury, and hemorrhaging may occur during or immediately after the procedure and should be assessed for before and during transport. Other common complications with feeding tubes include tube-site infections, leakage at the tube site, catheter occlusion, and catheter dislodgement. If obstruction or dislodgement occurs during transport, feeding should be discontinued immediately and the feeding tube clamped to prevent retrograde flow of fluid into the tube. Feeding tube replacement, although a relatively simple procedure when the tube tract is intact, should not be attempted during transport, but left for a physician at the receiving facility. An occlusive dressing can be placed over the open stoma during transport.

NASOINTESTINAL TUBES TO CORRECT BOWEL OBSTRUCTION

Anderson, Miller-Abbott, and Cantor tubes are long (up to 10 feet), wide-diameter tubes used to clear obstructions of the small bowel in patients who are considered high-risk surgical candidates. The tube has a weighted distal end that is pulled along the intestinal tract by peristalsis, and low continuous suction is applied to aid in the removal of impacted fecal material. In addition, irrigation can be utilized to facilitate breakup and removal of impacted material. The older Miller-Abbott (double-lumen) and Cantor (single-lumen) tubes were weighted by a mercury-filled balloon; these tubes are rarely used today because of the health risk associated with the introduction of mercury into the intestinal tract should the balloon rupture. The newer double-lumen Anderson tube has a tungsten tip, which adds weight without the health risk. One lumen is attached to low continuous suction, while the second lumen is available for irrigation if needed.

Transport considerations for a patient with any of these types of tubes are similar to those for NG and nasointestinal tubes. The patient should be kept NPO, and frequent changes of position may be required to ensure that the tube can advance in the bowel. Because the goal is to allow the tube to advance in the intestinal tract, it should not be secured to the nare prior to transport.

Anderson, Miller-Abbott and Cantor tubes long (up to 10 feet), wide-diameter tubes used to clear obstructions of the small bowel in patients considered high-risk surgical candidates.

T-TUBE

A **T-tube** derives its name from its shape, and is used to collect bile from the gallbladder after liver transplant, cholecystectomy, or other surgery of the common bile duct. (See Figure 24-19 ■.) One end of the crossbar of the tube is placed in the common bile duct, and the proximal end is brought out through the incision site in the upper right quadrant of the abdomen and attached to a collection bag. The production of 700–1,200 mL per day of dark gold to green bile is normal, and necessitates frequent draining of the collection bag. T-tubes are frequently left in for up to 6 weeks, and secured with a suture.

Transport considerations for patients with T-tubes consist of ensuring that the tube is patent and adequately secured. The collection bag should be drained or replaced prior to transport, especially if it is almost filled to capacity. This will allow for easier recording of flow during transport and will avoid the situation of a filled bag during transport. The insertion site should be checked for infection or drainage; bile is highly irritating to skin, and every effort should be made to prevent the two from coming in contact.

T-tube a tube used to collect bile from the gallbladder after liver transplant, cholecystectomy, or other surgery of the common bile duct.

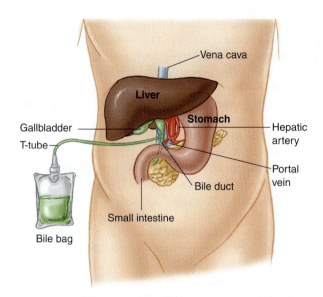

ESOPHAGEAL TUBES

The Sengstaken-Blakemore (often referred to as the Blakemore) tube and the Minnesota tube are NG tubes frequently used to control bleeding from esophageal and gastric varices. The **Sengstaken-Blakemore tube** is a triple-lumen tube with ports for the inflation of an esophageal balloon, inflation of a gastric balloon, and gastric aspiration. (See Figure 24-20 ■.)

The Sengstaken-Blakemore tube is inserted through a nare, down the esophagus, and into the stomach, where a gastric balloon is inflated to apply pressure at the cardioesophageal junction. This directly compresses gastric varices, and inflation of the esophageal balloon compresses esophageal varices. Traction is applied at the proximal end of the tube to hold the tube in place; traction can be maintained with a pulley system, or by taping the tube to the chin guard of a football helmet placed on the patient's head. Gastric contents, including blood, can be aspirated via the gastric port by gastric lavage or low-pressure intermittent suction. Swallowing is inhibited with the gastric balloon inflated, and secretions will accumulate above the balloon, requiring the insertion of a Salem sump or Levine tube and the application of low-pressure intermittent suction.

■ Figure 24-20 Sengstaken-Blakemore tube.

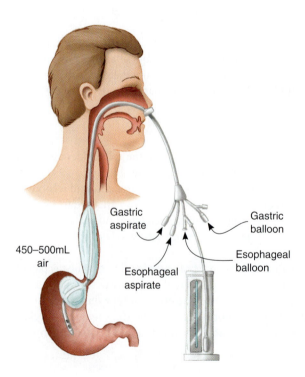

The **Minnesota tube** is similar to the Sengstaken-Blakemore tube, but also has an esophageal aspiration lumen that allows for the suctioning of collected esophageal secretions. Therefore, it does not require the additional placement of an NG tube.

Transport considerations for patients with Sengstaken-Blakemore and Minnesota tubes revolve around airway maintenance. Frequent suctioning of esophageal secretions is necessary to prevent aspiration. Placement of an endotracheal tube should be considered in all patients prior to esophageal tube insertion. Airway obstruction secondary to esophageal tube balloon inflation is always a major concern, and all balloons should be deflated immediately if respiratory compromise develops. Continued traction to the proximal end of the tube will be required during transport, and a plan developed to ensure that it is provided. Finally, remember that the various balloons used on many of these devices, may be subject to altitude changes during fixed-wing transports where atmospheric pressure may alter the pressure within the balloon or cuff.

OSTOMY COLLECTION BAGS

An intestinal resection is a procedure in which a part of the small or large intestine is excised, and two outcomes are possible. The preferred outcome is removal of the diseased portion of intestine and the attaching of the remaining proximal and distal ends, preserving the normal defecation process. The less desirable outcome is removal of the diseased bowel, and the attaching of the proximal bowel to the surface of the abdomen, forming an **ostomy.** Normal defecation is thus not preserved, and must instead take place through this opening. The opening is termed an *ileostomy* when the ileum is involved, and a *colostomy* when the colon is involved.

Because defecation through an ostomy is uncontrollable, the use of a collection bag is required. The critical care paramedic should ensure that the collection bag is emptied and secure prior to transport. In addition, gas buildup in the collection bag, especially during flight, may necessitate venting during transport, and crew members should ensure that the collection bag in place allows for such procedures.

RECTAL TUBES

Rectal tubes are employed as temporary measures to control and collect liquid stool. They are usually 25–35 cm long, 18–30 French in diameter, and may or may not have a distal balloon to keep them in place. If a distal balloon is used, care must be taken to prevent pressure necrosis of the rectal mucosa.

The critical care transport team should ensure that a collection system is securely in place and empty prior to transport. If a balloon is inflated to secure the tube, periodic deflation to prevent pressure necrosis may be warranted. If a rectal tube was placed immediately prior to transport, the crew should frequently assess for signs of rectal perforation and hemorrhaging, an uncommon but potentially deadly complication. Because consistency of fecal material can vary, obstruction of the rectal tube may occur and must be assessed for frequently.

SURGICAL WOUND DRAINAGE SYSTEMS

During surgery, a surgeon may elect to place a tube in the wound to aid in the removal of blood, pus, or other fluid that may accumulate at the surgical site. Methods that rely on gravity to facilitate drainage are termed passive drainage, and methods that utilize suction are considered active drainage.

A **Penrose drain** is a flat, 0.5- to 1.0-inch-diameter, single-lumen tube inserted into a surgical site to promote drainage of large amounts of fluid. (See Figure 24-21 ■.) It is a passive drainage method, relying on gravity to move fluid into a collection container. The Penrose drain is usually held in place with layers of absorbent dressings.

Two commonly used active drainage systems are the Jackson-Pratt and Hemovac systems. Both are used when small amounts of drainage are expected. With both systems, tubing is placed at or near the surgical incision site, and the proximal end attached to a suction device. The **Jackson-Pratt drainage system** is a hand-grenade-sized bulb that is compressed and then attached to the proximal end of the drainage tube, creating a closed, low-pressure system. The **Hemovac drainage system** has a more rigid plastic housing with internal springs; compressing the device, attaching the proximal

Minnesota tube *similar to the Sengstaken-Blakemore, but also has an esophageal aspiration lumen that allows for suctioning of collected esophageal secretions.*

Transport considerations for patients with Sengstaken-Blakemore and Minnesota tubes revolve around airway maintenance. Frequent suctioning of esophageal secretions is necessary to prevent aspiration. Placement of an endotracheal tube should be considered in all patients prior to esophageal tube insertion.

ostomy *removal of the diseased bowel, and surgical attachment of the proximal bowel to the surface of the abdomen with a portal that facilitates defecation.*

rectal tubes *tubes, 25–35 cm long and 18–30 French, that may have a distal balloon to keep them in place; used for temporary measure and collection of liquid stool.*

Penrose drain *a flat, 0.5–1.0 inch diameter, single-lumen tube inserted into a surgical site to promote drainage of large amounts of fluid.*

Jackson-Pratt drainage system *tubing placed at or near a surgical incision site with the proximal end attached to a "hand-grenade"-sized compressed bulb creating a closed, low-pressure drainage system.*

Hemovac drainage system *rigid plastic housing with internal springs that is compressed and attached to the proximal end of a drainage tube, thereby plugging a vent hole and creating a closed, low-pressure system.*

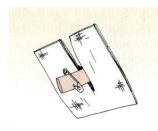

Sump tubes are basically Penrose tubes with a double-lumen sump tube inserted inside, resulting in a triple-lumen drainage tube.

peritoneal dialysis catheter
a flexible, siliconized rubber catheter surgically placed into the abdominal cavity to facilitate the administration and removal of dialysate solutions.

end of the drainage tube, and plugging a vent hole creates a closed, low-pressure system. Both the Jackson-Pratt and Hemovac devices have graduations on the collection chamber, making accurate measurement of drainage volume possible. As with the Penrose drain, the Jackson-Pratt and Hemovac drainage tubes are often held in place only with absorbent dressings. (See Figure 24-22 ■.)

Sump tubes are basically Penrose tubes with a double-lumen sump tube inserted inside, resulting in a triple-lumen drainage tube. These tubes are often inserted into the abdominal compartment, and are useful in draining large abscesses and large amounts of fluid and debris. One port is connected to low continuous suction, another to air to prevent the buildup of large suction pressures and subsequent tissue damage, and the third port to slow, continuous irrigation if needed.

Transport considerations for patients with these devices include ensuring that the tubes are patent and emptying the collection chambers prior to transport. Because Penrose, Jackson-Pratt, and Hemovac tubes are often held in place with dressings only, extreme care must be taken to ensure that they are not accidentally removed during transport. If a collection chamber must be emptied during transport, the drainage tube should be clamped, the drainage chamber removed, emptied, then reattached, and the clamp removed to continue suctioning. The amount of discarded drainage should be recorded.

PERITONEAL DIALYSIS CATHETERS

The most commonly used **peritoneal dialysis catheter,** the Tenckhoff catheter, is a flexible, siliconized rubber catheter surgically placed into the abdominal cavity to facilitate the administration and removal of dialysate solutions. (See Figure 24-23 ■.) A cuff is placed into the subcutaneous layer of the skin, and scarring around the cuff firmly anchors it in place.

Transport considerations for a newly placed catheter include assessing for external and intra-abdominal bleeding, and ensuring that the tube is properly secured during transport. The Tenckhoff catheter should be capped when not in use.

TUBE CHECKLIST

Regardless of the type of tube encountered by the critical care transport crew, the following checklist can be utilized to ensure that all pertinent considerations are addressed prior to transport:

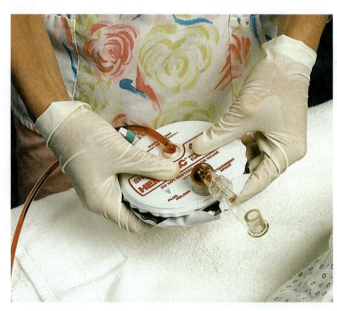

■ **Figure 24-22** Compress Hemovac by pushing top and bottom together.

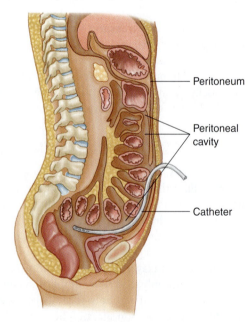

Peritoneum

Peritoneal cavity

Catheter

■ **Figure 24-23** Peritoneal dialysis catheter. This should never be mistaken for a feeding tube.

★ What is the tube's purpose?

★ Has proper placement been confirmed?

★ Is it patent?

★ Is it properly secured?

★ What amount and type of drainage can be expected?

★ How and with what frequency should the tube and equipment be assessed?

★ What are the potential complications?

★ What are the instructions for the care and maintenance of the tube during transport?

★ What information needs to be documented?

Summary

A thorough understanding of the complex GI tract is imperative if the critical care paramedic wishes to adequately address and treat any dysfunctions. This starts with a complete assessment of the patient, focusing on abdominal assessment and findings as necessary. To gain a complete picture, the critical care paramedic must review the patient's history, complete a thorough physical exam, and analyze available laboratory data. In addition, a review of any invasive and/or noninvasive diagnostic procedures will aid in identifying the disorder and allow a more accurate care plan to be developed.

Review Questions

1. What lab value is most useful in the diagnosis of pancreatitis?

2. Of the following, which is NOT an acceptable method of controlling bleeding in cases of esophageal varices?

   a. IV administration of a broad-spectrum antibiotic

   b. use of a Sengstaken-Blakemore tube

   c. IV octreotide

   d. administration of whole blood

3. Why are abdominal radiographs of no (or little) use in the diagnosis of acute pancreatitis?

4. What intravenous medication can be considered for fulminant hepatic failure?

5. Potential complications of liver failure include all of the following EXCEPT:

   a. volume depletion secondary to third spacing of fluids.

   b. loss of consciousness secondary to encephalopathy.

   c. hemorrhage secondary to a perforated hepatic vein.

   d. coagulation abnormalities secondary to decreased hepatic synthesis of clotting factors.

6. What is the most common cause of lower GI hemorrhage?

7. You are caring for a patient with a lower GI tract bleed. The following lab values are obtained prior to departure. What can be interpreted from these?

   Hematocrit: 19%   Hemoglobin: 6

   WBC: 22,000   Platelets: 45,000

   Na: 138   K: 3.9

   Cl: 110   Bicarb: 19

   BUN: 42   Creatinine: 1.0

8. What are some various GI disorders that may be discernible on a CT?

9. Why is the continued evacuation of stomach acid preferable in the patient with an upper GI disturbance?

See Answers to Review Questions at the back of this book.

Further Reading

Beejay U, Wolfe MM. "Acute Gastrointestinal Bleeding in the Intensive Care Unit. The Gastroenterologist's Perspective." *Gastroenterology Clinics of North America*, Vol. 29, No. 2 (June 2000): 309–336.

Bowyer MW. "Acute Pancreatitis." In *Critical Care Secrets*, 3rd ed. Parsons PE, Wiener-Kronish JP, editors. Philadelphia: Hanley & Belfus, 2003.

Broder JS, Rawden E. "Hepatic Disorders and Hepatic Failure." In *Emergency Medicine: A Comprehensive Study Guide*, 6th ed. Tintinelli JE, Kelen JD, Stapczynski JS, editors. New York: McGraw-Hill, 2004.

Brozenec SA, McAndrews CA, Monahan FD. "Knowledge Basic to the Nursing Care of Adults with Gastrointestinal Dysfunction." In *Nursing Care of Adults*. Monahan FD, Drake T, Neighbors M, editors. Philadelphia: W. B. Saunders, 1994.

Fallah MA, Prakash C, Edmundowicz S. "Acute Gastrointestinal Bleeding." *Medical Clinics of North America*, Vol. 84, No. 5 (September 2000): 1183–1208.

Hooker EA. "Complications of Gastrointestinal Devices." In *Emergency Medicine: A Comprehensive Study Guide*, 6th ed. Tintinelli JE, Kelen JD, Stapczynski JS, editors. New York: McGraw-Hill, 2004.

Kennedy MM. "Common Gastrointestinal Disorders." In *Critical Care Nursing: A Holistic Approach*, 7th ed. Hudak CM, Gallo BM, Morton PG, editors. Philadelphia: Lippincott-Raven Publishers, 1998.

Marino PL. *The ICU Book,* 2nd ed. Baltimore, MD: Williams & Williams, 1998.

Nobel KA. "Name That Tube." *Nursing,* Vol. 33, No. 3 (March 2003): 56–62.

Overton DT. "Gastrointestinal Bleeding." In *Emergency Medicine: A Comprehensive Study Guide*, 6th ed. Tintinelli JE, Kelen JD, Stapczynski JS, editors. New York: McGraw-Hill, 2004.

Perlstein J, Bowyer MW. "Hepatitis and Cirrhosis." In *Critical Care Secrets*, 3rd ed. Parsons PE, Wiener-Kronish JP, editors. Philadelphia: Hanley & Belfus, 2003.

Peter DJ, Dougherty JM. "Evaluation of the Patient with Gastrointestinal Bleeding: An Evidence Based Approach." *Emergency Medicine Clinics of North America*, Vol. 17, No. 1 (February 1999): 239–261.

Polio J, Groszmann RJ, Taylor MB. "Acute Management of Portal Hypertensive Hemorrhage from the Upper Gastrointestinal Tract." In *Gastrointestinal Emergencies*, 2nd ed. Taylor MB, editor. 131–150. Philadelphia: Lippincott Williams & Wilkins, 1997.

Velayos F. "Upper and Lower Gastrointestinal Bleeding in the Critically Ill Patient." In *Critical Care Secrets*, 3rd ed. Parsons PE, Wiener-Kronish JP, editors. Philadelphia: Hanley & Belfus, 2003.

Vissers RJ, Abdu-Laban RB. "Acute and Chronic Pancreatitis." In *Emergency Medicine: A Comprehensive Study Guide*, 6th ed. Tintinelli JE, Kelen JD, Stapczynski JS, editors. New York: McGraw-Hill, 2004.

Chapter 25

Renal and Acid–Base Emergencies

Timothy Duncan, RN, CCRN, CEN, CFRN, EMTP

Objectives

Upon completion of this chapter, the student should be able to:

1. Describe the anatomical structures of the renal system. (p. 751)
2. Understand the basic physiology of the renal system. (p. 752)
3. Identify three major causes of renal failure. (p. 755)
4. Describe emergent treatment of renal failure. (p. 756)
5. Describe the kidney's role in acid–base physiology. (p. 758)
6. Discuss the varying etiologies of acid-base disturbances. (p. 760)
7. Define the MUDPILES mnemonic and its effect on acid–base balance. (p. 761)

Key Terms

actual acidosis, p. 760
actual alkalosis, p. 760
anion gap, p. 762
blood urea nitrogen (BUN), p. 757
chronic renal failure (CRF), p. 756

continuous ambulatory peritoneal dialysis (CAPD), p. 756
creatinine, p. 757
filtration, p. 753
hemodialysis, p. 756
intrarenal failure, p. 755

lactic acidosis, p. 766
MUDPILES, p. 761
post-renal failure, p. 755
prerenal failure, p. 755
relative acidosis, p. 760
relative alkalosis, p. 760
uremia, p. 763

Case Study

A 13-year-old male with a past medical history of insulin-dependent diabetes was brought by EMS from home to a small receiving hospital in a neighboring city. Shortly thereafter, the decision was made by the medical personnel initially caring for the boy to summon your critical care transport service to move this patient to your referral center. After an uneventful flight to the community hospital, the critical care crew is escorted to the emergency department where the staff provides a brief synopsis of the boy's history and current clinical state. Following this, you and your partner enter the young patient's exam room and find the patient somnolent but arousable, with a Glasgow Coma Score of 13 (E=3, V=4, M=6). Vitals signs on assessment are:

- ★ Heart rate: 140
- ★ Blood pressure: 84/40
- ★ Respiratory rate: 30
- ★ Pulse oximetry: 100% on 2 liters per nasal cannula

Furthermore, you are provided with a copy of his current lab findings which include:

- ★ Hemoglobin: 15.4
- ★ Hematocrit: 45.2
- ★ White cell count: 14,000
- ★ BUN: 88
- ★ Creatinine: 2.2
- ★ Potassium: 6.5
- ★ Sodium: 155
- ★ Blood glucose: 444 mg/dL

The results of the arterial blood gas (ABG) analysis are:

- ★ pH: 7.01
- ★ PCO_2: 30
- ★ PO_2: 224
- ★ HCO_3^-: 12

The working diagnosis by the ED staff is diabetic ketoacidosis (DKA). He has an intravenous line in place of 0.9% NaCl, and has received 200 mL of intravenous fluid. Additionally, they have administered 10 units Humulin R insulin IVP and are preparing an insulin drip.

The patient is moved to the helicopter and the transport is uneventful. Blood glucose levels are monitored every 30 minutes because of the insulin drip and the blood glucose level steadily falls. Upon arrival at the receiving hospital, the patient has received approximately 800 mL of normal saline. His blood glucose is now 230 mg/dL, his pH has improved to 7.2, and his potassium is now 5.1 mEq/L. He is evaluated by multiple specialties and he and his family undergo additional diabetic education.

INTRODUCTION

Regardless of the reason why you are transporting a patient, all medical and trauma problems are heavily dependent on renal function to help maintain normal homeostasis. Beyond their role in fluid and electrolyte balance, the kidneys are also needed for blood pressure regulation, red blood cell (RBC) synthesis, metabolic waste removal, and medication metabolism. The inadequacy of this system, by way of renal failure, can surface as an acute or chronic change in kidney function from various etiologies such as direct and indirect trauma, toxic ingestion, and medical conditions that have altered renal physiology and function. While critical care paramedics may not be able to provide definitive treatment for renal emergencies or acid–base disturbances, they can provide emergent interventions to stabilize acid–base disturbances until hemodialysis can be performed.

This chapter will address some of the renal emergencies and acid–base disturbances that require critical care transport to a tertiary care or trauma center. First, by understanding renal physiology, the critical care paramedic can better understand the emergent needs of the critical care patient. It is the intent of this chapter to answer these as well as additional questions pertaining to acid–base disturbances seen in the critical care environment. Following this chapter, additional questions that pertain to a brief case study will be provided so that the critical care paramedic can apply lessons learned in this chapter.

RENAL ANATOMY

Normally, the kidneys are located in the retroperitoneal space at the area near the costovertebral angle. Blood that enters the kidneys does so through the renal artery at a rate of 1,200 mL/min, which equals about 25% of cardiac output. The kidney's main anatomical structures are the renal capsule, renal cortex, renal medulla, and renal pelvis. (See Figure 25-1 ■.) The renal cortex contains tiny, tubular structures that stretch across the surface of the kidneys. These functional structures of the

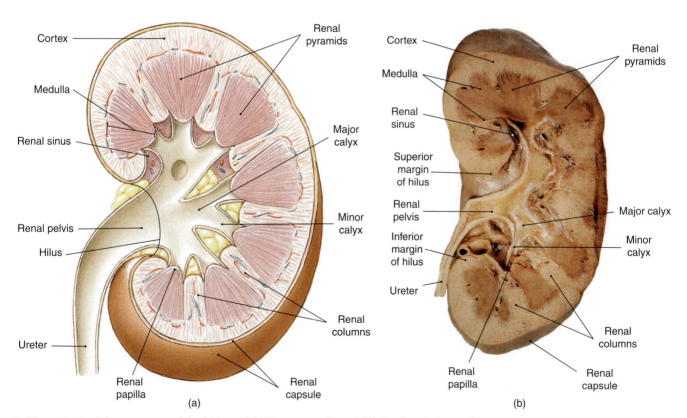

■ **Figure 25-1** The structure of the kidney. (a) Diagrammatic and (b) Sectional views of a frontal section through the left kidney. *(a from Fig. 19-3, p. 520, from* Essentials of Anatomy & Physiology, *2nd ed., by Frederic H. Martini, Ph.D. and Edwin F. Bartholomew, M.S. Copyright © 2000 by Frederic H. Martini, Inc. Published by Pearson Education, Inc. Reprinted by permission. b from Ralph T. Hutchings)*

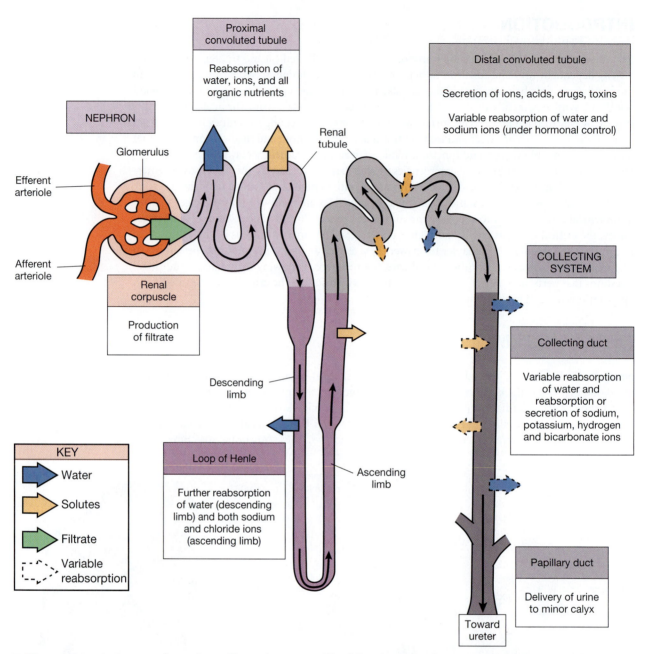

Proximal convoluted tubule

Reabsorption of water, ions, and all organic nutrients

Distal convoluted tubule

Secretion of ions, acids, drugs, toxins

Variable reabsorption of water and sodium ions (under hormonal control)

NEPHRON

Glomerulus

Renal tubule

Efferent arteriole

Afferent arteriole

Renal corpuscle

Production of filtrate

COLLECTING SYSTEM

Descending limb

Ascending limb

Collecting duct

Variable reabsorption of water and reabsorption or secretion of sodium, potassium, hydrogen and bicarbonate ions

KEY

Water

Solutes

Filtrate

Variable reabsorption

Loop of Henle

Further reabsorption of water (descending limb) and both sodium and chloride ions (ascending limb)

Papillary duct

Delivery of urine to minor calyx

Toward ureter

■ **Figure 25-2**   A representative nephron. The major structures and functions of each segment of the nephron and collecting system. *(Fig. 19-4, p. 521, from* Essentials of Anatomy & Physiology, *2nd ed., by Frederic H. Martini, Ph.D. and Edwin F. Bartholomew, M.S. Copyright © 2000 by Frederic H. Martini, Inc. Published by Pearson Education, Inc. Reprinted by permission.)*

kidneys, called nephrons, number about 1 million in each kidney. Each nephron contains a glomerulus (Bowman's capsule), proximal tube, loop of Henle, distal tubule, and collecting duct. (See Figure 25-2 ■.) Through a unique blood supply that maintains constant perfusion to renal cells (glomerular filtration rate), the nephron is the base unit of the renal system, responsible for filtration, reabsorption, and secretion of fluids, electrolytes, and waste products through the formation of urine.

RENAL PHYSIOLOGY

Along with the skin and respiratory systems, the kidneys serve as one of the body's primary excretory organs. Through a selective process of eliminating and retaining substances according to bodily needs, the renal system maintains the fragile internal ionic and fluid balance of the body. Without the renal system, the body can only survive for several days. Owing to its complexity, the kidneys not only maintain internal balance, but secrete hormones to stimulate the production of new red blood cells necessary to help ensure adequacy of end-cell and end-organ perfusion.

FILTRATION

Twenty percent of circulating blood flow passes through the capillaries of the glomerulus and Bowman's capsule and is filtrated. (See Figure 25-3 ■.) The filtrate is composed of water, ions (sodium, chloride, and potassium), glucose, and small proteins. The types of molecules filtered through Bowman's capsule are dependent on ionic charge, concentration, and size. Positively charged, smaller molecules will be allowed to pass through the capsule more readily without filtration than those that carry a negative charge or are molecularly larger. Additionally, the more concentrated the substances of the blood are, the more filtration that subsequently occurs. This process, called the glomerular filtration rate (GFR), occurs at a rate of 125 mL/min. At the normal GFR rate, circulatory blood volume is filtrated 20 to 25 times per day. **Filtration** occurs through a complex arrangement of capillaries that maintain pressure through the glomerulus during transient fluctuations in systemic blood pressure.

filtration *filtration of blood through a complex arrangement of capillaries that maintain pressure through the glomerulus during transient fluctuations in systemic blood pressure.*

REABSORPTION

Once the filtrate flows into the proximal tubule, smaller molecules are reabsorbed from the filtrate. Glucose, amino acids, and ions are grabbed by specialized proteins called *transporters* that are located on the membranes in various cells of the nephron. Each transporter grabs only one specific type of molecule from the filtrate as it passes. Water is reabsorbed passively by osmosis in response to the buildup of reabsorbed sodium in spaces that form the wall of the nephron. The reabsorption of most substances relies on the reabsorption of sodium, either directly through the sharing of a transporter, or indirectly through a process called solvent drag. As water passes through the proximal tubule of the nephron, some molecules are caught up in the flow of water and are passively reabsorbed.

If the transporters become overwhelmed with molecules, the excess molecules will "spill over" into urine. For example, when glucose transporters become saturated, as in uncontrolled diabetes, glucose will become detectable in a urine specimen. GFR will also affect the time available for transporters to reabsorb molecules. Approximately two-thirds of sodium, chloride, calcium, and bicarbonate ions are reabsorbed in the proximal tubule, and 25% of the same ions are reabsorbed at the loop of Henle. The distal tubule reabsorbs approximately 8% of the sodium, chloride, and bicarbonate.

SECRETION

Those substances that are not reabsorbed are transported by cells of the nephron into the distal collecting tubule for secretion in the form of urine. Urine, a substance comprised of 95% water and 5% solid material, is secreted according to the body's volume needs and hormonal release (e.g., aldosterone, antidiuretic hormone, and parathyroid hormone). The kidney has the ability to concentrate or dilute urine and regulate electrolyte balance based on physiological determinants. For example, when a patient consumes fluids, the body's fluid volume is increased and the kidneys recognize the need to secrete more urine in order to maintain the same intravascular volume. Conversely, during sleep when no fluid is being consumed and intravascular volume needs to be more conserved, antidiuretic hormone is released, formation of urine is lowered, and fewer urges to urinate result. Given this complex system, normal urine production and output should be greater than 500 mL per day. If urinary output is less than 500 mL/day (oliguria), regardless of etiology, renal insufficiency or renal failure should be considered until an alternative cause is diagnosed and appropriately managed.

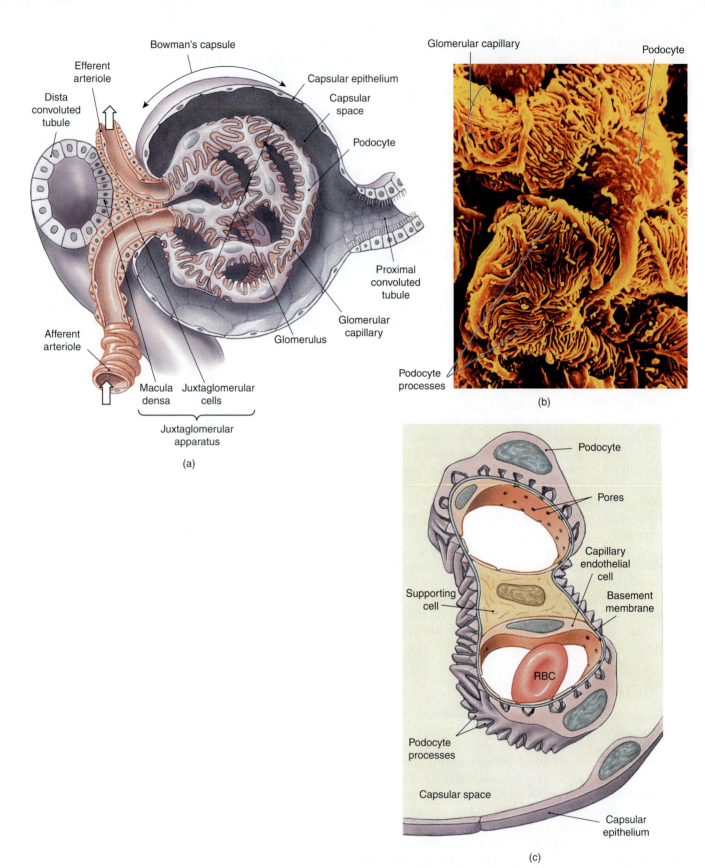

Figure 25-3 The renal corpuscle. (a) The renal corpuscle, showing important structural features. (b) Electron micrograph of the glomerular surface, showing individual podocytes and their processes. (c) A section of a glomerulus, showing the composition of the filtration membrane. *(a and c from Fig. 19-5, p. 522, from* Essentials of Anatomy & Physiology, *2nd ed., by Frederic H. Martini, Ph.D. and Edwin F. Bartholomew, M.S. Copyright © 2000 by Frederic H. Martini, Inc. Published by Pearson Education, Inc. Reprinted by permission. b from David M. Phillips/Visuals Unlimited)*

EMERGENCIES OF RENAL FAILURE

Renal failure, defined as failure of the kidneys to cleanse the blood with a resulting buildup of waste products, can occur acutely as a result of significant illness or serious injury, or slowly, usually as a result of a chronic condition from some other body system failure. Because of the various causes of renal failure, it is further subdivided and classified by the origin of its effects into three types of failure: prerenal, intrarenal, and post-renal.

PRERENAL FAILURE

Prerenal failure is caused by the decrease or loss of perfusion to the kidney, causing ischemic changes that become reflected in loss of renal function. Prerenal failure can occur as a result of hypovolemia, secondary to dehydration or blood loss, or can be a result of cardiac pump failure (regardless of volume status) such as would be expected in congestive heart failure. When perfusion is altered, the GFR decreases, and waste products begin to build in the bloodstream. Most notably, blood urea nitrogen (BUN) and creatinine levels will begin to rise as a result of decreases in GFR from inadequate renal perfusion.

Treatment of prerenal failure is aimed at finding and treating the causative agent(s) that initially allowed the poor renal perfusion to occur. For example, by ensuring proper long-bone immobilization, controlling external hemorrhage, and increasing myocardial preload by intravenous fluids, the critical care paramedic may decrease the amount of blood loss and maintain adequate perfusion in the traumatized patient and avoid prerenal failure. Administration of intravenous crystalloids (such as normal saline and lactated Ringer's) or transfusions of packed red blood cells will increase intravascular volume and result in enhanced perfusion to the kidneys. Treatments of prerenal failure resulting from cardiac pump abnormalities include the administration of diuretics such as furosemide (Lasix) or bumetanide (Bumex), inotropic agents such as dobutamine (Dobutrex), and other preload reducing agents such as nitroglycerin (Tridil).

The salient theme to be remembered by the critical care paramedic is that if perfusion to the kidneys is acutely or chronically altered and becomes insufficient, the GFR will drop and renal failure will ensue. As such, treatment should be geared at finding and treating the offending etiology.

prerenal failure *a decrease or loss of perfusion to the kidney, causing ischemic changes that are reflected in the subsequent loss of renal function.*

INTRARENAL FAILURE

Intrarenal failure results from direct damage to kidney parenchyma. Trauma, infection, or disease can cause damage to kidney tissues. Traumatic injuries to the kidneys can cause ischemic episodes that reduce kidney efficiency. Infectious organisms or diseases such as glomerulonephritis or renal tumors decrease GFR and cause acute tubular necrosis, an abrupt and progressive decrease in the function of the glomeruli and renal tubules. Nephrotoxic drugs such as tobramycin, gentamycin, and amphotericin B also can cause direct kidney injury leading to failure. As a critical care paramedic, treatment of direct parenchymal damage is causative. If trauma is the cause, transfer to definitive care while monitoring hemodynamic status, blood loss, and urinary output as the primary intervention.

intrarenal failure *trauma, infection, or disease that causes direct damage to kidney parenchyma; causes disruption of normal kidney function and can result in total organ failure.*

POST-RENAL FAILURE

Post-renal failure is caused by clinical conditions that cause obstruction to urine flow. Prostatic hypertrophy (benign or malignant), renal stones, bladder neck obstructions, or bladder tumors may obstruct normal blood flow. If this occurs, urine will back up in the ureters and will subsequently cause increased urine buildup within the kidney. Over time, the buildup of urine will result in actual nephron damage and intrarenal parenchymal damage.

Treatments of post-renal causes of renal failure include Foley catheter placement and the administration of analgesics such as fentanyl, morphine, or ketorolac to relieve ureteral spasm. If a Foley catheter is already in place, the critical care paramedic may have to replace the catheter to ensure optimum urinary output capabilities.

post-renal failure *result of clinical conditions that cause obstruction to urine flow.*

ACUTE EMERGENCIES IN CHRONIC RENAL FAILURE

chronic renal failure (CRF) *disruption of normal kidney function that results in patient use of artificial means to filter blood and maintain electrolyte and fluid balance.*

hemodialysis *external process for filtering waste products from the blood stream by means of scheduled and continuous ambulatory peritoneal dialysis (CAPD).*

continuous ambulatory peritoneal dialysis (CAPD) *also known as hemodialysis.*

In patients with **chronic renal failure (CRF),** the use of artificial means of filtration is essential to maintain electrolyte and fluid balance. **Hemodialysis,** or **continuous ambulatory peritoneal dialysis (CAPD),** done at scheduled times, is an external process for filtering waste products from the bloodstream. If the patient fails to complete treatments as prescribed, the physiological changes that occur can be life threatening. Additionally, if noncompliance is carried over to dietary restrictions, fluid restrictions, and medication administration, the risk for fluid volume overload, electrolyte imbalances, and cardiopulmonary compromise is high, because the chronic renal failure patient cannot rely on renal function to "kick in" if a dialysis treatment is missed. Fluid volume overload, hyperkalemia, acidosis, and hypoxia secondary to pulmonary edema can also occur.

DIALYSIS

Dialysis is a method of removing toxic substances (impurities or wastes) from the blood when the kidneys are unable to do so. Dialysis is most frequently used for patients who have kidney failure, but may also be used to quickly remove drugs or poisons in acute situations. Hemodialysis works by circulating the blood through special filters. The blood flows across a semipermeable membrane (the dialyzer or filter), along with solutions that help remove toxins. Hemodialysis requires a substantial blood flow, and a normal IV tube in an arm or leg will not support that volume of blood flow. Special forms of accessing the circulatory system are required. These access points can be temporary or permanent. Temporary access takes the form of dialysis catheters. These are large-bore catheters placed in large veins that can support acceptable blood flows. Most catheters are used in emergency situations, for short periods of time. However, catheters called tunneled catheters can be used for prolonged periods of time, often weeks to months. Permanent access when warranted is created by surgically joining an artery to a vein. This allows the vein to receive blood at high pressure, leading to thickening of the vein's wall. Now this "arterialized vein" can sustain repeated puncture and also provides excellent blood flow rates. The connection between an artery and a vein can be made using blood vessels (an arteriovenous fistula) or a synthetic bridge (arteriovenous graft). From this access point, blood is diverted to a dialysis machine. Here, the blood flows countercurrent to a special solution called the dialysate. The chemical imbalances and impurities of the blood are corrected and the blood is then returned to the body. Typically, most patients undergo hemodialysis for three sessions every week. Each session lasts 3–4 hours.

CONTINUOUS VENO-VENOUS HEMOFILTRATION (CVVH)

CVVH is another type of dialysis that may be seen by the critical care paramedic in the hospital. It is a short-term treatment, used in patients with kidney failure who are hemodynamically unstable (although the kidney failure may be new or already present). The CVVH machine will be located beside the patient and has several IV bags hanging under it. The machine contains a board that houses the various display panels and controls that manipulate the flow of blood, fluid removal, and replacement.

Similar to a regular dialysis machine, a dialysis catheter is first placed in one of the larger veins of the body. This catheter has two separate lines. Blood flows out of the catheter into the CVVH machine, which then goes into a filter where waste fluid is taken off. Fluids and electrolytes (such as sodium and potassium) are replaced, and then the blood is returned to the patient through the second line and into the catheter.

DIALYSIS-RELATED COMPLICATIONS

When the kidneys stop working, other bodily systems become taxed and do not typically work as efficiently as well. Unfortunately, this leads to complications, including the following:

★ *Anemia.* Anemia may occur due to a lack of erythropoietin, a hormone made by healthy kidneys that initiates the production of red blood cells. It can also be caused by low levels of iron that result from the patient's diet restrictions, poor absorption of iron, or removal of iron and vitamins by dialysis.

★ *Bone diseases.* People who receive dialysis typically experience changes in how well their bodies absorb calcium, phosphorus, and vitamin D. This can lead to renal osteodystrophy, osteomalacia, osteitis fibrosis, and calcium-phosphorous deposits.

★ *High blood pressure (hypertension).* Patients with kidney disease may experience difficulty in maintaining normal blood pressure due to complications of regulating salt and water balance.

★ *Fluid overload.* If patients neglect to follow their treatment plans, such as by drinking more liquid than is recommended, they will likely retain too much fluid in the body. Chronically this can lead to congestive heart failure or pulmonary edema.

★ *Pericarditis.* Pericardial inflammation may be caused by insufficient dialysis.

★ *High potassium levels (hyperkalemia).* Because of the difficulty in regulating electrolytes, the potassium level may become dangerously elevated and interfere with normal electrical conduction and depolarization in the heart.

★ *Peripheral neuropathy.* High levels of waste products in the body, diabetes, vitamin B$_{12}$ deficiencies, or other diseases may cause peripheral neuropathy.

★ *Infection.* Individuals receiving hemodialysis regularly can develop complications at their venous access site, such as blockage from blood clotting and poor blood flow. But the most serious problem at the venous access site is infection. About 15% to 20% of deaths among hemodialysis patients are due to infection, with the majority related to the venous access site.

Treatment of the chronic renal failure patient by the critical care paramedic must be focused on the side effects or physical symptoms caused by missed treatment(s) until dialysis can be performed. Hyperkalemia, which is common to CRF patients, entails interventions geared to antagonizing the effects of potassium on the heart, promoting the movement of potassium back inside the cells, and eventually removing excess potassium from the body. Antagonizing the effects of potassium is achieved with intravenous calcium gluconate or chloride and is the first priority. Intracellular movement of potassium is done as a temporizing intervention until removal from the body can be executed. Means to shift potassium into the cell include IV insulin and dextrose administration, and the use of intravenous bicarbonate administration. Continuous nebulized albuterol, with its beta-adrenergic stimulation, can also be used to shift potassium intracellular, but high doses are needed (10 to 20 times the dose for bronchotherapy). To eliminate potassium from the body, diuretic administration and the use of potassium exchange resins can be considered. If these measures fail to control hyperkalemia, dialysis must then be considered.

Keep in mind also that dextrose may be warranted in order to eliminate the risk of hypoglycemia, which may present with chronic renal failure. For this reason, measurement of blood glucose levels is necessary. For acidotic changes, the administration of sodium bicarbonate is indicated, and finally the critical care paramedic must also monitor for signs of hypomagnesemia.

DIAGNOSTIC FINDINGS OF ACUTE RENAL FAILURE

During transport, the critical care paramedic can garner information from lab values to assist with treatment priorities. Blood urea nitrogen and creatinine levels are hallmark diagnostic tests for the determination of renal function. Understanding what BUN and creatinine levels are will aid in interpreting the lab values for these markers of renal function.

As proteins are metabolized in the body, a waste product known as urea nitrogen is formed by the liver and carried to the kidneys for excretion. If the kidneys are not functioning properly, an excess amount of urea nitrogen will accumulate in the bloodstream. A **blood urea nitrogen** (BUN) test measures the amount of urea nitrogen present in the bloodstream. This test is used as a gross index of the filtration efficiency of the kidneys. However, since BUN values can be affected by the patient's hydration status, the creatinine clearance test is a much more sensitive indicator of declining renal function.

Creatinine is a protein that is produced by muscle tissue and released into the bloodstream. Muscle, for the most part, uses ATP for its energy needs. A substance known as creatine phosphate

blood urea nitrogen (BUN) *a diagnostic test for the determination of renal function that measures the amount of urea nitrogen present in the bloodstream.*

creatinine *protein that is produced by muscle tissue and released into the bloodstream.*

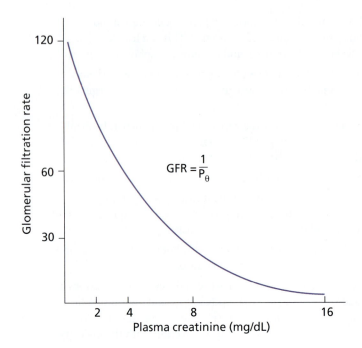

■ **Figure 25-4** Glomerular filtration rate (as a function of plasma creatinine levels).

$$GFR = \frac{1}{P_\theta}$$

is present in muscle as a backup for energy needs in case the available ATP is depleted. Over time, the creatine phosphate molecule degrades and creatinine is formed. There is nothing the body can do with creatinine, so it is filtered out of the blood by the kidneys. If kidney function is poor, the creatinine will not be filtered out efficiently and the levels will rise. Creatinine levels are dependent on the patient's muscle mass, which is much more stable from day to day than is the hydration status. For this reason, creatine clearance tests are much more sensitive indicators of kidney function than the BUN.

Normal values for BUN are 5–25 mg/dL, and normal creatinine values are 0.5–1.5 mg/dL. A ratio of BUN to creatinine levels should be maintained by the body at approximately 20:1. If the BUN-to-creatinine ratio exceeds 30, the most likely cause is prerenal in nature, and the critical care paramedic must utilize the patient's clinical presentation and past medical history to determine treatment choices. As mentioned earlier, creatinine is the best indicator of renal function. As the number of functioning nephrons falls, the GFR falls. The relationship of declining GFR to increasing creatinine is not linear. (See Figure 25-4 ■.) By the time the creatinine reaches 3–4 mg/dL, GFR has declined by 50%. Renal function is further determined by other tests—both blood and urine.

Other lab values that may be available include urinalysis, serum protein, serum albumin, and complete blood count. Urinalysis may be indicative of intrarenal or post-renal origin if proteinuria is present. If ketonuria (ketones) or glycosuria (glucose) is present in the urine, or if the specific gravity of the urine is elevated, a prerenal origin is suspected. Table 25–1 summarizes these diagnostic lab values as they pertain to the patient with renal failure.

ACID–BASE PHYSIOLOGY

In addition to the respiratory system, the renal system is also partially responsible for maintaining the body's acid–base balance. Utilizing carbon dioxide and bicarbonate from the respiratory and renal system, respectively, the body has the unique ability to adjust, or compensate for, any changes in systemic pH that cause the pH level to vary too far off the normal 7.35–7.45 range. In addition to these two organ systems, the utilization of the blood-buffering system also plays a role in the moment-to-moment regulation of the body's pH level, although the blood-buffering system can easily become overwhelmed if the acidic load becomes too great.

Table 25–1 | Diagnostic Lab Values for Patients with Renal Failure

Lab Test	Normal Value	Renal Failure	Reason
BUN	5–20 mg/dL	Increased	As the GFR decreases, the kidney's ability to excrete waste does the same. BUN and creatinine are measures of waste in the blood. These wastes will accumulate in the blood as the kidney function deteriorates, resulting in higher than normal lab values.
BUN/creatinine	10:1 to 20:1	Increased	
Creatinine	0.5–1.5 mg/dL	Increased	
Blood calcium (total)	8.5–10.5 mg/dL	Decreased	Calcium is decreased because, in a normally functioning kidney, vitamin D is metabolized to its active form. This active form of vitamin D is necessary for calcium to be absorbed from the GI tract. In kidney failure, vitamin D activation is compensated, resulting in decreased gut absorption of calcium, and a subsequent decrease in total blood levels.
Potassium	3.5–5 mEq/L	Increased	Potassium levels are increased in renal failure because of a decrease in the ability of the kidneys to excrete it. Also, with kidney failure, there is an increase in cellular destruction, with intracellular potassium released into extracellular spaces and tissue.
Phosphate	2.5–4.5 mg/dL	Increased	Phosphate levels are decreased because of the decreased GFR (resulting in a decreased ability for the kidneys to excrete phosphate).
Urine specific gravity	1.003–1.030	Decreased	The ability of the kidneys to concentrate urine is decreased.
pH	7.35–7.45	Decreased	Metabolic acidosis occurs because of impaired hydrogen ions (acid). There is also a decrease in the production and reabsorption of bicarbonate (an acid buffer).

BUFFERING SYSTEMS

Buffers are compounds added to solutions to prevent abrupt changes in pH. These buffers, usually weak acids, function as chemical "shock absorbers," either absorbing or releasing hydrogen ions to slow the rate of pH changes. Although response by the buffer system is immediate, it is limited. Compensation to changes in pH is limited to the degree of pH changes and the duration of the changes. The most common extracellular buffer is the bicarbonate ion (HCO_3^-), while the most common intracellular buffer is phosphate (PO_4^{3-}). One of the common types of blood buffering systems is the carbonic acid buffering system. In this system, carbonic acid is created as a product of carbon dioxide and water. It then separates into bicarbonate and hydrogen ions, which are manipulated by the body to either increase or decrease the pH as needed. This chemical reaction is shown here:

$$CO_2 + H_2O \rightarrow H_2CO_3 \rightarrow H^+ \text{ (hydrogen ion)} + HCO_3^- \text{ (bicarbonate ion)}$$

RESPIRATORY SYSTEM

The respiratory system also utilizes chemical receptors in the medulla of the brain to aid in pH regulation. These receptors are sensitive to pH levels within the cerebrospinal fluid (CSF), which reflects the body's $PaCO_2$ levels. If $PaCO_2$ levels within the bloodstream rise, the production of carbonic acid increases as the CO_2 is converted into hydrogen ions according to the preceding formula, and in turn causes the pH level to drop. The primary action of the respiratory system with this acidotic state is to increase respirations in order to improve alveolar ventilation and facilitate CO_2 elimination (i.e., "blow-off" carbon dioxide), therefore decreasing carbonic acid production.

The response of the respiratory system to changes in pH levels is immediate, regardless of the cause of the acidotic or alkalotic state. For example, a diabetic patient with diabetic ketoacidosis (DKA) will present with metabolic acidosis due to ketoacid metabolism. Although pH levels within CSF changes without fluctuations in $PaCO_2$ levels initially, hyperventilation in the form of Kussmaul's respirations occurs to compensate for the acidotic state.

RENAL SYSTEM

The renal system is the slowest of the three primary systems to balance pH levels. Through the excretion and/or reabsorption of bicarbonate (HCO_3^-) ions, the kidneys can raise or lower pH levels. Additionally, the excretion and reabsorption of phosphate ions and ammonia aid in adjusting pH levels, as hydrogen (H^+) ions follow with phosphate and ammonia. Although it is the most stable system for maintaining body pH levels, the renal system may take 24 to 48 hours to react to pH changes.

ACID–BASE IMBALANCES

Acid–base imbalances occur as the result of loss or gain of either an acid or base component. Relative imbalances occur as a result of a *loss* of an acid or base, whereas actual imbalances occur as a result of a *gain* in an acid or base component. (See Figure 25-5 ■.)

actual acidosis
overproduction of hydrogen ions.

actual alkalosis
overproduction of bicarbonate ions.

relative acidosis
overelimination of bicarbonate ions.

relative alkalosis
overelimination of hydrogen ions.

★ **Actual acidosis:** Overproduction of hydrogen ions
★ **Actual alkalosis:** Overproduction of bicarbonate ions
★ **Relative acidosis:** Overelimination of bicarbonate ions
★ **Relative alkalosis:** Overelimination of hydrogen ions

Imbalances can be categorized according to origin. Respiratory imbalances (discussed in Chapter 21) result from changes in carbon dioxide levels of the blood secondary to a decrease in alveolar ventilation. Metabolic imbalances result from changes in hydrogen and bicarbonate levels in the blood. Metabolic alkalosis (pH greater than 7.45) may occur from excessive bicarbonate ingestion (such as antacids) or a rapid and massive transfusion of blood, because the stored blood used for transfusion utilizes bicarbonate components as a preservative. Metabolic alkalosis, a much rarer syndrome, can occur from excessive hydrogen ion loss, as with vomiting, nasogastric suctioning, or drug therapy or abuse (laxative abuse, diuretic use, emetics). Metabolic acidosis (pH less than 7.35) may occur as a result of increased hydrogen ion production from a hypermetabolic state, anaerobic metabolism (lactic acidosis), and ketoacidosis from protein metabolism.

Acidosis can also occur as a result of underproduction of bicarbonate ions, such as with acute or chronic renal, hepatic, and pancreatic failure. Overelimination of bicarbonate ions, as with diarrhea, will also result in metabolic acidosis. The key for the critical care paramedic is to understand the origin of the acid–base imbalance and then set care priorities to normalize the pH level as

■ **Figure 25-5** Summary of acid–base disturbances and compensation. *(Fig. 20-29, p. 639, from* Principles of Human Physiology, *2nd ed., by William J. Germann and Cindy L. Stanfield. Copyright © 2005 by Pearson Education, Inc. Reprinted by permission.)*

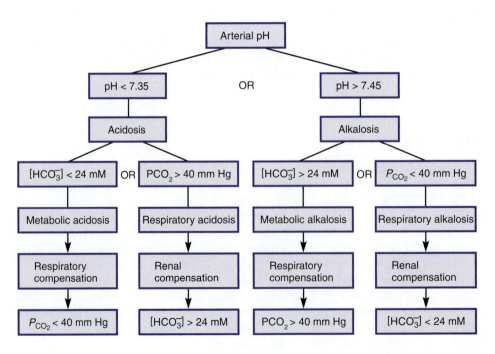

quickly as possible. Failure to do so may allow the development of pH levels that are not conducive to life (pH levels of less than 6.9 or greater than 7.8 are considered lethal). While metabolic alkalosis is not as common, metabolic acidosis occurs quite frequently, and can be a life-threatening event.

METABOLIC ACIDOSIS

To create a metabolic acidotic state, the amount of endogenous hydrogen ions produced is increased, the exogenous intake of hydrogen ions is increased, or the reabsorption of hydrogen ions is increased. Also contributory to the acidotic state could be a drop in the production of bicarbonate ions, diminishment in the exogenous intake of bicarbonate, or impaired reabsorption of bicarbonate ions.

While the leading cause of metabolic acidosis is anaerobic metabolism, usually from a low perfusion state, there are many causes of acute metabolic acidosis. The mnemonic **MUDPILES** identifies the most common causes of metabolic acidosis:

M:	Methanol
U:	Uremia
D:	Diabetic ketoacidosis
P:	Paraldehyde
I:	Infection
L:	Lactic acidosis
E:	Ethylene glycol
S:	Salicylates

These causes are discussed in the following sections.

MUDPILES *mnemonic used to identify the most common causes of metabolic acidosis, as in–Methanol; Uremia; Diabetic ketoacidosis; Paraldehyde; Infection; Lactic acidosis; Ethylene glycol; Salicylates.*

METHANOL

Methanol, or methyl alcohol, is an organic solvent found in cleaning materials, paints, varnishes, Sterno fuel, formaldehyde, antifreeze, gasohol, "moonshine" alcohol, windshield wiper fluid, and duplicating fluid. A central nervous system (CNS) depressant, methanol is rapidly absorbed and slowly metabolized. Methanol toxicity is usually a result of accidental ingestion, skin exposure, inhalation exposure in an industrial setting, and sometimes intentional "huffing" to experience its inebriating effects. Toxicity can occur with as little as a single mouthful. When metabolized by enzymes secreted by the liver, methanol forms formaldehyde and formic acid. Formic acid is the primary toxin that accounts for the anion gap, metabolic acidosis, and organ system sequelae because formaldehyde has a short half-life (lasting only minutes). The liver metabolizes 90% to 95% of methanol levels in the blood.

The primary clinical manifestations of methanol toxicity are CNS depression and cardiovascular collapse from lactic acidosis, and visual disturbances to formic acid-induced edema of the axons of the optic disk. The primary presentation includes visual disturbances (50%), CNS complaints (headache, vertigo), and GI symptoms (abdominal pain, nausea, vomiting). Physical symptom severity does not correlate well with the amount of ingestion. Onset of symptoms is variable, depending on the amount of ingestion and size of the patient. Symptoms may be evident within 40 minutes to up 72 hours after exposure. Simultaneous ingestion of ethanol (ethyl alcohol) will bring about the symptoms of toxicity more quickly and will prolong its half-life.

Diagnostic Evaluation

Lab data may be available in addition to clinical presentation and history to assist the critical care paramedic with treatment decisions. In acute methanol toxicity, the following lab data may be available:

★ *Blood glucose levels:* May be low (helpful to rule out DKA)

★ *BUN/creatinine:* May be elevated (late finding)

★ *Anion gap:* Elevated. The **anion gap** is an indirect measurement of phosphates, sulfates, and organic acids. Increases in the anion gap are seen with excessive acid production (H^+ ions), or the addition of exogenous acids.

To calculate anion gap: $[Na^+] - ([HCO_3^-] + [Cl^-])$. The normal anion gap is 12–16 mEq/L. For example, assume a patient has the following lab values:

– Na^+ = 140 mEq/L

– Cl^- = 106 mEq/L

– HCO_3^- = 22 mEq/L

For this example, the total number of sodium cations is 140 mEq and the total number of chloride and bicarbonate ions (added together) is 128 mEq. Thus, 140 mEq − 128 mEq = 12 mEq.

★ *Arterial blood gases:* Marked metabolic acidosis with low pH and low HCO_3^-

★ *Complete blood count:* Anemia may be present

★ *Urinalysis:* May have the odor of formaldehyde

★ *Methanol concentrations of blood alcohol content (BAC):*

– 0–20 mg/dL—usually asymptomatic

– 20–150 mg/dL—toxic; treatment required

– 150+ mg/dL—potentially fatal if untreated

Emergent Treatment of Methanol Toxicity

For the critical care paramedic, the treatment of methanol toxicity is primarily based on patient presentation. Definitive treatment will be hemodialysis, which is usually the reason for critical care transport. In addition to airway management and maintenance, primary treatment priorities include seizure control with the administration of intravenous benzodiazepines as needed. If available immediately after ingestion, the use of ipecac may be considered but is not being used currently by many clinicians (consult with your medical director regarding this). Naturally though, if CNS depression is evident, then the use of emetics is contraindicated.

The placement of a nasogastric tube and gastric decompression, followed by gastric lavage, has proven to be effective if used within 1 hour of ingestion. Activated charcoal administration is ineffective unless other substances are suspected. Intravenous ethanol administration is a primary treatment of methanol toxicity, because the hepatic enzyme alcohol dehydrogenase has a much greater affinity (10 to 20 times) for ethanol. By administering ethanol, either orally or intravenously, methanol's conversion to formaldehyde and formic acid is blocked, allowing for renal and pulmonary elimination of the unchanged, less toxic parent compound. Indications for intravenous ethanol therapy include significant methanol ingestion, the presence of symptoms following methanol ingestion, and documented elevations in the anion gap indicating metabolic acidosis. To prepare a 10% ethanol solution for patient management, remove 100 mL of fluid from 1 liter of D_5W and replace with 100 mL of absolute alcohol; or, remove 50 mL of fluid from 1 liter of commercially available 5% ethanol in D_5W solution, and add 50 mL of absolute alcohol.

The goal in the administration of intravenous ethanol is to obtain a blood alcohol level (BAC) of 100 mg/dL, so infusion rates will be based on patient's size, preexisting medical conditions (such as hepatic insufficiency), and whether ethanol was ingested in addition to methanol. Typical infusion rates are 7.6–10 mL/kg over 30 minutes, followed by a maintenance dose of 1.4 mL/kg/hour continuously.

Intravenous bicarbonate administration is indicated for arterial pH levels of less than 7.25 and serum bicarbonate levels of less than 15 mEq/L. The critical care paramedic may administer 50 mEq of 8.4% sodium bicarbonate every 30–60 minutes as needed during transport. The amount of sodium bicarbonate needed will depend on the amount of methanol ingested or methanol levels, if available.

Another treatment available in the treatment of methanol toxicity is fomepizole (Antizol). This drug is classified as an antidote to methanol poisoning, where it antagonizes alcohol dehydrogenase, the enzyme that begins the metabolism of methanol to its toxic metabolites. Fomepizole can be used alone or in combination with dialysis. The following outlines the drug profile for fomepizole:

Fomepizole (Antizol)

Contraindications: Allergy to fomepizole and its additives; not recommended for pediatric patient.

Side effects: Allergic reaction, bradycardia, hypotension, excessive sweating, disseminated intravascular coagulation, pain at injection site.

Dosage: 15 mg/kg IV over 30 minutes, followed by 10 mg/kg IV over 30 minutes every 12 hours for four doses; then 15 mg/kg IV over 30 minutes every 12 hours until ethylene glycol level is less than 20 mg/dL. In patients undergoing hemodialysis, doses should be given every 4 hours, with return to normal dosage pattern after hemodialysis is completed. The drug is supplied as 1.5 g/mL vials for reconstitution.

Pediatric dosage: Not established.

UREMIA

Uremia, meaning "urine in the blood," is a complex syndrome of clinical assessment and metabolic derangements. Due to hormonal, electrolyte, and fluid imbalances, uremia is generally associated with chronic renal failure. However, uremia may also be associated with acute renal failure if renal function deteriorates rapidly.

When hormonal production, acid–base metabolism and regulation, fluid balance, electrolyte regulation, and waste-product elimination processes are altered, clinical abnormalities such as anemia, acidosis, hyperkalemia, malnutrition, and hypertension may occur. Initial symptoms are vague in nature, and may be attributed to viral illness, gastroenteritis, and even depression. Initial symptoms include nausea, vomiting, weight loss, muscle cramps, and change in mental status. Primary causes of uremia include diabetes, hypertension, glomerulonephritis, cystitis, and cancer. Diabetes accounts for up to 40% of newly diagnosed uremia patients in the United States.

uremia *the accumulation of urea and other nitrogen–containing waste products in the blood.*

Diagnostic Evaluation

The diagnosis of uremia is primarily based on abnormal lab data, specifically elevations in BUN and serum creatinine levels. Other lab data include elevations in potassium, phosphorus, and parathyroid hormone (PTH), and decreased calcium, magnesium, serum bicarbonate, and hemoglobin levels. Arterial blood gases reveal metabolic acidosis with decreased pH and bicarbonate levels. Urinalysis may show the presence of protein, ketones, hemoglobin, glucose, and myoglobin. Urine creatinine clearance may be obtained to measure GFR. If acute renal failure is suspected, renal ultrasound may be obtained to evaluate for acute hydronephrosis or obstruction.

Emergent Treatment of Uremia

The definitive treatment for uremia, whether acute or chronic in presentation, is dialysis. The critical care paramedic's main treatment priorities beyond airway and ventilatory management will focus on individual patient presentation. Hyperkalemia that affects heart rate and rhythm can be treated emergently with intravenous calcium chloride or calcium gluconate. Hyperkalemia may also be corrected by correcting acidemia. The administration of intravenous sodium bicarbonate, or the administration of intravenous insulin, may help to lower serum potassium levels as identified earlier. (However, the critical care paramedic must remember to administer glucose with insulin administration to avoid a hypoglycemic episode.) Anemia may require transfusions of packed RBCs, but the critical care paramedic must again be cautious about overloading the uremic patient with excessive volume. Transfusion therapy is normally reserved for the symptomatically anemic patient, not just the anemic patient.

DIABETIC KETOACIDOSIS

Diabetic ketoacidosis is a potentially life-threatening condition characterized by hyperglycemia, dehydration, and ketoacid production in the insulin-dependent diabetic population. DKA patients normally present with blood glucose levels of over 300 mg/dL, bicarbonate levels of less than 15 mEq/L, a pH level of less than 7.39, and the presence of ketone bodies in the urine and blood.

In DKA, the absence of insulin prevents tissues (muscle, fat) from taking up glucose normally. Counterregulatory hormones, such as glucagons, then break down triglycerides into free fatty acids and glucose, causing an increase in serum glucose levels and the formation of ketone bodies. In short, carbohydrate metabolism is lost and fat metabolism occurs, similar to a fasting state. The buildup of free fatty acids decreases extracellular acid buffers (bicarbonate), causing acidosis. The increase in serum glucose levels produces hyperglycemia-induced diuresis, and sodium, phosphorus, potassium, and water are lost. Glucose and ketone bodies, abundant in quantity, are also lost. The water loss can be as much as 3 liters if left untreated. Primary causes of DKA are new-onset diabetes mellitus, noncompliance in insulin therapy, or the diabetic patient with an infectious condition, such as a urinary tract infection or gastroenteritis. Diabetic ketoacidosis is seen most often in younger patients (less than 19 years of age) with juvenile-onset insulin-dependent diabetes mellitus (IDDM), but can occur with any insulin-dependent patient.

Diagnostic Evaluation

As mentioned earlier, the classic signs of DKA are hyperglycemia and acidosis. Serum glucose levels in these patients are normally 300 mg/dL or greater. Glucose will be present in the urine as well. Arterial blood gases commonly reveal metabolic acidosis with a low pH (<7.30), low bicarbonate levels (<15 mEq/L), and low $PaCO_2$ (usually less than 30 mmHg). Decreases in $PaCO_2$ levels are a compensatory mechanism to raise pH levels, and are typically seen as deep, rapid respirations (Kussmaul-type respirations). BUN and creatinine levels may be elevated, due to dehydration. Serum ketone levels, normally not present, will be found as will urine ketones. The production of ketone bodies will give the patient's breath a distinctive fruity odor. Because of the acidosis, intracellular potassium is "pushed" into extracellular spaces, indicating hyperkalemia. This is not a true measure of actual potassium stores, and the critical care paramedic must be very cautious of hypokalemia and its sequelae after fluid resuscitation and insulin administration, because acidosis will begin to correct and potassium shifts will normalize. Serum sodium and potassium levels commonly will be low.

Emergent Treatment of DKA

During the most acute phase of DKA, the critical care paramedic's primary treatment priority is volume replacement with isotonic normal saline. Because of the hyperglycemic diuresis, the DKA patient may present with hypotension, tachycardia, poor peripheral pulses, and other symptoms of hypovolemic shock. Intravenous access and the administration of repeated fluid boluses of 20 mL/kg is indicated, with as much as 6 liters necessary in the first few hours to normalize intravascular volume. Some physicians may use a modified Baxter-Parkland formula, used for burn resuscitation, to guide resuscitation needs. Once the fluid volume replacement is addressed, the critical care paramedic must then address the hyperglycemia/acidosis. Before the administration of exogenous insulin in the 1920s, the mortality rate of DKA was 100%. Presently, DKA mortality is 2%.

The administration of intravenous, short-acting insulin is indicated, with dosages dependent on serum glucose levels and the degree of acidosis that exists. Typical dosages of insulin range from 5 to 15 units IVP, followed by an insulin drip of 3–10 units/hour. (The administration of intravenous intermediate and long-acting insulin for the acute phase of DKA is not indicated.) Once intravenous, short-acting insulin has been administered, the critical care paramedic must monitor serum glucose levels as least every hour, adjusting insulin drip administration according to glucose levels. Once the patient's blood glucose level falls below 250 mg/dL, the critical care paramedic should become even more diligent in monitoring the glucose level in the body to avoid accidental hypoglycemia. This can be managed by either changing intravenous fluids to dextrose-containing solutions (more controversial), or administering dextrose in metered amounts to maintain normal glucose levels. As volume loss and acidosis are corrected, the critical care paramedic must then also address the postassium deficiency that occurred during the diuretic phase of DKA. The administration of insulin drives potassium intracellularly. Thus, initially, when the blood glucose level is high, the patient may be hyperkalemic (relatively). However, when insulin is administered and potassium is driven intracellularly, the serum potassium level may fall and the patient can actually become hypokalemic. The administration of intravenous potassium should be considered once the potassium level is below 5.0 mEq/L, even though the level is considered within normal limits. Potassium phosphate (KPO_4) is typically the additive of choice, because the DKA patient is normally hypophosphatemic as well. The administration of 40 mEq per liter of solution is a typical concentration. Potassium replacement may be required for as long as 24 hours, so serial electrolytes must be drawn every 1–2 hours. During transport, the critical care paramedic must monitor vital signs and cardiac rhythm closely. The risk of hypokalemia and cardiac dysrhythmia may occur during transport, especially after intravenous fluid resuscitation has begun. Airway management and ventilatory assistance may be needed if an altered level of consciousness is present. Insertion of a nasogastric tube may be indicated to decrease the risk of aspiration, especially if there is an altered level of consciousness. Foley catheter placement may be indicated to monitor urinary output during transport.

The administration of sodium bicarbonate is generally not indicated for the DKA patient, because it has been linked to development of cerebral edema, especially in the pediatric patient. With intravenous fluid resuscitation and insulin therapy, acidosis in the DKA patient typically normalizes without the need for bicarbonate administration.

PARALDEHYDE

Paraldehyde, classified as a sedative/hypnotic, has been available for more than 100 years for use as treatment for acute delirium tremors associated with alcohol withdrawal syndrome. Paraldehyde may also be administered as an anticonvulsant for seizures unresponsive to phenytoin or other anticonvulsants. Today, it is rarely used. When metabolized, paraldehyde turns into acetic acid and acetaldehyde. Similar to ethyl alcohol in its action, dosages of 120 mL of paraldehyde may cause acute CNS depression, coma, and even death. Additionally, the buildup of acetic acid and acetaldehyde places the patient at risk for acute metabolic acidosis.

Diagnostic Evaluation

Acidosis associated with paraldehyde administration will typically reveal elevated potassium levels and decreased pH and bicarbonate levels. Urinalysis may reveal lower pH levels, as well as the presence of acetic acid.

Emergent Treatment of Paraldehyde Acidosis

The treatment of acidosis due to paraldehyde administration is similar to that for many other causes of acidosis. The administration of intravenous sodium bicarbonate depends on the pH and bicarbonate levels. Administration of vasopressor agents (dopamine, norepinepherine) may be necessary if hypotension is present and is unresponsive to fluid resuscitation. The critical care paramedic must also be acutely aware of the action of paraldehyde. As a hypnotic/sedative, paraldehyde can quickly change the patient's level of consciousness, leading to potential airway loss and ventilatory changes. That concern is heightened if paraldehyde is used as an anticonvulsant, and the postictal patient is at greater risk for airway loss.

INFECTION

Any infectious syndrome can place the critically ill patient at risk for systemic inflammatory response syndrome (SIRS), a precursor to sepsis, and end-organ failure. When infection becomes overwhelming, a complex series of cells, known as cytokines, and white blood cells are released at the site of infection (and beyond) to begin phagocytosis. Anti-inflammatory cytokines are then released to maintain homeostasis and to minimize epithelial damage. Platelets are released into the area of infection, producing "clumping" and cellular ischemia. When ischemia develops, anaerobic metabolism takes place, and the buildup of lactic acid occurs. Metabolic acidosis occurs due to the buildup of lactic acid. Endotoxin release promotes vasodilation, causing hypotension and further ischemia, and increased capillary permeability allows fluid shifts from intravascular spaces.

Diagnostic Evaluation

As with any infection, the WBC count is typically elevated; however, if sepsis has developed, the critical care paramedic may notice a lower WBC count. Serum bicarbonate levels will be low, as well as pH levels. The patient may have elevated BUN and creatinine levels due to poor perfusion and relative hypovolemia. Serum lactate levels will be elevated. If available, the critical care paramedic should observe for cultures to determine the origin of infection.

Emergent Treatment of Infection

For the critical care paramedic, the emergent treatment of the patient with metabolic acidosis due to infectious processes is supportive. Airway management and ventilatory assistance are of highest priority to maximize oxygen delivery to end cells. Additionally, the administration of vasopressor agents (dopamine, norepinepherine), in addition to intravenous fluids, may be needed to maximize end-cell perfusion. Intravenous sodium bicarbonate is indicated based on arterial pH levels. Finally, with medical director consultation, the critical care paramedic may opt to administer broad-spectrum antibiotics such as vancomycin if cultures are not available.

LACTIC ACIDOSIS

lactic acidosis a common cause of metabolic acidosis; a result of abnormal conversion of pyruvate (pyruvic acid) into lactate during hypoxic or anaerobic states.

When the buildup of lactic acid exceeds 5 mmol/L and pH levels drop below 7.25, the syndrome of lactic acidosis develops. **Lactic acidosis** is one of the more common causes of metabolic acidosis. Elevations in lactic acid occur as a result of abnormal conversion of pyruvate (pyruvic acid) into lactate. When the bicarbonate buffer system is overwhelmed, lactemia develops. Poor tissue oxygenation ensues, caused by either poor perfusion status or hypoxia-induced anaerobic metabolism. Cardiopulmonary failure, side effects of drugs or toxins, and various other preexisting or congenital conditions can also lead to lactic acidosis. Lactic acidosis, when present, is commonly divided into two categories:

★ *Type A:* Associated with clinical evidence of poor tissue perfusion or oxygenation
★ *Type B:*

        B1—associated with underlying diseases

        B2—associated with drugs and toxins

        B3—associated with inborn errors in metabolism

Diagnostic Evaluation

As with many other causes of metabolic acidosis, lab data abnormalities are most commonly seen in serum electrolytes and arterial blood gases. Elevations in potassium levels are common. Arterial blood gases may reveal lowered pH and bicarbonate levels. Serum lactate levels will be elevated (normal range is less than 2 mmol/L). The critical care paramedic needs to be aware that specimen collection for serum lactate is unique in that specimens must be kept on ice until they reach the respective lab for testing, and that specimens must be measured as quickly as possible, ideally within 4 hours of collection. Other lab data will be collected and analyzed based on patient presentation and underlying causes for lactic acidosis.

Emergent Care of Lactic Acidosis

More than any other cause of metabolic acidosis, the emergent treatment of lactic acidosis is completely focused on perfusion status improvement. The critical care paramedic must maximize cardiac performance and tissue oxygenation in order to optimize organ performance (especially the liver, kidneys, and skeletal muscle) and metabolize and eliminate circulating lactate. Endotracheal intubation and mechanical ventilation may be necessary. The administration of intravenous fluid resuscitation and vasopressor agents (dopamine, norepinephrine) may also be required. The administration of sodium bicarbonate in lactic acidosis is indicated only if toxic ingestion (ethylene glycol, methanol) is the cause. If the cause of lactic acidosis is poor cardiopulmonary performance, the administration of sodium bicarbonate is contraindicated, because it causes a buildup of carbon dioxide and may lead to respiratory acidosis. Moreover, the administration of bicarbonate does not improve hemodynamics in the critically ill patient.

ETHYLENE GLYCOL

Ethylene glycol, a solvent found in common household and industrial materials (particularly antifreeze), is a clear, colorless, odorless, viscous liquid with a sweet taste. Also found in antifreeze and hydraulic brake fluid, ethylene glycol is a common cause of accidental ingestion in the pediatric population because of its sweet taste. In the adult population, it is a common cause of intentional ingestion, because larger quantities are tolerated without nausea. While similar to methanol in its presentation with ingestion, ethylene glycol is not readily absorbed in the skin, and does not cause systemic toxicity with skin exposure. The compound of ethylene glycol is relatively nontoxic.

Its toxicity occurs during metabolism after absorption. The same liver enzyme that converts methanol, alcohol dehydrogenase, converts ethylene glycol to glycoaldehyde. Glycoaldehyde is further metabolized in glycolic acid, glyoxylic acid, and oxalate. Glycolic acid is the greatest contributor to metabolic acidosis. Oxalate precipitates with calcium that may cause widespread injury to kidney, brain, and liver tissues. Acute ethylene glycol toxicity typically presents in three phases:

★ *Phase I* is considered the CNS depression phase. Occurring within 30 minutes and up to 12 hours after ingestion, phase I symptoms include nausea, vomiting, ataxia, nystagmus, and myoclonic jerks. All of the symptoms are similar to ethanol intoxication, but the smell of ethanol is not present. Depending on the amount of substance ingested, CNS depression may be as severe as seizure and coma.

★ *Phase II* is considered the cardiopulmonary toxicity phase. Typically occurring 12–72 hours after ingestion, phase II is most commonly associated with tachycardia, tachypnea, and mild hypertension. Phase II is thought to be caused by the accumulation of oxalate crystal within the lung tissue, vascular tree, and myocardium.

★ *Phase III* is considered the renal toxicity phase. As glycolic acid and oxalate levels build, acute tubular necrosis occurs, and manifests itself as oliguric renal failure. Flank and abdominal pain may also be evident.

Diagnostic Evaluation

Lab data used in the diagnosis of ethylene glycol toxicity are similar to those used for methanol. Serum electrolytes, urinalysis, arterial blood gases, anion gap, and ethylene glycol blood levels need to be evaluated by the critical care paramedic. The presence of calcium oxalate crystals may be present on urinalysis, and urine may have a fluorescent appearance when placed under a Wood's lamp, because fluorescein is added to ethylene glycol, especially antifreeze. Serum calcium levels may be decreased due to calcium oxalate binding.

Emergent Treatment of Ethylene Glycol Toxicity

Treatment of ethylene glycol toxicity is similar to that for methanol. While hemodialysis is considered definitive treatment, administration of intravenous crystalloid at 250–500 mL/hour is indicated to aid in renal clearance of toxins, and limits the deposit of oxalate crystals in renal tissues. The administration of intravenous sodium bicarbonate is indicated for pH levels of less than 7.25. Intravenous ethanol infusions are used, with goals similar to methanol toxicity. For the critical care provider, investigation regarding the type of substance, the amount of substance ingested, and the approximate time when the substance was ingested is essential.

Another treatment available in the treatment of ethylene glycol toxicity is fomepizole (Antizol). As discussed earlier, this drug is classified as an antidote to ethylene glycol poisoning because it serves as an antagonist of alcohol dehydrogenase, the enzyme that begins the metabolism of ethylene glycol to its toxic metabolites. Fomepizole can be used alone or in combination with dialysis.

SALICYLATE POISONING

Salicylates have been utilized for years for their anti-inflammatory, analgesic, and antipyretic properties. Until the development of childproof packaging in the 1970s, salicylate ingestion was a common cause of poisoning and death in children. Despite safe-proofing bottles for children, salicylate poisoning is still a common occurrence, usually because of intentional ingestion during a suicide attempt, although salicylate poisoning can occur with frequent, chronic use.

In salicylate toxicity, cyclic ATP production is decreased, and oxygen consumption, carbon dioxide production, and heat production are increased. The Krebs cycle is altered and carbohydrate metabolism leads to the accumulation of pyruvate, lactate, and acetoacetate, causing metabolic acidosis and an increased anion gap. Symptoms include tachycardia, fever, tachypnea, increased metabolic rate, and dehydration due to vomiting and insensible water loss. Tachypnea will reveal respiratory alkalosis initially, followed by metabolic acidosis. CNS changes can vary from mild confusion to coma, depending on the concentration of salicylates in brain tissue. Tinnitus, deafness, and dizziness can occur with salicylate toxicity, though ototoxicity is reversible. Gastrointestinal symptoms include nausea, vomiting, and abdominal pain. Because of the prolongation in prothrombin times, there is a greater risk for GI bleeding. In addition to changes in prothrombin time, salicylates can also alter platelet aggregation, increasing risk of bleeding.

Diagnostic Evaluation

The critical care paramedic is met with many pieces of lab data information in the patient suffering from acute salicylate poisoning. Arterial blood gases may reveal respiratory alkalosis or metabolic acidosis, depending on when the sample was drawn in relationship to when the salicylate was taken. Coagulation studies may reveal a prolonged prothromin time (normal range being 7–10 seconds) and a decreased platelet count (normal range being 250,000–400,000). Hypokalemia may be present due to water and electrolyte loss as discussed earlier. Urinalysis may reveal a lower pH level.

Salicylate levels are not only diagnostic to rule out other causes for presenting symptoms, but also will give the critical care paramedic an idea of the amount of salicylates that might have been taken. The normal salicylate level is 15–30 mg/dL. Patients are typically symptomatic at levels of 40–50 mg/dL, and levels of 100 mg/dL or more are considered life threatening. The critical care paramedic must keep in mind that salicylate levels may not give an accurate indication of salicylate toxicity, since peak salicylate levels may not be seen for 4–6 hours. Information regarding time of ingestion is important for the critical care paramedic to know in addition to salicylate levels to correlate symptoms with salicylate levels.

Emergent Treatment of Salicylate Poisoning

As with most poisonings causing metabolic acidosis, hemodialysis is the definitive treatment for salicylate poisoning. For the critical care paramedic, the treatment priorities include fluid resuscitation, urine alkalization, and GI decontamination after airway management and ventilatory maintenance have been ensured. There is conflicting research regarding the efficacy of gastric decontamination, so the critical care paramedic should consult on-line medical direction before attempting this intervention.

Dilution of circulating acids with intravenous crystalloids at 250–500 mL/hour may be indicated. Administration of sodium bicarbonate may also be indicated to alkalinize urine being excreted from the fluid resuscitation. Dosages of 100–150 mEq are typically added to each liter of intravenous solution. Potassium replacement is indicated for serum potassium levels monitored to be less than 3.5 mEq/L. Potassium chloride 20–40 mEq in each liter of intravenous solution may then be required until serum potassium levels of 4.5–5.0 mg/dL are achieved.

Nasogastric tube placement and gastric lavage may prove beneficial if the patient is seen within 1 hour of ingestion. Gastric decontamination with the administration of activated charcoal 1–2 g/kg through the nasogastric tube, if performed, is done in an attempt to limit further gut absorption by binding available salicylates. Repeated doses of activated charcoal may be required every 4 hours to further aid in salicylate elimination. Discontinue administration of charcoal after the patient begins to pass stool containing charcoal.

Summary

The renal system is a complex system that helps the body remain in a homeostatic state of "balance." Disease processes or toxic events, accidental or intentional, put that balance at risk. The critical care paramedic has a responsibility to maintain and optimize cardiopulmonary performance in order to maintain end-cell and end-organ perfusion, while treating symptoms of metabolic derangements until definitive treatment (i.e., hemodialysis) can be done. Understanding and applying the knowledge addressed in this chapter when presented with acid–base and renal derangements will assist in this goal.

Additional Case Studies

A 34-year-old female with a history of clinical depression presents to the emergency department after taking forty (40) tablets of aspirin (325-mg tablets) approximately 5 hours ago. Upon arrival to the ED, the vital signs are found to be:

- *Heart rate: 150*
- *Respiratory rate: 32*
- *Blood pressure: 98/56*
- *Temperature: 101.5° F*
- *Pulse oximetry: 99% on room air.*
- *Glasgow Coma Score: 13 (E=3, V=4, M=6)*

1. After assessing airway, the critical care paramedic would first do which of the following:
   a. Administer ipecac 30 mL.
   b. Insert a nasogatric tube and instill activated charcoal 2 g/kg.
   c. Establish intravenous access, draw labs, and adminster 20 mL/kg fluid bolus.
   d. Administer sodium bicarbonate 50 mEq IV over 10 minutes.

This patient's lab data reveal the following:

- *Potassium: 3.4*
- *Arterial blood gas: pH=7.29, PaO_2= 110, $PaCO_2$=29, HCO_3^- =16*
- *Salicylate level: = 79*
- *Prothrombin time: 23 seconds*

2. Given the information above, the critical care paramedic should avoid:
   a. arterial puncture or unnecessary invasive procedures.
   b. intravenous fluid resuscitation.
   c. intravenous sodium bicarbonate.
   d. a follow-up lab draw in 2 hours.

3. Given the information available, definitive treatment for this patient during transport is:
   a. hemodialysis.
   b. intravenous sodium bicarbonate 150 mEq in 1 L of solution at 250 mL/hour.
   c. intravenous vitamin K 10 mg slow IVP over 5 minutes.
   d. continued administration of activated charcoal 2–3 g via nasogastric tube every 4 hours until charcoal-containing stool is passed.

A 4-year-old male, presents with confusion and decreased coordination. The child's parent found the child in the garage approximately 1 hour ago, drinking from a container containing antifreeze. On arrival, the critical care paramedic finds the child intubated and being ventilated with a self-inflating bag. He is bradycardic, hypotensive, and has an oxygenation saturation of 70%.

4. Given the above information, the critical care paramedic must consider which of the following as the cause of the patient's condition?
   a. endotracheal tube displacement
   b. tension pneumothorax
   c. endotracheal tube obstruction
   d. all of the above

See Answers to Review Questions at the back of this book.

Further Reading

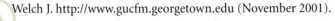

Barron SW. *Lactic Acidosis.* http//www.emedicine.com (July 2001).

Fencl V, Jabor A, Kazda A, Figge J. "Diagnosis of Metabolic Acid-Base Disturbances in Critically Ill Patients." *American Journal of Respiratory and Critical Care Medicine,* Vol. 162 (2000).

Likosky D. *Methanol.* http://www.emedicine.com (November 2001).

Morton P, et al. *Critical Care Nursing: A Holistic Approach,* 8th ed. Philadelphia: Lippincott Williams & Wilkins, 2005.

Priestley MA. *Metabolic Acidosis.* http://www.emedicine.com (October 2004).

Stillwell SB. *Mosby's Critical Care Nursing Reference,* 3rd ed. St. Louis, MO: Mosby, 2002.

Urden LD, et al. *Thelan's Critical Care Nursing: Diagnosis and Management,* 4th ed. St. Louis, MO: Mosby, 2001.

Welch J. http://www.gucfm.georgetown.edu (November 2001).

Infectious Disease Emergencies

Larry Johnson, NREMT-P, CCT, FP-C

Objectives

Upon completion of this chapter, the student should be able to:

1. Discuss the importance of infectious disease knowledge and prevention in the critical care setting. (p. 774)
2. Describe the basic types of disease-causing organisms including the following:
   - **A.** Bacteria (p. 774)
   - **B.** Viruses (p. 774)
   - **C.** Rickettsia (p. 775)
   - **D.** Fungus (p. 775)
   - **E.** Protozoa (p. 775)
   - **F.** Metazoa/helminths (p. 775)
   - **G.** Prions (p. 775)
3. Discuss the cycle of infectious disease transmission. (p. 775)
4. Detail the role of the critical care paramedic in infectious disease prevention. (p. 776)
5. Describe Universal Precautions and Body Substance Isolation Precautions as they pertain to critical care transport. (p. 776)
6. Detail the recommendations for vaccination of health care workers. (p. 785)
7. Discuss the etiology, transmission, pathophysiology, signs and symptoms, and treatment of the following epidemiologically important infectious diseases:
   - **A.** HIV/AIDS (p. 786)
   - **B.** Viral hepatitis (p. 787)
   - **C.** Respiratory infections (p. 789)

Key Terms

acquired immunodeficiency
   syndrome (AIDS), p. 786
airborne, p. 776
anthrax, p. 800
antibiotic-resistant organisms
   (AROs), p. 798
arenavirus, p. 803
bacteria, p. 774
Body Substance Isolation
   (BSI) Precautions, p. 776
botulism, p. 802
brucellosis, p. 804
chickenpox (varicella), p. 796
cholera, p. 803
epiglottitis, p. 789
filoviruses, p. 803
fungus, p. 775
gastroenteritis, p. 796
hantavirus, p. 803
hepatitis, p. 787

hosts, p. 775
human immunodeficiency
   virus (HIV), p. 786
infectious disease, p. 774
influenza (the flu), p. 790
measles (rubeola), p. 795
meningitis, p. 794
meningococcal infection,
   p. 794
metazoa/helminths, p. 775
mumps, p. 795
mycotoxins, p. 805
necrotizing fasciitis (NF),
   p. 798
plague, p. 801
pneumonia, p. 790
prions, p. 775
protozoa, p. 775
Q fever, p. 804
ricin, p. 804

rickettsia, p. 775
rubella, p. 795
saxitoxin, p. 805
septicemia, p. 797
severe acute respiratory
   syndrome (SARS), p. 792
smallpox, p. 801
sources, p. 775
staphylococcus enterotoxin
   B (SEB), p. 805
tetanus, p. 796
toxic shock syndrome (TSS),
   p. 797
tuberculosis (TB), p. 791
tularemia, p. 802
Universal Precautions, p. 776
vector-borne, p. 776
virus, p. 774

Case Study

An 18-year-old college student suddenly develops fever and chills on a Friday evening after attending a local high school football game. He had been in good health and had no risk factors for disease. When his roommate found him the next morning, he was unresponsive. EMS was summoned and the patient transported to a nearby community hospital.

Once there he was promptly evaluated. The patient could be aroused with painful stimuli but was incoherent. The emergency physician began an altered mental status workup. The CT of the head and CXR were negative. A second IV was started and the patient given D_5NS at 150 mL/hr. As the lab reports started to return, it was clear that the patient was suffering an infectious process. Blood cultures, urine cultures, and sputum cultures were ordered. The CBC revealed a WBC of 33.3 with a marked left shift. The chemistries were normal except for an elevated BUN and creatinine. Urine drug screen was clear.

A lumbar puncture was performed and cloudy spinal fluid was immediately noted. Three 1-mL tubes were taken and sent for cell count, differential, glucose, protein, India ink stain, Bactigen panel, cultures, sensitivity, and Gram stain. The physician hand-carried the tubes to the lab and looked at the Gram stain as soon as it was complete. There were a lot of neutrophils and gram-negative diplococci. The patient was immediately isolated.

Empiric intravenous antibiotic therapy was started with high-dose penicillin. The patient was intubated and mechanical ventilation begun. IV dexamethasone was administered as well.

The family requested the patient be moved to a tertiary care hospital closer to home and your unit was summoned to make the transport. On arrival you review the medical information and don appropriate protective gear. You assess the patient and transfer him to your equipment and stretcher. The transport is uneventful.

Fortunately, this patient received treatment quickly and, despite a stormy course, ultimately did well. The cultures and Bactigen panel confirmed *Neisseria meningitides* as the pathogen. Although your exposure was limited, you and your partner elect to complete a prophylactic course of ciprofloxacin.

INTRODUCTION

Health care workers have a professional responsibility to prevent the spread of infectious and communicable diseases.

Health care workers have a professional responsibility to prevent the spread of infectious and communicable diseases. This includes stopping (or minimizing) the spread of infection to and from patients, coworkers, themselves, and their families and friends. To fulfill this obligation, it is incumbent on every health care professional to be knowledgeable about the principles of infection control and the recognition and treatment of those infectious diseases that they may reasonably expect to encounter in their work.

This chapter has been developed to provide a broad overview of infectious and communicable diseases and to highlight some of the important aspects of infections as we understand them today. New advances in antimicrobial therapy and the emergence of new infectious agents and reemergence of old ones require constant attention on the part of all health care workers.

INFECTIOUS DISEASES

infectious disease *a condition caused by the invasion and multiplication of pathogenic microorganisms within the body.*

An **infectious disease** or condition is caused by the invasion and multiplication of pathogenic microorganisms within the body. Humans have several defense mechanisms to prevent disease-causing organisms from invading the body including the skin, which when intact, is virtually impervious to infecting microorganisms. Such things as the respiratory system's turbinates, nasal hairs, mucus, and mucociliary escalator all serve to trap and remove invading microorganisms. The normal bacterial flora of the gastrointestinal (GI) and genitourinary (GU) systems compete with pathogenic microorganisms for nutrients and space to grow, thus minimizing infection risks. Gastric acid in the stomach can destroy some microorganisms and their toxins, which are subsequently removed through the feces and urine.

If a disease-causing microorganism is able to penetrate these defenses, the body will respond by initiating an inflammatory response and an immune response (i.e., formation of antibodies). The inflammatory response, a normal protective physiological action, is responsible for many of the signs and symptoms associated with an infectious process.

CLASSIFICATIONS OF DISEASE-CAUSING AGENTS

Microorganisms capable of causing disease may be classified or grouped under several different categories.

Microorganisms capable of causing disease may be classified or grouped under several different categories including animal or plant, morphology, staining reactions, biochemical behavior, immunological characteristics, and cultural characteristics. For purposes of discussion within this chapter, pathogenic microorganisms will be described as follows:

bacteria *unicellular microorganisms that are round, spiral, or rod-shaped; capable of being pathogenic.*

★ *Bacteria.* **Bacteria** are unicellular microorganisms that are round, spiral, or rod-shaped and capable of being pathogenic. They live in soil, water, or organic matter or in the bodies of plants and animals. Antibiotics are especially effective against most bacterial infections.

   – *Aerobic bacteria.* Aerobic bacteria survive only in the presence of oxygen and can cause such diseases as streptococcal throat diseases (Group A Streptococi), syphilis (*Treponema pallidum*), tuberculosis (*Mycobacterium tuberculosis*), food poisoning (*Salmonella*), shigellosis (*Shigella sonnei*), meningococcal diseases (*Neisseria meningitidis*), plague (*Yersinia pestis*), pertussis (*Bordetella pertusis*), leprosy (*Mycobacterium aprae*, diphtheria (*Corynebacterium diphtheriae*), cholera (*Vibrio cholerae*), Legionnaire's disease (*Legionella pneumophila*), tularemia (*Francisella tularensis*), and typhoid fever (*Salmonella typhi*).

   – *Anaerobic bacteria.* Anaerobic bacteria survive in the absence of free oxygen and can cause such infections as colitis (*clostridium difficile*) tetanus (*clostridium tetani*), and abdominal infections (*bacteroides fragilis*).

virus *one of the smallest microorganisms; can only replicate and grow in the cell of another host or animal.*

★ *Virus.* A **virus** is one of the smallest microorganisms. Viruses grow and multiply only in living cells and cause a variety of very important diseases including AIDS, hepatitis, measles, rubella, viral hemorrhagic diseases, smallpox, herpes simplex, influenza, common cold, rabies, poliomyelitis, viral encephalitis, equine encephalitis, and yellow fever. They are not generally susceptible to antibiotics although some antiviral drugs have been developed. Some vaccines, however, have been developed or are under development to prevent some of the more important viral infections.

★ *Rickettsia.* **Rickettsia** are rod-shaped, coccoid, or diplococcus-shaped bacteria that live in lice or ticks and are transmitted to humans by the bite of these insects. They cause a number of serious diseases including typhus, rickettsialpox, Rocky Mountain spotted fever, scrub typhus, and Q fever. Most are responsive to antibiotic therapy.

★ *Fungus.* A **fungus** is a saprophytic and parasitic spore-producing organism that lacks chlorophyll. Fungi include molds, rusts, mildews, smuts, mushrooms, and yeasts. Those that are particularly important in man include actinomycetes (rat bite fever), dermatomycosis (ringworm), aspergillosis (infections of the external ear, pulmonary, sinus, and subcutaneous tissue), blastomycosis (abscesses of skin and subcutaneous tissue), coccidioidomycosis, histoplasmosis, cryptococcosis, candidiasis, and thrush. Numerous antifungal agents have been developed for many of these infections.

★ *Protozoa.* **Protozoa** are unicellular organisms including some pathogenic parasites that can infect humans includes amebiasis (*Entamoeba histolytica*, trypanosomiasis or sleeping sickness), leishmaniasis, trichomoniasis, malaria, and toxoplasmosis.

★ *Metazoa or helminth.* **Metazoa/helminths** are parasitic worms, including tapeworms, liver flukes, roundworms, and pinworms. Antihelmintics are available to treat many of these infections.

★ *Prions.* **Prions** are abnormal proteins that enter cells and convert normal cellular proteins into proteins just like themselves. These proteins disrupt normal cellular processes and are the cause of various infectious diseases of the nervous system such as scrapie and bovine spongiform encephalopathy (BSE) (also known as "mad cow disease"). Prions were formerly referred to as "slow viruses" although the term *prion* better describes them. No treatment is available for prion diseases.

★ *Other.* Other organisms that cause such problems as head lice, scabies, and malaria. Various treatment options are available.

HOW INFECTIOUS DISEASES OCCUR

SOURCE–HOST–TRANSMISSION

In order for a disease to be infectious or capable of being transmitted, three basic elements must be present: a source of infection, a susceptible host, and a means to transmit the infectious organism from the source to the host.

Sources of infection include persons with acute illnesses, those in the incubation period of a disease, and persons who are carriers of pathogenic microorganisms but are asymptomatic. Other sources of infection include one's own endogenous flora and inanimate objects that have become contaminated such as equipment, linens, and work surfaces.

Hosts are persons who may become infected with pathogenic microorganisms. A susceptible host is anyone who is capable of becoming infected with the disease being transmitted. Whether a person is susceptible to a particular pathogen is dependent on several factors including, but not limited to, their general health and hygiene, their immune status for various microorganisms, their age, the presence of any immunosuppressive diseases or therapies, and any break in the first lines of defense.

Microorganisms are passed from a source to a susceptible host through one of five *routes of transmission* including contact (direct and indirect), droplet, vehicle, vector-borne, and airborne. Some pathogens (e.g., chickenpox) are capable of being transmitted through more than one route. Also, with some diseases the infectious agent may make use of multiple transmission routes. Furthermore, in some cases diseases have been shown to mutate and "change" how they move both on an interspecies and on an intraspecies basis.

Direct contact is the ability of a pathogen to be transmitted from one person to another through direct personal contact, such as touching or kissing. *Indirect contact* occurs when a susceptible host becomes infected after contact with an object contaminated by the source organism, such as a contaminated needle or soiled dressings.

rickettsia *rod-shaped, coccoid, or diplococcus-shaped bacteria transmitted to humans by the bite of infected lice or ticks.*

fungus *a saprophytic and parasitic spore-producing organism that lacks chlorophyll; includes mold, rust, mildew, smut, mushroom, and yeast.*

protozoa *unicellular organisms, including some pathogenic parasites that can infect humans.*

metazoa/helminths *parasitic segmented worms; includes tapeworms, liver flukes, roundworms, and pinworms.*

prions *protein particles that lack nucleic acid; cause of various infectious diseases of the nervous system (formerly referred to as "slow viruses").*

In order for a disease to be infectious or capable of being transmitted, three basic elements must be present: a source of infection, a susceptible host, and a means to transmit the infectious organism from the source to the host.

sources *host or vector of infection; includes persons with acute illnesses, asymptomatic carriers of pathogenic microorganisms or diseases during incubation periods, endogenous flora and/or contaminated inanimate objects.*

hosts *persons or animals who may become (or are) infected with pathogenic microorganisms.*

Droplet transmission occurs when an infected individual sprays moist droplets into the air during coughing, sneezing, or speaking or during suctioning or bronchoscopy. In fact, nothing is quite better at producing the proper droplet size for infection in humans than sneezes and coughs. Organisms, capable of being transmitted by droplet spread infect a susceptible host when the droplet comes into contact with the mucous membrane of the host's mouth, nose, or eyes. It is possible for a host to facilitate the transmission by receiving the droplets on their hands and then immediately putting their hands to their eyes or mouth. Organisms transmitted on droplets are propelled for about 2–3 feet and will only remain in the air for a brief period of time before falling to the ground or other surface. The droplets will dry up quickly and the organism is no longer considered a source of infection.

Diseases that are spread by *vehicles* are transmitted through one or more of the following mediums: food, water, blood, drugs, and occasionally contaminated instruments or equipment. Examples of diseases that are transmitted through vehicles include typhoid fever, hepatitis A, and giardia lamblia.

Vector-borne diseases are transmitted through an intermediate host such as a fly, mosquito, or tick. These vectors can transmit the disease through simple mechanical means in which an organism from an infectious source will stick to the legs or body of the vector and is then deposited on the susceptible host or medium; or through biological transmission in which the infecting organism enters the intermediate host and will go through some form of life cycle change before being passed on to a susceptible host. This mechanism usually requires the intermediate host to bite or sting the susceptible host and inject the microorganism. Examples of diseases transmitted by vectors include Rocky Mountain spotted fever, bubonic plague, hantavirus, and malaria.

Airborne diseases are infections caused by microorganisms capable of being transmitted through the air as droplet nuclei or on dust particles. These organisms are very small and are capable of surviving in the air for a longer period of time and may be dispersed through air currents. Diseases that are spread through the airborne route include tuberculosis, chickenpox, and measles.

PREVENTION

Preventing the transmission of infectious agents requires practicing good infection control measures including general precautions and transmission-specific isolation precautions. Critical care providers should be knowledgeable in a variety of techniques and isolation precautions because they will encounter infections diseases through their work with different health care institutions.

The Hospital Infection Control Practices Advisory Committee (HICPAC) has published recommendations to prevent the transmission of infectious diseases in hospitals. They are recommending the adoption of Standard Precautions as the primary strategy for preventing the transmission of diseases regardless of a patient's diagnosis or presumed infection status. A second strategy is Transmission-Based Precautions intended for patients known or suspected to be infected by epidemiologically important pathogens spread by airborne or droplet transmission or by contact with dry skin or contaminated surfaces.

STANDARD PRECAUTIONS

Standard Precautions incorporate the major features of both Universal Precautions and Body Substance Isolation (BSI) Precautions and apply them to all patients. **Universal Precautions** were designed to reduce the risk of transmission of bloodborne pathogens and specifically were to be used to prevent contact with blood and/or body fluids that may contain blood. Universal Precautions, however, provide neither protection against diseases transmitted via body secretions or excretions not involving blood, nor against any diseases transmitted via droplet or airborne routes.

Body Substance Isolation (BSI) Precautions were designed to reduce the risk of transmission of diseases via moist body substances. Gloves are to be worn before any contact with mucous membranes, nonintact skin, or moist body substances. In addition, hospitals are to place a "Stop Sign Alert" on the room door of any patient who has an airborne-transmitted disease. BSI Precautions have been controversial in that they do not contain adequate provisions for diseases transmitted via droplet transmission (i.e., *Neisseria meningitidis*), direct or indirect transmission from dry skin or environmental surfaces (vancomycin-resistant enterococci), or true airborne transmission of infections (*Mycobacterium tuberculosis*) over long distances by floating droplet nuclei. In addition, BSI Precautions do not require that caregivers wash their hands after removing gloves.

---

vector-borne *diseases that are transmitted through an intermediate host such as a fly, mosquito, or tick.*

airborne *diseases transmitted by microorganisms capable of being transmitted as droplet nuclei or on dust particles through the atmosphere.*

Preventing the transmission of infectious agents requires practicing good infection control measures including general precautions and transmission-specific isolation precautions.

Standard Precautions incorporate the major features of both Universal Precautions and Body Substance Isolation (BSI) Precautions and apply them to all patients.

Universal Precautions *work practice controls designed to reduce the risk of transmission of bloodborne pathogens.*

Body Substance Isolation (BSI) Precautions *protective gear designed to reduce the risk of transmission of diseases via moist body substances.*

Table 26-1 — Infections and Conditions for Which Standard Precautions Are Indicated

Minor or limited draining abscess, actinomycosis, AIDS, amebiasis, anthrax (cutaneous and pulmonary), antibiotic-associated colitis, arthropod-borne viral encephalitides (eastern, western, Venezuelan equine encephalomyelitis; St. Louis, California encephalitis), arthropod-borne viral fevers (dengue, yellow fever, Colorado tick fever), ascariasis, aspergillosis, babesiosis, blastomycosis (North American, cutaneous and pulmonary), botulism, bronchiolitis, brucellosis, *Campylobacter* gastroenteritis, candidiasis, cat-scratch fever, chancroid, *Chlamydia trachomatis*, cholera (*Vibrio cholerae*), closed cavity infection, *Clostridium botulinum, C. perfringens,* coccidioidomycosis, Colorado tick fever, acute bacterial conjunctivitis, Creutzfeldt-Jakob disease, cryptosporidiosis, cysticercosis, cytomegalovirus infection, minor infected decubitus ulcer, dengue, echinococcosis, endometritis, enterobiasis (pinworm), enteroviral infections of adults, Epstein-Barr virus infection including infectious mononucleosis, erythema infectiosum, food poisoning (botulism, *Clostridium perfringens* or *welchii*, staphylococcal), gangrene (gas gangrene), gastroenteritis (*Campylobacter* species, cholera, *Cryptosporidium* species, *Escherichia coli* except enterohemorrhagic O157:H7 diapered or incontinent, *Giardia lamblia,* rotavirus unless diapered or incontinent, *Salmonella* species, *Shigella* species unless diapered or incontinent, *Vibrio parahaemolyticus,* viral unless covered elsewhere, *Yersinia enterocolitica*), gonococcal ophthalmia neonatorum, gonorrhea, granuloma inguinale, Guillain-Barré syndrome, *Hantavirus* pulmonary syndrome, *Helicobacter pylori,* hepatitis (type A, unless diapered or incontinent, type B-HBsAg positive, type C, and other unspecified non-A, non-B, type E), herpes simplex encephalitis or recurrent mucocutaneous, herpes zoster localized in normal patient, histoplasmosis, HIV, HIV infection, hookworm disease, infectious mononucleosis, Kawasaki syndrome, Legionnaires' disease, leprosy, leptospirosis, listeriosis, Lyme disease, lymphocytic choriomeningitis, lymphogranuloma venereum, malaria, melioidosis, meningitis (aseptic, gram-negative bacterial in neonates, fungal, *Listeria monocytogenes,* pneumococcal, tuberculosis), *Molluscum contagiosum,* mucormycosis, mycobacteria nontuberculosis (atypical), necrotizing enterocolitis, nocardiosis, Orf, pinworms, bubonic plague, pneumonia (*Chlamydia,* fungal, *Haemophilus influenzae* in adults, *Legionella,* pneumococcal, *Pneumocystis carinii, Pseudomonas cepacia, Staphylococcus aureus,* group A streptococcus in adults, viral in adults), poliomyelitis, psittacosis, Q fever, rabies, rat-bite fever, relapsing fever, acute respiratory infectious disease in adults, Reye's syndrome, rheumatic fever, rickettsial fevers, rickettsialpox, ringworm, Ritter's disease (staphylococcal scalded skin syndrome), Rocky Mountain spotted fever, roseola infantum, schistosomiasis, sporotrichosis, *Spirillum minus* disease, minor staphylococcal wound infections, staphylococcal (enterocolitis, pneumonia, scalded skin syndrome, toxic shock syndrome), *Streptobacillus moniliformis,* streptococcal diseases (minor skin wound or burn, endometritis purpura), strongyloidiasis, syphilis, tapeworm disease, tetanus, tinea, toxic shock syndrome, toxoplasmosis, trachoma, trench mouth, trichinosis, trichomoniasis, extrapulmonary tuberculosis, tularemia, typhus, urinary tract infections, Vincent's angina, adult viral respiratory diseases, minor wound infections, localized zoster in normal patient, zygomycosis.

The combination of Universal Precautions and BSI Precautions into Standard Precautions has resulted in precautions being applied to blood, all body fluids, secretions and excretions (except sweat), nonintact skin, and mucous membranes. Standard Precautions cover a variety of diseases (see Table 26–1) previously addressed by the Centers for Disease Control and Prevention (CDC) guidelines under category or disease-specific isolation precautions. In addition, Standard Precautions eliminate the need for the previous CDC categories of isolation precautions (strict isolation, contact isolation, respiratory isolation, tuberculosis isolation, enteric isolation), the drainage/secretion precautions, and the old disease-specific precautions, replacing these with the three Transmission-Based Precautions.

The HICPAC recommendations for preventing the transmission of infectious diseases include administrative controls that call for education and monitoring for adherence to precautions and using findings to identify opportunities for improvement.

Standard Precautions include the following:

★ *Hand washing.* Wash hands after touching blood, body fluids, secretions, excretions, and contaminated items whether gloves are worn or not; after removing gloves; between patient contacts; between procedures on the same patient; and when otherwise indicated to prevent transmission of organisms. Use a plain (non-antimicrobial) soap for routine hand washing. Use an antimicrobial agent under specific circumstances.

★ *Gloves.* Always wear approved gloves when touching blood, body fluids, secretions, excretions, or contaminated items. Nonlatex gloves should be available for health care workers with latex allergies.

★ *Mask, eye protection, face shield.* Wear a mask and eye/face protection during procedures that are likely to generate splashes or sprays of blood, body fluids, secretions, or excretions.

★ *Gown or outerwear protection.* Gowns and outerwear protection serve to protect skin and clothing from being soiled during procedures likely to generate sprays or splashes of blood, body fluids, secretions, or excretions.

★ *Patient care equipment.* Handle all patient care equipment so as to prevent contamination of hands or clean supplies with soiled items including the use of gloves and outerwear protection when indicated. Ensure that single-use equipment is appropriately disposed.

★ *Environmental control.* Ensure that adequate cleaning and disinfecting procedures are in place.

★ *Linen.* Handle soiled or contaminated linens so as to prevent cross-contamination to other patients or environment.

★ *Occupational health and bloodborne pathogens.* Always use caution to prevent injuries when using sharps including the use of safer medical devices, such as sharps with engineered sharps injury protection and needleless systems, work practice controls such as never recapping needles, proper disposal of sharps in puncture-resistant containers, and use of mouthpieces and resuscitation bags as an alternative to mouth-to-mouth resuscitation.

Airborne Precautions should be followed when caring for a patient with a known or suspected infectious disease that can be transmitted by airborne droplet nuclei that remain suspended in the air and can be widely dispersed. These precautions include:

★ *Transport.* CDC recommendations for transporting such patients in an ambulance include minimum 6–12 air exchanges per hour, venting to the outdoors or high-efficiency filtration of recirculated air, separate air circulation between cab and patient compartment, keeping door/window closed between cab and patient compartment, and airing out of vehicle after transporting.

★ *Respiratory protection.* Wear respiratory protection (N95 respirators) when entering room or location of a patient with known or suspected infectious pulmonary tuberculosis. Susceptible persons should not enter the room of patients known or suspected to have measles or varicella if other caregivers are available. If must enter, wear respiratory protection (N95 respirators). If respirators are used, a respiratory protection program should be developed and followed.

★ *Patient transport.* Limit movement to essential purposes only. Have patient wear surgical mask if possible and tolerated.

Droplet Precautions are used when caring for a patient who carries or is infected with pathogens capable of being spread by droplets that can be generated when sneezing, coughing, and talking or while performing procedures such as suctioning or bronchoscopy. These precautions include:

★ *Positioning.* Placement of patient to avoid contact within 3 feet of other persons.

★ *Mask.* Wear a mask when working within 3 feet of the patient.

★ *Patient transport.* Limit transport to essential purposes only. Place a surgical mask on the patient, if possible and tolerated.

Contact Precautions are used with patients who are infected with or colonized with epidemiologically important pathogenic organisms capable of being transmitted by contact including direct contact with the patient's dry skin or indirect contact with inanimate objects in the patient's environment or that have been contaminated by contact with the patient. These precautions include:

★ *Gloves and hand washing.* Wear gloves when entering patient's room. Change gloves when grossly contaminated or between procedures to prevent cross-contamination.

Wash hands with an antimicrobial agent or waterless antiseptic agent immediately upon removal of gloves and whenever hands touch a potentially contaminated surface.

★ *Gown or outerwear.* Wear a gown or other outerwear when entering patient's room if you anticipate having substantial contact with patient or potentially contaminated surfaces or objects in the room. Properly dispose of or decontaminate gown or outerwear per policy.

★ *Patient care equipment.* Dispose of nonreusable equipment appropriately. Nondisposable equipment must be cleaned and disinfected prior to being placed back in service.

★ Additional precautions are indicated for patients infected with vancomycin-resistant organisms.

Table 26–2 summarizes diseases that require additional precautions over the Standard Precautions described earlier.

With missions of the type that critical care personnel respond to, it is hoped that the diagnosis of or knowledge about the presence of an infectious disease is known. If not, the critical care provider must evaluate and react to symptomotology, selecting appropriate therapies and interventions. Critical care transport organizations may wish to adopt a list of signs and symptoms that would require the use of additional precautions designed to prevent the possible transmission of important infectious conditions. These precautions would be implemented in addition to Universal Precautions, Body Substance Isolation Precautions, or Standard Precautions depending on which of these systems the organization has adopted. A sample of a symptom-specific precautions system is provided in Table 26–3.

The Occupational Health and Safety Act (OSHA) requires qualified employers who have employees who may experience occupational exposure to bloodborne pathogens (29 CFR 1910.1030; see Table 26–4) and/or occupational exposure to *Mycobacterium tuberculosis* (general duty clause and 29 CFR 1910.135, Respiratory Protection) to develop and implement exposure control plans for these pathogens. The rules and the compliance directives for each of these plans provide specific guidance to employers regarding their obligations and the content of these plans. Additional guidance can be found in publications from the CDC, the OSHA rules on recordkeeping and reporting of injuries and illnesses (29 CFR1904 and 29 CFR 1910.1020), hazard communication (29 CFR 1910.1200), and the Needlestick Injury and Prevention Act (P.L. 106–430).

The bloodborne pathogen rule was revised in 2000 to provide for clarification of engineering controls to include review of available sharps with engineered sharps injury protection (SESIP) and needleless systems and the maintaining of a sharps injury log (see Table 26–5).

The CDC has published recommendations for the management of occupational blood exposures. Those recommendations may be found on the CDC website and include the following:

★ Provide immediate care to the exposure site.
★ Determine risk associated with exposure.
★ Evaluate exposure source.
★ Evaluate the exposed person.
★ Give PEP for exposures posing risk of infection transmission.
★ Perform follow-up testing and provide counseling.
★ HBV exposures.
★ HCV exposures.
★ HIV exposures.

Health care workers are at risk of exposure to many infectious diseases and should be immunized against those vaccine-preventable diseases they may encounter during the course of their work. The CDC has published recommendations for immunizations of health care workers and updates these periodically (see Table 26–6).

Table 26–2 | Transmission-Based Precautions

Infection/Condition	Type of Precaution	Duration
Abscess, draining, major	Contact	Duration of illness
Adenovirus in infants and young children	Droplet and Contact	Duration of illness
Cellulitis, uncontrolled drainage	Contact	Duration of illness
Chickenpox (varicella)	Airborne and Contact	Until all lesions are crusted. Exposed susceptible health care workers (HCWs) should be excluded from patient contact from the 10th to the 21st day (28 days if VZIG given) after exposure
Clostridium difficile, enterocolitis	Contact	Duration of illness
Congenital rubella	Contact	N/A
Conjunctivitis, acute viral (acute hemorrhagic)	Contact	Duration of illness
Decubitus ulcer, infected major with no dressing or dressing does not contain drainage adequately	Contact	Duration of illness
Diphtheria, cutaneous	Contact	Until off antibiotics and two cultures taken at least 24 hours apart are negative
Diphtheria, pharyngeal	Droplet	Until off antibiotics and two cultures taken at least 24 hours apart are negative
Ebola viral hemorrhagic fever	Contact	Duration of illness
Enterocolitis, *Clostridium difficile*	Contact	Duration of illness
Epiglottitis, due to *Haemophilus influenzae*	Droplet	Until 24 hours after initiation of effective therapy
Furunculosis-staphylococcal of infants and young children	Contact	Duration of illness
Gastroenteritis, *Vibrio cholerae*	Contact	Duration of illness
Gastroenteritis, *Clostridium difficile*		
Gastroenteritis, *Rotavirus*, diapered or incontinent		
Gastroenteritis, *Shigella*, diapered or incontinent		
Hemorrhagic fevers (i.e., Lassa and Ebola)	Contact	Duration of illness
Herpes simplex, neonatal or mucocutaneous, disseminated or primary, severe	Contact	Duration of illness
Herpes zoster (varicella-zoster), localized in immunocompromised patient, or disseminated	Airborne and Contact	Duration of illness. Persons susceptible to varicella are also at risk for developing varicella when exposed to persons with herpes zoster lesions
Impetigo	Contact	Until 24 hours after initiation of effective therapy
Influenza	Droplet	Duration of illness
Lassa fever	Contact	Duration of illness
Lice (pediculosis)	Contact	Until 24 hours after initiation of effective therapy
Marburg virus disease	Contact	Duration of illness
Measles (rubeola), all presentations	Airborne	Duration of illness
Meningitis, *Haemophilus influenzae*, known or suspected	Droplet	Until 24 hours after initiation of effective therapy
Meningitis, *Neisseria meningitidis* (meningococcal) known or suspected	Droplet	Until 24 hours after initiation of effective therapy
Meningococcal pneumonia or meningococcemia (meningococcal sepsis)	Droplet	Until 24 hours after initiation of effective therapy
Multidrug-resistant organisms, infection or colonization		
Gastrointestinal	Contact	Until off antibiotics and culture negative
Respiratory		
Skin, wound, or burn		

Table 26–2 | Transmission-Based Precautions *(continued)*

Infection/Condition	Type of Precaution	Duration
Mumps	Droplet	For 9 days after onset of swelling
Mycoplasma pneumonia	Droplet	Duration of illness
Parainfluenza virus infection, respiratory in infants and young children	Contact	Duration of illness
Parvovirus B19	Droplet	
Pediculosis (lice)	Contact	Until 24 hours after initiation of effective therapy
Pertussis (whooping cough)	Droplet	Until 5 days after patient is placed on effective therapy
Plague, pneumonic	Droplet	Until 72 hours after initiation of effective therapy
Pneumonia, adenovirus	Droplet and Contact	Duration of illness
Pneumonia, *Haemophilus influenzae* in infants and children (any age)	Droplet	Until 2 hours after initiation of effective therapy
Pneumonia, meningococcal	Droplet	Until 24 hours after initiation of effective therapy
Pneumonia, *Mycoplasma*, primary atypical pneumonia	Droplet	Duration of illness
Pneumonia, *Streptococcus*, group A in infants and young children	Droplet	Until 24 hours after initiation of effective therapy
Respiratory infectious disease, acute (if not covered elsewhere) in infants and young children	Contact	Duration of illness
Respiratory syncytial virus infection, in infants, young children, and immunocompromised adults	Contact	Duration of illness
Rubella (German measles)	Droplet	Until 7 days after onset of rash
Scabies	Contact	Until 24 hours after initiation of effective therapy
Staphylococcal (*S. aureus*) disease, skin, wound, or burn; major	Contact	Duration of illness
Streptococcal (group A streptococcus) disease, skin, wound, or burn; major	Contact	Until 24 hours after initiation of effective therapy
Streptococcal (group A streptococcus) disease, pharyngitis in infants and young children	Droplet	Until 24 hours after initiation of effective therapy
Streptococcal (group A streptococcus) disease, pneumonia in infants and young children	Droplet	Until 24 hours after initiation of effective therapy
Streptococcal (group A streptococcus) disease, Scarlet fever in infants and young children	Droplet	Until 24 hours after initiation of effective therapy
Tuberculosis, pulmonary, confirmed or suspected or laryngeal disease	Airborne	Discontinue precautions only after patient is on effective therapy, is improving clinically, and has three consecutive negative sputum smears collected on different days, or TB is ruled out
Varicella (chickenpox)	Airborne and Contact	Until all lesions are crusted. Exposed susceptible HCWs should be excluded from patient contact from the 10th to the 21st day (28 days if VZIG given) after exposure
Whooping cough (pertussis)	Droplet	Until 5 days after patient is placed on effective therapy
Wound infections, major	Contact	Duration of illness
Zoster (varicella-zoster), localized in immuno-compromised patient, disseminated	Airborne and Contact	Duration of illness Persons susceptible to varicella are also at risk for developing varicella when exposed to persons with herpes zoster lesions

Source: Adapted from the Public Health Service, U.S. Department of Health and Human Services, Centers for Disease Control and Prevention, Atlanta, Georgia; Garner JS. Hospital Infection Control Practices Advisory Committee. "Guidelines for Isolation Precautions in Hospitals." *Infect. Control Hosp. Epidemiol.,* Vol. 17 (1996): 53–80; *Am. J. Infect. Control,* Vol. 24 (1996): 24–52; http://www.cdc.gov/ncidod/hip/isolat/isolat.htm (updated February 18, 1997).

Table 26-3 | Sample Symptom-Specific Precautions System

Signs or Symptoms	Potential Infection or Pathogen	Additional Precautions
Diarrhea	*Clostridium difficile*	Contact
	E. coli (O) 157:H7	
	Rotavirus	
	Shigella	
Drainage or draining wounds not contained within a dressing	*S. aureus* or group A streptococcus	Contact
Fever in adults		
With no other symptoms	As below	Airborne and Contact
With rash	*Neisseria meningitidis*/varicella/measles	Airborne and Contact
With respiratory symptoms	*Mycobacterium tuberculosis*	Airborne
With neurologic symptoms	*Neisseria meningitidis*	Droplet
Fever in infants and children		
With no other symptoms	As below	Airborne and Contact
With rash	*Neisseria meningitides*/varicella/measles	Airborne and Contact
With respiratory symptoms	Respiratory syncytial or parainfluenza virus/staph or strept pneumonia, and so on	Airborne and Contact
With neurologic symptoms	*Neisseria meningitidis*	Droplet
Rashes	*Neisseria meningitidis*/varicella/measles	Airborne and Contact
Respiratory symptoms without other explanation	*Mycobacterium tuberculosis* or pneumonia or pertussis or respiratory syncytial or parainfluenza virus	Airborne and Contact
Special Note: if possibility of infection or colonization with multidrug-resistant microorganism	Resistant bacteria	Contact

In this example the author has chosen to default to the highest level of precautions to ensure adequate protection is provided in the event of a worst case scenario. Others may choose to describe more complex symptomatology and further differentiate the possible conditions and the appropriate precautions to be taken. The reader is referred to Table 2 of Garner JS, Hospital Infection Control Practices Advisory Committee, "Guideline for Isolation Precautions in Hospitals." *Infect. Control Hosp. Epidemiol.,* Vol. 17 (1996): 53–80; *Am. J. Infect. Control,* Vol. 24, (1996): 24–52; and http://www.cdc.gov/ncidod/hip/isolat/isolat.htm (updated February 18, 1997).

Unvaccinated health care workers or those who fail to maintain their immunity pose a risk to themselves, their patients, coworkers, family, and friends when they are exposed to infectious diseases.

Unvaccinated health care workers or those who fail to maintain their immunity pose a risk to themselves, their patients, coworkers, family, and friends when they are exposed to infectious diseases. While proper precautions will reduce the risk for transmission, often the exposure occurs prior to knowing or suspecting a patient has a communicable disease and, therefore, prior to implementing the appropriate precautions. This is especially true with diseases transmitted by the airborne or droplet route of transmission. It is important to remember that infected persons may be asymptomatic but most infectious during the incubation period and during carrier states.

The CDC has published recommendations for other immunobiologics that are or may be indicated for health care workers including hepatitis A immune globulin, hepatitis A vaccine, meningococcal polysaccharide vaccine (tetravalent A, C, W135, and Y), typhoid vaccine, and vaccinia vaccine (smallpox). Health care workers who may need protection against these vaccine-preventable diseases include individuals who travel internationally or work in laboratories where these microorganisms may be present.

The threat of biological weapon usage by terrorists may result in the CDC recommending additional vaccinations for emergency response workers and health care workers including anthrax, rabies, and plague. Critical care organizations will need to stay current with CDC and Department of Homeland Security recommendations for immunizations for health care workers in order to make the most informed decisions regarding their workforce's health and safety. Furthermore, as

Table 26–4	Bloodborne Pathogens Standard (29 CFR 1910.1030)

Major Provisions by Paragraph

(a) Scope

(b) Definitions

(c) Exposure Control Plan

(d) Methods of Compliance

    Universal Precautions

    Engineering and Work Practice Controls

    Personal Protective Equipment

    Housekeeping

       Regulated Waste

       Laundry

(e) HIV and HBV Research Labs

(f) Hepatitis B Vaccination and Post-Exposure Evaluation and Follow-Up

(g) Communication of Hazards

    Labels and Signs

    Information and Training

(h) Recordkeeping

    Medical Records

    Training Records

    Sharps Injury Log

Appendix A

    Hepatitis B Declination Form (Mandatory) (9)

the changing threat of bioterrorisim evolves, it is becoming more evident that there may be an ongoing and/or immediate (i.e., "on-the-fly") need to vaccinate EMS, critical care transport providers, and/or other emergency responders based on intelligence for a specific threat agent. This may also pertain to even specific geographic regions, as long as the threat of bioterrorism exists. (Refer to Chapter 33 for more on weapons of mass destruction.)

MANAGING PATIENTS WITH INFECTIOUS DISEASES

The management of patients with an infectious process will often include treatment to relieve the symptoms associated with the infection, treatment directed at eradicating the infecting organism, treatment to reduce or reverse the toxic effects of certain pathogens, general supportive care and the use of isolation precautions to prevent the spread of infection to other patients, and cross-contamination of the other body parts of the patient or of health care workers and family members.

Critical care personnel will care for patients with infectious diseases whose diagnosis may or may not be known at the time of contact. All health care workers have been taught to use Universal Precautions (or BSI or Standard Precautions) in the management of all patients regardless of diagnosis. The use of Universal Precautions reduces the risk of occupational exposure to bloodborne pathogens, but offers little protection for diseases that are transmitted by droplet, airborne, or contact routes. As such, it becomes important that critical care personnel recognize the potential for an infectious disease in the patients they treat, recognize the symptoms or patterns of illness suggestive of an infectious agent, and adopt appropriate precautions for the situation.

The first step in the management of potentially infectious patients is the recognition of signs and symptoms suggestive of the presence of an infection. In general, a high suspicion of an infectious process should occur with any of the general signs and symptoms discussed next.

Critical care personnel will care for patients with infectious diseases whose diagnosis may or may not be known at the time of contact.

Table 26–5	Bloodborne Pathogen Rules

Excepts from 29 CFR 1910.1030 revised January 18, 2001; effective date April 18, 2001:

(c)(1)(iv) The Exposure Control Plan shall be reviewed and updated at least annually and whenever necessary to reflect new or modified tasks and procedures which affect occupational exposure and to reflect new or revised employee positions with occupational exposure. The review and update of such plans shall also:

(c)(1)(iv)(A) reflect changes in technology that eliminate or reduce exposure to bloodborne pathogens; and

(c)(1)(iv)(B) document annually consideration and implementation of appropriate commercially available and effective safer medical devices designed to eliminate or minimize occupational exposure.

(c)(1)(v) An employer, who is required to establish an Exposure Control Plan shall solicit input from non-managerial employees responsible for direct patient care who are potentially exposed to injuries from contaminated sharps in the identification, evaluation, and selection of effective engineering and work practice controls and shall document the solicitation in the Exposure Control Plan. . .

(h)(5) **Sharps Injury Log.**

(h)(5)(i) The employer shall establish and maintain a sharps injury log for the recording of percutaneous injuries from contaminated sharps. The information in the sharps injury log shall be recorded and maintained in such manner as to protect the confidentiality of the injured employee. The sharps injury log shall contain, at a minimum:

(h)(5)(i)(A) the type and brand of device involved in the incident,

(h)(5)(i)(B) the department or work area where the exposure incident occurred, and

(h)(5)(i)(C) an explanation of how the incident occurred.

(h)(5)(ii) The requirement to establish and maintain a sharps injury log shall apply to any employer who is required to maintain a log of occupational injuries and illnesses under 29 CFR 1904.

(h)(5)(iii) The sharps injury log shall be maintained for the period required by 29 CFR 1904.6. (9)

According to Waldman and Kluge (1984), fever, one of the cardinal signs of infection, "is . . . the most primitive of the body's responses to disease and is the most constant of all clinical manifestations of infectious diseases . . . often absent in the very young or the very old . . . fever (is) important because the termination of febrile response is usually associated with improvement in the patient's clinical condition and recovery" (p. 9).

In addition to fever, other signs and symptoms of infection include redness, swelling, heat, pain, pus, enlarged lymph glands, headache, myalgia, malaise, loss of appetite, and delirium. As an organism attacks specific body organs or systems, symptoms related to dysfunction of those organs or systems may become apparent. Examples include the neurologic symptoms of seizure, impaired function of sensory or motor nerves, and vision and auditory symptoms that may be seen with meningitis or encephalitis or the vomiting and diarrhea often associated with gastrointestinal illnesses.

Space does not permit the inclusion in this chapter of every infectious disease and their accompanying signs and symptoms and management. Entire books have been written that address the topic more comprehensively than this author will be able to accomplish here, and the reader is referred to the Further Reading reference list at the end of this chapter for more information on specific disease entities. Instead, a brief overview of either commonly encountered or epidemiologically important infectious diseases is provided including signs and symptoms, prevention when available, and treatment. Precautions to be taken with various infectious agents or based on signs and symptoms have been previously discussed.

Table 26–6	CDC Immunization Recommendations for Health Care Workers			
Disease	**Route of Transmission**	**Vaccine**	**Vaccine Schedule**	**Indications**
Hepatitis B (HBV)	Percutaneous or permucosal exposure to blood or body fluids containing blood	Hepatitis B recombinant vaccine	Two doses IM 4 weeks apart; third dose 5 months after second; booster doses not necessary	HCWs at risk for exposure to blood or body fluids
		Hepatitis B immune globulin (HBIG)	0.06 mL/kg IM ASAP after exposure but no later than 7 days. A second dose should be administered 1 month later if the HB series has not been started	Postexposure for persons exposed to blood or body fluids containing HBsAg and who are not immune to HBV infection
Influenza	Airborne	Annual vaccination with current vaccine	IM per vaccine schedule	HCWs who have contact with patients at high risk for influenza or its complications; HCWs who work in chronic care facilities; HCWs with high-risk medical conditions or who are aged ≥65 years
Measles (rubeola)	Airborne	Measles live-virus vaccine. Measles–mumps–rubella (MMR) vaccine of choice if recipients likely to be susceptible to mumps or rubella as well as measles	One dose SC; second dose at least 1 month later	HCWs born during or after 1957 who do not have documentation of having received 2 doses of live vaccine on or after the first birthday or a history of physician-diagnosed measles or serologic evidence of immunity. Vaccination should be considered for all HCWs who lack proof of immunity, including those born before 1957
Mumps	Droplet and direct contact with saliva	Mumps live-virus vaccine. MMR vaccine of choice if recipients likely to be susceptible to measles or rubella as well as mumps	One dose SC; no booster	HCWs believed to be susceptible can be vaccinated. Adults born before 1957 can be considered immune
Rubella, German measles, three-day measles	Droplet and direct contact with nasopharyngeal secretions	Rubella live-virus vaccine. MMR vaccine of choice if recipients likely to be susceptible to measles or mumps as well as rubella	One dose SC; no booster	Indicated for HCWs who do not have documentation of having received live vaccine on or after their first birthday or laboratory evidence of immunity. Adults born before 1957, except women who can become pregnant, can be considered immune

(continued)

Table 26–6 | CDC Immunization Recommendations for Health Care Workers (continued)

Disease	Route of Transmission	Vaccine	Vaccine Schedule	Indications
Pneumococcal disease	Droplet spread, direct oral contact or indirectly through contact with items soiled with respiratory secretions	Pneumococcal polysaccharide vaccine (23 valent)	One 0.5-mL dose, IM or SC; revaccination recommended for those at highest risk ≥5 years after the first dose	Adults who are at increased risk of pneumococcal disease and its complications because of underlying health conditions; older adults, especially those age ≥65 who are healthy
Tetanus and diphtheria	Tetanus spores introduced into the body through contaminated puncture wounds. Contact with diphtheria patient or carrier or rarely contact with items soiled with discharges from lesions of infected persons	Tetanus and diphtheria (toxoids) Td	Two IM doses 4 weeks apart; third dose 6–12 months after second dose; booster every 10 years	All adults
Varicella, chickenpox or herpes zoster (shingles)	Direct contact, droplet, or airborne spread, indirect contact with items contaminated with discharges from vesicles or respiratory tract	Varicella zoster live-virus vaccine Varicella-zoster immune globulin (VZIG)	Two 0.5-mL doses SC 4–8 weeks apart if ≥13 years of age Persons <50 kg: 125 units/10 kg IM; persons >50 kg: 625 units	HCWs who do not have either a reliable history of varicella or serologic evidence of immunity

Source: Adapted from CDC "Immunization of Health-Care Workers: Recommendations of the Advisory Committee on Immunization Practices (ACIP) and the Hospital Infection Control Practices Advisory Committee (HICPAC)." *MMWR* (December 26, 1997): 46, RR-18.

COMMONLY ENCOUNTERED OR EPIDEMIOLOGICALLY IMPORTANT INFECTIOUS DISEASES

HUMAN IMMUNODEFICIENCY VIRUS AND ACQUIRED IMMUNODEFICIENCY SYNDROME

acquired immunodeficiency syndrome (AIDS) *a severe life-threatening disease caused by the Human Immunodeficiency Virus (HIV); the terminal clinical manifestation of HIV infection.*

human immunodeficiency virus (HIV) *a retrovirus that attacks the immune system, consisting of two identified types similar in epidemiologic characteristics; HIV-1 appears more pathogenic than HIV-2.*

Acquired immunodeficiency syndrome (AIDS) is a severe life-threatening disease caused by the **human immunodeficiency virus (HIV)**, a retrovirus. There are two identified types: type 1 (HIV-1) and type 2 (HIV-2). The two are similar in epidemiologic characteristics but HIV-1 appears more pathogenic than HIV-2. Worldwide, the predominant virus is HIV-1, and generally when people refer to HIV without specifying the type of virus they will be referring to HIV-1. The relatively uncommon HIV-2 type is concentrated in West Africa and is rarely found elsewhere.

Infection with HIV may demonstrate no symptoms initially but more often results in a mononucleosis-like viral illness that develops a couple of weeks after exposure. After the initial viral-like illness, other clinical manifestations of infection with HIV may not present for months to years. The virus attacks the immune system, rendering the person vulnerable to a variety of infectious diseases and cancers. AIDS is the late clinical manifestation of HIV infection. The average time from HIV infection to death is 10–12 years. However, more rapid rates of progression have been documented with individuals moving from HIV infection to death from AIDS in 6 months. What this seems to infer is that the virus may mutate and represent a severe change in disease progression.

General symptoms of disease development include fever, weight loss, loss of appetite, fatigue, chronic diarrhea, and lymphadenopathy. Later symptoms are related to the opportunistic infections or other manifestations the disease may take including *Pneumocystis carinii* pneumonia; Kaposi's sarcoma; cytomegalovirus (CMV) infections of the eyes, lungs; GI system or ventral nervous system; toxoplasmosis; cryptosporidiosis; candidiasis; disseminated herpes simplex; non-Hodgkin's lymphomas; symptoms of wasting disease; HIV dementia; and others.

AIDS was first described in 1981, and the World Health Organization reports that as of 2004 there were more than 39.4 million persons diagnosed and living with AIDS worldwide. There are approximately 4.9 million new cases annually. Approximately 3.1 million people died from AIDS in 2004, and 20 million have died since the virus was identified. The CDC has estimated that by the end of 2003 there were approximately 1.1 million persons in the United States living with AIDS although approximately 25 percent of these are undiagnosed and unaware of the infection.

HIV is transmitted through sexual contact with an infected person, by sharing needles and syringes with an infected person, through blood or blood product transfusions, or by exposure to blood or other potentially infectious materials (OPIM) such as semen, vaginal fluids, peritoneal fluid, pleural fluid, or other fluids with visible blood. Infants born to HIV-infected mothers may be infected before, during, or right after birth. Transmission has occurred with breast-feeding. Health care workers have been infected with HIV after sustaining a needle-stick or sharps injury or contact with the mucous membrane or nonintact skin with blood from an infected person. Every exposure does not result in infection. Studies indicate that the risk of developing infection after a single needle-stick that is contaminated with a known HIV-infected person's blood is less than 0.5% as compared with hepatitis B where the risk is about 25% with the same type of exposure.

Treatment of patients with HIV or AIDS is directed toward treating the opportunistic infection(s) or cancers. Several antiretroviral therapies have reduced the number of HIV-related illnesses and death and have proven effective in improving the quality of life of infected persons. Currently, however, there is no cure for HIV infection and no effective vaccine to prevent the infection. Prevention is directed at reducing or eliminating behaviors that put persons at risk for infection. Occupational exposures can be reduced by the development and adherence to an effective bloodborne pathogen plan and the use of Universal or Standard Precautions in the management of all persons regardless of diagnosis.

All exposed individuals, whether occupational exposure or other, should be referred for appropriate counseling, testing and follow-up. Postexposure prophylaxis for occupational exposures is available but individuals will need to receive information on the rationale for prophylaxis, the limitations of current knowledge of the efficacy of antiretroviral therapies, the toxicity associated with these agents and the need for close follow-up prior to making a decision to accept or refuse such treatments.

HEPATITIS

Hepatitis is an inflammation of the liver that can lead to failure. Hepatitis, specifically hepatitis B, poses a greater risk for critical care paramedics than HIV. Fortunately, an effective vaccine is available for hepatitis A and hepatitis B. The following information will detail the various types of hepatitis.

hepatitis An inflammation of the liver that can lead to organ failure and death.

Hepatitis, specifically hepatitis B, poses a greater risk for critical care paramedics than HIV.

Hepatitis A

Hepatitis A is a liver disease caused by the hepatitis A virus (HAV.) The disease produces symptoms that include nausea, diarrhea, jaundice, abdominal pain, fatigue, fever, and loss of appetite. Hepatitis A, unlike many of the other forms of hepatitis, has no long-term effects. Some persons may remain ill or relapse for a 6- to 9-month period, but chronic infection does not develop. Infection ensures lifelong immunity and it is estimated that one-third of all adults have antibodies to hepatitis A indicating a prior infection.

The disease is spread via the fecal–oral route of transmission. Most commonly, spread occurs by putting a hand in the mouth after it has been contaminated with feces (even if not visible) from an infected person; however, water supplies (wells) contaminated with sewage also serve as sources of infection. Standard Precautions are sufficient in most cases of infection with hepatitis A. Contact

Precautions may be needed with diapered or incontinent individuals. Hand washing after going to the bathroom, changing diapers, and before and after preparing food is the most effective means to prevent the spread of hepatitis A.

Treatment is supportive in nature, with attention to maintenance of fluid and electrolyte balance if diarrhea is severe and/or if oral intake is not tolerated. A vaccine is available and immune globulin may be indicated for exposed individuals.

Hepatitis B

Hepatitis B is a serious infection of the liver caused by the hepatitis B virus (HBV) and is responsible for 4,000 to 5,000 deaths annually from cirrhosis and liver cancer. Many of the persons infected with HBV (30%) will have no clinical symptoms of disease. In those who do develop clinical disease, the symptoms may include fatigue, loss of appetite, nausea and vomiting, abdominal pain, mild fever, occasionally a rash, and jaundice in about 30% to 50% of patients. This disease, unlike hepatitis A, may develop into chronic disease. Infants are at greatest risk for developing chronic hepatitis B (90% of those infected at birth) and persons over 5 years of age have a risk of about 6%. Chronic disease is a serious complication of infection with hepatitis B virus, with a mortality rate of 15% to 25%.

Hepatitis B is transmitted through exposure to blood or other body fluids. While the virus has been found in almost all body fluids, transmission has only occurred with exposure to infected blood, saliva, semen, and vaginal fluids. The most common routes of transmission are sexual intercourse and sharing of contaminated needles and syringes. Occupational exposure occurs through percutaneous or permucosal exposure to infected body fluids. Transmission has occurred from contaminated blood or blood product transfusions (rare today), dialysis, and childbirth. Because the organism can survive for days on inanimate surfaces, transmission from these surfaces can occur if there is exposure to open skin or mucous membrane or percutaneous injury. The presence of organic matter on an inanimate surface fosters the survival of these organisms. Appropriate cleaning and disinfecting reduces or eliminates this hazard. Standard Precautions should be followed for hepatitis B infection and, as always, safe handling of sharps.

Patients with hepatitis B may be asymptomatic and no treatment is indicated. A qualified physician should evaluate all persons infected with hepatitis B for liver disease. Supportive care is indicated. On occasion, hospitalization is necessary to treat the abdominal symptoms and/or if dehydration occurs or other more serious signs and symptoms. Alpha interferon and lamivudine may be indicated for chronic hepatitis B. Patients should be counseled to avoid drinking alcohol. A vaccine is available for hepatitis B and is recommended for all health care professionals. The vaccine is now routinely given to newborns.

Hepatitis C

Hepatitis C is a serious liver disease caused by hepatitis C virus (HCV). Hepatitis C progresses to chronic hepatitis in 75% to 85% of infected persons. The symptoms of infection with hepatitis C are similar to other forms of hepatitis: fatigue, abdominal pain, jaundice, dark urine, nausea, and loss of appetite. The disease is transmitted in a manner similar to that for hepatitis B including percutaneous or permucosal exposure to infected blood or blood products or OPIM, blood or blood product transfusions (rare today), injecting drug users, and infants born to infected mothers. Transmission can occur with sex, but less easily than with hepatitis B or HIV.

Treatment in addition to supportive care includes evaluation by a physician for liver disease and consideration for interferon and ribavirin singularly or in combination.

Hepatitis D (Delta Hepatitis)

Hepatitis D is a co-infection or a superinfection of hepatitis B and is caused by the hepatitis D virus (HDV). The modes of transmission of hepatitis D are similar to those for hepatitis B, with percutaneous transmission most efficient. Co-infection and superinfection of HBV with HDV can increase the severity of disease and increase the incident of development of chronic states. HDV is dependent on hepatitis B virus for replication, therefore prevention of hepatitis B will prevent infection with hepatitis D. There is no vaccine or preventive for hepatitis D, therefore, superinfections with hepatitis B depend on preventing transmission through risk reduction.

Table 26-7	Viral Hepatitis Comparison				
	Hepatitis A	**Hepatitis B**	**Hepatitis C**	**Hepatitis D**	**Hepatitis E**
Cause	HAV	HBV	HCV	HDV	HEV
Incubation period	15–50 days (average 30 days)	45–160 days (average 120 days)	2–25 weeks (average 7–9 weeks)	2–8 weeks	2–9 weeks (average 40 days)
Transmission	Fecal–oral	Contact with infected body fluids	Contact with infected body fluids	Contact with infected body fluids	Fecal–oral
Chronic disease	No	Yes	Yes	Yes	No
Vaccine	Yes	Yes	No	HBV vaccine prevents HDV	No

Hepatitis E

Hepatitis E is an infection of the liver caused by hepatitis E virus (HEV) and produces a disease similar to those caused by the other hepatitis viruses. Symptoms include abdominal pain, fatigue, anorexia, jaundice, dark urine, and occasionally pruritis and a rash. HEV is transmitted like hepatitis A through the fecal–oral route of transmission. Unlike hepatitis A, most cases occur as a result of drinking water contaminated with feces and few cases are transmitted person to person. Standard Precautions should be followed with consideration for Contact Precautions in persons who are diapered or incontinent.

Table 26–7 compares the various hepatitis infections.

RESPIRATORY INFECTIONS

Respiratory infections are a major cause of morbidity and mortality in the United States, and include the following conditions and/or signs and symptoms: common cold, sore throats, ear infections, conjunctivitis, laryngitis/croup, epiglottitis, tracheobronchitis, bronchiolitis, severe acute respiratory distress syndrome (SARS), and pneumonia. Upper respiratory infections (URIs) are the most common acute illnesses in the United States, usually causing a brief, mild illness but extreme morbidity. The average adult has two to five URIs per year lasting 5–7 days, more often if they have frequent contact with children. URIs result in millions of lost work and school days annually, accounting for 80% of lost days from school and 40% of the lost days from work.

Major complications from respiratory infections include the development of bacterial super-infections manifesting as bacterial sinusitis, otitis media, bronchitis, or pneumonia. Treatment of respiratory infections of viral origin is directed toward relief of symptoms. Antibiotics are not indicated unless the patient is at risk for or has developed a secondary bacterial or superinfection. Adequate oxygenation and hydration are important support measures. Route of transmission may be airborne, droplet, or contact for many of the causative agents of respiratory infections. Appropriate precautions would be the use of a surgical mask on the patient if appropriate and tolerated and the use of Airborne and Contact Precautions.

EPIGLOTTITIS

Epiglottitis is an inflammation of the epiglottis seen mostly in children between the ages of 2 and 6 but can be observed in adults. The epiglottis becomes inflamed and swollen secondary to a bacterial infection, resulting in a partial or total airway obstruction. The organism most often associated with epiglottitis in children is *Haemophilus influenzae* type B (HIB). Vaccination with HIB has greatly reduced the incidence of *H. influenzae* epiglottitis in children. Other causative agents include *Streptococcus pneumoniae, Pneumococcus, Staphylococcus aureus* or *Haemophilus parainfluenzae.*

Epiglottitis is a true emergency because it develops rapidly and results in a compromised airway. Death may occur if the patient is left untreated or managed incorrectly. Patients frequently present with respiratory distress of sudden onset, sitting upright, leaning forward with their jaw jutted

epiglottitis *An inflammation of the epiglottis secondary to a bacterial infection; seen mostly in children between the ages of 2 and 6, but has been observed in adults.*

forward and often drooling. Additional signs and symptoms include strider, hoarseness or muffled voice, sore throat, dysphagia, fever (>103 °F), perioral cyanosis, tachycardia, tachypnea, and retractions. They are often anxious but may appear lethargic or fatigued due to exhaustion from their efforts to breathe.

Health care professionals must maintain a high level of suspicion for epiglottitis. Patients with suspected or known epiglottitis must be treated cautiously but expeditiously. Every effort must be made to keep the child calm because any agitation or crying may lead to laryngospasm and complete airway obstruction. Patients with epiglottitis often require advanced airway management including intubation or tracheostomy. Intubating patients with epiglottitis can be very problematic due to the swelling of the epiglottis, which interferes with visualization of the vocal cords and placement of the tube. Patients are usually treated with antibiotics including cefotaxime, ceftriaxone, or ampicillin with sulbactam given intravenously. On occasion steroids are administered to help reduce swelling of the epiglottis. However, such treatment makes it more difficult to determine effectiveness of the antibiotics because it masks symptoms. Critical care transport personnel may want to contact medical direction for guidance on management of these fragile patients.

INFLUENZA

influenza (the flu)
dangerous respiratory infection caused by a virus that may lead to complications of pneumonia and death.

Influenza (the flu), like a cold, is a respiratory infection caused by a virus; however, the flu is a more dangerous infection that may lead to complications of pneumonia and death. Signs that help distinguish the flu from the common cold include sudden onset of symptoms, which appear more severe including headache, dry cough, and chills. Myalgia and high fever are common. The weakness and "washed out" feeling may last for several weeks.

Complications of the flu are responsible for the deaths of thousands of Americans every year and in the 1918–1919 pandemic 20 million people died. In the United States, significant influenza activity occurred during the winter seasons of 1999–2000 and 2003–2004. The CDC estimates that in excess of 20,000 deaths occur annually as a result of influenza virus.

Treatment for the flu, like the common cold, is supportive in nature including the use of decongestants, antitussives, expectorants, and pain relievers. Antibiotics are effective in treating these viral illnesses; however, each year a vaccine is prepared in anticipation of that year's expected causative viral agent. Caregivers should be vigilant for the development of bacterial or superinfections, including pneumonia, and initiate appropriate antibiotic treatment.

PNEUMONIA

pneumonia *swelling and obstruction of the lungs by fiberlike fluids and/or mucous; commonly contracted by inhalation of the* Dipplococcus pneumoniae *bacteria, rickettsiae, a virus, or a fungi.*

Patients with **pneumonia,** an infectious process that settles in the lungs, usually present with respiratory symptoms including crackles (rales) heard over the affected lobe(s), possibly an increase in tactile fremitus, and bronchial breathing. Purulent sputum may be seen with bacterial pneumonias; blood-tinged sputum may be seen with pneumococcal, *Klebsiella* or *Legionella* infections. Chest X-ray is required to make the diagnosis.

Atypical pneumonia may be treated with oral macrolides (erythromycin, clarithromycin, or azithromycin) or newer quinolones (Levaquin). Azithromycin or a newer quinolone may be indicated for *Legionella* or severe atypical pneumonias.

Bacterial community-acquired pneumonia (CAP) is usually caused by gram-positive *Streptococcus pneumoniae* or *Streptococcus pyogenes, Staphylococcus aureus* or *Moraxella catarrhalis.* Antibiotic therapy may include penicillin G or V, amoxicillin, cephalosporins, macrolides (Azithromycin) or quinolones (levofloxacin) for penicillin-resistant strep, gatifloxacin, or moxifloxacin. Antibiotic treatment is directed at the causative agent and may involve the use of any of the available antibiotics depending on sensitivity and resistance of the organism as well as patient tolerance of the selected therapies (see Table 26–8).

Supportive care should be provided including monitoring vital signs, using pulse oximetry, and administering oxygen as indicated and selected antibiotics. Patients requiring hospitalization often are elderly or have underlying disease complicating the situation. Any immunocompromised patient is at greater risk of acquiring pneumonia and having a more complicated course. Patients who

Table 26–8 — Antibiotic Classes

Class	Actions	Examples
Beta-lactams	Bacteriocidal—interferes with synthesis of bacterial cell walls resulting in cell lyses. The cell ruptures and is destroyed	Penicillins, amoxicillin-clavulanate, cephalosporins, carbapenems (meropenem and combinations of imipenem/cilastatin)
Fluoroquinolones (quinolones)	Bacteriostatic—interferes with bacterial cell reproduction by interfering with synthesis of nucleic acids	Ciprofloxacin (Cipro), levofloxacin, sparfloxacin, gemifloxacin, gatifloxacin, moxifloxacin, trovafloxacin, and clinafloxacin
Macrolides and azalides	Affect the genetics of bacteria	Erythromycin, azithromycin (Zithromax), clarithromycin (Biaxin), and roxithromycin (Rulid)
Tetracyclines	Inhibit bacterial growth	Doxycycline, tetracycline, and minocycline
Trimethoprim-sulfamethoxazole		Bactrim, Cotrim, Septra
Aminoglycosides	For very serious bacterial infections; have very serious side effects	Gentamycin, kanamycin, tobramycin, amikacin
Lincosamide	Prevents bacteria from reproducing	Clindamycin (Cleocin)
Glycopeptide	Used in *S. aureus* infections that are resistant to standard antibiotics	Vancomycin, teicoplanin
Ketolides		Telithromycin (Ketek)
Oxazolidinone	Effective against MRSA	Linezolid (Zyvox)
Streptogramins		Quinupristin/dalfopristin (Synercid)

Source: "What Antibiotics Are Used for Pneumonia?" *Well-Connected Reports.* http://content.health.msn.com/printing/article/1680.52940 (2001).

present with shock should be evaluated for other preexisting conditions and treated accordingly. It is important to try to differentiate other causes of the presenting symptoms including congestive heart failure, myocardial infarction, chronic bronchitis, drug hypersensitivity reactions, pulmonary embolism, cancer, or asthma.

TUBERCULOSIS

Tuberculosis (TB) is a major disease that occurs worldwide and is caused primarily by pulmonary infection with the bacillus *Mycobacterium tuberculosis.* Occasionally *M. africanum* and *M. bovis* have been identified as the causative agent. The World Health Organization estimates that 8.7 million people are infected worldwide. The disease is readily transmitted and exposure often results in infection but not necessarily active disease. Of persons infected with *M. tuberculosis* 90% to 95% will not develop symptoms or active disease during the initial infection. Instead the disease will enter a latent period during which it lies dormant, but may reactivate at any time, often when the patient is stressed or becomes immune suppressed. The other 5% to 10% of infected persons and nearly 50% of persons also infected with HIV will develop active disease shortly after infection. The disease most frequently develops as a pulmonary infection but extrapulmonary infection of lymph nodes, kidneys, pericardium, meninges, bones, joints, skin, GI tract, or eyes may occur.

Symptoms of pulmonary tuberculosis include fever, chills, cough (especially a productive cough), chest pain, hemoptysis, night sweats, loss of appetite, weight loss, and fatigue. Extrapulmonary tuberculosis symptoms are related to the organs or systems infected, such as back pain with spinal TB or bloody urine with TB of the kidney. TB is primarily transmitted through the airborne route with inhalation of droplet nuclei or dust particles carrying the infecting agent. Persons with active, infectious pulmonary or laryngeal TB expel the tubercle bacilli in droplet nuclei during coughing, speaking, singing, or sneezing. Unless there is a draining lesion, extrapulmonary TB (except laryngeal TB) is rarely communicable. TB has developed after exposure to cattle infected with TB or consuming milk or meat from infected cattle.

tuberculosis (TB) a potentially deadly pulmonary disease caused primarily by infection with the bacillus Mycobacterium tuberculosis.

Exposure may or may not result in infection and not all infections will result in active disease. After an exposure, a determination of infection can usually be determined by administering a skin test with intermediate-strength tuberculin. The determination of a positive or negative skin test is dependent on several conditions. Most persons who have competent immune systems would be considered infected and with a positive skin test if the area of induration was equal to or greater than 10 mm difference over 2 years. Very young patients, the elderly, and immune-compromised individuals might be considered TB skin test positive with an induration of only 5 mm, and persons at very low risk for TB infection may not be considered TB positive until the area of induration is 15 mm. Anergy testing and two-step testing may be indicated in certain situations. Only persons specifically trained in the Mantoux skin test should administer or read the test. Under no circumstances should a person self-read a skin test. Determination of active disease and infectiousness requires additional evaluation and diagnostic testing including chest X-rays, physical assessment, skin test results, history, and sputum (or other site) cultures.

Treatment of latent TB is recommended for those who have positive skin test results (>5 mm) and are HIV positive, who have a history of recent contacts with a TB case, who have fibrotic changes on X-ray consistent with old TB, and who are immunosuppressed or who have received organ transplants. In addition, other candidates for treatment for latent TB include persons with skin test results >10 mm and who are recent arrivals from countries with high rates of TB; IV drug users; persons with clinical conditions that make them high risk (HIV infection); residents or employees of high-risk settings including correctional facilities, health care settings, hospitals, nursing homes, or homeless shelters; young children; and persons who work in mycobacterial laboratories. Treatment usually involves a 2- to 9-month course of antimicrobials including isoniazid, rifampin, and rifampin and pyrazinamide given singularly or in combination.

Active TB (infectious) is usually treated for a period of 6–9 months depending on the drugs used, drug susceptibility tests, and the patient's response to therapy. The drugs should preferably be given once daily and include isoniazid and rifampin, plus pyrazinamide, ethambutol, or streptomycin. An initial course of a four-drug regimen is recommended in areas where multidrug resistance is prevalent.

Patients suspected or known to be infected with active, infectious tuberculosis should be cared for using Standard Precautions and Airborne Precautions. Health care professionals caring for these patients should wear NIOSH-approved particulate respirators (PR) with at least a 95% filtering efficiency (N95). All persons wearing particulate respirators should be appropriately trained and evaluated in compliance with the organization's respiratory protection plan before wearing any PR. HCWs who become infected and develop active TB should remain off work until they have initiated effective antimicrobial therapy as evidenced by three consecutive negative sputum tests taken at least 24 hours apart.

Tuberculosis infections in the United States were common until the late 1940s when effective antimicrobial therapy became available. It was hoped that aggressive treatment of infected persons and the use of effective isolation precautions would eliminate the disease from the United States. From 1953 to 1984 tuberculosis cases were on the decline. However, from 1985 through 1992, TB cases increased 20%. Since 1993 the incidence of newly diagnosed TB cases has again been on a downward trend. Increased surveillance, effective therapy, and adherence to respiratory precautions have promoted this turnaround and it is important that health care professionals stay alert and on guard to prevent another reoccurrence of this serious disease and to promote its eradication.

SEVERE ACUTE RESPIRATORY SYNDROME (SARS)

severe acute respiratory syndrome (SARS) *a potentially deadly coronavirus spread by close personal exposure or person-to-contaminated surface contact, via droplet method.*

Severe acute respiratory syndrome (SARS) is a viral respiratory illness that first appeared in southern China in November 2002. It became a global threat in March 2003 by spreading internationally via Hong Kong. Ultimately, 8,098 people worldwide were affected with SARS. Of these, 774 died. SARS entered Canada and several other countries and spread rapidly. Toronto, Ontario, was particularly affected. In fact, SARS placed a significant stress on the Toronto EMS system. During this event, four paramedics reportedly contracted SARS before mandatory personal protective equipment (PPE) measures were undertaken. SARS appears to be an ongoing threat because of the highly infectious nature of the illness.

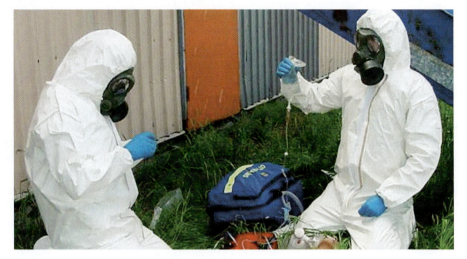

The virus that causes SARS was previously unrecognized and is called SARS-associated coronavirus (SARS-CoV). Coronaviruses play a major role in upper respiratory infections and the common cold. Preliminary studies indicated that the SARS-CoV may survive in the environment for several days. Other infectious agents may play a role in SARS as well. SARS is spread by close person-to-person contact. SARS-CoV is transmitted by respiratory droplets that are produced when an infected person coughs or sneezes. Disease transmission occurs when these droplets are deposited on the mucous membranes of the mouth, nose, and eyes of persons who are nearby. SARS-CoV can also be spread by touching a surface or objects contaminated by infectious droplets.

The incubation period (the time from exposure until the onset of symptoms) is generally 2–7 days although some cases have been as long as 10–14 days. People with SARS are considered to be contagious as long as they have symptoms. Furthermore, there have been no reported cases of disease transmission before the source patient develops symptoms. People with documented SARS should be quarantined to their home for at least 10 days after the fever has abated and symptoms cleared.

If a SARS outbreak has been identified, all personnel should use appropriate PPE on every call or as directed by local health authorities. If, in a non-SARS epidemic area, a case is encountered that has SARS-like symptoms, all involved should immediately don appropriate PPE (see Figures 26-1 ■ and 26-2 ■).

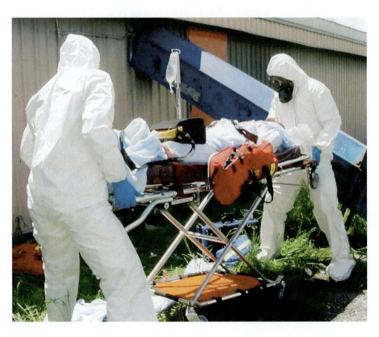

As with any respiratory illness, first address signs of severe respiratory distress. Look for altered mental status, 1–2 word speech dyspnea, cough, cyanosis, and hypoxia as documented by pulse oximetry. Patients with underlying respiratory disease (asthma, emphysema, chronic bronchitis) and those with chronic illnesses are at increased risk of SARS-related problems.

Signs and symptoms that have been associated with SARS include sore throat, rhinorrhea (runny nose), chills, rigors, myalgias (muscle aches), headache, and diarrhea. This can progress to cough, sputum production, respiratory distress, and, eventually, respiratory failure.

From a management standpoint, any patient suspected of SARS should be treated like any patient with suspected pneumonia or respiratory illness. Place the patient in a comfortable position and administer high-flow oxygen. Use pulse oximetry to assess the patient's oxygenation requirements. In severe cases, ventilatory assistance may be needed and endotracheal intubation may be required. Establish intravenous access and base fluid administration on the patient's hydration status. If the patient is wheezing, consider the administration of a nebulized bronchodilator. If SARS is suspected, notify the receiving hospital of your suspicions so that they can take appropriate measures for isolation of the patient and protection of other health care workers.

MENINGITIS

Viral, bacterial, fungal, and parasitic infections, intrathecal agents, foreign bodies, drugs or diseases such as leukemia and lupus may cause **meningitis,** which is a potentially life-threatening inflammation of the meningeal layers. Symptoms include fever, headache, stiff neck, photophobia, nausea and vomiting, and mental status changes including irritability, hallucinations, drowsiness, opisthotonos, positive Babinski reflex, and in infants a bulging fontanel. Diagnostic tests may include white blood count, C-reactive protein, throat cultures, lumbar puncture with culture of cerebrospinal fluid (CSF), CT scan, MRI, India ink stain, and rapid antigen panels.

Care of patients with viral meningitis is usually supportive in nature. Antibiotics are not usually indicated except in bacterial forms. The disease is usually self-limiting and full recovery is common. All patients with the diagnosis of meningitis regardless of cause should be provided with a quiet, darkened environment, with minimal movement to reduce the discomfort associated with meningeal irritation. Analgesics may be indicated.

Patients with bacterial meningitis may deteriorate rapidly and antibiotic therapy is often initiated before all tests are completed. If there are no contraindications for a spinal tap, one is performed and if the fluid is cloudy, treatment is started immediately. Patients should be monitored closely for neurologic signs and symptoms of increasing intracranial pressure. Blood gases should be monitored. Oxygen may be indicated. Intravenous therapy is usually initiated to provide fluid and electrolytes in severely ill patients and as a route for drugs including antibiotics, treatment for cerebral edema and seizure control, and drugs to support circulation.

Antibiotic therapy for bacterial meningitis varies depending on the causative agent, pathogen sensitivity, and patient tolerance and may include penicillins, cephalosporins, aminoglycosides, or glycopeptide. Patients receiving antibiotics should be monitored closely for sensitivity reactions and other untoward or side effects. Many antibiotics interact with other drugs and caregivers should be alert to the possibility and be aware of other drugs the patient may be taking and to observe for signs and symptoms of an incompatibility or synergistic effect.

While bacterial meningitis can be a life-threatening event, immediate treatment with appropriate antibiotics reduces the morbidity and mortality dramatically. Bacterial infections are associated with more complications than viral causes, but are often very responsive to therapy once diagnosed and treated promptly.

MENINGOCOCCAL INFECTIONS

Meningococcal infections are caused by a gram-negative diplococcus called *Neisseria meningitidis* and are responsible for several serious bacterial infections including meningococcal meningitis and meningococcemia. Symptoms of meningococcal infections include sudden onset of fever after several days of URI symptoms, severe headache, photophobia, stiff neck, nausea and vomiting, irri-

From a management standpoint, any patient suspected of SARS should be treated like any patient with suspected pneumonia or respiratory illness.

meningitis *potentially life-threatening inflammation of the meningeal layers; can be either bacterial or viral.*

meningococcal infections *caused by a gram-negative diplococcus bacteria called* Neisseria meningitidis; *responsible for several serious infections including meningococcal meningitis and meningococcemia.*

tability, altered level of consciousness, coma, and the development of a petechial skin rash that may progress to extensive ecchymosis.

The reservoir for meningococcal organisms is the nasopharynx of man and they are spread by droplet transmission. Exposed persons may become carriers of meningococcus and never develop clinical disease. Those who do become infected and develop disease may develop mild infection or a disease that rapidly develops into a life-threatening condition. Case fatality rates for meningococcal infections is about 10%, but can be 50% or higher for fulminant menigiococcemia. However, early recognition and treatment is usually very effective.

Treatment for meningococcal infections includes the prompt initiation of antibiotic therapy with penicillin G, ceftriaxone, chloramphenicol, or cefuroxime. Patients are considered noninfectious after 24 hours with effective antibiotic therapy. Additional therapy may include vasopressors, such as dopamine, to support circulation and drugs to treat developing disseminated intravascular coagulation (DIC). Additional supportive care includes providing patients with a quiet, darkened environment with little movement or other stimulation to reduce the discomfort associated with meningeal symptoms; intravenous fluids to maintain fluid and electrolyte balance, and as a route for administration of drugs until patient is able to tolerate oral fluids; and antiseizure medications. Analgesics may also be indicated. Patients should receive Standard Precautions and Droplet Precautions until at least 24 hours after initiation of effective therapy.

THE CHILDHOOD DISEASES

Measles, mumps, rubella, and chickenpox were once common diseases of childhood. With the development of effective vaccines, the incidents of these diseases have dropped dramatically since 1957 (including chickenpox). Occasional outbreaks continue to occur in young adults who live together in dormitory-like settings such as seen in universities. This is usually due to the ease of transmission of these diseases when persons live in proximity and are vulnerable to droplet spread diseases. Susceptible individuals may acquire the disease and then spread it to other susceptible persons before they realize they are infected, that is, before symptoms develop. The age group at risk is those persons who either were not immunized as children or did not receive adequate immunization when they were young and are now susceptible to these diseases.

The CDC recommends all children be immunized against these highly infectious diseases. In addition, the CDC further recommends that health care workers without documentation of immunity from acquired disease, serological evidence, or effective vaccination should be immunized per guidelines published in CDC publication *Morbidity and Mortality Weekly Report (MMWR)*.

(**Measles rubeola,** hard measles, red measles) is a highly contagious viral infection characterized by prodromal symptoms of cough, fever, conjunctivitis, coryza, malaise, and anorexia. An erythematous, maculopapular rash appears between the 3rd and 7th day after symptoms appear and lasts for 4 to 7 more days. Koplik spots can be seen on the buccal mucosa just prior to the rash developing. The incubation period may be 5–21 days after exposure. It is contagious from approximately 3 days before appearance of the rash until 7 days afterward. Measles is spread through droplet contact, direct contact with nasal and throat secretions, and indirect contact with items recently contaminated by secretions from the nose and throat of infected persons. The disease is self-limiting and treatment is supportive in nature. Vaccine or immune globulin may be indicated for exposed susceptible persons. Complications of measles include superinfections, pneumonia, and dehydration.

The **mumps** virus causes an acute infection with symptoms of fever, swelling, and tenderness of one or both parotid glands and sometimes the other salivary glands. Occasionally males will develop orchitis, and even more rarely, women may develop oophoritis secondary to the virus migrating down the oophoritis. Sterility rarely occurs. Some cases of mumps go undetected. Mumps is transmitted by droplet spread and direct contact with saliva of infected persons. The disease is self-limiting and treatment is supportive. The incubation period is 12–25 days, and susceptible persons who have been exposed should be considered infectious from the 12th to the 25th day after exposure. CDC recommends all health care workers be immunized against mumps.

Rubella (German measles, three-day measles) is a highly infectious viral disease that presents with mild fever and a diffuse maculopapular rash that resembles measles. While children usually

measles rubeola *a highly contagious viral infection characterized by prodromal symptoms of cough, fever, conjunctivitis, coryza, malaise, and anorexia. (sometimes called hard measles and/or red measles)*

mumps *a virus that causes an acute infection of one or both parotid glands (sometimes involves salivary glands), characterized by fever and swollen, tender glands.*

rubella *a highly contagious viral infection characterized by mild fever and a diffuse maculopapular rash. (sometimes called German or 3-day measles)*

have no other clinical symptoms, adults may develop low-grade fever, headache, and URI symptoms. Rubella is an important disease because it can cause numerous anomalies in developing fetuses. Rubella is transmitted by droplet spread or direct contact with infected persons. Exposed susceptible individuals should be considered infectious from the 5th through the 21st day after exposure or until 5 days after development of rash.

(**Chickenpox varicella,** herpes zoster, shingles) is a highly infectious disease caused by the human herpesvirus. The disease presents with rapidly developing mild symptoms including slight fever, some general symptoms, and a maculopapular rash that becomes vesicular and eventually pustular. The lesions are itchy and when scratched may become infected or cause additional scarring. Eventually the lesions will dry up and fall off. Lesions in various stages will appear during the course of the illness with more present on covered rather than exposed body areas. The patient is considered infectious from the 10th through the 21st day after exposure or until all lesions are dry. This disease is one of the most communicable of all infectious diseases and may be transmitted through direct or indirect contact with patient or items contaminated with secretions from the mouth, nose, or lesions, or by droplet contact or airborne. Treatment is supportive and a vaccine is available.

chickenpox varicella *a rapidly developing, highly infectious disease caused by the human herpesvirus. Presents with slight fever, general malaise, and maculopapular rash that becomes vesicular, then pustular, before crusting over (sometimes called chickenpox, herpes zoster or shingles depending upon the location on/in the body)*

GASTROENTERITIS (BACTERIAL)

gastroenteritis *an inflammation and infection within the GI tract.*

Gastroenteritis is an inflammation and infection within the GI tract. Agents responsible for gastroenteritis include Norwalk virus, rotovirus, hepatitis A, *Salmonella, Shigella, Staphylococcus, Campylobacter jejuni, Clostridium* (botulism), *Escherichia coli,* listeriosis, toxoplasmosis, *Vibrio, Yersinia* and others. The mode of transmission is through ingestion of foods contaminated with the one of the listed pathogens. The CDC estimates that food-borne diseases cause approximately 76 million illnesses and 5,200 deaths annually in the United States.

Symptoms of gastroenteritis include diarrhea, which may be watery or less commonly bloody, nausea and vomiting, abdominal pain, headache, fever, myalgia, and loss of appetite. Vital signs will vary with the degree of dehydration or discomfort and other effects of the infection. Children and the elderly are at special risk from the effects of gastroenteritis and should be observed closely for worsening condition.

Treatment includes ensuring adequate hydration with oral fluids or, if not tolerated or increasing symptoms, the administration of intravenous fluids and electrolytes to replace those lost with the diarrhea and vomiting; antibiotics as appropriate for the infecting pathogen and antiemetics may be indicated. While most patients will do well with supportive treatment, severe complications may occur especially in the very young, very old, and immunocompromised persons. Complications include hypotension and shock, kidney failure, necrotizing enteritis, and DIC. Close observation for signs and symptoms of these complications and early intervention may be lifesaving.

TETANUS

tetanus *infectious process resulting from exposure to exotoxins produced by the gram-negative, spore-forming, anaerobic bacilli,* Clostridium tetani.

Tetanus is caused by the exotoxins produced by the gram-negative, spore-forming, anaerobic bacilli, *Clostridium tetani.* The bacillus is a harmless, normal inhabitant of the intestines of mammals, including horses and humans. Tetanus bacilli reside in soil contaminated with feces. The organism will form a spore and is especially hardy to hostile environments. Tetanus becomes infectious when it is transmitted to the body through open wounds (often deep, puncture wounds) that are contaminated with soil, dust, or feces.

Tetanus manifests with uncontrolled muscular contractions that are extremely painful. The contractions usually involve the muscles of the neck first and then progress to the trunk region of the body. Abdominal rigidity is a common early symptom. Patients often assume an opisthotonic position as they develop spasmodic contractions triggered by sensory stimulation. Evidence of a puncture or infected wound may or may not be present.

Any wound, even trivial wounds, may become infected with the tetanus bacilli. To prevent infection with tetanus, persons should maintain their immunity by receiving tetanus toxoid (DPT, Td) vaccine on the CDC recommended schedule. In the event of an injury, careful assessment of the patient's immunity status, as well as the nature of the injury and whether the wound is contaminated or not, must be done. Based on that assessment, recommendations for tetanus toxoids or antitoxin therapy may be given.

All wounds should be thoroughly cleaned, removing all debris or foreign objects, and antibiotic therapy administered as appropriate. Patients who have received tetanus toxoids within the last 10 years and whose wounds are minor and not contaminated will not usually require a tetanus booster. If the wound is deep or contaminated, tetanus toxoid should be given if a booster has not been given in the last 5 years. For persons who have not completed their primary immunization schedule, a dose of tetanus toxoid should be give as soon as possible and consideration for administering human tetanus immune globulin (TIG) considered. Patients whose tetanus immune status is unknown or who have never received at least three doses of tetanus toxoids should be treated with TIG or tetanus antitoxin (animal origin).

Patients who develop tetanus will require hospitalization and intensive care where monitoring and support of cardiorespiratory functions can be given. As the disease progresses, respiratory muscle contractions will lead to respiratory failure. Attempts to ventilate the patient are difficult, due to the rigidity of the muscles. Patients usually require sedation and oftentimes neuromuscular blockade to permit intubation and mechanical ventilation with a respirator. Of special note, these patients may remain on neuromuscular blocking agents for extended periods of time and may be conscious with intact sensory nerves. Careful attention to the airway, eyes, skin, body positioning, vital signs, and the patient's environment are important care issues, because the patient will not be able to indicate when he is feeling pain and will not be able to move voluntarily including blinking eyelids, coughing, or swallowing, and will not be able to protect himself.

Patients who develop tetanus will require hospitalization and intensive care where monitoring and support of cardiorespiratory functions can be given.

SEPTICEMIA AND TOXIC SHOCK SYNDROME

Septicemia is a symptomatic condition in which bacteria are actively multiplying in the bloodstream, causing an overwhelming infection. Identifying the site of infection is important for adequate treatment to be initiated. Various organ systems may be involved and organ failure can lead to a variety of symptoms. An elevated temperature (>102 °F) is often seen with septicemia but low body temperature may be observed. Signs and symptoms of hypoperfusion may be present, impaired mental function, and pain with various organ involvement or at the site of the primary infection.

septicemia *a potentially lethal condition in which bacteria are spread from an infected part of the body via the bloodstream causing an overwhelming infection.*

Septicemia may be caused by the introduction of pathogens into the body via intravenous catheters or other devices; during surgical or diagnostic procedures; by perforations or rupture of intra-abdominal or pelvic organs or structures (appendix, ovaries, bladder); bladder or other urinary tract infections; by infections of the pancreas, gallbladder, prostate gland; or from abscesses, meningococcal infections, wound infections, and many other conditions.

Treatment is directed at identifying the source and cause of the infection and initiating effective antimicrobial therapy. When abscesses or infected tissue or organs are involved, drainage or surgical removal of the infected site may be required. Patients will require care aimed at supporting the various organs or body systems involved in the infectious process and sustaining overall hemodynamics. Specific attention is given to supporting the cardiorespiratory systems. Empiric broad spectrum antibiotics are used initially until the causative agent is identified. Then, antibiotics specific for the pathogen are used.

Toxic shock syndrome (TSS) results from an infection with a toxin-producing pathogen that overwhelms the body causing multisystem failure. Toxins produced from staphylococci and streptococci are responsible for most cases of TSS. The first reported cases of TSS were associated with the use of tampons during menstruation and the presence of staphylococci in the vagina.

toxic shock syndrome (TSS) *potentially lethal systemic infection resulting from toxins produced by Staphylococcus aureas.*

Symptoms of TSS caused by staphylococci include fever, erythroderma, chills, diarrhea, myalgia, headache, malaise, sore throat, fatigue, vomiting, reddened conjunctiva, decreased level of consciousness, abdominal pain, and/or vaginal discharge. Symptoms of TSS caused by streptococci may include "flu-like" symptoms, fever, chills, vomiting, and diarrhea. Patients may develop renal failure, respiratory failure, or coagulopathies as complications of TSS.

Staphylococcal TSS is diagnosed when the following are determined: temperature >38.9 °C, systolic BP < 90 mmHg, presence of a rash with desquamation, involvement of three or more organ systems (GI, muscular, mucous membranes, renal, hepatic, hematologic, or CNS), and a negative serology test for Rocky Mountain spotted fever, leptospirosis, and measles.

Streptococcal TSS is diagnosed when the following findings are present: isolation of group A streptococci from blood, spinal fluid, pleural fluid, peritoneal fluid, tissue biopsy, throat, vagina, sputum or skin lesions; hypotension; and involvement of two or more of the following—renal impairment, coagulopathy, liver abnormalities, acute respiratory distress syndrome, soft tissue necrosis, or generalized erythematous macular rash.

Treatment of TSS includes aggressive fluid therapy including the use of albumin or vasopressors, removal of potential sources (tampon, wound packing), use of intravenous immunoglobulin, surgical debridement of necrotic tissue, appropriate antibiotic treatment (clindamycin, vancomycin, and penicillin alone or in combinations), intensive care support that may require renal dialysis, ventilatory support, and correction of coagulopathy.

NECROTIZING FASCIITIS

necrotizing fasciitis (NF)
an insidious soft tissue infection characterized by widespread fascial necrosis.

Necrotizing fasciitis (NF) is an insidious soft-tissue infection characterized by widespread fascial necrosis. Etiologically it has been found that numerous bacteria in isolation or as a polymicrobial infection can cause NF. Although group A beta-hemolytic streptococci is often linked with NF, *Haemophilus aphrophilus* and *Staphylococcus aureus* have also been identified as causative agents.

Organisms that cause NF migrate from subcutaneous tissue along the superficial and deep fascial planes. The progressing infection causes vascular occlusion, ischemia, and eventual tissue necrosis. During this process superficial nerves are damaged, which produces characteristic localized anesthesia. With the worsening of the infection, septicemia can occur with resultant systemic toxicity. NF is seen most commonly in young people who were previously healthy, and carries with it a mortality rate as high as 25%. In cases of NF with sepsis and renal failure, the mortality rate climbs to 70%.

NF tends to begin with fever and chills. After 2–3 days, erythema is noted to the skin and supralesional vesiculation or bullae formation ensues. From the rapidly advancing erythema, painless ulcers appear as the infection spreads along the fascial planes. The borders of the affected area may be identified by black necrotic tissue. As the condition worsens, the patient can display blistering necrosis, cyanosis, elevated core temperature, tachycardia, hypotension, and altered consciousness. As mentioned previously, septicemia is typical and leads to severe systemic toxicity and rapid death unless appropriately treated.

On diagnosis, the treatment must begin immediately for optimal outcomes. The patient is often moved to a surgical intensive care unit where management proceeds with the administration of antibiotics, hyperbaric oxygen (HBO), intravenous immunoglobulin, and surgical debridement of the site. It is for this reason that the critical care paramedic may encounter the patient with NF. The patient may be transported to a health care facility that is more experienced with this diagnosis or that has the ability to administer HBO.

ANTIBIOTIC-RESISTANT ORGANISMS AND MULTIDRUG-RESISTANT ORGANISMS

antibiotic-resistant organisms (AROs) *multidrug resistant pathogenic microorganisms, including methicillin-resistant* Staphylococcus aureus *and vancomycin-resistant enterococcus (VRE).*

Several antibiotic-resistant strains of pathogenic microorganisms have developed during the past several years including methicillin-resistant *Staphylococcus aureus* (MRSA) and vancomycin-resistant enterococcus (VRE). Infection or colonization with AROs has become a challenge both for the patient whose treatment is dependent on eradication of an infectious pathogen and for the health care institutions that must manage these patients within their organization. Many health care professionals are uninformed or misinformed about AROs and believe these organisms to be more virulent. **Antibiotic-resistant organisms (AROs)** are of special concern because they are multidrug resistant and therefore have limited treatment options. Patients who are colonized or infected with an ARO will often be managed with Standard Precautions and Contact Precautions.

All health care organizations should have an infection control plan with policies and procedures in place for managing persons colonized or infected with AROs including patients and employees. Infection control plans may include any or all of the following elements.

Infection or colonization with AROs has become a challenge both for the patient whose treatment is dependent on eradication of an infectious pathogen and for the health care institutions that must manage these patients within their organization.

- ★ Identifications of AROs
  - – Colonization and infection
  - – Reservoirs
  - – Transmission
  - – Risk factors
  - – Procedures for obtaining cultures for identifying AROs
- ★ Decolonization
  - – Infection control measures
    - ▪ Standard Precautions
    - ▪ Contact Precautions
    - ▪ Termination of precautions
- ★ Communication
- ★ Surveillance
- ★ Training and education
- ★ Employee health

INFECTIOUS AGENTS AND BIOTERRORISM

September 11, 2001, saw the worst terrorist attacks in U.S. history. In little more than an hour four commercial airlines had been hijacked. Three of those aircraft were deliberately flown into targeted buildings including the twin towers of the World Trade Center in New York City and the Pentagon in Washington, D.C. The fourth airline was prevented from reaching its target when passengers attacked the hijackers and the airliner crashed into the woods in Pennsylvania. Close to 4,000 lives were lost in total including 3,000 in the collapse of the Twin Towers.

Acts of terrorism are not new and occurred long before the French Revolution (1789–1799) when the term was first phrased (Reign of Terror). The Federal Bureau of Investigation (FBI) defines terrorism as "The unlawful use of force or violence against persons or property to intimidate or coerce a government, the civilian population, or any segment thereof in furtherance of political or social objectives."

History provides us with many examples of terrorism. Adolf Hitler, Benito Mussolini, Joseph Stalin, and Saddam Hussein each used terrorism to control their subjects and maintain their hold over their respective governments. The citizens of Northern Ireland have for decades lived in fear of both Roman Catholic and Protestant extremists who use terrorism in either opposition to or support of British rule. A Jewish group conducted a campaign of terror until Israel was established, and today Palestinian groups including Hamas and Hezbollah engage in terrorist tactics in an attempt to reestablish a Palestinian homeland and in opposition to U.S. involvement in Middle Eastern affairs.

The United States has seen terrorism firsthand both domestically and internationally including the Ku Klux Klan, which used terrorism against African Americans; the 1995 bombing of the Murrah Federal Building in Oklahoma City, Oklahoma, by two Americans that killed 168 and wounded more than 500 others; the 1983 bombing of the barracks in Beirut, Lebanon, that killed 241 U.S. Marines and the 1984 bombing of the U.S. Embassy annex in Beirut that killed 16 persons; the 1988 bombing of Pan Am 103 over Lockerbie, Scotland, that killed 270; the 1993 bombing of the World Trade Center that killed six people and injured more than 1,000; the 1996 bombing of the U.S. barracks in Dhahran, Saudi Arabia, that killed 19 Americans and injured 500 people; the 1998 twin bombings at the U.S. embassies in Nairobi, Kenya, and Dares Salaam, Tanzania, that killed 224 people and wounded thousands; and the 2000 bombing of the USS *Cole* in Yemen's Aden Harbor that killed 17 sailors and wounded 39 others; and the most recent and worst terrorist act in U.S. history, the September 11, 2001, hijacking of four planes.

Bioterrorism is the use of biological agents and/or their toxins as weapons of intimidation or mass destruction. These weapons are intended to injure or kill people, animals, or crops. The use of biological agents as a weapon of war is not a new strategy, but dates back to at least the 14th century when the corpses of bubonic plague victims were thrown into the enemy's cities. The British exposed Native Americans to the blankets of smallpox victims during the French and Indian wars.

During the past century, many countries including the United States developed and stockpiled various biological agents for use as both offensive and defensive weapons. In 1969, then President Richard Nixon pledged the United States would never use biological weapons against an enemy even if that enemy used biological weapons first, and he ordered the destruction of all biological agent stockpiles.

In 1972, an international treaty was drafted that has been signed by more than 120 nations banning the development or use of biological agents in war. And while most nations honor this treaty, some nations continue to manufacture and stockpile offensive biological agents. These agents may become weapons of terrorists. All health care professionals must be aware of this very real hazard and be prepared to recognize the signs of and take appropriate actions in the event of a potential biological threat.

Shortly after September 11, 2001, the United States faced another terrorist attack on its citizens but this time a biological weapon was used, anthrax. Several letters laden with anthrax spores were mailed to various governmental offices and media companies. While the exact numbers of infected persons is not known at this time, at least 22 people became ill with cutaneous or inhalation anthrax including a 10-month-old baby and at least six persons died of inhalation anthrax.

The CDC, in their bioterrorism guidance materials for health care providers and public health officials, have identified the following biological agents as having the most concern from a public health standpoint:

★ *Bacillus anthracis* (anthrax)

★ *Yersinia pestis* (plague)

★ Variola major (smallpox)

★ *Clostridium botulinum* toxin (botulism)

★ *Francisella tularensis* (tularemia)

★ Filovirus (Ebola hemorrhagic fever, Marburg hemorrhagic fever)

★ Arenaviruses (Lassa fever), Junin (Argentine hemorrhagic fever), and related viruses

The National Emergency Response and Rescue Training Center includes the following biological agents (in addition to those listed with the CDC guidance) in their training programs: *Vibrio cholerae* (cholera), *Coxiella burnetii* (Q fever), Venezuelan equine encephalitis, ricin, saxitoxin, staphylococcal enterotoxin B, brucellosis, *Burkholderia mallei* (glanders), *Burkholderia pseudomallei* (melioidosis), *Salmonella typhi* (typhoid fever), *Rickettsia typhi* (typhus), Chikungunya virus, Congo-Crimean hemorrhagic fever virus, dengue fever, Rift Valley fever virus, and yellow fever.

ANTHRAX

anthrax *an acute bacterial infection caused by* Bacillus anthracis, *a gram-positive, encapsulated, spore-forming rod.*

Anthrax is an acute bacterial infection caused by *Bacillus anthracis,* a gram-positive, encapsulated, spore-forming rod. Herbivores are the usual reservoir of anthrax, however, humans and other carnivorous animals may become infected. The bacilli are shed from the host animal usually at death or when bleeding. On exposure to air, they will form spores that are very resistant to environmental conditions including disinfectants. Anthrax spores can survive in the soil for years. The hides and skin of infected animals, where spores survive, remain an important source of transmission of anthrax worldwide.

Cutaneous anthrax is transmitted from contact with the tissues, skin, hide, wool, or hair of infected animals, contact with contaminated soil or bone meal, and possibly by biting flies that fed on infected animals. Animals may become infected from contaminated soil or feed. Ingesting contaminated meat may transmit anthrax; however, there are no reported cases of transmission from milk. Inhalation anthrax occurs when spores are inhaled, and is usually associated with working in tanneries or wool or bone processing industries. There have been no reported cases of transmission of anthrax from person to person.

Symptoms of cutaneous anthrax include initial itching of exposed skin, followed by the development of one or more lesions that progress from papular to vesicular to the formation of a black eschar. The skin around the lesion(s) is usually red and swollen and additional vesicles may form. Untreated, the infection may spread to the lymph and bloodstream causing a severe septicemia. Occasionally meningeal symptoms will develop. Fatalities may occur 5% to 20% of the time in untreated cutaneous anthrax, but when treated, fatalities are rare.

Inhalation anthrax often presents with mild flu or URI symptoms. Within a few days, symptoms of severe respiratory distress, cyanosis, fever, and shock develop. X-rays will often demonstrate a widening mediastinum. Death usually occurs shortly thereafter. Early recognition and treatment of inhalation anthrax can be very effective; however, anthrax is rarely included in the differential diagnosis unless there is a high index of suspicion.

Intestinal anthrax is very rare. Symptoms of abdominal distress resemble those of food poisoning and include abdominal pain, nausea and vomiting, diarrhea, loss of appetite, dehydration, and fever. Patients rapidly progress to septicemia and death. The CDC has recommended the use of Standard Precautions in managing patients with anthrax.

The incubation period for anthrax is a few hours to 7 days, with most cases presenting symptoms within 48 hours after exposure. Penicillin is the antibiotic of choice for anthrax and is given for 5–7 days. Other effective antibiotics include tetracyclines, erythromycin, or chloramphenicol. Postexposure prophylaxis for anthrax may include ciprofloxacin 500 mg po BID for 60 days or doxycycline 100 mg po BID for 60 days. A vaccine has been developed for anthrax and U.S. production levels have been increased, as well as efforts to develop additional vaccines that may prove more effective and with fewer side effects.

SMALLPOX

Smallpox is a viral disease caused by the variola virus. Smallpox was totally eradicated from the world in 1977 when the last naturally occurring case was diagnosed. The World Health Organization (WHO) certified global eradication 2 years later. Various countries have kept stocks of variola vaccine as a defense in the event a new outbreak of disease were to occur. Additionally, some countries have maintained stocks of variola virus in an effort to develop offensive or defensive biological weapons.

smallpox *a disease caused by the variola virus.*

Smallpox disease begins with an acute viral illness with symptoms that resemble the flu including fever, myalgia, headache, vomiting, and chills. A rash develops predominantly on the face and extremities, initially papular in appearance, progressing to vesicular (fluid filled) and eventually becoming pustular. Eventually the lesions become dry and scab over. As the scabs fall off, they leave a permanent pockmark (scar). The lesions of chickenpox look similar to smallpox but are more prominent on the trunk, and in various stages of development. Classical smallpox carried a 30% mortality, while variola minor has a case fatality rate closer to 5%.

The disease is transmitted through the airborne and contact routes, both direct contact with lesions, drainage, or scabs and indirect contact with materials contaminated with the lesions or mucous membrane of the patient. The incubation period is 12–14 days and patients are infectious from the period when symptoms are just beginning to develop until all lesions have dried and fallen off.

Treatment for smallpox patients is supportive in nature. Patients should be treated with Standard Precautions and Airborne and Contact Precautions. A vaccine is available; however, due to the disease being eradicated as a natural infection and the risk of complications from the vaccine while rare may be severe, the United States has not been routinely vaccinating persons since 1972. In the event an outbreak of smallpox were to occur, the United States has vaccine available, which may be given prior to exposure or within 3 days of exposure. Due to the risk of smallpox being used as a biological weapon, the United States is increasing production of vaccine to ensure adequate supplies are available.

PLAGUE

The bacillus *Yersinia pestis* causes **plague.** The disease is carried by fleas on rats and other rodents and is transmitted by fleas to man through a bite, contact with infected animal tissues, or airborne droplets from rodents or other infected animals or materials. Rodents (rats) are the primary reservoir for

plague *a viral disease caused by the bacillus,* Yersinia pestis.

plague. The pneumonic form of plague can be transmitted from person to person through airborne droplets. Bubonic plague is usually not transmitted from person to person, unless direct contact with infected fluid from the buboes (infected lymph nodes) occurs.

The incubation period for plague is 1–7 days with pneumonic plague having the shortest incubation period (1–3 days). Symptoms of plague include fever, chills, headache, malaise, myalgias, and swollen and painful lymph nodes. Primary septicemia plague will usually present additionally with gastrointestinal symptoms and signs and symptoms of shock and coma. Pneumonic plague progresses rapidly with signs and symptoms that include productive cough that becomes bloody and difficulty breathing that may lead to respiratory failure.

Untreated bubonic plague has a case fatality rate of 50% to 60%; untreated septicemia plague and pneumonic plague are almost always fatal. Early and appropriate treatment of bubonic plague reduces mortality dramatically. Septicemia plague and pneumonic plague may also respond to therapy, but case fatality rates are higher than with treated bubonic plague.

Treatment of plague victim includes supportive care and antibiotics (streptomycin, doxycycline, gentamycin, tetracyclines, and chloramphenicol). Postexposure prophylaxis for pneumonic plague includes doxycycline or ciprofloxacin. A vaccine is available to persons at high risk for exposure: three initial doses, three booster doses every 6 months and then boosters every 1–2 years for persons at continued risk of exposure. The vaccine does not appear to be effective against aerosolized plague bacilli.

BOTULISM

botulism *a spore-forming anaerobic bacillus caused by Clostridium botulinum.*

Food-borne, wound, and infant **botulism** is caused by *Clostridium botulinum,* a spore-forming anaerobic bacillus. The diseases and symptoms are caused by toxins (types A, B, E; rarely F and G).

Ingesting food in which toxins have formed causes food-borne botulism. Improper processing or canning of foodstuffs usually is responsible. Consumption of the following have been responsible for botulism cases: improperly home-canned vegetables and fruit, uneviscerated fish, and improperly prepared baked potatoes, pot pies, sautéed onions, garlic, smoked meats and salmon, eggs, and preserved meats.

The incubation period for botulism is between hours and days after ingesting the bacteria or the toxin. Usually the earlier the symptoms develop, the more severe the symptoms and the fatality rate. Symptoms include blurred or double vision, descending weakness or paralysis, dysphagia, dry mouth, vomiting, and constipation or diarrhea.

Wounds contaminated with soil or gravel or from improperly treated compound fractures can cause wound botulism. The symptoms are the same as for toxins that are ingested.

Infant botulism occurs when infants ingest botulism spores and the toxins develop in the GI tract. The condition develops in infants under 1 year of age and presents with symptoms of constipation, lethargy, poor feeding, difficulty swallowing, developing generalized weakness with difficulty holding the head up, drooping eyelids, and flaccid extremities and may progress to respiratory failure and arrest.

Treatment of botulism includes administration of antitoxin if diagnosed early (except infant botulism), supportive care especially respiratory support, debridement of wound if present, and administration of antibiotics.

TULAREMIA

tularemia *febrile syndrome caused by the bacterium,* Francisella tularensis *(formerly* Pasturella tularensis) *a gram-negative coccobacillus (also known as "Rabbit fever" and "deer-fly fever").*

Tularemia (rabbit fever, deer-fly fever) is caused by the bacteria *Francisella tularensis* (formerly *Pasturella tularensis*), a gram-negative coccobacillus. The disease is transmitted by the bite of infected ticks and deer-flies; by contact with mucous membrane or skin with contaminated blood, tissue, water; by eating contaminated meat or drinking contaminated water; or by the bites of animals that have recently eaten infected animals. Incubation period is 1–14 days. It is not usually transmitted from person to person, but that does not mean that it cannot spread easily. For example, an incident occurred where lawn care workers were exposed to tularemia from infected rabbits via the aerosolization of fecal matter and blood from revolving mower blades. This is only one example of how easily an infective aerosol can be created.

Symptoms of tularemia may include an ulcer at the entrance site of the infection, swollen and painful lymph nodes, painful pharyngitis, nausea and vomiting, abdominal pain, diarrhea, painful purulent conjunctivitis, and signs and symptoms of septicemia and pneumonia.

Inhalation tularemia is possible and is considered a likely method of dissemination as a biological weapon. Symptoms of inhalation of *F. tularensis* include febrile illness followed by later development of pleuropneumonitis.

Treatment for tularemia includes supportive measures and antibiotic therapy as with plague.

FILOVIRUSES

Ebola fever and Marburg fever are two serious often fatal viral hemorrhagic fevers due to **filoviruses.** These bloodborne pathogens are transmitted through direct contact with infected blood, secretions, organs, or semen. Standard Precautions and Contact Precautions are indicated with patients with known or suspected Ebola or Marburg fever.

Symptoms of Ebola and Marburg fever include sudden onset of fever, malaise, weakness, myalgias, headache, vomiting, diarrhea, maculopapular rash, and bleeding from gums and mucous membranes progressing to hemorrhaging. Patients rapidly develop shock, and mortality is as high as 70%. Ribavirin is available for treatment. Supportive care is required.

filoviruses *class of viruses, such as the Ebola and Marburg fevers, that cause systemic hemorrhage and are often fatal.*

ARENAVIRUSES

Lassa fever is another hemorrhagic fever or **arenavirus.** Transmission is similar to that of the filoviruses but also includes aerosol or direct contact with excreta of infected rodents and contact with pharyngeal secretions of infected persons. Symptoms are similar to Ebola and Marburg and treatment is the same. Ribavirin is available and should be administered within the first 6 days of illness. Standard, Airborne, and Contact Precautions are indicated. There have been few reported cases of Ebola fever, Marburg fever, or Lassa fever in the United States.

arenavirus *class of viruses, such as Lassa fever; another hemorrhagic fever with symptoms similar to Ebola and Marburg.*

HANTAVIRUS

Hantavirus was first recognized in the United States in 1993 when several cases of Hantavirus pneumonia were diagnosed in the Four Corners area of the Southwest. Since that time several dozen more cases have been identified in primarily the western United States and Canada. In each of these cases the infection manifested as a respiratory disease (Hantavirus pneumonia, Hantavirus adult respiratory distress syndrome). The disease presents with fever, GI symptoms, and myalgia and progresses rapidly to severe respiratory failure and cardiogenic shock. The mortality rate is approximately 50%.

Hantavirus pneumonia, like its counterpart Hantavirus-caused hemorrhagic fever with renal syndrome, is transmitted through the aerosolization of rodent excreta. The virus has been found in the urine, feces, and saliva of rodents.

Hantavirus pneumonia requires hospitalization and intensive care with very close monitoring of respiratory status. Respiratory and circulatory support are frequently required. Caution must be exercised with fluid resuscitation to avoid overloading and further impairing respiratory function. Standard Precautions are recommended.

hantavirus *group of viruses that cause potentially lethal respiratory syndromes in humans; transmitted by respiratory exposure to the aerosolized feces of infected mice.*

CHOLERA

Cholera is caused by the bacteria *Vibrio cholerae* which produces an enterotoxin resulting in explosive diarrhea. The disease is characterized by sudden onset of painless explosive diarrhea that may rapidly lead to dehydration and, if untreated, death. Cholera is transmitted by ingesting food or water contaminated with the feces or vomitus of infected persons or from water sources that are natural reservoirs for cholera. The organism is readily killed with heat (dry, steam, boiling) or chlorination.

Most U.S. cases are related to eating raw or undercooked seafood that has been contaminated with *V. cholerae*. There is presumed to be a natural reservoir of this organism in the estuaries and

cholera *debilitating syndrome attributed to enterotoxins produced by the bacteria* Vibrio cholerae; *transmitted through infected food or water.*

coastal waters off Louisiana and Texas. Contact Precautions are indicated when patients are incontinent or diapered; otherwise Standard Precautions are sufficient.

Treatment is aimed at the rapid replacement of the fluids and electrolytes lost with diarrhea. Oral administration is usually effective in mild to moderate cases; however, in more severe cases IV therapy is required. Tetracycline is usually an effective antibiotic; others include ciprofloxacin or erythromycin, trimethoprim or sulfamethoxazole depending on patient age and drug resistance. A vaccine is available that is given in two doses, 4 weeks apart, and then boosters every 6 months. Compliance and efficacy of this vaccine has caused the U.S. military to no longer give it to their personnel. Newer vaccines are being developed.

Q FEVER

Q fever *an acute illness caused by the rickettsia* Coxiella burnetii, *a spore-forming, gram-negative coccobacillus.*

Q fever is an acute illness caused by the rickettsia *Coxiella burnetii* a spore-forming, gram-negative coccobacillus. It is characterized by sudden onset of fever, chills, headache, malaise, weakness, dry cough, dyspnea, nausea and vomiting, abdominal pain, myalgia, and maculopapular rash. Fatalities are rare in treated cases and are usually related to the development of complications such as endocarditis.

Q fever is found worldwide in reservoirs including mammals, birds, and ticks. Transmission is usually airborne with exposure to infected animals, especially farm animals. Humans inhale dust and particles contaminated by animal by-products such as occurs with the processing of animals for food or hides. Direct contact with infected animals or products contaminated by infected animals or persons can also transmit the organism. Blood transfusions have also transmitted disease. The organism is considered a target for terrorists due to its hardy nature and ease of production. Only one organism need be inhaled to produce disease and at least mild symptoms.

Q fever is usually a self-limiting disease with 2% to 4% mortality. In addition to supportive treatment, antipyretics, antitussives, and expectorants, the organism is responsive to antibiotic therapy including tetracycline, doxycycline, chloramphenicol, rifampin, and ciprofloxacin. A new vaccine has been developed that appears to provide excellent protection against Q fever but may have serious side effects in immune individuals and is not yet readily available.

BRUCELLOSIS

brucellosis *debilitating illness caused by the gram-negative, rod-shaped, non-spore-forming bacilli,* Brucella (suis, melitensis, abortus).

Brucellosis is caused by a gram-negative rod-shaped non-spore-forming bacilli, *Brucella* (*suis, melitensis abortus*). Humans contract brucellosis after contact with infected animals including cattle, sheep, goats, swine, and occasionally with infected elk, deer, bison, and sometimes dogs and coyotes. Direct contact with blood, tissue, urine, or birth by-products or ingestion of raw milk has been a means of transmission of brucellosis. Airborne transmission has occurred in animal pens, laboratories, and abattoirs.

Symptoms may include fever that may be intermittent or variable, weakness, lethargy, diaphoresis, anorexia, weight loss, myalgias, depression, abdominal pain, arthralgia, and headache.

Antibiotic treatment may include combinations of the following drugs depending on age and response to therapy: rifampin, doxycycline, streptomycin, gentamycin, and trimethoprim-sulfamethaoxazole. Antibiotic therapy may continue for months and adherence to the treatment regime is essential to ensure eradication of the infecting agent.

TOXINS

RICIN

ricin *an extremely lethal cytotoxin derived from a component of the castor bean. It is transmitted by ingestion, injection or inhalation, and kills cells upon contact.*

The cytotoxin **ricin** is made from the mash left during the processing of castor oil from castor beans. Experience with ricin is limited with few cases of poisoning by this agent. The toxin inhibits cellular protein synthesis, which leads to cell death. It is theorized that it could be introduced into persons via ingestion, injection, or inhalation. In each case, the tissue or cells contacted by the toxin would be destroyed, leading to various organ failures and presumably death.

There is no specific treatment for ricin poisoning. No vaccine or antidote exists. Patients should receive supportive care including respiratory and circulatory support in the event of organ failure.

SAXITOXIN

Saxitoxin is a neurotoxin produced by marine dinoflagellates, blue-green algae, crabs, and blue-ringed octopus. It has been weaponized for years with the CIA holding a large supply. It was destroyed in 1970 under President Nixon's order although some of the toxin was sent to research facilities. Shellfish poisoning occurs worldwide and is a life-threatening condition. Symptoms include numbness and tingling of mouth, lips, and tongue, progressing to the neck and extremities, including the fingertips. Patients complain of lightheadedness, dizziness, visual disturbances, aphasia, and progressive neurologic symptoms. Death is usually secondary to respiratory paralysis. Treatment is aimed at trying to eliminate the agent by inducing vomiting and supportive care, especially respiratory support. Atropine is contraindicated in cases of saxitoxin poisoning and may increase fatalities.

saxitoxin *a neurotoxin produced by marine dinoflagellates, blue-green algae, crabs, and blue-ringed octopus; transmitted by ingestion, can cause respiratory paralysis.*

SEB

Staphylococcus enterotoxin (B) (SEB) is an agent responsible for food poisoning. Symptoms include nausea, vomiting, and diarrhea. If the agent were to be aerosolized and inhaled, the symptoms would be more severe and include cough, fever, chills, myalgia, and headache. No vaccine or antitoxin is available for SEB poisoning, and treatment is supportive. If patients become severely compromised, respiratory and circulatory support with intubation and mechanical ventilation and intravenous therapy are indicated.

staphylococcus enterotoxin (B) (SEB) *an agent responsible for food poisoning; transmitted by ingestion or inhalation, causes severe, debilitating syndromes.*

MYCOTOXINS

Trichothecene **mycotoxins** are produced by filamentous fungi. The toxin may be inhaled, ingested, or absorbed through the skin and mucous membranes. Absorbed toxin appears to be more effective than inhaled toxin. Symptoms begin with burning of the tissues contacted by the toxin, redness, pain, blistering, and eventually necrosis and sloughing of exposed tissue. With involvement of the respiratory tract, symptoms can include sneezing, itching and pain of the nares, rhinorrhea, epistaxis, bloody sputum, dyspnea, wheezing, and coughing. Ingested toxins can cause oral burning, bleeding, vomiting, bloody diarrhea, and bloody saliva. Neurologic symptoms include dizziness, weakness, and loss of coordination. Symptoms may progress to tachycardia and hypotension and death may occur.

mycotoxins *agents, Trichothecene mycotoxins, produced by filamentous fungae; may be inhaled, ingested, or absorbed through the skin and mucous membranes.*

No vaccine or antitoxin currently exists for mycotoxin exposures and treatment is supportive in nature. Patients should be monitored closely for progressive symptoms and appropriately treated.

INFORMATION SOURCES ON BIOLOGICAL/ CHEMICAL WEAPONS

The publication "Interim Recommendations for Firefighters and Other First Responders for the Selection and Use of Protective Clothing and Respirators against Biological Agents" provides guidance in managing incidents involving the use of aerosolized biological agents and includes the following recommendations:

1. "Responders should use NIOSH-approved, pressure-demand SCBA in conjunction with a Level A protective suit in responding to a suspected biological incident where any of the following information is unknown or the event is uncontrolled:

   —The type(s) of airborne agent(s);

   —The dissemination method;

   —If dissemination via an aerosol-generating device is still occurring or it has stopped but there is no information on the duration of dissemination, or what the exposure concentration might be.

2. Responders may use a Level B protective suit with an exposed or enclosed NIOSH-approved pressure-demand SCBA if the situation can be defined in which:

—The suspected biological aerosol is no longer being generated;

—Other conditions may present a splash hazard.

3. Responders may use a full facepiece respirator with a P100 filter or powered air-purifying respirator (PAPR) with high-efficiency particulate air (HEPA) filters when it can be determined that:

—An aerosol-generating device was not used to create a high airborne concentration;

—Dissemination was by a letter or package that can be easily bagged.

These types of respirators reduce the user's exposure by a factor of 50 if the user has been properly fit tested."

The publication goes on to state: "Care should be taken when bagging letters and packages to minimize creating a puff of air that could spread pathogens. It is best to avoid large bags and to work very slowly and carefully when placing objects in bags. Disposable hooded coveralls, gloves, and foot coverings also should be used. NIOSH recommends against wearing standard firefighter turnout gear into potentially contaminated areas when responding to reports involving biological agents."

"Decontamination of protective equipment and clothing is an important precaution to make sure that any particles that might settle on the outside of protective equipment are removed before taking off the gear. Decontamination sequences currently used for hazardous material emergencies should be used as appropriate for the level of protection employed. Equipment can be decontaminated using soap and water, and 0.5% hypochlorite solution (one part household bleach to 10 parts water) can be used as appropriate or if gear had any visible contamination. Note that bleach may damage some types of firefighter turnout gear (one reason why it should not be used for biological agent response actions). After taking off gear, response workers should shower using copious quantities of soap and water."

Additional information regarding bioterrorism can be found by accessing the following entities: U.S. Departments of Defense, Homeland Security, and Health and Human Services, Centers for Disease Control and Prevention, the Occupational Safety and Health Administration, the National Institute for Occupational Safety and Health, and state and local governments.

Summary

The world and its nations are changing, opening their borders and becoming more global in business, travel, and immigration policies. Diseases believed eradicated in all or parts of the world and those confined to distant regions will begin to cross borders. In addition, terrorists are now using biological weapons in their arsenal of fear. Health care workers, including critical care transport personnel, must be vigilant and prepared to respond to any indications of emerging or changing prevalence of infections.

Review Questions

1. Discuss the importance of infectious disease knowledge and prevention in the critical care setting.

2. Detail the various guidelines for personal protection.

3. What are some of the currently epidemiologically important infectious diseases?

4. Discuss precautions that should be taken for patients with childhood diseases.

5. Name some older agents that are now important because of the increased risk of bioterrorism.

See Answers to Review Questions at the back of this book.

Further Reading

"Acute Upper Airway Obstruction." Adam.com. http://content.health.msn.com/printing/asset/adam_disease_acuteupperairway_obstruction (1999).

Abuhammour W, Nashar K. "Brucellosis." *eMedicine*, Vol. 2, No. 9 (2001). http://www.emedicine.com.

"Bacterial Gastroenteritis." http://content.health.msn.com/printing/asset/adam_disease_infectious_diarrhea. (1999).

Bartlett JG, Breiman RF, Mandell LA, File TM. "Community-Acquired Pneumonia in Adults: Guidelines for Management." *Clinical Infectious Diseases,* Vol. 26 (1998): 811–838.

Berstein D. "Diagnosis and Management of Hepatitis C." *Gastroenterology Clinical Management.* Vol. 1. http://nurses.medscape.com/Medscape/gastro/ClinicalMgmt/CM.v01/pnt-CM.v01.html.

Carson-DeWitt RS. "Epiglottitis." *Gale Encyclopedia of Medicine.* Farmington Hills, MI: Gale Research, 1999.

Centers for Disease Control and Prevention. "Appendix A. Practice Recommendations for Health-Care Facilities Implementing the U.S. Public Health Service Guidelines for Management of Occupational Exposures to Bloodborne Pathogens." *Morbidity and Mortality Weekly Report,* Vol. 50, No. RR11 (2001): 43–44.

Centers for Disease Control and Prevention, "Appendix B. Management of Occupational Blood Exposures." *Morbidity and Mortality Weekly Report,* Vol. 50, No. RR11 (2001): 45–46.

Centers for Disease Control and Prevention. "Appendix C. Basic and Expanded HIV Postexposure Prophylaxis Regimens." *Morbidity and Mortality Weekly Report,* Vol. 50, No. RR11 (2001): 47–52.

Centers for Disease Control and Prevention. *HIV and Its Transmission.* http://www.cdc.gov/hiv/pubs/facts/transmission.htm.

Centers for Disease Control and Prevention. "Immunization of Health-Care Workers." *Morbidity and Mortality Weekly Report,* Vol. 46, No. RR18 (1997).

Centers for Disease Control and Prevention. *Interim Recommendations for Firefighters and Other First Responders for the Selection and Use of Protective Clothing and Respirators against Biological Agents.* http://www.bt.cdc.gov/DocumentsApp/Anthrax/Protective/10242001Protect.asp (October 14, 2001).

Centers for Disease Control and Prevention. *Interim Smallpox Response Plan and Guidelines.* http://www.cdc.gov/nip/diseases/smallpox/default.htm (November 26, 2001).

Centers for Disease Control and Prevention. *Preventing Occupational HIV Transmission to Healthcare Personnel.* http://www.cdc.gov/hiv/pubs/facts/hcwprev.htm.

Centers for Disease Control and Prevention. "Recognition of Illness Associated with the Intentional Release of a Biologic Agent." *Morbidity and Mortality Weekly Report,* Vol. 50, No. 41 (2001): 893–897.

Centers for Disease Control and Prevention. *"Recommendations for Preventing Transmission of Human Immunodeficiency Virus and Hepatitis B Virus to Patients During Exposure-Prone Invasive Procedures."* Vol. 36 (suppl. No. 2S):6S–7S.

Centers for Disease Control and Prevention. "Revised Guidelines for HIV Counseling, Testing and Referral: Technical Expert Panel Review of CDC HIV Counseling, Testing and Referral Guidelines." *Morbidity and Mortality Weekly Report,* Vol. 50, No. RR19 (2001): 1–58.

Centers for Disease Control and Prevention. "Update: Investigation of Anthrax Associated with Intentional Exposure and Interim Public Health Guidelines." *Morbidity and Mortality Weekly Report,* Vol. 50, No. 41 (2001): 889–893.

Centers for Disease Control and Prevention. "Update: Investigation of Bioterrorism-Related Anthrax and Interim Guidelines for Exposure Management and Antimicrobial Therapy." *Morbidity and Mortality Weekly Report,* Vol. 50, No. 42 (2001): 909–919.

Centers for Disease Control and Prevention. "Updated U.S. Public Health Service Guidelines for Management of Occupational Exposures to HBV, HIV and Recommendations for Postexposure Prophylaxis." *Morbidity and Mortality Weekly Report,* Vol. 50, No. RR11 (2001): 1–42.

Centers for Disease Control and Prevention. *Viral Hepatitis A Fact Sheet.* http://www.cdc.gov/ncidod/diseases/hepatitis/a/fact.htm (May 29, 2001).

Centers for Disease Control and Prevention. *Viral Hepatitis B Fact Sheet.* http://www.cdc.gov/ncidod/diseases/hepatitis/b/fact.htm (December 12, 2001).

Centers for Disease Control and Prevention. *Viral Hepatitis C Fact Sheet.* http://www.cdc.gov/ncidod/diseases/hepatitis/c/fact.htm (August 25, 2001).

Centers for Disease Control and Prevention. *Viral Hepatitis D Fact Sheet.* http://www.cdc.gov/ncidod/diseases/hepatitis/slideset/hep_d/slide_1.htm (May 29, 2001).

Centers for Disease Control and Prevention. *Viral Hepatitis E Fact Sheet.* http://www.cdc.gov/ncidod/diseases/hepatitis/slideset/hep_e/slide_1.htm (May 29, 2001).

Centers for Disease Control and Prevention, Division of Tuberculosis Elimination. *Core Curriculum on Tuberculosis: What Every Clinician Should Know,* 4th ed. 2000. http://www.cdc.gov/nchstp/tb/pubs/corecurr/default.htm.

Chin J, editor. *Control of Communicable Diseases Manual,* 17th ed. Washington, DC: American Public Health Association, 2000.

"Colds and Flu: Time Is the Only Sure Cure." http://content.health/msn.com/printing/article/1680.50946 (May 1999).

"The Common Cold." http://content.health.msn.com/printing/article/3624.127 (1998).

Cunha BA. "Community-Acquired Pneumonia (CAP)." *eMedicine,* Vol. 2, No. 5 (2001). http://www.emedicine.com.

"Current Treatment Considerations in Community-Acquired Pneumonia in Older Patients." *Drugs and Therapy Perspectives,* Vol. 17, No. 21 (2001): 5–8.

DeLorenzo RA, Porter RS. *Weapons of Mass Destruction Emergency Care.* Upper Saddle River, NJ: Pearson Prentice Hall, 2000.

Dhawan VK. "Toxic Shock Syndrome." *eMedicine,* Vol. 2, No. 7 (2001). http://www.emedicine.com.

"Epiglottitis." Adam.com. http://content.health.msn.com/printing/asset/adam_disease_epiglottitis (1999).

Faust S, Nadel S. "Aseptic Meningitis." *eMedicine,* Vol. 2, No. 9 (2001). http://www.emedicine.com.

Fennelly G. "Measles." *eMedicine,* Vol. 2, No. 9 (2001). http://www.emedicine.com.

Frazier MS, Dryzmkowski JW. *Essentials of Human Diseases and Conditions,* 2nd ed. Philadelphia: W. B. Saunders, 2000.

Gannon JC. *The Global Infectious Disease Threat and Its Implications for the United States.* http://www.odci.gov/cia/publications/nie/report/nie99-17d.html, NIE 99-17D (January 2000).

Garner JS. Hospital Infection Control Practices Advisory Committee. *Guideline for Isolation Precautions in Hospitals.* Centers for Disease Control and Prevention, 2000. http://www.cdc.gov/ncidod/hip/isolat/isolat.htm.

Gordon JE. *Control of Communicable Diseases in Man,* 10th ed. New York: American Public Health Association, 1965.

Ho H, Amin H. Vibrio. *eMedicine,* Vol. 2, No. 7 (2001). http://www.emedicine.com.

Hoffman TA. "Meningococcal Disease." *eMedicine,* Vol. 2, No. 7 (2001). http://www.emedicine.com.

"Immunity." http://content.health.msn.com/printing/asset/miller_keane_16960.

"Infection." http://content.health.msn.com/printing/asset/miller_keane_17210.

Kaufman HL, Flanagan K. "Vaccinia." *eMedicine,* Vol. 2, No. 5 (2001). http://www.emedicine.com.

Krause PJ, Gross PA, Barrett TL, et al. "Quality Standards for Assurance of Measles Immunity among Health Care Workers." *Clinical Infectious Diseases,* Vol. 18 (1994): 431–436.

Maryland Department of Health and Mental Hygiene, Epidemiology and Disease Control Program. "Guidelines for Control of Methicillin-Resistant *Staphylococcus aureus* in Long-Term Care Facilities." *Infection Control in Long Term Care,* Vol. 11, No. 1 (2000): 1–5.

"Meningitis." http://content.health.msn.com/printing/asset/adam_disease_viral_meningitis (1999).

"Meningitis; meningococcal." http://content.health.msn.com/printing/asset/adam_disease_meningitis_ meningococcal (1999).

Migala AF, Neumann L. "Q Fever." *eMedicine,* Vol. 2, No. 9 (2001). http://www.emedicine.com.

"Occupational Exposure to Bloodborne Pathogens; Needlesticks and Other Sharps Injuries; Final Rule." Federal Register, 29 CFR 1910.1030 (January 18, 2001).

Occupational Safety and Health Administration. "Protecting the Workplace Against Anthrax." http://www.osha.gov/bioterrorism/anthrax/matrix/index.html (November 26, 2001).

Phelan D, Jacobson RM, Poland GA. "Current Adult and Pediatric Vaccine Recommendations." *Infections in Medicine,* Vol. 18, No. 85 (2001): FV6–FV14.

San Antonio Uniformed Services HEC Pediatric Residency, Department of Pediatrics. "Epiglottitis." *Pediatric Emergency Manual.* Virtual Naval Hospital. http://www.vnh.org/ PediatricEmergencyManual/Epiglottitis.html (2001).

Santer DM, D'Alessandro MP. "Acute Epiglottitis." *Virtual Children's Hospital.* http://www.vh.org/ Providers/Textbooks/ElectricAirway/Text/Epiglottitis.html. 2001.

Schleiss MR. "Streptococcus Pyogenes." *eMedicine,* Vol. 2, No. 9 (2001). http://www.emedicine.com.

Schremmer RD. "Plague." *eMedicine,* Vol. 2, No. www.emedicine.com. 2001;2(4).

Sidell FR, Patrick WC, Dashiell TR. *Jane's Chem-Bio Handbook.* Alexandria, VA: Jane's Information Group, 1999.

Tolan RW, Whitner ML. "Viral Hemorrhagic Fevers." *eMedicine,* Vol. 2, No. 5 (2001). http://www.emedicine.com.

Waldman RH, Kluge RM. *Textbook of Infectious Disease.* New York: Medical Examination Publishing, 1984.

"What Antibiotics Are Used for Pneumonia." *Well-Connected Reports.* http://content.health.msn. com/printing/article/1680.52940 (2001).

Zimmerman L, Neuman M, Jurewicz D. *Infection Control for Prehospital Care Providers,* 2nd ed. Grand Rapids, MI: Mercy Ambulance, 1993.

Pediatric Medical Emergencies

William S. Krost, NREMT-P

Objectives

Upon completion of this chapter, the student should be able to:

1. Discuss why the critical care paramedic must remain aware of the special concerns surrounding the assessment and management of the pediatric patient. (p. 812)
2. Understand the physiological differences between the adult and the pediatric patient. (p. 813)
3. Recognize how the pediatric patient suffering from common medical emergencies may present with differing symptomatology as compared to the adult. (p. 814)
4. Understand the importance of maintaining proficiency in supporting the pediatric patient's airway, breathing, and circulatory function. (p. 814)
5. Be able to discuss the pathophysiology of respiratory complications in the pediatric patient. (p. 818)
6. Understand the pathophysiology of congenital heart disease that is common to the pediatric patient. (p. 832)
7. Discuss the steps of the initial assessment when caring for a pediatric patient. (p. 834)
8. Discuss the pathophysiology of hypoglycemia in the pediatric patient. (p. 836)
9. Summarize the common denominator present in the majority of pediatric arrest situations. (p. 837).

Key Terms

bronchiolitis, p. 827
cardiogenic shock, p. 830
congenital heart defects, p. 833
croup (laryngotracheo-bronchitis), p. 821

distributive shock, p. 829
epiglottitis, p. 824
nondistributive shock, p. 829
obstructive shock, p. 830
respiratory distress, p. 819

respiratory failure, p. 820
respiratory syncytial virus (RSV), p. 827

Case Study

After working a long 24-hour shift that ends at 0700 hours, the phone rings and it is one of the incoming crew members who tells you they will be "a little late" getting into the base site. You volunteer to hang over, and hope that a mission does not come in during the extra few minutes you remain on duty. But as fate would have it, about 5 minutes later, your pager goes off for an interhospital transport. You ask dispatch to call your spouse to let her know you'll be late and then start to gather the equipment and head toward the aircraft.

You learn your patient is an 8-year-old male found unresponsive in his bed this morning by his mother. EMS was called and the EMS providers initiated care and then transported the patient to the closest emergency department facility. Because none of the neighboring hospitals has a dedicated pediatric ED, nor provides specialty care for pediatrics, performing critical care transport missions for this age bracket is a common occurrence for your flight program. During the flight you review with your partner the pediatric algorithm for an unknown unresponsive presentation, the potential causes of this (AEIOU-TIPS), and medication dosages. Prior to starting your final descent to the helipad located on the roof of the hospital, you find the Broselow tape in the jump-bag, pull it out, and stuff it in your flight suit pocket.

The pilot gently sets the EC 135 down on the ground, and you receive the go-ahead from the pilot to exit the aircraft as he shuts down the twin turbine engines. You and your partner strap your pediatric bag, monitor, IV pumps, and drug bag on your portable stretcher and start the trek off the helipad and down the elevator toward the emergency department.

Upon arrival at the ED, the staff there briefs you as to the patient's status, which correlates with what you were told by your communications specialist. As you walk toward the exam room, the ED staff also updates you on the patient and advises you that the patient's condition continues to worsen.

The initial assessment reveals a thin 8-year-old male lying on the stretcher with sinus tachycardia present on the monitor, the skin extremely pale, slight inward contraction of the hands, and the mother frantically sobbing "Please help him. . . . Please help him." The security officer who led you down from the helipad escorts the mother out of the room. The respiratory therapist in the room tells you she just started positive-pressure ventilation (PPV) since the patient's breathing never improved, and he eventually became fatigued.

After ensuring that the oropharynx is devoid of any fluid or foreign bodies, you visualize chest rise and fall and auscultate equal breath sounds bilaterally. You find the carotid pulse to be weak and rapid with peripheral pulses faint to palpation. Upon assessment of the mental status, your patient only moans to painful stimuli.

The physician, now standing at your side while the respiratory therapist resumes positive-pressure ventilation, begins to cover the medical history of the child and the history of the present chief complaint. You learn that the patient was an apparently healthy child, no allergies, no medications, no past medical history. Mom thought the child had the "flu" for the past few days because he has had a decreased appetite, nausea, vomiting, and was just not "acting right." Mom stated that the child went to bed at 2000 last night and she couldn't awaken him at 0630 this morning.

While listening to the report from the physician you, and your partner notice the following parameters on the attached patient monitors: BP 68/40 mmHg, sinus tachycardia at 160 bpm in Lead II, respiratory rate of 24 (via PPV with 100% oxygen), and an O_2 saturation of 98%. In addition, you confirm posturing of the hands in response to noxious stimuli.

Treatment immediately consists of rapid-sequence intubation (RSI) and fluid resuscitation. You follow your pediatric RSI protocol, and base the fluid resuscitation on a 45-kg patient (totaling 1,000 mL). Orotracheal intubation is complicated by an anterior and cephalad glottic opening, and the presence of edema and blood from the previous intubation attempts. However, after the physician provides cricoid pressure on the patient, the glottic opening drops into clear view and you successfully pass a 6.5 ETT, with confirmation of equal breath sounds bilaterally. Initial end-tidal capnography readings are 50 mmHg.

While discussing further treatments with the MD, the first set of blood work is handed to you. You notice that the patient's sodium is 155 mEq, glucose is 880 mg/dL, potassium 3.3, and the pH on the ABG is 7.28. An initial diagnosis of new-onset diabetic ketoacidosis is suspected.

Treatment now includes fluid resuscitation, an insulin bolus and drip, potassium supplementation, hyperventilation, and sodium bicarbonate administration in an attempt to reverse the hyperglycemia, stabilize the intracellular environment, and reverse the acidosis.

Before leaving you allow the mother and father to quickly kiss and say good-bye to their son as you prepare for transport to the pediatric hospital. Before flight you perform a quick I-Stat and find the patient's BGL now to be 600, Na^+ of 150, K^+ of 3.5, and pH of 7.32. The patient's vital signs are BP 94/60, HR of 140, and respirations of 24 per minute (assisted). For continued mechanical ventilation you paralyze the patient with vecuronium and sedation with fentanyl.

In flight you continue fluid resuscitation based on HR and urinary output (from the Foley catheter). The patient develops occasional PVCs and PACs, which you attribute to the electrolyte and fluid imbalance, as well as the acidotic environment. On arrival at the pediatric hospital your vitals are BP 98/76, HR 135 per minute, with respirations still at 24 per minute assisted. The patient is admitted to the pediatric ICU after a brief stay in the emergency department. Three days later on follow-up you find the patient and family doing well, diagnosis of new-onset IDDM was made, and the patient/family education has begun. About a week later, you are contacted by your service's medical director who asks you to prepare this mission as a case study to be presented at your next internal continuing education program.

INTRODUCTION

Evaluation of the infant, child, or adolescent must be comprehensive and includes both physical and psychological factors. The need to understand the pediatric patient population and pathophysiology is great because more than 20,000 pediatric deaths occur each year in the United States. In addition, an increasing number of ill and injured pediatric patients are requiring the services of the critical care transport team. As such, the ability for the critical care paramedic to properly assess and manage the critical pediatric patient cannot be overstated. Providing optimum care to these young patients can only be achieved by obtaining an appropriate clinical history and then coupling it with an effective physical exam. In fact, the critical care transport team must be capable of providing care to the pediatric patient in essentially the same manner that care would be delivered in a pediatric intensive care unit (PICU). In the transport of pediatric patients, the critical care transport should be treated as an extension of the PICU.

RELATIVE ANATOMY AND PHYSIOLOGY

The critical care paramedic student should have a good understanding of pediatric anatomy and physiology. We will review and update aspects of these as they pertain to the presented material.

PHYSIOLOGY OF METABOLISM AND THERMOREGULATION

One of the first concerns that the critical care paramedic should remember when dealing with pediatric patients, long before the consideration of any advanced skills, is that the pediatric body surface area-to-volume ratio is four times that of an adult, whereas its heat production is only one and a half times as high. This predisposes the pediatric patient to a greater risk for accidental hypothermia that can easily result in significant physiological compromise. Additionally, the pediatric patient's muscle tone and nervous system may yet be underdeveloped and immature and as a result cannot effectively induce muscular shivering as an effective mechanism for thermogenesis. Compounding this heat production/ maintenance concern is that these patients also generally have smaller amounts of adipose tissue, which contributes to additional difficulty in maintaining core body temperature. Heat loss in the pediatric patient occurs, like in the adult patient, as the result of evaporation, convection, conduction, and radiation. While the majority of heat loss in the infant and pediatric occurs from evaporation, heat loss through convection can also easily occur if the pediatric patient is in either a cool hospital room or one with excessive air flow. Pediatric patients often kick off sheets and blankets while sleeping, and although a seemingly harmless action, this can be contributory to the subtle onset of a lowered core body temperature. Certainly the care provider should not allow an excessive ambient temperature that is too warm or too cool. If the critical care paramedic finds a room (or patient compartment of the transporting vehicle or aircraft) to be at a "comfortable" temperature, then this may be too cool for the critically ill pediatric patient. Exercise caution regarding the maintenance of normothermia in the pediatric patient.

Pediatric patients also have another physiological difference that may bear on treatment considerations when providing transport. They have a higher basal metabolic rate characteristic than do adults. An infant's consumption of oxygen occurs at almost twice the rate of an adult (the younger the patient, the higher the metabolic rate). This translates into heightened concerns about oxygen maintenance and the prevention of hypoxemia. Although the pediatric patient may be able to maintain impaired pulmonary function at the expense of heightened respiratory effort for a period of time, as soon as either system starts to fail, the onset of hypoxemia and hypercapnia will occur at a much faster rate.

GLUCOSE REQUIREMENTS

Infants and small children are at a greater risk for the development of acute hypoglycemia because of (1) decreased glycogen stores; (2) the inability to stimulate the release of stored glycogen from an immature liver; (3) an increased metabolic rate (as mentioned previously), resulting in the utilization of large quantities of serum glucose; or (4) a known history of diabetes. Stress may induce hypoglycemia, and a bedside glucose level should be evaluated in all infants regardless of the diagnosis. Certainly a bedside glucose determination should be made if the presentation included seizures or dehydration, and in the setting of a post-arrest pediatric patient of any age, glucose level monitoring is a must.

Indications of hypoglycemia in the pediatric patient may include twitching, seizures, limpness, eye-rolling, apnea, irregular respirations, or objective determination with a Glucometer. The onset of hypoglycemic symptoms can be rapid and, as a result, requires emergent intervention to prevent cerebral injury. When performing an assessment on a pediatric patient, blood sugar evaluation should be done on arrival in order to plan for any appropriate glucose administration, and during

The greater body surface area and various other factors predispose the pediatric patient to a greater risk for accidental hypothermia that can easily result in significant physiologic compromise.

Pediatric patients have a higher basal metabolic rate than do adults. Because of this, an infant's consumption of oxygen occurs at almost twice the rate of an adult.

Infants and small children are at a greater risk for the development of acute hypoglycemia because of (1) decreased glycogen stores; (2) the inability to stimulate the release of stored glycogen from an immature liver; (3) an increased metabolic rate (as mentioned previously), resulting in the utilization of large quantities of serum glucose; or (4) a known history of diabetes.

transport as well because the onset of hypoglycemia may be insidious and rapid. Glucose monitoring equipment must always be readily available.

AIRWAY ANATOMY AND PHYSIOLOGY

Pediatric patients are unique and have very different anatomical and physiological qualities as compared to adults. The tongue exhibits one of the most obvious anatomical differences seen between the adult and the pediatric patient. The pediatric tongue is larger than an adult's in relationship to the amount of free space in the oropharynx. The large tongue creates a significant probability for airway occlusion in the obtunded patient, and leaves little room for airway swelling should it occur. In addition, the external nares, which constitute the primary route for ventilation in infants, are proportionally smaller and any occlusion or partial occlusion from edematous nasal mucosa (or hemorrhage) can easily contribute to difficulties in maintaining adequate ventilations. The airway may also be subject to partial occlusion from tissue hypertrophy common to adenoidal hypertrophy or polyps in the nasopharyngeal region. The infant may also have a history of congenital choanal stenosis or atresia, both of which may present with apnea, dyspnea, or cyanosis at rest that is relieved by crying because the pediatric patient uses the mouth for breathing while crying. Eventually, as the pediatric patient ages, the nasopharyngeal diameter continually enlarges and dependence on nasal breathing gives way to more oronasal reliance as seen with the adult. (See Table 27–1.)

As discussed in greater detail in Chapter 29, "Neonatal Emergencies," the pediatric trachea is much more pliable than the adult's. Infant and younger pediatric patients may not yet have fully developed tracheal rings (with the exception of the first tracheal ring), and the resultant increased pliability of the trachea can be troublesome should hyperextension and/or hyperflexion of the neck occur because this may lead to occlusion of the airway. As was also mentioned about the external nares, the small diameter of the trachea is subject to becoming easily occluded should even a small degree of swelling be present.

The pediatric epiglottis is larger, not as well supported by its cartilaginous structure, and more U- or Ω (omega)-shaped or oblong than the adult's, which makes it more difficult to manipulate during orotracheal intubation attempts. For this reason, pediatric intubation should be performed using a straight (Miller) blade versus a curved (MacIntosh) blade. Whereas the curved blade fits into the vallecular space and indirectly lifts the epiglottis, the straight blade directly lifts the epiglottis,

Table 27–1	Summary of Pediatric vs. Adult Physiologic and Anatomic Differences
Physiologic/Anatomic Difference	**Impact on Assessment and Treatment**
Larger tongue	Easily blocks airway, requires good airway positioning, complicates intubation
Epiglottic positioning	Complicates visualization for intubation
Epiglottic structure	Necessitates use of straight intubation blade
Funnel-shaped larynx	Use of uncuffed intubation tubes
Obligate nose breathers	Nasopharyngeal occlusion can be critical
Reduced size of airway	Small amounts of edema can occlude airway
Abundant secretions	Contributes to airway blockage
Proportionately larger head	Supine positioning can flex neck and block airway
Diaphragmatic breathers	Air in stomach or pressure on the abdomen can restrict breathing
Short, narrow trachea	Can close off with overextension of neck
Faster respiratory rate	Can fatigue muscles, leading to distress
Faster metabolic rate	Reduced oxygen intake leads to significant cellular hypoxia and hypercapnia quickly

which is more advantageous given its more pliant characteristic, and allows for better visualization of the vocal cords.

The adult larynx sits at about the level of the fourth or fifth cervical vertebrae and the pediatric larynx sits roughly at the level of the first or second cervical vertebrae. This is important to realize because the higher the larynx is, the more anterior the glottic opening is as well. To be successful in managing a pediatric patient's airway, it should always be assumed that the airway is anterior, and the critical care paramedic should employ techniques and equipment that will make his first attempt at intubation, his best.

An additional difference between these airways is that the narrowest portion of the adult airway is at the glottic opening and the narrowest portion of the pediatric airway is subglottic—at the level of the cricoid ring. The airway in a pediatric patient, to draw an analogy, is shaped like an inverted cone, whereas the adult airway is cylindrical. (See Figure 27-1 ■.) The clinical relevance of this is that the subglottic space is exceedingly susceptible to edema from viruses, allergies, burn trauma, or direct trauma, all of which can lead to airway occlusion. Additionally, this is why pediatric and infant patients are intubated commonly with an uncuffed endotracheal (ET) tube. The cricoid ring, when using an appropriately sized ET tube, will serve as a physiological cuff to help isolate the trachea and lungs from fluid present in the upper airway or gastric juices that may be regurgitated from the stomach.

The adult larynx sits at about the level of the fourth or fifth cervical vertebrae and the pediatric larynx sits roughly at the level of the first or second cervical vertebrae. This is important to realize because the higher the larynx is, the more anterior the glottic opening is as well.

The cricoid ring, when using an appropriately sized ET tube, will serve as a physiological cuff to help isolate the trachea and lungs from fluid present in the upper airway or gastric juices that may be regurgitated from the stomach.

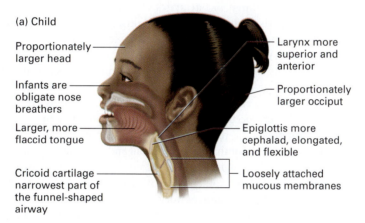

(a) Child

Proportionately larger head

Infants are obligate nose breathers

Larger, more flaccid tongue

Cricoid cartilage narrowest part of the funnel-shaped airway

Larynx more superior and anterior

Proportionately larger occiput

Epiglottis more cephalad, elongated, and flexible

Loosely attached mucous membranes

Infants and young children rely on the diaphragm to breathe more than adults do.

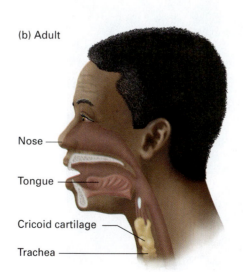

(b) Adult

Nose

Tongue

Cricoid cartilage

Trachea

■ **Figure 27-1**

Understanding the unique aspects of a child's airway makes it possible to adapt techniques learned for managing the adult airway appropriately for the pediatric patient. (A) Child. (B) Adult.

PULMONARY ANATOMY AND PHYSIOLOGY

The anatomy of the pediatric chest results in differences in how respiratory compromise will be observed. The bones of the pediatric thoracic cage are not yet completely calcified and tend to be flexible. This causes a relative inability to support the lungs when intrathoracic pressure becomes more negative during heightened ventilation attempts. When a pediatric patient suffers some form of respiratory compromise, he or she must then attempt to increase the volume of air entering the chest through the utilization of accessory muscles. Compounding this is the fact that the pediatric ribs are positioned in such a way that the ribs are more horizontal than rounded, as seen in adults. The horizontal nature of the ribs provides for very little leverage to increase the anterior and posterior diameter of the chest by intercostal muscle contraction. Thus, there is not the provision of necessary lift that is needed to increase the volume of air within the chest, when it is needed most. Some pediatric patients (the younger the more prominent) also have less well developed accessory muscles, which then makes it difficult to maintain heightened ventilatory effort when the accessory muscles are being employed. This lack of accessory muscles combined with the increased pliancy of the ribcage is the reason many pediatric patients in respiratory distress will present with significant diaphragmatic breathing.

The sternum of a neonate is also very pliable. When the accessory muscles are being stretched, they will pull on various bony structures, including the sternum. The increased pliancy of the sternum also contributes to the neonate's inability to create a strong negative intrathoracic pressure, thereby inhibiting the efficiency of the inspiratory effort.

Infants and children, like neonates, also have a lower pulmonary reserve capacity than do their adult counterparts. To better understand this, the critical care paramedic need only review a normal pediatric chest X-ray. Here it will be easy to appreciate the relative amount of space the heart occupies within the mediastinal cavity of the thorax. (See Figures 27-2 ■ and 27-3 ■.) Children have a reduced ability to increase the volume within the lungs because the lungs can only expand according to the degree to which space is available to expand. Since the heart is larger, and the ribs and sternum fail to adequately support the lungs, the net result is a diminishment in the space in which lung expansion can occur. In the end, this contributes to a more rapid development of hypoxemia and hypercapnia should the neonate suffer some type of pulmonary compromise.

The pediatric abdominal cavity is small and has relatively large abdominal organs compressed within the cavity. Although the intra-abdominal cavity will enlarge as the body develops into young adulthood, a significant problem with overcrowding still exists for pediatric patients that results in a negative effect on the compensatory mechanism for ventilation. Since the pediatric patient cannot rely on the thoracic cavity participating much in promoting enhanced air exchange, she must

> Infants and children, like neonates, also have a lower pulmonary reserve capacity than do their adult counterparts.

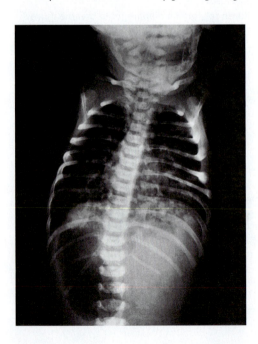

■ **Figure 27-2** Chest X-ray indicating pneumonia in an infant. *(© Lester V. Bergman/CORBIS)*

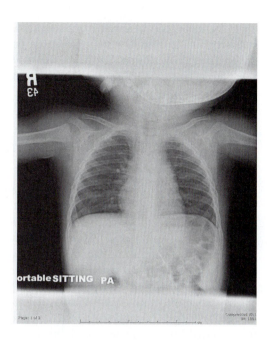

■ **Figure 27-3** Normal infant chest X-ray. *(Kathy Altergott, BSN, MBA, CRA. Banner Good Samaritan Medical Center, Phoenix, AZ)*

instead rely on exaggerated diaphragmatic movement. Since the diaphragm must displace the abdominal contents inferiorly during contraction, the relative size of the abdominal organs naturally impedes the diaphragmatic excursion. This also underscores the reason why the pediatric patient with significant respiratory distress (or on a mechanical ventilator) should have a nasogastric tube placed to ensure the stomach is properly decompressed. By keeping the stomach decompressed, the work of the diaphragm is greatly reduced and allows for more efficient intrathoracic cavity elongation to enhance the ventilatory effort.

The final difference regarding the physiology of the pediatric pulmonary system is that it must be competent enough to maintain the higher metabolic rates common to this age group. From birth through childhood, pediatric patients consume oxygen in the bloodstream at nearly double the rate of the adult patient. A smaller pulmonary reserve capacity coupled with a higher metabolic demand for oxygen leaves the pediatric more predisposed to hypoxemia at the cellular level, despite the presence of spontaneous ventilatory efforts. Hypoxemia in the pediatric patient develops very insidiously with disastrous effects, should the critical care paramedic not stay attuned to the pulmonary functioning of the patient.

CARDIOVASCULAR ANATOMY AND PHYSIOLOGY

Although the pediatric and adult heart share identical anatomy, several important distinctions need to be made between the adult and pediatric cardiovascular systems for the critical care paramedic. The first distinction is that the adult myocardium has the ability to increase its cardiac output by enhancing both inotropy and chronotropy should the output drop (due to, for example, hypovolemic shock). In contrast, the pediatric myocardium can only increase the heart rate efficiently in an attempt to improve cardiac output and not the stroke volume. The pediatric heart has low compliance as it relates to volume and therefore cannot compensate by increasing stroke volume. Consequently, heart rate should be viewed as a significant clinical marker when monitoring cardiac output in the pediatric patient. When the pediatric patient becomes bradycardic, you should assume that the patient's cardiac output has been drastically reduced.

The second distinction that should be made pertains to the ability of the child to alter peripheral vascular resistance. Since the degree of arterial tone is the other determinant of perfusion pressure (systemic perfusion = cardiac output × systemic vascular resistance), the critical care paramedic should remember that this age group has the ability to promote vigorous arterial vasoconstriction. The end result is the maintenance of "acceptable" systolic blood pressure in the face of diminished end-organ perfusion. The critical care team should recall that blood pressure is a

When the pediatric patient becomes bradycardic, it should be assumed that the patient's cardiac output has been drastically reduced.

relatively nondescriptive variable in assessing the quality of peripheral perfusion. By the time there is a recognizable drop in systolic perfusion pressure, there will have already been a significant change in organ perfusion. The key is to maintain a high index of suspicion for conditions that may alter peripheral perfusion, and treat these conditions aggressively with fluids, medications, and the like in an attempt to thwart any diminishment of end-organ perfusion *before* it becomes clinically evident or physiologically significant.

GENERAL PATHOPHYSIOLOGY IN THE PEDIATRIC PATIENT

Causes of respiratory compromise may include mechanical obstruction of the airway by foreign bodies, edema, or bronchospasm. (See Figure 27-4 ■.) Other causes that do not directly affect the airway but can still have untoward effects include congenital heart defects, and trauma or infection resulting in chest wall compromise. It is important to remember at all times with neonatal, infant, and pediatric patients that the leading cause of cardiopulmonary arrest is airway and breathing insufficiency. If the airway and ventilatory systems are not carefully monitored and managed appropriately when compromises arise, the pediatric patient will degrade rapidly into cardiopulmonary failure and arrest, which carries with it even more abysmal rates for successful resuscitation than seen in the adult population. If early identification and treatment for a failed body system were ever to be stressed, it would involve the ability to maintain airway and ventilations in pediatrics.

RESPIRATORY DISTRESS, FAILURE, AND ARREST

The critical care paramedic will probably care for more pediatrics with a respiratory problem during interfacility transports than any other condition. If fact, respiratory problems are the leading cause of cardiopulmonary arrest in children. The common feature to all pulmonary problems in the pediatric patient is respiratory distress signs and symptoms. With respiratory distress findings present, the critical care team must realize that the pediatric patient is employing physiological mechanisms designed to maximize pulmonary function. Although the pediatric patient may still be achieving adequate alveolar ventilation for oxygenation and carbon dioxide elimination, it is usually just a matter of time until these compensatory mechanisms fail and the patient deteriorates into respiratory failure.

■ Figure 27-4   Effects of edema on airway resistance in the infant and adult.

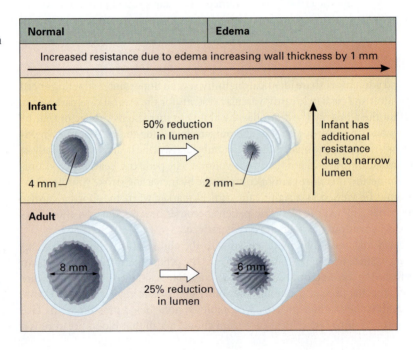

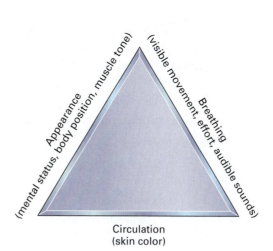

■ **Figure 27-5** The pediatric assessment triangle. *(Used with permission of the American Academy of Pediatrics.)*

Appearance (mental status, body position, muscle tone)

Breathing (visible movement, effort, audible sounds)

Circulation (skin color)

In assessing for, describing, and ultimately treating these findings, the critical care paramedic must be precise in the use of the terms *respiratory distress, respiratory failure,* and *respiratory arrest.* This distinction dictates how aggressive transport personnel need to be in the management of the acutely ill pediatric patient. (See Figure 27-5 ■.) Failure to recognize the prearrest states of respiratory distress and failure will allow patient deterioration to a clinical state where the loss of physiological function may not be remediable. The key, then, is to provide appropriate basic as well as advanced life support resuscitative interventions early in the progression of complete cardiopulmonary failure.

> Respiratory problems are the leading cause of cardiopulmonary arrest in children.

CLINICAL PRESENTATION OF RESPIRATORY DISTRESS AND FAILURE

As mentioned previously, a pediatric patient with **respiratory distress** is one who is utilizing several compensatory mechanisms in order to achieve adequate alveolar ventilation. And although this maintenance is good, the indications of this increased work of breathing (WOB) should be readily identified so that concern at finding the cause of distress can be isolated and managed. Failure to do so will allow this compensated respiratory distress to progress into a worse clinical condition. Although numerous respiratory emergencies may present with similar symptomatology initially, the critical care paramedic should not disregard these findings. The findings of compensated respiratory distress, when the pediatric patient is still achieving adequate alveolar ventilation at the expense of a heightened WOB, include:

> **respiratory distress**
> *breathing difficulty hallmarked by inadequate alveolar gas exchange.*

- ★ Tachypnea (to include "quiet" tachypnea)
- ★ Use of accessory respiratory muscles
- ★ Nasal flaring
- ★ Diaphoresis
- ★ Tachycardia (as defined by patient's age)
- ★ Irritability
- ★ Inspiratory retractions
- ★ Excessive abdominal motion
- ★ Grunting (physiological positive end-expiratory pressure)
- ★ Pulse oximetry and end-tidal capnography changes
- ★ Alterations to normal breath sounds

In addition to these findings of compensated respiratory distress and increased WOB, disease-specific findings may also be present; these are presented in greater details under the "Pulmonary Disorders" section later in this chapter.

The clinical symptoms of **respiratory failure,** if present, are an ominous sign of impending respiratory arrest (cessation of breathing) and present themselves from the worsening of tissue hypoxia and metabolic acidosis. Eventually there will be evidence of end-organ dysfunction and, without appropriate and aggressive management for the failing pulmonary system, the progression to arrest is rapid. Findings consistent with respiratory failure include:

★ Altered mental status (as appropriate for age)
★ Muscular hypotonia
★ Tachycardia giving way to bradycardia
★ Diminishment in systolic perfusion pressure
★ Pallor and eventual cyanosis
★ Loss of vesicular breath sounds
★ Irregular respirations

It is important to note that the etiology of respiratory compromise may not readily be available or even identifiable to transport personnel in all pediatric interactions. The goal in managing respiratory compromise is to identify a set of causes and treat the patient based on the most likely causes. (See Table 27–2.)

PULMONARY DISORDERS

Respiratory distress and failure may occur in the pediatric patient for a multitude reasons. (See Table 27–3.) These problems will result in either a primary respiratory condition—one that is caused by a direct deficiency in the airway—lung parenchyma, or thoracic bellows action—or through a secondary respiratory condition, which is a process in which the failure of the pulmonary

Table 27–2	Clinical Manifestations of Respiratory Failure and Imminent Respiratory Arrest
Physiologic Cause	**Clinical Manifestations**
These signs occur because the child is attempting to compensate for oxygen deficit and airway blockage. Oxygen supply is inadequate; behavior and vital signs reflect compensation and beginning hypoxia.	***Respiratory failure—Initial signs*** Restlessness Tachypnea Tachycardia Diaphoresis
The child attempts to use accessory muscles to assist oxygen intake; hypoxia persists and efforts now waste more oxygen than is obtained.	***Respiratory failure— Early decompensation*** Nasal flaring Retractions Grunting Wheezing Anxiety and irritability Mood changes Headache Hypertension Confusion
These signs occur because oxygen deficit is overwhelming and beyond spontaneous recovery. Cerebral oxygenation is dramatically affected; central nervous system changes are ominous.	***Imminent respiratory arrest— Severe hypoxia*** Dyspnea Bradycardia Cyanosis Stupor and coma

Table 27–3 | Clinical Manifestations of Apparent Life-Threatening Events

Etiology	Clinical Manifestations	Clinical Therapy
Functional or structural airway problem or immaturity	Apnea of 20 seconds or longer; accompanied by bradycardia or cyanosis	Cardiorespiratory monitoring, sleep study, pneumogram, sepsis workup
Aspiration as a result of dysfunctional swallowing or gastroesophageal reflux	Choking, coughing, cyanosis, vomiting	Barium swallow, esophageal pH probe
Cardiac problems	Tachycardia, tachypnea, dyspnea	Cardiorespiratory monitoring, electrocardiogram, echocardiogram, arterial blood gases
Drug toxicity or poisoning; maternal history of ingestion	Central nervous system depression, hypotonia	Serum magnesium level, toxicity screen
Environmental, thermoregulation problem	Lethargy, tachypnea, hypothermia or hyperthermia	Cardiorespiratory and temperature monitoring, environmental temperature level (ambient air temperature)
Impaired oxygenation, respiratory disease (pulmonary edema, atelectasis, pneumonia)	Cyanosis, tachypnea, respiratory distress, anemia, choking, coughing	Oximetry, chest radiograph, arterial blood gases, complete blood count, upper airway evaluation, sleep study, serum electrolytes
Acute infection (sepsis, meningitis, necrotising enterocolitis)	Feeding intolerance, lethargy, temperature instability	Complete blood count, cultures when appropriate, C-reactive protein, chest and abdominal radiographs
Intracranial pathology (intraventricular hemorrhage, ventricular dilation, CNS anomalies, meningitis)	Abnormal neurologic examination, seizures	Cranial ultrasound, computed tomography scan, electroencephalogram, magnetic resonance imaging, cerebrospinal fluid evaluation
Metabolic disorders	Jitteriness, poor feeding, lethargy, central nervous system depression or irritability, hypotonia	Serum electrolytes (potassium, sodium, chloride), glucose, calcium, arterial blood gases

Note: Modified from Theobald, K., Botwinski, C., Albanna, S., & McWilliam, P. (2000). Apnea of prematurity: Diagnosis, implications for care, and pharmacologic management, *Neonatal Network, 19*(6), 17–24; and Eichenwald, E., & Stark, A. (1992). Apnea of prematurity: Etiology and management. *Tufts University School of Medicine Reports on Neonatal Respiratory Diseases, 2*(1), 1–11.

system is due to a disease or disorder that has caused failure elsewhere in the body (CNS dysfunction, cardiovascular dysfunction, and so on).

CROUP (LARYNGOTRACHEOBRONCHITIS)

Croup (**laryngotracheobronchitis**) is a viral infection primarily found in children and is most common in children with a recent history of upper respiratory infections (URIs). Regarding the epidemiology of croup, it has an annual peak incidence of 50 new cases per 1,000 children during the second year of life and decreases substantially after the 6th year. Croup typically occurs in late fall and early winter, and if the diagnosis is made in children older than 6 years, it should arouse suspicion for an underlying anatomical abnormality. The recurrence rate for croup is 5%.

Since the narrowest portion of the pediatric airway is directly beyond the glottic opening, the distal airways may be directly affected by edema and fluid accumulation secondary to croup exacerbation. The typical presentation of croup includes respiratory distress findings as discussed earlier, along with croup's hallmark "barking cough," which may be accompanied by stridor and a low-grade fever. Historically, the critical care paramedic will find that the children have commonly

croup (laryngotracheobronchitis) *a viral pulmonary infection most common in children with a recent history of upper respiratory infections (URIs).*

The typical presentation of croup includes respiratory distress findings as discussed earlier, along with croup's hallmark "barking cough," which may be accompanied by stridor and a low-grade fever.

been sick for between 1 and 5 days before the onset of croup. The diagnosis of croup is made by observing physical findings coupled with a significant history of illness. (See Table 27–4.)

Although the typical presentation for epiglottitis is rapid onset of a fever, sore throat, and unwillingness to eat or drink (as will be discussed in the next section), the child with croup will have no difficulty in eating or drinking because the point of irritation is below the level of the glottis, and neither food nor fluid will cause direct irritation of the subglottic tissues.

Treatment of croup is aimed at preventing airway obstruction.

Treatment of croup is aimed at preventing airway obstruction. The first treatment step is the administration of oxygen and moisture, ideally humidified oxygen because it is better tolerated by the child. Another overriding goal of all critical care providers should be to promote and ensure an environment around the patient that leads the child to remain calm. Since differentiating between epiglottitis and croup may be difficult at times for the critical care paramedic, it is not recommended that an inspection of the child's airway be attempted in order to make a more definitive field impression. Suffice it to say that the majority of treatment for a patient with either croup or epiglottitis is similar enough that neither will be inappropriately managed if the transport team follows basic treatment procedures common to any type of clinical respiratory distress.

If the child is suspected of having croup, and is found to be acutely ill with humidified oxygen not effective in reducing airway edema, expedited transport to the receiving hospital must be initiated. The emergency management of croup, which may be initiated either prior to departing the ED or performed en route to the second destination, is the administration of racemic epinephrine. Racemic epinephrine works similarly to epinephrine in that it stimulates vascular constriction. Aerosolizing the epinephrine reduces swelling of airway tissues by vessel constriction in the edematous tissues. The greatest complication associated with racemic epinephrine is rebound swelling of the airways once the epinephrine has worn off. The risk for rebound swelling makes the utilization of steroids critically important in the croup patient who has received racemic epinephrine.

If the child does not respond to racemic epinephrine, the critical care paramedic must consider the need to protect the airway by endotracheal intubation. Intubating these children should be avoided unless all other options have been exhausted. Table 27–5 details the staging of croup severity.

Alternative therapies for this condition include the use of corticosteroids to reduce airway inflammation. Routine use of corticosteroids in the management of croup remains controversial; however, they are administered on occasion for severe or moderate croup. Dexamethasone has been shown effective in relieving the symptoms from mild or moderate croup. Additionally, the use of inhaled corticosteroids (especially budesonide), has been shown to be effective. Administration of nebulized budesonide has been shown to decrease croup symptoms substantially within 2–4 hours of administration when compared to nebulized saline.

■ Figure 27-6 The phrase "thumb sign" has been used to describe this enlargement of the epiglottis. Note the stiff, enlarged "thumb" sign in this lateral neck X-ray?

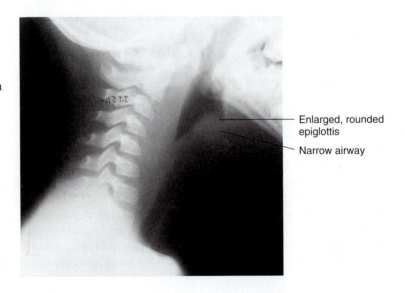

Enlarged, rounded epiglottis

Narrow airway

Table 27-4 | Summary of Croup Syndromes

	Viral Syndromes		Bacterial Syndromes	
	Acute Spasmodic Laryngitis (Spasmodic Croup)	Laryngotracheitis	Bacterial Tracheitis	Epiglottitis (Supraglottitis)
Severity	Least serious	Most common[a]	Laryngotracheo-bronchitis: Most serious; progresses if untreated	Guarded; requires close observation	Most life threatening (medical emergency)[a]
Age affected	3 months to 3 years	3 months to 8 years	3 months to 8 years	1 month to 13 years[a]	2 years to 8 years
Onset	Abrupt onset; peaks at night, resolves by morning (recurs)[a]	Gradual onset; starts as URI, progresses to moderate respiratory difficulty	Gradual onset; starts as URI, progresses to symptoms of respiratory distress	Progressive from URI (1–2 days)	Progresses rapidly (hours)[a]
Clinical manifestations	Afebrile; mild respiratory distress; barking-seal cough	*Early:* mild fever [<39.0 °C (102.2 °F)]; hoarseness; barking-seal, brassy, croupy cough; rhinorrhea; sore throat; stridor; apprehension (inspiratory) *Progressing to* labored respirations	*Early:* mild fever; [<39.0 °C (102.2 °F)]; barking-seal, brassy, croupy cough; rhinorrhea; sore throat; stridor (inspiratory); apprehension; restless/irritable *Progressing to* retractions (progressive); increasing stridor; cyanosis	High fever [>39.0 °C (102.2 °F)]; URI appears as viral croupy cough; croup initially; stridor (tracheal); purulent secretions	High fever [>39.0 °C (102.2 °F)]; URI; intense sore throat; dysphagia[a] drooling[a], increased pulse and respiratory rate; prefers upright position (tripod position with chin thrust)[a]
Etiology	Unknown; suspect viral with allergic/emotional influences	Parainfluenza, types I and II, RSV, or influenza	Parainfluenza, types I and II, RSV, or influenza	Staphylococcus	Haemophilus influenzae

[a] Classic parameter or key point (distinguishes condition).

Table 27–5	Croup Scale to Identify the Severity of Croup			
	Severity Score			
Signs	**0**	**1**	**2**	**3**
Stridor	None	Mild	Moderate at rest	Severe, on inspiration and expiration
Retractions	None	Mild	Suprasternal, intercostal	Severe, may see sternal retractions
Color	Normal	—	—	Dusky or cyanotic
Breath	Normal sounds	Mildy decreased	Moderately decreased	Markedly decreased
Level of consciousness	Normal	Restless when disturbed	Anxious, agitated	Lethargic

Scoring: To quantify the severity of croup, add the individual scores for each of the sign categories. A score between 0 and 15 is possible. The rating of mild, moderate, and severe is as follows: 4–5 is mild, 6–8 is moderate, >8 or any sign in the severe category is severe.

Note: Modified from Davis, H. W., Gartner, J. C., Galvis, A. G., Michaels, R. H., and Mestad, P. H. (1981). Acute upper airway obstruction: Croup and epiglottitis. *Pediatric Clinics of North America, 28*(4), 859–880.

EPIGLOTTITIS

epiglottitis *an acute, severe, life-threatening disease characterized by inflammation and edema of the epiglottis and surrounding connected tissues.*

Epiglottitis is an acute, severe, life-threatening disease of the upper airway. (See Figure 27-6 ■.) The epiglottis and the structures connected to or immediately surrounding it become inflamed and edematous, leading to a compromised airway at the level of the epiglottis and resultant respiratory compromise.

Epiglottitis has been predominantly referred to as a disease of children ages 2–7; this is not necessarily the case anymore. There has been vast progress in the reduction of epiglottitis since the mid-1980s, and this is primarily attributed to the introduction of the Hib (*Haemophilus influenzae* type B) vaccine. Recent epidemiological studies show a decreased incidence in children from 3.47 cases per 100,000 people in 1980 to 0.63 cases per 100,000 people in 1990. Since the majority of epiglottitis cases have been caused by Hib, as a result of the Hib vaccine, epiglottitis is being seen more in young adults than in children.

The typical presentation for epiglottitis is rapid onset of a fever that may or may not be accompanied by a sore throat. The child will likely refuse to eat or drink because of the irritation this may cause, and will eventually be unable to tolerate his own secretions, which leads to the characteristic drooling seen in these patients. The child may also develop signs of upper airway obstruction with inspiratory stridor and some degree of respiratory compromise. The older child will tend to remain in a sitting position with his neck extended in a sniffing position. This position is maintained to assist the child in optimizing the amount of open airway. This child will typically avoid coughing, because this further irritates the inflamed tissue.

Treatment of epiglottitis is focused on preventing airway obstruction.

Treatment of epiglottitis is focused on preventing airway obstruction. The first treatment step is the administration of high-flow, high-concentration oxygen through a blow-by mask, as tolerated by the child. As with the croup patient, the maintenance of a calm and quiet environment will lead the child to remain calm and lessen the respiratory distress burden. Finally, there is absolutely no need to force an inspection of the child's airway as long as he is adequately exchanging air, thus it should not be attempted. Attempting oral intubation in a child with epiglottitis is only warranted in those extreme cases of respiratory occlusion from the edema to the airway structures. (Orotracheal intubation commonly fails in these patients, and the stimulation created by the failed intubation attempt usually results in a worsening of the glottic edema.)

If the child continues to clinically deteriorate and ultimately requires assisted ventilations with a bag-valve-mask device, remember to use a slow ventilation sequence. If this is not effective in ventilating the child, the critical care provider will face a situation of complete airway obstruction at the level of the epiglottis and will then need to consider a needle or surgical cricothyrotomy. With severe cases, intubation may need to be performed in the hospital where brochoscopy is readily available.

Antibiotic therapy is necessary but should be initiated after securing the airway. Prior to receiving culture results, use antibiotics covering the most likely organisms. Following trauma to the epiglottis, *Staphylococcus aureus* should be suspected. With the presence of white patches, *Candida albicans* should be suspected. Antibiotics such as ceftriaxone, cefuroxime, and ampicillin have been used with success.

ASTHMA

In the year 2000, there were 14 million people with asthma, of which 4.8 million were under 18 years of age. A more astounding and disturbing statistic than this is that from 1983 to 1996, the adverse outcomes and deaths related to asthma have tripled. In 2003, asthma in children accounted for a loss of 12.8 million school days annually.

Asthma is a long-term inflammatory process that targets the lower airways. (See Figure 27-7 .) The causes of asthma may be intrinsic or extrinsic. Regardless, the end result is bronchial narrowing from edema and inflammation of the bronchiole wall. This is complicated by increased mucus production and plugging which further reduce the diameter of the airway lumen.

The narrowing of the airway diameter is further complicated by bronchiole spasms (also referred to as bronchoconstriction or bronchospasms). All bronchial airways are wrapped with smooth muscle capable of contraction and relaxation. These tiny muscles respond to local triggers and to a variety of substances that can be inhaled. This is important because it explains the mechanics of bronchospasms and the therapy utilized to treat wheezing. This constriction contributes to the increased airway resistance through the bronchioles and translates into a greater work of breathing. As the bronchiole smooth muscle contracts and the airways are narrowed, air moves forcefully and more turbulently through the tiny passages, and that process produces the wheezing that is heard through the stethoscope. (See Table 27–6.)

Treatment of asthma is focused on reversing bronchospasm, correcting hypoxia, airway inflammation, and reducing the amount of mucous plugging the bronchiole airways. Asthma is a disease of ventilation, so asthma patients will not become hypoxic until ventilation has been severely compromised. (See Table 27–7.) Many patients describe symptomatic improvement with supplemental oxygen, so an initial treatment step is the administration of oxygen. Most patients will benefit from oxygen administered by cannula, but if the pulse oximeter reading is below 92%, the patient is still displaying significant pulmonary dysfunction, so oxygen would be administered at 100% by nonrebreather mask. Note, however, that oxygen will work to correct the hypoxia, but it will not reverse bronchospasm or inflammation. To alleviate these symptoms, inhaled beta-agonists and/or anticholinergics should be used. Nonspecific alpha- and beta-agonists may also be administered by subcutaneous injection, particularly for those patients in severe distress at presentation who may not have a deep enough tidal volume to inhale the medications for topical absorption on the bronchiole smooth muscle. The use of subcutaneous treatment may promote initial bronchodilation, particularly in the pediatric patient, and therefore make inhalation treatments with beta-agonists even more effective. Corticosteroids may also be used to help decrease inflammation within the airways after the acute bronchospasm has been relieved, but since they may take several hours to begin working, they should not be viewed as an emergent airway treatment modality. Common medications used for an acute asthma exacerbation include the following:

Beta-Agonists

★ Albuterol (Proventil, Ventolin)

★ Levalbuterol (Xopenex)

★ Metaproterenol (Alupent)

★ Terbutaline (Brethine)

★ Epinephrine

★ Isoproterenol (Isuprel)

Corticosteroids

★ Methylprednisolone (Solu-Medrol)

★ Dexamethasone (Decadron)

★ Hydrocortisone Sodium (Solu-Cortef)

The end result from asthma is inflammation of the bronchiole wall that is complicated by increased mucous production, which causes an acute narrowing of the airway lumen.

Methylxanthines

★ Aminophylline

Anticholinergics

★ Ipratropium (Atrovent)

★ Atropine

■ **Figure 27-7** What can cause an asthma attack? Some asthma triggers are exercise, infection, and allergies. Shown is how asthma obstructs airflow through constriction and narrowing of the airway along with increased production of mucus.

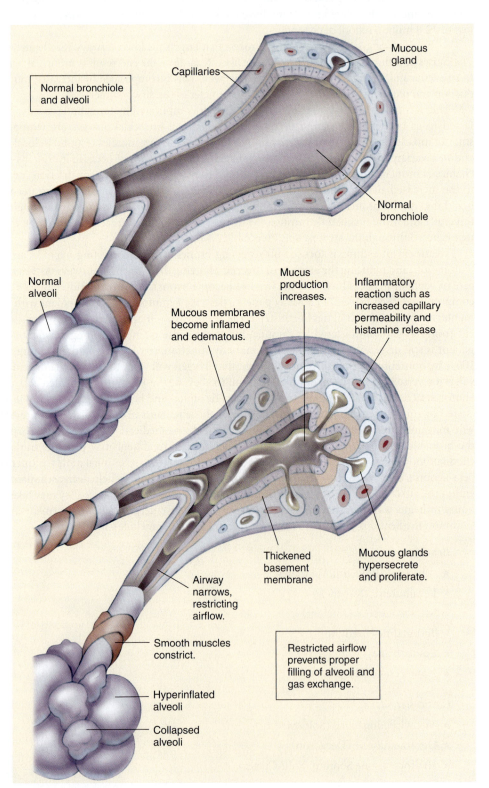

Normal bronchiole and alveoli

Capillaries

Mucous gland

Normal bronchiole

Normal alveoli

Mucous membranes become inflamed and edematous.

Mucus production increases.

Inflammatory reaction such as increased capillary permeability and histamine release

Thickened basement membrane

Mucous glands hypersecrete and proliferate.

Airway narrows, restricting airflow.

Smooth muscles constrict.

Restricted airflow prevents proper filling of alveoli and gas exchange.

Hyperinflated alveoli

Collapsed alveoli

Table 27–6 — Clinical Manifestations of Asthma in Children by Severity of Acute Exacerbations

Assessment Criteria	Mild	Moderate	Severe
PEFR[a]	70%–90% predicted or personal best	50%–70% predicted or personal best	<50% predicted or personal best
Respiratory rate, resting or sleeping	Normal to 30% increase above the mean	30%–50% increase above mean	Increase over 50% above mean
Alertness	Normal	Normal	May be decreased
Dyspnea[b]	Absent or mild; speaks in complete sentences	Moderate; speaks in phrases or partial sentences; infant's cry softer and shorter; has difficulty sucking and feeding	Severe; speaks only in single words or short phrases; infant's cry softer and shorter; stops sucking and feeding
Pulsus paradoxus[c]	<100 mmHg	10–20 mm Hg	20–40 mmHg
Accessory muscle use	No intercostal to mild retractions	Moderate intercostal retractions with tracheosternal retractions; use of sternocleidomastoid muscles; chest hyperinflation	Severe intercostal retractions, tracheosternal retractions with nasal flaring during inspiration; chest hyperinflation
Color	Good	Pale	Possibly cyanotic
Auscultation	End-expiratory wheeze only	Wheeze during entire expiration and inspiration	Breath sounds becoming inaudible
Oxygen saturation	>95%	90%–95%	<90%
P_{CO_2}	<35	<40	>40

Note: Within each category, the presence of several parameters, but not necessarily all, indicate the general classification of the exacerbation.
[a] For children 5 years of age or older.
[b] Parents or physicians' impressions of degree of children's breathlessness.
[c] Pulsus paradoxus does not correlate with phase of respiration in small children.
Note: From National Asthma Education and Prevention Program. (1994) *Acute exacerbations of asthma: Care in a hospital-based emergency department* (p. 13). Bethesda, MD: National Heart, Lung, and Blood Institute, National Institutes of Health.

In severe cases, those in which it is difficult to break the bronchospasms, the need to artificially ventilate and intubate may become necessary. The concern with this is that the continued bronchospasms result in air trapping because the body cannot force the air out (exhale) as efficiently as the inspiratory effort. The provision of positive-pressure ventilation will worsen this and promote continued air trapping and carbon dioxide accumulation. Although there is no real way to get around this, it must be stressed that for the child in severe respiratory distress, it is imperative that aggressive therapy be initiated to prevent having to get to the point where intubation and ventilation become necessary. Finally, rehydration of the severe asthmatic patient will correct any dehydration present as well as contribute to expectoration by hydrating the mucous plugs in the smaller airways.

Treatment of asthma is focused on reversing bronchospasm, correcting hypoxia, and treating airway inflammation.

BRONCHIOLITIS

Bronchiolitis is an acute infectious process of the lower respiratory tract common in children under 24 months of age. Bronchiolitis typically occurs in children between 2 and 24 months in age, and is most commonly caused by a virus. Annual incidence is 11.4% in children younger than 1 year and 6% in those ages 1–2 years. The illness accounts for 4,500 deaths and 90,000 hospital admissions per year. Prevalence may be higher in urban areas. In children 2 years old, approximately 95% have serologic evidence of past infection with the predominant causative agent, **respiratory syncytial virus (RSV)**.

Symptoms of bronchiolitis include a fever, tachycardia and/or tachypnea, shortness of breath, chest tightness, wheezing, and coughing. Just like the older child who suffers inflammation of the lower airways, the bronchiolitis patient will experience increased production of mucus and an acute narrowing of the airways through inflammation of bronchiole tissue and clogging of the airway with infectious by-products.

bronchiolitis *an acute infectious process of the lower respiratory tract common in children under 24 months of age; most often attributed to respiratory syncytial virus or Mycoplasma pneumoniae.*

respiratory syncytial virus (RSV) *a highly contagious subgroup of myxoviruses that are the predominant causative agent for bronchial infections in children.*

Table 27-7 | Revised Asthma Severity Classification

Classification (Steps)	Description	Clinical Therapy
Step 1: Mild intermittent	Brief exacerbations with symptoms no more often than twice a week. Nighttime symptoms less than twice a week. PEFR ≥80% of predicted with variability <20%.	Quick relief bronchodilator as needed. If needed more than twice a week, move to next level.
Step 2: Mild persistent	Exacerbations more than twice a week, but less than once a day. May affect activity. PEFR ≥80% of predicted.	Daily anti-inflammatory medication. Quick relief bronchodilator as needed.
Step 3: Moderate persistent	Daily symptoms. Daily use of inhaled short-acting beta-agonist. Exacerbations at least twice a week that may last for days; nighttime symptoms more than once per week. Affects activity. PEFR >60% but <80% of predicted with variability >30%.	Daily anti-inflammatory medication, medium dose. Bronchodilator as needed up to three times a day.
Step 4: Severe persistent	Continuous symptoms, limited physical activity. Frequent exacerbations and frequent nighttime symptoms. PEFR ≤60% of predicted with variability >30%.	Daily anti-inflammatory medication, high dose. Systemic corticosteroid. Bronchodilator as needed for symptoms up to three times a day.

Note: From National Asthma Education and Prevention Program, (1997). *Expert panel report II: Guidelines for the diagnosis and management of asthma* (NIH Publication No. 97-4051, pp. 45–48). Bethesda, MD: National Institutes of Health.

The bronchiolitis patient will typically present in the same way the asthma patient does, with a few variations. The major differences are that the bronchiolitis patient will likely have a fever and a relatively slow onset of symptoms. The findings of general respiratory distress, as discussed earlier, will be present. Just as the physical assessment is key to determining the degree of respiratory distress present, gathering a thorough history from the primary care provider will help point the field impression to that of bronchiolitis.

Treatment of bronchiolitis is focused on correcting hypoxia, reversing bronchospasm, treating airway inflammation, and, if possible, identifying and treating the causative pathogen. The first treatment step is the administration of high-flow, high-concentration oxygen by mask. Oxygen will work to correct the hypoxia but will not correct the bronchospasm or inflammation. To alleviate these symptoms, inhaled beta-agonists are used, however their use is controversial. These agents relieve reversible bronchospasm by relaxing smooth muscles of the bronchi. Meta-analyses of clinical studies show little benefit from treatment with inhaled beta-adrenergic agents (with or without ipratropium bromide). Drugs and dosages are the same as those for asthma. Nebulized epinephrine may occasionally be useful. Although often used, the majority of clinical trials have demonstrated that corticosteroids have no benefit in the treatment of bronchiolitis. Because RSV is the most often implicated cause, the critical care paramedic may find the patient to be receiving ribavirin. This drug is used for inpatients who have, or who are at high risk for, severe RSV infection.

The decision to assist ventilations to prevent respiratory failure is pivotal to the overall outcome of the child. While a more conservative approach to invasive airway management is preferred for reasons discussed earlier, in the infant with RSV, periods of apnea are not uncommon so endotracheal intubation may be necessary.

Treatment of bronchiolitis is focused on correcting hypoxia, reversing bronchospasm, treating airway inflammation, and, if possible, identifying and treating the causative pathogen.

FOREIGN BODY AIRWAY OBSTRUCTION (FBAO)

According to the National Safety Council, a total of 3,200 deaths (1.2 per 100,000 people per year) from airway obstruction caused by unintentional ingestion or inhalation of food or other objects occurred in the United States in 1998. Children younger than 4 years had the highest mortality rate at 0.7 per 100,000 people per year. The overall risk of death from foreign body aspiration is estimated to be 0.66 per 100,000 people per year. Even if the patient does not succumb, symptoms develop immediately. Morbidity increases if extraction of the object is delayed beyond 24 hours.

Airway obstruction is a true medical emergency. If immediate steps are not taken to clear a patient's airway, he will surely die. Identifying and clearing an airway obstruction takes precedence over any other emergent treatment. To put it simply, failure to maintain a patent airway will doom all other efforts to failure.

Remember that clinically, the patient with a complete airway obstruction will be unable to breath, talk, or cough. The first phase of managing an FBAO is the implementation of basic airway maneuvers such as back blows and chest thrusts in infants and the Heimlich maneuver in older children. If the foreign body is expelled from the airway at any time, the critical care provider should (if it is visible) remove the object from the victims mouth. As has been taught several times over, it is imperative that a blind finger sweep not be performed on the pediatric airway because inserting a finger into the posterior pharynx may lodge the object further into the airway or cause soft-tissue trauma with resultant hemorrhage. If basic maneuvers do not work to dislodge the obstruction, several advanced level interventions may be employed.

Advanced interventions that may be successful in the pediatric patient with an obstructed airway include direct laryngoscopy of the airway to visualize the obstruction and, if it is visible, removal of the obstruction with Magill forceps. If after laryngoscopy, the airway is not open or the obstruction is not visible, the next step would be to attempt to insert an ET tube through the vocal cords in hopes that the foreign body would move down into one of the mainstem bronchi. If the foreign body does move (usually into the right mainstem bronchi), the left bronchus will be opened and the patient may be ventilated through it. This will allow for the emergent exchange of gases and oxygenation of the tissues. This maneuver will not always work and, as a result, the critical care provider may need to consider a surgical cricothyrotomy. A needle cricothyrotomy could be considered also, but the drawback of only providing oxygenation with this technique without adequate ventilation leaves it less desirable in the critical care setting.

HYPOPERFUSION SYNDROMES

As with the adult, but more significantly, pulmonary performance is inextricably linked to the proper functioning of the cardiovascular system. A cardiovascular deficiency that results in a hypoperfusive state (as discussed later) can result in the development of secondary respiratory failure. Chronic cardiac conditions also stress the body, which causes the body to be less tolerant of mild pulmonary illnesses and encourages development of primary respiratory failure. Other conditions beyond that of cardiac, such as acidosis, sepsis, anemia, heat emergencies, and certain toxins, can precipitate respiratory failure.

As with the adult, but more significantly, pulmonary performance is inextricably linked to the proper functioning of the cardiovascular system.

NONDISTRIBUTIVE SHOCK

In **nondistributive shock,** circulating volume is lost and the primary problem is a lack of fluid within the vascular space. This can be seen with hypovolemic and hemorrhagic shock syndromes, as well as with fluid loss from excessive vomiting or diarrhea. The dilemma in nondistributive shock is that the pump eventually is unable to efficiently maintain an adequate forward flow of blood through the vasculature due to volume loss and massive sympathetic mediated vasoconstriction. Because volume is the issue, management must be geared toward the replenishment of this lost volume (through isotonic crystalloids or blood products, as appropriate).

nondistributive shock *also known as hypovolemic or hemorrhagic shock, the circulating volume is diminished or lost from within the vascular space.*

distributive shock *characterized by the body's inability to maintain cardiovascular tone; results in a deficit of oxygenated perfusion throughout the body.*

DISTRIBUTIVE SHOCK

In **distributive shock,** pediatric patients, like adult patients, may have sufficient amounts of volume and an effective myocardial pump, but lack the ability to allow good perfusion pressures due to the body's inability to regulate vascular tone. The end result is an insufficient pressure gradient between the left ventricular ejection and the vascular system. Without an appropriate pressure gradient, there is nothing to allow the blood within the vessels to move forward as the heart ejects another stroke volume into the aortic root. The result is, again, inadequate tissue perfusion. Etiologies of distributive shock include anaphylaxis, sepsis, and neurogenic shock. The goal then for this condition is the careful induction of vasoconstriction via the use of sympathomimetic drugs with alpha stimulatory properties as supportive therapy until the offending mechanism (sepsis, anaphylaxis, and so on) can be eliminated and the body can again control its arterial tone.

CARDIOGENIC SHOCK

cardiogenic shock
characterized by the heart's inability to eject an adequate stroke volume, resulting in relative hypovolemia, and compromised oxygenation.

The third form of hypoperfusion that may be seen by the critical care transport team is cardiogenic shock. In **cardiogenic shock,** the culprit of inadequate blood flow is the heart itself. In this form of shock, the body has an adequate volume with a normal control of vasculature tone, but despite the normality of these two components, the heart simply cannot eject an adequate stroke volume. In the pediatric patient, cardiogenic shock will likely be caused by some form of cardiac injury that prevents/damages cardiac muscle contraction or secondary to significant cardiac dysrhythmias. Finally, there may be an as-yet undiagnosed cardiac defect that has remained subclinical due to the ability of the heart and/or the vascular system to compensate. Conditions such as undiagnosed aortic stenosis or ventricular septal defects may not present acutely in a neonate, but as the child matures and the demands of the heart become greater, they may then become clinically evident. With these situations there is usually a history of unusual fatigability at this young age, exertional dyspnea, and potential syncope or postural syncope. There may also be a history of congestive heart failure (CHF), tachypnea, respiratory distress, or lethargy. On closer examination at this time, it is not uncommon to find cardiomegaly and increased pulmonary vascular markings on chest X-rays, and an ECG that demonstrates ventricular hypertrophy. The management of the pediatric patient at this stage is to maintain oxygenation and create an optimal environment for the myocardium to pump blood with careful use of fluids and inotropic agents. These patients, as seen by the critical care paramedic, are probably being transported to specialty pediatric hospitals with the surgical capability to correct these newly diagnosed cardiac defects.

OBSTRUCTIVE SHOCK

obstructive shock
characterized by the body's inability to pump blood due to some form of mechanical obstruction or compression to the heart.

Obstructive shock is most commonly caused by a traumatic mechanism and includes specific etiologies such as cardiac tamponade, tension pneumothorax, or a pulmonary embolism. The etiology behind this type of shock is somewhat dependent on the mechanism, but each has the salient characteristic of an inability to pump blood due to some form of mechanical obstruction or compression to the heart. For example, cardiac tamponade and tension pneumothoracies both result in excessive mechanical compression of the heart, which inhibits the heart's ability to accept an adequate preload. With a pulmonary embolism, the pulmonary vasculature is obstructed to such a degree that the right ventricle fails in its job to perfuse the lungs and provide adequate preload to the left side of the heart. The management for obstructive mechanisms usually involves the correction of the initial defect causing the obstruction (i.e., decompression or pericardiocentesis). These traumatic mechanisms and their appropriate management are defined in better detail in Chapter 22.

In summarizing the etiologies of pediatric hypoperfusion, the critical care team must remember that the overriding goal is to provide maximum oxygenation to a patient in circulatory compromise, and also to create the most favorable environment for the heart to pump blood effectively within. The etiology for circulatory compromise needs to be identified and the specific dysfunction must usually be corrected first in order for the perfusion to return to pre-event levels. (See Tables 27–8 and 27–9.)

SEPSIS

Sepsis is a life-threatening infection of the bloodstream resulting in systemic toxicity.

Sepsis is a life-threatening infection of the bloodstream resulting in systemic toxicity. In the pediatric patient, the presentation of sepsis is typically subtle and may be difficult to distinguish from a noninfectious pathology. In addition, the primary site of infection may often be difficult to identify in the septic patient. As sepsis progresses, hypoperfusion may develop as a result of the release of

Table 27–8 | Drugs Used in Pediatric Advanced Life Support*

Drug	Dose	Remarks
Adenosine	0.1–0.2 mg/kg Maximum strength dose 12 mg	Rapid IV bolus
Amiodarone	5 mg/kg IV/IO	Rapid IV bolus
Atropine sulfate	0.02 mg/kg per dose	Minimum dose 0.1 mg Maximum single dose: 0.5 mg in child; 1.0 mg in adolescent
Calcium chloride 10 percent	20 mg/kg per dose	Give slowly
Dopamine hydrochloride	2–10 mcg/kg per minute	Adrenergic action dominates at ≥15–20 mcg/kg per minute
Epinephrine *for bradycardia*	IV/IO 0.01 mg/kg (1:10,000) ET: 0.1 mg/kg (1:1,000)	Be aware of effective dose of preservatives administered (if preservatives are present in epinephrine preparation) when high doses are used
for asystolic or pulseless arrest	*First dose:* IV/IO: 0.01 mg/kg (1:10,000) ET: 0.1 mg/kg (1:1,1000) Doses as high as 0.2 mg/kg may be effective *Subsequent doses:* IV/IO/ET: 0.1 mg/kg (1:1,000) Doses as high as 0.2 mg/kg may be effective	Be aware of effective dose of preservatives administered (if preservatives are present in epinephrine preparation) when high doses are used
Epinephrine infusion	Initial at 0.1 mcg/kg per minute Higher infusion dose used if asystole present	Titrate to desired effect (0.1–1.0 mcg/kg per minute)
Lidocaine	1 mg/kg per dose	Rapid bolus
Lidocaine infusion	20–50 mcg/kg per minute	
Sodium bicarbonate	1 mEq/kg per dose or 0.3 × kg × base deficit	Infuse slowly and only if ventilation is adequate

*IV indicates intravenous route; IO, intraosseous route; ET, endotracheal route.

Table 27–9 | Preparation of Infusions

Drug	Preparation*	Dose
Epinephrine	0.6 × body weight (kg) equals milligrams added to diluent† to make 100 mL	Then 1 mL/hr delivers 0.1 mcg/kg per minute; titrate to effect
Dopamine/dobutamine	0.6 × body weight (kg) equals milligrams added to diluent† to make 100 mL	Then 1 mL/hr delivers 0.3 mcg/kg per minute; titrate to effect
Lidocaine	120 mg of 40 mg/mL solution added to 97 mL of 5 percent dextrose in water, yielding 1200 mcg/mL solution	Then 1 mL/kg per hour delivers 20 mcg/kg per minute

*Standard concentration may be used to provide more dilute or more concentrated drug solution, but then individual dose must be calculated for each patient and each infusion rate:

$$\text{Infusion Rate (mL/h)} = \frac{\text{Weight (kg)} \times \text{Dose (mcg/kg/min)} \times 60 \text{ min/h}}{\text{Concentration (mcg/mL)}}$$

† Diluent may be 5 percent dextrose in water, 5 percent dextrose in half-normal, normal saline, or Ringer's lactate.

bacterial endotoxins causing dilation of the vasculature. The dilation of the blood vessels is so significant that the body cannot create an adequate pressure gradient to fill the vascular space and hypoperfusion ensues.

During the early phases of pediatric sepsis, common clinical signs include respiratory distress, pulmonary hypertension, hypoxemia, severe shock, and disseminated intravascular coagulation (DIC). Although rare, meningitis may also occur as the infection spreads.

Treatment of sepsis is generally centered on antibiotic therapy and pressure support. Pediatric patients have immature renal and hepatic systems and, as a result, the administration of antibiotics should be done judiciously and with regard for potential complications related to drug clearance. Sepsis that is refractory to antibiotic therapy may be caused by a virus rather than bacteria. If the sepsis is related to a virus, central nervous system and hepatic function will most likely be compromised.

DROWNING AND NEAR-DROWNING

More than 1,500 children die in the United States each year from drowning. For every drowning death in this country, an estimated 4 additional hospitalizations and 14 emergency department visits are due to submersion injuries. Approximately 1 in 8 males and 1 in 23 females experience some form of water-associated accident but are saved and never seek medical attention.

When describing the age of pediatric patients who drown versus those who experience a near-drowning, two age brackets emerge. Children younger than 4 years and adolescents ages 15–19 years are at highest risk for drowning. This occurs predominantly in males (as mentioned earlier), who have a much higher incidence of submersion injuries during adolescence than females. The location of injury also differs between these two groups. Most toddlers drown in swimming pools and bathtubs, whereas most adolescents drown in natural bodies of water.

While more of a traumatic event than a medical complaint, drowning is classified as death within 24 hours of submersion, whereas near-drowning is recognized as submersion with greater than 24-hour survival time, regardless of long-term survival.

When involuntarily immersed in water and/or unable to surface, a child will experience extreme panic, hold her breath, and struggle for air. When the child is no longer capable of holding her breath, she may gasp and aspirate fluid into the lungs. If a significant amount of fluid enters the lungs, the resulting death is referred to as a wet drowning, which accounts for the majority of all pediatric drownings.

A dry drowning occurs when laryngospasm occurs as a protective reflex, and prevents fluids from entering the lungs. Although this laryngospasm may prevent fluids from entering the lungs, cellular hypoxia is sustained. If this spasm persists throughout the event, the resulting death is referred to as a dry drowning.

Management for this emergency follows traditional recommendations for airway, breathing, and circulatory support. First, if a concern exists about cervical or spinal trauma, all procedures must be performed with cervical-spinal precautions taken. Constantly monitor for vomiting, and suction the airway as necessary. The airway should be secured with endotracheal intubation should the gag reflex be absent, and initiation of positive-pressure ventilation with high-flow, high-concentration oxygen implemented as needed. Assess for a central and peripheral pulse; in their absence institute cardiopulmonary resuscitation. Remember to be diligent with pediatric patients with suspected or diagnosed drops in core temperature; they may still be resuscitatable once the core temperature is elevated. If the pediatric is not in arrest, support any lost function of airway, breathing, oxygenation, or hemodynamics as needed during transport.

Congenital anomalies, many of which are cardiac in origin, are the number one cause of death in children less than a year of age.

CONGENITAL HEART DISEASE

Congenital anomalies, many of which are cardiac in origin, are the number one cause of death in children less than a year of age. Incidence of congenital heart disease (CHD) has been reported as 2–10 per 1,000 live births. Although the mortality rate resulting from CHD has been decreasing because of improved surgical repair techniques, CHD remains the leading cause of death in all congenital defects.

Many types of congenital anomalies exist. These may affect a single organ or structure or may affect many organs or structures. Congenital anomalies are the leading cause of death in infants—causing approximately one-quarter of infant deaths. Several recognized patterns, called *syndromes*, occur. It is not within the scope of this text to discuss all of the various congenital anomalies. However, there are a few congenital anomalies that may make resuscitation of the neonate more difficult. Among the congenital anomalies encountered, congenital heart defects are among the most common. The cause of these is largely unknown. **Congenital heart defects** are often classified by whether or not they increase pulmonary blood flow, decrease pulmonary blood flow, or obstruct blood flow.

Some congenital heart problems result in increased pulmonary blood flow. These include cases where the *ductus arteriosus* fails to close—a condition referred to as *patent ductus arteriosus* (also called *persistent ductus arteriosus*). (See Figure 27-8 ■.) Also, *septal defects* (a hole between the atria or the ventricles) can result in increased pulmonary blood flow. With an *atrial septal defect* there is a hole between the atria that allows the comixing of blood. (See Figure 27-9 ■.) With a *ventricular septal defect*, there is a hole between the two ventricles that allows comixing of blood. (See Figure 27-10 ■.) An increase in pulmonary blood flow can lead to congestive heart failure.

Other congenital anomalies can lead to decreased pulmonary blood flow, thus decreasing the ability of the lungs to oxygenate the blood. These include *tetralogy of Fallot*, which is a combination of four congenital conditions. (See Figure 27-11 ■.) In addition, a condition called *transposition of the great vessels* can occur whereby normal outflow tracts of the right and left ventricles are switched. (See Figure 27-12 ■.)

Finally, some congenital anomalies can result in obstruction of blood flow. Causes of blood flow obstruction include *coarctation of the aorta* (see Figure 27-13 ■); *aortic*, or *mitral* (*tricuspid*) or *pulmonary stenosis/atresia* (see Figures 27-14 ■ through 27-18 ■); and *hypoplastic left heart syndrome* (see Figure 27-19 ■.) With *coarctation of the aorta*, the aorta is narrowed in the arch of the aorta, thus obstructing blood flow. Problems with either the mitral or aortic valve can cause blood flow obstruction—a condition called *mitral* or *aortic stenosis*. With *hypoplastic left heart syndrome*, the left side of the heart is underdeveloped—a condition that is usually fatal by 1 month of age if untreated.

Some noncardiac congenital anomalies are of note. For example, some children may be born with a defect in the diaphragm that allows some of the abdominal contents to enter the chest through the defect. This abnormality is referred to as a *diaphragmatic hernia*. If you suspect a diaphragmatic hernia, do not treat the infant with bag-valve-mask ventilation. This procedure will cause stomach distention, which protrudes into the chest cavity, thus decreasing ventilatory capacity. Instead, immediately intubate the infant.

congenital heart defects
congenital abnormalities of the heart, often classified by increased pulmonary blood flow (PDA, ASD), decreased pulmonary blood flow (tetralogy of Fallot), or obstructed blood flow (coarctation of the aorta, aortic, or mitral (tricuspid) or pulmonary stenosis/atresia, and hypoplastic left heart syndrome).

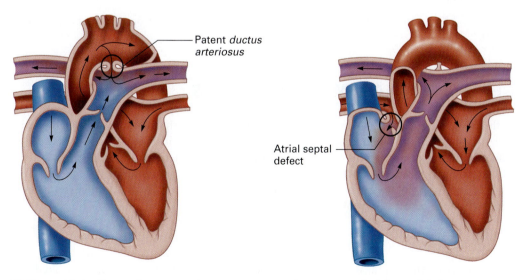

■ **Figure 27-8**   Patent ductus arteriosus.

■ **Figure 27-9**   Atrial septal defect.

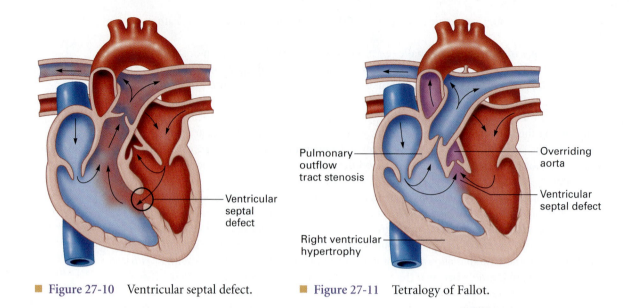

■ **Figure 27-10**   Ventricular septal defect.

■ **Figure 27-11**   Tetralogy of Fallot.

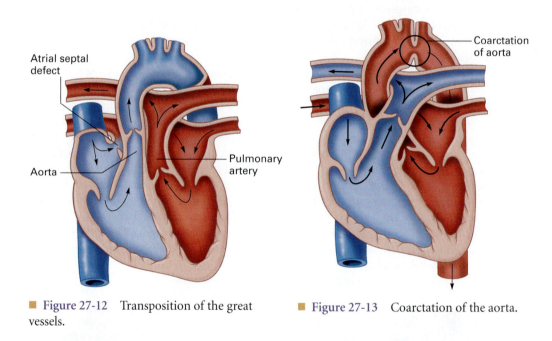

■ **Figure 27-12**   Transposition of the great vessels.

■ **Figure 27-13**   Coarctation of the aorta.

GENERAL MANAGEMENT CONCERNS

To this point, each subsection of the medical problems common to the transport of critically ill children have included basic management principles with which the critical care paramedic should be familiar. The following section identifies some additional concerns about pediatric management that would be applicable to all of the aforementioned medical conditions. The critical care paramedic should incorporate the following discussions into the general care interventions whenever responsible for a pediatric patient.

AIRWAY

Airway management is of the utmost importance in the pediatric patient and must be secured and maintained as early as possible. Rapid-sequence induction (RSI) as discussed in the airway chapter is a common practice in the critical care transport environment and should be considered as the

Airway management is of the utmost importance in the pediatric patient and must be secured and maintained as early as possible.

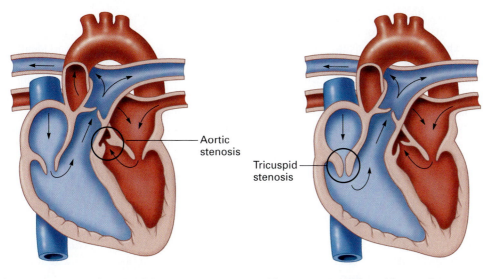

■ **Figure 27-14** Aortic stenosis.

Aortic stenosis

■ **Figure 27-15** Tricuspid stenosis.

Tricuspid stenosis

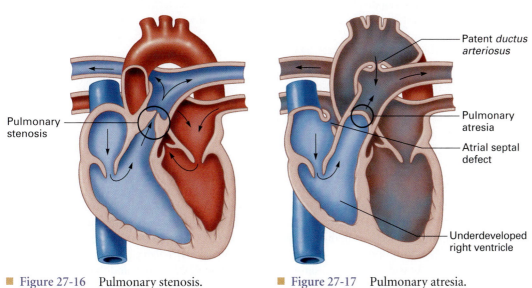

■ **Figure 27-16** Pulmonary stenosis.

Pulmonary stenosis

■ **Figure 27-17** Pulmonary atresia.

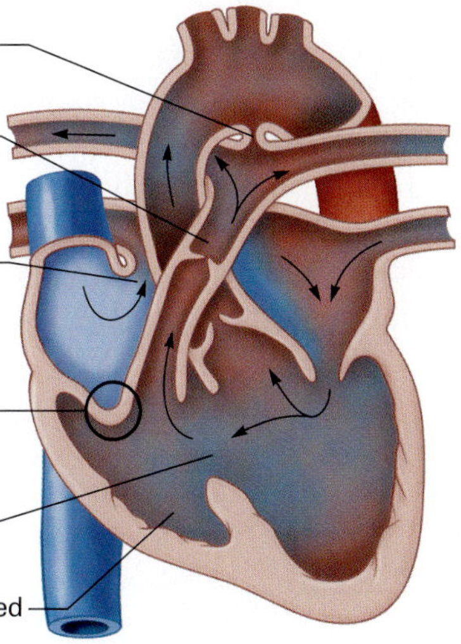

Patent *ductus arteriosus*

Pulmonary atresia

Atrial septal defect

Underdeveloped right ventricle

Patent *ductus arteriosis*

Hypoplastic pulmonary artery

Atrial septal defect

Tricuspid atresia

Ventricular septal defect

Underdeveloped right ventricle

■ **Figure 27-18** Tricuspid atresia.

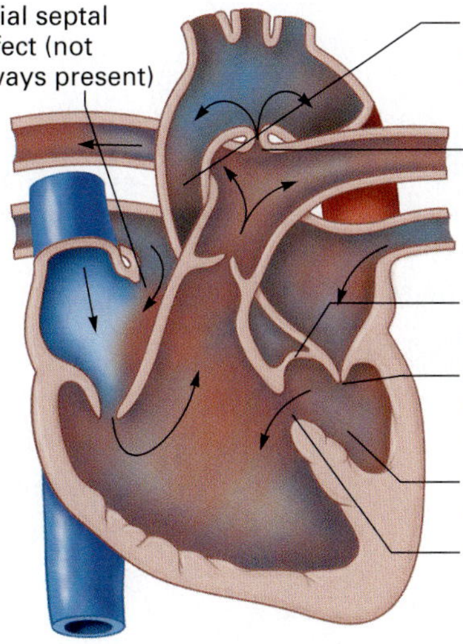

Atrial septal defect (not always present)

Hypoplastic ascending aorta

Patent *ductus arteriosis* (beginning to close)

Aortic valve atresia

Mitral atresia (may be present)

Hypoplastic left ventricle

Ventricular septal defect

■ **Figure 27-19** Hypoplastic left heart.

optimal method for securing an airway in a child who has an intact gag reflex but is unable to meet the ventilatory needs of the body.

The single most frequent respiratory complication in the pediatric patient is accidental extubation. Properly securing an ET tube is necessary, but will not guarantee that the tube will not become accidentally dislodged during patient movement or during other care interventions. In addition to standard tube securing measures once the tube is placed, the use of sedatives and paralytics may be helpful. Using a lateral restraint on the pediatric patient's head will minimize the mobility of the airway and thus also reduce the risk of accidental extubation. Lateral restraint can be accomplished in the same manner that traumatic cervical-spine restraint is employed.

Regarding the RSI process, common intubation and ventilation equipment, and the use of pharmacologic agents as sedatives, please refer to Tables 27–10 through 27–12.

VASCULAR ACCESS

Venous access should be of paramount concern in managing the critically ill pediatric patient. Due to the small anatomical size of the vasculature, obtaining access can be very difficult for even the most skilled health care provider.

Venous access should be of paramount concern in managing the critically ill pediatric patient. Due to the small anatomical size of the vasculature, obtaining access can be very difficult for even the most skilled health care provider. Vascular access should not be delayed in the ill infant, and in fact should be secured aggressively and expeditiously. It is imperative that critical care transport personnel have multiple vascular access options since standard access techniques may be difficult to secure. The access options should employ both venous and intraosseous routes.

TEMPERATURE REGULATION

Maintaining the core body temperature of pediatric patients is critically important and should be done as soon as possible.

Maintaining the core body temperature of pediatric patients is critically important and should be done as soon as possible. Temperature regulation is initially treated by preventing heat loss while promoting strategies for aggressive warming. In preparation for transport, temperature maintenance should be accomplished quickly and aggressively.

HYPOGLYCEMIA

Pediatric hypoglycemia should be managed aggressively using a solution of 25% dextrose and water.

Pediatric hypoglycemia should be managed aggressively using a solution of 25% dextrose and water. The administration of $D_{50}W$ is contraindicated in the pediatric patient because this solution can cause significant increases in the plasma osmolarity. This increase in osmolarity may then lead to hypernatremia and ultimately cerebral and systemic cellular edema. To administer $D_{25}W$ (if prepackaged $D_{25}W$ is not available), simply dilute $D_{50}W$ with water first, and then administer the solution at a dose of 0.5–1 g/kg.

Table 27–10	Drugs for Pharmacologically Assisted Intubation	
Premedication	Sedation	Paralysis
Atropine	Thiopental	Succinylcholine
Glycopyrrolate	Ketamine	Rocuronium
Lidocaine	Etomidate	Vecuronium
	Fentanyl	Pancuronium
	Diazepam	
	Midazolam	
	Propofol	

Table 27-11 | Characteristics of Sedative Agents

Agent	Dose (IV/IO)	Onset	Duration	Adverse Effects
Thiopental	2.0–4.0 mg/kg	10–20 sec	5–10 min	Respiratory depression, hypotension
Ketamine	1.0–2.0 mg/kg	1–2 min	10–30 min	Secretions, increased intraocular and intracranial pressure, increased blood pressure, emergence reactions
Etomidate	0.2–0.3 mg/kg	1 min	3–12 min	Respiratory depression, fasciculations
Fentanyl	2.0–4.0 mcg/kg	1 min	1–2 hours	Respiratory depression, hypotension
Midazolam	0.1–0.2 mg/kg	1–2 min	1–2 hours	Respiratory depression, hypotension but less than other agents
Propofol	2.0–2.5 mg/kg	30–60 sec	10–15 min	Respiratory depression, hypotension

Table 27-12 | Characteristics of Paralytic Agents

Characteristics of Paralytic Agents

Agent	Dose	Onset	Duration
Succinylcholine	2.0 mg/kg <10 kg or <12 mo	30–60 sec	3–5 min
	1.0 mg/kg >10 kg or >12 mo	30–60 sec	3–5 min
Rocuronium	0.6 mg/kg (low range)	60–90 sec	30–40 min
	1.2 mg/kg (high range)	30–60 sec	60–90 min
Vecuronium	0.1 mg/kg (low range)	2–3 min	30–60 min
	0.2 mg/kg (high range)	30–90 sec	90–120 min

Summary

The common denominator for deaths seen in the pediatric population is hypoxia secondary to airway and breathing deficits. Medical conditions that can precipitate this encompass a very diverse group of illnesses, including infectious diseases, congenital heart diseases, and pulmonary compromise. Healthy pediatric patients maintain pulmonary and cardiovascular function until they become extremely deranged, so the critical care paramedic must stay acutely aware of subtle changes and early indications of respiratory distress and early respiratory failure. The goal during the critical care transport of an acutely ill pediatric patient is to preserve or support airway, pulmonary, and cardiovascular function. Failure to do so will cause rapid decompensation of the pediatric patient's condition and lead to cardiopulmonary arrest. Once arrested, the rate of successful resuscitation from arrest in this patient population is dismal. Focus should remain on preventing the arrest.

Review Questions

1. Why are pediatric patients at a higher risk for hypoglycemic episodes?
2. What are three anatomical differences between a pediatric airway and an adult airway that would make intubation a more challenging task?
3. What is the leading cause of cardiopulmonary arrest in children?
4. Describe the difference between respiratory distress and respiratory failure as far as presenting signs and symptoms.

5. Describe the difference in clinical presentation between epiglottitis and croup in a pediatric patient.

6. Describe the difference in presentation between asthma and bronchiolitis in a pediatric patient.

7. What common medications are used in the treatment of an acute asthma attack in a pediatric patient?

8. What are the four etiologies for hypoperfusion (shock) as discussed in this chapter.

9. Briefly describe the difference between a wet and dry drowning.

See Answers to Review Questions at the back of this book.

Further Reading

American Academy of Pediatrics. *Pediatric Education for Prehospital Professionals.* Sudbury, MA: Jones and Bartlett, 2000.

American Academy of Pediatrics. *Textbook of Pediatric Resuscitation,* 4th ed. Elk Grove Village, IL: Author, 2000.

American College of Surgeons, Committee on Trauma. *Advanced Trauma Life Support Course: Student Course Manual.* Chicago: Author, 1997.

American Heart Association. *PALS Provider Manual.* Dallas, TX: American Heart Association, 2002.

Bledsoe BE, Porter RS, Cherry RA. *Paramedic Care: Principles & Practice, Volume 5—Special Considerations.* 2nd ed. Upper Saddle River, NJ: Pearson Prentice Hall, 2005.

Bledsoe BE, Porter RS, Cherry RA. *Paramedic Care: Principles & Practice, Volume 4—Trauma.* 2nd ed. Upper Saddle River, NJ: Pearson Prentice Hall, 2005.

Crain EF, Gershel JC. *Clinical Manual of Emergency Pediatrics.* New York: McGraw-Hill, 2003.

Dietrich AM, Shaner S, John E., Campbell JE, editors. *Pediatric Basic Trauma Life Support,* 2nd ed. Oak Terrace, IL: Basic Trauma Life Support International, 2002.

Edgren AR. "*Pediatric Jaundice.*" In *Gale Encyclopedia of Medicine.* Farmington Hills, MI: Gale Research, 1999.

Gomella TL, Cunningham MD, Eyal FG, Zenk KE. *Neonatology: Management, Procedures, On-Call Problems, Diseases, and Drugs.* New York: McGraw-Hill, 2004.

Holleran RS. *Air and Surface Patient Transport, Principles and Practice.* St. Louis, MO: Mosby, 2003.

Jaimovich DG, Vidyasagar D. *Handbook of Pediatric and Pediatric Transport Medicine,* 2nd ed. Philadelphia: Hanley and Belfus, 2002.

Krost WS. "Epiglottitis, Bronchiolitis, and Bigwheels: Pediatric Pulmonary Emergencies." *Emergency Medical Services* (January 2004).

Limmer D, Krost W, Mistovich J. "Asthma: Prehospital Pathophysiology Column." *Emergency Medical Services* (April 2004).

Markenson DS. *Pediatric Prehospital Care.* Upper Saddle River, NJ: Pearson Prentice Hall, 2002.

Martini FH, Bartholomew EF, Bledsoe BE, *Anatomy and Physiology for Emergency Care.* Upper Saddle River, NJ: Pearson Prentice Hall, 2002.

Morris FC, Levin DL. *Essentials of Pediatric Intensive Care,* 2nd ed. New York: Churchill-Livingston, 1997.

National Safety Council. http://www.nsc.org/ (last updated June 1, 2005).

Park MK. *Pediatric Cardiology for Practitioners,* 4th ed. St. Louis, MO: Mosby, 2002.

Paneth N, Kiely JL. "Newborn Intensive Care and Pediatric Mortality in Low-Birth-Weight Infants. A Population Study." *New England Journal of Medicine,* Vol. 307 (1982):149.

Pollack MM, Alexander SR, Clark N, et al. "Improved Outcomes from Tertiary Center Pediatric Intensive Care: A Statewide Comparison of Tertiary and Nontertiary Care Facilities." *Critical Care Medicine*, Vol. 19 (1991)150.

Siberry GRI. *The Harriet Lane Handbook.* St. Louis, MO: Mosby, 2000.

Taussig LM, Landau LI. *Pediatric Respiratory Medicine.* St. Louis, MO: Mosby, 1999.

Tintinalli JE. *Emergency Medicine: A Comprehensive Study Guide.* New York: McGraw-Hill, 2000.

Williams LJ, Shaffer TH, Greenspar JS. "Inhaled Nitric Oxide Therapy in the Near-Term or Term Pediatric Patient with Hypoxic Respiratory Failure." *Pediatric Network: The Journal of Pediatric Nursing*, Vol. 23 (2004)1.

High-Risk Obstetrical/ Gynecological Emergencies

Scott R. Snyder, B.S., CCEMTP

Objectives

Upon completion of this chapter, the student should be able to:

1. Describe the anatomy and physiology of the organs and structures of the female reproductive system and fetal gestation. (p. 843)
2. Describe the physiological changes that occur in the pregnant female. (p. 847)
3. List the components of a general assessment of the obstetric patient. (p. 848)
4. Describe the evaluation assessment of fetal heart rate patterns. (p. 851)
5. Describe the pathophysiology, assessment, and management of various OB-GYN emergencies to include:
   A. Fetal distress (p. 857)
   B. Vaginal hemorrhage during pregnancy (p. 857)
   C. Abruptio placentae (p. 858)
   D. Placenta previa (p. 859)
   E. Preterm labor (p. 860)
   F. Breech presentation (p. 862)
   G. Dystocia (p. 863)
   H. Umbilical cord prolapse (p. 865)
   I. Uterine rupture (p. 865)
   J. Postpartum hemorrhage (p. 866)
   K. Hypertension in pregnancy (p. 867)
   L. Preeclampsia (p. 867)
   M. Eclampsia (p. 869)
   N. Gestational diabetes (p. 869)
   O. Embolism (p. 870)

Key Terms

Case Study

You, a critical care paramedic, and your RN partner are performing your phlebotomy duties in the emergency department of your base hospital when your pagers simultaneously go off, indicating that you have a transport call. You walk quickly over to the dispatch center, where the dispatcher is just hanging up the phone after taking the information from the caller. "High-risk OB transfer from General back here, she's a direct admit to the unit," the dispatcher tells you. "Cool" you think, as this means that you and your partner will have help on this trip in the form of an RN from the OB floor. It is hospital protocol for an RN from the OB unit to assist the flight team with all high-risk transports.

"Have a nice drive" the pilot says as she reviews the latest weather radar on the Internet "because there's too much in the way of thunderstorms between here and there." In a way, you don't really mind, as the BO 105 your service uses gets a bit cramped with the extra person in the patient care compartment. You give a quick call down to the garage and tell the driver to prepare the mobile intensive care equipped ambulance for a transport. You and your partner prepare your equipment, and are met by the OB RN, Karen, on the way to the garage. You all exchange pleasantries, load your equipment into the ambulance, and are on your way.

During the 30-minute drive to General Hospital, Karen phones the transferring physician and gets a patient report. After finishing the call, she informs the team that you are transporting a 46-year-old female who is at 30 weeks' gestation and is experiencing tearing abdominal pain and a minimal amount of dark red vaginal hemorrhaging. She is G5-P3 (4,1,0,3), is a smoker, has had numerous STDs in the past, and has admitted to cocaine use this morning. In addition, the physician reported that she has not received any prenatal care and appears malnourished. "In other words, this patient has hit about seven of the risk factors for preterm labor," your partner says, as Karen smiles knowingly.

You arrive on scene in 28 minutes and, after entering the emergency department and introducing yourselves to the staff, head into the examination room with your partner to perform a patient assessment. While Karen speaks with the attending physician, you introduce yourselves and ask the patient if it is OK to perform a physical exam and switch her over to your equipment; she agrees. As your partner performs the assessment, you switch the patient from a nasal cannula to a nonrebreather mask with a 15-lpm flow of 100% oxygen. You note that the patient is not having any respiratory distress, but does appear anxious, is slightly pale, and is diaphoretic. You place her on your cardiac monitor, and flush the established 16-gauge angiocath placed in her right antecubital area. You listen as your partner walks her through a history and physical exam, and note how she described an acute onset of sharp, constant abdominal pain that woke her from sleep this morning. She came to the ED for evaluation after the pain did not subside on its own. She has not experienced any contractions and did not notice any vaginal bleeding while at home, but the ED physician did note some about half an hour ago; "just a little bit" she says, holding her thumb and pointer finger together for emphasis. Your partner advises you that her abdomen is nonrigid, and he is able to palpate the uterus and feel fetal movement. She winces a bit when he palpates deeply, and he keeps his hand on her uterus for a while, checking for contractions that do not occur. As you place the patient on the fetal heart rate monitor and tocodynamometer, your partner finishes taking the patient's vital signs, and Karen returns with the available lab values. They are:

Vital Signs
- ★ HR = 110
- ★ BP = 112/70
- ★ RR = 16
- ★ SpO_2 = 100%

Blood Gases
- ★ PO_2 = 96
- ★ PCO_2 = 30
- ★ pH = 7.4
- ★ HCO_3^- = 25
- ★ Na^+ = 140
- ★ K^+ = 4.3

Fetal Heart Rate
- ★ Baseline of 150 bpm
- ★ Short- and long-term variability present
- ★ Accelerations noted with fetal movement and agitation
- ★ No decelerations noted
- ★ Tocodynamometer indicates that no contractions are present

The physician walks into the room and reports that an ultrasound was negative for placenta previa, and a cautious vaginal exam with a speculum revealed intact membranes and some slight dark red vaginal bleeding. You, your partner, and Karen are momentarily dumbfounded—and pleasantly surprised—at the collected results. The patient sees the looks on your faces, and nervously asks "Is everything ok?" "Actually," Karen says, "everything is absolutely wonderful!" "Yeah," you reply. "As the doctor has already told you, based on the story you told and the clinical exam findings, we thought that you might have what is called abruptio placentae. However," you continue, "all of your lab values are fine, your vital signs are good, and most important, your baby is doing great right now."

The patient breathes a sigh of relief and says, "So I don't have to go to the other hospital." You and your partners then explain how she needs to go to your facility for an evaluation by a specialist in high-risk obstetric care, and she agrees.

You and your partners concur that the management during transport will consist of a 250-cc bolus of normal saline, continued fetal heart rate and uterine monitoring with EFM, and a nice, easy ride back to your hospital. You all agree that a tocolytic agent such as terbutaline or magnesium sulfate is not needed at this time, but will reevaluate that decision if contractions develop. Should the abruption and bleeding worsen, you could administer the packed red blood cells you procured from the transferring facility. You transport the patient without incident to the OB unit at your hospital.

INTRODUCTION

Complications of pregnancy that will result in the need for critical care transport can have multiple etiologies. While some complications may be related to preexisting medical conditions, others may be precipitated by the pregnancy and still others by the fetus itself.

It is imperative that the critical care paramedic be able to perform a proper physical assessment of both the mother and the fetus, form a differential diagnosis and treatment plan, and anticipate the risks and possible complications involved with any given scenario so as to ensure the proper care and best possible outcome of both the mother and the fetus.

ANATOMY AND PHYSIOLOGY

The female reproductive system consists of two ovaries and the female reproductive tract: the paired fallopian tubes, the uterus, and the vagina. This system functions to produce and secrete sex hormones and viable gametes and to support, protect, and deliver a developing fetus. After birth, the female reproductive system will provide nourishment to the newborn infant. This review of anatomy and physiology will concentrate on prenatal development and the changes that take place in maternal and fetal anatomy and physiology. It assumes that the reader has an understanding of the female reproductive system.

Gestation is the time between fertilization of an oocyte until birth, and in a human averages 266 days. A gestation of less than 37 weeks is considered premature, and a gestation of greater than 42 weeks is considered postmature. The gestational period is often broken down into three trimesters, each three months in duration.

gestation *the time between fertilization of an oocyte until birth; in humans the average is 266 days.*

The gestational period is often broken down into three trimesters, each three months in duration.

FERTILIZATION AND THE FIRST TRIMESTER

The first trimester is a period of rapid embryonic and fetal development. It is during this time that rapid cell division occurs, implantation of the zygote in the uterine wall takes place, development of the placenta is completed, and the foundations of all the major organ systems are developed.

Fertilization, if it occurs, usually takes place in the distal one-third of the fallopian tube. After fertilization, the egg is termed a *zygote,* and contains the normal human compliment of 46 chromosomes. The zygote continues its travel down the length of the fallopian tube to the uterus, with cell division within the zygote starting immediately.

After the fertilized egg reaches the uterine cavity, it will continue to divide, forming a hollow sphere of cells called the blastocyst. (See Figure 28-1 ■.) The blastocyst adheres to the endometrium of the uterus, usually at the body or the fundus, and the cells in this area differentiate into a layer called the syncytial trophoblast. The syncytial trophoblast releases an enzyme, hyaluronidase, which erodes a path through the epithelial cells of the endometrium into the functional zone. During the first few days of implantation, human chorionic gonadotropin (HCG) is produced and stimulates the corpus luteum to continue the release of progesterone, which further prepares the uterus for pregnancy, and prevents the start of new ovarian and menstrual cycles during pregnancy.

By day 9, the syncytial trophoblast has spread into the surrounding endometrium, surrounding and eroding endometrial capillaries. (See Figure 28-2 ■.) Maternal blood leaking from the eroded capillaries flows through channels, called lacunae, in the syncytial trophoblast. From days 9 through 21, fingerlike projections called chorionic villi form on the trophoblast and extend into the endometrium. Embryonic blood vessels develop within the villi, and circulation within these vessels begins. As larger endometrial blood vessels become involved, maternal blood flow through the lacunae increases, and the first exchange between fetal and maternal blood takes place. These are the first steps in the creation of the placenta.

By the end of week 4, the embryo is about 5 mm long, weighs about 0.02 g, has a heartbeat, and the trachea, lungs, intestinal tract, liver, pancreas, eyes, and ears have begun to develop. By the end of week 8 of gestation, the diaphragm, intestinal subdivisions, kidneys, axial and appendicular cartilage, and axial musculature have started to develop. It is at this point, the end of week 8, that the embryo is termed a fetus. (See Figure 28-3 ■.)

The first trimester is a period of rapid embryonic and fetal development.

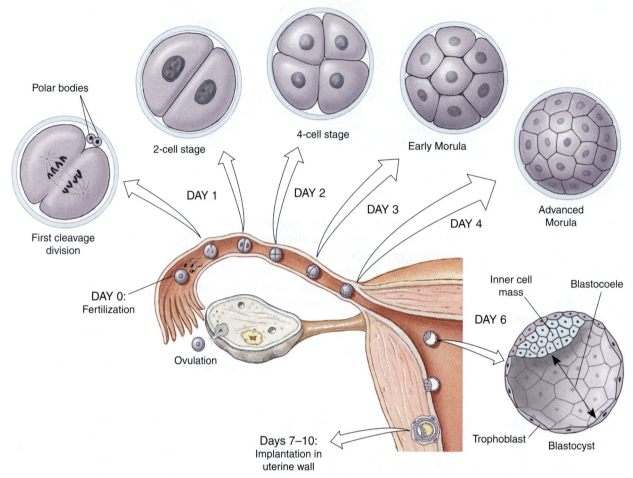

Polar bodies

2-cell stage

4-cell stage

Early Morula

DAY 1

DAY 2

DAY 3

DAY 4

Advanced Morula

First cleavage division

DAY 0:
Fertilization

Ovulation

Inner cell mass

Blastocoele

DAY 6

Days 7–10:
Implantation in uterine wall

Trophoblast

Blastocyst

■ **Figure 28-1** Cleavage and blastocyst formation. *(Fig. 21-2, p. 580, from* Essentials of Anatomy & Physiology, *2nd ed., by Frederic H. Martini, Ph.D. and Edwin F. Bartholomew, M.S. Copyright © 2000 by Frederic H. Martini, Inc. Published by Pearson Education, Inc. Reprinted by permission.)*

placenta *the blood-rich structure that facilitates the exchange of nutrients and wastes between the mother and fetus; also produces hormones necessary for the maintenance of pregnancy and fetal development.*

By the end of the first trimester (week 28), the gallbladder, gonads, brain, spinal cord, and appendicular musculature start to develop, and the fetus in about 80 mm in length and weighs about 25 g. The **placenta** has fully developed and is normally located in the fundal or body region of the uterus. The typical human placenta is about 20 cm in diameter, 2.5 cm thick, and weighs about 500 g, and its primary functions are to facilitate the exchange of nutrients and wastes between the mother and fetus and to produce hormones necessary for the maintenance of pregnancy and fetal development. Blood flows between the fetus and placenta via the umbilical cord, which contains the paired umbilical arteries and single umbilical vein. The developing fetus represents a significant demand to the mother; a significant amount of maternal blood flow is redirected to the placenta. During the second and third trimesters, the placenta acts as an endocrine organ, and will take over progesterone-releasing duties from the corpus luteum. In addition, the placenta produces the hormones HCG, estrogen, human placental lactogen, and relaxin.

It is during the second trimester that the development of organ systems nears completion, and the fetus continues to mature rapidly.

THE SECOND AND THIRD TRIMESTERS

It is during the second trimester that the development of organ systems nears completion, and the fetus continues to mature rapidly. The fetus is moving by the end of week 16, and by the end of the second trimester, the developing fetus has taken on distinctive human characteristics. By this time the eyebrows and eyelashes are well formed, and all eye components are developed. The fetus has a hand and startle reflex, footprints and fingerprints are forming, and alveoli are developing in lungs.

Early in the third trimester, the majority of organ systems have matured and become fully functional. In addition, the third trimester is characterized by rapid growth of the fetus: At week 24 it

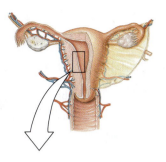

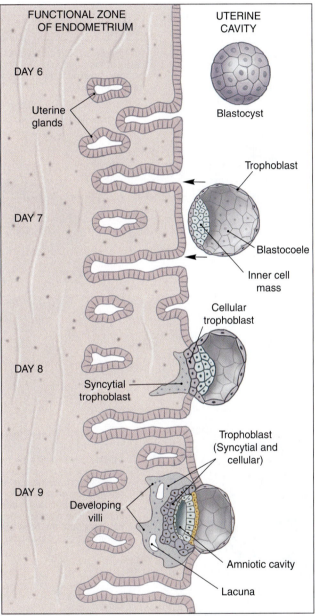

■ **Figure 28-2** Stages in the implantation process. *(Fig. 21-3, p. 581, from* Essentials of Anatomy & Physiology, *2nd ed., by* Frederic H. Martini, Ph.D. *and Edwin F. Bartholomew, M.S. Copyright © 2000 by Frederic H. Martini, Inc. Published by Pearson Education, Inc. Reprinted by permission.)*

FUNCTIONAL ZONE OF ENDOMETRIUM

UTERINE CAVITY

DAY 6

Uterine glands

Blastocyst

DAY 7

Trophoblast

Blastocoele

Inner cell mass

DAY 8

Cellular trophoblast

Syncytial trophoblast

DAY 9

Trophoblast (Syncytial and cellular)

Developing villi

Amniotic cavity

Lacuna

was approximately 230 mm in length and 0.65 kg in weight. By the third trimester, it has grown to a length of about 345 mm and weighs about 3.2 kg at full gestation. Other developmental markers to note during this phase are rapid deposition of body fat; rhythmic breathing movements (but lungs are not fully mature); fully developed bones, although they are still soft and pliable; and the storage by the fetus of iron, calcium, and phosphorus. A baby born at 36 weeks has a high chance of survival, but may require some medical interventions, and is considered full term during weeks 37 through 40.

Early in the third trimester, the majority of organ systems have matured and become fully functional.

Anatomy and Physiology   **845**

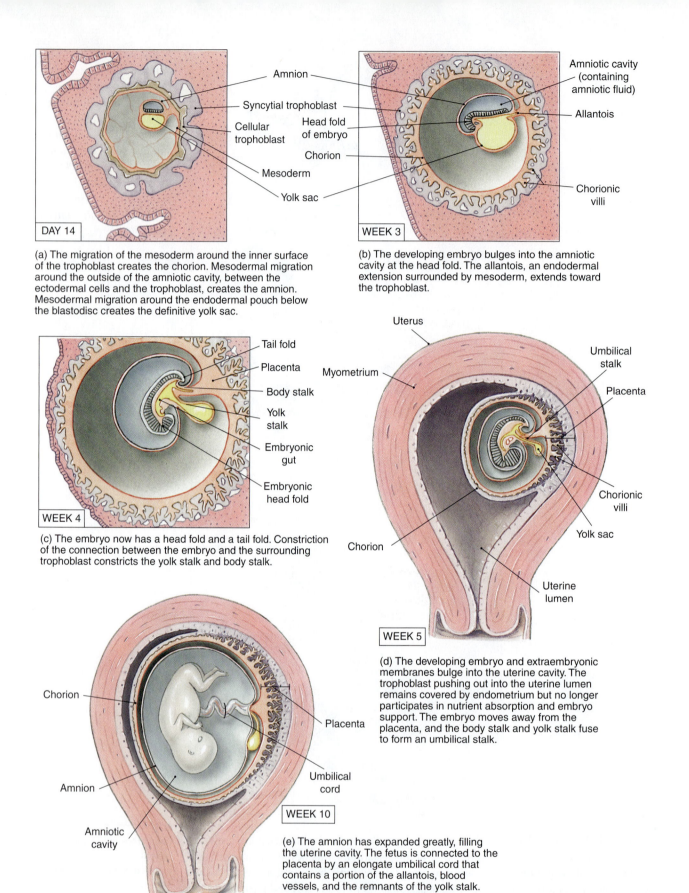

Amnion

Syncytial trophoblast

Cellular trophoblast

Mesoderm

Yolk sac

DAY 14

(a) The migration of the mesoderm around the inner surface of the trophoblast creates the chorion. Mesodermal migration around the outside of the amniotic cavity, between the ectodermal cells and the trophoblast, creates the amnion. Mesodermal migration around the endodermal pouch below the blastodisc creates the definitive yolk sac.

Amniotic cavity (containing amniotic fluid)

Head fold of embryo

Allantois

Chorion

Chorionic villi

WEEK 3

(b) The developing embryo bulges into the amniotic cavity at the head fold. The allantois, an endodermal extension surrounded by mesoderm, extends toward the trophoblast.

Tail fold

Placenta

Body stalk

Yolk stalk

Embryonic gut

Embryonic head fold

WEEK 4

(c) The embryo now has a head fold and a tail fold. Constriction of the connection between the embryo and the surrounding trophoblast constricts the yolk stalk and body stalk.

Uterus

Myometrium

Chorion

Umbilical stalk

Placenta

Chorionic villi

Yolk sac

Uterine lumen

WEEK 5

(d) The developing embryo and extraembryonic membranes bulge into the uterine cavity. The trophoblast pushing out into the uterine lumen remains covered by endometrium but no longer participates in nutrient absorption and embryo support. The embryo moves away from the placenta, and the body stalk and yolk stalk fuse to form an umbilical stalk.

Chorion

Placenta

Amnion

Umbilical cord

Amniotic cavity

WEEK 10

(e) The amnion has expanded greatly, filling the uterine cavity. The fetus is connected to the placenta by an elongate umbilical cord that contains a portion of the allantois, blood vessels, and the remnants of the yolk stalk.

■ **Figure 28-3** Extraembryonic membranes and placenta formation. (*Fig. 21-5, p. 584, from Essentials of Anatomy & Physiology, 2nd ed., by Frederic H. Martini, Ph.D. and Edwin F. Bartholomew, M.S. Copyright © 2000 by Frederic H. Martini, Inc. Published by Pearson Education, Inc. Reprinted by permission.*)

Table 28–1	Physiological Changes of Pregnancy	
System	**Item**	**Change**
Cardiovascular	Blood volume	Increases by 40% to 50%
	Blood constituents	RBC mass increased by 20% to 30%
	Cardiac output	Increases by 30% to 40%
	Cardiac size	Enlarged by both chamber dilation and hypertrophy
	ECG	Left axis deviation, flattening or inversion of T wave in Lead III
	Blood pressure	Slight decline in both systolic and diastolic pressure
	Venous distention	Increases by 150%
Respiratory	Respiratory tract	Engorgement and swelling of the mucosa
	Lung volumes	Slight decrease in lung volume
	Ventilation	Up to 40% rise in tidal volumes and increase in rate by 2–3 breaths per minute, thus increasing minute volume by 50%
Gastrointestinal	Mechanical	Enlarging uterus displaces abdominal organs toward the head
	Physiological	Delayed gastric emptying; gastric motility reduced
Renal	Kidneys	Dilate by 1.0–1.5 cm; GFR increases by 50%
	Bladder	Displaced upward; volume increases due to relaxation of bladder muscle tone
Endocrine	Pituitary	Increases in size by 30%; body water increases by 8.5 L
	Thyroid	Increases in size; all metabolic processes increased
	Parathyroid	Increase in vitamin D metabolism
	Pancreas	Increases in size of islets of Langerhans; increased number of insulin receptors; increased tendency for hypoglycemia
Dermatologic	Skin	Increased pigmentation (linea nigra) and "mask of pregnancy"

CHANGES IN MATERNAL PHYSIOLOGY

The developing fetus is dependant on the maternal organ systems for the provision of nourishment and oxygen, and the removal of metabolic waste. This places a significant strain on the mother, especially in the third trimester, and compensatory changes take place in maternal physiology. It is important for the critical care paramedic to be familiar with these changes and incorporate this knowledge to better assess and manage a pregnant patient. Systems affected in pregnancy include the cardiovascular, respiratory, reproductive, gastrointestinal, and urinary systems. (See Table 28–1.)

Changes in the cardiovascular and respiratory system occur because the mother is, for all practical purposes, pumping blood and breathing for two. Blood flow to the placenta and uterus greatly reduces the volume available for systemic maternal circulation. In addition, fetal metabolism results in a decrease in the maternal PO_2 and an increase in PCO_2. As a result, renin and erythropoietin production increases, resulting in an increased blood volume and red blood cell production. Volume increase is more pronounced than red blood cell increase, resulting in the dilutional edema common in pregnancy. Toward the end of gestation, maternal blood volume has increased by 40% to 50%, resulting in an increased resting heart rate, increased cardiac output, and flow murmurs

The developing fetus is dependant on the maternal organ systems for the provision of nourishment and oxygen, and the removal of metabolic waste.

Changes in the cardiovascular and respiratory system occur because the mother is, for all practical purposes, pumping blood and breathing for two.

that may be appreciated on auscultation. In addition, slight decreases in peripheral vascular resistance result in a slight decrease in blood pressure during the first and second trimesters, which rises to pre-pregnancy levels during the third trimester. In addition, intravascular fluid shifts into the intracellular space in dependant areas, especially the limbs, resulting in edema.

Although not a true physiological change, a transient decrease in venous return to the heart and subsequent hypotension can occur when the gravid uterus compresses the inferior vena cava (IVC), most often when the pregnant female is laid supine. This condition, **supine hypotensive syndrome,** can be avoided by placing the pregnant female in a left lateral recumbent position during transport, allowing the gravid uterus to displace to the left, away from the IVC located to the right of the spinal column.

Changes in blood chemistry also occur in the gravid female. Pregnancy results in a hypercoagulable state, secondary to an increase of clotting factors and a decrease in fibrinolytic activity, and an increase in platelet activation and venous stasis. As a result, a pregnant female has a five times increased risk of venous thromboembolism, which is the most common cause of maternal mortality in the United States.

A number of changes in the maternal respiratory system meet the increased needs for oxygen delivery and CO_2 removal. Maternal O_2 demand increases during pregnancy, and a 10% to 20% increase in O_2 consumption is typical. To help meet this demand, progesterone secretion results in weakening of the costal cartilage, allowing greater movement of the rib cage and a 35% to 40% increase in tidal volume. In addition, a mild increase in respiratory rate occurs; this, together with the increase in tidal volume, results in an increased minute volume. As a result, a mild, compensated respiratory alkalosis is often present, creating a greater CO_2 gradient between fetal and maternal circulation and greater diffusion of CO_2 between the two.

The most obvious and significant change in the reproductive system, to the critical care paramedic, occurs in the uterus. For the first 14 weeks of pregnancy, estrogen and progesterone influence uterine enlargement, after which time the developing fetus stretches and enlarges the uterus to its full gestational size of about 30 cm in length, 1,000 g in weight, and 5 liters in volume. Considering that the nongravid uterus has a length of about 7.5 cm, a weight of about 60 g, and volume of 10 mL, this represents an enormous increase in both size and volume. By the end of gestation, the uterus receives about 15% of the maternal blood volume. Obviously, any insult to the uterus can result in significant, if not fatal, maternal blood loss.

The increased size of the uterus results in the compression and displacement of the abdominal organs, making the assessment of the abdomen challenging. In addition, peristalsis is slowed, delaying gastric emptying, which makes bloating, nausea, and constipation common. Maternal nutritional requirements increase 10% to 30% during pregnancy as a result of fetal metabolic demands.

As a result of the increase in maternal blood volume, the glomerular filtration rate (GFR) increases by about 50%, accelerating the renal excretion of fetal metabolic waste. As a result of increased GFR, glucose may not be sufficiently reabsorbed in the proximal tubule and subsequently excreted in the urine. The resulting glucosuria may be normal, and not indicative of the development of gestational diabetes; as such, urine glucose is a poor indicator of serum glucose levels in a pregnant patient, and blood glucose levels should be obtained for a better appreciation of glucose control. Increased GFR, along with uterine compression of the bladder, results in increased urinary frequency in the gravid female.

GENERAL ASSESSMENT OF THE OB/GYN PATIENT

HISTORY

Ascertaining the age of the patient is important, because both a low or an increased age predispose the obstetric patient to complications. A past medical history should include not only an exploration of the obstetric history, but the entire medical history. Past medical histories (PMHs) such as diabetes, seizure disorders, heart disease, hypertension, and neuromuscular disorders can be exacerbated by or complicate pregnancy. Medications and allergies to medications should be identified and recorded.

A specific obstetric history is of great importance, because it may have some predictive value for the outcome of the current pregnancy, and should include an exploration of past pregnancies

---

supine hypotensive syndrome *a transient decrease in venous return to the heart when the gravid uterus compresses the inferior vena cava (IVC); occurs most often when the pregnant female is supine.*

Table 28–2	Gravida/Para Status: G/P T-P-A-L				
Gravida "G"	Para "P"	Full-Term Infants "T"	Preterm Infants "P"	Number of Abortions "A"	Number of Living Children "L"
Total number of pregnancies, including current	Total number of deliveries after 20 weeks' gestation	Number of full-term infants delivered	Number of preterm infants delivered	Number of abortions	Number of currently living children

as well as the present one. The patient's gravida/para (G/P) status should be determined, and is written as "G/P T-P-A-L," where gravida is the total number of pregnancies (including the present one), para is the number of deliveries after 20 weeks of pregnancy, and "T-P-A-L" is the number of full-term infants, number of preterm infants, number of abortions, and number of living children, respectively. (See Table 28–2.) Also, how many living children does she have? Has she experienced any complications with previous pregnancies or deliveries? If so, what? Has she had any preterm deliveries and, if so, at what gestational age and what was the outcome? Has she ever had an elective or spontaneous abortion and was a dilation and curettage performed? **Dilation and curettage (D&C)** is a procedure used to diagnose or treat abnormal bleeding from the uterus. Dilation means to stretch the opening of the cervix to make it wider. Curettage involves removing a sample of the endometrium to be examined later. Have all previous births been vaginal, or has a cesarean section been performed in the past? Has the patient delivered vaginally after a cesarean section? Despite what the patient reveals, examine for the presence of surgical scars that may suggest cesarean section, and inquire as to the origin of all scars noted. When was her last labor and what was its length?

> **dilation and curettage (D&C)** *a surgical procedure used to diagnose or treat abnormal bleeding from the uterus; involves* dilation *of the cervix and* curettage *of endometrial tissue for later examination.*

With regard to the current pregnancy, what is the estimated date of confinement (EDC)? Has the patient received adequate, limited (defined as three or fewer visits), or no prenatal care? Has any problem with this pregnancy been identified and, if so, what? Have diagnostic tests such as ultrasound been performed? If so, what were the results? Is the patient taking any medications for obstetric or nonobstetric reasons? If so, what medication, what dose, and has she been compliant? Is drug or alcohol abuse suspected and, if so, what substances, with what frequency, and when was the last use? Does the patient smoke? Has she experienced a normal weight gain with the pregnancy, or does she appear malnourished or obese? Is the patient presently having contractions and, if so, when did they begin and what are the frequency and duration? Is there an urge to defecate? Has the patient's amniotic sac ruptured and, if so, at what time, and was it a trickle or a gush of fluid? Was meconium present in the fluid or did it have a foul odor? Has the patient experienced any vaginal bleeding and, if so, is it painless or is there pain? If there is pain, is it associated with contractions or constant? Has the patient or transporting facility used sanitary napkins or other absorbent devices to soak up blood? If so, how much was collected?

PHYSICAL EXAM

While the abdominal exam in a pregnant patient is basically identical to that of a nonpregnant patient, the displacement and compression of abdominal organs by the gravid uterus will make identification of familiar abdominal landmarks challenging. The critical care paramedic can, however, palpate for pain, tenderness, guarding, masses, and uterine contractions.

During uterine contractions, the fundus should be palpated for strength, frequency, and duration of contractions. This can be done in concert with a subjective assessment by the patient, who will usually be able to anticipate the start, describe and compare the intensity, and announce the end of a contraction. In addition, a **tocodynamometer,** or intrauterine pressure-monitoring catheter, can be utilized during assessment and transport to detect and record uterine contractions. An external tocodynamometer evaluates uterine contractions in a nonquantitative manner; the frequency and duration of uterine contractions can be recorded, but not the intensity. This is a monitor that uses a pressure-sensitive device that is strapped to the patient's abdomen by using either elastic adjustable belts or a wide elasticized band. The pressure-sensitive component of the device records the strength, duration, and time between contractions. This is recorded and printed out constantly while the patient is hooked up to the monitor.

> While the abdominal exam in a pregnant patient is basically identical to that of a nonpregnant patient, the displacement and compression of abdominal organs by the gravid uterus will make identification of familiar abdominal landmarks challenging.

> **tocodynamometer** *an intrauterine pressure-monitoring catheter utilized to detect and record uterine contractions.*

Palpation of the uterus, as described earlier, is probably just as effective as external uterine monitoring, and provides some information with regard to contraction intensity. As the name implies, an intrauterine pressure-monitoring catheter measures the pressure change, in mmHg, that occurs in the uterus during each contraction. As such, it is useful for determining the frequency, duration, and intensity of uterine contractions.

The fundal height (FH) of the uterus should be measured, in centimeters, from the symphysis pubis to the most superior portion of the fundus.

The fundal height (FH) of the uterus should be measured, in centimeters, from the symphysis pubis to the most superior portion of the fundus. (See Figure 28-4 ■.) Each centimeter of FH corresponds roughly to the gestational age in weeks. (See Figure 28-5a and b ■.) In addition, the position of the fetus can be determined by palpating the uterus for the head and buttocks, and the fetal spine can often be palpated as well.

A visual examination of the external genitalia is encouraged in all critical care transports, and special attention should be given to preparing the patient for such an exam and protecting her modesty during it. The external genitalia should be examined for discharge, blood, mucus, a prolapsed cord, or crowning. It is helpful to evaluate for crowning during a contraction, as the fetus's head may be located in the vaginal canal, almost to the external anatomy, but moves in and out of the examiner's view between contractions. Unless trained to do so, an internal vaginal exam is not normally within the scope of practice of the critical care paramedic and should not be performed. Prior to transport, physician examination of the patient's cervix may be warranted to better appreciate what stage of labor the patient is currently in.

Vital signs including pulse, blood pressure, respiratory rate, temperature, and SpO_2 should be assessed every 15 minutes or as frequently as the situation warrants. All obstetric patients who display signs of poor perfusion (supine hypotensive syndrome) while lying supine should be placed in the left lateral recumbent position during transport and have vital sign determination taken serially to eliminate the situation whereby the gravid uterus obstructs the vena cava and alters hemodynamics. If the patient can tolerate a Fowler's position comfortably, and there is no overriding reason not to use this position, the patient can assume this position of comfort during transport.

As described earlier, the fetus's location in the uterus can be determined by palpation, and its hemodynamic status evaluated through the assessment of fetal heart tones (FHT), and monitoring should occur throughout transport. FHTs are commonly assessed and monitored via Doppler auscultation, although a stethoscope can be used, or by electronic fetal heart rate (FHR) monitoring. Obviously, many critical care transport environments exclude the possibility of auscultation due to ambient noise. The evaluation and monitoring of uterine contractions and fetal heart rate with electronic methods is termed **electronic fetal monitoring (EFM).**

electronic fetal monitoring (EFM) *the electronic evaluation and/or monitoring of uterine contractions and fetal heart rate by Doppler wave or other methods.*

■ **Figure 28-4** The use of a measuring tape to measure a pregnant woman's fundal height as she lies supine on an examination table.

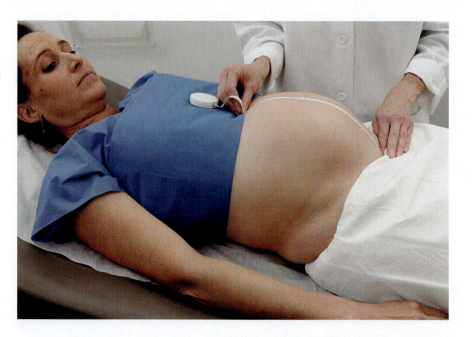

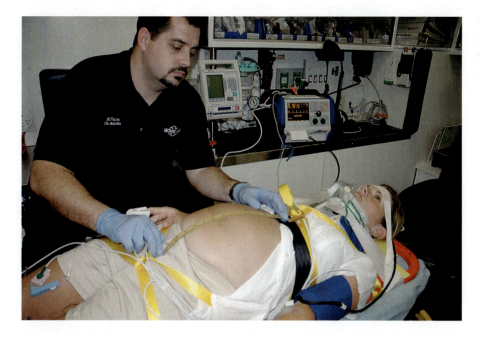

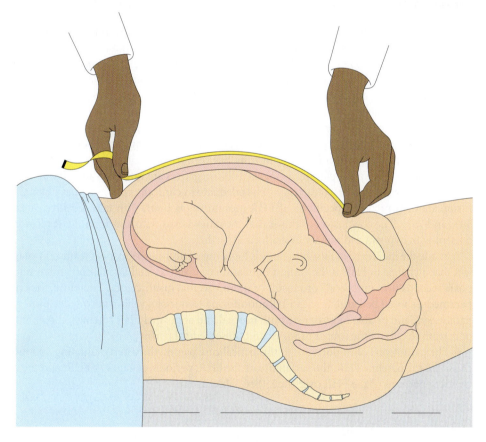

■ **Figure 28-5B** A cross-sectional view of estimating fetal gestational age when using a measuring tape.

INTRAPARTUM FETAL HEART RATE MONITORING

Intrapartum FHR monitoring was introduced as a method of preventing intrapartum fetal compromise, death, and asphyxia-induced brain damage. While the number of intrapartum stillbirths has been reduced significantly since the advent of FHR monitoring, there has been virtually no reduction in asphyxia-induced brain damage (such as cerebral palsy) associated with its inception.

Table 28–3	A Systematic Approach to Reading Fetal Heart Rate Recordings

1. Evaluate recording—is it continuous and adequate for interpretation?
2. Identify type of monitor used—external versus internal, first-generation versus second-generation.
3. Identify baseline fetal heart rate and presence of variability, both long-term and beat-to-beat (short-term).
4. Determine whether accelerations or decelerations from the baseline occur.
5. Identify pattern of uterine contractions, including regularity, rate, intensity, duration, and baseline tone between contractions.
6. Correlate accelerations and decelerations with uterine contractions and identify the pattern.
7. Identify changes in the FHR recording over time, if possible.
8. Conclude whether the FHR recording is reassuring, nonreassuring, or ominous.
9. Develop a plan, in the context of the clinical scenario, according to interpretation of the FHR.
10. Document in detail the interpretation of FHR, clinical conclusion, and plan of management.

Note: FHR = fetal heart rate. Source: Modified from: Swetia A, Hacker TW, Nuovo J. "Interpretation of the Fetal Heart Rate during Labor. *American Family Physician.* Vol. 59, No. 9 (1999): 2487–2491.

We should mention that <10% of cerebral palsy can be attributed to intrapartum hypoxia. This means that >90% of cases are caused *in utero* prior to birth.

Indications for the use of a FHR monitor include the presence of antepartum risk factors such as multiple gestation, preeclampsia, chronic hypertension, and maternal diabetes. Intrapartum risk factors include cases of active or suspected abruptio placentae, placenta previa, meconium staining, prematurity, and the documentation of past abnormal FHR patterns. FHR monitoring is also suggested in cases of active labor with the use of analgesia, anesthesia, or oxytocin.

Asphyxia is said to have occurred when hypoxia with a resulting metabolic acidosis is present, and continuous intrapartum FHR monitoring has very good sensitivity (about 90%) in detecting those fetuses at risk for developing asphyxia. False-negatives are rare, meaning that in the vast majority of cases a normal FHR tracing will be adequate to clinically conclude that normal fetal perfusion status is present. Specificity of FHR monitoring is poor, with false-positive rates between 50% and 75%. The conclusion of this is that most newborns with abnormal FHR records will not present with hypoxia and metabolic acidosis at birth.

While the incidence of false-positives is high, the critical care transport team cannot ignore the fact that a change in FHR is the earliest indication of insult to fetal circulation and developing hypoxia secondary to umbilical cord insult or uteroplacental insufficiency. Therefore, the critical care paramedic should be familiar with FHR monitoring terminology, have knowledge of normal FHR parameters, and be able to recognize both normal and abnormal FHR tracings, allowing the transport team to correct the source of insult and preserve fetal perfusion.

The parameters of importance to the critical care paramedic when evaluating and monitoring FHRs are the baseline FHR, the variability of the FHR, periodic changes in FHR, and the change in trending patterns of the FHR over time. (See Table 28–3.)

BASELINE RATE

The baseline FHR is the average FHR during a 10-minute period rounded off to the nearest 5 beats per minute (bpm). For baseline FHR to be established, there must be at least 2 minutes out of the 10-minute period where there are no instances of episodic changes, periods of significant FHR variability, or segments of the baseline with differences greater than 25 bpm. Normal baseline FHR is 110–160 bpm. Figure 28-6 ■ shows a normal FHR tracing.

Bradycardia is said to exist when the FHR is less than 110 bpm for greater than 10 minutes. It is not uncommon, though, for a term or postmature fetus to have baselines between 100 and 110 bpm, owning to their more mature neurologic and cardiovascular systems. Bradycardia occurs sec-

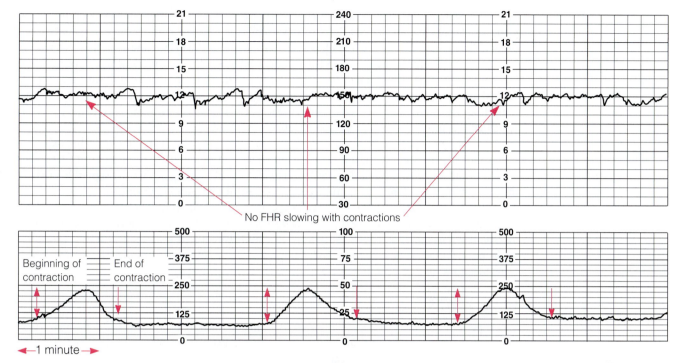

■ **Figure 28-6** Normal FHR range is from 110–160 bpm. The FHR tracing in the upper portion of the graph indicates an FHR range of 140–155 bpm. The bottom portion depicts uterine contractions. Each dark vertical line marks 1 minute, and each small rectangle represents 10 seconds. The contraction frequency is about every 2½ minutes, and the duration of the contractions is 50–60 seconds.

ondary to increased fetal parasympathetic tone and results in decreased cardiac output, hypoxia, and eventual metabolic acidosis.

Bradycardia can occur secondary to umbilical cord compression or occlusion, maternal hypotension, uterine hyperstimulation resulting in increased intrauterine pressure during contractions (as with the use of oxytocin), and chronic hypoxia. In cases of chronic hypoxia, fetal bradycardia is a late, ominous sign. Maternal pushing during contractions during the second stage of labor can also result in fetal bradycardia, and delivery usually follows shortly thereafter. In addition, what appears to be fetal bradycardia may actually be inadvertent measurement of the maternal pulse.

Tachycardia is defined as a FHR of greater than 160 bpm for more than 10 minutes. Tachycardia, as in adults, occurs as a result of an increase in sympathetic tone and is an early, immediate compensatory reaction to increase cardiac output in instances of hypoxia. Significantly less variability in heart rate usually occurs during episodes of tachydardia. Causes of fetal tachycardia include transient fetal hypoxia, fetal anemia, maternal fever, maternal or fetal infections, smoking, sympathomimetic drugs such as terbutaline, and chorioamnionitis.

A sinusoidal wave pattern may be appreciated in cases of fetal anemia, erythroblastosis, or hypovolemia and is indicative of severe fetal hypoxia. Maternal use of narcotics may also result in a sinusoidal wave pattern, but is not an indication of fetal distress. The normal presentation is a frequent, wavelike pattern of regularly occurring increases and decreases of FHR over a range of 5–20 beats from baseline.

VARIABILITY

Variability in baseline FHR is normal, and indicates an adequately oxygenated and normally functioning autonomic nervous system. Variability of FHR occurs as the sympathetic and parasympathetic nervous systems alternate in exerting influence on the fetal heart rate, and can be described as short term and long term. Short-term variability is the beat-to-beat changes in FHR, is usually irregular in rate and frequency, and is greatly influenced by the parasympathetic branch, which is more susceptible to hypoxia than is the sympathetic branch.

variability *variability of FHR (Fetal Heart Rate) occurs as the sympathetic and parasympathetic nervous systems alternate short- or long-term influence on the fetus; abnormalities can indicate differing levels of fetal distress.*

As a result, the cessation of normal, short-term variability may be the first indicator of fetal hypoxia. Conversely, the presence of short-term variability is associated with normal oxygenation status at delivery. Long-term variability has been described as a broad "waviness" of the FHR tracing over time and can range from 5 to 25 beats above and below the baseline; less than 5 beats over 1 minute is considered short. Long-term variability differs from the sinusoidal wave pattern described above in that its waves occur with much less frequency, or over a longer period of time. Long-term variability is influenced by the sympathetic nervous system, as opposed to the parasympathetic nervous system's influence over short-term variability.

Absent or minimal variability, both long and short term, can be the result of fetal hypoxia, maternal narcotic use, smoking, administration of magnesium sulfate, extreme prematurity, fetal neurologic insult, and normal fetal sleep cycles. Increased variability can be an early sign of hypoxia or the result of the use of an ultrasound transducer. Ultrasound transducers are notorious for erroneously high variability readings in the critical care transport environment, and they are the most likely measuring devices to be used by a transport team, due to their noninvasive nature. In scenarios where true evaluation of FHR short-term variability is required, placement of a fetal scalp electrode by a physician is recommended. Long-term variability is accurate with an ultrasound transducer, and should be monitored and recorded during transport.

PERIODIC CHANGES IN FHR

Short, periodic changes that may occur in FHR include accelerations and decelerations. These changes are often normal, but can be the result of fetal distress and should evoke concern on the part of the critical care transport team.

An **acceleration** is an obvious, abrupt increase (less than 30 seconds from onset to peak rate) in FHR with a peak rate 15 bpm above baseline that lasts for greater than 15 seconds and less than 2 minutes from onset to return to baseline. An acceleration that lasts greater than 2 minutes is considered prolonged, and greater than 10 minutes is considered a change in baseline. Accelerations can occur secondary to uterine contractions or fetal movement, and indicate that the fetus has an intact central nervous system and a normal pH. As such, the presence of accelerations strongly suggests a normal fetal pH. However, an acceleration can also be the harbinger of fetal hypoxia, occurring before a change in pH has occurred. Therefore, the critical care transport team should ensure that fetal movement or contractions accompany all accelerations. This can be accomplished by asking the mother if movement or contractions are taking place, palpating the uterus during the acceleration, or identifying contractions on a tocodynamometer.

FHR decelerations can be classified as early, late, or variable. An early deceleration is an obvious, gradual (greater than 30 seconds from onset to nadir) decrease and return of FHR from baseline during a uterine contraction. The nadir of the deceleration occurs simultaneously with the peak of the uterine contraction, and in most cases the progression of the deceleration is a mirror image of the contraction. **Deceleration** during uterine contraction is considered normal, and most likely represents a vagal response secondary to fetal head compression. Early decelerations are not associated with fetal hypoxia or acidosis, and no intervention is required. (See Figure 28-7 ■.)

A late deceleration begins at the peak of a uterine contraction, and then returns to the FHR baseline after the contraction is finished. Late decelerations are a more serious sign than early decelerations, usually indicating hypoxia and acidosis secondary to uteroplacental insufficiency; that is, inadequate oxygen exchange is taking place across the placenta during uterine contractions. (See Figure 28-8 ■.) Causes of uteroplacental insufficiency include abruptio placentae and previa, uterine

acceleration *during uterine contraction, an abrupt increase in FHR of 15 bpm (or more) above baseline, lasting from 15 seconds to 2 minutes.*

deceleration *during uterine contraction, a normal, gradual decrease in FHR below baseline of greater than 30 seconds duration, then gradual return to baseline.*

■ **Figure 28-7** Early deceleration.

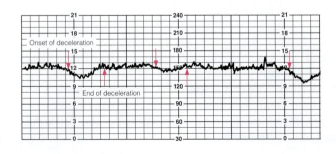

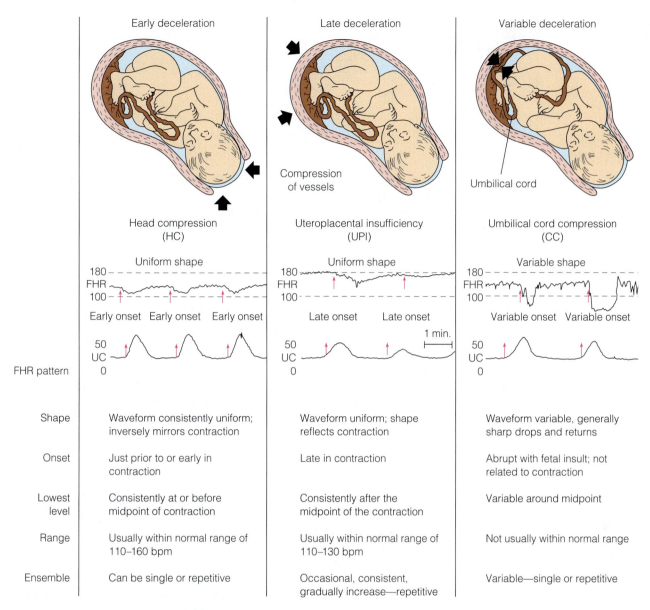

	Early deceleration	Late deceleration	Variable deceleration
	Head compression (HC)	Uteroplacental insufficiency (UPI)	Umbilical cord compression (CC)
Shape	Waveform consistently uniform; inversely mirrors contraction	Waveform uniform; shape reflects contraction	Waveform variable, generally sharp drops and returns
Onset	Just prior to or early in contraction	Late in contraction	Abrupt with fetal insult; not related to contraction
Lowest level	Consistently at or before midpoint of contraction	Consistently after the midpoint of the contraction	Variable around midpoint
Range	Usually within normal range of 110–160 bpm	Usually within normal range of 110–130 bpm	Not usually within normal range
Ensemble	Can be single or repetitive	Occasional, consistent, gradually increase—repetitive	Variable—single or repetitive

Figure 28-8 Types and characteristics of early, late, and variable decelerations. *(Hon, E. [1976]. An Introduction to Fetal Heart Rate Monitoring [2nd ed., p. 29]. Los Angeles: University of Southern California School of Medicine).*

hypertonicity secondary to oxytocin administration, maternal hypotension and smoking, diabetes, and postmaturity (See Figure 28-9 ■.)

The degree of deceleration is proportional to the strength of the contractions. Two mechanisms are responsible for late decelerations: First, a CNS-induced reflex bradycardia secondary to hypoxia occurs and, second, metabolic acidosis exerts a direct effect on the myocardium, resulting in myocardial depression. In cases of severe hypoxia, subtle late depressions will be appreciated with a lack of short-term variability, in other words, a flat FHR baseline.

Variable decelerations can occur any time during a contraction or independent of contractions, and are caused by umbilical cord compression and occlusion secondary to uterine contraction or fetal movement. They are typically characterized by an abrupt decrease in FHR below baseline greater than 15 bpm and lasting between 15 seconds and 2 minutes. Morphology may be in the shape of an inverted V, or sometimes present as a very short acceleration followed by a rapid, longer deceleration, then a rapid rise above the FHR baseline for a short acceleration prior to return the FHR baseline, resembling the shape of an M. The short accelerations on either side of the deceleration are termed *shoulders,* and their appearance is thought to be caused by a partial,

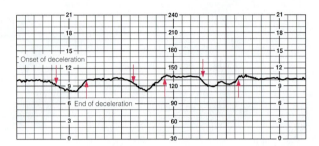

■ **Figure 28-9** Late deceleration.

rather than complete, cord occlusion. It is not uncommon for variable deceleration morphology to change from contraction to contraction.

Cord compression is more likely to occur after membrane rupture and loss of amniotic fluid, when there is less fluid to cushion the umbilical cord, and can also occur in instances of nuchal cord, short cord, and cord entanglement. Variable decelerations are the most common decelerations seen in labor, and while not an ominous sign when isolated, should arouse concern when they are deep and of long duration, are accompanied by decreased FHR variability, are slow to return to baseline, or when the baseline FHR increases or becomes tachycardic. In addition, "smoothing out" of the decelerations or loss of shoulders is also indicative of fetal distress.

In summary, accelerations are usually benign, and can occur during episodes of fetal movement or contractions. Acceleration in the presence of an absence of fetal movement, however, may be the first indication of developing hypoxia. Likewise, early decelerations are benign and a normal fetal response to the rise in intrauterine pressure that occurs during a uterine contraction. Late decelerations are suggestive of fetal distress secondary to uteroplacental insufficiency and are proportional to the strength of the contraction; the greater the contraction, the greater the deceleration. Variable decelerations signify umbilical cord compression, and can be an indication of fetal distress if they are slow to return to baseline, are accompanied by a rising FHR baseline (tachycardia), are deep and of long duration, lose their shoulders, or flatten out.

CHANGES IN TRENDING PATTERNS OF FHR

The chances are good that at some point during a high-risk OB transport in which the FHR is being monitored, some type of event will take place. The question for the critical care paramedic then becomes "Is this event significant?"; in other words, is fetal distress present or is this event a normal variant from baseline? A significant event is one in which there are grounds to believe that the fetus is in danger of developing hypoxia and metabolic acidosis, and these events required immediate intervention. To rule out fetal distress, the critical care transport team can ask the following questions in an attempt to identify those variants that suggest fetal well-being:

1. Is the FHR baseline within a normal range? If the baseline is between 110 and 160 bpm, the fetus is maintaining an adequate cardiac output and metabolic acidosis is not present. Remember that some fetuses, especially those that are postmature, may have a normally decreased baseline HR; this should have been identified and recorded prior to transport.

2. Is adequate variability present? If so, the fetus is being adequately oxygenated. If hypervariabilty is present, it may be due to the ultrasound transducer. In addition to hypoxia, decreased variability, both long and short term, can be secondary to the administration of magnesium sulfate or narcotics, or to normal fetal sleep patterns.

3. Are accelerations present? Accelerations can only occur in the absence of metabolic acidosis, therefore their presence is reassuring. The caregiver can encourage FHR acceleration with fetal scalp stimulation or vibroacoustic stimulation. An acceleration in response to a stimuli is as reassuring as an unprovoked one.

4. Is the event an early deceleration? If so, it is a normal, benign event that can be expected to occur with each uterine contraction. It is very important to be able to differentiate an early deceleration from a late deceleration, because late decelerations are an indicator of fetal distress, as are variable decelerations.

Table 28–4	Nonreassuring and Ominous Patterns

Nonreassuring Patterns	Ominous Patterns
Fetal tachycardia	Persistent late decelerations with loss of beat-to-beat variability
Fetal bradycardia	Nonreassuring variable decelerations associated with loss of beat-to-beat variability
Saltatory variability	Prolonged severe bradycardia
Variable decelerations associated with a nonreassuring pattern	Sinusoidal pattern
Late decelerations with preserved beat-to-beat variability	Confirmed loss of beat-to-beat variability not associated with fetal quiescence, medications, or severe prematurity

5. If tachycardia or bradycardia is present, are accelerations and adequate variability present? If so, metabolic acidosis is not present.

6. If late or variable decelerations are present, are accelerations and adequate variability present? If so, the fetus is tolerating the events well and metabolic acidosis is not present.

Signs that the fetus is not tolerating the event well and may be developing hypoxia and acidosis include a gradual, significant, uncorrected decrease in baseline FHR over time, a fluctuating baseline over time, tachycardia or bradycardia with reduced short- and long-term variability, reduced variability as labor progresses, and late decelerations that "smooth out" over time. These signs, or any combination of these signs, indicate fetal distress and will require intervention on the part of the critical care transport team. (See Table 28–4.)

MANAGEMENT OF FETAL DISTRESS

When fetal distress is suspected, intrauterine resuscitation measures need to be employed, the goal being to improve uterine blood flow and increase fetal oxygenation. After ensuring that the patient is breathing adequately and has a pulse, ensure that high-flow, 100% oxygen is administered, preferably via a nonrebreather mask. Confirm that she is in a proper left lateral recumbent position. Even if she has been previously placed, the uterus may have shifted during transport or the patient may have moved herself into a more comfortable posture, requiring readjusting of her position. If maternal hypotension still exists, consider repeated fluid boluses until hypotension is corrected. Perform an external vaginal exam to ensure that there is no vaginal hemorrhage, especially if the patient was high risk for abruptio placentae or placenta previa. Also ensure that umbilical cord prolapse is not a factor in the fetal distress. If prolapse is present, take action to ensure that no part of the cord is obstructed by any presenting fetal anatomy. If the fetal distress occurs secondary to hypertonic contractions resulting from oxytocin infusion, discontinue the infusion immediately. In addition, a tocolytic agent such as terbutaline 0.25 mg subcutaneous or 0.125–0.25 mg intravenous can be administered to relax the uterus.

In addition, amnioinfusion may be performed in cases of hemodynamically significant variable decelerations as well as meconium staining. Amnioinfusion is a process in which normal saline or lactated Ringer's solution is infused into the uterus during labor. In instances of variable decelerations, the infused fluid helps to cushion the umbilical cord and decrease cord compression and occlusion. Amnioinfusion's role in meconium staining is discussed later in the meconium section.

When fetal distress is suspected, intrauterine resuscitation measures need to be employed, the goal being to improve uterine blood flow and increase fetal oxygenation.

PATHOPHYSIOLOGY, ASSESSMENT, AND MANAGEMENT OF SPECIFIC OB/GYN EMERGENCIES

VAGINAL HEMORRHAGE DURING PREGNANCY

Life-threatening etiologies of vaginal hemorrhages that occur during the second half of pregnancy include abruptio placentae, placenta previa, and premature labor. The critical care transport team should recognize the seriousness of vaginal bleeding in the pregnant patient, because one-third of all cases of vaginal bleeding occurring after the 20th week of gestation result in fetal death. Abruptio placentae and placenta previa will be discussed here, and preterm labor and premature labor will be addressed in the section titled "Complications of Labor and Delivery." For clarity in the use of obstetrical terms, the critical care paramedic should be reminded that preterm labor is labor prior to 37 weeks' gestation, whereas premature labor is rupture of membranes before the onset of labor (contraction/cervical dilation and effacement). During the course of this discussion it is assumed that a general obstetric assessment, as detailed earlier, has already been performed, as has an assessment of the fetus.

ABRUPTIO PLACENTAE

abruptio placentae *the premature separation of a normally implanted placenta from the uterine wall.*

Abruptio placentae is the premature separation of a normally implanted placenta from the uterine wall, and occurs in about 0.83% (1/120) of all deliveries. Risk factors associated with abruptio placentae include chronic or gestational hypertension (most common factor), cocaine use, smoking, trauma, increasing maternal age (over 35 years), multiparity, and uterine scarring from surgeries, past curettage, or infection. In addition, a past incidence of abruptio placentae increases the risk of a second.

Fetal death occurs in 0.4% of all abruptions, and approaches 100% when 50% to 100% of the placenta is involved. Besides death, fetal complications also include hypoxia, anoxia, anemia, and CNS compromise. Maternal complications include the development of hemorrhagic shock, the development of disseminated intravascular coagulation (DIC), and end-organ failure.

Pathophysiology

Abruption begins with arterial hemorrhaging into the decidua basalis, and hematoma formation and progression can result in an expanding abruption. As abruption continues, a greater number of vessels become involved, further contributing to the expanding retroplacental hematoma. Because the decidua is rich in thromboplastin, encouragement of rapid clot formation may help attenuate the hemorrhage. Separation of the placenta can be partial (marginal) or complete, and an abruption with vaginal bleeding is termed an external hemorrhage (90% of all abruptions). If no vaginal bleeding is appreciated on physical exam, the abruption is said to be concealed (10% of all abruptions). Blood loss is impossible to estimate based on external observation alone, because significant amounts of blood can remain in the uterus, trapped behind the placenta. Most of the blood loss that occurs in abruptio is maternal in origin, although it is possible for the fetus to hemorrhage as well. In reaction to the insult, the uterus will often contract during an abruptio episode. (See Figure 28-10 ■.)

Assessment

Due to the different types of placental separations that can occur in abruptio placentae, clinical presentations can vary. The classic signs are considered to be the presence of abdominal pain (50%),

■ **Figure 28-10** Abruptio placentae (premature separation).

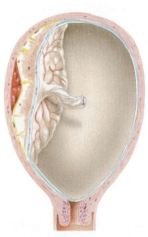
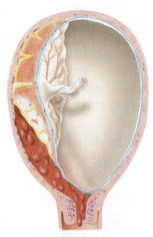
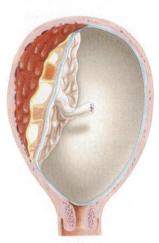

Partial separation (concealed hemorrhage)   Partial separation (apparent hemorrhage)   Complete separation (concealed hemorrhage)

uterine contractions (>90%), vaginal bleeding (90%), uterine tenderness to palpation, and fetal demise. Remember that in cases of concealed abruptio, vaginal bleeding will not be present (10%). Pain symptoms can range from mild abdominal tenderness in cases of mild, partial abruptions to severe, tearing abdominal pain in cases of central abruptio. Uterine contractions can vary in duration, intensity, and frequency, varying from normal contractions to hypertonic to tetanic. Tetanic contractions result in a rigid, boardlike abdomen on palpation and are indicative of severe abruption. In severe cases of abruptio, a patient can develop hemorrhagic shock; because a healthy gravid woman can lose up to 25% (about 1500 mL) of her blood volume before the clinical signs are evident, their appearance suggests the need for aggressive volume replacement.

Ultrasound cannot diagnose the presence or absence of abruptio placentae itself, although it can demonstrate a placental hematoma that is consistent with abruption. Retroplacental hematomas may be recognized in 2% to 25% of all abruptions, but recognition of a retroplacental hematoma depends on the severity of hematoma and on the operator's skill level. Ultrasound can, however, rule out placenta previa as a cause of vaginal bleeding by determining the location of the placenta. As such ultrasound does have a place, albeit limited, in the assessment of the high-risk OB-GYN patient. Labs ordered should include a CBC, type and cross-match, coagulation profile, and renal function studies.

Patients should also be assessed for signs associated with DIC, which include bleeding from IV or catheter sites, hypotension, and increased ventilatory resistance. A fibrinogen level of less than 150 mg/dL is suggestive for DIC, and the administration of fresh frozen plasma should be performed to facilitate initial coagulopathy. The only treatment for DIC is delivery, after which resolution usually occurs.

Management

Immediate attention to oxygenation and perfusion is a priority in the treatment of abruptio placentae, especially in cases where the signs and symptoms of shock are present. At the very least, 100% oxygen should be supplied at 15 lpm via a nonrebreather mask. Assisted ventilations with a bag-valve mask (BVM) or endotracheal intubation may be required if level of consciousness (LOC) and respiratory drive are affected by developing hemorrhagic shock. Two large-bore IVs, or a central line, should be initiated, and volume resuscitation begun with crystalloid solution in cases of mild abruptio. If hemorrhagic shock is present, aggressive volume replacement should be initiated with a crystalloid and packed RBCs. The critical care transport team should procure additional packed RBCs from the transporting facility for infusion during transport. An indwelling urinary catheter should be inserted to allow for monitoring of urinary output; an output of greater than 0.5 mL/kg/hr is desired, and is suggestive of adequate intravascular volume and renal perfusion. Finally, in cases of hypertonic or tetanic uterine contractions, the use of tocolytics may help prevent the expansion of a developing abruption.

PLACENTA PREVIA

Placenta previa occurs when the placenta implants and develops in the lower third of the uterus, totally or partially covering the cervical os. The incidence of placenta previa at 18 weeks is about 5% to 15%, but about 90% of these cases will resolve by the end of gestation, with about 0.5% (1/200 deliveries) still present at delivery. About 20% of all cases of vaginal bleeding occurring in the second half of pregnancy are a result of placenta previa.

Risk factors contributing to placenta previa include advanced maternal age (>35 years), smoking (doubles risk compared to nonsmokers), cocaine use, prior history of previa, multiparity, multifetal gestations, and previous cesarean section or curettage.

Maternal complications associated with previa include the need for a cesarean delivery, postpartum hemorrhage, and the development of hemorrhagic shock. Fetal complications include hypoxia, anoxia, and death.

Physiology

Placenta previa occurs when the placenta implants in the lower one-third of the uterus, rather than the fundus or body of the uterus, covering the cervical os. It has been suggested that decreased perfusion of the decidua of the fundus and body results in the implantation in the lower uterus. Compared

placenta previa occurs when the placenta implants and develops in the lower third of the uterus, totally or partially covering the cervical os.

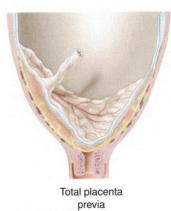 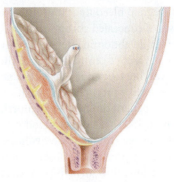

■ **Figure 28-11** Placenta previa (abnormal implantation).

Total placenta previa

Partial placenta previa

to the fundus and body, the lower uterus has less vascularization; to preserve adequate perfusion, a thinner placenta covering more surface area develops, increasing the possibility of cervical os occlusion. About 90% of cases identified at 18 weeks' gestation resolve by delivery, probably due to the fact that as the uterus elongates upward into the abdomen to accommodate the developing fetus, the placenta grows and migrates superiorly toward the fundus, away from the cervical os.

For the 10% of cases that do not resolve and continue to the end of gestation, three types of presentation are possible. A marginal previa occurs when the edge of the placenta lies adjacent to, but does not cover, the cervical os. A partial previa is characterized by a placenta that partially covers the cervical os, and a complete previa completely covers the cervical os. (See Figure 28-11 ■.)

Complications occur when cervical effacement and dilation take place prior to the onset of labor. These cervical changes manipulate the placenta, tearing it from the uterine wall, disrupting blood vessels, and resulting in hemorrhage. In addition, hemorrhage may result from tearing of the placenta as the fetus's head enters the birth canal, or by digital or speculum inspection.

Assessment

The hallmark of previa is the acute onset of painless, bright red bleeding in the late second or third trimester.

The hallmark of previa is the acute onset of painless, bright red bleeding in the late second or third trimester. In addition, a history of recent vaginal exam, sexual intercourse, or onset of labor should increase suspicion, but is not necessary for previa to occur. The abdominal exam is usually benign, though uterine contractions may be present. Digital or speculum examination is to be avoided in all cases of suspected placenta previa. Diagnosis of previa is confirmed with transabdominal ultrasound, which has an accuracy of 93% to 98% and a false-negative rate of about 7%.

Management

The management of placenta previa mirrors that of abruptio placentae, as discussed earlier.

COMPLICATIONS OF LABOR AND DELIVERY

This section will explore some of the more frequent complications of labor and delivery likely to be faced by the critical care transport paramedic including preterm labor, breech presentation, shoulder dystocia, cord prolapse, and postpartum hemorrhage. When possible, the critical care transport team should include a neonatal nurse or physician if delivery is a possibility, because the management of the complications of labor and delivery is a specialized division of medicine and best administered by those individuals who deal with it through daily practice. During the course of this discussion it is assumed that a general obstetric assessment, as detailed earlier, has already been performed, as has an assessment of the fetus.

PRETERM LABOR

A big risk factor associated with premature labor is premature rupture of membranes (PROM).

Labor is the occurrence of uterine contractions resulting in progressive cervical dilation and effacement. (See Figure 28-12 ■.) Preterm labor is defined as frequent uterine contractions resulting in progressive cervical dilation or effacement between the 20th and 37th weeks of gestation. Preterm

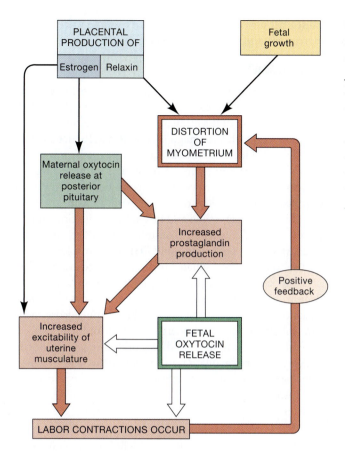

■ **Figure 28-12** Interacting factors during labor and delivery. *(Fig. 21-10, p. 592, from* Essentials of Anatomy & Physiology, *2nd ed., by Frederic H. Martini, Ph.D. and Edwin F. Bartholomew, M.S. Copyright © 2000 by Frederic H. Martini, Inc. Published by Pearson Education, Inc. Reprinted by permission.)*

labor occurs in about 10% to 15% of all pregnancies, complicates 10% to 12% of all births, and is responsible for about 85% of all neonatal deaths not due to genetic or congenital abnormalities. A big risk factor associated with premature labor is **premature rupture of membranes (PROM),** with 50% of premature patients going into labor within 24–48 hours of PROM. Additional risk factors include smoking, cocaine use, poor nutritional status, maternal age >35 years or less than 20 years, previous preterm delivery, abruptio placentae or previa, infection, dehydration, uterine abnormalities, cervical incompetence, and STDs such as *Chlamydia,* gonorrhea, and syphilis.

Maternal complications of premature labor include endometritis, septicemia and septic shock secondary to PROM, and chorioamnionitis. Fetal consequences of premature labor include preterm birth, which accounts for about 100 neonatal deaths for every 100,000 live births in the United States. The majority of neonatal mortality occurs in infants delivered prior to 28 weeks' gestation.

premature rupture of membranes (PROM) *a significant risk factor associated with premature labor and can lead to endometritis, septicemia and septic shock, chorioamnionitis, premature delivery, and fetal or neonatal death.*

Pathophysiology

Numerous physiological factors can contribute to the development of preterm and premature labor. Many hormonal influences can contribute to the premature onset of labor, such as the prostaglandin release associated with bacterial infections, abdominal trauma, and PROM. High levels of oxytocin are present in meconium-stained amniotic fluid, which facilitates the onset of labor.

A decrease in uteroplacental blood flow will result in an increase of uterine irritability, activity, and the onset of labor. Maternal dehydration, secondary to infection, fever, vomiting, diarrhea, or blood loss, can lead to hypotension and a subsequent decrease in uteroplacental blood flow. Maternal hypertension can also compromise uteroplacental blood flow, as can overdistention of the uterus, smoking, cocaine use, cardiovascular disease, and placental abruption or previa.

Physiological abnormalities that affect the cervix or uterus and can result in preterm labor include congenital defects and those caused by trauma. Cervical incompetence, in which the cervix is unable to support the developing fetus and intrauterine structures of pregnancy, can result in PROM and rapid delivery. Possible etiologies of cervical injuries that lead to cervical incompetence include injury from previous childbirth or gynecological procedures. Any uterine abnormalities that restrict uterine expansion can also result in preterm labor. Possible etiologies include previous cesarean section, scarring from STD infection or curettage, or congenital abnormalities.

Assessment

Preterm labor should be suspected in cases where there is a history of uterine contractions 10 minutes apart or less for greater than 1 hour. When suspected, the critical care transport team should assess for evidence of the numerous etiologies of preterm labor, including the presence of fever, dehydration, vaginal hemorrhaging, and PROM. Particular attention should be directed to the history with the goal of identifying risk factors such as age, previous history of preterm labor, social history, and such. A speculum examination should be performed by an appropriately trained health care provider to assess for cervical dilation or membrane rupture. In the absence of a trained individual, suspected amniotic fluid can be tested with nitrazine paper (pH > 6.5 is positive for amniotic fluid) or swabbed on a glass slide and inspected for ferning, indicating amniotic fluid, though the presence of blood will render both of these tests useless. In addition, the fundal height should be determined, fetal weight estimated, and FHR and contractions monitored via EFM.

Lab studies to be evaluated include a CBC to evaluate for leukocytosis and low hematocrit, urinalysis to assess the degree of dehydration and rule out infection, and cervical cultures for *Chlamydia*, gonorrhea, and group B streptococcus. A urine toxicology screen can be considered if substance abuse is suspected. In addition, serum glucose and potassium should be determined prior to the initiation of beta-adrenergic agonists for tocolysis.

Particular attention should be paid to the pattern of contractions, status of membranes, and the degree of cervical dilation to determine the stage of labor. This allows for an informed decision on the part of the transport crew as to whether the transport should be delayed to allow delivery at the transporting facility.

Management goals during transport include maintaining uteroplacental perfusion and suppressing labor.

tocolytic agents
medications used to help limit or stop contractions in patients who present in preterm labor between 24 and 36 weeks gestation.

Management

Management goals during transport include maintaining uteroplacental perfusion and suppressing labor. The patient should be placed in the left lateral recumbent position and administered 100% oxygen at 15 lpm via a nonrebreather mask. IV access should be obtained, and volume replacement initiated if dehydration is suspected.

Tocolytic agents are used in patients who present in preterm labor between 24 and 36 weeks' gestation, and are used to help limit or stop contractions. These agents are not only used to "buy time" and prevent delivery during interfacility transport of the patient, but are commonly used to prevent delivery for up to 2 days, allowing time for corticosteroid therapy to hasten fetal lung development. Beta-adrenergic agonists, magnesium sulfate, calcium channel blockers, and prostaglandin synthetase inhibitors are the agents most commonly used for tocolysis, with IV terbutaline or magnesium sulfate commonly utilized by critical care transport teams. Terbutaline is administered as an IV infusion starting at 2.5 mg/min, titrated every 10 minutes to tocolysis with a maximum dose of 50 mg/min. Serum glucose and potassium levels should be determined prior to the initiation of beta-adrenergic agonists, because they result in the movement of potassium into the intracellular space and glucose into the intravascular space, and can worsen existing hypokalemia and hyperglycemia, respectively. Magnesium sulfate is commonly administered as a 4- to 6-g bolus over 20 minutes followed by a 2–4 g/hr drip titrated to tocolysis.

BREECH PRESENTATION

Delivery usually occurs with the fetus presenting in the vertex position. Breech presentation is the term used to describe the situation in which the fetus's buttocks or legs present first. To be specific, a frank breech presentation, the most common type, occurs when both legs are extended upward, with both hips flexed and both knees extended. A complete breech occurs when the buttocks descend first, both hips are flexed, and one or both knees flexed, resulting in one of both feet presenting with the buttocks. If either hip is extended, leading to a foot or knee initially being presented, an incomplete breech is said to occur. Breech presentations occur in 3% to 4% of all term pregnancies (higher incidence prior to 34 weeks' gestation) and have a morbidity rate 3–4 times than that of cephalad presentations. Entrapment of the head in an incompletely dilated cervix is a major concern in breech presentation, and occurs when the body passes through a cervix that is not sufficiently dilated to allow passage of the head.

Risk factors that predispose a fetus for breech presentation include a previous breech delivery, grand multiparity, multiple gestation, uterine tumors and congenital abnormalities, placenta previa, and hydrocephaly. In addition, a fetus of less than 34 weeks has a large head in comparison to its body and is in the cephalad position, favoring a breech birth should premature labor begin.

Because of the atypical presentation of breech delivery, maternal trauma is common. In the infant, prolapsed cord, cord compression, and cord entanglement are common complications, and birth trauma is likely to occur. In addition, the breech fetus is at higher risk for hypoxia, acidosis, and anoxia than is an infant delivered in the cephalad position.

Management

The main point to remember during a breech birth is to refrain from touching the fetus and let the delivery happen on its own. Breech delivery can be a frightening experience for the critical care transport team, who must resist the temptation to do too much. It is certainly appropriate to support the legs and be ready to catch the fetus should the head delivery quickly, but the birth should be allowed to progress on its own, with no traction applied to the fetus. Not until the umbilical cord has delivered should the critical care paramedic assist in the freeing of the legs, if necessary. At this point the fetus can be wrapped in a towel, and rotated so the shoulders are in an anterior-posterior position. As the shoulders become visible, a finger can be used to hook each arm and apply gentle downward traction to remove each one, or, upward traction can be applied to facilitate the delivery of the posterior shoulder, and downward traction for the anterior shoulder. After the shoulders have been delivered, the body is rotated so the back is anterior, and flexion of the head is maintained by placing the index and middle fingers over the fetus's maxilla. With the body resting on the forearm of the same arm and the opposite hand supporting the head and shoulders, upward traction can be applied to the body while an assistant applies suprapubic pressure to encourage the delivery of the head with as little traction as possible.

DYSTOCIA

In cases of shoulder dystocia, delivery of the fetal head is followed by impaction of the fetal shoulders against the pubic symphysis and sacrum, within the pelvis. (See Figure 28-13 .) The complication becomes obvious when the head retracts slightly as it is pulled down against the perineum (turtle sign). Shoulder dystocia occurs in 0.6% to 1.4% of all vaginal deliveries, with high birth weight greater than 4,000 grams being the most common risk factor. Other risk factors include maternal diabetes, maternal obesity, operative delivery, and a contracted maternal pelvis.

Management

Once shoulder dystocia has been recognized, the immediate draining of the urinary bladder and a generous mediolateral episiotomy may facilitate delivery. Pressure to the fetus's anterior shoulder should be applied by one crew member to dislodge the anterior shoulder from the pubic symphysis; the anterior shoulder can be palpated in the maternal suprapubic area. DO NOT apply pressure to the fundal area, because this will further impact the shoulders on the pelvic rim. At the same time, gentle downward traction can be applied to the fetal head by another crew member. If this maneuver is unsuccessful, other maneuvers can be attempted.

McRobert's maneuver involves sharply flexing the maternal legs against the abdomen in an attempt to stretch the pelvic joints and increase the diameter of the pelvis, allowing for passage of the fetal shoulders. (See Figure 28-14 ■.) The Woods corkscrew maneuver requires the critical care transport paramedic to rotate the posterior shoulder of the fetus 180 degrees in a corkscrew fashion in an attempt at freeing the posterior shoulder. The Rubin maneuver involves displacing the anterior shoulder toward the chest of the fetus within the pelvis, effectively reducing the shoulder width and facilitating delivery. Even more undesirable is the deliberate fracture of the fetal clavicles. As a last resort, the Zavanelli maneuver involves flexing the fetal head and placing the fetus back into the uterine cavity and then removing the fetus via emergent cesarean section.

Because of the atypical presentation of breech delivery, maternal trauma is common.

In cases of shoulder dystocia, delivery of the fetal head is followed by impaction of the fetal shoulders against the pubic symphysis and sacrum, within the pelvis.

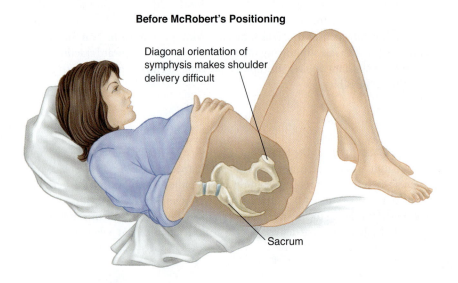

Normal

Shoulder Dystocia

Anterior shoulder impacted behind pubic symphysis

Dangers Include:

• Entrapment of cord
• Inability of child's chest to expand properly
• Severe brain damage or death if child is not delivered within minutes

■ Figure 28-14   McRobert's maneuver.

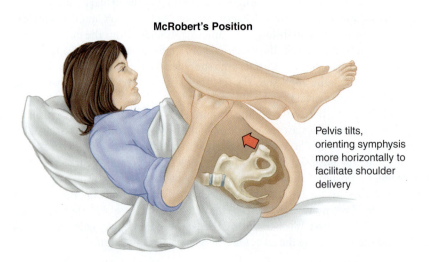

Before McRobert's Positioning

Diagonal orientation of symphysis makes shoulder delivery difficult

Sacrum

McRobert's Position

Pelvis tilts, orienting symphysis more horizontally to facilitate shoulder delivery

UMBILICAL CORD PROLAPSE

Overt umbilical cord prolapse occurs when the cord enters the vaginal canal or presents externally prior to the fetus. Occult cord prolapse occurs when the cord slips into or near the pelvis and is occluded by a presenting part; it is not visible or palpable on exam. A prolapsed cord occurs about 1 time in every 250 deliveries. Risk factors include PROM, transverse lie of the fetus in the uterus, breech presentation, large fetus multiparity, multiple gestations, preterm labor, and a long cord. The major concern with a prolapsed cord is cord compression and occlusion, and fetal complications can include hypoxia, acidosis, anoxia, and death.

Assessment

While the assessment findings of an overt umbilical cord prolapse are straightforward, the occult prolapse can be much more insidious and requires a careful examination on the part of the critical care transport team. Clinical signs include evidence of fetal distress including the absence of short- and long-term variability, fetal bradycardia, and recurrent variable decelerations that do not respond to maternal positioning, oxygen administration, or fluid administration.

While the assessment findings of an overt umbilical cord prolapse are straightforward, the occult prolapse can be much more insidious and requires a careful examination on the part of the critical care transport team.

Management

If the umbilical cord presents externally or can be visualized in the vagina, two fingers of a gloved hand should be used to prevent any presenting part of a delivering fetus from occluding the cord. The cord can be assessed for a pulse, but should not be compressed by the critical care paramedic. A presenting cord should never be pulled or replaced into the uterus, though it should be allowed to retract if it does so spontaneously. The cord should be kept free of pressure for the duration of transport, and the mother can be placed in a Trendelenburg or knee-chest position to further decrease pressure on the cord.

After umbilical cord pressure has been relieved, 100% oxygen should be supplied via a non-rebreather mask at 15 lpm and an IV of normal saline started. Delivery should be stopped with the use of a tocolytic agent such as terbutaline in an effort to further alleviate compression on the umbilical cord. If a prolapsed cord does not spontaneously resolve, definitive treatment is cesarean section.

UTERINE RUPTURE

Uterine rupture is the complete disruption of all layers of the uterine wall, allowing communication between the uterine and abdominal cavities, the majority of which occur in women who have undergone previous cesarean section. The risk of rupture is greatest (4% to 7%) with an inverted T-shaped (classic) scar, 1% to 7% with a low vertical scar, and less than 1% with a low transverse scar. *It is important to remember that the scar on the skin tells you nothing about the scar on the uterus.*

Uterine rupture is the complete disruption of all layers of the uterine wall, allowing communication between the uterine and abdominal cavities.

In addition to previous cesarean section, factors increasing the risk of uterine rupture include overdistention of the uterus, grand multiparity, previous rupture, and trauma. Uterine rupture can occur before or during labor, and in the total absence of any risk factors. Fetal complications include hypoxia, acidosis, anoxia, and death.

Pathophysiology

Uterine rupture usually involves separation of an old incision scar, resulting in total transection of the uterine wall and violation of the membranes. Bleeding can be significant, and fetal parts may travel into the peritoneal cavity. A uterine dehiscence is an incomplete disruption of the uterine wall, commonly a defect in the uterine muscle with an overlying serosal patch. A dehiscence does not involve the fetal membranes, involves minimal or no bleeding, and typically has no clinical significance. A dehiscence may, however, rupture with uterine contractions or trauma.

The extent of bleeding and fetal compromise depends on the location and severity of the rupture. Complete ruptures often result in fetal mortality, and ruptures involving large blood vessels will obviously have higher morbidity and mortality associated with them.

Assessment

The acute onset of sharp, severe abdominal pain and the signs and symptoms of hypovolemic shock are indicative of uterine rupture. In addition, rebound tenderness, the palpation of extrauterine fetal parts, and distention may be appreciated on palpation of the abdomen if complete rupture has occurred. Palpation of the uterus can reveal hypertonic contractions, normal contractions, or cessation of contractions. Vaginal bleeding may be present, though most bleeding tends to be intraabdominal. Signs and symptoms of hypovolemic shock may develop if hemorrhage is significant.

Laboratory studies of immediate use include a CBC, type and cross-match, and a coagulation profile.

If the uterine rupture compromises uteroplacental blood flow, evidence of fetal distress including the absence of short- and long-term variability, fetal bradycardia, and recurrent variable decelerations that do not respond to maternal positioning, oxygen administration, or fluid administration will be evident.

Management

Definitive care for uterine rupture is surgical repair, and the critical care paramedic's primary goals should be to ensure proper maternal airway control, oxygenation, and circulatory integrity in order to preserve uteroplacental perfusion. The patient should be placed in the left lateral recumbent position and administered 100% oxygen at 15 lpm via a nonrebreather mask. Large-bore IV access should be obtained, and volume replacement with a crystalloid solution initiated if blood loss is significant. If hypovolemic shock is present, aggressive volume replacement should be initiated with a crystalloid and packed RBCs. The critical care transport team should procure additional packed RBCs from the transporting facility for infusion during transport. An indwelling urinary catheter should be inserted to allow for monitoring of urinary output; an output of greater than 0.5 mL/kg/hr is desired, and is suggestive of adequate intravascular volume and renal perfusion. Uterine contractions can be encouraged with the administration of 20–40 units of oxytocin 1,000 mL at 100 mL/hr, and may attenuate bleeding via blood vessel constriction.

POSTPARTUM HEMORRHAGE

The loss of greater than 500 mL of blood after a vaginal delivery or greater than 1,000 mL of blood after a cesarean section is considered a postpartum hemorrhage (PPH). PPH occurs in about 5% of all deliveries, is implicated in almost 30% of all pregnancy-related deaths, and most hemorrhages occur within 24 hours of delivery. The most common cause of PPH is uterine atony, and retained placental fragments and birth canal trauma are additional causes. Risk factors for uterine atony include retention of placental fragments, overdistention of the uterus, multiparity, polyhydramnios (an abnormal amount of amniotic fluid), chorioamnioitis (an infection of the placental tissue membranes and amniotic fluid), prolonged or obstructed labor, use of general anesthesia, and magnesium tocolysis. A major risk factor for retained placenta is the development of placenta accreta.

Pathophysiology

Normally, post-labor platelet aggregation and clot formation in the decidua are complemented by myometrial contraction that constricts and occludes blood vessels torn when the placenta disassociates from the uterine implantation site. Because the blood flow to the uteroplacental boundary is about 600 mL/min, the potential for significant hemorrhage exists if uterine contraction does not take place. As any of the etiologies described earlier prevent uterine contraction, blood accumulates and clots within the uterus, further preventing uterine contraction and worsening bleeding.

A retained placenta can also result in postpartum hemorrhage, and is said to occur when the placenta has not delivered within 30 minutes after the onset of the third stage of labor. A common cause of retained placenta is placenta accreta, a condition in which the Nitabuch's layer does not form between the trophoblastic layer of the developing placenta and the myometrium, allowing the placenta to invade the myometrium. Formation of the cleavage plane between the placenta and the uterine wall does not take place, and the placenta is wholly or partially retained. Applying traction to the cord in an attempt to facilitate delivery of the placenta results in tearing of the uterine wall and worsening hemorrhage.

The loss of greater than 500 mL of blood after a vaginal delivery or greater than 1,000 mL of blood after a cesarean section is considered a postpartum hemorrhage (PPH).

In addition, trauma to the birth canal can result in PPH. Though lacerations of the lower uterus, cervix, vaginal canal, and perineum seldom result in massive hemorrhage, continuous, slow hemorrhaging over hours or days can result in significant blood loss.

Coagulation abnormalities such as DIC and von Willebrand's disease (a hereditary bleeding disorder) should also be considered as causes of PPH.

Assessment

Uterine atony can be identified by a lack of uterine contractions and a flaccid uterus on palpation. Vaginal bleeding should be apparent, but external blood loss may not be representative of total blood loss, much of which may be sequestered in the uterus. Signs and symptoms of shock, rather than estimates of total blood loss, should be assessed to evaluate the hemodynamic status of the patient. An external examination of the reproductive anatomy may reveal lacerations to the perineal region and vaginal vestibule, and an internal exam, performed by a properly trained individual, may reveal trauma to the vaginal canal, cervix, and lower uterus.

Laboratory results useful to the critical care transport paramedic include a CBC, type and cross-match, and hematocrit to aid in the administration of blood products. Coagulation studies can help rule out DIC.

Treatment

Administer 100% oxygen at 15 lpm via a nonrebreather mask. Large-bore IV access should be obtained, and volume replacement with a crystalloid solution initiated if blood loss is significant. If hypovolemic shock is present, aggressive volume replacement should be initiated with a crystalloid and packed RBCs. A urinary catheter should be placed in order to monitor urinary output and allow for contraction of the lower uterus.

Uterine fundal massage may help stimulate uterine contractions, as will the administration of oxytocin 20–40 units at 1,000 mL at 100 mL/hr. The drug carboprost tromethamine (Hemabate) can be used for the treatment of postpartum hemorrhage due to uterine atony that has not responded to conventional methods of management. Prior to the use of this drug, treatment should include the use of intravenously administered oxytocin and manipulative techniques such as uterine massage. Clinical studies have shown that use of carboprost tromethamine has resulted in satisfactory control of hemorrhage when used correctly. The drug is administered by deep intramuscular injection at a dose of 250 mcg. If persistent hemorrhage continues despite aforementioned medical management, the situation will have to be corrected in the OR.

MEDICAL COMPLICATIONS OF PREGNANCY

HYPERTENSION IN PREGNANCY

With the American College of Obstetricians and Gynecologists' adoption of the National High Blood Pressure Education Program Working Group's 2002 revision of the classification of hypertension during pregnancy, four categories are now recognized: chronic hypertension, gestational hypertension, preeclampsia, and chronic hypertension with preeclampsia. A pregnant female is considered hypertensive when she has a systolic blood pressure above 140 mmHg or a diastolic blood pressure above 90 mmHg. Chronic hypertension is hypertension that predates pregnancy or is identified prior to 20 weeks' gestation. Gestational hypertension occurs after 20 weeks' gestation and is not accompanied by proteinuria. **Preeclampsia** is said to exist when hypertension and proteinuria (greater than 300 mg in a 24-hour urine collection or, less formally, a urine dipstick positive for protein) coexist. Chronic hypertension with superimposed preeclampsia exists when a female with known hypertension develops worsening hypertension and proteinuria.

Preeclampsia occurs in 6% to 8% of all live births. The exact cause or causes of preeclampsia are unknown, but many theoretical models exist that include immunologic responses, increased sensitivity to endogenous vasoconstrictors, endothelial damage with prostacyclin and thromboxane A_2 production, chronic DIC, and genetic predisposition. One common thread among practically all of these models is an increase in vasoconstriction, peripheral vascular resistance, and subsequent hypertension. Known risk factors include an age greater than 35 years and less than 15

preeclampsia *potentially life-threatening (both mother and fetus) syndrome of combined hypertension and proteinuria in the third trimester of pregnancy.*

Preeclampsia occurs in 6% to 8% of all live births.

years, history of preeclampsia in a previous pregnancy (25% chance of recurrence), multiparity (multiparity plus previous preeclampsia has a recurrence rate of 50%), preexisting renal or cardiovascular disease, diabetes, family history, and African American descent.

Fetal risks associated with preeclampsia include uteroplacental hypoperfusion, placental infarction, abruptio placentae, inhibited fetal growth, oligohydramnios, and fetal demise. Maternal risks include renal failure, hepatic failure, DIC, seizures and strokes, and death. The maternal mortality rate is 2% to 4% in eclampsia or when hemolysis, elevated liver enzymes, and low platelets syndrome complicates preeclampsia.

Pathophysiology and Assessment Findings

The primary complication of hypertension in pregnancy is decreased perfusion to, and function of, all major body organs and systems and the development of eclampsia. A decrease in renal blood flow results in a decrease in GFR and, therefore, urinary output. Damage to the glomerular capillary endothelial cells results in the loss of protein (albumin) in the urine, and decreased kidney function. As a result, water and sodium are retained, and uric acid, urea nitrogen, and creatinine excretion diminish, resulting in elevated plasma levels.

Reduction in hepatic blood flow results in a decrease in liver function and an elevation of liver enzymes. Capsular edema and subcapsular hemorrhage can occur to such a degree that the liver capsule can rupture with resultant hemorrhage into the peritoneal space.

A relative hemoconcentration occurs in pregnancy-induced hypertension (PIH) as a result of a loss of plasma volume into the intravascular space. This loss of volume occurs when the normal oncotic pressure is upset by the loss of albumin in the urine. Blood plasma then moves from the intravascular to the intracellular space, resulting in an increased hematocrit and a worsening of the normal edema commonly seen in pregnancy. Hemolysis of red blood cells occurs when they pass through the scarred, constricted microvasculature, resulting in hyperbilirubinemia. In addition, consumptive thrombocytopenia unaccompanied by any other coagulopathies is characteristic of progressive hypertension in pregnancy.

While cerebral perfusion is not impaired, vasospasm of the cerebral arteries results in headaches, nausea and vomiting, seizures, and cerebral edema. In the lungs, changes in pulmonary capillary permeability can result in pulmonary edema.

Preeclampsia can be classified as mild or severe. Severe preeclampsia is said to exist when any of the following clinical or laboratory exam findings are present:

- ★ SBP >160 mmHg or DBP >110 mmHg two times at least 6 hours apart
- ★ Proteinuria >5 g in 24 hours
- ★ Cerebral or visual symptoms
- ★ Oliguria, 500 mL over 24 hours
- ★ Pulmonary edema
- ★ Right upper quadrant pain
- ★ Elevated liver enzymes
- ★ Low platelet count (<100,000/mm^3)
- ★ Restricted fetal growth

The **HELLP** syndrome is an acronym for **H**emolysis, **E**levated **L**iver function tests, and **L**ow **P**latelets, and is thought to be a subcategory of severe preeclampsia. Patients exhibiting the HELLP syndrome often experience a rapid, degenerative course, and many physicians elect for prompt delivery before the onset of eclampsia. Preeclampsia is termed mild when findings are present but do not meet the criteria established for severe preeclampsia. Eclampsia, the most serious manifestation of PIH, is said to be present when the patient has a seizure.

Management

After ensuring that the patient has a patent airway, is breathing adequately, and has a pulse, she should be placed on 100% oxygen via a nonrebreather mask, and large-bore IV access should be established. An indwelling urinary catheter should be placed and urine output monitored. A urine dipstick can be used to assess for proteinuria.

To aid in patient comfort and the prevention of seizure activity, care should be taken to ensure that the transport environment is as quiet and as low lit as possible. Planning and preparation should take place as to what action shall be taken by which crew members should seizures develop. Advanced airway supplies and magnesium sulfate should be readily available should this occur.

If pulmonary edema is present, IV morphine 2–5 mg and IV furosemide 20–120 mg can be administered, and CPAP or endotracheal intubation may be required in severe cases of respiratory distress. Diuretics should only be used if absolutely needed, because they can worsen the vasoconstriction and vascular depletion characteristic of preeclampsia.

Significant elevations in blood pressure (DBP >110 mmHg, MAP > 125 mmHg) can be treated with antihypertensives such as magnesium sulfate, hydralazine, or labetalol. If the patient becomes **eclamptic,** broadly defined as seizure activity or coma unrelated to other cerebral conditions in an obstetrical patient, additional management is warranted. As with any seizure, the initial management is to ensure a clear airway and provide high-flow, high-concentration oxygen. The patient should be positioned in the left lateral position to help improve uterine blood flow and obstruction of the vena cava by the gravid uterus. The patient should be protected against maternal injury during the seizure, and secretions should be suctioned from the patient's mouth.

eclamptic *broadly defined as seizure activity or coma unrelated to other cerebral conditions in an obstetrical patient; usually associated with preeclampsia.*

No attempt should be made to control initial seizure activity. If seizures are prolonged or recur, administration of 2–4 g of magnesium sulfate IV or IM should be considered. Although magnesium sulfate may cause respiratory depression, by the time the patient reaches this level of criticality the airway is likely already being controlled. Ongoing and/or ultimate management for the eclamptic patient is delivery of the infant after proper stabilization. If the patient is undelivered, no attempt should be made to deliver the infant either vaginally or by cesarean delivery until the acute phase of the seizure or coma has passed. The mode of delivery should be based on obstetric indications but should be chosen with an awareness of the fact that vaginal delivery is preferable from a maternal standpoint with preeclampsia.

GESTATIONAL DIABETES MELLITUS

Gestational diabetes mellitus (GDM) is a term used to identify those cases of diabetes, regardless of severity or insulin requirements, that initially present during pregnancy. GDM can be a true initial onset of Type I or Type II diabetes, or may represent a previously unrecognized case, worsened by the increased demand placed on the mother by the developing fetus. The incidence of GDM varies between less than 1% to 15% of all pregnancies. The pathogenesis of GDM mimics that of Type II non–insulin-dependent DM, in that impaired insulin secretion and increased insulin resistance are present in both. Most cases of GDM resolve after pregnancy, though there is a 32% lifetime risk of developing Type II DM after GDM.

gestational diabetes mellitus (GDM) *diabetes, regardless of type, that initially presents during pregnancy, and usually resolves postdelivery.*

Risk factors for developing GDM include maternal obesity, previous infant over 4,000 g birth weight, history or family history of DM, history of preeclampsia, maternal age over 30 years, and excessive weight gain during pregnancy (>40 lb). Pregnant women considered high risk are given a 3-hour oral glucose tolerance test (OGTT) during their first prenatal visit.

Maternal complications include preterm labor, preeclampsia, pyelonephritis, and the need for cesarean section. Fetal complications include increased perinatal morbidity and mortality, shoulder dystocia, stillbirth, operative delivery, and macrosomia (a newborn with an excessive birth weight).

Most cases of GDM are controlled with diet and frequent glucose monitoring, though if diet is unsuccessful after 2 weeks insulin may be used to maintain euglycemia. Pregnant patients taking insulin to control their diabetes often have wider variations in their sugar levels than do nonpregnant diabetics. Especially in the first trimester, when morning sickness may prevent adequate food intake, hypoglycemia is common among patients with fixed insulin doses.

Assessment

Any patient who has a preexisting history of diabetes, GDM, or presents with an altered mental status or decreased LOC should have her blood glucose determined. Because the clinical signs and symptoms of hypoglycemia can widely vary, the best idea is to get into the habit of establishing a blood glucose on every patient with which you come in contact. In addition to altered mental status and decreased LOC, signs of sympathetic nervous system activation are common in cases of hypoglycemia, including tachycardia and pale, diaphoretic skin.

Management

The management of a diabetic emergency in the pregnant patient is the same as in the nonpregnant patient. After ensuring that the airway is patent, breathing is adequate, and your patient has a pulse, 100% oxygen should be administered via nonrebreather mask at 15 lpm, an IV of normal saline established, and blood glucose determined. If hypoglycemia is present, administer 25–50 g of dextrose IV. If hyperglycemia is present, administer insulin subcutaneously.

Because of the increased metabolic demands, patients in active labor with GDM should have their blood glucose levels checked every hour. Patients with preterm labor being controlled with beta-adrenergic agonists are at a higher risk for hypoglycemia and should be monitored carefully. If blood glucose levels drop below 80 dL/mg, a continuous infusion of D_5W, at 125 mL/hr can be initiated. For insulin-dependent patients in labor, a continuous insulin infusion should be considered.

EMBOLISM

Thromboembolic disorders occur secondary to numerous reasons, many of which are related to the physiological changes seen in pregnancy, as already discussed. For the female patient, the greatest risk for developing a pulmonary embolism is in the time immediately following birth of the baby, especially if a cesarean section was performed. Of those who experience death secondary to a pulmonary embolism following birth of the baby, two-thirds die within 30 minutes of the initial embolism state. The assessment, management, and complications associated with a pulmonary embolism are essentially the same as the nonpregnant patient experiencing a pulmonary emboli; however, the differential diagnosis of amniotic fluid embolism must be considered.

Amniotic fluid embolism (AFE) is rare, but when it occurs it is associated with mortality rates between 80% and 90%. The majority of those deaths occur within the first few hours of the event. In an attempt to better understand the pathophysiology, risk factors for AFE have been identified and include large fetus, maternal age >32 years old, multiparity, premature separation of the placenta, tumultuous labor, and placental abruption.

The pathophysiology behind AFE shares many of the same features as anaphylactic and septic shock. There is a release of cellular chemical mediators such as prostaglandins, histamines, and leukotrienes, which are associated with many of the manifestations of AFE. It is believed that when the amniotic sac tears, there is a release of fluid into the maternal venous circulation, which then travels to the lungs. Vasospasm occurs, which causes transient pulmonary hypertension and subsequent right ventricular failure, pulmonary edema, and severe hypoxia. DIC is a common process with this emergency and is thought to be the result of activation of the fibrinolytic system by the amniotic fluid.

Suspicion of AFE is made when the patient has an acute onset of symptoms during or after delivery. They typically have acute respiratory distress, shock findings out of proportion to the actual blood loss, chills, shivering, diaphoresis, and fever. Pulmonary edema is present in worsening cases and is followed closely by acute cardiovascular collapse. In a subset of this population, the initial finding may be a seizure.

Suspicion of AFE is made based on symptomatology, and is confirmed by the presence of fetal squamous cells, vernix, meconium, and mucin from blood aspirated from the pulmonary artery. Obtaining a chest X-ray may demonstrate pulmonary edema, plural effusions, and cardiac silhouette enlargement. Management includes ensuring oxygenation, supporting inadequate breathing, and providing for cardiovascular support. The use of inotropics, fluid therapy, and blood are commonly used. Additional therapies may include bronchodilators, low-dose heparin, and steroids.

Summary

This chapter was designed to provide the critical care paramedic with necessary knowledge regarding the related anatomy and physiology, pathophysiology, symptomatology, and management techniques appropriate for a female patient with a high-risk OB/GYN condition. Furthermore, it behooves the health care provider in this environment to stay abreast of current literature regarding the assessment and management of these patients because the medical science used to treat OB/GYN emergencies is continually evolving. By reading this chapter and employing the knowledge gained within, it is hoped that the high-risk OB/GYN patient will enjoy the same high level of patient care as others do who utilize the critical care transport systems.

Review Questions

1. The HELLP syndrome is an acronym for _____, and is thought to be a subcategory of _____.

2. Four medications that can be utilized in the critical care transport environment to achieve tocolysis include:

   _____

   _____

   _____

   _____

3. Diuretics, such as furosemide, should be used with caution in the treatment of pulmonary edema secondary to severe preeclampsia because _____.

4. If uterine massage proves ineffective for correcting uterine atony and controlling postpartum hemorrhage, the critical care paramedic can consider the administration of _____ at _____ mL/hr via _____.

5. Once shoulder dystocia has been recognized, the immediate _____ and a _____ may facilitate delivery of the fetus when combined with suprapubic pressure and downward traction on the fetal head.

6. Which of the following is NOT a sign of fetal well-being?
   a. accelerations
   b. late decelerations
   c. short-term variability
   d. long-term variability

7. Which of the following is NOT a sign of fetal distress?
   a. early decelerations
   b. variable decelerations
   c. late decelerations
   d. lack of long-term variability

8. Which of the following findings meets the criteria of severe preeclampsia?
   a. proteinuria, 4.8 g in 24 hours
   b. SBP > 150 mmHg
   c. platelet count of 10,000/mm^3
   d. 600 mL of urine output over 24 hours

9. All of the following are appropriate actions for the management of fetal distress EXCEPT:
   a. administration of terbutaline if hypertonic uterine contractions are causing the fetal distress
   b. discontinuing an oxytocin infusion if the fetal distress is secondary to hypertonic contractions
   c. amnioinfusion in cases of premature membrane rupture
   d. the evaluation of abruptio placenta with transabdominal ultrasonography

10. Which of the following should be avoided in suspected cases of placenta previa?

    a. vaginal examination with a speculum

    b. administration of a tocolytic agent

    c. delivery via cesarean section

    d. evaluation and diagnosis via ultrasound

See Answers to Review Questions at the back of this book.

Further Reading

Bader TJ, Day LD. "Hypertension in Pregnancy." In *OB/GYN Secrets, updated,* 3rd ed. Bader TJ, editor. Phildelphia: Elsevier Mosby, 2005.

Bledsoe BE, Porter RS, Cherry RA. *Paramedic Care: Principles & Practice,* 2nd ed. Upper Saddle River, NJ: Pearson Prentice Hall, 2005.

Forouzan I. "Pathophysiology of the Placenta." In *OB/GYN Secrets, updated* 3rd ed. Bader TJ, editor. Phildelphia: Elsevier Mosby, 2005.

Gill A. "Antepartum Bleeding." In *OB/GYN Secrets, updated,* 3rd ed. Bader TJ, editor. Phildelphia: Elsevier Mosby, 2005.

Holleran RS. *Air & Surface Patient Transport: Principles & Practice,* 3rd ed. St. Louis, MO: Mosby, 2003.

Kuhn GJ. "Emergencies during Pregnancy and the Postpartum Period." In *Emergency Medicine: A Comprehensive Study Guide,* 6th ed. Tintinelli JE, Kelen JD, Stapczynski JS, editors. New York: McGraw-Hill, 2004.

Maiolatesi CR. "The Critically Ill Pregnant Women." In *Critical Care Nursing: A Holistic Approach,* 7th ed. Hudak CM, Gallo BM, Morton PG, editors. Philadelphia: Lippincott-Raven Publishers, 1998.

Martini FH, Timmons MJ, McKinley, MP. *Human Anatomy,* 3rd ed. Upper Saddle River, NJ: Pearson Prentice Hall, 2000.

Pare E. "Intrapartum Fetal Surveillance." In *OB/GYN Secrets, updated,* 3rd ed. Bader TJ, editor. Philadelphia: Elsevier Mosby, 2005.

Simhan HN. "Diabetes in Pregnancy." In *OB/GYN Secrets, updated,* 3rd ed. Bader TJ, editor. Phildelphia: Elsevier Mosby, 2005.

Simhan HN. "Preterm Labor." In *OB/GYN Secrets, updated,* 3rd ed., Bader TJ, editor. Phildelphia: Elsevier Mosby, 2005.

Sokol RJ, Larsen JW, Landy HJ, et al. "Methods of Assessment for Pregnancy at Risk." In *Current Obstetric and Gynecologic Diagnosis and Treatment,* 7th ed., Pernoll ML, editor, pp. 269–299. East Norwalk, CT: Appleton and Lange, 1991.

VanRooyen MJ, Fortner KB. "Emergency Delivery." In *Emergency Medicine: A Comprehensive Study Guide,* 6th ed. Tintinelli JE, Kelen JD, Stapczynski JS, editors. New York: McGraw-Hill, 2004.

Neonatal Emergencies

William S. Krost, NREMT-P

Objectives

Upon completion of this chapter, the student should be able to:

1. Appreciate the physiological differences between the adult and the neonate. (p. 876)
2. Discuss the pathophysiology of respiratory complications in the neonate. (p. 880)
3. Discuss the pathophysiology of meconium aspiration. (p. 882)
4. Discuss the step wise procedure used to manage a neonate who presents with meconium aspiration. (p. 882)
5. Discuss the pathophysiology of congenital heart disease in the neonate (p. 884)
6. Describe the initial steps and ongoing management in the assessment and management of the neonate. (p. 891)
7. Discuss the importance of, and how to assure normothermia in the neonatal patient during transports (p. 892).
8. Discuss the pathophysiology of hypoglycemia in the neonate. (p. 893)

Key Terms

atrial septal defect (ASD), p. 885
bilirubin, p. 890
cyanotic heart defects, p. 887
ductus arteriosus (DA), p. 879
ductus venosus, p. 879

extrauterine, p. 879
foramen ovale, p. 879
intrauterine, p. 879
jaundice, p. 890
necrotizing enterocolitis (NEC), p. 890
neonatal respiratory distress syndrome, p. 882

persistent pulmonary hypertension of the newborn (PPHN), p. 881
surfactant, p. 882
transient tachypnea of the newborn (TTN), p. 882
ventricular septal defect (VSD), p. 885

Case Study

You and your partner are working an overnight shift at the regional neonatal and pediatric referral center. Around 0130 your pager activates, and directs you to the helipad for a mission. By the time you and your partner have retrieved the refrigerated drugs and completed your preinspection around the aircraft, the pilot is already in the helicopter and is warming up the engines. You climb into the aircraft and secure the drugs and mobile equipment when the pilot informs you that you are going to a rural ED about 70 miles northeast of the city. This referral center is one of the network institutions that is affiliated with your base hospital and flight program, and is the largest consumer of the critical care flight program. Approximately 8 minutes into your flight you receive the following information across your pager "36-year-old female, 36 weeks' gestation. Transport back to high-risk OB unit due to decreased amniotic fluid noted on ultrasound." This seems like a rather routine mission for you and your partner, and about 20 minutes later you touch down on the helipad of the referral facility. There, you are met by security, and they escort you to the emergency department while the pilot stays with the aircraft.

Upon arrival in the ED, the patient's nurse advises you that the mother is gravida IV, para III, had no prenatal care, and just delivered the baby, despite some difficulty in doing so. The newborn, she advises you, responded slowly and had an initial APGAR of 4, and a 5-minute APGAR of 7. She then adds there was a fair amount of meconium staining noted in the amniotic fluid.

As you walk into the patient's room, you see the mother lying on the bed in obvious emotional distress as she watches the other care providers work on her baby now lying under the radiant warmer. The baby, from what you've seen thus far, looks very limp and ashen in color. You glance back at the RN and ask if they updated the receiving facility of this change in patient status. The RN responds she hasn't had a chance to yet because things "happened so fast," but she would do that now. You then ask her to ensure that the receiving facility knows that the infant is premature and is not responding appropriately.

As you approach the neonate, a few of the hospital staff step to the side so you can get access to the young infant lying on the small area of bedding beneath the radiant warmer. The female neonate has skin that is cool to the touch, you see only moderate flexing of the major muscle groups, and you note that there is some laborious effort to the neonate's breathing pattern. Cyanosis is noted to the hands and feet of the newborn. As your partner starts to gather medical documentation and speaks to the mother, you focus more intently on the neonate's airway and oxygenation status.

The neonate has an intact airway, and the ED resident present states there was a small amount of meconium evident during birthing, but none was noted in the oropharynx. The mother denies any history of drug abuse or other drug ingestion prior to delivery. Despite ongoing oxygenation, stimulation, and blow-by oxygen, the neonate is still not responding as well as you'd like. The decision is made to test the neonate's blood glucose level (BGL). While this is being performed, you consult with your partner about the need for an isolette for transport back to your facility. The only viable option is to alert another helicopter and have them bring one to you at your present location. The problem you conclude is that this will add a considerable amount of time overall to the transport.

The ED resident alerts you that the neonate's BGL level is 38 mg/dL. There is consensus between you and the ED physician to administer a 5 mL/kg bolus of 10% dextrose in water after initiating an intravenous line with crystalloid solution (via umbilical vein access). Shortly following these therapies, the neonate was noted to initiate more spontaneous movements of the flexor and extensor muscles, began to cry, and had a noted improvement in skin color. After about another 5 minutes of observation, the infant's APGAR has reached a numeric value of 10.

Pleased with the status of the infant's condition, you and your partner elect to carefully bundle the infant in warmed blankets and place her with her mother on your portable cot. Due to the prematurity of the infant, and the lack of prenatal care, the decision to transport the mother and child back to your facility is upheld by your medical control physician. You carefully secure the both of them, apply warmed humidified oxygen, and take careful measures to ensure the warmth of both the mother and infant. You radio ahead to your pilot to ready the aircraft and ensure the heater in the patient compartment is turn on high heat.

You load the aircraft and start the uneventful transport back to the receiving facility where the neonatal heath care providers were awaiting your return.

INTRODUCTION

In 2002 there were 4,021,726 births in the United States. It is estimated that roughly 6% of all newborns require life support in the ED or delivery room. Of those who have a birth weight of less than 1,500 g, the need for resuscitation rises to 60%. Additionally, those neonates that are birthed at 24 weeks' gestation have an approximate viability rate of only 20% to 30%.

Morbidity and mortality of these premature and other critically ill neonates decreases when these neonates are cared for in specially designed neonatal intensive care units (NICUs). As care for these neonates has evolved and specialty care centers have progressed, the capabilities of the critical care transport personnel have also continued to evolve out of necessity. Critical care transport teams should be capable of providing care to the neonate in essentially the same manner that care would be delivered in an NICU. The transport environment, in this situation, should be treated as an extension of the neonatal intensive care unit.

Gestational age will determine the potential problems the neonate will have in making the transition from intrauterine to extrauterine life. Table 29–1 illustrates gestational age classification and some of the more common complications associated with each of these gestational ages.

The discussion in this chapter of pertinent anatomy and physiology precedes any discussion on pathophysiology. Following the review of the neonatal anatomy, the common emergencies seen by the critical care paramedic will be grouped under the headings of pulmonary and cardiovascular pathophysiology. Following this, we will discuss a few general emergencies that may be seen by the critical care transport team that do not fit in either category. Then, following the specific emergencies, a section on general assessment considerations and management principles will be provided

Table 29–1	Gestational Age	
Classification	**Gestation**	**Potential Complications**
Preterm infant	Less than 37 weeks	Thermoregulation, IRDS, sepsis
Term	38–42 weeks	Pneumonia, birth asphyxia, meconium aspiration, sepsis
Post-term infant	More than 42 weeks	Asphyxia-related complications, sepsis

that could be applied to multiple situations of neonatal transport since it is impossible to entertain all types of problems that could occur.

RELATIVE ANATOMY AND PHYSIOLOGY

PHYSIOLOGY OF THERMOREGULATION

At birth, the neonatal body surface area-to-volume ratio is four times that of an adult, while their heat production (thermogenesis) is only one and a half times as high. This leaves the neonate at significant risk for hypothermia with resultant physiological compromise. Despite the larger surface area, the neonate has little adipose tissue and as a result, a limited ability to maintain core body temperature. Additionally, neonatal muscle tone is immature and cannot effectively induce shivering to promote heat generation. Heat loss in the neonate, as in the adult, occurs as the result of evaporation, convection, conduction, and radiation. The majority of heat loss in the neonate occurs from evaporation, especially in the moments just following birth. Heat loss through convection (the room ambient temperature) is dependent on the environment in which the neonate is born. A cold room or a room with excessive air flow should be considered problematic in the preparation for delivery of the newborn, and hence avoided. Generally speaking, if the care provider is "comfortable" in the temperature of the room, then it is too cold for the neonate. Steps should be taken to ensure the ambient temperature for the infant is as close to normal core temperature as possible.

Generally speaking, if the care provider is "comfortable" in the temperature of the room, then it is too cold for the neonate.

GLUCOSE REQUIREMENTS

Newborns are at significant risk for the development of acute hypoglycemia because of (1) poor glucose stores, (2) inability to stimulate the release of glucose stores from the immature neonatal liver, or (3) increased metabolism that results in the utilization of large quantities of available glucose. Neonatal glucose levels should be assessed within 1–2 hours after birth and repeated every 30 minutes to 1 hour thereafter until normal glucose levels have been attained. Normal blood glucose levels (BGLs) in the neonate should be maintained above 70–80 mg/dL.

Neonatal mentation may be very difficult to assess so the ability to recognize the clinical signs and symptoms of hypoglycemia is imperative for the critical care paramedic. Signs of hypoglycemia in the neonate may include twitching, seizure activity, muscular hypotonia (limpness), eye-rolling, a high-pitched cry, respiratory apnea, or irregular respirations. Should any of these indications be present, normal assessment and management of the neonate would include glucose testing and administration of 10% dextrose as warranted.

Newborns are at significant risk for the development of acute hypoglycemia because of (1) poor glucose stores, (2) inability to stimulate the release of glucose stores from the immature neonatal liver, or (3) increased metabolism that results in the utilization of large quantities of available glucose.

AIRWAY ANATOMY AND PHYSIOLOGY

Neonates are unique and have very different anatomical and physiological qualities as compared to adults. The tongue exhibits one of the most obvious anatomical differences seen between the adult and the neonate. The neonatal tongue is larger than an adult's (owing to the need for breast-feeding) in relationship to the amount of free space in the oropharynx. The large tongue creates a significant probability for airway occlusion in the depressed neonate, and additionally there is very little room should there be any type of airway edema. (See Figure 29-1 ■.)

The neonatal trachea is much more pliable than an adult's. Neonates do not have completed cartilaginous tracheal rings (with the exception of the first tracheal ring). The increased pliability of the trachea can be troublesome in the neonatal patient because hyperextension and/or hyperflexion of the neck may lead to complete or partial occlusion of the airway because of kinking. This small diameter of the trachea is the primary reason why even small amounts of swelling cause significant compromises of airflow.

The neonatal epiglottis is large and more U- or Ω-shaped or oblong than an adult's. It is also more pliable from the incomplete cartilaginous support, making it more difficult to manipulate when attempting orotracheal intubation. For this reason, neonatal laryngoscopy should be per-

Neonates are unique and have very different anatomical and physiological qualities as compared to adults.

The neonatal trachea is much more pliable than an adult's.

Neonatal intubation should be performed using a straight (Miller) blade versus a curved (MacIntosh) blade.

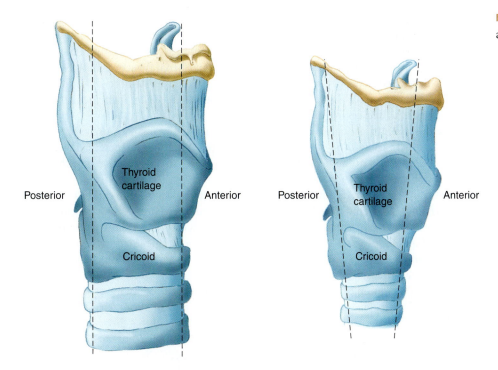

Posterior   Thyroid cartilage   Anterior   Posterior   Thyroid cartilage   Anterior

Cricoid   Cricoid

Adult and Infant Airways

formed using a straight (Miller) blade versus a curved (MacIntosh) blade. The reason for this preference is attributed to the unique shape of the epiglottis. The curved blade fits into the vallecula and indirectly lifts the epiglottis out of the way while the straight blade gets under the epiglottis and directly elevates it for visualization of the vocal cords. The epiglottis of the neonate may still rest posterior despite the curved blade exerting pressure to the glossoepiglottic ligament, and cause visual obstruction of the glottic opening. The use of the straight blade will directly lift the epiglottis and expose the vocal cords.

Another factor of concern regarding the neonatal airway is the position of the larynx. It is located both more anterior and cephalad as compared to the adult. The adult larynx sits at about the level of the fourth or fifth cervical vertebrae, and the neonatal larynx sits at about the level of the first or second cervical vertebrae. This is important to realize because the higher the larynx is, the more anterior the airway is, and the harder it is to achieve a single plane view needed for orotracheal intubation. To be successful in managing a neonate's airway, you should always assume that the airway is anterior, and you should utilize laryngoscopy techniques beneficial to providing an unobstructed view of the glottis (use of a straight blade, adequate displacement of the tongue, and posterior displacement of the larynx by implementing cricoid pressure with the tip of one finger).

Another anatomical difference in the neonate that makes airway maintenance a concern is that the mainstem bronchi are at less of an angle than an adult's and, as a result, aspiration can occur to either the left or right mainstem bronchi. As neonates grow, the chest diameter and the angle of the left bronchi will increase to a position more characteristic of the adult patient.

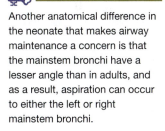

Another anatomical difference in the neonate that makes airway maintenance a concern is that the mainstem bronchi have a lesser angle than in adults, and as a result, aspiration can occur to either the left or right mainstem bronchi.

PULMONARY ANATOMY AND PHYSIOLOGY

The anatomy of the neonatal chest results in differences in how respiratory compromise will be observed. The bones in neonates are not completely calcified and tend to be flexible. When a neonate suffers some form of respiratory compromise, he will attempt to increase the volume of air entering the chest through the utilization of accessory muscles; however, the result of the increased inspiratory effort may not equal the degree of air flow.

First, the neonatal ribs are more horizontal than they are rounded (as seen in adults). The horizontal nature of the ribs provides for very little leverage to increase the anterior and posterior diameter of the chest. This results in the relative inability to provide the degree of lift that is necessary to increase the volume of the chest cavity on inspiration, when it is needed most. Neonates also have less well developed accessory musculature, which also makes it more difficult to increase the strength of ventilations. This lack of accessory muscles is one reason many neonates in respiratory distress present with excessive diaphragmatic breathing.

The sternum of a neonate is also very pliable. When the accessory muscles are being stretched, they will pull on various bony structures, including the sternum. The increased pliancy of the sternum also contributes to the neonate's inability to create a strong negative intrathoracic pressure, thereby inhibiting the efficiency of the inspiratory effort.

Neonates also have a diminished pulmonary reserve capacity compared to their adult counterparts.

Neonates also have a diminished pulmonary reserve capacity compared to their adult counterparts. To better understand this, the critical care paramedic need only review a normal neonatal chest x-ray. Here it will be easy to appreciate the relative amount of space the heart occupies in the thoracic cavity. Neonates have less ability to increase the volume within the lungs because the lungs can only expand according to the degree to which space is available for expansion. Since the heart is larger, and the ribs and sternum fail to adequately support the lungs, the net result is a diminishment in the space in which lung expansion can occur. In the end, this contributes to a more rapid development of hypoxemia and hypercapnia should the neonate suffer some type of pulmonary compromise.

Neonates are also primarily abdominal breathers. This means that they rely heavily on diaphragmatic motion (again a consequence of immature intercostal muscles and pliable ribs) for the work of breathing. The problem here is that the neonatal abdominal cavity is small and has relatively large abdominal organs compressed within it. This overcrowding of the neonatal abdominal cavity is a significant problem since it has a negative effect on the compensatory mechanisms for ventilation in neonates. In situations of excessive gastric insufflation, or issues of increased abdominal pressure, there is a limiting effect on diaphragmatic excursion. The inability of the diaphragm to lower during inhalation against increased intra-abdominal pressure has a direct negative effect on the quality of inspiratory volumes. Since neonates rely heavily on changing the respiratory rate to maintain minute ventilation rather than tidal volume (due to the relative inability to change tidal volume as a result of the aforementioned problems), an increase in the rate of respiration for compensation may not be sufficient if the diaphragm cannot move down against the abdominal contents.

The final difference that bears discussion is that neonates have a higher metabolic rate than adults, and they consume oxygen in the bloodstream at nearly double the rate of the adult. A smaller pulmonary reserve capacity coupled with a higher metabolic demand for oxygen leaves the neonate more predisposed to hypoxemia at the cellular level, despite the presence of spontaneous ventilatory effort. Hypoxemia in the neonate is a problem that can develop rapidly with disastrous effects should the critical care paramedic not stay attuned to the pulmonary functioning of the patient.

Neonates have a higher metabolic rate than adults, and they consume oxygen in the bloodstream at nearly double the rate of the adult.

A summary of the airway and pulmonary differences that impact the quality of ventilation and respiration in a neonate can be summarized as follows. First, the larger tongue and pliable epiglottis allow for the development of airway occlusion in the obtunded neonate very easily. In addition, they both serve as a formidable challenge when providing orotracheal intubation. Second, the pliancy of the thoracic bony structure fails to provide needed lift and support to the lung tissue to allow inhalation, especially in situations of heightened ventilatory effort. Third, the nature of the neonate being primarily an abdominal breather is diminished by any situation in which intra-abdominal pressure is elevated, thereby limiting diaphragmatic motion. Fourth, because the neonatal musculature is still relatively weak, it will fatigue easily in situations where ventilatory effort is markedly higher. Last, the higher metabolic consumption of oxygen at the cellular level in neonates will result in a faster onset of hypoxemia from an airway or ventilatory deficit. All of these contribute to the nature of the neonate to rapidly decompensate from hypoxemia and hypercapnia induced by a pulmonary dysfunction.

CARDIOVASCULAR ANATOMY AND PHYSIOLOGY

Several distinctions can be made between the adult and neonatal cardiovascular systems. The first distinction is that in the adult, gas exchange occurs at the alveolar-capillary level of the lungs. While this is also true for the neonate following birth, while still *in utero*, the fetus receives its oxygenation through the placenta. The important realization for the critical care paramedic is that should there be a disturbance to the alveoli following birth, then the critical care paramedic must deal with the nonfunctional alveoli immediately. If the neonate is expected to live, the alveolar dysfunction needs to be remedied almost immediately (oxygenation dysfunctions to the neonate will be discussed later in the chapter).

Another significant distinction is that the adult heart increases its stroke volume by increasing contractile force and heart rate when a higher cardiac output is demanded by the body. In contrast, the neonatal heart is usually only capable of increasing its rate in order to improve cardiac output (and systemic perfusion pressures). The neonatal heart has a low compliance as it relates to volume, and therefore cannot compensate by increasing stroke volume through inotropic changes. Consequently, the heart rate should be seen as a significant clinical marker when monitoring cardiac output in a distressed neonate. When the neonatal patient becomes bradycardic, it should be assumed that the patient's cardiac output has been drastically reduced.

The majority of physiological changes that occur to the neonatal cardiovascular system occur in the first minutes after delivery. The most significant of these physiological changes occurs when the umbilical cord is clamped and circulation is shifted from intrauterine (placental) to extrauterine (lungs). Once pulmonary circulation has been established, placental circulation ceases. The interruption of low-resistance, placental blood flow from the umbilical cord causes an increase in systemic vascular resistance. The lack of blood returning from the placenta forces the **ductus venosus** (vessel that leads directly into the vena cava, which allows some oxygenated blood and nutrients to be pumped out of the body without passing through the kidneys) to close due to pressure changes. The closure of the *ductus venosus* results in perfusion of the kidneys and initiates renal filtration of the blood. (See Figure 29-2 ■.)

Once pulmonary circulation has been established, the lungs will expand and a new physiological cascade is initiated. The first changes occur when then neonate takes its first breath and the lungs expand, causing a reduction in pulmonary vascular resistance (from negative intrathoracic pressure). This promotes an increase in pulmonary blood flow (more blood going into the lungs) and a reduction in pulmonary artery pressures (less arterial blood pressure inside the lungs). Because of these pressure changes, a shift occurs that causes the left heart to assume higher pressures than the right side of the heart and as a result, the **foramen ovale** (the opening between the left and right atria that while in *utero* allows blood to enter the left atrium of the heart from the right atrium) closes. The closure of the foramen ovale is what completes the wall of the septum between the left and right atria. Once the left- and right-sided heart borders have been established, normal circulation will commence.

Once the left side of the heart begins to receive oxygenated blood from the lungs, it is ejected from the left ventricle and into the aortic root. Here, it passes the sinus for the **ductus arteriosus (DA)**. The DA is a vascular structure that is open during fetal development and serves as a connection between the pulmonary artery and the aorta. It allows blood ejected out of the right ventricle to bypass the lungs by flowing through the DA and into the aorta (for systemic perfusion), rather than perfusing the nonfunctional lungs. After birth (and the systemic pressure in the aorta increases), it forces a portion of blood flow from the aorta into the still patent DA (in an opposite blood flow direction). When blood begins to move through the DA in this situation, it is now highly oxygenated. The high levels of oxygen in the blood passing through the DA from the aorta serve as a stimulant for vascular constriction of the ductal smooth muscle, which in turn leads to closure of the DA. In most full-term infants the ductus closes spontaneously in the first hours to weeks following birth.

Following the closure of this structure, there is now finally normalcy between how blood flows in the neonate and how it occurs in the adult. The important thing to note, however, is that this changeover of perfusion patterns from **intrauterine** (growth and development within the uterus) to **extrauterine** (life and growth outside the uterus) life is fraught with complications should some irregularity occur. One such reason is failure of the foramen ovale (within the atrial septum) to close. This allows mixture of deoxygenated blood from the right side of the heart to mix with oxygenated blood of the left atrium. While other abnormalities exist, many of them correctable with modern-day surgical techniques, it still does not relieve the critical care paramedic of having to assess and treat these dysfunctions should they be noted in your newborn patient.

The majority of physiological changes that occur to the neonatal cardiovascular system occur in the first minutes after delivery.

ductus venosus *vessel that leads directly into the vena cava that allows some oxygenated blood and nutrients to be pumped directly out of the body, bypassing the kidneys.*

foramen ovale *during fetal development, an opening between the left and right atria that allows blood to enter the left atrium of the heart from the right atrium.*

ductus arteriosus (DA) *during fetal development, a vascular connection that joins the right ventricle and pulmonary artery directly to the descending aorta, bypassing the immature lungs.*

intrauterine *growth and development within the uterus.*

extrauterine *life and growth outside the uterus.*

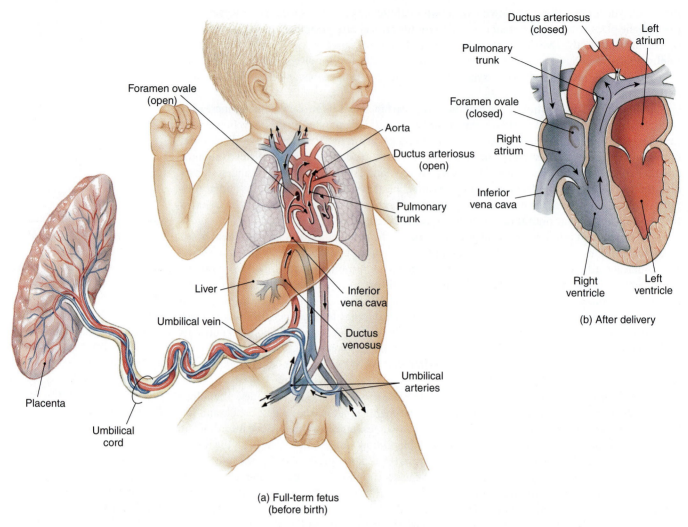

Foramen ovale
(open)

Aorta

Ductus arteriosus
(open)

Pulmonary
trunk

Liver

Inferior
vena cava

Umbilical vein

Ductus
venosus

Placenta

Umbilical
arteries

Umbilical
cord

(a) Full-term fetus
(before birth)

Ductus arteriosus
(closed)

Left
atrium

Pulmonary
trunk

Foramen ovale
(closed)

Right
atrium

Inferior
vena cava

Right
ventricle

Left
ventricle

(b) After delivery

■ **Figure 29-2** Fetal circulation. (a) Blood flow to and from the placenta. (b) Blood flow through the neonatal (newborn) heart. *(Fig. 14-22, p. 403, from* Essentials of Anatomy & Physiology, *2nd ed., by Frederic H. Martini, Ph.D. and Edwin F. Bartholomew, M.S. Copyright © 2000 by Frederic H. Martini, Inc. Published by Pearson Education, Inc. Reprinted by permission.)*

GENERAL PATHOPHYSIOLOGY: PULMONARY

ASSESSMENT OF RESPIRATORY DISTRESS

The general approach to the neonate by the critical care paramedic includes the assessment of the maternal and perinatal history, a focused physical examination of the neonate, and the use of diagnostic transport monitors. Causes of respiratory compromise may include mechanical obstruction of the airway by meconium, edema, or bronchospasm. Other causes that do not directly affect the airway but can still have untoward effects include congenital heart defects, thoracic trauma, or infection resulting in poor lung compliance.

RESPIRATORY DISTRESS, FAILURE, AND ARREST

Critical care paramedics who transport neonates need to be precise in the use of terms describing respiratory distress, respiratory failure, and respiratory arrest. This distinction commonly dictates how aggressive the critical care team needs to be in the management of the acutely ill neonate. It is important to note, however, that the etiology of respiratory compromise may not be readily available or identifiable to the critical care providers in all neonatal interactions. So the first goal is to provide care to any lost function of the airway or breathing components. Once this is assured, the

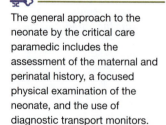

The general approach to the neonate by the critical care paramedic includes the assessment of the maternal and perinatal history, a focused physical examination of the neonate, and the use of diagnostic transport monitors.

The first goal of neonatal care is to provide care to any lost function of the airway or breathing components.

critical care team then needs to turn its attention to identifying potential causes of the hemodynamic and/or respiratory compromise. The goal in managing respiratory compromise in the critical care environment is to identify a set of causes, and treat the patient based on the most likely etiology.

Respiratory distress indicates that the patient still has the ability to compensate and maintain adequate minute ventilation spontaneously. However, the signs and symptoms seen indicate that the neonate is struggling harder to breathe, and further pulmonary deterioration will probably occur if left untreated. Respiratory failure is considered to be present when the patient has exhausted all of his compensatory mechanisms, and the respiratory effort present is now insufficient for meeting the metabolic oxygenation and carbon dioxide elimination demands being made by the body. It is important to understand that at this point, the neonate may still be breathing spontaneously, however the ventilatory effort is insufficient for the body's needs. A patient in respiratory distress can progress to respiratory failure rapidly, and a patient in respiratory failure will progress to respiratory arrest if management is not rapid and aggressive. For clarity and ease of review, the symptoms consistent with respiratory distress, respiratory failure, and respiratory arrest are summarized in Table 29–2.

PERSISTENT PULMONARY HYPERTENSION OF THE NEWBORN

Persistent pulmonary hypertension of the newborn (PPHN) is a clinical syndrome in which pulmonary vascular resistance is elevated in the presence of changes in pulmonary vessel reactivity. This change in the pulmonary circulation leads to sustained fetal circulation, meaning that the *ductus arteriosus* and *foramen ovale* remain open.

Respiratory distress indicates that the patient still has the ability to compensate and maintain adequate minute ventilation spontaneously.

Respiratory failure is considered to be present when the patient has exhausted all of his compensatory mechanisms, and the respiratory effort present is now insufficient for meeting the metabolic oxygenation and carbon dioxide elimination demands being made by the body.

persistent pulmonary hypertension of the newborn (PPHN) *a clinical syndrome in which the ductus arteriosus and foramen ovale remain open after birth, increasing pulmonary vascular resistance and causing cardiorespiratory distress.*

Table 29–2	Summary of the Symptoms Consistent with Respiratory Distress, Respiratory Failure, and Respiratory Arrest
Physiologic Cause	**Clinical Manifestations**
These signs occur because the child is attempting to compensate for oxygen deficit and airway blockage. Oxygen supply is inadequate; behavior and vital signs reflect compensation and beginning hypoxia.	*Respiratory failure—Initial signs* Restlessness Tachypnea Tachycardia Diaphoresis
The child attempts to use accessory muscles to assist oxygen intake; hypoxia persists and efforts now waste more oxygen than is obtained.	*Respiratory failure—Early decompensation* Nasal flaring Retractions Grunting Wheezing Anxiety and irritability Mood changes Headache Hypertension Confusion
These signs occur because oxygen deficit is overwhelming and beyond spontaneous recovery. Cerebral oxygenation is dramatically affected; central nervous system changes are ominous.	*Imminent respiratory arrest—Severe hypoxia* Dyspnea Bradycardia Cyanosis Stupor and coma

PPHN can occur from multiple etiologies but is most commonly associated with severe hypoxia, meconium aspiration syndrome, or congenital diaphragmatic hernia. The clinical presentation of PPHN mirrors many of the signs and symptoms seen with congenital heart diseases so unless heart defects have been diagnosed previously, it may be difficult to assess in the aeromedical or ground transport environment. PPHN is most commonly a clinical sign of another problem and is considered to be a disease process in and of itself.

The treatment of PPHN is aimed at maintaining oxygenation and, if a clear diagnosis is made, maintaining an alkalotic state through the administration of IV sodium bicarbonate. Past recommendations have suggested that hyperventilation may promote alkalemia; however, current literature suggests that hyperventilation reduces cerebral blood flow and thus has untoward effects on neonatal cerebral perfusion and development. Alternative therapies that have been used include the administration of inhaled nitric oxide. This has been shown to promote pulmonary vascular dilation, thereby decreasing the significance of PPHN by restoring the pulmonary and systemic perfusion pressures back to a closer-to-normal state, allowing closure of the fetal vascular structures. Additional studies have also suggested that magnesium sulfate and adenosine are effective as pulmonary vasodilators. The use of traditional pulmonary vasodilators like prostaglandin E_1, nitroglycerin, and nitroprusside have been shown to cause significant systemic hypotension because of their roles in systemic vasodilation and are not currently recommended for transport of the PPHN patient.

MECONIUM ASPIRATION SYNDROME

Meconium is a dark green-black substance that is found in the intestinal tract of full-term infants. Meconium is typically expelled as the first bowel movement of the delivered fetus. In 10% to 15% of all deliveries, however, meconium is expelled prematurely and may be distributed to the neonatal airways prior to delivery. Of these patients only 2% to 10% will aspirate the meconium into the lower airways, but when this does occur, the results can be life threatening. The meconium, once delivered to the respiratory tract of the neonate, may cause airway obstruction and, if obstruction is not immediately evident, may contribute to the inactivation of alveolar surfactant.

There are no known aspiration prevention strategies to date but it is believed that nasopharyngeal and endotracheal suctioning of the patient prior to delivery of the thoracic cavity may limit the extent of meconium aspiration into the lower airways. (See Figure 29-3 ■.)

TRANSIENT TACHYPNEA OF THE NEWBORN

transient tachypnea of the newborn (TTN) *a normally self-limiting syndrome of neonatal acute respiratory distress caused by delayed clearing of excess fluid in the lungs; also called "wet lung," or "Type II Respiratory Distress Syndrome" (RDS).*

Transient tachypnea of the newborn (TTN) is a cause of acute respiratory distress in the newborn. TTN may also be called *wet lung* or *Type II respiratory distress syndrome* (RDS). TTN is typically a self-limiting process that auto-resolves within 48–72 hours from birth and is caused by delayed clearing of fluids in the lungs.

Oxygen support should be provided and may need to be delivered by endotracheal intubation if the infant appears to be poorly oxygenating. It is common and appropriate to transport infants with the diagnosis of TTN on antibiotics until the diagnosis of sepsis or pneumonia is ruled out.

NEONATAL RESPIRATORY DISTRESS SYNDROME

neonatal respiratory distress syndrome *a lack of pulmonary surfactant causes significant difficulty in breathing; also known as hyaline membrane disease.*

surfactant *a mixture of phospholipids and proteins with a primary function of reducing surface tension within the alveoli and increasing lung compliance.*

Neonatal respiratory distress syndrome is also known as hyaline membrane disease. This disorder is one that primarily affects the lungs of premature infants and causes significant difficulty in breathing. Neonatal respiratory distress syndrome affects 10% of all premature infants and is rarely seen in full-term infants. This disease is caused by a lack of pulmonary surfactant in the alveoli. **Surfactant** is a mixture of phospholipids and proteins that is produced by the body from approximately 24 weeks of gestation onward. The primary and most relevant function of surfactant is that it reduces surface tension within the alveoli and increases lung compliance. The reduction in surface tension within the alveoli due to adequate surfactant levels keeps them from collapsing and allows them to inflate and reinflate more easily. In infant respiratory distress syndrome (IRDS) the problem is that, in the absence of sufficient alveolar surfactant, the alveoli collapse (causing atelec-

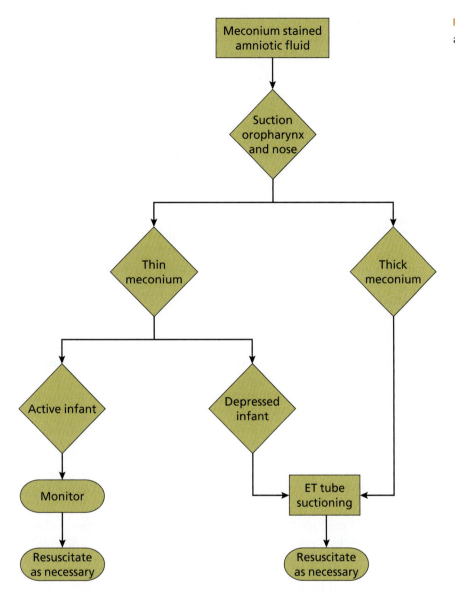

■ **Figure 29-3**   Meconium aspiration.

tasis), and the difficulty encountered in trying to reinflate them by neonatal ventilatory effort results in ineffective gas exchange with resultant hypoxia and hypercapnea.

Symptoms of IRDS include tachypnea, accessory muscle use, sternal retractions, shortness of breath, grunting, and nasal flaring. As the disease progresses, the infant may experience respiratory arrest from muscle fatigue, overwhelming hypoxemia, and acidosis. With respiratory arrest, cardiac arrest should be expected shortly.

The treatment for IRDS is focused around prompt recognition of the syndrome, followed rapidly by assessment and management of the ABCs. In transport, the most significant intervention that could be performed is the administration of high concentrations of oxygen. Infants with mild symptoms and adequate ventilatory efforts may be given supplemental oxygen by way of an oxygen mask. Those neonates with severe symptoms (respiratory failure or arrest) are managed best with bag-valve-mask (BVM) ventilation. Utilization of oxygen with BVM ventilation promotes alveolar inflation, oxygenation, and carbon dioxide elimination.

Although supportive ventilatory support during transport is the most appropriate initial management for IRDS, it is important to realize that premature lungs with a surfactant deficiency can still only maintain oxygenation for a limited period of time. The presence of surfactant is necessary for gas exchange to occur at the alveolar-capillary level as well. During transport by the critical care team, the focus is not on providing curative treatment to the patient, but on supporting ventilations until the patient can be delivered to the receiving hospital for definitive care. Long-term management for IRDS includes surfactant replacement therapy.

CONGENITAL DIAPHRAGMATIC HERNIA

Diaphragmatic herniation is a complication in which the bowel has protruded from the abdominal cavity to the thoracic cavity through an interruption of the diaphragm.

Diaphragmatic herniation is a complication in which the bowel has protruded from the abdominal cavity to the thoracic cavity through an interruption of the diaphragm. In the neonate, this would occur as the result of a congenital anomaly. During the first trimester, the diaphragm fails to close completely and allows a shift of abdominal contents into the thoracic cavity. This is most common to the left dome of the diaphragm; in fact, 85% of all congenital diaphragmatic herniations occur to the left side of the body. A mortality rate between 40% and 60% has been experienced in patients with congenital diaphragmatic herniation.

Although it involves the abdominal contents, the signs and symptom of congenital diaphragmatic herniation usually cause a compromise to pulmonary function due to a decrease in overall chest capacity. The abdominal contents that have invaded the thorax prevent full lung expansion in the affected hemithorax, and pulmonary compromise ensues. The clinical manifestations of diaphragmatic herniation include respiratory distress, unequal lung sounds, and a scaphoid-shaped abdomen. It is important to note that the finding of a scaphoid abdomen is rare immediately following birth, but will likely present shortly after birth—commonly the time when a critical care transport team becomes involved with patient care.

Treatment of diaphragmatic herniation centers around ensuring the neonate is adequately oxygenated and ventilated.

Treatment of diaphragmatic herniation centers around ensuring the neonate is adequately oxygenated and ventilated. To effectively ventilate this patient, the stomach must be decompressed to allow for maximum lung expansion after nasogastric tube insertion. Additionally, if artificial ventilation is required, the patient should be pharmacologically sedated and paralyzed, and an endotracheal tube inserted. The use of face-to-mask ventilation will promote gastric distention and thereby further decrease functional lung capacity. Surgical repair of the defect is the definitive treatment modality in diaphragmatic herniation syndromes.

GENERAL PATHOPHYSIOLOGY: CARDIOVASCULAR

The incidence of congenital heart disease in the United States is approximately 8 per 1,000 live births, or roughly 40,000 neonates born each year with a heart defect. Although the causes of congenital heart defects are generally not known, several risk factors or predispositions have been shown to increase the risk of a neonate being born with a heart defect. Table 29–3 lists the breakdown of congenital heart defect types in the United States.

Many congenital heart defects do not produce significant hemodynamic compromise. Some defects cause abnormalities in volumes and/or pressures in the atria or ventricles. Others can cause mixing of venous and arterial blood, and many produce inadequate cardiac output and promote poor systemic perfusion. Also, multiple defects may be present at the same time in the same neonate.

Table 29–3	Breakdown of Congenital Heart Disease
Ventricular septal defect (VSD)	25%
Atrial septal defect (ASD)	12%
Patent ductus arteriosus (PDA)	12%
Coarctation of the aorta (COA)	12%
Tetrology of Fallot (TOF)	9%
Transposition of great arteries (TGA)	9%
Pulmonary stenosis (PS)	6–9%
Aortic stenosis (AS)	8%

LEFT-TO-RIGHT SHUNT DEFECTS

In left-to-right shunt defects, oxygenated blood is shifted from the left side of the heart to the right side. This type of defect is considered to be acyanotic because the oxygenated blood received by the left side of the heart remains in the left side and there is no right-sided (venous) blood mixture. The pressure in the left heart is so high that unoxygenated blood from the right heart cannot be pushed to the left side and mixed with the oxygenated systemic blood.

ATRIAL SEPTAL DEFECT

In an **atrial septal defect (ASD),** the significance of the defect is directly related to the size of the opening. With ASD, the atrial septum (the dividing wall between the left and right atria of the myocardium) is not complete, or it has a hole in it. This is most commonly seen at the foramen ovale, and may actually be caused by incomplete closure of the foramen ovale. This will, on diagnosis, become the "patent" foramen ovale. In this type of defect, oxygenated blood enters the left atria from the pulmonary vein, and since the left atrial pressure exceeds the right atrial pressure, the existing pressure gradient causes a shift of blood volume to the right side of the heart. This will eventually cause right atrial and ventricular enlargement. (See Figure 29-4 ■.)

> **atrial septal defect (ASD)** *a hole in the atrial septum thought to be from incomplete closure of the foramen ovale.*

Although history is the most reliable identifier of ASD, the majority of ASD patients present with essentially no clinically significant findings. Although relatively rare, the most clinically significant finding in ASD is symptoms of congestive heart failure (CHF). Definitive treatment for an ASD includes patching the hole in the septum once the infant reaches school age, unless CHF is present. If CHF is present, patching should occur as quickly as possible. The patching can be done in either the cardiac catheterization lab or the operating room depending on the size and location of the defect.

VENTRICULAR SEPTAL DEFECT

In a **ventricular septal defect (VSD),** the clinical significance is also directly related to the size of the defect. In VSD, the ventricular septum (the dividing wall of the myocardium between the left and right ventricles) is not complete, or it has a hole in it. The size of the defect has a significant impact on the variables present in the clinical presentation of the VSD. In a small VSD, there tends to be little pulmonary vascular congestion or right chamber enlargement. This usually means that it is initially more difficult to diagnose via traditional measures. In large VSD, there are two major presentation types. The first type of large VSD is clinically recognizable in the early stages, shortly after birth, and is generally evident by the identification of global chamber enlargement. The second type of large VSD presentation is common to the chronic environment (i.e., may take years to

> **ventricular septal defect (VSD)** *a hole in the ventricular septum between the left and right ventricles.*

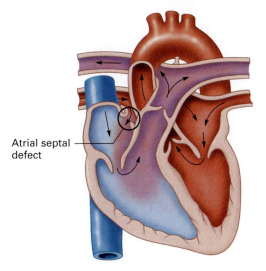

■ Figure 29-4 Atrial septal defect.

Atrial septal defect

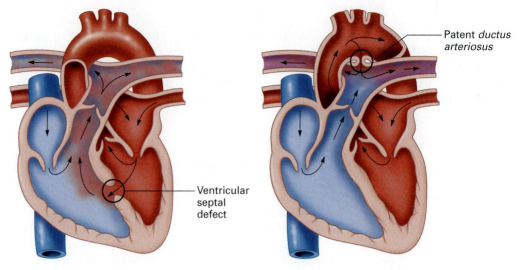

■ Figure 29-5   Ventricular septal defect.   ■ Figure 29-6   Patent ductus arteriosus.

develop clinically), and is characterized by nearly equal pulmonary vascular resistance and systemic vascular resistance. When these pressures are equal, all heart chambers return to almost normal size, with the absence of a significant pressure gradient and equal mixing of arterial and venous blood (there will be left-right and right-left shunting). (See Figure 29-5 ■.)

The clinical presentation of the neonatal VSD patient may include increasing respiratory rate and effort, fatigue and diaphoresis at feedings, a history of poor weight gain (or weight loss), and eventually CHF as the condition worsens. If the critical care paramedic finds himself transporting a VSD patient, who is symptomatic for CHF, then treatment centers around administration of diuretics and fluid restriction. Definitive treatment includes patching the hole on the septum in infancy prior to the neonate becoming increasingly symptomatic for CHF and/or pulmonary hypertension. The surgical repair is essentially always done in the operating room.

PATENT DUCTUS ARTERIOSUS

PDA as a disease process is essentially failure of the ductus arteriosus to close after pulmonary circulation has been initiated.

Patent *ductus arteriosus* (PDA) is similar to VSD and ASD in that size is the determining factor for magnitude of illness. PDA as a disease process is essentially failure of the ductus arteriosus to close after pulmonary circulation has been initiated. The diameter and length of the ductus is very important in determining how much resistance will be present and, therefore, how much blood volume will be shifted between the aorta and the pulmonary artery. Because there is such a large pressure difference between the aorta and the pulmonary artery, there is a constant flow of blood volume during systole and diastole. Pulmonary hypertension and hypertrophy of the myocardium are the greatest complications in PDA. (See Figure 29-6 ■.)

The clinical presentation of the PDA patient may include increasing respiratory rate and effort, increasing heart rate, bounding pulses, widening pulse pressures, and fatigue at feedings times. As such, gathering a thorough history of the medical complaints from the primary care providers is as important as a thorough assessment of the neonatal patient.

Initial treatment for a PDA includes treatment with indomethacin (a prostaglandin inhibitor) to close the ductus arteriosus. If indomethacin is ineffective, the PDA can be closed in either the cardiac catheterization lab using coils or in the operating room by ligating the ductus closed.

OBSTRUCTIVE HEART DEFECTS

Obstructive defects are defined by either a complete or partial blockage of blood flow. The blockage is most commonly caused by a structural deformity, and signs and symptoms are secondary to the cardiovascular structures involved.

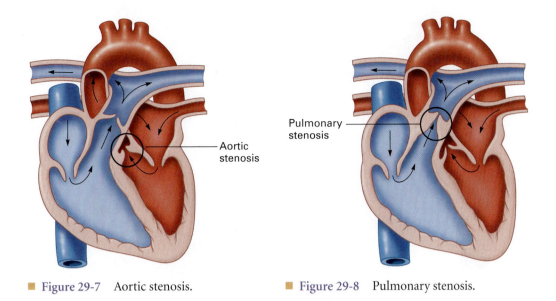

Pulmonary
stenosis

■ Figure 29-7   Aortic stenosis.   ■ Figure 29-8   Pulmonary stenosis.

AORTIC AND PULMONARY VALVE STENOSIS

Aortic or pulmonary valve stenosis is a defect in which the valve itself is narrowed and blood flow is impeded as it passes through it. Depending on the pressure against which the ventricle must pump to clear the valve, there may be significant enlargement of the ventricle secondary to the increased systolic pressure. Additionally, because of the significant pressure exerted on the aorta or pulmonary artery, respectively, there may also be dilation of the great vessel from prolonged stretching of the vascular walls.

The clinical presentation of the aortic stenosis (AS) (see Figure 29-7 ■) or pulmonic stenosis (PS) (see Figure 29-8 ■) patient includes increasing respiratory rate and effort, increasing heart rate, weak pulses, hypotension, and fatigue at feedings. Treatment for an AS and PS patient includes either balloon valvuloplasty or angioplasty within the valve. If the critical care paramedic finds himself transporting a patient with either AS or PS, the treatment will likely be continuation of the oxygenation and pharmacologic adjuncts currently being rendered. The goal of the therapy is to create the most favorable environment for the heart to pump blood within, given the defect, until a surgical remedy can be performed.

COARCTATION OF THE AORTA

Coarctation of the aorta (COA) is a localized narrowing of the aorta near the distal aspect of the aortic arch (after the generation of the brachiocephalic, left common, and left subclavian arteries). (See Figure 29-9 ■.) Because of the narrowing of the aorta, the left ventricle has more resistance to work against and, as a result, becomes hypertrophied under this consistently elevated afterload. In addition to elevated workload on the left ventricle, there is also a risk for the development of a stroke due to the increased systolic pressure exerted on the blood vessels of the cerebral cortex.

The clinical presentation of the COA patient may include increasing respiratory rate and effort, increasing heart rate, bounding pulses in the upper extremities with thready or absent pulses in the lower extremities, and fatigue at feedings. Initial treatment for a COA includes treatment with prostaglandins to open the aorta and diuretics to treat CHF if present. Definitive treatment includes either balloon angioplasty or a surgical resection of the aorta.

CYANOTIC HEART DEFECTS

The final group of defects to be discussed in this chapter is known as **cyanotic heart defects.** In these types of defects, the offending problem is somehow related to a diminishment of pulmonary blood flow. The result is cyanosis due to poor pulmonary perfusion and inadequate oxygenation. More

cyanotic heart defects
systemic cyanosis due to poor pulmonary perfusion, shunting of deoxygenated blood from right to left, or structural deformity of the heart.

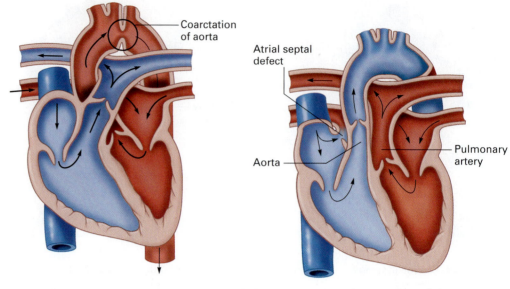

■ **Figure 29-9**   Coarctation of the aorta.

■ **Figure 29-10**   Transposition of the great vessels.

specifically, these defects may cause one or more of the following conditions: difficulty in pumping blood out of the right side of the heart, a greater pressure gradient from the right to the left side of the heart that promotes a shunting of blood to the left side (leading to unoxygenated blood being returned to the left heart), blockage of pulmonary blood flow, or structural deformity. Regardless of the cause, the common denominator is cyanosis. Poorly oxygenated blood is pumped throughout the systemic circulation and, as a result, the tissues are hypoxic and maintain a bluish discoloration.

COMPLETE TRANSPOSITION OF THE GREAT VESSELS

In complete transposition of the great vessels (TGV), the great vessels are positioned abnormally. (See Figure 29-10 ■.) The pulmonary artery leaves the left ventricle and the aorta exits the right ventricle without communication between the systemic and pulmonary circulations. The problem with TGV is that hypoxemic blood is circulated systemically and oxygenated blood is circulated through the pulmonary vasculature. Also present in up to 80% of the TGV patients, is the coexistence of ASD, VSD, and/or PDA. Although these are also abnormal cardiac conditions, these defects actually allow intracardiac mixing of blood. Without these defects also being present, the infant would certainly die because of the presence of closed parallel circuits.

The clinical presentation of the TGV patient may include increasing respiratory rate and effort, increasing heart rate, and cyanosis. The treatment of choice for a TGV is a surgical repair in which the great vessels are detached and the aorta is reattached to the left ventricle while the pulmonary artery is reattached to the right ventricle. This procedure should be performed within the first few weeks of life. The procedure is designed to reestablish normal circulation.

The problem with TGV is that hypoxemic blood is circulated systemically and oxygenated blood is circulated through the pulmonary vasculature.

TETRALOGY OF FALLOT

Tetralogy of Fallot (TOF) is the most common cyanotic heart defect seen in children beyond infancy. Tetralogy of Fallot is a complex of anatomical abnormalities arising from the maldevelopment of the right ventricular infundibulum. In 1888, Fallot described the anatomy as consisting of a subaortic ventricular septal defect, right ventricular infundibular stenosis, aortic valve positioned to override the right ventricle, and right ventricular hypertrophy (RVH). To make a diagnosis of TOF, the VSD must be large enough to equalize right and left ventricular pressures. In addition, there must be an obstruction of outward flow from the right ventricle from pulmonary stenosis. The primary problem with TOF is that there is systemic distribution of blood from both ventricles; as such, the systemically perfused blood is a mixture of oxygenated and deoxygenated blood. (See Figure 29-11 ■.) In the ma-

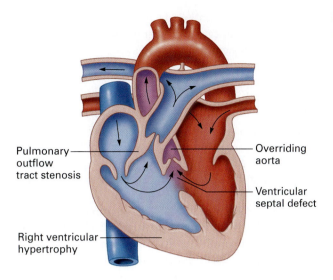

Pulmonary outflow tract stenosis

Overriding aorta

Ventricular septal defect

Right ventricular hypertrophy

jority of cases, there is also pulmonary stenosis (as mentioned previously), which impedes blood flow to the lungs and decreases the amount of oxygenated blood available to the left side of the heart.

The clinical presentation of the TOF patient may include increasing respiratory rate and effort, increasing heart rate, clubbing of the nails, and fatigue at feedings. Initial treatment for a TOF is designed to open any stenosed vessels through the use of prostaglandins and surgical or interventional closure of the VSD.

Tetralogy of Fallot (TOF) is the most common cyanotic heart defect seen in children beyond infancy.

TRANSPORT CONSIDERATIONS FOR CONGENITAL HEART DEFECTS

In accordance with the standard of care, it is vital to ensure that the patient has an intact airway and is being adequately oxygenated and ventilated. An infant with a recent diagnosis of a cyanotic defect that presents with hypoxia and cyanosis should be treated as having an acute hypoxic event. During transport, it is always recommended that high concentrations of oxygen be administered when treating these neonatal CHD patients. The variables in a cyanotic presentation include a heart rate and respiratory rate within normal limits, and normal display regarding the effort needed to breathe. When these clinical signs are normal, it can be assumed that the patient has been effectively compensating for the hypoxia, the clinical presentation is chronic, and the infant does not require more aggressive oxygenation.

After addressing any airway or breathing concerns, consider circulatory compromise. Treatment of circulatory collapse is similar to the treatment used in adult patients. For example, in an adult patient with signs and symptoms of hypovolemic shock, IV crystalloid solutions should be administered to maintain core organ perfusion. Frequent reassessment is also necessary to ensure the patient does not develop pulmonary edema. In neonatal patients, especially those diagnosed with a CHD disorder, the treatment for hypoperfusion is identical. The critical care paramedic should carefully use IV crystalloids to maintain core organ perfusion, and provide ongoing pulmonary assessments that can help to ensure that pulmonary edema does not develop. If CHF develops (as evidenced by acute pulmonary edema or cardiogenic shock), treatment is consistent with care provided to the adult CHF patient, to include diuretics and vasopressors such as dopamine.

GENERAL PATHOPHYSIOLOGY: OTHER NEONATAL EMERGENCIES

To be inclusive of every neonatal emergency, this chapter would turn into a multiple-volume series. The focus, however, is on the critical care transport of neonatal patients, so the emergencies described in these pages reflect the most common things seen by the critical care paramedic. As expected, the aforementioned emergencies that fit this description have either fit into the heading of a pulmonary or cardiovascular problem. The exceptions are the two problems to be discussed next, necrotizing enterocolitis and sepsis.

NECROTIZING ENTEROCOLITIS

necrotizing enterocolitis (NEC) *ischemic damage to the lining of the stomach and/or intestines and bacterial growth that results in acute inflammation of the large intestine with subsequent necrosis of the intestinal mucosa.*

Necrotizing enterocolitis (NEC) is the most commonly seen serious abdominal emergency in neonates that requires emergency surgical intervention. The etiology of NEC is not known in most cases, but does have some coexisting factors. These factors include ischemic damage to the lining of the stomach and/or intestines and bacterial growth. Both of these seem to be required for the development of NEC. Ultimately, NEC results in an acute inflammation of the large intestine leading to necrosis of the intestinal mucosa.

Signs and symptoms of NEC include abdominal distention, decreased or absent bowel sounds, vomiting, bloody diarrhea, lethargy, poor feeding habits, and a depressed core body temperature. If the necrotic enterocolitis results in bowel perforation, the patient will likely develop peritonitis, and is at further risk for the development of sepsis.

Treatment of NEC includes keeping the patient NPO, nasogastric tube insertion and decompression, maintenance of acid–base and electrolyte balance, IV fluid maintenance, and antibiotic therapy. If intestinal perforation has occurred, surgical intervention is likely to be required.

SEPSIS

Neonatal sepsis, similar to sepsis occurring in the adult patient, is a life-threatening infection of the bloodstream resulting in systemic toxicity.

Neonatal sepsis, similar to sepsis occurring in the adult patient, is a life-threatening infection of the bloodstream resulting in systemic toxicity. In the neonate, the presentation of sepsis is typically subtle and may be difficult to distinguish from a noninfectious pathology. The most common etiology for sepsis in the neonate is maternal gastrointestinal or genital infections, although the primary site of infection may often be difficult to identify in the septic neonate. As the sepsis progresses in the neonate, shock may develop.

Septic shock is caused by the release of bacterial endotoxins, which results in dilation of the vasculature. The dilation of the blood vessels can be so significant that the body cannot create an adequate pressure gradient to fill the vascular space, and a form a distributive shock ensues.

During the early phases of neonatal sepsis, common clinical signs include respiratory distress, pulmonary hypertension, hypoxemia, severe hypoperfusion, and disseminated intravascular coagulation (DIC). Although rare in occurrence, meningitis may also become evident.

Treatment of sepsis is generally centered on antibiotic therapy and blood pressure support. Neonates have immature renal and hepatic systems; as a result, the administration of antibiotics should be done judiciously and with regard for potential complications related to drug clearance. Sepsis that is refractory to antibiotic therapy may be caused by a virus rather than bacteria. If the sepsis is related to a virus, central nervous system and hepatic function will most likely be compromised.

GENERAL NEONATAL ASSESSMENT FINDINGS AND CONSIDERATIONS

SKIN COLOR

jaundice *results from high serum bilirubin levels (due to immature liver function) in neonates; presents as a yellowish discoloration of the skin and the sclera of the eyes.*

Cyanosis of the hands and feet is a common finding in the newborn and is an insignificant finding when the infant is crying. If the infant is not crying and cyanosis is present, it is important to assess the respiratory and circulatory stability of the neonate. The neonate's hands and feet may turn blue because of a lack of oxygen and decreased blood supply to the extremities caused by constriction or spasm of the vasculature.

bilirubin *by-product of red cell destruction, the liver processes and removes the bilirubin from the blood, excreting it in the stool.*

Jaundice presents as a yellowish discoloration of the skin and the sclera of the eyes. Neonatal jaundice is related to high serum bilirubin levels. **Bilirubin** is formed when the body breaks down old red blood cells. The liver usually processes and removes the bilirubin from the blood and excretes it in the stool. Jaundice in babies usually occurs because their immature livers are not efficient at removing bilirubin from the bloodstream. While in the uterus, fetal bilirubin is broken down through the mother's blood and hepatic systems. Once delivered, the neonate's liver has to take over the task of processing bilirubin on its own, and as a result, almost all neonates will develop high levels of bilirubin (to some degree) within the first week of extrauterine life. Infant jaundice, when present, is related to a rapid breakdown in red blood cells, short-lived liver enzyme insufficiency, and reabsorption of toxins through hepatic circulation. In most cases of newborn jaundice, the condition will resolve without the need for medical intervention. If bilirubin levels are extremely high for a prolonged period, however, the infant may need to be treated with phototherapy by exposing the infant's skin to fluorescent light. The bilirubin in the infant's skin will absorb the light and be altered into a substance that can be easily excreted through the urine. If unresponsive to phototherapy, and serum bilirubin levels remain extremely high, the infant may require a blood transfusion.

VITAL SIGNS

The normal vital signs of a neonate are different from that of the adult and the child. The neonatal vital signs are represented by elevated numerical values and vary substantially from what would generally be thought of as normal. These variations make it extremely important for transport personnel to have readily available reference materials when dealing with the neonatal patient. In addition to the pediatric Broselow tape, it is helpful to carry a pocket card with documentation of normal vital sign parameters for the neonate, infant, and child. Finally, although a blood glucose level is not typically considered to be a vital sign in the adult patient, it should be in the neonate. Blood sugar levels in the neonate should be above 70–80 mg/dL to be considered nonhypoglycemic.

GENERAL NEONATAL TREATMENT CONSIDERATIONS

Throughout this chapter, several references have been made about the need to maintain an adequate airway, ventilatory sufficiency, and perfusion status in the neonatal patient. The following section is designed to discuss these considerations during neonatal transport. Important to remember is that the aforementioned emergencies and their specific treatment modalities must occur in concert with continued attention to airway, breathing, and circulation.

AIRWAY

Airway management is of the utmost importance in the neonate, and must be secured and maintained as early as possible. In critical care transport of the adult patient, providing rapid-sequence induction (RSI) for continued airway control is a rather common occurrence. However, in the transport of neonatal patients, this skill is infrequently used and commonly unnecessary. This is not to say that pharmaceuticals should not be used in this patient population, but the induction medications may be utilized to promote relaxation in the anxious infant. This will often calm the neonate and lessen the amount of work needed for breathing.

When intubation is warranted, however, the single most frequent respiratory complication of this process is accidental extubation that is not immediately recognized. Properly securing an endotracheal tube is important, but does not guarantee that the tube will not become accidentally dislodged. In addition to standard tube-securing measures, the use of sedatives and paralytics in this situation may prove beneficial. Using cervical and lateral immobilization devices for the neonate's head will minimize the mobility of the airway and thus reduce the risk of accidental extubation.

If, however, the need to rapidly obtain and secure the airway in a decompensating neonate becomes clinically evident (by demonstration of ventilatory inadequacy in the presence of an intact gag reflex), neonatal RSI should be instituted.

When intubation is warranted, the single most frequent respiratory complication of this process is accidental extubation.

VASCULAR ACCESS

Venous access should be of paramount concern in managing the critically ill neonate. Due to the small anatomical size of the vasculature, obtaining access can be very difficult for even the most skilled health care provider. Vascular access should never be delayed in the ill infant and should be secured aggressively and expeditiously. It is imperative that the critical care paramedic have multiple

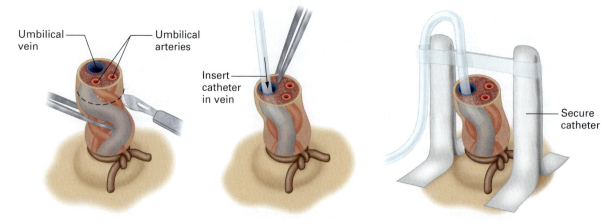

■ **Figure 29-12** Umbilical vein anatomy and catheter insertion technique.

Labels in figure: Umbilical vein; Umbilical arteries; Insert catheter in vein; Secure catheter

In addition to the access routes that are currently practiced by emergency medical personnel (IV and IO routes), umbilical catheterization should be considered.

vascular access options available since standard access techniques may be difficult to obtain. The access options should employ both venous and intraosseous routes.

In addition to the access routes that are currently practiced by emergency medical personnel (IV and IO routes), umbilical catheterization should be considered. Catheterization of the umbilical vein should only be performed by adequately trained personnel. Significant complications associated with umbilical catheterization may consist of infections, liver failure, or liver necrosis. When the umbilical line is placed, it should be inserted into the umbilical vein, not into either of the two umbilical arteries. Additionally, when inserting the catheter, caution should be taken to ensure that the catheter tip is not inserted into the liver or portal circulation. Figure 29-12 ■ outlines the basic steps taken when umbilical catheterization is warranted.

TEMPERATURE REGULATION

Maintaining the core body temperature of neonates is critically important and should be consistently ensured during the entire transport scenario. Temperature regulation is maintained by preventing heat loss while promoting strategies for aggressive warming. In preparation for transport, temperature maintenance should be accomplished by the utilization of a radiant warmer when available. If a radiant warmer is not available, specially designed insulated blankets and sheets should be used. In the critical care transport setting, a transport incubator, when available, should always be used and is considered to be the current standard of care. (See Figure 29-13 ■.)

■ **Figure 29-13** Modern transport isolette. *(Scott and White Hospital and Clinic)*

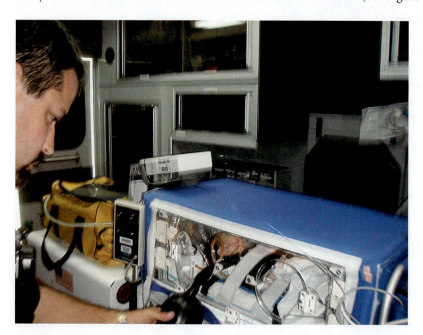

HYPOGLYCEMIA

Neonatal hypoglycemia should be managed aggressively using a solution of 10% dextrose and water. The administration of $D_{25}W$ or $D_{50}W$ is contraindicated in the neonate because these solutions can cause significant increases in the plasma osmolarity. This increase in osmolarity may lead to hypernatremia and ultimately cerebral and systemic cellular edema. To administer $D_{10}W$, simply dilute the $D_{50}W$ five times with water and administer 0.5–1 g/kg (or 5–10 mL/kg) of $D_{10}W$ solution. If a glucose infusion is necessary, $D_{10}W$ should be infused at a maintenance rate of 80 cc/kg/day.

Neonatal hypoglycemia should be managed aggressively using a solution of 10% dextrose and water.

Summary

The common denominator for unexpected deaths in neonates is hypoxia. This encompasses a very diverse group of illnesses, including infectious diseases, congenital heart disease, and pulmonary compromise. Healthy neonates maintain cardiovascular function until they become extremely hypoxic, so a high index of suspicion and diligent monitoring for rapid decompensation are always warranted. Since the neonate's rapid metabolism requires high oxygen levels, and failure of the airway and ventilatory systems are the most contributory factors to neonatal death, they should remain at the forefront of the critical care paramedic's assessment and treatment concerns. Failure to do so will allow airway/pulmonary compromise that ultimately progresses to cardiovascular compromise and death.

After managing any pulmonary deficits, CHD-specific emergencies should then be addressed. The key to successful critical care transport management of CHDs is identification of the cardiac anomaly, obtaining an effective history and physical assessment, and providing supportive care as necessitated for the offending disturbance. Realizing that most transport care providers are not well versed in the various CHDs, and are not likely to have a great deal of experience in working with CHD patients, conferring with medical direction prior to the initiation of any treatments is strongly encouraged. The transport care for the CHD patient is primarily supportive, but in certain cases may require substantial intervention. Transport personnel should not be concerned with diagnosing specific defects but should be aware of the global effects that various defects have on normal perfusion.

Finally, the critical care paramedic should realize that only the most commonly seen congenital heart defects have been reviewed here; multiple other defects exist that may be seen in the critical care transport environment. It is the responsibility of the individual care provider to stay abreast of common neonatal emergencies, and current standards of care for each.

Review Questions

1. Discuss the anatomical differences in the neonatal airway that makes airway control particulary difficult as compared to the adult.

2. Why is temperature maintenance so important to the neonatal patient?

3. What is the difference in clinical symptomatology between respiratory distress, failure, and arrest in the neonate?

4. What is neonatal respiratory distress syndrome, and what is the appropriate management for this condition?

5. List the common left-to-right shunt defects (acyanotic) seen in neonatal emergencies.

6. What are the common cyanotic defects seen in neonates, and what is their salient pathological characteristic?

7. A preterm infant is one who is less than how many weeks' gestation?

8. PPHN can occur from multiple etiologies but is most commonly associated with all of the following EXCEPT:
   a. severe hypoxia.
   b. hypoglycemia.

c. meconium aspiration syndrome.

d. congenital diaphragmatic hernia.

9. Describe the general treatment parameters for a neonate with sepsis.

See Answers to Review Questions at the back of this book.

Further Reading

American Academy of Pediatrics. *Pediatric Education for Prehospital Professionals.* Sudbury, MA: Jones and Bartlett, 2000.

American Academy of Pediatrics. *Textbook of Neonatal Resuscitation,* 4th ed. Elk Grove Village, IL: Author, 2000.

American College of Surgeons, Committee on Trauma. *Advanced Trauma Life Support Course: Student Course Manual.* Chicago: Author, 1997.

American Heart Association. *PALS Provider Manual.* Dallas, TX: Author, 2002.

Bledsoe BE, Porter RS, Cherry RA. *Paramedic Care: Principles & Practice, Volume 5—Special Considerations, 2nd ed.* Upper Saddle River, NJ: Pearson Prentice Hall, 2005.

Crain EF, Gershel JC. *Clinical Manual of Emergency Pediatrics.* New York: McGraw-Hill, 2003.

Dietrich AM, Shaner S, Campbell JE, editors. *Pediatric Basic Trauma Life Support,* 2nd ed. Oak Terrace, IL: Basic Trauma Life Support International, 2002.

Edgren AR. "*Neonatal Jaundice.*" In *Gale Encyclopedia of Medicine.* Farmington Hills, MI: Gale Research, 1999.

Gomella TL, Cunningham MD, Eyal FG, Zenk KE. *Neonatology: Management, Procedures, On-Call Problems, Diseases, and Drugs.* New York: McGraw-Hill, 2004.

Holleran RS. *Air and Surface Patient Transport, Principles and Practice.* St. Louis, MO: Mosby, 2003.

Jaimovich DG, Vidyasagar D. *Handbook of Pediatric and Neonatal Transport Medicine, 2nd ed.* Philadelphia: Hanley and Belfus, 2002.

Markenson DS. *Pediatric Prehospital Care.* Upper Saddle River, NJ: Pearson Prentice Hall, 2002.

Martini FH, Bartholomew EF, Bledsoe BE. *Anatomy and Physiology for Emergency Care.* Upper Saddle River, NJ: Pearson Prentice Hall, 2002.

Morris, FC, Levin DL. *Essentials of Pediatric Intensive Care.* New York: Churchill-Livingston, 1997.

Park MK. *Pediatric Cardiology for Practitioners,* 4th ed. St. Louis, MO: Mosby, 2002.

Paneth N, Kiely JL. "*Newborn Intensive Care and Neonatal Mortality in Low-Birth-Weight Infants. A Population Study.*" *New England Journal of Medicine* Vol. 307 (1982): 149.

"Pediatrics: Heart Disease & Health." Available at http://www.americanheart.org

Pollack MM, Alexander SR, Clark N, et al. "*Improved Outcomes from Tertiary Center Pediatric Intensive Care: A Statewide Comparison of Tertiary and Nontertiary Care Facilities.*" *Critical Care Medicine,* Vol. 19 (1991): 150.

Siberry GRI. *The Harriet Lane Handbook.* St. Louis, MO: Mosby, 2000.

Taussig LM, Landau LI. *Pediatric Respiratory Medicine.* St. Louis, MO: Mosby, 1999.

Tintinalli JE. *Emergency Medicine : A Comprehensive Study Guide.* New York: McGraw-Hill, 2000.

Williams LJ, Shaffer TH, Greenspan JS. (2004). "Inhaled Nitric Oxide Therapy in the Near-Term or Term Neonate with Hypoxic Respiratory Failure." *Neonatal Network: The Journal of Neonatal Nursing,* Vol. 23 (2004): 1.

Environmental Emergencies

Philip M. DaVisio, BS, NREMT-P, PA-C, David G. Patterson, BBA, MA, EMT-P, and
Bryan E. Bledsoe, DO, FACEP

Objectives

Upon completion of this chapter, the student should be able to:

1. Describe the pathophysiology associated with the varying levels of heat-related emergencies. (p. 898)
2. List the factors that contribute to the heat-related emergencies. (p. 899)
3. Describe the methods of thermoregulation in the body. (p. 900)
4. Determine, based on clinical presentation, the different levels of heat-related emergencies. (p. 903)
5. Define the appropriate treatment modalities for heat exhaustion. (p. 904)
6. Define the appropriate treatment modalities for heatstroke. (p. 905)
7. Describe the pathophysiology of hypothermia. (p. 905)
8. Describe the impact of hypothermia on neurologic, cardiovascular, and respiratory systems. (p. 906)
9. Understand how hypothermic events should be addressed in the presence of other etiologies. (p. 907)
10. Determine, based on clinical presentation and assessment, the appropriate treatment modalities for hypothermic patients. (p. 909)
11. Understand the various treatment modalities, applied in the critical care setting, for the management of cold-related injuries. (p. 909)
12. List the signs and symptoms of frostbite and describe the appropriate treatment. (p. 909)
13. List the different types of mechanisms for drowning and near-drowning. (p. 912)
14. Explain the pathophysiology associated with drowning. (p. 912)
15. Discuss the short- and long-term effects of hypoxia associated with drowning and near-drowning. (p. 912)
16. Explain the cardiovascular, neurologic, and respiratory impact of drowning and near-drowning. (p. 913)
17. List and discuss the treatment modalities for drowning and near-drowning. (p. 914)

Key Terms

Case Study

You and your partner are on standby for a massive wildfire that has already consumed more than 61,000 acres of timber. More than 500 firefighters are involved and the outside temperature is approaching 100°F. While watching the red glow from the fire over the mountain top, the radio crackles with a call that a firefighter needs transport. Your unit is next up. You depart the staging area and go to the designated drop zone.

Upon arrival EMT first responders are taking the bunker gear off of a 39-year-old volunteer firefighter from a neighboring community. He was actively involved in making a fire break with a shovel and collapsed. He has been confused and somewhat combative.

You begin your assessment. The patient is arousable and confused—at times combative. The EMTs are removing his gear. He is now wearing only a T-shirt and underwear. He is warm and dry to touch and looks somewhat sunburned. He is obese at approximately 110 kg. An EMT attempts to take a tympanic temperature and cannot get a reading. You call for the ice chest from your critical care ground unit, and ask an EMT to retrieve the hyperthermic thermometer. While your partner covers the patient with a single dry sheet and starts applying ice to the patient's axilla, neck, and chest, you lubricate the thermometer and insert it into the patient's rectum. The mercury quickly climbs to 106.2°F. You ask for additional ice and start an IV of normal saline at a wide-open rate. You check the blood glucose during the IV stick and find it to be 88 mg/dL. The EMTs get vital signs. His blood pressure is 100/60 mmHg, pulse is 140, respirations 30 per minute, SpO$_2$ of 96% on room air.

The patient is moved to the portable cot and taken to the ambulance. Once in the ambulance, the ECG monitor is attached and reveals a sinus tachycardia. Ten minutes after your first reading, you retake the rectal temp and find it to be 104.3°F. You look in the ice chest and find it empty. Knowing you still have a considerable amount of time prior to reaching the hospital, you yell at your partner to stop at a convenience store for more ice. After stopping briefly at a convenience mart, he returns with two 20-pound bags of ice.

You continue icing the patient until his rectal temp is 101°F and then cease the active cooling. Since you are still about 20 minutes from the destination hospital, you remove the wet sheet the patient is lying on and place a dry one. His heart rate is now 100 and he is alert and oriented. The IV is slowed to 100 mL/hr and the remainder of the transport is uneventful.

INTRODUCTION

Environmental emergencies can be the most challenging conditions health care professionals face. Once there is a disruption in the body's ability to maintain a regulated core temperature, the processes of cellular respiration are significantly disrupted. It is important that critical care providers thoroughly understand the pathophysiology behind these processes so that patients affected by these conditions can be identified and treated appropriately. The treatment provided must address correcting the temperature abnormality and managing the metabolic obstacles as they arise. Unlike trauma, there is no opportunity to practice proactive medicine; most of the approach is "reactive"—catching up to and trying to stay ahead of the condition.

Based on information from the National Oceanic and Atmospheric Administration (NOAA), heat-related disorders account for approximately 175–200 deaths each year in the United States. From the years 1979–1997, the National Centers for Health Statistics (NCHS) reported a total of 7,046 heat-related deaths, an average of 371 per year. As one would expect, the number of fatalities significantly elevates during a heat wave (i.e., the heat wave of July 1995 resulted in 465 deaths in Chicago alone). Note, however, that the patient's outcome is greatly affected by several comorbid factors such as underlying pathology, age, and amount and condition of exposure.

Cold-related injuries are not as statistically tracked as are heat-related emergencies. Information suggests that most cases are seen in urban areas and are usually secondary to another process. For the years 1979–1995, the average annual mortality from hypothermia was in excess of 700 patients a year. Several comorbid factors will be discussed.

PATHOPHYSIOLOGY

Generally speaking, temperature management is nothing more than balancing heat loss with heat production. (See Figure 30-1 ■.) When heat loss exceeds heat production, hypothermic conditions begin and the inverse produces hyperthermic conditions.

The temperature of the human body is closely maintained between 35.6°–37.8°C (96°–100°F) and averages 36.8°C (98.2°F). If temperatures exceed these limits for a protracted amount of time, enzymes cease to function, proteins denature, and cellular metabolism is hampered. When the upper extremes of these conditions are met the **critical thermal maximum** is reached, that is, a core temperature equal to or greater than 43°C (109.4°F).

The homeostatic management of temperature regulation begins in the anterior portion of the hypothalamus. The **hypothalamus** is a portion of the diencephalon and is located immediately superior to the brainstem and inferior to the thalamus. It is responsible for many functions, but of paramount importance is its management of body temperature regulation and the regulation of water balance and thirst.

The thermostat for the body is located in the **preoptic region** (see Figure 30-2 ■) of the hypothalamus; this area is the principal center for thermoregulation. Several **thermoreceptor** sites monitor information about the current temperature of the body. These sites are located in the skin

Once there is a disruption in the body's ability to maintain a regulated core temperature, the processes of cellular respiration are significantly disrupted.

Generally speaking, temperature management is nothing more than balancing heat loss with heat production.

critical thermal maximum
a core temperature equal to or greater than 43°C (109.4°F).

The temperature of the human body is closely maintained between 35.6°–37.8°C (96°–100°F) and averages 36.8°C (98.2°F).

hypothalamus   *a portion of the diencephalon, located immediately superior to the brainstem and inferior to the thalamus. Primarily responsible for regulation of body temperature, water balance, and thirst.*

preoptic region   *located in the hypothalamus, this area is the principal center for thermoregulation.*

thermoreceptor
temperature sensors located in the skin (peripheral thermoreceptors), the body core, interior vessel walls (central thermoreceptors), and in the hypothalamus itself.

■ Figure 30-1   Body temperature scale is a balance between heat-generation and heat-loss.

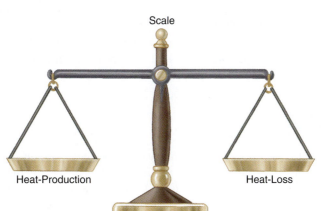

Scale

Heat-Production   Heat-Loss

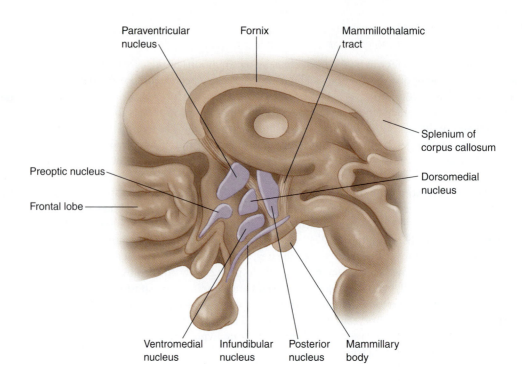

■ Figure 30-2
Hypothalamic anatomy.

Paraventricular nucleus

Fornix

Mammillothalamic tract

Splenium of corpus callosum

Preoptic nucleus

Frontal lobe

Dorsomedial nucleus

Ventromedial nucleus

Infundibular nucleus

Posterior nucleus

Mammillary body

set point *the internal temperature that the body "wants" to maintain and controlled in the hypothalamus.*

As long as these feedback mechanisms for heat gain and heat loss are working properly, a stable internal temperature will be maintained.

(peripheral thermoreceptors), the core of the body, interior vessel walls (central thermoreceptors), and the hypothalamus itself. Information from each of these locations is integrated and analyzed in the preoptic region. Based on the thermostatic **set point** that the hypothalamus has (which refers to the internal temperature that the body wants to maintain) versus the relative temperature of the body, certain compensatory mechanisms are set in motion.

As long as these feedback mechanisms for heat gain and heat loss are working properly, a stable internal temperature will be maintained. However, certain conditions can alter the normal functioning of the regulatory process and predispose the patient to temperature-related emergencies. Some of these factors include, but are not limited to, the following:

★ *Age of patient.* Pediatric and geriatric patients tolerate less temperature variation because regulating mechanisms are less responsive. Elderly patients can be hypothermic in only mildly cool temperatures.

★ *Health of the patient.* Diabetics become hyperthermic quicker because of autonomic neuropathy, which interferes with thermoregulatory input. Hypothyroidism suppresses metabolism. Malnutrition, hypoglycemia, Parkinson's disease, and fatigue can interfere with the body's ability to produce heat.

★ *Medications.* Diuretics worsen hyperthermia, beta-blockers interfere with vasodilation and interfere with thermoregulatory input, psychotropics interfere with thermoregulation. Narcotics, alcohol, phenothiazines, barbiturates, antiseizure medications, and various pain medications interfere with heat production.

★ *Exposure time.* Amount of time the patient has been exposed to the hot or cold environment.

heat *the kinetic energy of molecules in motion.*

absolute zero *the temperature at which molecular motion stops, described as "−460°F" or "−273°C."*

HEAT

Heat is actually the kinetic energy of molecules in motion. The greater the molecular motion, the greater the heat. Molecular motion totally stops when the temperature of the object reaches **absolute zero** (−460°F or −273°C). Although an object can approach absolute zero, it can never actually reaches absolute zero due to factors described by the *third law of thermodynamics.* Thus, although there is no limit on how hot an object can get, no object can be cooled below absolute zero.

The difference in temperature between two objects is called the **thermal gradient.** The warmer object will transfer heat to the cooler object until a steady state, called **thermal equilibrium,** is reached. For example, if you drop an ice cube into a glass of room-temperature water, a thermal gradient exists between the water and the ice cube. Because the molecules in the water have more kinetic energy than do the molecules in the ice, heat will be transferred from the water to the ice until both are at the same temperature (thermal equilibrium).

HEAT PRODUCTION

Heat production arises primarily as a result of many of the biochemical processes that normally occur within the body. Most of the body's heat production occurs within the deep organs of the body, especially the liver, brain, and heart. During physical activity, the skeletal muscles produce heat that is subsequently transferred to the deep organs and tissues via the circulatory system. The circulatory system plays a major role in the transfer of heat throughout the body.

Heat is a common by-product of many biochemical processes. The rate of heat production is referred to as the *metabolic rate of the body*. The rate of heat production while the body is at rest is a function of the **basal metabolic rate (BMR).** The BMR refers specifically to the amount of energy needed to maintain homeostasis when the individual is at digestive, physical, and emotional rest.

In addition to heat production from normal metabolic activities, heat can also result from enhanced metabolic processes—most often occurring in muscles. When necessary, the body can activate specialized biochemical pathways known as **futile cycles.** Unlike the other biochemical processes of the body, a futile cycle uses energy to generate heat as the principal effect (**chemical thermogenesis**). This heat production augments that occurring in the normal metabolic processes. In addition, alternating contraction and relaxation of muscle fibers, commonly called *shivering*, also serves to produce heat when needed. Shivering augments the body's other heat-producing mechanisms.

HEAT LOSS

When the body needs to be cooled, heat is transferred from the deeper structures to the skin. Blood vessels within the skin are dilated, allowing heat to be transferred to the skin. Once there, it is lost to the air and other surroundings. The rate of heat loss is determined by how rapidly heat can be conducted from the deep tissues to the skin and how rapidly heat can be transferred from the skin to the environment.

While the skin can be used to transfer heat to the environment, it is also important in retaining heat. The skin and the fatty subcutaneous tissues immediately under the dermis serve as an effective heat insulator for the body. In fact, the fatty subcutaneous tissues conduct heat significantly less efficiently than other tissues. Because of this, the skin serves as an insulator, thus allowing the body to maintain a normal core temperature even though the temperature of the skin approaches that of the surrounding environment.

Heat is lost from the skin by four methods: *radiation, conduction, convection,* and *evaporation.*

Radiation

60% of heat loss that occurs can do so via the skin due to **radiation** in an unclothed person. This heat loss is in the form of infrared rays (a type of electromagnetic waves). All objects not at absolute zero temperature will radiate heat into the environment. Other objects in the environment (walls, trees, furniture) also radiate heat because they too are not at absolute zero. In summary, the greater the temperature difference between the body and the environment, the greater the heat loss.

Conduction

Conduction is the loss of heat from the body through direct contact of the skin with another, cooler solid object. As mentioned earlier, heat flows from higher temperature matter to lower temperature matter. However, only about 3% of body heat is lost through this mechanism. Heat is also conducted to the air (provided the temperature of the ambient air is less than the body temperature). Loss of heat by conduction to air represents approximately 15% of total body heat loss.

Convection

convection *heat loss from air currents passing over a surface.*

Heat loss from air currents passing over the body is called **convection.** Heat, however, must first be conducted to the air before being carried away by convection currents. Some convection almost always occurs because air adjacent to the skin becomes heated by the body. When heated, the air rises, allowing cooler air to take its place and thus repeating the cycle. Even without gross air movement, an unclothed person will lose approximately 15% of his body heat through conduction of the heat to the air and subsequent loss of the heat through convection.

Both environmental temperature and wind velocity affect cooling. The greater the difference between the body temperature and the environmental temperature, and the greater the wind velocity, the greater the cooling effect. This is the basis for the development of wind chill factor (WCF) tables. (See Figure 30-3 ■.)

Evaporation

evaporation *heat loss that occurs as water changes from a liquid to a vapor.*

Evaporation is the change of a liquid to a vapor. Evaporative heat loss occurs as water evaporates from the skin. When water evaporates from the skin, heat is lost along with the water. Even when a person is not sweating, water still evaporates from the skin. This loss is typically called the *insensible loss.* In addition, a great deal of heat loss occurs through evaporation of fluids in the lungs. Water normally evaporates from the skin and lungs at a rate of approximately 600 mL/day.

heat index *system based on the Fahrenheit scale; allows an accurate measure of how it really feels when relative humidity is added to actual air temperature.*

When the relative humidity of the environment is increased, evaporation becomes a less effective cooling mechanism. This important consideration is the basis for the development of the heat index used in the warmer climates and during summer months. (See Figure 30-4 ■.) The **heat index** (measured in degrees Fahrenheit) is an accurate measure of how it really feels when the relative humidity is added to the actual air temperature. That is, the greater the air temperature and the greater the relative humidity, the less effective the body's cooling mechanisms.

THERMOREGULATION

When the peripheral or central thermoreceptors sense an increase in temperature, a series of involuntary and voluntary responses is set in motion. Involuntarily, there is activation of the sebaceous glands and sweat is produced. Activation of sweat glands (sudoriferous and merocrine) usually occurs at temperatures greater than 32.8°C (91°F). Second, there is dilation of the capillaries in the skin. These two mechanisms allow the body to decrease its overall temperature by moving the blood closer to the surface of the skin (radiation) and cooling the skin by the production of sweat (evap-

■ **Figure 30-3** Wind chill.

Temperature (°F)																	
Calm	40	35	30	25	20	15	10	5	0	−5	−10	−15	−20	−25	−30	−35	−40	−45
5	36	31	25	19	13	7	1	−5	−11	−16	−22	−28	−34	−40	−46	−52	−57	−63
10	34	27	21	15	9	3	−4	−10	−16	−22	−28	−35	−41	−47	−53	−59	−66	−72
15	32	25	19	13	6	0	−7	−13	−19	−26	−32	−39	−45	−51	−58	−64	−71	−77
20	30	24	17	11	4	−2	−9	−15	−22	−29	−35	−42	−48	−55	−61	−68	−74	−81
25	29	23	16	9	3	−4	−11	−17	−24	−31	−37	−44	−51	−58	−64	−71	−78	−84
30	28	22	15	8	1	−5	−12	−19	−26	−33	−39	−46	−53	−60	−67	−73	−80	−87
35	28	21	14	7	0	−7	−14	−21	−27	−34	−41	−48	−55	−62	−69	−76	−82	−89
40	27	20	13	6	−1	−8	−15	−22	−29	−36	−43	−50	−57	−64	−71	−78	−84	−91
45	26	19	12	5	−2	−9	−16	−23	−30	−37	−44	−51	−58	−65	−72	−79	−86	−93
50	26	19	12	4	−3	−10	−17	−24	−31	−38	−45	−52	−60	−67	−74	−81	−88	−95
55	25	18	11	4	−3	−11	−18	−25	−32	−39	−46	−54	−61	−68	−75	−82	−89	−97
60	25	17	10	3	−4	−11	−19	−26	−33	−40	−48	−55	−62	−69	−76	−84	−91	−98

Wind (mph) is the left vertical axis.

Frostbite Times ☐ 30 minutes ☐ 10 minutes ☐ 5 minutes

Wind Chill (°F) = $35.74 + 0.6215T - 35.75(V^{0.16}) + 0.4275T(V^{0.16})$

Where, T = Air Temperature (°F)   V = Wind Speed (mph)

Figure 30-4 Heat index.

°F	90%	80%	70%	60%	50%	40%
80	85	84	82	81	80	79
85	101	96	92	90	86	84
90	121	113	105	99	94	90
95		133	122	113	105	98
100			142	129	118	109
105				148	133	121
110						135

Temperature (°F) versus Relative Humidity (%)

HI	Possible Heat Disorder:
80°F - 90°F	Fatigue possible with prolonged exposure and physical activity.
90°F - 105°F	Sunstroke, heat cramps, and heat exhaustion possible.
105°F - 130°F	Sunstroke, heat cramps, and heat exhaustion likely, and heatstroke possible.
130°F or greater	Heat stroke highly likely with continued exposure.

oration). Voluntary mechanisms that can reduce the amount of heat in the body are the decision to limit amount of activity, moving to a cooler environment, or removing and/or changing into lighter clothing. This process is a **negative feedback loop.** The response generated by the hypothalamus reacts in a negative manner on the initial stimulus, in this case increased body temperature. This process will continue until the temperature of the body is returned to the set point defined by the hypothalamus. (See Figure 30-5 ■.)

negative feedback loop *a response that continually reacts in a negative manner to a particular stimulus.*

If there is a decrease in the core temperature, voluntary and involuntary mechanisms occur to help manage this event. Involuntarily responses are the stimulation of the hypothalamus to constrict peripheral blood vessels and to stimulate the adrenal cortex that increases the production and release of epinephrine. This production is initiated by the stimulation of the hypothalamic axis, ultimately resulting in the release of thyroxine from the thyroid gland. Thyroxine stimulates the release of thyroid hormone into the bloodstream. Thyroid hormone stimulates the adrenal medulla to produce epinephrine, resulting directly in the increase in the BMR.

The amount of energy needed to carry out essential tasks can be increased by the effects of thyroxine. The normal BMR is 50–60 kcal/hr/m^2; however, this value can vary significantly. Factors such as age, height, weight, relevant pathology, and gender affect this measurement. Males tend to have a higher metabolic rate than females due to the presence of greater muscle mass on the male frame. Unopposed, the BMR can raise the temperature of the body 1.1°C/hr. For example, in an environment where humidity is 100%, the body loses its ability to decrease it temperature via the evaporation of sweat.

Epinephrine from the adrenal medulla increases the muscle tone, causing shivering, and also produces peripheral vasoconstriction. Vessel constriction helps to preserve heat by decreasing radiation, and shivering produces heat via kinetic energy.

The voluntary responses are the addition of heavier clothing, the increase of activity (stomping feet), or the reduction of exposed surface area help to maintain body temperature. This entire process is also a negative feedback loop that is active until the temperature matches that of the hypothalamic set point.

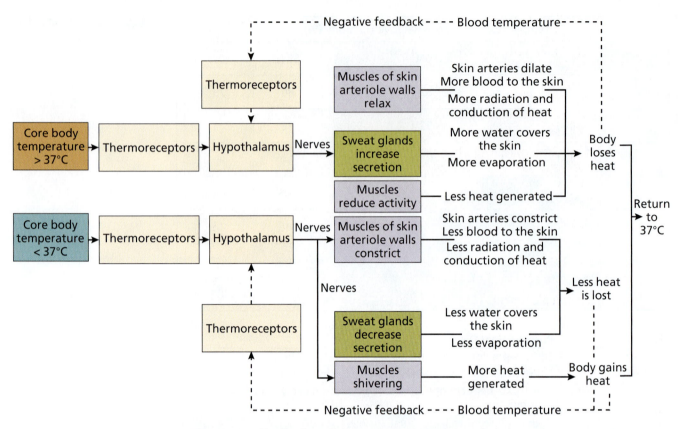

Figure 30-5 Feedback mechanisms in temperature regulation.

MECHANISMS THAT DECREASE BODY TEMPERATURE WHEN THE BODY IS TOO WARM

The body uses three physiological mechanisms to reduce the body temperature when it becomes too great:

1. *Vasodilation.* Almost immediately, the blood vessels in the skin become dilated due to inhibition of sympathetic nervous system function by the hypothalamus. This vasodilation results in the almost immediate transfer of heat to the skin and subsequently to the environment. Clinically, this is seen as red, warm skin.

2. *Sweating.* An increase in body temperature results in the production of sweat. When stimulated by the hypothalamus via the sympathetic nervous system, specialized glands (sweat glands) within the skin begin to secrete a fluid on the skin surface that is similar to that of blood plasma—but without the plasma proteins. Clinically, this is seen as perspiration.

3. *Decreasing heat production.* Cooling of the body also occurs through inhibition of mechanisms that cause excess heat production, namely, shivering and chemical thermogenesis. Inhibition of these mechanisms is somewhat slow to occur.

MECHANISMS THAT INCREASE BODY TEMPERATURE WHEN THE BODY IS TOO COLD

When the body temperature is too cold, various mechanisms are instituted to return the body temperature to normal including:

1. *Vasoconstriction of blood vessels in the skin.* To conserve heat, blood vessels to the skin are constricted through activation of components of the sympathetic nervous system. Clinically, this results in pale skin that is cool to the touch.

2. *Piloerection.* **Piloerection** causes what most people refer to as "goose bumps" or "goose flesh." Piloerection causes hairs in the skin to stand erect. This occurs through sympathetic stimulation of small muscles (*arrector pili*) that are attached to the hair fibers within the hair follicle. The purpose of piloerection is to trap a layer of "insulating air" next to the skin in order to diminish heat loss. Piloerection is an evolutionary remnant from a time in our distant past when humans were covered with hair. Today, it is much less effective in humans, but remains very important in the lower animals.

3. *Increase in heat production.* As discussed previously, heat production can be increased by sympathetic stimulation of heat-generating processes and by release of thyroxine from the thyroid gland. These mechanisms include activation of chemical thermogenesis pathways and shivering.

HYPERTHERMIC CATEGORIES

Hyperthermia can result in several clinical conditions:

★ Heat tetany

★ Heat cramps

★ Heat syncope

★ Heat exhaustion

★ Heatstroke

Hyperthermia is an abnormal elevation in body temperature. Unlike fever, it is not a normal physiological response. Factors that lead to the development of hyperthermia can either be environmental or result from problems within the body.

Changes in the environment are a common reason persons develop hyperthermia and heat-related illnesses. Any increase in the environmental temperature will decrease the rate at which the body can cool itself. Likewise, other factors such as increased humidity and still air can further decrease the effectiveness of the body's cooling mechanisms. Heat waves occur regularly throughout the United States. However, in areas of the country where excessive heat is uncommon, heat waves can be particularly devastating. Persons living in these areas often do not have access to air conditioning or other facilities where they can seek respite from the heat. Likewise, people living in these areas have not had time to adjust to the sudden change in temperature. It was factors like these that lead to the 1995 Chicago heat wave where more than 600 persons died of heatstroke and heat-related illness. Any factor that inhibits heat loss or causes heat production predisposes a person to hyperthermia. These include exercise and improper hydration. Over time, persons adjust to a warm environment through a process called **acclimatization,** where the body learns to better adjust its physiological processes to maximize normal heat loss and improve heat tolerance (or vice versa when in cooler climates).

The two most common manifestations that will be encountered are heat exhaustion and heatstroke. Both of these conditions arise out of an inability to balance heat production with heat loss. Heat exhaustion when not treated can and will progress to heatstroke.

Hyperthermia can result in several clinical conditions.

HEAT TETANY

In extremely warm environments, persons tend to hyperventilate as an additional cooling mechanism (similar to panting in a dog) and as a result of metabolic acidosis. Persons who suddenly start to hyperventilate develop a respiratory alkalosis (elevated pH) and tend to develop spasms of their fingers and toes (carpopedal spasms). This problem, called **heat tetany,** is self-limited and disappears when the hyperventilation ceases—often when the patient is moved to a cooler environment.

HEAT CRAMPS

Heat cramps are brief, yet painful muscle cramps that are a frequent complication of heat exhaustion. They are more common in athletes and workers exposed to an unusually hot environment. Salt depletion and other electrolyte problems are often associated with heat cramps. They are self-limited and treatment is symptomatic.

HEAT SYNCOPE

Heat syncope is a form of postural hypotension that results from the massive peripheral vasodilation that occurs when the body attempts to rapidly cool itself, coupled with dehydration. It usually occurs in persons not yet acclimatized to the heat and during the early stages of heat exposure. Treatment is symptomatic and similar to that provided for any syncope victim.

HEAT EXHAUSTION

A more severe heat-related illness is **heat exhaustion.** It results from cardiovascular strain as the body strives to maintain a normal temperature. Heat exhaustion is an ill-defined syndrome that usually develops over several days. Most commonly, derangements in bodily functions start to occur at temperatures between 39.4°–40°C (102.9°–104°F). However, this is a rather unreliable finding and EMS personnel should rely on the physical assessment to make the determination as to whether a patient is suffering heat exhaustion. The symptoms of heat exhaustion include dizziness, headache, fatigue, irritability, anxiety, chills, nausea, vomiting, and heat cramps. On physical examination the skin is commonly found to be diaphoretic; there will also be tachycardia, hyperventilation, and hypotension. In some cases, syncope is seen. Heat exhaustion is treated by removing the patient from the warm environment, providing rest, and replacing fluids and electrolytes.

Heat exhaustion is most commonly seen in athletes, but the elderly and pediatric populations can also be affected. The elderly are at risk due to underlying pathology, medications, and ineffective thermoregulatory mechanisms. The pediatric population is at risk because of an inability to communicate thirst and an incomplete development of thermoregulatory mechanisms.

Heat exhaustion is usually associated with hot air temperatures, which results in fluid loss due to excessive sweating. The fluid loss is complicated by the loss of sodium and these mechanisms give rise to the symptoms commonly seen in heat exhaustion. This imbalance creates a mildly hyponatremic and hypovolemic state and puts excessive strain on the cardiovascular system and overall produces the findings shown in Table 30–1.

Heat exhaustion is most commonly seen in athletes, but the elderly and pediatric populations can be affected also.

Heat exhaustion is usually associated with hot air temperatures, which results in fluid loss due to excessive sweating.

Table 30–1	Heat Exhaustion Complications
Core temperature 37.5°–39°C (99.5°–102.2°F)	
Tachycardia	
Normal to low blood pressure	
Possible hypovolemia	
Orthostasis	
Profuse diaphoresis	
Nausea and/or vomiting	
Headache	
Fatigue and weakness	
Muscle cramps and myalgias	
Pale, cool, clammy skin	
Lab values consistent with hypovolemia ($\uparrow Na^+$, $\uparrow BUN$)	

HEATSTROKE

Heatstroke is a life-threatening emergency defined as the following triad of signs and symptoms:

- ★ Core temperature greater than 40.5°C (104.9°F)
- ★ Loss of sweating (anhidrosis)
- ★ Altered mental status (CNS dysfunction)

It is important to point out that anhidrosis may not be present for various reasons. However, any patient with the combination of an elevated temperature and altered mental status should be assumed to have heatstroke until proven otherwise.

Heatstroke represents a total failure of temperature regulation. That is, the body's cooling mechanisms have collectively failed. Survival and prognosis may depend on duration of the event and how high the core temperature climbed. Heatstroke can be rapidly fatal and emergency treatment measures should be initiated as soon as possible. These include CPR, fluid and electrolyte administration, and immediate cooling. The goal of cooling is to get the body temperature to 40°C (104°F). The preferred method of cooling the heatstroke victim is immersion cooling in a cold water or ice water bath. Care must be taken to remove the patient from the bath as soon as the target temperature is reached. Cooling the patient below the target temperature (40°C or 104°F) can cause the development of shivering and peripheral vasoconstriction that can result in a rebound rise in body temperature. Evaporative cooling through the use of cool wet sheets and ice packs can be utilized, but are generally less effective than immersion therapy.

Heatstroke has two broad classifications: exertional and nonexertional. In either condition the normal thermoregulatory mechanisms have failed to meet the needs of the body. The clinical definition of heatstroke is core temperature greater than 41.1°C (106°F) and anhidrosis (inability to produce sweat) associated with an altered sensorium. However, some patients can retain the ability to sweat even in this condition.

When temperatures approach the critical thermal maximum of 43°C (109.4°F), metabolic processes break down and irreversible organ death occurs. When core temperatures reach these levels, cellular respiration (energy production) is impaired, specifically psychotic due to uncoupling during oxidative phosphorylation. This uncoupling increases the permeability of cell membranes to sodium. There is heightened activity on the part of the cell requiring more ATP, which increases energy expenditures by the body and enhances heat production and further potentiates the condition. If temperatures persist or rise, proteins in the body begin to denature and tissue necrosis begins.

Exertional heatstroke is differentiated from nonexertional heatstroke by age of the individual and the presence of an intact thermoregulatory mechanism. Exertional heatstroke is usually seen in a younger healthy population working or exercising in a warm environment and usually has a sudden onset. Nonexertional heatstroke is usually seen in elderly people, children, or chronically ill populations and usually has an onset over a period of several days. Nonexertional heatstroke is usually responsible for the fatalities seen during heat waves. The presence of ineffective or underdeveloped thermoregulatory systems and underlying cardiac, neurologic, or pulmonary disease places these populations at risk. Also the medication used to treat the underlying pathology can predispose the patient to heat stroke. See Table 30–2.

Patients may present with an altered mental status from mildly delusional to psychosis. This finding is present in 80% of cases. Anhidrosis may or may not be present; it should be considered a late finding. The presentation of an obtunded or comatose patient is not uncommon. The patient may also be hyperventilating giving rise to a respiratory alkalosis. The hypoventilation may be due to a disruption in the respiratory center in the brain and/or an attempt to reduce temperature. Other symptoms include pulmonary edema, syncope, seizures, and posturing (decorticate or decerebrate) in extreme cases.

HYPOTHERMIC CATEGORIES

Hypothermic events can be broken down into central and peripheral categories. Central events have been classically described as hypothermia and peripheral have been defined in the various degrees of frostbite.

heatstroke *a life-threatening emergency described by a triad of signs and symptoms that include a core temperature greater that 104.9°F (40.5°C), anhidrosis, and CNS dysfunction.*

Heatstroke represents a total failure of temperature regulation.

Table 30–2	Medications That Increase the Risk of Heatstroke	
Drug	**Effect**
Phenothiazines	Inhibition of sweating
Tricyclic antidepressants	
Antihistamines	
Antiparkinsonian medications	
Beta-blockers	Depress cardiovascular performance
Antihypertensives	
Diuretics	Depress cardiovascular performance, produce an underlying dehydration

HYPOTHERMIA

hypothermia *defined as a body core temperature of less than 95°F (35°C).*

wind chill factor *refers to the increased body heat lost from convection on windy days, especially in the cold.*

Hypothermia, defined as a core temperature of less than 35°C (95°F), occurs because the body can no longer generate sufficient heat to maintain body functions. It is usually classified as mild or severe. Mild hypothermia is defined as a core temperature less than 35°C (95°F) and greater than 32.2°C (90°F). Severe hypothermia is defined as a core temperature less than 32.2°C (90°F). The body's response to hypothermia varies significantly among individuals. Outdoor accidents and injury are associated with a risk of hypothermia that can be exacerbated by the use of cold IV fluids and prolonged exposure of the patient for examination. Hemorrhagic shock secondary to trauma can worsen hypothermia. The speed of onset for hypothermia can also be influenced by the **wind chill factor.** This refers to the increased heat lost on windy days as more body heat is lost due to convection. Wind chill can make a fairly moderate winter day equivalent to a much colder one—sometimes dangerously so. For example, a day with a temperature of 30°F might seem of little concern, but combined with winds of 10 miles per hour, it can feel like it is only 16°F.

Initially, as hypothermia develops, there is an excitation phase where the body's heat-conserving and heat-generating mechanisms are maximally activated. In this phase, the heart rate, blood pressure, and cardiac output all rise. Typically, though, the patient with mild hypothermia will usually exhibit:

★ Shivering (from attempted thermogenesis)

★ Lethargy (from CNS depression)

★ Lack of coordination (from CNS depression)

★ Cool, dry, pale skin (from massive peripheral vasoconstriction)

Later, when body temperature drops below 32.2°C (90°F), this gives way to slowing of the body's physiological functions. Metabolism slows and the body begins to utilize less oxygen and to produce less carbon dioxide. In this later phase the cardiac output, blood pressure, and pulse rate begin to fall. The patient is often lethargic, exhibits poor muscle coordination, and usually has cool pale skin (from massive peripheral vasoconstriction). When the temperature drops below 32.2°C (90°F), ECG abnormalities may develop. The typical signs and symptoms of severe hypothermia include:

★ Lack of shivering

★ Dysrhythmias

★ Loss of voluntary muscle control

★ Hypotension

★ Undetectable pulse and blood pressure

★ Cardiac arrest

Treatment of hypothermia is dependent on the severity. Generally speaking, all wet garments should be removed and the patient protected from additional heat loss. The patient should be maintained in a horizontal position. Particular care should be taken to avoid handling the patient in a rough manner because this may trigger a dysrhythmia. If possible, measure and monitor the core temperature as well as the ECG and vital signs.

If protocols allow it, the patient should be rewarmed. Patients with mild hypothermia should receive rewarming with active external methods (blankets, heat packs, and occasionally warm water immersion). Now, with the advent of portable IV fluid warmers, active internal rewarming with heated IV fluids can be initiated. Internal rewarming is much more effective than external rewarming. If available, warmed humidified oxygen can be administered. Patients with severe hypothermia tend to develop numerous complications during the rewarming process. Most patients who die during active rewarming of hypothermia do so from ventricular fibrillation. Because of this, rewarming of the severe hypothermia patient is best deferred to a hospital setting using a predefined protocol. However, if transport times exceed 15 minutes, rewarming may need to be started in the field. Always follow medical direction regarding the treatment of hypothermia.

Conditions that arise from ineffective hypothermia can be further divided into the following conditions, accidental and secondary (or intentional).

Accidental hypothermia is the spontaneous decrease in core temperature to less than 35°C (95°F), usually as a direct result of exposure to a colder environment. In this scenario the patient has an intact thermoregulatory system and no contributory pathology (i.e., underlying medical condition or medication).

Secondary (intentional) hypothermia is usually characterized by a compromised thermoregulatory mechanism or induced by medications or procedures. An example of an induced hypothermic condition is best demonstrated by the cooling of a patient during bypass surgery. Contributory factors for secondary hypothermia are listed in Table 30–3.

Several groups are susceptible to hypothermia, specifically because they all lack intact or have incompletely developed thermoregulatory mechanisms: infants, elderly people, chronic alcohol abusers and binge drinkers, and trauma victims.

Whether accidental or secondary, hypothermia impacts most if not all organ systems. Conduction, convection, radiation, and evaporation are all mechanisms of heat loss. When there is an extreme condition or an underlying disease process, these mechanisms become unopposed. Examples of mechanisms of heat loss are detailed in Table 30–4. Overall heat loss slows enzyme metabolism

Patients with mild hypothermia should receive rewarming with active external methods (blankets, heat packs, and occasionally warm water immersion).

Patients with severe hypothermia tend to develop numerous complications during the rewarming process.

accidental hypothermia *a spontaneous decrease in core temperature that falls below 35°C (95°F); usually a direct result of exposure to a colder environment.*

secondary (intentional) hypothermia *characterized by a compromised thermoregulatory mechanism, a side effect of medications or induced by medical procedures.*

Whether accidental or secondary, hypothermia impacts most if not all organ systems.

Table 30–3	Conditions That Increase the Risk of Hypothermia
Alcoholism	Encephalopathy
Severe burns	Myxedema (hypothyroidism)
Chemotherapy	Sepsis
CNS disturbances	Shock

Table 30–4	Mechanisms of Heat Loss
Mechanism	**Example**
Conductive	Water (immersion)
	Snow
	Damp ground
Convection	Wind
	Wind chill factors (see Figure 30–3)
Radiation	Outside temperature less than body temperature
Evaporation	Burns
	Damp clothing

and causes uncoupling of oxygen-dependent metabolism (producing an anaerobic state), but of primary concern is its impact on the cardiovascular, respiratory, and central nervous systems.

In the cardiovascular system hypothermia decreases the inotropic, dromotropic, and chronotropic characteristics of the heart. This directly affects the mean cardiac output and increases irritability. (Up to 90% of all hypothermic patients have some type of ECG abnormality.) Patients can present with bradycardias that are *not* vagally mediated and therefore refractory to atropine. Other common findings are atrioventricular blocks, prolonged QT intervals, widened QRS complexes, and T-wave inversion. The most documented and utilized criteria is the presence of the **J (or Osborne) wave** which "gives the impression that the beginning of the ST segment has been hitched up and it probably represents a distortion of the earliest stage of repolarization" (Maririott, 1988). These waves can be seen most often in the precordial leads and the size of the wave seems to be directly proportional to the level of hypothermia (Asystole and ventricular fibrillation can present spontaneously at temperatures at or below 25°C (77°F).

The respiratory impact of hypothermia is directly related to the overall slowing of the metabolism. A decrease in the respiratory rate decreases the amount of oxygen available to the tissues. The slowing of the metabolism, the decrease in cardiac output, and the decrease in the delivery of oxygen produce anaerobic conditions that result in lactic acid production. Together this will lead to a respiratory and metabolic acidosis.

Central nervous system disturbances can serve to increase the overall survivability of the patient. Dramatic temperature decreases drop cerebral oxygen requirements. This decrease can be 6% to 7% for each 1°C of decline until the temperature of 25°C (77°F) is reached. In lower temperatures the oxygen requirement of the patient can be as much as 25% to 50% less than normal. This mechanism serves to facilitate survivability by decreasing the amount of anoxic damage.

An alternate system classifies hypothermia into three categories instead of two. The classifications are:

Mild hypothermia 34°–35°C (93.2°–95.0°F)

Moderate hypothermia 29°–32°C (84.2°–89.6°F)

Severe hypothermia <29°C (84.2°F)

STAGES OF MILD HYPOTHERMIA

Mild hypothermia is the first "stage" of hypothermia. At this level there is an increase in the metabolic rate to produce heat. The thermoregulatory mechanisms are still intact and the outward signs of heat production are apparent: shivering, increase in heart rate, and cardiac output. In the later stages, shivering ceases, there is impairment of the CNS, a loss of fine motor control, a drop in the level of consciousness, and the patient may become lethargic.

If left untreated, moderate hypothermia may develop. As the process continues, the patient develops delirium, has a marked decrease in reflexes, has a dramatic decrease in the metabolic rate, the liver ceases to function, and cardiac dysrhythmias can be seen.

Severe hypothermia is characterized by the absence of shivering, unresponsiveness, respiratory depression, decreased cardiac output and decreased heart rate, and ECG disturbances.

One item of note is the consideration of how fast a patient moves through the three stages of hypothermia. If the progression is slow, there is a good chance that hypoglycemia may develop. Shivering requires a large amount of energy and this energy is liberated from glucose. If the patient remains in mild to moderate hypothermic states for long periods of time, their blood glucose level will be low. Conversely, if there is rapid progression through these stages there will not be enough time for shivering to expend the glucose reserves, and instead the patient reaches a point of metabolic failure and insulin fails to function. This can artificially drive up the glucose level and the patient may present with hyperglycemia.

FROSTBITE

Frostbite is freezing of the distal extremities (See Figure 30-6 ■.) Most commonly the hands and feet are involved. A freezing environment is not a prerequisite for frostbite; it may be facilitated by

A freezing environment is not a prerequisite for frostbite; it may be facilitated by wetness, winds and high altitude.

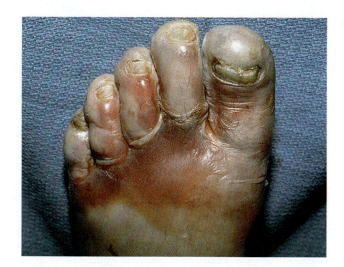

wetness, winds, and high altitude. The peripheral vasoconstriction found in hypothermia can contribute to the presence of frostbite. Outdoor enthusiasts and soldiers can be at greater risk for frostbite as well as populations who have underlying pathology that results in decreased cardiac output and/or poor peripheral circulation.

Cold exposure causes formation of ice crystals in the extracellular compartments, cellular dehydration, abnormal cell wall permeability, capillary damage, and pH changes. Capillary damage can lead to the leaking of serum into the tissues and increasing the viscosity of blood. This increase in viscosity further impairs the circulation, eventually leading to cessation of blood flow to the body part. As the extremity becomes hypoxic, the patient may complain of stinging, burning, or numbness.

Frostbite is classified through four degrees. Each increase in degree describes an increase in the depth of an injury. First-degree frostbite is superficial freezing only with edema; there are no blisters or vesicles and the skin has a waxy erythematous appearance. Some level of sensory deficit will be noted. Second-degree frostbite has vesicle formation with clear fluid noted; the skin is less waxy but still presents with erythema and edema. Third-degree frostbite is only differentiated from second degree by the presence of blood-filled blisters. Fourth-degree frostbite is considered a full-thickness injury. There is death of the dermal tissue, and extension into muscles, tendons, and bones can be seen.

TREATMENT FOR HYPERTHERMIC CONDITIONS

Without superceding the need for airway or circulatory management, treatment modalities should focus on removing the patient from the environment and initiating cooling measures. This must be done immediately and can be done in any number of modalities. Immediate management can decrease the mortality rate associated with heatstroke. In mild cases of heat exhaustion, cooling measures and some oral fluids may allow the condition to resolve.

One of the easiest and most convenient methods of heat reduction is placing cold packs over areas that have prominent superficial blood vessels, for example, the anteriolateral aspects of the neck, the axillae, and in the groin. Other methods include lightly spraying the patient with lukewarm water and allowing a fan to blow across the patient. Lukewarm water is utilized because it will vaporize faster, thus cooling the skin and improving dissipation of heat. The most effective method of heat reduction is ice water immersion; however, this practice can be problematic and is not practical in the transport setting. In extreme cases, cold IV fluids and gastric or peritoneal lavage with cold water can be effective. Whatever technique is utilized it must be discontinued when the patient's temperature reaches 40°C (104°F). This will prevent the possibility of an iatrogenic hypothermia. The placement of an indwelling rectal or esophageal thermometer can also help to avoid this condition and allows monitoring of the effectiveness of current therapy.

Without superceding the need for airway or circulatory management, treatment modalities should focus on removing the patient from the environment and initiating cooling measures.

During active cooling the patient may present with shivering, seizures, or vomiting. Shivering is a method of heat production and decreases the effectiveness of cooling. Benzodiazapines can be utilized in the management of shivering. Lorazepam (Ativan) is the drug of choice. It can be administered IV or IM and has a rapid onset of action. Dosage is 0.044 mg/kg IV, maximum rate is 2 mg per minute repeat q15min until a maximum dose of 8 mg is given. If not available, chlorpromazine (Thorazine) can be utilized. Adult dosage is 25–50 mg IV. If the patient has received other CNS depressants, anticholinergics, or anticonvulsants, these may potentiate a synergistic response. The efficacy of chlorpromazine has come into question because it is associated with a decrease in the seizure threshold and may produce hypotension.

Airway management is indicated in the patient who is unable to control his own airway. Endotracheal intubation is the method of choice, keeping in mind that the patient may have an underlying respiratory alkalosis. Therefore, ventilatory rates and volumes must be adjusted accordingly.

Hypotension in the presence of heatstroke should not initially be treated with aggressive fluid management. Hypotension should resolve with a decrease in body temperature producing a decrease in peripheral vasoconstriction. If cooling mechanisms are ineffective, fluid administration may be necessary. Administration of a crystalloid solution with careful monitoring may be the best approach. Monitoring of central venous pressure, pulmonary wedge pressure, systemic vascular resistance, and cardiac index (via a Swan-Ganz catheter) are the best methods to avoid overhydration.

In extreme cases of heatstroke, rhabdomyolysis may develop. Rhabdomyolysis is a process by which destruction of skeletal muscles occurs and results in kidney dysfunction. Evidence of rhabdomyolysis includes the development of dark-colored urine (due to myoglobin) and tender, swollen muscles. The best management of this condition includes aggressive fluid management and alkalization of the urine. The administration of sodium bicarbonate can help prevent acute renal failure due to myoglobin. Dosage is 2–3 amps added to 1,000 cc of D_5W infused at 200 cc/hr to maintain a urine pH of 7.5–8.0. Mannitol (Osmitrol) may also be used to improve renal perfusion and enhance filtration. It will also help with urine production. It should be administered in dosages of 25–100 g IV over 1–2 hours.

TREATMENT FOR HYPOTHERMIC CONDITIONS

Differentiation must be made between mild, moderate, or severe hypothermia. If the patient presents with cardiac dysrhythmias or a core temperature of less than 30°C (86°F) rewarming must begin as soon as possible. If the patient's core temperature continues to fall, the myocardium may become refractory. As in hyperthermic conditions, removing the patient from the environment is the best first step. This includes the removal of any wet or damp clothing.

In mild cases rewarming may be as simple as covering the patient with blankets and placing the patient in a warm environment. Rewarming in this fashion will increase the temperature of the patient 1°C per hour, which is considered a slow rewarming technique. Other approaches include IV solutions heated to 45°C (113°F) and/or heated humidified oxygen administered via mask. (See Figure 30-7 ■.)

As the acuity of the patient increases, more aggressive rewarming techniques must be utilized. The application of thermal blankets and utilization of heated baths and IV solutions heated to 65°C (149°F) can be used. Patients presenting with moderate hypothermia (without dysrhythmias) may benefit from these approaches. However there is the possibility of an afterdrop (1°–2°C) in the core-temperature after rewarming has been initiated. It is theorized that this is because colder blood in the extremities reaches the heart and decreases the threshold for ventricular fibrillation.

Profoundly hypothermic patients must be handled carefully because of cardiac irritability and are in need of aggressive rewarming techniques. Warmed thoracic lavage, warmed peritoneal lavage, and cardiopulmonary bypass are examples of aggressive rewarming.

Management of airway or cardiovascular conditions must be tempered. Endotracheal intubation must be performed carefully. Excess force or stimulation may precipitate ventricular fibrillation in the hypothermic patient. Preoxygenation without hyperventilation can decrease the potential for fibrillation. Cardiac dysrhythmias may or may not respond to treatment based upon temperature. At temperatures <30°C (86°F) the myocardium becomes refractory to most medications. In the setting

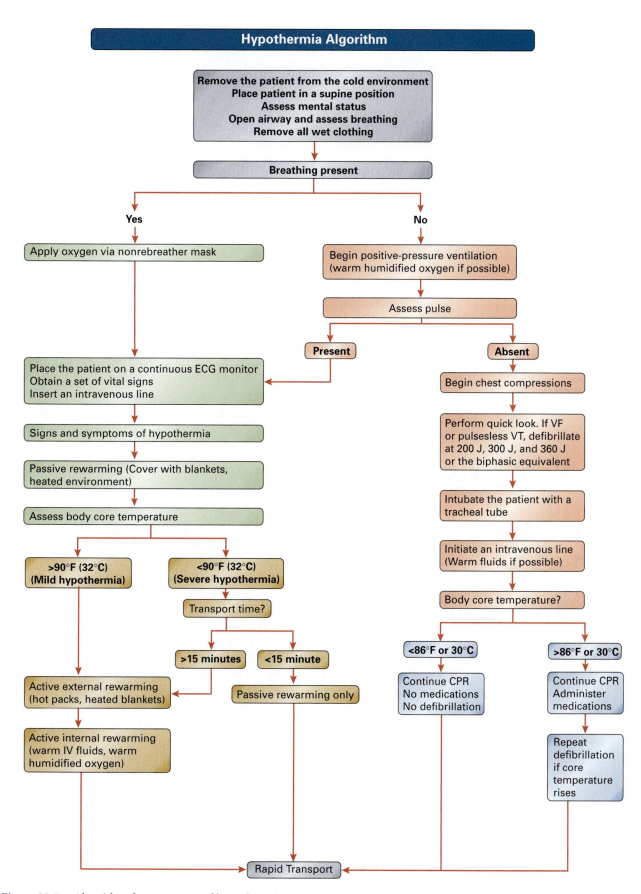

Figure 30-7 Algorithm for treatment of hypothermia.

of ventricular fibrillation and a core temperature less than or equal to 28°C (82.4°F), defibrillation should be done a maximum of twice and then suspended until the patient's temperature has increased.

The hypothermic patient who presents in cardiac arrest should be resuscitated until the core temperature of the body rises above 32°C (89.6°F). Throughout the resuscitation, aggressive rewarming techniques must be utilized. The decision to continue resuscitative efforts must take into consideration the presence of underlying pathology and the amount of downtime.

Pharmacological management of severe hypothermia is a source of great debate. One item that is clear is that caution and restraint must be practiced in the administration of medications. Because of decreased blood flow and peripheral pooling the medications may not reach the core of the patient until rewarming has occurred. The sudden bolus of multiple medications may have a deleterious effect.

The hypothermic patient who presents in cardiac arrest should be resuscitated until the core temperature of the body rises above 32°C (89.6°F).

FROSTBITE

Frostbite can occur by itself or it may be a component of a moderate to severe hypothermic event. Life threatening conditions must be managed first.

Rewarming of the affected area must begin immediately unless there is the possibility of refreezing, in which case it should be deferred. Rewarming can be accomplished by utilizing a warm bath (39°–42°C or 102.2°–107.6°F). Do not rub the affected part as that may increase tissue damage. The affected area should be completely thawed in 20–40 minutes. This can be confirmed by blanching of the distal tip of the extremity.

The main consideration for the patient during this process will be pain management. Rewarming can be exceedingly painful and can be mitigated by the administration of morphine or fentanyl.

SPECIAL CONSIDERATIONS: DROWNING AND NEAR-DROWNING

Each year in the United States about 1,500 children drown. In 1998 drowning was the second leading cause of death in children 1 to 14 and the 5th leading cause of death in all age groups. The highest drowning rates have been reported for children 1–5 years old and young adults age 15–24 years. The annual cost of care per year in a chronic care facility for the impaired survivor of a near-drowning event is approximately $100,000 and lifetime cost attributed to the management of near-drowning and drowning patients yearly is $384 million.

drowning *death from suffocation due to submersion in a liquid within 24 hours of insult.*

near-drowning *survival of suffocation due to submersion in a liquid past the 24-hour point of insult.*

Drowning can be divided into two categories: d*rowning* and *near-drowning*. **Drowning** is defined as death from suffocation due to submersion in a liquid within 24 hours of insult. Survival past the 24-hour point is categorized as **near-drowning.** Drowning events can occur almost anywhere; however, the data suggest that there is a correlation with age and location in the younger populations.

PATHOPHYSIOLOGY

The principal insult in drowning is hypoxia.

The principal insult in drowning is hypoxia. Once immersion occurs there is a natural tendency to hold your breath. The panic and hysteria that accompany these events make this an arduous task. At some point the victim will succumb to the situation and gasp for air; this will occur when the stimulus to breathe overrides the voluntary effort of breath holding. This gasping and the sudden influx of fluid will cause either laryngospasm or inhalation of fluid. This etiology differentiates a "wet drowning" from "dry drowning."

Wet drowning is due to aspiration and collection of fluids in the airway while dry drownings are secondary to airway spasm. Statistically up to 15% of drownings are dry and the remaining 85% are wet.

Once fluid is taken into the lungs, pulmonary vasoconstriction develops, which in turn produces hypertension. If the event occurs in cold water, core body functions begin to slow down and hypothermic states can develop. Blood is shunted to coronary and cerebral circulation.

As mentioned previously, the principal insult is hypoxia directly due to the loss of adequate gas exchange at the alveolar level. The type of fluid, saltwater versus freshwater, can play a role in the pathophysiology of the metabolic processes but ultimately the management of hypoxia can be the best determinate of prognosis.

In a freshwater drowning, the water moves from the alveolar space into the vascular space due to osmotic pressures. This movement causes destruction of surfactant, which leads to an increase of surface tension on the alveolar walls, resulting in atelectasis. Ultimately this causes intrapulmonary shunting and produces a ventilation perfusion mismatch. In saltwater, immediate washout of surfactant occurs. Because of the chemical structure of surfactant it reacts with the saltwater to exudate in the smaller airways. This produces a physiological shunting because of the accumulation of fluid in the alveoli. The longer the patient remains submerged, survival options dwindle. Another factor that affects outcome is the mammalian diving reflex. When exceedingly cold water hits the face it can produce this phenomenon, most notably in children. This reflex can cause apnea, bradycardia, and vasoconstriction and facilitates the slowdown of metabolic activities previously described. This decrease can be attributed with the increased survival rates associated with cold-water immersion. (See Table 30–5.)

Depending on the specific mechanism of injury, the patient may be at risk for a spinal cord insult and this must be factored into the assessment. While maintenance of the hypoxic event is paramount, it must be done cautiously to prevent further damage. The provider must also be careful not to allow the presentation of the patient to fool him. The patient can present anywhere from awake and alert to unconscious. The duration of the event, possibility of neurologic trauma, and amount of cerebral hypoxia are obviously factors in determining the prognosis of the patient.

Cardiac complications are usually secondary to hypoxic events. Rhythms borne out of hypoxic etiologies are common, namely, atrial fibrillation, PVCs, and in extreme cases ventricular tachycardia/fibrillation.

If there is a significant increase in the intravascular volumes, there can be dilution and hemolysis of the blood. This coupled with the hypoxic event can lead to renal impairment or failure. However, this complication is rare and not usually seen in the clinical setting.

Drowning and near-drowning patients can be classified into four distinct categories: asymptomatic, symptomatic, cardiopulmonary arrest, and obviously dead. Even in the asymptomatic patient great care must be taken to determine the history of the event including duration of exposure, mechanism of injury, and a review of systems.

Symptomatic patients can present from mild to severe. Any alteration in vital signs, respiratory disturbances, tachypnea, dyspnea, or hypoxia regardless of severity classify the patient as symptomatic. Neurologic deficit may be due to the event or the presence of another mechanism (i.e., ETOH or drug use, or head injury). In either case always assume that it is a result of the event.

Cardiopulmonary arrest due to drowning is no different than other causes and is managed accordingly. Pay attention to the core temperature of the patient. Cold-water drownings that do not present as obviously dead (rigor mortis, diffuse tissue degradation, lividity, devastating physical trauma, normothermic, and asystolic) should be resuscitated until a normothermic state is reached.

Table 30–5	Locations of Drownings by Age Group
Age of Victim	**Location of Event**
>1 year old	Bathtubs, buckets
1–4 years old	Home or apartment swimming pools
15–19 years old	Lakes, ponds, rivers, and pools

These data are not suggestive of variations by geographic location, gender, or season.

TREATMENT

Special attention must be given to the maintenance of a patent airway for these patients. Vigilant monitoring of breath sounds and a review of blood gas values should be obtained. Serial blood gasses may be utilized in the symptomatic patient to accurately monitor ventilation status. Utilization of pulse oximetry will be dependent on the core temperature of the patient. Indications for ET intubation are the inability to maintain a PO_2 greater than 60–70 mmHg with 100% oxygen. The presentation of fluid in the airways is best managed by positive end-expiratory pressure (PEEP) starting at 5 cm H_2O. PEEP can improve ventilating patterns by shifting interstitial pulmonary water into capillaries, increasing lung volume, mitigating atelectasis, providing better alveolar ventilation, and increasing airway diameter.

Other indications of the need for intubation are any signs of impending respiratory failure, decreasing level of consciousness, inability to maintain a patent airway, one- to two-word dyspnea, and accessory muscle use. Such indications should be watched for and managed swiftly.

Decompression of the stomach can be accomplished via NG/OG tube. The increased amount of fluid in the stomach will cause a decrease in tidal volumes and hamper effective oxygenation. In cold-water drowning patients can present with cold-induced bronchorrhea. A beta$_2$-agonist can best manage this event.

Removal of excess fluid can be accomplished by the utilization of a diuretic. It is important to note that the effect of this treatment in the hypothermic patient is questionable. Administration once the patient has returned to a normothermic status is advisable.

Cold-water drowning should be rewarmed by any of the previously described methods. Using warmed and humidified oxygen, warmed IV fluids, and bladder and stomach lavage can be effective in the unconscious patient. If the patient presents in cardiac arrest, warmed peritoneal lavage and thoracotomy with warm mediastinal lavage may be utilized.

Summary

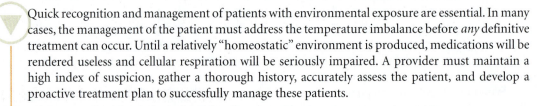

Quick recognition and management of patients with environmental exposure are essential. In many cases, the management of the patient must address the temperature imbalance before *any* definitive treatment can occur. Until a relatively "homeostatic" environment is produced, medications will be rendered useless and cellular respiration will be seriously impaired. A provider must maintain a high index of suspicion, gather a thorough history, accurately assess the patient, and develop a proactive treatment plan to successfully manage these patients.

Review Questions

1. Describe the concept of thermostatic control of body temperature.
2. Describe physiological processes used by the body to generate and retain heat.
3. Describe physiological processes used by the body to lose heat.
4. Describe the basal metabolic rate.
5. Detail assessment and management of heat exhaustion.
6. Detail emergencies related to hypothermia.
7. Describe the assessment and treatment of the hypothermic patient.
8. Describe the various classification schemes for hypothermia.
9. Discuss the benefits and limitations of active rewarming.
10. Describe the physiology and treatment of drowning.

See Answers to Review Questions at the back of this book.

Further Reading

American Academy of Pediatrics. *Drowning in Infants, Children and Adolescents.* Washington, DC: Author, 2001.

Bledsoe BE, Herterlendy A, Romig LE. "Disorders of Temperature Regulation: Prehospital Implications." *Journal of Emergency Medical Services (JEMS),* Vol. 28, No. 3 (2003): 36–50.

Braunwald E, Fauci AS. *Harrison's Principles of Internal Medicine.* New York: McGraw-Hill, 2001.

CDC, Center for Injury Prevention and Control. *Drowning Prevention.* Atlanta, GA: Author, 2000.

Conrad S. "Respiratory Distress Syndrome, Adult." *eMedicine Journal,* Vol. 2, No. 2, http://www.emedicine.com (2001).

Curley FJ, Irwin RS. "Disorders of Temperature Regulation." In *Intensive Care Medicine,* Rippe JM, et al., editors. Boston: Little, Brown, 1985.

Decker W. "Hypothermia." *eMedicine Journal,* Vol. 2, No. 8, http://www.emedicine.com (2001).

Golden L, Bennett JC. *Cecil Textbook of Medicine.* Philadelphia: W. B. Saunders, 2000.

Helman RS. "Heatstroke." *eMedicine Journal,* Vol. 2, No. 7, http://www.emedicine.com (2001).

Huether S, McCance C. *Understanding Pathophysiology.* St. Louis: Mosby, 2000.

Knochel JP. "Heat Illness." In *Current Therapy in Emergency Medicine.* Philadelphia: BC Decker, 1987.

Kunihiro A. "Heat Exhaustion and Heat Stroke." *eMedicine Journal,* Vol. 2, No. 6, http://www.emedicine.com (2001).

Lee G. *Flight Nursing Principles and Practice.* New York: Mosby-Year Book, 1996.

Marieb E. *Understanding Anatomy and Physiology.* Menlo Park: Benjamin/Cummins Science Publishing, 1998.

Maririott HJL. *Practical Electrocardiography,* 8th ed. Baltimore: Williams & Wilkins, 1988.

McElroy C, Auerbach PS. "Heat Illness: Current Perspectives." In *Management of Wilderness and Environmental Emergencies.* New York: Macmillan, 1987.

Mechem C. "Frostbite." *eMedicine Journal,* Vol. 2, No. 4. http://www.emedicine.com (2001).

National Institutes of Health, National Institute of Child Health and Human Development. *National Study Examines Sites Where U.S. Children Drown.* Baltimore, MD: Author, 2001.

Nettina SM. *The Lippincott Manual of Nursing Practice.* Philadelphia: Lippincott Williams & Wilkins, 2000.

O'Brian DJ. "Heat Illness." *Journal of Aeromedical Healthcare* (May/June 1985): 6.

Shepherd S. "Submersion Injury: Near Drowning." *eMedicine Journal,* Vol. 2, No. 8, http://www.emedicine.com (2001).

Diving Emergencies

Jeff McDonald, AA, NREMT-P

Objectives

Upon completion of this chapter, the student should be able to:

1. Describe physical laws that affect gas pressure and depth (physics of diving). (p. 919)
2. Describe the effects on the body at depth in an underwater environment (physiology of depth). (p. 920)
3. Identify diving environments. (p. 920)
4. Identify diving equipment. (p. 921)
5. Describe the pathophysiology, assessment, management, and critical care considerations of:
   A. Ear, sinus, pulmonary, and other significant barotrauma (p. 922)
   B. Nitrogen narcosis (p. 923)
   C. Decompression sickness (p. 923)
   D. High-pressure neurologic syndrome (HPNS) (p. 925)
   E. Hypoxia and gas toxicity (p. 926)
6. Discuss aquatic concerns associated with diving:
   A. Drowning (p. 927)
   B. Saltwater aspiration syndrome (p. 927)
   C. Cold and hypothermia (p. 927)
   D. Infection (p. 927)
   E. Dangerous animals (p. 927)
7. Identify causes of medical emergencies related to diving:
   A. Hearing loss (p. 930)
   B. Disorientation (p. 930)
   C. Unconscious divers (p. 930)
   D. Diver deaths (p. 930)
   E. Sudden death syndrome (p. 930)

8. Understand hyperbaric medicine. (p. 931)
9. Identify concerns for females who dive and for stress associated with diving. (p. 932)
10. Discuss the role of the CCP in diving emergency support situations. (p. 933)

Key Terms

Case Study

It is 1600 hours on a Sunday afternoon and you are working your part-time job as an on-call critical care paramedic for a fixed-wing air medical service. Your pager goes off alerting you to a flight. You immediately don your flight suit and head for the airport.

On arrival you are met by the pilot who tells you that you have a flight to a hospital in Cancun, Quintana Roo, Mexico, to pick up an American citizen who had some problems while diving in Cozumel. As you are heading toward the jet to start preparing for the flight, the on-call flight nurse pulls up. He is quickly briefed on the flight. The only information available is that the person is a 47-year-old male who developed an unknown complication while diving. The medical evacuation was set up through American Express. The contact person provides a phone number for the hospital and the attending physician in Cancun—but that is it. You check to make sure you have the satellite phone and will try to contact the physician or hospital en route.

En route you make contact with the hospital and speak with a pleasant English-speaking nurse. The patient is stable and developed chest pain while diving. Although they feel the problem is not related to the diving, they are being cautious in returning the patient to his home in Shreveport, Louisiana. The pilot settles into a cruising altitude and you doze off. The next thing you hear is the sound of the landing gear opening as you approach the airport. The area is dark—but you can make out the lights of the hotels and resorts in the distance.

You land and are allowed to taxi to the main terminal. Mexican customs officials enter the plane and take a brief look at your passports and look around the plane. You are then allowed to deplane. A small Cruz Roja ambulance meets you and transports the nurse and you to the hospital. The hospital is modern and seems well equipped. You are met by a security guard who leads you to the *cuarto de cuidado intensivo* (intensive care room).

The physician presents the patient and reports that five minutes into his first dive, he developed tightness in his chest. The tightness got worse as he tried to continue. He returned to the dive boat and was taken to the docks where an ambulance took him to the hospital. The patient has a family history of heart disease. He has hypertension and hyperlipidemia. His medications include Zestoretic and Zocor. He has had some brief episodes of chest tightness in the hospital that cleared with morphine.

You complete your assessment and review the chart. The 12-lead ECGs have been nonspecific and the cardiac enzymes normal. There was nothing abnormal about the dive—in fact, the patient had not gotten below 10–15 feet deep. Despite this, you cannot exclude a diving-related problem. A repeat ECG with your equipment reveals some nonspecific ST-T wave changes, but is otherwise negative.

The patient is packaged and taken to the ambulance and you are driven to the airport. At the airport, the driver is waved through up to the plane. The patient is moved to the plane and you thank your cohorts from Cruz Roja. The pilot closes the door and prepares for departure as you finish preparing the patient for flight. The patient remains pain free and stable all the way to Shreveport where he is delivered to the care of his family physician.

In a routine follow-up you learn that the patient underwent coronary angiography and had diffuse coronary artery disease. He underwent a coronary artery bypass graft (CABG) and is expected to do well.

INTRODUCTION

For the critical care paramedic, care for victims of diving-related injuries will be mostly supportive. Transportation from local hospital facilities to hyperbaric chambers where recompression can be accomplished as the definitive treatment will be all that is required in most cases.

For the critical care paramedic, care for victims of diving-related injuries will be mostly supportive. Transportation from local hospital facilities to hyperbaric chambers where recompression can be accomplished as the definitive treatment will be all that is required in most cases. However, when emergencies do arise in transport, an understanding of how diving-related injures arise can mean the difference between the right decision and sudden death. An understanding of the diving environment is important in understanding the extent of injury and the importance of timely treatment.

HISTORY OF DIVING

SCUBA or scuba *self-contained underwater breathing apparatus.*

Self-contained underwater breathing apparatus (SCUBA or scuba) has obvious limitations. One is the amount of time a diver can remain underwater—eventually the compressed air cylinder becomes empty. Multiple tanks can extend dive time, but doing so carries additional complications related to compression/decompression and decreased mobility underwater.

Professional divers, with a need for extended deep dives, have developed elaborate tables and specifications for mixing oxygen, air, nitrogen, helium, and other gases. By combining gases, the risks of decompression sickness, nitrogen narcosis, and other underwater conditions are substantially reduced. As expected, however, other complications can occur, especially in the hands of improperly trained or inexperienced divers.

Saturation diving is a method of placing divers in an underwater habitat for extended periods of time, often to depths exceeding 1,000 feet. These divers may spend as much as a month underwater, living in pressurized structures and leaving through open bottoms to work on the ocean floor. Saturation diving is a common practice in the offshore oil industry where divers work stabilizing deep-water pilings and help to maintain the integrity of the drilling site. This sort of diving is not without consequences. Although the divers often earn as much as $1,000 per hour, their effective working time is very limited. The return to the surface can take as much as 48 hours. Effects of excessive pressure can have long-term effects on the bones and soft tissues of the body. *Dysbaric osteonecrosis* is a condition leading to the death of bone tissues, resulting in unexpected fractures, bone degeneration, and devastating arthritis often requiring the surgical placement of artificial joints.

Today diving occurs in both professional and recreational circles. As the popularity of diving increases, so does the need for understanding the medical-related conditions that are associated with the sport. In the United States today, more than 8.5 million people are certified divers, approximately one-quarter of which are women. Florida, California, Hawaii, and Texas lead the list of states with large numbers of divers. Through research and training, diving is considerably safer than it was just a few years ago. Although some injuries and deaths occur from factors we still do not understand, the majority are the result of divers pushing limits or failing to properly use and care for their equipment.

Today diving occurs in both professional and recreational circles. As the popularity of diving increases, so does the need for understanding the medical-related conditions that are associated with the sport.

DIVING PHYSICS

It is a simple fact that man cannot breathe underwater, at least not without assistance. (See Figure 31-1 ■.) In the case of scuba diving, the device compensates for one problem but opens the human body to additional physiological strains. One of these strains is pressure. Pressure is the relationship between force and area:

$$\text{Pressure} = \frac{\text{Force (F)}}{\text{Area (A)}}$$

Pressure is measured in several units:

$$\frac{\text{Pound (lb)}}{\text{Square inch (in.}^2)} = \text{pounds per square inch (psi)} \qquad \frac{\text{Newtons (N)}}{\text{Square meters (m}^2)} = \text{Pascals (Pa)}$$

It can also be measured in atmospheres (atm), millimeters of mercury or torr (mmHg), kilopascals (kPa), or centimeters of water (cm/H_2O). For example, at sea level, the pressure from the atmosphere can be measured as:

$$1 \text{ atm} = 14.7 \text{ lb/in.}^2 = 760 \text{ mmHg} = 760 \text{ torr} = 101.3 \text{ kPa} = 1{,}033 \text{ cm/H}_2\text{O}$$

As the force increases or the area decreases, the pressure increases. Two types of pressure are a factor for divers: atmospheric pressure, exerted by almost 500,000 feet of molecules at the surface, and hydrostatic pressure, exerted by water at depth.

An understanding on the relationship between volume and pressure is essential to the understanding of dive-related medicine. Refer to Chapter 4 (Altitude Physiology) for a review of important gas laws.

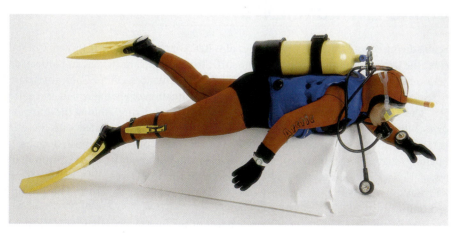

■ Figure 31-1   A well-equipped modern SCUBA diver. *(Steve Shott/Dorling Kindersley)*

GASES OF DIVING

Breathing compressed air seems to be the safest means of maintaining normal bodily function in an underwater environment. It is however, fraught with perils. Both oxygen and nitrogen have toxic effects on the body when under pressure.

Oxygen, necessary for normal metabolism, is toxic at pressures above 0.21 **atmospheres of absolute pressure (ATA)** for long periods of time. Deep divers breathe a mixture of oxygen with nitrogen or helium aimed at reducing the percentage of oxygen in the total mixture.

Nitrogen, considered an "inert gas" on the body at the surface, has specific dangers at depth. Under pressure, nitrogen has narcotic effects that can lead to dangerous behavioral changes underwater. The absorption of nitrogen at depth causes problems on surfacing that can lead to decompression sickness. To avoid this, divers are now adding oxygen to regular air to allow for a more lengthy dive with a reduced risk of decompression sickness. However, this practice increases the risks of oxygen toxicity if deep depths are reached.

The practice of compressing air also has its risks. Unreliable air-fill stations may have faulty filters and exhausts that place unwanted gases or contaminants in the scuba cylinder. Gases from these sources can contain contaminants such as carbon monoxide, hydrocarbons, and rust. All of these can have fatal effects with inhalation.

BUOYANCY

Buoyancy is determined by the density of an object and the specific gravity of the liquid in which it is suspended. Density is determined by the mass per unit volume. In other words the more material you can get into the smaller amount of space, the denser the object. **Specific gravity** is determined by the density of an object compared to the density of freshwater, which has a specific gravity of 1.0. An object that has a specific gravity of less than 1.0 will float, while an object with a specific gravity of more than 1.0 will sink.

The human body has a specific gravity of slightly more than 1.0, making it sink in most cases. However, fat has a specific gravity of less than 1.0 as does air. People with high fat content or with full lungs tend to float better than people with little body fat or those with no air in their lungs.

The Greek mathematician Archimedes discovered that an object placed in water will displace an amount of water equal to the weight of water displaced by the object. This is known as Archimedes' principle. It is the explanation of why an object that weighs less than the water it displaces will float, and an object that weighs more that the water it displaces will sink. Divers generally weigh less than the water they displace when dressed in dive gear so the addition of dive weights is necessary to achieve proper buoyancy at depth. Because the specific gravity of freshwater is lower than that of saltwater, more weight is required when diving in oceans than in lakes.

DIVING ENVIRONMENTS

Scuba diving is not limited to large bodies of water, nor to calm bodies of water. Coastal divers often enter the water by simply walking into the surf. Strong surge, large waves, and unseen objects hidden below the foam combine to create potentially fatal consequences. Off the California coast, large forests of sea kelp can entangle an unwary diver, creating a situation of entanglement and entrapment.

There is a growing interest in specialty and technical diving. Among these are confined space dives, which include ice, wreck, and cave diving. One danger associated with these environments is the lack of easy egress should a problem arise. Divers often must push a scuba tank through openings slightly larger that the diameter of a person. With no place to turn around, it is often necessary to back out, feeling the way with the feet or fin tips. Caves and wrecks often have still waters that can easily silt up as a diver swims, decreasing visibility to zero and obscuring any possible exit opportunity.

For divers descending deeper than 100 feet or for those who remain underwater for extended periods of time, decompression becomes a serious concern. To prevent post-diving injuries, divers

---

atmospheres of absolute pressure (ATA) *describes underwater pressure; includes the weight of the water plus the atmospheric pressure at the surface. Every 33 feet of depth is equal to 1 atmosphere (or 14.7 psi in pressure); surface pressure is also equal to 1 atmosphere. (A diver at a depth of 33 feet is at an ATA of 2 atmospheres.)*

Nitrogen, considered an "inert gas" on the body at the surface, has specific dangers at depth.

buoyancy *determined by the density of an object and the specific gravity of the liquid in which it is suspended.*

specific gravity *determined by the density of an object compared to the density of freshwater (which has a specific gravity of 1.0).*

Scuba diving is not limited to large bodies of water, nor to calm bodies of water. Coastal divers often enter the water by simply walking into the surf.

For divers descending deeper than 100 feet or for those who remain underwater for extended periods of time, decompression becomes a serious concern.

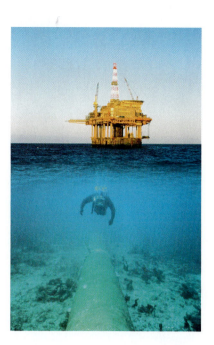

■ **Figure 31-2** A commercial diver swims along a pipeline beneath an offshore oil platform. *(Terje Rakke/Getty Images, Inc.)*

must ascend slowly and make frequent stops at predetermined increments. These stops may range from 3 to 20 minutes, and require divers to plan ahead to make sure they will have sufficient air supply to properly decompress. (See Figures 31-2 ■ and 31-3 ■.)

A factor important to divers is the effects of pressure during high-altitude dives, those dives which occur above 10,000 feet. Diving in mountain lakes and rivers require a recalculation of standard dive tables. Although the pressure underwater has not significantly changed, the pressure above the surface causes decompression injuries to occur more easily.

DIVING EQUIPMENT

Recreational scuba divers breathe compressed air. This normal mixture of 79% nitrogen and 21% oxygen is an appropriate breathing gas within the limits of normal sport diving depths, that is, less than 120 feet deep. At deeper depths, however, both of these gases have toxic effects. To combat

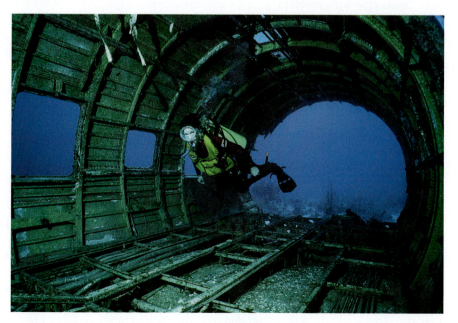

■ **Figure 31-3** A scuba diver investigates the hollow interior of the fuselage of an airplane wrecked under the ocean near South Caicos Island. *(Fred Bavendam/Peter Arnold, Inc.)*

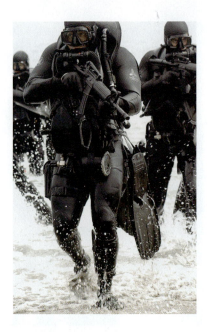

■ **Figure 31-4** Special forces diver with scrubber. *(Courtesy of HMCM Michael Beske [WARCOM]. Photo cleared by Naval Special Warfare Command Public Affairs Office)*

these effects, commercial divers use mixed gases. Combinations of oxygen, helium, nitrogen, and other inert gases are blended to reduce the risks of toxicity and to improve the safety in underwater operations.

Some diving operations, usually military, utilize a method of rebreathing exhaled air. (See Figure 31-4 ■.) These systems include small canisters of compressed oxygen and *scrubber* canisters, which remove excess carbon dioxide. The advantage of these systems is an almost complete removal of exhaled bubbles, which is important for covert military maneuvers and is also useful for scientists interested in becoming less intrusive in the study environment. Injuries can occur, however, from the use of these rebreathers. The majority of these are caused by a failure of the oxygen mixer or the carbon dioxide scrubber, resulting in either oxygen toxicity or hypoxia.

An important piece of diving equipment, probably second only to the equipment that delivers oxygen, is the exposure suit. Known by most people as a wet suit, exposure suits can be either wet or dry. The purpose of both types of suits is to protect the diver from heat loss. Water cools the body 20 times faster than air. Thus, even in relatively warm water, heat can be lost from the unprotected body. Divers experience problems in exposure suits when not properly oriented to the operation of these suits at depth where compression changes the functional protection. Dry suits are extremely prone to operator error when failure to purge the suit can cause a rapid rise in trapped air volume. This increases the diver's buoyancy and can send him rapidly to the surface. Overexpansion injuries are common in such mishaps.

INJURIES ASSOCIATED WITH DESCENT

As a diver descends below the surface, pressure changes occur almost immediately.

As a diver descends below the surface, pressure changes occur almost immediately. Most people have felt the effects of pressure changes on their ears when they swim to the bottom of a neighborhood swimming pool. Even at these shallow depths, the effects of pressure changes can have serious effects. The ear is most often affected, but problems with the sinuses and blood vessels of the eye are also possible.

The tympanic membrane experiences pressure changes when the eustachian tube is compressed and no longer allows equalization of the pressure in the middle ear. Divers learn to purge the pressure by exhaling against closed nostrils. However, if infection or inflammation exists in the inner ear or eustachian tube, purging becomes difficult or impossible. As depth increases, purging becomes increasingly more difficult, because the pressure closes the eustachian tube ever tighter. Failure to purge can result in tears or ruptures of the tympanic membrane, which will be seen as severe pain in the affected ear and blood coming from the auditory canal. While underwater the pain caused by the pressure is often relieved when the membrane tears. A cold sensation is also felt as water enters the middle ear. Depending on the size of the tear, the diver may experience temporary hearing loss. Without proper care, the loss may become permanent. Vertigo is often present.

A similar condition can exist when the weak point of the ear is the oval or round window leading from the middle ear to the inner ear. Pressure in the middle ear can literally drive the stapes through the round window and force water into the cochlea of the ear, disrupting the auditory sensibility. Deafness, temporary or permanent, can result.

Sinuses are also frequently injured when inflammation combines with pressure changes. Allergies, colds, decongestant medication rebound, smoking, and infections are some of the possible causes of sinus inflammation. When air in the sinus becomes trapped during the diver's descent, the shrinking volume is replaced by fluids or blood from the sinus linings. Known as a **sinus squeeze,** the diver will experience pressure or pain in the areas above the eye, over the upper teeth, or from deep in the skull. This will eventually dissipate during the dive and return on ascent, usually accompanied by bleeding from the nose. After ascent the increased fluid and blood leakage produce a rich bed for bacterial growth, promoting severe sinus infections. Headaches after a dive are common with a sinus squeeze. Because decompression sickness also presents with a headache, the diver should be monitored closely for the development of additional symptoms.

sinus squeeze *pressure or pain in the areas above the eye, over the upper teeth, or from deep in the skull, while diving at depth.*

INJURIES ASSOCIATED WITH DEPTH AND DECOMPRESSION

NITROGEN NARCOSIS

Nitrogen narcosis is an intoxicating effect that occurs to a diver at depth. Specific physiological actions are not clear, but it appears that pressurized nitrogen affects the brain in a manner similar to alcohol or narcotics. Divers are affected at different rates and at different depths, with most cases occurring at depths greater than 100 feet. Also known as "raptures of the deep," it should come as no surprise that some divers actually seek the buzz associated with nitrogen narcosis. This may lead to a diving emergency that requires critical care paramedics to respond.

nitrogen narcosis *an intoxicating effect of unclear etiology that appears to affect the brain in a manner similar to alcohol or narcotics, and affects diver judgment.*

Signs and symptoms of nitrogen narcosis include deficits in reasoning, judgment, memory, and perception. With greater depth, symptoms worsen and may eventually lead to unconsciousness—a lethal condition underwater. A feeling of calmness and well-being give the diver a false sense of security and comfort. This feeling of comfort may lead to a feeling of panic or stress as the narcotic effects wear off during ascent. Injuries and deaths are not caused by the narcosis itself, but rather by the lack of judgment and attention to surroundings. It is possible for narcotic divers to forget to breathe, or to ascend at a rapid and uncontrolled rate, which can be detrimental. If the individual is diving with a buddy, the buddy also commonly experiences similar narcotic effects, creating a team of irrational divers, and unfortunately potential problems for both.

Divers can reduce the effects of narcosis through acclimatization, which helps to develop a tolerance similar to the development of a tolerance for alcohol. Focusing on a specific task can also ward off narcotic effects. Use of alcohol or other depressant (including anti-seasickness medications) or hallucinogenic drugs can increase the rate and effects of narcosis, as can hypothermia, fatigue, and poor visibility.

decompression sickness *a condition caused by the expansion of nitrogen in the tissues following a dive of significant depth and duration. Also known as; "caisson disease," the "bends," "diver's paralysis," and "dysbarism."*

Treatment for nitrogen narcosis is not necessary because it is self-correcting on ascent. However, it may be necessary to treat any injuries that result from the loss of judgment at depth. Often the lack of judgment results in a failure to monitor the air supply, leaving the divers with no choice but to make an emergency ascent, which can cause pulmonary barotrauma and decompression sickness. Decompression sickness as an emergency and how to properly manage it are discussed next.

caisson disease *also known as "decompression sickness," the "bends," "diver's paralysis," and "dysbarism."*

DECOMPRESSION SICKNESS

Decompression sickness is also known as **caisson disease,** the "**bends,**" *diver's paralysis,* and *dysbarism.* This condition is caused by the expansion of nitrogen in the tissues following a dive of significant depth and duration. Although seldom considered in normal physiology, nitrogen also

"bends" *also known as decompression sickness, "caisson disease," "diver's paralysis," and "dysbarism."*

diffuses into the bloodstream along with oxygen, and travels to the tissues and cells of the body. Under pressure, the nitrogen dissolves at a rate greater than normal and saturates into the body's tissues. The greater the pressure, the more the nitrogen dissolves and the greater the tissue saturation.

This has special significance for scuba divers because the effects of depth change the volume and pressure of nitrogen being inhaled. As a diver descends, more and more nitrogen is absorbed into the tissues of the body. The longer the diver remains submerged and the deeper the dive, the greater the tissue saturation becomes. On ascent the volume of nitrogen in the lungs decreases. Unfortunately for divers, the rate in which nitrogen leaves the alveoli and the rate it leaves the tissues are greatly different, creating a state of disequilibrium. The nitrogen trapped in tissues is released considerably slower than the nitrogen in the alveoli. On release into the bloodstream, nitrogen expands on ascent producing microbubbles, which can affect all the tissues of the body. These microbubbles cause occlusions of capillary systems and produce states of tissue ischemia. Because of the supersaturated state that occurs at depth, release of nitrogen and the subsequent bubble formation may not occur for several hours after surfacing.

The signs and symptoms of decompression sickness start small and worsen as small bubbles expand and combine to form larger bubbles. This causes occlusions of larger blood vessels, affecting greater tissue fields. Tissue ischemia and occasionally infarction can occur.

Pain in the joints and muscles occurs in the majority of patients. Most often the pain is located in the shoulder, but the elbow, wrist, hip, and knee are also commonly involved. This pain can be debilitating and often results in a contorted posture that provides the source of the term "bends." The pain often starts as simple pressure or discomfort, but eventually leads to an intense burning or throbbing pain. Movement usually worsens the condition but slight pressure may create relief. Although injury or arthritis can create similar symptoms, it is important to consider decompression sickness when these symptoms occur 24–48 hours after surfacing from a dive.

Additional signs and symptoms occur in more severe cases of decompression sickness. These include nervous system injuries that can lead to sensation impairment, headache, vertigo, loss of muscle coordination or paralysis, seizures, and coma. Most of these conditions are temporary and transient. However, paralysis may be permanent for patients with severe decompression sickness who do not get proper treatment in a timely manner.

A severe manifestation of the condition, known as the **"chokes,"** is seen in some worst case scenarios. This is the result of pulmonary capillary occlusions. Patients will complain of chest pain and dyspnea and will have moderate to severe pulmonary edema. Death may occur.

The definitive treatment for decompression sickness is recompression in a hyperbaric chamber so that the nitrogen in the body can safely exit over time. (See Figures 31-5 ■ and 31-6 ■.) It is

The signs and symptoms of decompression sickness start small and worsen as small bubbles expand and combine to form larger bubbles.

"chokes" *a potentially lethal condition hallmarked by chest pain, dyspnea, and pulmonary edema, secondary to pulmonary capillary occlusions.*

The definitive treatment for decompression sickness is recompression in a hyperbaric chamber.

■ Figure 31-5 Hyperbaric chamber. *(Courtesy of NASA)*

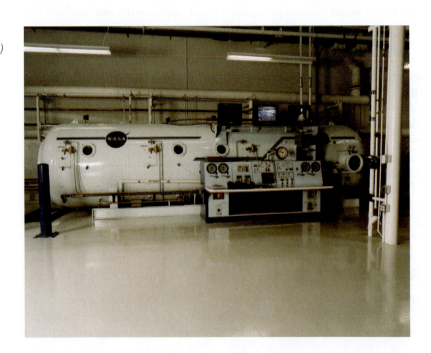

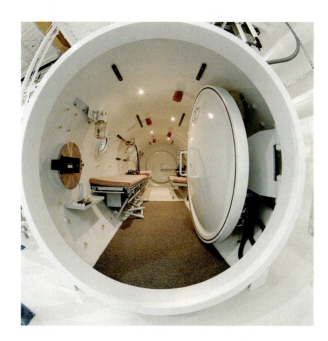

■ **Figure 31-6** Interior of hyperbaric chamber. *(Courtesy of NASA)*

the transport to the recompression chamber that will commonly find the critical care paramedic involved. Critical care transport by ground will require little more than supportive care in most cases. Air transportation is more risky since higher altitudes may allow nitrogen to exit the tissues at a faster rate, complicating matters. It is important that air transportation of these patients occur at low altitudes or within a pressurized aircraft.

The administration of oxygen should be considered so as to reduce the effects of tissue ischemia. Since breathing compressed air results in general dehydration, an IV of normal saline or lactated Ringer's should be titrated to blood pressure or to treat any signs of dehydration. An initial bolus of 300–500 mL is recommended for this purpose. Diazepam or midazolam should be given to treat seizures or severe cramping. Placement of the patient in a left-sided Trendelenburg position is a traditional treatment for all dive-related injuries, but has no real basis in research. Supine positioning or the recovery position is equally beneficial. Monitor the ECG and oxygen saturation, and be prepared for more aggressive therapy should the patient's condition deteriorate and lost airway, breathing, or circulatory compromise becomes evident.

HIGH-PRESSURE NEUROLOGIC SYNDROME

In the commercial diving industry deep dives are performed utilizing mixed gases in place of compressed air. When oxygen and helium are used at depths exceeding 400 feet, a condition known as **high-pressure neurologic syndrome (HPNS)** can develop. Also known as helium tremors, HPNS is the result of breathing helium and may be more related to the effects of helium on nervous tissues than the pressurization of helium itself.

HPNS starts with a tremor in the hands and arms similar to shivering, and difficulty in general muscle coordination. As the diver continues to descend, alterations in level of consciousness may occur. Confusion, unconsciousness, and seizures are possible. Difficult breathing develops as the muscles lose more coordination.

As an understanding of the effects of depth increased, it was found that giving a slight sedative to the diver would decrease the effects of HPNS. The dive industry now induces a slight and controlled nitrogen narcosis to prevent tremors in deep divers. Tri-mix gas is the mainstay for deep diving and includes oxygen, helium, and nitrogen.

Direct management for HPNS is the same as that for nitrogen narcosis discussed earlier. The role of critical care personnel is to treat the results of any mishaps that occurred during the disorientation period. This may include treating overexpansion injuries and decompression sickness. Contacting and coordinating efforts with recommendations made by the **Divers Alert Network (DAN)** is highly recommended.

high-pressure neurologic syndrome (HPNS) *also known as "helium tremors," HPNS is the result of breathing pressurized helium and oxygen at depths exceeding 400 feet.*

Divers Alert Network (DAN) *a nonprofit medical and research organization dedicated to the safety and health of scuba divers.*

DAN is a nonprofit medical and research organization dedicated to the safety and health of scuba divers and associated with Duke University Medical Center. Founded in 1980, DAN has served as a lifeline for the scuba industry by operating diving's only 24-hour emergency hotline, which is an emergency service for injured divers. Additionally, DAN operates a diving medical information line, conducts vital diving medical research, and develops and provides a number of educational programs for everyone from beginning divers to medical professionals. What DAN can do in support of the critical care paramedic's role is provide emergency medical advice and assistance for underwater diving injuries. The Divers Alert Network should be contacted for referral to hyperbaric chambers worldwide, and can be of great benefit in arranging transportation and technical assistance.

HYPOXIA AND GAS TOXICITY

As mentioned earlier, in an attempt to increase underwater time, divers have developed a practice of mixing gases. As seen already with nitrogen, helium, and oxygen, all gases have their risks when inhaled under pressure. The greatest risk of mixing gases is the onset of hypoxia. A failure to include sufficient oxygen to allow normal cell physiology can be a fatal mistake. Carbon monoxide toxicity is a rare occurrence today. However, poorly maintained, vented, or older gasoline-powered air compressors have a tendency to suck their own exhaust, allowing the entrance of carbon monoxide (CO) into scuba cylinders. At depth it takes relatively little carbon monoxide to produce symptoms. Sadly, victims of CO poisoning at depth have a poor prognosis.

All gases, under pressure and inhaled at depth, have a tendency to affect the body in a negative way.

All gases, under pressure and inhaled at depth, have a tendency to affect the body in a negative way. It is important to remember that any change in normal physiology will alter the normal operation of our cells and tissues. In nearly all cases these alterations are harmful, and rarely if ever beneficial.

INJURIES ASSOCIATED WITH ASCENT

Ascent injuries are associated with improper exhalation as the diver ascends or with air trapped in tissues. Pulmonary barotrauma, the most serious of ascent injuries, can produce a variety of presentations depending on the weak spot of the pulmonary tissue. Pulmonary barotrauma is also known as *pulmonary overexpansion injury.*

Ascent injuries are associated with improper exhalation as the diver ascends or with air trapped in tissues. Pulmonary barotrauma, the most serious of ascent injuries, can produce a variety of presentations depending on the weak spot of the pulmonary tissue.

Failure to properly exhale during ascent can cause the pulmonary tissue to rupture from the expansion of gases. Pneumothorax is common when the rupture is to the apical or lateral areas of the lung. Under most cases these are simple pneumothoraces, but tension cases are possible because the breathing of compressed air accelerates development. Hemothorax is also possible.

mediastinal emphysema *described as a tear in pulmonary tissues along the central area of the mediastinum. Symptoms can include dysphasia and tracheal pressure; extreme cases may present as cardiac tamponade.*

When the tear in pulmonary tissues occurs along the central area of the lungs, a condition known as **mediastinal emphysema** will develop. Divers will complain of difficulty swallowing and tracheal pressure. In extreme cases symptoms similar to cardiac tamponade can develop, because air trapped in the mid-thoracic space expands and makes cardiac contraction difficult.

arterial gas embolism (AGE) *a serious overexpansion syndrome, secondary to air being forced into the capillary system of the alveoli. Gases combine in the circulatory system to form larger "bubbles" that block arterial vasculature of the heart.*

The most serious condition seen in overexpansion is an **arterial gas embolism (AGE).** An AGE occurs when air is forced into the capillary system of the alveoli. The air bubbles filter through the circulatory system, combine to form larger bubbles, and pass through the heart into the general circulation of the body. Myocardial infarction, stroke, renal failure, and blindness are some of the conditions that can develop because these bubbles occlude the circulation into important tissues. Divers may loose consciousness immediately. Stroke victims may complain of, or be seen with, an inability to control kicks and swim strokes.

Signs and symptoms of pulmonary overexpansion injuries are usually apparent soon after surfacing.

Signs and symptoms of pulmonary overexpansion injuries are usually apparent soon after surfacing. Although an AGE may be delayed slightly, dyspnea from the pulmonary injury is usually immediate. Dyspnea, altered consciousness, difficulty in coordination of movement, chest pain, bleeding from the nose or ears, weakness, and fatigue should be clues that an overexpansion injury exists. Often the diver must have help getting out of the water, and the history of the dive and medical presentation must come from fellow divers or rescuers.

The management of pulmonary overexpansion injuries is best performed in a decompression chamber. The possibility that decompression sickness may accompany ascent barotrauma is very real. But, more importantly, hyperbaric therapy can reduce the size of the air bubble and potentially break up the occlusion and return normal blood flow to the affected tissues. As with a heart attack, time is essential. The critical care paramedic should transport these patients either by ground or at a cabin pressure that is as close to 1 atmosphere as physically possible. Treatment of occlusions with fibrinolytics or blood thinners is not indicated in most cases. Anecdotal evidence has suggested that the administration of aspirin may be beneficial in the treatment of AGE. The placement of the patient in a left lateral Trendelenburg position is another ancient and outdated approach that has no medical basis to show any benefit to the patient. Without appropriate and expedient management, the prognosis of serious overexpansion injuries is poor.

AQUATIC DISEASES ASSOCIATED WITH DIVING

A frequent misconception by nondivers is that divers can swim, and a misconception by divers is that swimming is not necessary. Realizing this, *drowning* then seems less out of place than it first appears. Although divers enter the water with a presumably full scuba cylinder, a wide range of factors can make that cylinder simply a fashion accessory. Running out of air at depth, medical emergencies underwater, panic, euphoria, and stupidity all make the list of reasons divers drown. Of these, panic is probably the biggest contributor. Functioning in an alien environment can be a frightening experience for even the most avid diver. When underwater conditions make the diver uneasy, panic often takes over and obscures rational thought. Without quick action of fellow divers or a sudden focus on the problems at hand, the panic can turn deadly.

Faulty regulators or leaking seals can allow small amounts of water to enter the diver's lungs leading to a condition known as **saltwater aspiration syndrome.** This condition can produce pneumonia-like symptoms including dyspnea, cough, hemoptysis, and even radiographic changes. A similar condition can be expected from diving in freshwater that is not "fresh," such as stagnant ponds, pools, and sediment-rich runoff areas. Rest, oxygen and occasionally antibiotics are included in the treatment of these patients.

Hypothermia is a condition that can occur in relatively warm water. Because water conducts heat 20 times faster than air, divers who are not properly insulated can experience hypothermia in water we would normally consider warm. This is a factor that should be considered in the care and transport of every diver experiencing an emergency.

saltwater aspiration syndrome *faulty regulators or leaking seals allow small amounts of water to enter the diver's lungs, producing dyspnea, a labored cough, and hemoptysis.*

DANGEROUS MARINE ANIMALS

The underwater world allows opportunities for people to come as close to nature as anywhere else on earth. The diversity and beauty of marine animals are what draw many divers to the sport of scuba. Unfortunately not all of these encounters are without danger. Marine organisms have developed defensive and predatory strategies that have potentially life-threatening consequences for divers. An understanding of these strategies is essential for avoiding and treating injuries from marine animals.

ANIMALS THAT BITE AND CAUSE TRAUMA

Large predatory animals cause injury through the simple act of biting. Sharks, barracuda, and moray eels are most often associated with these injuries, but seals, sea lions, octopuses, and groupers have been known to cause severe bites. Dolphins and smaller toothed whales also have the ability to bite if threatened. Generally these bites are not fatal from the initial attack, but the trauma can be devastating. It is important that the patient be removed from the water as soon as possible and that all bleeding be controlled. Although blood loss is the most apparent cause of death, marine infections are another life-threatening concern.

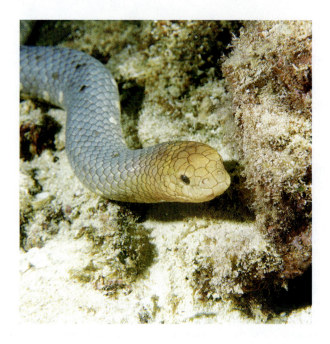

ANIMALS THAT BITE AND ENVENOMATE

Marine animal envenomation occurs through many mechanisms. Sea snakes, the blue-ringed octopus, and cone snails inject venom through a bite. (See Figure 31-7 ■.) The definitive treatment is antivenom. However, an attempt should be made to deactivate the venom by submersion in hot water as soon as possible for 30–90 minutes. The venom from these animals is primarily a neurotoxin that can cause muscle rigidity and respiratory paralysis. To prevent burns, the water should be between 105° and 115° F. If no thermometer is immediately available, use the patient's tolerance of heat. Be careful not to administer pain medications without knowing the temperature of the water. The definitive treatment is the administration of antivenom. Ventilation and chest compressions may be required for extended periods of time in the arrested patient until the appropriate antivenom can be administered. It is important to remember that the toxin is a neuromuscular blocker similar to that used in rapid- sequence induction. Ventilations and chest compressions should be continued until absolute assurance that the toxin has worn off. Some clinicians advocate the use of the "pressure-immobilization technique" to contain the toxin before severe effects begin. This procedure involves the placement of a folded gauze bandage over the bite site and wrapping with enough pressure to form an indentation in the skin over the bite site.

ANIMALS THAT PUNCTURE

Accidently stepping on or touching many marine animals can lead to intense pain and even death. Puncture envenomation occurs from contact with the spine of a stingray; the dorsal spines of lionfish, scorpionfish, stonefish, or hardhead catfish; or the thorns of a sea urchin. (See Figure 31-8 ■.) Other types of fish also have spines that can inject venom.

ANIMALS THAT STING

Cnidaria *stinging marine animals belonging to the phylum coelenterates. Includes jellyfish, Portugese man-of-war, hydroids, fire coral, and sea anemones.*

Of the five different phyla that stinging marine animals belong to, the phylum **Cnidaria** (coelenterates) includes jellyfish, Portugese man-of-war, hydroids, fire coral, and sea anemones. (See Figure 31-9 ■.) The mechanism of injury from these animals is a small inverted cell called a nematocyst. A nematocyst is a small organelle that lines the tentacles of cnidarians and then unravel on contact. They shoot out a thin, threadlike fiber which invades the tissues and releases a venom which causes im-

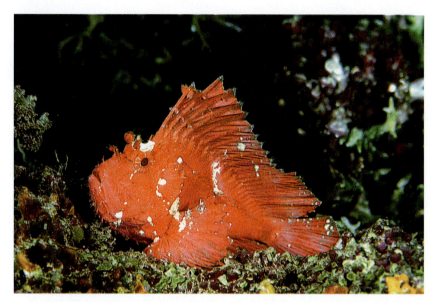

■ **Figure 31-8** Bright red leaf scorpionfish, with thin spiny dorsal fin, nestled in algae-covered coral reef. *(Fred Bavendam/Peter Arnold, Inc.)*

mense irritation, pain, and other symptoms including death. Different animals have different abilities to invade tissues. Venom from the sea wasp or box jellyfish (*Chironex fleckeri*) of Australia, considered the most deadly animal in the world, has the ability to invade blood vessels and cause death within seconds. (See Figure 31-10 ■.)

Treatment for a Cnidaria sting is to immediately remove as many remaining tentacles as possible by rinsing with seawater. Freshwater will cause remaining nematocysts to discharge, worsening the situation. Apply vinegar over the affected area to deactivate the stinging cells. Continuous application may be necessary for severe stings. If vinegar is not available, one-quarter strength ammonia, baking soda solution, or alcohol may be used. The uric acid in urine may be applied as a last resort but is not recommended for initial treatment. It may be necessary to remove the tentacles by applying shaving cream over the affected area and shaving the tentacles away.

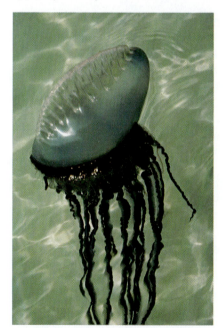

■ **Figure 31-9** Portuguese man-of-war with an inflated float and helical tentacles. *(©O.S.F./Animals Animals/ Earth Scenes)*

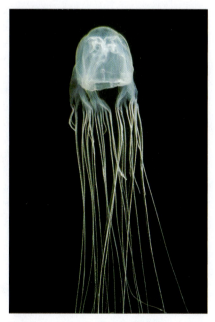

■ **Figure 31-10** Box jellyfish.

AQUATIC-LIFE BORNE DISEASE

Divers who engage in the sport of underwater hunting open themselves to eating tainted fish and crustaceans. Although most fish are safe, some species provide certain risks and should be eaten with caution.

Ciguatera is an accumulated toxin encountered in reef-dwelling fish. It is found in small planktonic organisms that are food for small fish. As larger fish eat smaller fish, the toxin is concentrated in the tissues, growing stronger with each contaminated fish eaten. The toxin can be found in any number of reef-dwelling and ocean-going species including groupers, snappers, jacks, barracuda, dorado (mahi mahi), swordfish, and eel. No testing has been found to determine the presence of ciguatera. Occasionally patrons of restaurants will be served contaminated fish and may develop symptoms.

Signs and symptoms of ciguatera poisoning develop within 15 minutes to 3 hours from ingestion, with symptoms worsening at 12–24 hours. Initially, nausea, abdominal pain, vomiting, and diarrhea will occur. A tingling sensation in the lips and mouth and running down the extremities is followed in a few days by itching to the soles and palms. Other signs include fatigue, blisters, skin rash, difficulty walking, leg and arm pain, headache, vision disturbances, sweating, insomnia, hypotension, irregular cardiac rhythms, dyspnea, seizures, and coma. An interesting and classic symptom is the reversal of hot and cold perception. This condition causes hot objects to feel cold and cold objects to feel hot. This may continue for up to a year.

The treatment of ciguatera in the prehospital and critical care settings is supportive. IV fluids can be helpful in preventing the dehydration associated with vomiting and diarrhea. Diphenhydramine may help to relieve the itching sensation.

Scombroid poisoning is found in tuna and related species and is the result of improper preservation. The muscles of the fish experience decomposition from the growth of bacteria. A chemical reaction occurs in the tissues and develops histamines, leading to allergic reactions on ingestion.

The initial indication of a tainted fish is a metallic or peppery taste. Symptoms develop within 90 minutes and mimic those of an allergic reaction with a headache, abdominal cramps, cardiac irregularities, and hypotension. Treatment should start with diphenhydramine and include the management of severe nausea and pain.

OTHER MEDICAL CONDITIONS ASSOCIATED WITH DIVING

Hearing loss is a frequent complication seen in avid divers. Repeated damage to the tympanic membrane and the round or oval windows can result in the development of scar tissue, which disrupts sound determination. A single incident of tympanic rupture or disruption of cochlear function can lead to permanent damage in the affected ear.

Disorientation underwater occurs when the vestibular system fails to compensate for the effects of pressure and buoyancy. Vertigo is often the result, causing the diver to lose the ability to maintain a straight and level swim pattern. This can have disastrous consequences if the diver swims down instead of up, ending up below safe depths.

Divers who experience unconsciousness while underwater are unlikely to reach the surface alive. When this condition occurs on land, the victim maintains the ability to breathe as long as the airway stays open. While underwater, however, the diver's regulator will most likely not remain in the mouth. Even if the regulator remains in place, the natural breathing tendency would be unlikely to pull air from the scuba system. A dive buddy with enough presence of mind to remain calm and slowly ascend while using the purge system on the regulator of the unconscious diver may be the only hope of survival. Even so, the risks of pulmonary barotrauma would be extremely high. The role of the critical care paramedic in the care of these patients would be the rapid transport to a recompression chamber.

CAUSES OF DEATH IN DIVERS

For those who view recreational scuba diving as a relatively safe sport, consider the fact that many medical insurance policies deny benefits for any illness or injury encountered while participating in

---

ciguatera *an accumulated toxin encountered in large, reef-dwelling fish that feed on small planktonic organisms and other smaller fish, thus concentrating the toxin.*

scombroid *toxin created by improper preservation of tuna and related species. Bacterial growth causes decomposition of the muscle in the fish and triggers a chemical reaction that releases histamines. Ingestion of affected fish will cause allergic reactions.*

Divers who experience unconsciousnes while underwater are unlikely to reach the surface alive.

scuba activities. In fact, scuba diving is fraught with dangers, any number of which can be fatal. The average number of deaths from diving worldwide is difficult to determine, but an estimate of 1 death for every 100,000 dives has been made. The majority of these deaths occur when a problem occurs underwater that the diver is unable to overcome. Panic and poor decision making can individually be fatal errors; combined, there may be no escape. In studies of deceased divers, 95% were found to still have their weight belts in place. One of the most fundamental techniques for treating underwater emergencies is removing the weight belt.

Additionally, 86% of deaths occurred to divers who were either diving alone or who got separated from their dive buddies. Twenty-five percent of divers who died experienced problems at the surface. Of these, 50% died on the surface.

As more and more divers become certified each year, more inexperienced divers and potentially unfit divers enter the water. Although many certifying agencies require a medical certificate before beginning scuba lessons, few doctors are qualified and experienced in determining medical fitness in regard to diving. Worse, divers who were fit when they began diving continue to dive after a diagnosis of asthma, heart disease, diabetes, seizures, stroke—often against medical advice.

An interesting statistic is that women, who make up approximately 25% of divers, account for only 10% of deaths.

The majority of factors related to diving deaths can be separated into three groups (listed in order of most common causes): human error, environmental causes, and equipment failure. Human error includes diving with a disqualifying medical condition, panic, fatigue, buoyancy problems, low-on-air or out-of-air situations, failure to ditch the weight belt in difficult situations, ignoring the buddy system, and improper use of equipment. Adverse sea conditions, water movement, and extreme temperatures make up the list of environmental factors. Finally, failure of the equipment itself may be the cause of death, but has been a factor in amazingly few cases.

Despite the risk of death to the recreational diver, professional divers face an even greater risk. Because they make deeper dives, are more dependent on surface support equipment, and are often in an inhospitable working environment, professional divers face a rate of death approaching 5 per 1,000, approximately 30% of which are related to decompression sickness or arterial gas embolism.

As divers age, the possibility of *sudden death syndrome* becomes greater. Approximately 20% to 25% of diver deaths are related to heart disease and related conditions. Divers who exhibit significant cardiac risk factors should reconsider their future in diving.

HYPERBARIC MEDICINE

Recompression in a hyperbaric chamber is the definitive treatment for both decompression sickness and arterial gas embolism. It is essential for a good prognosis that treatment begin as soon as possible; however, the reality is that a delay is inevitable. A **hyperbaric chamber** is a medical device into which the patient is placed, and then the device repressurizes the patient to a certain level. Transportation to a hyperbaric chamber has no specific challenges for ground units. Transportation by air elevates the possibility of worsening the condition because increased altitude will further expand gas bubbles in the body. Aircraft such as helicopters should fly at the lowest possible altitude safety will allow. Pressurized aircraft should maintain a cabin pressure as close to the departure altitude as possible. (See Figure 31-11 ■.)

Transport hyperbaric units are bulky and not common in the civilian world. Made primarily for use in utility helicopters like the military UH-1 or the civilian 212 or 412, they can be used in larger aircraft, again mostly in military configurations.

Hyperbaric chambers are made in a wide variety of sizes. Single-patient models allow the patient to either sit or lay down in a small box with all attendants on the outside of the unit. Should a problem arise with the patient that requires attention, the unit must be brought back to atmospheric pressure before opening. Multiple-place units allow an attendant to sit with the patient and care for any problems as they occur without changing pressures. Larger units have lockout chambers that allow attendants to move in and out of the chamber through pressurized portals. Because of the dangers associated with treating both decompression sickness and arterial gas embolism, it is in the best interest of the patient to transport him or her to a multiple-place attended chamber.

In studies of deceased divers, 95% were found to still have their weight belts in place, indicating a fundamental failure to perform the most basic technique for handling an emergency underwater.

Despite the risk of death to the recreational diver, professional divers face an even greater risk.

As diver's age, the possibility of *sudden death syndrome* becomes greater. Approximately 20% to 25% of diver deaths are related to heart disease and related conditions.

hyperbaric chamber *a medical device used to recompress internal gases in patients suffering from decompression sickness or AGE, as well as injuries related to necropsy in diabetes, and so on.*

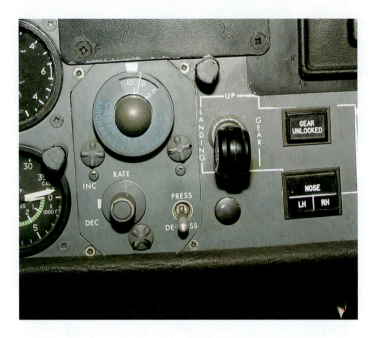

■ **Figure 31-11** Cabin pressure control on airplane.

Once inside the chamber, the patient will be placed at a pressure of 2 to 3 atmospheres for several hours. Eventually, as the patient's symptoms subside the pressure will be reduced and eventually returned to normal. The time duration from injury to treatment will have a great bearing on the success of treatment. For short intervals full recovery can be expected. Long intervals between injury and recompression may relieve minor symptoms but, paralysis and brain deterioration will most likely remain for the remainder of the person's life.

The critical care paramedic may encounter hyperbaric therapy used for other medical conditions. Most prevalent in the critical care environment is the hyperbaric treatment of carbon monoxide poisoning and occasionally cyanide poisoning. Gas gangrene, problem wound healing, intracranial abscess, skin grafts, radiation injury, and thermal burns are other areas where hyperbaric therapy has shown a benefit. These conditions actually benefit from the pressurized oxygen entering the tissues. Although oxygen is essential to the injured diver, it is the pressure that makes the most difference.

SPECIAL CONSIDERATIONS FOR FEMALES IN DIVING

Female divers typically have a smaller muscle mass, smaller lungs, lighter frame, and greater fat distribution. The smaller muscle mass means that the equipment worn by divers can make it more difficult to maneuver above the surface. The smaller lungs of women combined with the smaller muscle mass equate to an air consumption rate that is considerably less than that of men. This allows female divers to stay underwater longer and dive deeper than the average man. Unfortunately, that also increases the risk of decompression sickness.

Having a greater fat distribution means that, pound for pound, women are more buoyant, requiring a greater amount of weight to achieve neutral buoyancy. It also means that women are more prone to store nitrogen, increasing the risk of decompression sickness.

The only study concerning women in diving relates to decompression sickness, indicating that they are three times more likely to suffer from this condition. Many theories have been developed to explain this mismatch. With proportionally more fat as one factor, other factors include increased fluid retention during menstruation and the use of birth control pills.

Some concern exists for women who dive following the placement of breast implants. Although the silicone implants do not suffer from compression like a gas-filled bag would, there is evidence that they absorb significant nitrogen. On ascent a slight increase in breast size has been reported, returning to normal after a short surface time.

ROLE OF THE CRITICAL CARE PROVIDER IN SUPPORT SITUATIONS

Drowning is the third most common cause of accidental death for adults, and the second most common cause of unintentional injury death among children and young adults in the United States. Every year, new rescue and recovery dive teams are formed to find drowning victims. They are formed by fire and law enforcement departments, the military, sometimes EMS squads, and even people outside the public safety community. The critical care service may be called on to support an ongoing event that deals with an emergency that either involves a diver who is in trouble or the use of diving teams for some water-related event. Situations of this nature may include a downed aircraft over a body of water, a recreational or commercial ship that has sunk, swimming and/or water-skiing emergencies, diving emergencies (commercial and recreational), and the occasional motor vehicle that has crashed (or was driven) into a body of water.

Considerations that the critical care paramedic should be advised of other than the number of potential patients include the characteristics of the diving emergency. Is the situation a search and rescue or a body recovery? Is the water deep or shallow? Is the water temperature warm, cold, or icy? Is the scenario one of fast water diving, hazardous materials, diving, or black-water diving? Does it involve underwater cave diving or underwater vehicle extrication? Are those participating in the dive novice or experienced? How long was the person(s) underwater? Remember too that you may be waiting for the recovery of a person, but one of the divers involved in the recovery process may experience a diving emergency and become your patient.

For all of these reasons, diving teams use different diving techniques and equipment. The common theme with all of these is the utilization of public safety diving, and the role of the critical care provider during these events is one of support. Critical care services may provide rehabilitation during the event (this is analogous to EMS providing rehab at a fire scene for a fire department), or they may be responsible for the treatment and transport of patient(s) involved in the mishap. In the latter role the critical care paramedic should treat the patient using the principles addressed in this chapter. Do not forget to treat the patient as a whole; you may be caring for a diving victim, but there may be more involved (as the opening case study inferred). You could have a diving emergency in conjunction with a traumatic event, a medical emergency, or other concerns that will play a role in your treatment and transport decisions.

The critical care service may be called on to support an ongoing event that deals with an emergency that either involves a diver who is in trouble or the use of diving teams for some water-related event.

Summary

Diving-related emergencies are relatively uncommon. For the critical care paramedic, care for victims of diving-related injuries will be mostly supportive and usually involves transportation from a local hospital facility to a hyperbaric chamber where recompression can be accomplished. Emergencies, however, can arise during transport. Because of this, a thorough understanding of diving-related injures can mean the difference between the right decision and sudden death. An understanding of the diving environment is important in understanding the extent of injury and the importance of timely treatment.

Review Questions

1. Describe diving-related injuries associated with descent.
2. Describe decompression sickness, including its signs, symptoms, and treatment.
3. Discuss high-pressure neurologic syndrome (HPNS).
4. Describe diving-related illnesses usually associated with ascent.
5. Describe ciguatera poisoning, including its signs and symptoms and treatment.

6. Describe the most common cause of deaths in divers.

7. Detail the role and importance of recompression therapy for selected dive-related problems.

8. List sources of information that pertain to diving emergencies, including the Divers Alert Network.

See Answers to Review Questions at the back of this book.

Further Reading

Auerbach PS. *A Medical Guide to Hazardous Marine Life,* 3rd ed. Jacksonville, FL: Progressive Printing, 1997.

Edmonds C. *Dangerous Marine Animals.* New South Wales, Austrailia: Reed Books, 1989.

Edmonds C, McKenzie B, Thomas R. *Diving Medicine for Scuba Divers.* Melborne, Australia: JL Publications, 1992.

Guyton AC, Hall JE. *Textbook of Medical Physiology,* 11th ed. Philadelphia: W. B. Saunders, 2006.

Chapter 32

Toxicological Emergencies

Matthew Bonner, M.D., and Daniel E. Brooks, M.D.

Objectives

Upon the completion of this chapter, the student should be able to:

1. Describe the epidemiology of toxic emergencies. (p. 938)
2. Briefly describe the role of the poison control center (PCC) to include how to contact them in case of emergency. (p. 938)
3. Define the following:
   ★ Drug or substance abuse (p. 938)
   ★ Drug addiction (p. 938)
   ★ Drug dependency (physical and psychological) (p. 938)
   ★ Drug withdrawal (p. 938)
4. Discuss the presentation of the following toxidromes:
   ★ Hallucinogens (p. 939)
   ★ Sympathomimetics (p. 939)
   ★ Opiates (p. 940)
   ★ Sedative (p. 940)
5. Describe how the clinical manifestation and basic management techniques for the following toxic emergencies by prescription class:
   ★ Cardiac medications (p. 940)
   ★ Psychiatric medications (p. 941)
   ★ Anticonvulsants (p. 942)
   ★ OTC medications (p. 943)
   ★ Herbal medications (p. 944)
6. Explain how caustic injuries can affect the body. (p. 944)
7. Discuss ethanol and toxic alcohol emergencies. (p. 945)
8. Discuss toxic emergencies regarding industrial exposures. (p. 946)
9. Explain the two major categories of warfare agents. (p. 948)
10. List common findings seen in a toxic emergency involving plants and mushrooms. (p. 951)

11. What are some common findings in toxic emergencies from envenomations and stings. (p. 952)
12. Recognize scene and environmental indicators that may identify that a toxicological emergency has occurred or may occur. (p. 955)
13. Describe such issues as initial evaluation, toxin decontamination and transportation issues as they pertain to toxicological emergencies. (p. 955)

Key Terms

addiction, p. 938
drug abuse, p. 938
hazardous materials, p. 946
herbal medications,
  p. 944
lacrimators, p. 949

Material Safety Data Sheet
  (MSDS), p. 946
organophosphate (OP)
  compounds, p. 949
physical dependence,
  p. 938

poison control center (PCC),
  p. 938
tolerance, p. 938
toxic alcohols, p. 945
toxidrome, p. 938
withdrawal syndrome, p. 938

Case Study

It's the middle of January and you are working a 24-hour shift. Your ship is down for the first 8 hours due to a heavy snowfall. Around 1500 hours, dispatch calls and asks if you can check weather conditions for a pending transfer from a small emergency department for an overdose. The pilot states that he should be able to complete the flight under IFR, so you and your partner prepare for flight. En route, you are advised by air traffic control that the cold weather is resulting in freezing at higher altitudes. Discussion then continues among the crew regarding options for alternative transport if the weather closes in while you are packaging the patient at the hospital.

The pilot communicates with dispatch prior to your final descent to the hospital helipad, and requests that a local ambulance company be dispatched to meet the crew at the hospital to provide transport with the critical care crew. After landing and exiting the aircraft with your equipment, you are escorted by hospital security to the emergency department where you are then led to the trauma bay by the unit clerk. Inside you observe an 18-year-old male actively vomiting charcoal. As you step inside, the patient wretches and copious amounts of black vomitus erupt from his mouth. The vomit is thick and black from the activated charcoal with the texture of chewed pizza and the smell of alcohol.

Your partner quickly helps the staff roll the patient onto his side and begins clearing the assessment. The MD relays the following patient information: 18-year-old male taken from his girlfriend's home after a fight with his parents. Social dynamics surrounding this incident illustrate that he was arguing with his parents because they did not approve of his current girlfriend, and they demanded he stop seeing her. Hours after the argument the patient arrives at the girlfriend's home in a "drunken state." His girlfriend decided to call EMS when, after arrival, he started to become unresponsive. The only additional history available from the girlfriend is that the patient stated something to the extent of "I took all my Mom's psycho pills."

On arrival in the ED, he was unresponsive to external noxious stimuli. Vitals included a heart rate of 43 beats per minute, respirations of 8, and a blood pressure of 52/40. Initial management by the staff included placement of a nasal airway, IV access, placement of an OG catheter, and administration of activated charcoal. The staff was still trying to reach the parents in order to ascertain what the medication was that the patient ingested.

While awaiting arrival of the transporting ambulance and further information on the type of toxic overdose, you converse with your partner and the ED staff about continued patient management options. The decision is made to secure the airway by endotracheal intubation due to the possibility of the airway becoming compromised. To help prevent potential aspiration you perform a BURP maneuver (backwards, upwards, rightward pressure) to the larynx while administrating sedation and paralytic agents for elective intubation. The patient is successfully intubated with a 7.5-mm endotracheal tube, and placed on your transport ventilator in SIMV mode with a ventilatory rate of 16, V_t of 650, PS of 10, and PEEP of 5 cm/H_2O. The pre-intubation ABG results just handed to you reveal a pH of 7.18, PaO_2 of 78 torr, $PaCO_2$ of 44 torr, and an HCO_3^- of 12 mEq/L. You conclude from these values that the patient is displaying uncompensated metabolic acidosis.

Your attention is suddenly drawn to the audible alarm of the cardiac monitor as you identify an idioventricular rhythm at a rate of 40. Making matters worse, as you attempt to medicate the bradycardic rhythm, the patient begins to seize. The seizure fails to respond to repeated diazepam administration; however, it finally terminates after initiation of phenytoin. A repeat blood gas is performed about 10 minutes later and reveals the following values: pH 7.23, PaO_2 of 178 torr, $PaCO_2$ of 40 torr, and an HCO_3^- level of 10. Further lab results are noncontributory.

Currently the heart rate is 42 (sinus bradycardia with a wide QRS), and the blood pressure is 48/22 mmHg. Further attempts at increasing the heart rate fail, as you and your partner await the arrival of the transporting ambulance. Since you still have a few minutes, you decide to contact your medical direction. After a brief review of the patient history, events, vital signs, lab values, and treatment rendered thus far, medical direction concludes that the toxic overdose is probably a tricyclic antidepressant (TCA) agent. At this point you are requested to give 2 ampules of sodium bicarbonate, 1 mg of glucagon, and initiate a Levophed drip.

As you review this case with the on-line physician, you now recognize the metabolic acidosis, widened QRS, and seizure activity as hallmark signs of a tricyclic overdose. You recall how TCAs block sodium channels, which then impairs conduction through the His-Purkinje system leading to the widening QRS as well as diminished muscular contraction, and conclude the patient's seizure activity is most likely a secondary result of uncontrolled neural firing due to the sodium imbalance.

Regarding the patient management, the sodium bicarbonate is used to alkalinize the blood while glucagon is used to help elevate intracellular levels of cyclic-AMP, which in turn increases the binding and release of calcium. Finally the needed elevation in the patient's blood pressure is achieved by the alpha-adrenergic property of Levophed, which promotes vasoconstriction.

As the medical director's treatments are initiated, the ambulance that will transfer you and the patient arrives. The patient's HR is now 78 bpm and the blood pressure has increased to 96/40 mmHg. After attaching the patient to your mobile equipment and securing him to the ambulance cot, the EMS crew loads the patient and you are all off to the destination hospital. The rest of the 90-minute transport is uneventful as you reassess the patient and work on your interhospital transfer paperwork. On arrival, the patient is taken directly to the medical ICU where you provide the staff an oral report of the patient's conditions and you relinquish patient care to them.

INTRODUCTION

In 2003, there were almost 2.4 million human toxin exposures reported to U.S. poison control centers. This number includes accidental and intentional drug use, drug abuse, and environmental exposures (envenomations, plant ingestions, and so on). In more than 90% of exposures, when they occurred at a residence, EMS was involved in the initial evaluation or transportation to a health care facility. Over 125,000 cases resulted in a moderate or major medical effect, and 1,106 fatalities were reported. Over 75% of cases involved ingestion, 7.5% dermal exposure, 5.8% inhalational exposure, and 3.5% envenomation. It is important to realize that countless other exposures and deaths went unreported and are therefore not included in these data. Given the magnitude of these numbers, and the trend for certain geographical areas to be more prone to these types of emergencies, it is not an impossible type of emergency to be seen by the critical care paramedic. The critical care team may be responsible for stabilizing and transporting this type of emergency from either a remote scene flight, or a mission that has the flight crew responsible for transporting a patient to a higher level care facility.

At the completion of this chapter, the critical care paramedic should be better able to assess the poisoned patient, develop an initial treatment strategy, and correctly intervene if the patient suddenly decompensates. One of the many roles of a U.S. **poison control center** (PCC) is to assist with the triage and management of patients with (potentially) toxic exposures. Critical care paramedics should take full advantage of the knowledge and resources available through consultation of a poison control center. They can be contacted at 800-222-1222.

DRUG ABUSE DEFINED

Many cases of drug exposures involve the intentional abuse of medication or illicit drugs. Key terms involved in the discussion of **drug abuse** include addiction, physical dependence, and tolerance. The American Society of Addiction Medicine has approved the following definitions. An **addiction** is characterized by one or more of the following behaviors: "impaired control over drug use, compulsive use, continued use despite harm, and craving," and the condition's development and manifestations are influenced by genetic, psychosocial, and environmental factors. **Physical dependence** is "a state of adaptation that is manifested by a drug class–specific withdrawal syndrome that can be produced by abrupt cessation, rapid dose reduction, decreasing blood level of drug, or administration of an antagonist." **Tolerance** is "a state of adaptation in which exposure to a drug induces changes that result in a diminution of one or more of the drug's effects over time."

Withdrawal syndrome requires both a preexisting physical adaptation (i.e., tolerance) to a specific drug with continued exposure necessary to prevent withdrawal, and decreasing concentrations of that drug to cause the withdrawal. The specific clinical manifestations of withdrawal syndrome are determined by the drug's underlying physiological actions (i.e., effects on neurotransmission). A withdrawal syndrome will usually manifest symptoms exactly opposite those the drug manifests. For example, alcohol withdrawal is characterized by hallucinations, jitteriness, insomnia, tremors, and seizures. Opiate withdrawal is characterized by anxiety, insomnia, diarrhea, vomiting, coughing, runny nose, and pain.

TOXIDROMES

Toxidromes (or *tox-syndrome*) are clinical syndromes that are essential for the successful recognition of poisoning patterns. A **toxidrome** is a constellation of clinical signs and symptoms that, together, reliably suggest an exposure to a specific drug class. Many patients, when exposed to an adequate dose of a drug, display the specific clinical effects of that drug class. A list of toxidromes with examples of responsible agents and clinical manifestations can be found in Table 32–1.

SPECIFIC DRUGS OF ABUSE

Illicit and prescription medications are abused for many purposes including relief from pain, treatment of anxiety, self-medication for psychiatric disorders, or to modify consciousness ("to get high"). The major illicit drug groups include hallucinogens, sympathomimetics (cocaine, amphetamines), narcotics (opioids), sedative-hypnotics (benzodiazepines, GHB), and marijuana.

---

poison control center (PCC) *information banks that assist with the triage and management of patients with (potentially) toxic exposures.*

drug abuse *the intentional abuse of medication or illicit drugs; includes addiction, physical dependence, and tolerance.*

addiction *characterized by one or more behaviors that may include impaired control over drug use, compulsive use, continued use despite harm, and cravings.*

physical dependence *a syndrome wherein withdrawal syndromes can be produced by abrupt cessation, rapid dose reduction, decreasing blood level of drug, or administration of an antagonist.*

tolerance *a state of adaptation in which exposure to a drug induces changes that result in a diminution of one or more of the drug's effects over time.*

withdrawal syndrome *requires both a preexisting physical adaptation (i.e. tolerance) to a specific and decreasing concentrations or availability of that drug.*

toxidrome *clinical syndromes essential for the successful recognition of poisoning patterns; a constellation of clinical signs and symptoms that together, reliably suggest an exposure to a specific drug class.*

Table 32–1   Toxidromes

Toxidrome	Toxin	Signs/Symptoms	Treatment
Cholinergic	Organophosphates (i.e., diazinon) and nerve agents (i.e., sarin, soman), pilocarpine, muscarine	Salivation, diarrhea, abdominal cramps, miosis, urinary incontinence, ataxia, seizures, coma (SLUDGE)	Atropine Pralidoxime (2-pam) Glycopyrrolate
Anticholinergic	Tricyclic antidepressants (i.e., amitriptyline), atropine, scopolamine, antihistamines (diphenhydramine)	Dry skin and mucous membranes, tachycardia, agitation, delirium, mydriasis, hyperthermia	Benzodiazepines Physostigmine
Opioid (narcotic)	Codeine, heroin, meperidine, morphine, oxycodone, propoxyphene, hydromorphone	Respiratory depression, CNS depression (sedation), myosis	Naloxone
Sympathomimetic	Cocaine, (meth-)amphetamines, methylphenidate, epinephrine	Hypertension, tachycardia, tremor, hyperthermia, seizures	Benzodiazepines Active cooling
GABA-agonist withdrawal	Withdrawal from alcohol, benzodiazepines, barbiturates	Tremor, agitation, delirium, seizure, tachycardia, hyperthermia, hypertension	Benzodiazepines (or restart the original GABA-agonist)
Opioid withdrawal	Withdrawal from any opioid (i.e., heroin)	Nausea, diarrhea, abdominal cramps, yawning, anxiety, piloerection, restlessness	Methadone (or other long-acting opioid) Control of symptoms (i.e., antiemetics)
Hypoxia/hypoxemia	Asphyxiation, carboxyhemoglobin, methemoglobin	Headache, nausea, confusion, ataxia, tachycardia, syncope; multiple victims possible	Remove from exposure Supplemental oxygen Methylene blue (consider other victims)

Hallucinogens are compounds that typically involve serotonergic effects and lead to distorted sensorium, hallucinations, and entactogenic ("to touch within") effects. Commonly abused agents include lysergic acid diethylamide (LSD), psilocybin ("magic mushrooms"), mescaline (from the peyote cactus), and 3,4, methylenedioxy-amphetamine (MDMA or Ecstasy) or other hallucinogenic amphetamines. Clinical effects include altered sensorium (confusion), ataxia, bruxism (involuntary clenching of teeth), and labile emotions. Agents that also produce sympathomimetic effects (such as hallucinogenic-amphetamines) may produce diaphoresis, tremor, tachycardia, and hypertension.

Sympathomimetics are a class of drugs that mimic the effects of endogenous catecholamines (epinephrine and norepinephrine) and produce effects by stimulating adrenergic receptors in the nervous system. These agents, both illicit (like cocaine, amphetamine, and methamphetamine) and over-the-counter or prescription medications (like ephedrine and phenylpropanolamine), lead to tachycardia, hypertension, delirium, and agitation. Toxic effects can include intracranial hemorrhage, seizure, myocardial infarction, and hyperthermia.

Opiates are a group of naturally occurring compounds (e.g., morphine, codeine) derived from the poppy plant (*Papaver somniferum*). Opioids include these compounds and all other synthetic derivatives, such as fentanyl and hydrocodone. In general, opioids work by stimulating opiate receptors in the central and peripheral nervous systems. The classic opioid toxidrome presents clinically with myosis (pinpoint pupils), respiratory depression, and sedation. Other effects include apnea and noncardiogenic pulmonary edema. Seizures are associated with meperidine, propoxyphene, or tramadol abuse. Patients suffering from opioid toxicity typically respond to an opioid antagonist, like naloxone. Small doses of naloxone (0.4 mg IV), repeated as necessary, should be used in all nonintubated patients suspected of an opioid overdose. The use of naloxone after intubation should be done cautiously to minimize adverse effects, especially if a narcotic agent is being used to maintain patient sedation. Being cautious at this time will allow the critical care paramedic the opportunity to administer alternative pharmacological agents if necessary.

Sedative-hypnotics include a wide range of medications used for the treatment of anxiety and insomnia. This group of medications includes several subgroups, each with different mechanisms of action. The largest group includes agents that increase concentrations of gamma-aminobutyric acid (GABA), the main neuroinhibitory transmitter in the central nervous system. Agents that enhance GABA activity include benzodiazepines, barbiturates, gamma-hydroxybutyrate (GHB), chloral hydrate, propofol, and meprobamate. Other subgroups of the sedative-hypnotics include antihistamines (i.e., diphenhydramine), skeletal muscle relaxants (methocarbamol and cyclobenzaprine), and even certain antidepressants (i.e., trazodone) used for their sedating effects. The clinical effects, despite the underlying mechanism of action, include drowsiness, ataxia, nystagmus, and respiratory depression. After a larger ingestion the degree of sedation increases and can be associated with coma, bradycardia, hypotension, and respiratory arrest.

Marijuana itself is not associated with acute toxicity but can lead to severe effects if it is mixed with other drugs. Some common adulterants of marijuana, intentionally or otherwise, include scopolamine, PCP, cocaine, and LSD. Clinical effects depend on the amount of adulterant.

The practice of mixing or coadministering illicit drugs is not isolated to marijuana. A speedball is a mixture of cocaine and heroin. Typically the opiate effects dominate the clinical picture in these situations. If these patients receive naloxone, the reversal of the opiate effects may produce unopposed sympathomimetic (cocaine) effects and lead to patient agitation, tachycardia, and hypertension. The co-ingestion of cocaine should be considered in any patient who initially presents with an opioid toxidrome (miosis, CNS and respiratory depression) but immediately develops severe agitation and a hyperadrenergic state after receiving naloxone.

Initial management of the drug-abusing patient includes securing an airway, assisting with ventilations, and correcting abnormal vital signs. Minimizing agitation and preventing patient or rescuer harm should be a priority.

SPECIFIC PRESCRIPTION DRUGS

The abuse of prescription medications can lead to significant toxicity and is associated with significant morbidity and mortality every year. Although we cannot discuss all medications, several important drug classes will be discussed in this chapter. These include cardiac-related (calcium channel blockers, beta-blockers, and digoxin) and psychiatric (tricyclic antidepressants, monoamine oxidase inhibitors, selective serotonin reuptake inhibitors, and lithium) medications.

CARDIAC MEDICATIONS

Cardiac medications can significantly decrease cardiac output and lead to profound bradycardia, hypotension, or dysrhythmias. Calcium channel blockers (CCBs, or calcium-antagonists) are dangerous in overdose with clinical effects complicated by sustained-release preparations. There are three main types of CCBs:

★ Dihydropyridines (nifedipine, amlodipine)

★ Benzothiapines (diltiazem)

★ Phenylalkylamines (verapamil)

Clinical manifestations include hypotension, bradycardia or other bradydysrhythmias, metabolic acidosis, pulmonary edema, and coma. Some agents, particularly the dihydropyridines, primarily affect the systemic vascular resistance and lead to hypotension without affecting the heart rate. Patients who overdose on a CCB may present with significant hypotension and a rapid heart rate (reflex tachycardia). In a massive overdose, which occurs occasionally, the patient will develop both hypotension and bradycardia.

Beta-blocker (BB) overdose typically manifests with bradycardia, hypotension, or dysrhythmias (often associated with ECG changes such as a prolonged PR interval). Severe toxicity can cause hypoglycemia (particularly in children), pulmonary edema, or coma. Propranolol toxicity can lead to QRS widening and seizures, due to sodium channel blockade.

Digitalis is a widely used cardiac medication with a narrow therapeutic window. Minimal elevations in blood concentrations can lead to toxicity. Digoxin produces toxicity by poisoning the sodium-potassium pump and allowing more sodium and calcium to enter cells. This causes increased excitability of the cells and subsequently induces premature ventricular contractions (PVCs) and tachydysrhythmias. Atrial tachycardia with an associated block and bidirectional ventricular tachycardia are the characteristic ECG findings, but PVCs are the most common finding. Digoxin also increases vagal tone and can lead to heart blocks and bradydysrhythmias. Additionally, digoxin poisoning can present with subtle complaints, such as nausea, vomiting, generalized malaise, visual disturbances, or mental status changes, with or without cardiac effects.

The initial management of a patient who overdoses on a cardiac medication should focus on supporting cardiac function. After securing the airway, patients should receive intravenous fluids for hypotension, and have any dysrhythmias identified and controlled with standard advanced cardiac life support (ACLS) medications. It is important to focus on the blood pressure more than the heart rate. For instance, a patient with bradycardia may be maintaining a normal blood pressure, and only require close monitoring with pacing pads and atropine ready to use if needed during transport. Alternatively, another patient's tachycardia may be supporting blood pressure and therefore should not be controlled unless it is known to be causing hypotension.

For CCB or BB toxicity, hypotension and bradycardia may respond to IV calcium chloride (1 ampule) or glucagon (up to 10 mg). Often, the hypotension present in these patients will only respond to the use of vasoactive pressors, such as norepinephrine, and should be used if available. Dysrhythmias and hypotension associated with QRS widening, and propranolol-induced seizures, respond well to IV boluses of sodium bicarbonate. Patients suffering from digoxin toxicity should not receive boluses of calcium because of the risk of rapidly increasing the intracellular calcium levels, leading to cardiac arrest.

Subsequent critical care decisions may include the treatment of electrolyte abnormalities. Significant digoxin toxicity (i.e., shock, hemodynamically significant heart block, or hyperkalemia) may be treated with Digibind. Intravenous pacing, intra-arterial balloon pumps, and cardiac bypass are other potential options for patients in cardiovascular shock.

PSYCHIATRIC MEDICATIONS

Acute, intentional overdoses involving antidepressant or antipsychotic drugs are common because these drugs are often available to patients who, by nature of their underlying depression or psychiatric illness, are at higher risk for suicide attempts. Tricyclic antidepressants (TCAs, cyclic antidepressants) and monoamine oxidase inhibitors (MAOIs) are considerably more toxic than selective serotonin reuptake inhibitors.

Examples of TCAs include amitriptyline, nortriptyline, desipramine, and amoxapine. Pathophysiological effects include blockade of sodium channels, alpha-adrenergic blockade, inhibition of neuronal catecholamine uptake, and anticholinergic effects. The most important toxic effect is the sodium channel blockade, which causes QRS prolongation, dysrhythmias, and seizures. Hypotension occurs from the alpha-adrenergic blockade. These patients may also develop anticholinergic effects, manifested by agitation and delirium, tachydysrhythmias, acidosis, hypotension, seizures, or coma (again refer to Table 32–1). There is a well-known mnemonic for TCA overdose patients, which underscores the toxidrome's most common findings: "three Cs and an A," which stands for coma, convulsions, cardiac dysrhythmias, and acidosis.

The initial treatment of TCA toxicity includes airway support, IV access and rehydration, glucagon administration, and the use of sodium bicarbonate for QRS widening (greater than 114 msec) and acidosis. Seizures, if present, can be initially managed by benzodiazepine administration.

A second class of toxic antidepressants are the monamine oxidase inhibitors, which are rarely used because of numerous food and drug interactions and the severe toxicity in overdose. MAOIs were the first type of antidepressant in use, dating back to the 1950s. MAOIs relieve depression by preventing the enzyme monoamine oxidase from metabolizing the neurotransmitters norepinephrine, serotonin, and dopamine in the brain. As a result, these levels remain high in the brain, elevating the patient's mood.

MAOIs can, however, adversely interact with selective serotonin reuptake inhibitors, amphetamines, and tyramine-containing food (certain wines, cheeses, beer, and so on). Patients with overdose can present with neurologic, autonomic, and neuromuscular instability. Neurologic manifestations include lethargy, ataxia, headache, confusion, disorientation, mumbling speech, seizures, and coma. Autonomic instability can lead to flushing, diaphoresis, hypertension, tachycardia, and ventricular dysrhythmias. Neuromuscular complications include tremor, nystagmus, myoclonus, fasciculations, and generalized rigidity.

The prehospital treatment of an MAOI overdose is mainly supportive care (ABCs). Benzodiazepines are used for severe agitation and seizures, while cardiac toxicity is treated with typical ACLS protocols.

Selective serotonin reuptake inhibitors (SSRIs) work by interfering with the normal reuptake of serotonin in the brain. SSRI medications that are widely used agents for the treatment of psychiatric illness include venlafaxine, fluoxetine, paroxetine, trazadone, buproprion, olanzapine, sertraline, and mirtazapine. These medicines increase the availability of serotonin or other neurotransmitters (i.e., dopamine or norepinephrine) in the central nervous system. Mild overdoses lead to nausea, lethargy, tremors, and mild to moderate hypotension typically associated with reflex tachycardia. Massive overdoses can present with significant hypotension, severe agitation, tremor, or seizures. Respiratory distress (from hypoventilation or aspiration) and coma are possible.

Bupropion is specifically associated with tremor, tachycardia, and seizure. In an overdose situation, olanzapine can lead to an anticholinergic-like syndrome, with tachycardia, agitation, and delirium. The co-ingestion of several different pro-serotonergic medications can lead to a more severe disease complex, *serotonin syndrome*. SSRIs, MAOIs, lithium, amphetamines, dextromethorphan, meperidine, and many other drugs all lead to increased serotonin levels. Patients with a serotonin syndrome present with altered mental status (delirium, agitation, seizures), autonomic instability (fever, tachycardia, hypertension, or hypotension), and neuromuscular derangements (myoclonus and rigidity). Patients with true serotonin syndrome often require hemodynamic monitoring, IV hydration, active control of hyperthermia, and benzodiazepines for rigidity. Paralysis and intubation may be necessary to achieve adequate oxygenation and ventilation in the compromised patient.

Lithium is a common drug used to treat bipolar disease and other psychiatric disorders. Due to its narrow therapeutic window, toxicity can develop with minimal changes in blood concentrations. In fact, patients can present with lithium toxicity despite normal lithium levels. Toxicity is caused by excessive levels in tissue, particularly the brain, and is not caused by elevated blood levels. For this reason, a patient chronically taking lithium, who then has an acute overdose, can present with severe toxicity due to increased tissue levels. Patients with mild toxicity can present with nausea, tremor, ataxia, and rigidity. Moderately affected patients present with delirium, vomiting and diarrhea, and myoclonus. Severe toxicity leads to hypotension, seizures, and coma.

Prehospital and critical care transport evaluation and management include airway support, IV hydration, and close monitoring. As with all ingestions, establishing the number, timing, current medications, and possible co-ingestions is critically important in the care of the lithium toxic patient. Ultimate treatment may include the use of hemodialysis.

ANTICONVULSANTS

Many prescription medications are used to control and prevent seizures. The anticonvulsants will be discussed as groups based on their mechanisms of action or toxic effects. These groups include the benzodiazepines and barbiturates, phenytoin, valproic acid, carbamazepine, and the "newer" anticonvulsants.

Benzodiazepines (e.g., lorazepam) and barbiturates (e.g., phenobarbital) act by stimulating gamma-aminobutyric acid (GABA) receptors in the central nervous system (CNS) leading to depression of neuronal activity. Clinically this increase in GABA concentrations leads to CNS depression, decreased respiratory effort, decreased motor activity, hypothermia, and progressive stupor and coma.

Phenytoin (Dilantin) is used to treat generalized and partial complex seizures, and cardiac dysrhythmias. Phenytoin undergoes slow and erratic absorption following oral ingestion. Toxic effects can also occur from chronic, excessive ingestion or IV administration. Clinical effects include nausea, tremor, nystagmus, ataxia, delirium, and sedation. Massive overdose can lead to stupor, coma, and even seizures. Rapid IV administration can lead to hypotension, bradycardia, or cardiac arrest.

Carbamazepine (Tegretol) has numerous clinical indications for use, including seizures, chronic pain, and psychiatric illness. Systemic absorption can be delayed for over 24 hours following the acute overdose of an extended-release formulation. Carbamazepine has a similar structure to tricyclic antidepressants and can lead to anticholinergic effects in overdose (see Table 32–1). Clinical effects include ataxia, nystagmus, myoclonus, and respiratory depression. Massive overdose can lead to seizure, coma, and hypotension. During recovery, the patient may experience cyclic coma with recurrent symptoms after a massive ingestion.

Valproic acid (Depakote®) is commonly used to control seizures, bipolar disorder, migraines, and chronic pain syndromes. In overdose it can lead to gastritis (nausea and vomiting), confusion, coma, and respiratory failure. Paradoxical seizures, pancreatitis, and encephalopathy (due to elevated ammonia) may occur as well.

The "newer" anticonvulsants are a heterogeneous group of agents including felbamate, gabapentin, tiagabine, and vigabatrin. These agents are typically more benign in overdose, leading to CNS and respiratory depression, and mild to moderate hypotension. The patient may present with nausea and vomiting or reflex tachycardia.

Emergent care for anticonvulsant-induced toxicity includes securing the airway, obtaining IV access, and hemodynamic support. Blood glucose levels should also be checked in all patients with altered sensorium. Benzodiazepines should be used as the agent of choice to control seizures.

OVER-THE-COUNTER MEDICATIONS

Acetaminophen (APAP, or Tylenol) is one of the most common over-the-counter (OTC) medications used in the United States. Due to APAP's availability and the common underestimation of its potential toxicity by laypersons, suicide gestures result in significant morbidity and mortality. In overdose APAP overwhelms normal hepatic metabolism and leads to cellular toxicity. Clinical effects can be divided into four stages, though there is significant overlap. In stage one (0.5–24 hours after the ingestion) patients develop nausea, vomiting, and abdominal pain. Stage two (24–48 hours after ingestion) is associated with an improvement of gastrointestinal symptoms but right upper quadrant pain may develop. In stage three (2–3 days after ingestion) hepatic and renal failure, coagulopathy, jaundice, hypoglycemia, and shock may develop. Stage four (2 days to 8 weeks after ingestion) is associated with either recovery or fulminant hepatic failure and potential death.

Determining the exact time of ingestion is very important. Remember that prehospital personnel gathers history and evidence from the scene to pass onto future care providers, including the critical care transport team. Initial evaluation and care during this time will have consisted of gathering information about the time of ingestion, amount, and possible co-ingestions, followed by supportive care. Definitive treatment involves the administration of *n*-acetylcysteine (Mucomyst) in a monitored setting.

Salicylates (aspirin or ASA) are found in numerous OTC and prescription medications as well as other compounds, including oil of wintergreen and Peptobismol. In overdose, ASA acts as a cellular poison disrupting energy production and causing metabolic acidosis. Dehydration occurs from tachypnea, vomiting, and diaphoresis. Acutely poisoned patients present with tinnitus (ringing in their ears), nausea, tachycardia, and tachypnea. As the poisoning progresses the patient can develop marked tachypnea and tachycardia, diaphoresis, and agitation. Severe toxicity leads to delirium, hyperthermia, cardiac dysrhythmias, pulmonary edema, and seizures. Patients with chronic, excessive ASA use develop nausea, dehydration, and mental status changes.

Critical care evaluation and management include bedside glucose monitoring with appropriate treatment, IV hydration, and possible administration of sodium bicarbonate after medical consultation. All chemically sedated patients (including those with ASA-induced CNS depression) need to be intubated and provided with controlled hyperventilation in order to minimize systemic acidosis. Definitive treatment includes maintenance of the above interventions, with the addition of hemodialysis.

Nonsteroidal anti-inflammatory drugs (NSAIDs) such as ibuprofen (Motrin) are common in intentional overdose, with most patients developing only minimal symptoms. Patients can have a myriad of signs and symptoms including metabolic acidosis. Severe toxicity can lead to coma, respiratory depression, and renal insufficiency.

Management consists of assisting with ventilation (if needed) and IV hydration. Again, gathering as much information from the scene and witnesses, including the time of ingestion, amount, and other co-ingestions, will help determine definitive therapy. Further treatment by the critical care team will be based on the specific agent involved, lab findings, and patient response to therapy.

Dextromethorphan is a common ingredient in numerous OTC medications and is metabolized to a compound that activates glutamate receptors, leading to CNS excitation. Recently, adolescents have started to intentionally abuse dextromethorphan-containing medications in attempts to alter sensorium and produce hallucinations. Clinical effects of dextromethorphan toxicity include ataxia, dizziness, nystagmus, mydriasis, and seizures. Hyperthermia, rhabdomyolysis, and serotonin syndrome are possible with these overdoses as well.

Initial care includes limiting external stimuli to minimize agitation, rehydration with intravenous fluids, and the use of benzodiazepines for severe agitation or seizures.

HERBAL MEDICATIONS

herbal medications
"natural" products that may not have been subjected to the rigors of scientific testing, as are prescription or other over-the-counter (OTC) drugs.

The availability of **herbal medications** has rapidly increased since the passage of the Dietary Supplement Health and Education Act in 1994. Since then, dietary supplements (including herbal medications) have not been stringently regulated by the FDA or other government agency. Therefore, these "natural" products do not undergo any scientific testing and are potentially dangerous for several reasons: first, no verification of ingredients; second, no testing for biological effects; and third, no knowledge of drug interactions. These potential dangers are increased for those patients with significant underlying disease and those taking prescription medications. Common prescription drugs with herbal interactions include warfarin, digoxin, and several anticonvulsants. Furthermore, the manufacture of herbal medications is not regulated and there have been numerous reports in the literature about herbal medications being contaminated with other compounds, microbes, medications, or heavy metals.

Some of the more commonly used herbal medications in the United States include aloe, bilberry, echinacea, garlic, *Ginkgo biloba,* ginseng, grape seed extract, green tea, saw palmetto, and St. John's wort. Their effectiveness in disease prevention or cure has not been definitively shown.

Taking this information into account, it is nearly impossible to predict what medical effects or toxicity can be expected from either acute or chronic use of herbal medications. Because most of these products are ingested, expected toxic effects include gastroenteritis with nausea, vomiting, and diarrhea. Other toxic effects can involve metabolism or excretion of the herbal preparation and therefore may lead to hepatic or renal dysfunction. Some Chinese herbal medications have been found to contain digoxin-like compounds and can lead to cardiac dysrhythmias, which are successfully treated with digoxin-specific Fab. Digoxin-specific Fab antibody fragments are indicated normally for treatment of potentially life-threatening digitalis intoxication with severe ventricular dysrhythmias, progressive bradycardia, second- or third-degree heart block not responsive to atropine, and/or hyperkalemia. Other herbal medications have been associated with chronic effects including hepatitis and neuropathy.

Evaluation of a patient with a possible herbal medication-induced toxicity begins with a record of current and past medical illnesses and an accurate list of current prescription, OTC, and herbal medications. The critical care paramedic should attempt to bring all available pill containers to the admitting hospital along with the patient.

CAUSTICS

Caustic injuries result from the ingestion of, inhalation of (as gases), or dermal exposure to corrosive compounds that can lead to tissue irritation, burn, and deep tissue injury. A large number of chemical agents are capable of causing corrosive injury, including acids, alkalis, oxidizing agents, and some hydrocarbons. The extent of mucosal and dermal injury, airway compromise, and permanent scarring varies depending on several factors. These include the alkalinity, concentration, and volume of the corrosive material, and the duration of exposure.

Alkali ingestions make up the leading cause of death from nonpharmaceutical exposures. Common alkali agents include Drano, bleach (sodium hypochlorite), ammonia, hair dyes, and cement (lime). When an alkali compound comes into contact with tissue, proteins and cell membranes are emulsified and deep tissue penetration is possible. This process is called liquefaction necrosis. Additionally, acids such as hydrofluoric acid and phenol cause skin and tissue to undergo coagulation necrosis in which an eschar forms; this limits the extent of deep tissue penetration.

Patients who ingest a corrosive compound can present with burns to the face and lips, mouth, upper gastrointestinal tract, and upper airway. Signs and symptoms include pain, drooling, stridor, refusal to swallow, and dysphagia. When the upper airway is involved patients may display a cough, stridor, or hoarse voice. These patients can rapidly develop airway compromise. Significant ingestions can lead to esophageal or gastric rupture, causing chest or abdominal pain, metabolic derangements, and cardiovascular shock. Airway establishment and continued patency are of paramount concern in these patients.

Dermal exposure to a corrosive agent can lead to pain, erythema or blanching, edema, and tissue destruction. Inhalation of a corrosive gas can lead to dermal, mucous membrane, and airway irritation and to burns and scarring. Airway compromise is a main concern in these patients as well. Ocular exposures can lead to conjunctivitis, corneal ulceration, full-thickness burns, and blindness.

Emergent treatment of corrosive injuries should immediately focus on airway issues due to the fact that a patient may rapidly develop severe airway compromise. Decontamination includes removal of contaminated clothing, and copious irrigation of exposed dermal and ocular tissue. Care providers should protect themselves from secondary contamination by ensuring appropriate Body Substance Isolation (BSI) Precautions and personal protective equipment (PPE), are used accordingly. Supplemental oxygen should be administered and IV access obtained. Consultation with a poison control center may help identify unique medical concerns associated with individual corrosive agents. This consultation should not however, delay transport.

Ingestion of a button battery may also cause a corrosive injury and typically involves children less than 5 years of age. These batteries can cause tissue necrosis by leakage of their contents, minute electric currents, and mechanical pressure. The corrosive effects are increased if the battery is lodged in an area of the patient's nose, mouth, or esophagus. These patients may present with pain, drooling, dysphagia, odynophagia (pain on swallowing), or refusal to eat. Emergent management includes airway protection, history gathering as to the size and type of battery, and transport.

ETHANOL AND TOXIC ALCOHOLS

For the purpose of this section, the term *alcohols* will refer to ethanol, methanol, ethylene glycol, and isopropanol; and the term **toxic alcohols** will refer only to methanol, ethylene glycol, and isopropanol.

The abuse of ethanol and the toxic alcohols is a serious medical issue and is associated with significant morbidity and mortality. The toxic alcohols are common ingredients in many commercial and industrial products and are therefore readily available for accidental or intentional ingestions. (See Table 32–2.) All significant alcohol intoxications result from oral ingestion and lead to shared clinical effects: gastritis, altered sensorium (euphoria, inebriation, coma), impaired judgment, and ataxia. Hypoglycemia may occur, particularly among children and malnourished abusers. All intoxicated patients are at increased risk for trauma-related injuries.

The effects of ethanol depend on several factors, including the amount ingested, rate of ingestion, co-ingestions, and tolerance. Acute clinical effects include those just listed, as well as nystagmus, loss of social inhibitions, agitation, and aggressive behavior. Profound ethanol intoxication can lead to coma, respiratory depression, and loss of airway reflexes. Aspiration and respiratory distress are possible. Chronic ethanol abuse can lead to liver disease (including coagulopathy), gastrointestinal bleeding, cardiac dysrhythmias, and central or peripheral neuronal disorders. Some of these effects are worsened by chronic malnutrition or repeated trauma.

Isopropanol (isopropyl alcohol) is found in rubbing alcohol and occasionally abused as a substitute for ethanol. Isopropanol is associated with significant gastritis and CNS depression (leading to respiratory depression and coma). Isopropanol is metabolized to acetone, which can prolong the duration of CNS and respiratory depression but does not cause a metabolic acidosis. Initial

toxic alcohols *methanol, ethylene glycol, and isopropanol; ingestion of these is associated with significant mortality.*

Table 32–2	Ethanol and the Toxic Alcohols
Toxic Alcohol	**Common Sources**
Ethanol	Beer, wine, liquors (i.e., whiskey), colognes, mouthwash, food flavorings
Methanol	Windshield washer fluid/antifreeze, paint removers, a contaminant in moonshine
Ethylene glycol	Automotive antifreeze
Isopropanol (isopropyl alcohol)	Rubbing alcohol, disinfectant solutions

management of an isopropanol ingestion situation centers on securing the airway, assisting with ventilation, and evaluating for hypoglycemia and hypotension.

Methanol can be found in windshield washer fluid or as a contaminant in the production of moonshine. After ingestion a patient initially develops an ethanol-like intoxication, with gastritis, ataxia, and inebriation. Methanol, however, is ultimately metabolized to a toxin (formic acid) that leads to severe metabolic acidosis, blindness, seizure, coma, and death.

Ethylene glycol (found in antifreeze) also initially presents with inebriation and ataxia, but is metabolized to acidic compounds that lead to a metabolic acidosis, respiratory distress, seizures, and renal failure. Without appropriate interventions the patient will develop severe acidosis and death.

The initial management of the intoxicated patient involves maintaining an airway, correcting hypoglycemia, and evaluating for trauma-related or environmental injuries (i.e., hypothermia). A chronic alcoholic may also present with similar findings (i.e., altered sensorium and agitation) when withdrawing from ethanol. It is important to consider the possibility of underlying substance abuse (i.e., alcoholism), psychiatric disorder, or suicide attempt in all intoxicated patients.

INDUSTRIAL EXPOSURES

hazardous materials
describes the significant danger from chemicals and/or biological agents, with regard to type, volume, and concentrations of such agents.

The majority of tox-related industrial injuries develop after a dermal or inhalational exposure and may involve multiple patients. Industrial exposures to **hazardous materials** are associated with significant danger due to the vast number of chemicals and biological agents as well as the larger volumes and higher concentrations of chemicals (when compared to commercial products) that are available. Acute exposures to industrial agents typically cause respiratory, dermal, CNS, and gastrointestinal effects. Other chemicals, including agents that are known carcinogens and neurotoxins, are capable of causing illness and disease but only after prolonged or chronic exposures. A list of general groups of industrial hazards can be found in Table 32–3.

Material Safety Data Sheet (MSDS) *federally mandated product descriptions that contain specific information about an individual product, including the chemical name, brand name, health effects, and the Chemical Abstracts Service number (CAS#).*

All hazardous materials used or transported for industrial purposes are required to be accompanied by a **Material Safety Data Sheet (MSDS).** The MSDS contains specific information about an individual product, including the chemical name, brand name, health effects, and the Chemical Abstracts Service number (CAS#). Specific product information can also be obtained by contacting the Occupational Safety and Health Administration (OSHA, 1-800-321-OSHA) or your regional PCC at 1-800-222-1222.

As with any hazardous material scene, care providers must protect themselves, and others, from becoming secondary victims prior to engaging in rescue attempts. A careful scene survey is mandatory. It is most important to remember that an optimal treatment plan can only be established after correctly identifying the chemical(s) involved in the exposure.

Although it is impossible to discuss all known industrial chemicals, a few of the more notorious industrial toxins, including asphyxiants, such as carbon monoxide, hydrogen sulfide, and cyanide, and caustics, such as hydrofluoric acid, will be covered.

Table 32–3	Industrial Hazards
Industrial Hazard Group	**Common Examples**
Biological agents	Bacteria, viruses, fungi, blood, body wastes
Gases	Carbon monoxide, hydrogen sulfide, natural and chlorine gas
Solvents	Hydrocarbons, acetone, xylene, toluene
Heavy metals	Lead, arsenic, mercury, cadmium, beryllium
Pesticides	Organophosphates, fungicides, arsenicals
Cleaning agents	Ethylene oxide, glycol ethers
Corrosives	Acids (hydrofluoric acid), alkalis (ammonium)
Irritants	Isocyanates, chlorine, nitrogen dioxide
Carcinogens	Hexavalent chromium, vinyl chloride, benzene
Neurotoxins	*N*-Hexane, acrylamide

Asphyxiants are agents that interrupt the normal delivery of oxygen to tissue, leading to hypoxia. The two classes include simple asphyxiants (compounds that simply displace oxygen in the atmosphere and decrease the percentage of inhaled oxygen) and chemical, or systemic, asphyxiants (agents that interfere with the transportation or utilization of oxygen within the body). Examples of simple asphyxiants include carbon dioxide, methane, and butane. Examples of chemical (systemic) asphyxiants include carbon monoxide, hydrogen sulfide, and cyanide.

Carbon monoxide (CO) results from incomplete combustion and can be encountered near any source of combustion, including fires, generators, and space heaters. However, the most common source of CO exposure is automobiles. CO is a colorless, odorless, nonirritating gas that when inhaled is rapidly absorbed into blood and tissue. These characteristics are dangerous because exposed persons may not realize that they are being poisoned. The amount of CO absorbed depends on the ambient CO concentration and the length of exposure. Once absorbed, CO inhibits the delivery and cellular utilization of oxygen, leading to hypoxia at the cellular level. The clinical effects are nonspecific and can mimic many medical conditions, including viral illnesses. Signs and symptoms of CO toxicity include headache, dizziness, nausea/vomiting, and confusion. The clinical effects moderately correlate with CO blood levels. (See Table 32–4.)

The initial treatment of CO poisoning involves removal from exposure, administration of 100% oxygen via a tight-fitting nonrebreather facemask, intubation (if required), and rapid transport to an ED by EMS providers. The critical care transport team may be called on to maintain this therapy as they transport the patient to a secondary facility that is capable of providing hyperbaric oxygen (HBO) therapy.

Hydrogen sulfide (also known as "sewer," "pit," or "swamp gas") is a by-product of the natural breakdown of organic material. It is a highly lethal gas that smells like rotten eggs and is heavier than air, accumulating in low-lying pits, trenches, or containers (e.g., sewers). Hydrogen sulfide is rapidly absorbed after inhalation and inhibits the cellular use of oxygen. Clinical effects include burning eyes, cough, headache, nausea, dizziness, and the rapid development of coma. Massive or prolonged exposure can lead to seizures, cardiovascular shock, and death. The cellular effects are so rapid that hydrogen sulfide can lead to rapid unconsciousness and is known as a "knockdown agent." Fortunately, its obnoxious smell and mucous membrane (eye, mouth, and throat) irritation allow for early, though transient, warning properties.

All rescuers must protect themselves from potential exposure, so the use of a self-contained breathing apparatus may be warranted. Initial patient management involves removal from the exposure, providing 100% oxygen, and assisting with ventilation. A patient may spontaneously recover once he is removed from the source and receives fresh air or supplemental oxygen. Theoretically, the use of nitrites (contained in a cyanide antidote kit) or HBO may assist in the treatment of a patient with severe poisoning.

The cellular toxicity of cyanide is similar to that of hydrogen sulfide and therefore leads to similar clinical effects. After cyanide exposure, the patient rapidly develops severe hypoxia and metabolic acidosis, leading to abrupt coma, cardiovascular collapse, and death. The management of

Table 32–4	Clinical Effects of Carbon Monoxide (CO) Toxicity
CO Blood Level (%)	Signs and Symptoms
<10	None
10–20	Headache, dyspnea
20–30	Headache, dizziness, nausea
30–40	Headache, ataxia, confusion
40–50	Syncope, delirium
50–60	Syncope, seizure, coma
60–70	Coma, hypotension, dysrhythmia, death
>70	Rapid death

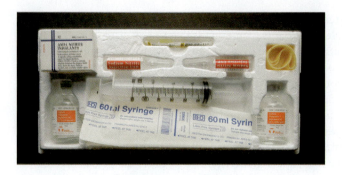

■ **Figure 32-1** Cyanide antidote kit. (© *Jeff Forster*)

cyanide toxicity includes aggressive control of the airway, supporting circulation, treatment of seizures, and the immediate administration of a cyanide antidote. (See Figure 32-1 ■.)

Hydrofluoric (HF) acid is a highly reactive corrosive commonly found in commercial and industrial products, including rust removers and glass etching compounds, and in the manufacture of semiconductor chips. Clinical effects vary depending on the route of exposure (inhalation, dermal, or ingestion), HF acid concentration, and amount of tissue exposed (i.e., total body surface area). An exposure to a low (<15%) concentration of HF acid may have minimal, if any, immediate symptoms. Highly concentrated (>40%) solutions lead to immediate, severe effects and may cause systemic toxicity, even if only involving a small amount of tissue.

Inhalation of hydrogen fluoride gas leads to mucous membrane (ocular, nasal, and oropharyngeal) irritation, bronchospasm (wheezing and coughing), and, with larger exposures, a chemical pneumonitis or pulmonary edema. The degree and onset of symptoms depend on the concentration and duration of exposure.

The dermal effects of HF acid include burning pain, erythema or blanching, and edema. The degree and speed of onset of symptoms depends on the concentration of the involved product; the higher the concentration the sooner the onset of more severe symptoms. Exposure to a low concentration of HF acid may not produce symptoms (i.e., pain or erythema) for more than 12 hours. It is important to realize that with this type of exposure, a patient may experience excruciating pain without any obvious signs of dermal burn.

Small dermal exposures to highly concentrated HF acid solutions can lead to systemic toxicity. Systemic HF acid toxicity involves deep tissue penetration, which can lead to destruction, hypocalcemia, hyperkalemia, cardiac dysrhythmias, acidosis, and shock.

Treatment of HF acid toxicity depends on the route of exposure. Dermal burns may react to the topical application of calcium-containing gels (e.g., mixing calcium gluconate with a water-based lubricant such as K-Y Jelly®). Ocular exposures should be flushed with copious amounts of water and immediately evaluated by a physician. A patient with inhalation exposure requires removal from the source and airway support. Bronchospasm may respond to humidified oxygen, bronchodilators (i.e., albuterol), or inhaled calcium gluconate via nebulizer.

All patients with significant exposures should be placed on cardiac monitoring and observed for dysrhythmias. Cardiac dysrhythmias (secondary to acute hyperkalemia) may respond to intravenous calcium. Following an acute ingestion of HF acid, patients with an intact airway should receive any calcium or magnesium-containing substances, such as milk or calcium carbonate. Further treatment of HF acid burns involves the use of subcutaneous or intra-arterial injections of calcium gluconate. During transport the critical care team may need to continue this type of supportive therapy.

WARFARE AGENTS

Modern warfare agents include two general groups, biological and chemical agents. Biological agents include anthrax, botulinum toxins, plague, smallpox, and tularemia. Chemical agents include nerve agents, vesicants, lacrimators, and incapacitating agents. Although all these are presented in greater detail in Chapter 33 (Weapons of Mass Destruction), they are mentioned first here for completeness of discussion.

Biological agents produce toxicity by causing infectious disease. Signs and symptoms can range from mild viral-like syndromes, with cough, fever, and myalgias, to severe sepsis and shock. Of main concern with biological agents are the complications of a mass casualty incident and the secondary, widespread contamination of other victims and rescuers. If there is any suspicion that a biological incident, has occurred, immediate contact with medical direction, regional EMS coordinators, and the police department or FBI is mandatory.

Nerve agents, including tabun, sarin, soman, and VX, are considered **organophosphate (OP) compounds** and are potent examples of warfare agents. OPs, and carbamate insecticides like Malathion® and Chlormephos®, inhibit the enzyme acetylcholinesterase (AChE), leading to an increase in acetylcholine activity. This excess acetylcholine stimulates receptors in the CNS and at neuromuscular junctions, resulting in a cholinergic (crisis) syndrome. (See Table 32–1.) Toxicity is possible after inhalational or dermal exposure, with secondary contamination to other victims or rescuers possible.

organophosphate (OP) compounds *potent warfare agents that may be lethal to humans; includes nerve agents (such as tabun, sarin, soman, and VX).*

The clinical effects of an OP-induced cholinergic crisis can be remembered by using the mnemonic *SLUDGE:* salivation (with airway compromise), lacrimation, urinary incontinence, diarrhea, gastric upset (emesis, diarrhea, and abdominal cramps), and excessive (airway) secretions. Other effects include miosis, muscle fasciculations, and bronchospasm. Morbidity and mortality are associated with airway compromise due to excessive secretions and resultant hypoxia.

Decontamination and airway support are the main concerns when caring for patients with OP toxicity. The use of water-impermeable garments, neoprene gloves, weak bleach wipes, and the removal of clothes will limit secondary contamination and aid in decontamination. Emergent treatment of patients includes airway, ventilatory, and circulatory support as well as the administration of an anticholinergic agent such as atropine (in doses of 1–2 mg IV, repeated every 2–3 minutes) as needed until airway secretions are controlled and hemodynamics are improved.

Vesicants (i.e., mustard and lewisite) are warfare agents that produce dermal toxicity and lead to vesicles (blisters) and tissue corrosion. Clinical effects of these gases include ocular and upper airway irritation, cough, dyspnea, and a chemical pneumonitits. Prehospital, ED, and critical care transport efforts should focus on rapid, copious decontamination, airway support, and establishing IV access for pain control and rehydration.

Lacrimators are irritant gases and solutions, such as tear gas and capsaicin (or pepper spray), that are typically used as riot control agents. These agents cause mucous membrane irritation, affecting the eyes, nose, and upper airway (and lower airway to a lesser extent). Ocular effects include eyelid spasm, tearing, and conjunctivitis. The upper airway effects include coughing, wheezing, and increased secretions; gagging, retching, or vomiting may occur.

lacrimators *irritant gases and solutions (i.e., tear gas and capsaicin spray); induce temporary debilitation by means of irritation to the mucous membranes and respiratory tree, as well as uncontrolled watering of the affected eyes(s) and the nose.*

Decontaminate the patient by removing him from the source, removing and bagging his clothing, and irrigating exposed tissue with copious amounts of water or saline. Although these agents' effects are designed to be self-limited, some patients can have lasting ocular, dermal, or pulmonary injuries. Acute allergic reactions are possible and can lead to severe respiratory compromise. Closely monitor the airway and respiratory effort during transportation.

OTHER POTENTIALLY TOXIC AGENTS

Several potentially toxic agents deserve specific discussion, including warfarin, hydrocarbons, and heavy metals.

Warfarin is an anticoagulant that inhibits the body's ability to stop bleeding. Warfarin and other natural anticoagulants are found in prescription medications (Coumadin), plant-derived (herbal) medications, and rodenticides. The effects of these anticoagulants can last for days to months, leaving the patient at risk for trauma-induced and spontaneous bleeding. Small, unintentional ingestions may be evaluated in a routine manner after consultation with a PCC or the patient's physician. However, all patients with a large or intentional ingestion require immediate medical evaluation.

Hydrocarbons (HCs), including alcohols, are derived from petroleum distillates and are common ingredients in many products, including solvents, fuels, and lubricants. Examples include motor oil, kerosene, lamp oil, and turpentine. The main risk after ingestion involves pulmonary aspiration and respiratory distress. Pulmonary aspiration is possible with even small, accidental ingestions and may lead to a chemical pneumonitis. Any sign of respiratory distress, such as cough, wheeze, or tachypnea, suggests an aspiration. After ingestion, nausea, vomiting, and diarrhea may develop. Some HCs are also irritating to skin, eyes, and mucous membranes; dermal decontamination should be done as soon as possible.

Intentional abuse of volatile HCs, such as toluene and xylene, can include inhalation of paints, glues, polishes, or nail polish removers in attempts to alter sensorium. The inhalation of these products can be done in several ways: huffing (inhaling the HC from a soaked rag), sniffing (inhaling the HC from a container), or bagging (inhaling the HC from a bag, intermittently placed over the patient's head). HC abuse can lead to hypoxemia, chemical pneumonitits, or respiratory and cardiac arrest. Abuse of halogenated hydrocarbons (i.e., Freon®) can sensitize the heart to catecholamines (i.e., epinephrine) and lead to tachydysrhythmias or asystole. Patients found with severe tachycardia or asystole after a hydrocarbon exposure should be treated with a beta-blocker and the use of epinephrine should be avoided.

Heavy metal toxicity is very complicated and usually presents after a chronic exposure. Chronic toxicity can develop after prolonged ingestion, inhalation, or dermal exposure to many different metals. Clinical effects include dermatitis, gastritis, liver or kidney failure, and neuropathy. Metals involved in chronic poisonings include lead, gold, manganese, and mercury. An acute ingestion of certain metals can lead to significant toxicity. Metals capable of causing acute effects include arsenic, cadmium, iron (possibly from iron-containing vitamins), lead, mercury, nickel (contact dermatitis from nickel-containing jewelry), and thallium. Some metals can cause both acute and chronic toxicity.

Another metal-associated toxic syndrome is metal fume fever. This is caused by inhaling the fumes (fine particles) of metal oxides. Compounds containing zinc, cadmium, magnesium, or manganese (among others) can lead to an acute syndrome characterized by fever, headache, and myalgias. Respiratory irritation is also possible, manifested by cough, wheeze, or dyspnea. The symptoms are typically transient and respond well to removal from the source, supplemental oxygen, and bronchodilators.

FOOD POISONING

Food poisoning is caused by the ingestion of bacteria or preformed bacterial toxins contained in food. The resulting illness typically produces mild to moderate symptoms and is self-limited with recovery expected within 48 hours. The onset of symptoms can be rapid (within 1 hour) if the ingested food contained preformed bacterial toxins, or delayed (up to several days) if the bacteria need to invade the host's tissue to cause symptoms. Several organisms are commonly associated with specific foods, so an accurate history of recent meals may be helpful.

The classic symptoms of food poisoning are nausea, vomiting, diarrhea, and abdominal pain. Systemic effects, such as fever, myalgias, and bloody stool are more common with invasive organisms, such as *Shigella*. Some invasive organisms can lead to serious systemic toxicity, including meningitis or renal failure.

Initial treatment involves IV fluid resuscitation and antiemetics. The use of antibiotics or antidiarrheal agents is not routinely indicated and should be discussed with medical direction prior to their use by the critical care paramedic.

Botulism is an infectious disease caused by the neurotoxin produced by the bacterium *Clostridium botulinum*. The infection may develop by ingesting food containing the organism or its preformed toxins, or through wound contamination. A modern example of wound botulism involves skin-popping (subcutaneously injection) of illicit drugs, typically "black tar" heroin. Botulin toxin prevents the release of acetylcholine at neuromuscular junctions and leads to muscle weakness. Clinical effects include gastritis (nausea and abdominal pain) and subsequent muscle weakness with descending paralysis. Classically, the muscles of the head and neck are first affected, leading to diplopia (double vision), ptosis (drooping eyelids), dysarthria (difficulty speaking), and dysphagia (difficulty swallowing). Aggressive supportive care (to prevent death secondary to respiratory failure) and the use of an antitoxin can allow complete recovery.

A variety of unique toxins are associated with fish and shellfish ingestion. Several of these toxins (ciguatera, paralytic shellfish poisoning, neurotoxic shellfish poisoning, and tetrodotoxin) involve gastroenteritis and neurologic complaints, such as paresthesias, weakness, or myoclonus. All patients with neurologic complaints require immediate medical evaluation.

Another common fish-derived toxin is scombroid, caused by eating poorly refrigerated deep-water fish, such as tuna or mahi-mahi. The unrefrigerated meat produces elevated concentrations of histamine, leading to gastroenteritis, flushing, and a rash that typically involves the face, neck, and chest. Treatment of scombroid poisoning involves antihistamines (i.e., diphenhydramine) and antiemetics.

PLANTS AND MUSHROOMS

The ingestion of plants and mushrooms (including berries, leaves, or roots) is a common human exposure, typically involving an accidental ingestion by a child. These cases involve exposures ranging from decorative (nontoxic) houseplants to exotic species with well-established toxicity. Although there is a wide range of clinical effects, gastrointestinal distress (nausea, vomiting, and diarrhea) are the most common finding. The vast majority of these exposures are limited to self-resolving gastroenteritis. However, some plants and mushrooms are capable of causing systemic toxicity, with an occassional delay in the onset of clinical effects. (See Table 32–5.) Other species are capable of inducing irritant or allergic reactions leading to dermatitis or airway difficulties.

In general, the sooner the onset of gastroenteritis, the less likely it is that systemic toxicity will develop, particularly with mushrooms. If nausea and abdominal pain start within 6 hours of a mushroom ingestion, the effects are almost always limited to isolated gastroenteritis.

Initial treatment of a patient with a plant or mushroom ingestion involves airway support, if needed, rehydration, and control of nausea. Proper identification of the involved plant or mushroom may help determine optimal treatment. Discussion with a regional poison center may help identify those patients who require transfer or immediate medical evaluation.

Table 32–5	Examples of Toxic and Nontoxic Plants and Mushrooms	
Plant/Mushroom Species	Systemic Toxicity	Clinical Effects
Christmas cactus (*Schlumbergera* spp.)	No	None
Holly (*Ilex* spp.)	No	Gastroenteritis
Philodendron (*Philodendron* spp.)	No	Dermal/mucous membrane irritation, gastroenteritis
Poison ivy (oak and sumac)	No	Contact dermatitis
Castor bean (*Ricinus communis*)	Yes	Gastroenteritis and multiple-organ system failure
Oleander (*Thevetia* and *Nerium* spp.)	Yes	Cardiac dysrhythmias
Water hemlock (*Cicuta maculata*)	Yes	Seizures
Pokeweed (*Phytolacca americana*)	Yes	Severe gastroenteritis
Jimsonweed (*Datura stramonium*)	Yes	Anticholinergic poisoning
Typical "little brown mushroom" (i.e., *Chlorophyllum molybdites*)	No	Gastroenteritis
"Magic mushrooms" (*Psilocybin* spp.)	No	Hallucinations, gastroenteritis
"Death cap" mushroom (*Amanita phalloides*)	Yes	Gastroenteritis and hepatic failure
False morel mushrooms (*Gyromitra esculenta*)	Yes	Seizures, hepatic failure

ENVENOMATIONS AND STINGS

More than 85,000 cases of stings and envenomations were reported to U.S. poison centers in 2002. These include human encounters with arthropods (i.e., spiders and scorpions), hymenoptera (i.e., bees, wasps, and ants), fishes, snakes, and other reptiles. Fire ants are a particular problem in the South. Originally imported from South America in the 1930s, they have spread to 10–15 states now. Not all envenomations lead to life-threatening effects or require immediate medical attention.

SNAKES

The venomous snakes endemic to North America include the pit vipers (*Crotalinae* family, includes rattlesnakes) and coral snakes (*Elapidae* family). (See Figure 32-2 ■.) Many other exotic species can be found in zoos and private collections. Snakebites typically occur in an extremity and involve varying amounts of venom and clinical effects. Some bites are considered "dry" and lead to no significant effects due to a lack of envenomation.

Some snakes' venom, such as rattlesnakes and copperheads, causes significant pain, edema, myonecrosis (tissue destruction), and coagulopathy. Other snakes, such as coral snakes and cobras (not endemic to North America), have venom that causes pain and neurologic effects (fasciculations and weakness). Depending on the species involved and the amount of venom injected, patients can present with pain, muscular weakness (including respiratory paralysis), or cardiovascular collapse. Although rare, an immediate allergic reaction to the venom is possible. The onset of some effects, such as muscle weakness or coagulopathy, can be delayed for many hours.

It is seldom necessary to identify the involved snake, so the risks in attempting to do so should be considered by initial EMS responders. Intravenous access should be established, preferably in a nonenvenomated limb because of the potential for subsequent edema. The affected limb should be immobilized and elevated above the heart with a noncompressive, straight splint. The use of a tourniquet, ice, or suction kit is contraindicated.

The patient should be monitored closely for signs of shock or airway compromise. Most patients will benefit from an intravenous fluid bolus, analgesics, and antiemetics. Patients receiving antivenin (including a skin test) are at risk for anaphylaxis and require close monitoring during interfacility transfer by the critical care paramedic.

HYMENOPTERA

Hymenoptera is a large, diverse order of animals that includes bees, wasps, and ants. Their bites and stings are common human exposures and can lead to significant local or systemic effects. Their venom is typically weak yet capable of inducing severe local pain and inflammation, as well as inducing anaphylaxis in susceptible individuals.

Common effects from hymenoptera stings/bites include localized pain, edema, and erythema. Systemic effects such as urticaria, wheeze, hypotension, airway compromise, or anaphylaxis are possible. It is important to realize that prior reactions to a hymenoptera envenomation (i.e., bee sting) do not accurately predict subsequent reactions. Massive exposures are occasionally encountered and may involve attacks by species such as fire ants or Africanized bees. These patients are at risk for systemic effects due to an anaphylactoid reaction, leading to hypotension or respiratory arrest.

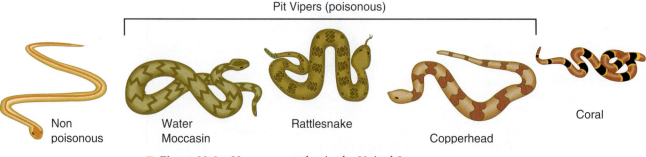

■ Figure 32-2   Venomous snakes in the United States.

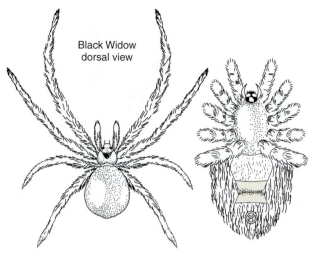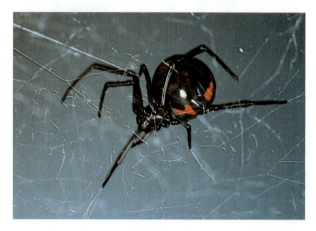

Black Widow
dorsal view

Initial treatment of hymenoptera envenomations includes gently removing any retained stingers, which is best done by scraping with a hard, flat surface like a credit card. The area should be irrigated or washed, and a cool compress may help alleviate pain. Patients with clinical evidence of a systemic reaction (i.e., bronchospasm or hypotension) require more aggressive interventions, including IV access, breathing treatments, antihistamines, and epinephrine.

ARTHROPODS: SPIDERS AND SCORPIONS

Black widow spiders (*Latrodectus spp.*) can be found in all regions of the continental United States and throughout the world. (See Figure 32-3 ■.) A black widow envenomation (also termed Latrodectism) is considered the most important spider envenomation in the world. These spiders are typically encountered on webs in solitary environments, often spun from the undersurface of low-lying structures (e.g., a bench). The venom's active protein is a potent neurotoxin that stimulates the release of neurotransmitters, including acetylcholine and norepinephrine.

The initial bite of a black widow spider is often described as a transient pinprick but may go unrecognized. The bite site may reveal two small puncture wounds with minimal erythema or inflammation and is called a "target lesion." Other localized effects (pain, diaphoresis, or piloerection isolated to the bite site) typically begin within 60 minutes of the envenomation. A severe envenomation will progress to involved diffuse pain, muscle cramps (typically of the abdomen or back), tachycardia, and hypertension. Additional effects include nausea, headache, fever, tremor, and weakness. Rarely reported are periorbital edema/ecchymosis, priapism, cardiac dysrhythmias (including reflex bradycardia), or paralysis.

Emergent treatment for a black widow spider envenomation includes IV hydration and analgesics. Severe pain agitation can be treated with benzodiazepines. An antivenin is available but is not often necessary and its use is reserved for intensive care settings. Consultation with medical authorities by the critical care paramedic should be done prior to the use of the antivenin.

Brown recluse spiders (*Loxosceles reclusa*) are found throughout the United States, typically encountered in dark, isolated environments. (See Figure 32-4 ■.) Their envenomations lead to varying amounts of local vascular injury and dermonecrosis. Classically, the site of the body where the spider has bitten develops into a necrotic wound within 4 days of envenomation. (See Figure 32-5 ■.) An eschar then forms, falls off, and the wound heals slowly over several weeks. Systemic effects, termed Loxoscelism, are rare but possible and typically develop 1–2 days after the envenomation. Clinical findings include nausea, fever, and myalgias. Serious effects include significant skin deterioration, exudates from the bite site, systemic hemolysis, renal failure, and death. It is important to realize that many arthropods are capable of causing a necrotic skin lesion; therefore, not all of these wounds are caused by brown recluse envenomation.

Initial management of a brown recluse spider envenomation involves local wound care, immobilization, and analgesics. The routine use of antibiotics, corticosteroids, or early surgical

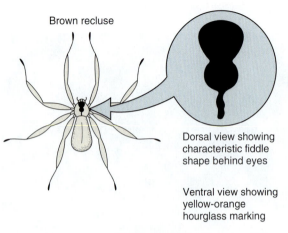

Brown recluse

Dorsal view showing characteristic fiddle shape behind eyes

Ventral view showing yellow-orange hourglass marking

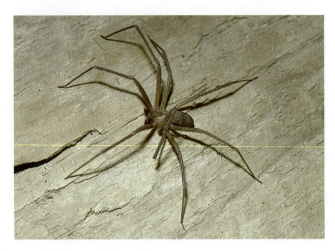

■ Figure 32-4   Brown recluse spider.

■ Figure 32-5   Brown recluse spider bite 24 hours after bite. Note the bleb and surrounding white halo. *(Courtesy of Scott and White Hospital and Clinic)*

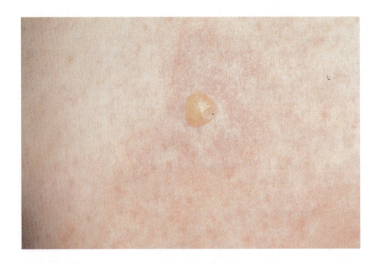

debridement has not been proven beneficial and therefore not routinely recommended. The use of delayed cosmetic surgery may be required to decrease scar formation.

There are numerous poisonous scorpions throughout the world, but only the bark scorpion (*Centruides spp.*) is endemic to North America. The bark scorpion's venom contains a neurotoxin that increases the release of several neurotransmitters. Clinical effects include immediate pain and paresthesias at the sting site. Larger envenomations may progress to involve diffuse pain, paresthesias, and muscle fasciculations. Severe envenomations progress to involve cranial nerve dysfunction and cause rotatory nystagmus, hypersalivation, and difficulty swallowing. The patient's airway may be compromised, and immediate management by the emergency staff will then be warranted. Despite these effects the patient is awake and alert but may have difficulty speaking due to venom-induced dysarthria.

Prehospital and critical care transport therapy includes providing oxygen therapy, establishing IV access, providing analgesics, and monitoring the airway. Consider the use of benzodiazepines to control severe fasciculations. Subsequent hospital care may include the administration of an antivenin (only available in Arizona), or sedation and intubation for airway support.

MARINE ANIMAL

Marine animal envenomations encompass a wide variety of organisms and clinical presentations. Poisonous species include jellyfish, fire coral, sea urchins, sea snakes, stingrays, and various fishes (i.e., lionfish, scorpionfish, and stonefish). These organisms inject their venoms through several mechanisms: bites (sea snakes), barbs (i.e., stingrays, lionfish, sea urchins), or dermal contact with nematocysts (tiny pressure-sensitive capsules containing venom barbs, found in many species including jellyfish).

Sea snake envenomations lead to pain and muscle weakness that may progress to cause paralysis and respiratory failure. The majority of other envenomations lead to local pain, erythema, and edema. The extent of pain can be overwhelming and contribute to weakness, nausea, and autonomic instability. Exposures to nematocysts can lead to ongoing toxin exposure until the affected area is properly decontaminated. Stingrays and fish envenomations can involve a retained barb capable of causing a local, deep tissue infection or necrosis. All such wounds require exploration to remove retained foreign bodies.

Emergency treatment includes decontamination of the venom site with seawater or 5% acetic acid (vinegar). If the envenomation involves nematocysts, irrigation with freshwater must be avoided to prevent remaining nematocysts from releasing toxin. Talcum powder or shaving cream can then be applied to remove adhered nematocysts by gently scraping them off. Lionfish and other fish contain toxins that are neutralized by heat. These wounds should be immersed in hot water (up to 115° F or 46° C) for 30 minutes to alleviate pain. Further treatment should include IV access, hydration, pain control, and recognition of anaphylactic reactions.

INITIAL EVALUATION

An in-depth scene survey is paramount to initiating optimal care while ensuring rescuer safety. Prehospital providers may be the only health care professionals capable of uncovering important information necessary to determine the cause for the patient's condition and thereby impacting the treatment plan. Items such as pill bottles, product containers (e.g., antifreeze bottle), suicide notes, or bystander interviews can provide immediate information that is relevant to patient care and would otherwise be missed. The need to gather as much information from the scene without delaying transport cannot be overemphasized.

DECONTAMINATION

Decontamination involves minimizing a patient's exposure to a noxious or toxic material. After ensuring rescuer safety, the initial step involves removing the patient(s) from the source of toxicity. Mechanical decontamination involves attempts to remove any toxins from physical contact with the patient. All solid substances (i.e., powders) should be removed by carefully wiping them off. Care should be taken not to scrub the patient's skin because small abrasions can allow increased dermal absorption. All contaminated clothing should be removed and bagged for proper disposal.

After removing the bulk of the toxin and contaminated clothing, copious irrigation with water should be done; a priority should be placed on the eyes. Contact lenses should be removed and then the eyes should be irrigated with low-pressure water. Care should be taken to avoid runoff from surrounding skin into the patient's eyes, ears, or mouth. Although rescuer safety can never be compromised, decontamination techniques should not delay life-saving interventions. Physical decontamination and copious irrigation should not be delayed while attempts to find specific agents (M291 resin kit or 0.5% hypochlorite solution) are made, particularly when water or normal saline is available. Always contact medical direction with any significant exposure should the critical care paramedic be called to an exposure site, and initiate HAZMAT procedures as necessary. Finally, ensure there is adequate ventilation of the patient compartment during transport to avoid accidental inhalational contamination by the critical care providers.

GASTRIC DECONTAMINATION

Gastric decontamination (GD) techniques include administering syrup of ipecac, activated charcoal, and gastric lavage. Although GD is not a "life-saving" intervention per se, it does help limit further absorption of the toxin via the GI tract during the first couple hours post exposure. As such, it does have some utility in the initial and ongoing management of many ingested poisons. Ipecac is no longer recommended due to limited effects and the risk of nausea, vomiting, and aspiration.

The use of activated charcoal is potentially beneficial but is only recommended if it can be given within 1 hour of an acute ingestion. Activated charcoal should not be given to any patient with nausea or abdominal pain. The use of activated charcoal is contraindicated in patients who have (or may develop) airway compromise or CNS depression (with loss of airway reflexes) due to the risk of aspiration and respiratory distress.

TRANSPORTATION ISSUES

Finally, we look at some general principles to keep in mind during the critical care transport of a poisoned patient. Consider intubating the patient (in a controlled environment) prior to transport if the history suggests the potential for increasing CNS depression and airway compromise, or there is a concern for severe agitation. This may prevent patient decompensation or procedural complications during transportation. Be judicious with the use of naloxone in the opiate-sedated, intubated patient due to the potential reversal of sedation, subsequent agitation, and potential loss of the secured airway. During the interfacility transport of an agitated patient, the use of chemical restraints (e.g., sedation with a benzodiazepines) while protecting the airway, rather than physical restraints, may be more beneficial and tolerable by the patient. The practice of "hog-tying" a patient in a prone position in order to "control" them can compromise the airway and cardiovascular status or lead to mechanical-type injuries.

Pregnant patients should be managed in the same manner as nonpregnant patients, with generalized support focused on the mother. In the vast majority of cases, fetal compromise is directly due to maternal illness and therefore the tested axiom "treat the baby by treating the mother" stands true.

Some toxins (e.g., salicylates, methanol, ethylene glycol) are associated with metabolic derangements and can lead to a severe metabolic acidosis. Such patients may benefit from boluses of intravenous fluids, sodium bicarbonate, and (if intubated) hyperventilation to maintain a low-to-normal $PaCO_2$. Contact medical command or a regional poison center for uncertainty surrounding ingestions in pretransport decision making.

Finally, all patients with overt or suspected psychiatric illness require medical evaluation at an emergency department or psychiatric facility. Patients who appear to have had a nontoxic exposure but are actively depressed or suicidal require immediate transport for evaluation. For the prehospital EMS provider, if a suicidal patient refuses transport, medical direction or police should be notified.

Summary

Providing care for a poisoned patient often presents a number of challenges to health care providers. As stated throughout the chapter, the optimal treatment of an overdose or environmental toxin requires the rapid and accurate identification of the medication(s) or toxin(s) involved. Because every patient is unique, a discussion with your regional poison center (1-800-222-1222), medical direction, or a medical toxicologist may help to establish the best treatment approach. During the interfacility transport of these patients by the critical care team, management is still largely supportive of lost function due to the toxic exposure. These interventions include airway skills (to include medication-assisted intubation), ventilatory support, circulatory management by way of IV fluids and vasopressor, and the continued management of lethal dysrhythmias.

Finally, further information on all of these topics can be found in multiple medical toxicology, industrial, or environmental textbooks. If the critical care paramedic finds himself working in an environment where toxicological emergencies are more prevalent, these textbooks could prove to be an invaluable asset to the provider's personal library.

Review Questions

1. What are your general treatment priorities in the toxicologically ill patient?

2. Describe the main routes of exposure for toxic substances, and explain how you would limit the amount of continued toxin absorption for each type of exposure.

3. Describe the general clinical indications that would lead the critical care paramedic to suspect that a patient is experiencing a toxicological emergency.

4. Describe what scene characteristics would lead you to believe your patient is experiencing a toxicological emergency.

5. Why do herbal supplements have a much greater potential for misuse than do prescription drugs?

6. If a patient accidentally takes a toxic dose of a beta-blocking agent, what initial and ongoing treatment regimes should be provided by the critical care paramedic?

7. What are the clinical implications for utilizing a cyanide antidote kit for a toxic exposure?

8. When should a PCC be contacted regarding a toxic exposure, and what type of information will the PCC specialist need prior to offering management techniques?

See Answers to Review Questions at the back of this book.

Further Reading

Auerbach PS. *Wilderness Medicine.* St. Louis, MO: Mosby, 2001.

Balit CR, Lynch CN, Isbister GK. "Bupropion Poisoning: A Case Series." *Medical Journal of Australia,* Vol. 178, No. 2 (2003): 61–63.

Bent S, Ko R. "Commonly Used Herbal Medications in the United States: A Review." *The American Journal of Medicine,* Vol. 116 (2004): 478–485.

Callaway CW, Clark RF. "Hyperthermia in Psychostimulant Overdose." *Annals of Emergency Medicine,* Vol. 24, No. 1 (1994): 68–76.

Chan K. "Some Aspects of Toxic Contaminants in Herbal Medicines." *Chemosphere,* Vol. 52, No. 9 (2003): 1361–1371.

Chyka PA, Seger D. "Position Statement: Single-Dose Activated Charcoal. American Academy of Clinical Toxicology; European Association of Poison Centers and Clinical Toxicologists." *Journal of Toxicology—Clinical Toxicology,* Vol. 35, No. 7 (1997): 721–741.

Curry SC, Vance MV, Ryan PJ, Kunkel DB, Northey WT. "Envenomation by the Scorpion *Centruroides sculpturatus.*" *Journal of Toxicology—Clinical Toxicology,* Vol. 21, No. 4–5 (1983): 417–449.

Ford MD, Delaney KA, Ling LJ, Erickson T. *Clinical Toxicology.* Philadelphia: W. B. Saunders, 2001.

Fugh-Berman A. "Herb–Drug Interactions." *Lancet,* Vol. 355 (2000): 134–138.

Goldfrank LR, Flomenbaum NE, Lewin NA, Howland MA, Hoffman RS, Nelson LS. *Goldfrank's Toxicologic Emergencies.* New York: McGraw-Hill, 2002.

Greenberg MI. *Occupational, Industrial, and Environmental Toxicology.* St. Louis, MO: Mosby, 2003.

Hardy KR, Thom SR. "Pathophysiology and Treatment of Carbon Monoxide Poisoning." *Journal of Toxicology—Clinical Toxicology,* Vol. 32, No. 6 (1994): 613–629.

Heit HA. "Addiction, Physical Dependence, and Tolerance: Precise Definitions to Help Clinicians Evaluate and Treat Chronic Pain Patients." *Journal of Pain and Palliative Care Pharmacotherapy,* Vol. 17, No. 1 (2003): 15–29.

Jelinek G. "Widow Spider Envenomation (Latrodectism): A Worldwide Problem." *Wilderness and Environmental Medicine,* Vol. 8, No. 4 (1997): 226.

Krenzelok EP, McGuigan M, Lheur P. "Position Statement: Ipecac Syrup." *Journal of Toxicology—Clinical Toxicology,* Vol. 35, No. 7 (1997): 699–709.

Olson KR. *Poisoning and Drug Overdose.* New York: McGraw-Hill, 2004.

Palenzona S, Meier PJ, Kupferschmidt H, Rauber-Luethy C. "The Clinical Picture of Olanzapine Poisoning with Special Reference to Fluctuating Mental Status." *Journal of Toxicology—Clinical Toxicology,* Vol. 42, No. 1 (2004): 27–32.

Pizon A, Brooks DE. "Fentanyl Patch Abuse: Naloxone Complications and Extracorporeal Membrane Oxygenation Rescue." *Veterinary and Human Toxicology,* Vol. 46, No. 5 (2004): 256–257.

Sullivan JB, Krieger GR. *Clinical Environmental Health and Toxic Exposures.* Philadelphia: Lippincott Williams & Wilkins, 2001.

Watson WA, Litovitz TL, Klein-Schwartz W, et al. "2003 Annual Report of the American Association of Poison Control Centers Toxic Exposure Surveillance System." *American Journal of Emergency Medicine,* Vol. 22, No. 5 (2004): 335–404.

Weapons of Mass Destruction

Glenn A. Miller, BSAS, NREMT-P, and Brandon W. Graham, BS, Licensed Paramedic

Objectives

Upon completion of this chapter, the student should be able to:

1. Discuss how to ensure personal protection in situations involving weapons of mass destruction. (p. 959)
2. Define CBRNE agents. (p. 962)
3. Describe the concept and importance of decontamination. (p. 963)
4. Describe the characteristics, clinical effects, and critical care interventions for the following chemical agents:
   A. Nerve agents (p. 964)
   B. Pulmonary agents (p. 967)
   C. Cyanide (p. 967)
   D. Vesicants (p. 968)
   E. Incapacitating and irritant agents (p. 970)
5. Describe the characteristics, clinical effects, and critical care interventions for the CDC Category A biological agents:
   A. Bacterial agents
      i. Anthrax (p. 972)
      ii. Plague (p. 973)
      iii. Tularemia (p. 974)

Key Terms

acute radiation syndrome (ARS), p. 980

agents of opportunity, p. 963

anthrax, p. 972

botulinum toxin, p. 977

CBRNE agents, p. 962

incapacitating and irritant agents, p. 970

ionization, p. 979

nerve agents, p. 964

plague, p. 973

pulmonary agents, p. 967

smallpox, p. 975

toxic industrial chemicals (TICs), p. 964

tularemia, p. 974

vesicants, p. 968

viral hemorrhagic fevers (VHFs), p. 975

Case Study

You are drawn to the television news networks as you try to piece together the events of the day. Current national news reports that a small device, disguised as a briefcase, was left in the food court of a shopping mall in a residential community approximately 60 miles away from you. At approximately 10:00 A.M. this morning, the briefcase released an unknown liquid substance onto the floor. It seems that within a matter of minutes several of the customers in the food court began to feel ill, complaining of dizziness, photophobia, rhinorrhea, and mild difficulty breathing. One of the patrons, while attempting to flee the area, apparently slipped in the liquid, falling to the floor and came into direct contact with the substance. Several others went to the aid of this victim and attempted to render care. The fallen patron, lying in the puddle of liquid, lost consciousness within 2 minutes and began to seize. Two of those who were attempting to assist this victim also lost consciousness within minutes. As panic ensued in the mall, the majority of mall patrons self-extricated to the parking lot areas. Many of the victims who were in the food court at the time of this incident got into their personal vehicles and proceeded to go to either of the two community hospitals in the immediate area. On initial arrival of EMS, 15 minutes had elapsed and a full evacuation of the mall had been initiated by the shopping center's security personnel.

The initial EMS crew, acting on the pleas of the witnesses, entered the shopping mall to assess the victims in the food court. Reports indicate that they found seven nonambulatory victims remaining in the food court. Three of the victims appeared to be deceased, two were experiencing active generalized seizure activity, and two were experiencing extreme shortness of breath and muscle fasciculations. The EMS crew made the decision to self-evacuate and await assistance from the fire department and hazardous materials team.

Following their preestablished standard operating guidelines, the fire department donned full turnout gear, SCBAs, and gloves—taping up cuffs and seams with duct tape—and proceeded to make entry into the food court area. Allowing only 3 minutes for their initial recon and recovery efforts, the entry team extricated the only two live victims they located, reporting to EMS command that they located an additional five deceased victims. As the incident progressed, the entry team was decontaminated, the hazardous materials team arrived, and the entire shopping mall was secured and searched. . . . . . . BEEP . . . . . . BEEP . . . . . . BEEP . . . . . . Flight Alert . . . . . . Your tones sound at 1847 hours indicating that it's time to tear yourself away from the news coverage and go on your next flight.

Strangely enough, you soon discover that you are being sent to transport one of the surviving victims of this morning's events. You proceed as directed to one of the community hospitals that received the initial victims from the shopping mall incident. Your patient is located in the ICU, and transport to a larger tertiary facility has been requested. While en route to the sending facility, you receive an update from communications that your patient is unresponsive, intubated, and on a ventilator. On arrival at bedside you learn that the patient was in the food court at the time of the incident, and was one of the two victims removed by the fire department. The patient has no significant past medical history. On arrival, the patient was suffering from acute dyspnea with hypoxia, requiring intubation. The sending facility staff also indicates that the patient suffered a brief generalized seizure approximately 25 minutes after arrival. Since that time, the patient has not regained consciousness. Your physical assessment shows the following:

- Heart rate: 168/min, sinus tachycardia
- Respiratory rate: 16/min
- Blood pressure: 164/104 mmHg
- Temperature: 37.8° C (100.0° F)
- Pulse oximetry: 94%
- Lung sounds: Rhonchi and wheezing bilaterally; diminished bilateral bases
- Heart tones: Slightly rapid, regular, distant
- Continuous IV meds: Atropine at 2 mg/hr
      Midazolam at 2 mg/hr
      D_5W in 0.9% NaCl at 50 mL/hr

Since the patient is sedated and intubated, you note the ventilator settings so you can preset these values into your transport ventilator:

- Vent mode: SIMV
- Demand ventilatory rate: 12/min
- Tidal volume: 800 mL
- Flow rate: 45 L/min
- FiO$_2$ 0.4
- PEEP   10 cm/H$_2$O

You and your partner start the process of moving the patient's medications infusions to your syringe pumps and placing the patient on your transport ventilator. The staff at the sending hospital assures you that adequate decontamination was performed on the patient and that no special personal protective measures are necessary. After completing the preparation of the equipment, the patient is moved to your cot, and the medical records and appropriate transfer documents obtained. You proceed to your aircraft and complete the transport without incident.

INTRODUCTION

Chemical, biological, radiological, nuclear, and explosive agents, often referred to as *Weapons of Mass Destruction,* have received extensive public media and emergency service attention in recent years as potential agents of terrorist use.

Chemical, biological, radiological, nuclear, and explosive (CBRNE) agents, often referred to as *weapons of mass destruction* (WMD), have received extensive public media and emergency service attention in recent years as potential agents of terrorist use. Training programs and textbooks related to the initial response of these potentially catastrophic events have proliferated, and yet very little attention has been paid to the extended care of the individual victims, especially in the critical care transport realm. Although the consequences of an effective use of certain CBRNE agents can be widespread and devastating to a community, the likelihood of isolated incidents affecting just one or a handful of patients is even greater. In this chapter, the critical care paramedic will learn the basics of CBRNE agents, the similarities they have when compared to other more common substances, and appropriate considerations to take during critical care transport of CBRNE agent victims.

The field of CBRNE response has been subject to much fallacy during the past several years. It is often assumed that any use of CBRNE agents will yield mass fatalities and will leave in its wake many victims who will be seriously ill or injured. In addition to this widespread illness and death, other results would include community-wide panic and grave economic losses due to the costs of medical care, decontamination, law enforcement, and loss of commerce. Although it is true that the possibility of such a scenario exists, history has shown that the more likely scenario is a very different picture. Low-fatality, low-impact events are historically much more common, even in situations in which CBRNE agents are intentionally employed. It is the job of the critical care paramedic to weed through the misinformation and understand the individual effects and pathologies of the likely agents. This knowledge, coupled with a solid understanding of physiology, pharmacology, infectious disease processes, and toxicology will prepare the critical care paramedic to effectively and safely provide care during transport of CBRNE victims. During the course of this chapter, it will be assumed that hours, days, or in some cases even weeks have passed since the initial response to the CBRNE event or recognition of the covert use of an agent.

CBRNE agents *defined as chemical, biological, radiological, nuclear, and/or explosive agents or substances that can cause illness or injury to exposed victims.*

CBRNE agents are defined as chemical, biological, radiological, nuclear, and explosive agents or substances that possess the ability to cause illness or injury to exposed victims. In this context, it is typically accepted that these agents will be intentionally disseminated into a target population with the primary goal of inflicting harm on that population. The array of agents varies widely, and includes chemical weapons such as nerve agents and sulfur mustard, industrial chemicals such as cyanide and anhydrous ammonia, bacterial agents such as plague and anthrax, viral agents such as smallpox and Ebola, and radioactive substances. Obviously, the impact of these varied agents will differ greatly from one another, so we will approach the agent classes separately and group them in such a manner as to ease understanding.

Of significant importance as you review this chapter is the realization that the critical care paramedic may very well encounter patients suffering from conditions similar to CBRNE agents even when an intentional dissemination has not occurred. Many of the agents we will discuss are either very similar to, or exactly the same as, other substances or diseases that may be naturally encountered in today's society. Nerve agents, for instance, are nearly identical in structure and effect to the organophosphate pesticides used in agriculture. Chlorine, the first military chemical agent used in modern warfare, is also used for water treatment as well as for numerous other industrial uses. Bubonic plague infections still occur naturally in the southwestern United States, and the pneumonic form of the plague presents in a manner very similar to tuberculosis. Finally, radioactive substances are used in the industrial, research, and medical fields every day. The principles discussed will assist in preparing the critical care paramedic for other emerging threats and diseases that can only be imagined as of today. The treatment modalities employed during the transport of a pneumonic plague, smallpox, or inhalational anthrax victim are likely to be no different than those which may be necessary for a SARS or avian influenza victim. The reality is that victims of exposure to CBRNE agents, or substances similar to them, are likely to require critical care transport regardless of the initial route of exposure or potential that the patient was the victim of an intentional attack using a CBRNE agent.

With the heightened awareness in the post-9/11 era, toxicological and WMD experts now believe that many of the most likely threats of chemical terrorism involve so-called **agents of opportunity.** Both common and unusual industrial agents may pose a considerable threat as potential terrorist weapons. While an understanding of the traditional military chemical weapons (e.g., nerve agents) remains essential, an appreciation of the myriad of other potential toxic chemicals readily available in our society is crucial if we are to optimally prepare for, identify, and defend against chemical threats.

With the heightened awareness in the post-9/11 era, toxicological and WMD experts now believe that many of the most likely threats of chemical terrorism involve so-called agents of opportunity.

agents of opportunity
describes both common and unusual industrial agents, along with a myriad of other potential toxic chemicals, readily available in our society.

PERSONAL PROTECTION

The first priority for the critical care paramedic is the safety of the crew and the patient. And an important component of this priority is the separation of what can be considered operational and clinical issues. From an operational standpoint, the critical care paramedic will not usually, if ever, be involved in the actual rescue of a patient subjected to a CBRNE event. Not until the individual has been safely extricated from the situation by experts and has received appropriate decontamination will he become a clinical patient for the critical care paramedic, who becomes involved during the assessment and management phases.

To ensure that the crew is not exposed to any hazardous substances, any casualty of a CBRNE or toxic industrial chemicals (TIC)/toxic industrial materials (TIM) TIC/TIM incident must be thoroughly decontaminated and must not be a risk for off-gassing. Off-gassing is the emanation of vapor, usually from chemicals trapped in clothing or on the patient's body. In rare cases of toxic substance ingestion, off-gassing may also emanate from the GI or pulmonary tract. For the purposes of this text, it is assumed that the patient has been thoroughly and adequately decontaminated by either the emergency personnel at the scene or the staff of the medical facility to which the patient self-transported. With few exceptions, patients adequately decontaminated during initial care will not pose a threat to the critical care paramedic providing care for the patient during interhospital transport missions. The primary concern of these exceptions is the patient who has ingested or aspirated a hazardous substance that may off-gas through the gastrointestinal or respiratory tracts, respectively. Additionally, there are a small number of toxicants which are so toxic that metabolism and excretion do not alter the chemicals before they are eliminated via exhalation, perspiration, lacrimation, defecation, urination, or vomiting. In these rare instances, the critical care paramedic must wear appropriate chemical protective equipment and treat the patients as though they are still contaminated. Following care of these patients, it is critical to ensure that all personnel, equipment, supplies, and vehicles are free of contamination before being returned to service.

The first priority for the critical care paramedic is the safety of the crew and the patient.

To ensure that the crew is not exposed to any hazardous substances, any casualty of a CBRNE or TIC/TIM incident must be thoroughly decontaminated and must not be a risk for off-gassing.

CHEMICAL AGENTS

Modern chemical weapons (CWs), a side effect of the Industrial Revolution, have widely proliferated since the beginning of the 20th century. Use of chlorine, phosgene, and mustard agent in World War I caused hundreds of thousands of casualties on the battlefields in Europe, and though CWs were not deployed in World War II, the participating countries had enough stockpiled to kill millions of people. Since the end of World War II, there have been few changes to CW agents, because most technological improvements have focused primarily on delivery of the agents. In the 1980s, sarin and mustard agents were used during the Iran–Iraq war, causing widespread casualties against civilian and military targets. Tens of thousands of tons of CWs remain available throughout the world, as some nations attempt to destroy their stockpiles while other nations and groups secretly build their own arsenals.

There are literally thousands of toxic industrial chemicals that could be used as CWs. Even the classic CW agents can be covertly manufactured using the existing chemical infrastructure, domestically or internationally. This production could be accomplished without detection, under the disguise of an operation of legitimate commercial use. The Aum Shinrikyo, a cult in Japan, proved in the 1990s that CWs are no longer solely a military concern when they employed the use of sarin against civilian targets at Matsumoto City and in the Tokyo subway system. Though the number of critical injuries from these incidents was relatively low, scores of patients emerged from these incidents in need of immediate and follow-up critical care. This incident demonstrated the potential for the use of chemicals as weapons against civilian populations.

Military CWs, like all other hazardous materials, may exist as solids, liquids, or gases, depending on the temperature and pressure. When used as weapons, most are disseminated as liquids and aerosols. The clinical effects of CW use are wide ranging and present a challenge to the critical care paramedic who will very rarely, if ever, encounter patients affected by CWs. The critical care team is far more likely to encounter patients injured in an industrial hazardous materials accident or the use of **toxic industrial chemicals (TICs)** otherwise known as toxic industrial materials (TIM) as a weapon than they are to encounter use of a true CW. Though these industrial chemicals are less toxic than CWs, the sheer volume of quantities available makes them an effective potential weapon. Nearly 1 million businesses in the United States use, store, or produce hazardous materials, and there are more than 100 individual sites in the United States that each have the volume of TICs needed to kill or severely injure more than 1 million people. To address both military CWs and TICs, this text will concentrate on key similarities in these agents and on groups of clinical syndromes that are likely to be encountered as a result of incidents ranging from a small hazardous materials spill to a large-scale CW attack on an urban target.

NERVE AGENTS

CWs or industrial chemicals that affect the ability of the nervous system to function properly by inhibiting acetylcholinesterase (AChE) are referred to as **nerve agents.** Classic military nerve agents such as tabun (GA), sarin (GB), soman (GD), cyclosarin (GF), and the very persistent V nerve agents, such as VX, are all extremely potent agents that are lethal in very small doses. For the critical care paramedic, however, long-term management of nerve agent casualties will differ very little from the clinical management of patients affected by an exposure to organophosphate or carbamate pesticides. To understand the management of these patients, it is critical that the provider understand the basic pathophysiology of these agents related to the nervous system. (See Figure 33-1 ■.)

Acetylcholine (ACh) is a neurotransmitter that has its effects on the nicotinic and muscarinic receptors within the nervous system. Nicotinic receptors are responsible for skeletal muscle movement, while muscarinic receptors control, among other things, the function of glands and the smooth muscles of the gut. Acetylcholinesterase is the enzyme that performs the deactivation and breakdown of this neurotransmitter after it has performed its function. Agents in this class cause a disturbance in normal neural activity, as discussed next.

During a nerve impulse, ACh leaves the presynaptic neuron and crosses the synaptic cleft to the postsynaptic cholinergic receptor site. Binding of the ACh to this site results in the transmission of

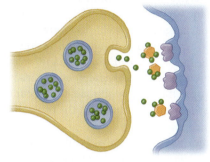

Acetylcholine crossing
synapse

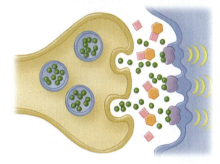

Acetylcholine binding to receptor
initiating postsynaptic transmission

Cholinesterase binding to
acetylcholine

Cholinesterase inactivated due to
binding with nerve agent

■ **Figure 33-1** Nerve agent at the neuromuscular junction.

the appropriate neural impulse. Under normal conditions, AChE, which is resident on the postsynaptic membrane, breaks down ACh into acetic acid and choline. This degradation process removes the ACh from the receptor site, thereby ceasing transmission of the neural impulse and resetting the cholinergic receptor to its prestimulated condition. ACh is immediately regenerated and prepared for the next signal transmission opportunity.

Organophosphorous compounds, such as nerve agents, bind with the AChE, rendering it unable to function. This reduces the body's ability to deactivate and degrade the ACh in the synapse. This excess ACh then remains in the synaptic cleft and continues to interact with the cholinergic receptor, resulting in a constant, uncontrolled stimulation of the receptor site.

If this binding of the nerve agent to the AChE is not reversed through timely treatment, a process known as "aging" can occur. Aging is a biochemical process that results in a permanent binding of the nerve agent to the AChE, refractory to all clinical intervention attempts. Once aging occurs, the AChE is rendered permanently useless, and the clinical effects of the resultant ACh overstimulation will remain until new AChE enzyme is produced. The aging time for CW nerve agents is relatively short. In fact, in the case of soman (GD), aging can occur in as little as 2–6 minutes. The approximate aging times for the other military CW agents are:

★ GA (tabun)—14 hours

★ GB (sarin)—5 hours

★ VX—48 hours

The aging process represents an important difference between organophosphate compounds (including nerve agents) and carbamate pesticides. Organophosphate pesticides, for instance, function in a similar manner to the military nerve agents, and aging will occur at rates that vary depending on the specific pesticide used. With carbamate casualties, however, AChE aging does not ever completely occur and the effects are almost always reversible.

Significant exposure to organophosphorous compounds, such as nerve agents, results in clinical effects associated with the resultant uncontrolled stimulation of the smooth muscles, the skeletal muscles, the CNS, and the exocrine glands. The patient will exhibit signs of increased

Significant exposure to organophosphorous compounds, such as nerve agents, results in clinical effects associated with the resultant uncontrolled stimulation of the smooth muscles, the skeletal muscles, the CNS, and the exocrine glands.

perspiration, miosis, lacrimation, rhinorrhea, increased salivation/drooling, bronchorrhea, bronchoconstriction, and associated respiratory distress, nausea, vomiting, diarrhea, skeletal muscular fasciculation, and altered level of consciousness. Patients exposed to higher doses of the substance will experience more significant CNS effects, including loss of consciousness, seizures, and respiratory arrest. Close attention to airway maintenance and ventilatory support during the treatment of these severe cases is paramount.

The treatment of patients with significant exposure to organophosphorous compounds will be aimed primarily at airway maintenance and prevention of ACh receptor site overstimulation. During the emergency care immediately following exposure, it is likely that the patient will have received advanced airway management, atropine sulfate, pralidoxime chloride (2-PamCl), and diazepam. (See Figure 33-2 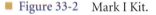.) Atropine is given to competitively inhibit the effects of the uncontrolled ACh effects at the receptor site. While atropine is very effective in reducing the muscarinic effects of organophosphate toxicity, it is less effective on the nicotinic effects. 2-PamCl, an oxime, can be effective in breaking the bond between the nerve agent and the AChE, which effectively reactivates it for use again. Once this bond is broken, the AChE is able to return to its normal function of hydrolyzing ACh. Oxime therapy should be initiated within the first 48 hours following the exposure, but will not be effective once aging has occurred. Diazepam, and/or other benzodiazepines, may be administered to control seizure activity. Benzodiazepines may also be effective in reducing the long-term CNS effects that result from the hypoxic episodes that occur during seizure activity. Clinicians should be prepared to treat for seizures throughout the treatment of the nerve agent patient.

If aging has occurred, then the use of oximes will be ineffective. In these cases, it will likely be necessary to maintain a therapeutic dose of atropine for a prolonged period of time, until new AChE is generated. This has specific implications for the critical care paramedic, because repeated atropine boluses or a continuous atropine infusion may be required during transport. The dose of atropine in these cases is based on clinical presentation, but may be as high as 2.0 mg IV every 5–15 minutes. If atropine is administered as a continuous intravenous infusion, the dosage should be titrated primarily to control the patient's respiratory secretions and ease of ventilation. Although less important, heart rate should be maintained at no higher than 100 bpm. Extreme cases of exposure to organophosphorous compounds, especially when ingestion of commercial pesticides has occurred, may result in the need for IV dosages as high as 5 mg every 10 minutes for the first 24 hours. In these cases, atropine infusions may need to be continued for several weeks, with doses ranging from 0.5–2.4 mg/kg/hr. Other than the pharmacologic therapies indicated earlier, the remainder of the treatment for nerve agent exposures is supportive in nature. It is possible that a pa-

■ Figure 33-2 Mark I Kit.

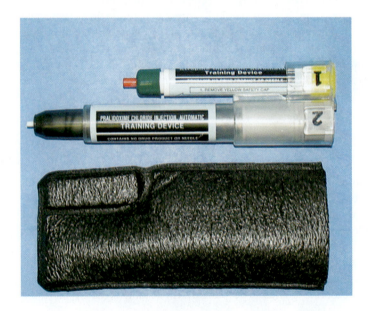

tient who survives a significant organophosphorous compound exposure may be ventilator dependent for a prolonged period of time.

PULMONARY AGENTS

Pulmonary agents, such as chlorine and phosgene, were first used as weapons during World War I. In fact, these agents were used extensively during this conflict, and accounted for 80% of the war's chemical casualties. Many of these chemicals also have multiple industrial uses, and they are currently mass produced and mass transported worldwide. Due to the fact that large quantities of these chemicals may be so easily found in our society, their potential for accidental release or intentional use as a weapon is very high.

Pulmonary agents are commonly distributed as a vapor, and may be lethal in relatively low concentrations since they can be readily absorbed across pulmonary tissue. Chlorine, for example, is considered to be immediately dangerous to life or health (IDLH) in concentrations as low as 1.0 part per million (ppm). The degree of injury that a pulmonary agent casualty receives is based on the concentration, solubility, and reactivity of the specific chemical involved. As the chemical vapor enters the respiratory system, it reacts with the water present in the respiratory tract, causing direct damage to the affected structures.

Chlorine, for instance, rapidly reacts with water to form both hypochlorous and hydrochloric acids. As it is inhaled, it immediately reacts with the moisture in the tissues of the airway, resulting in chemical burns caused by the acid formation. In lower concentrations, most of the chlorine reaction will occur in the upper airways, causing damage to the nasopharynx, oropharynx, and trachea. In higher concentrations, however, chlorine may cause damage to both the upper and lower airways—causing not only upper airway damage, but also extensive damage to the structures of the central and peripheral airways, including the bronchi, bronchioles, and alveoli. Direct damage to the alveoli may cause an increase in pulmonary capillary permeability, allowing fluid to enter the alveoli and resulting in the development of noncardiogenic pulmonary edema. Depending on the severity of exposure, onset of this condition can occur within minutes to hours.

Phosgene, in comparison, causes similar sequelae to the alveolar-capillary membrane. The chemical reaction converting phosgene to hydrochloric acid, however, is much slower. Onset of airway and respiratory symptoms in phosgene casualties, therefore, is likely to be delayed when compared to those exposed to chlorine.

It is likely that clinical management by the critical care paramedic will be the same regardless of the specific pulmonary agent involved. Advanced airway and ventilatory management are of paramount importance. The need to perform frequent tracheal suctioning, in order to remove upper airway secretions and mucosal tissue that has sloughed off, is common. Supplemental oxygen should be administered in order to maintain an SpO_2 of greater than 95%. Additionally, in patients experiencing pulmonary edema, strict fluid management should be considered. Ventilatory support is commonly required, often while maintaining increased positive end-expiratory pressure (PEEP). Because this pulmonary edema is noncardiogenic in nature, the use of diuretics is typically considered to be contraindicated.

Treatment of bronchospasm may include administration of beta-2 specific bronchodilators such as albuterol or metaproterenol. Aerosolized terbutaline has also been demonstrated to yield benefits in these patients. If administered early in treatment, corticosteroids may also have the effect of preventing short-term airway inflammation. Though it is very common for pulmonary agent casualties to present with bacterial infections 3–5 days following the exposure, empiric use of antibiotics is not recommended.

CYANIDE

Cyanide exposure can occur from a variety of sources including smoke inhalation from residential or industrial fires. Cyanide compounds also have many industrial and commercial applications, and are used in the metal industry, mining, electroplating processes, and during X-ray film recovery. In

pulmonary agents
chemicals that can be readily absorbed across pulmonary tissue; commonly released as a vapor and may be lethal in relatively low concentrations.

Due to the fact that large quantities of these chemicals may be so easily found in our society, their potential for accidental release or intentional use as a weapon is very high.

Cyanide exposure can occur from a variety of sources including smoke inhalation from residential or industrial fires.

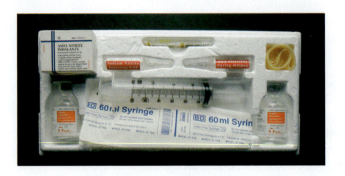

■ **Figure 33-3** Cyanide antidote kit. *(© Jeff Forster)*

addition, cyanide has also been developed and used as a battlefield CW. There are many forms of cyanide, including gaseous hydrogen cyanide (HCN or AC) and numerous cyanide salts. Cyanogen compounds, such as cyanogen chloride (CK), may also release cyanide during metabolism following entry into the body.

Cyanide affects almost every body tissue by inactivating cellular enzymes necessary for normal aerobic metabolism. This results in a disruption of cellular respiration within the mitochondria, despite the presence of adequate oxygen levels. As a result, the cells can no longer produce adenosine triphosphate (ATP), and all biochemical processes depending on ATP cease to function. The resulting anaerobic cellular respiration will produce severe lactic acidosis. Widespread cellular degradation leads to tissue and organ failure, which will ultimately result in death.

Clinical effects progress quite rapidly following a significant exposure to cyanide, potentially culminating in death in less than 10 minutes. Most of the clinical signs are a result of the effects of cellular asphyxiation in the central nervous system. Patients will initially present as tachypneic, hypertensive, and tachycardic. With a large dose or continued exposure, these signs may progress quickly to seizures, respiratory arrest, and cardiac arrest.

If rapidly removed from the environment, cyanide inhalation casualties who do not exhibit immediate signs of toxicity will most likely recover without intervention. Because the body systems are normally able to metabolize and eliminate low cyanide concentrations, patients have the ability to naturally combat and survive low-concentration exposures. In the event of higher dose exposure, immediate emergency medical care will be required to effectively reverse cyanide toxicity.

Cyanide antidote kits are available to treat acute exposures to cyanide. They typically consist of 0.3 cc/kg of a 3% sodium nitrite solution, which is administered via slow IV push (maximum 10 cc), and 12.5 g of sodium thiosulfate, which is given as a very slow IV push over 10 minutes. The sodium nitrite is given in order to convert hemoglobin into methemoglobin. The cyanide in the affected cells is strongly attracted to methemoglobin, which irreversibly binds the cyanide to form a compound known as cyanmethemoglobin. Sodium thiosulfate is then administered, reacting with the newly formed cyanmethemoglobin to form thiocyanate, which is then excreted by the kidneys. Other pharmacologic agents have also proven effective in combating cyanide toxicity. In Europe, there has been widely documented success with the use of hydroxocobalamin and dicobalt EDTA as cyanide antidotes. Figure 33-3 ■ shows one such antidote kit.

Despite successful emergency care of the cyanide victim, a significant lactic acidosis may still occur. This is the result of anaerobic cellular respiration and may require follow-up administration of sodium bicarbonate to correct an acid–base imbalance. The critical transport phase for these patients will consist of standard supportive measures including the continuation of sodium thiosulfate, ventilator management, and the treatment of acid–base disorders.

VESICANTS

vesicants *potentially lethal chemical agents that cause severe blistering of human and animal tissue, both internally and externally (i.e., "sulfur mustard").*

Vesicants, the most well known of which is sulfur mustard, are blister-producing substances. Chemicals of this class have posed a military threat since their battlefield introduction during World War I, and more recently were used in the 1980s during the Iran–Iraq war. The vesicants include both mustard agents and lewisite (L). Phosgene oxime (CX) is also typically classified as a vesicant, although it is actually a corrosive urticant agent.

Vesicants pose not only a potential military threat, but also may be a threat to civilian populations. Because they are relatively easy to synthesize and manufacture, they are a likely choice for groups that decide to develop a capacity for CWs. Vesicants may be delivered by a variety of methods including liquid spray or aerosolization. They represent both a vapor and a liquid threat to all exposed skin and mucous membranes.

The effects of mustard agents are delayed, appearing hours after exposure. Lewisite's and phosgene oxime's effects, however, will be observed almost immediately. The organs most commonly affected by vesicants are the skin, eyes, and airways. Common signs seen following exposure are erythema, large vesicles, conjunctivitis, and respiratory distress. Significant exposure to the respiratory system may lead to necrotic hemorrhage of the airway mucosa and tissues.

MUSTARD

During exposure to mustard, the agent penetrates the skin and distributes to other tissues of the body. Within minutes of exposure, the mustard agent forms a highly reactive substance that binds to DNA, RNA, and proteins, causing cellular damage. Despite the speed of its damage, clinical effects are not typically observed for several hours. Commonly, these effects are seen within 4 to 6 hours, but can be delayed for as much as 48 hours. At high doses, systemic mustard distribution can affect the kidneys, liver, intestines, and lungs and also damage the bone marrow precursor cells, which can lead to significant compromise of the immune system. The GI tract may also be damaged by vesicants, resulting in severe vomiting and diarrhea.

There is no specific treatment or antidote for mustard casualties. Treatment of these casualties is largely supportive and symptomatic. The most common clinical effect of mustard exposure is eye damage. If this occurs, it is critical to maintain ophthalmic moisture. The skin damage caused by these agents will also leave these patients prone to secondary infection. Prophylactic antibiotics are often administered following exposure to prevent this occurrence. In addition to systemic antibiotics, topical antibiotics may be applied to the vesicles and erythematous areas of the skin, and ophthalmic antibiotics may also be considered. Patients will require frequent flushing of the wounds and occasionally debridement of damaged skin. Fluid replacement therapy should be administered to maintain normal hemodynamic status. Aggressive analgesia is also often considered. Figure 33-4 ■ shows the cutaneous effects of mustard gas during military conflict.

In the presence of inhaled mustard vapor, significant damage to the epithelial lining of the airway may occur. This will result in significant respiratory distress and the need for the critical care paramedic to more aggressively manage the patient's airway. Bronchodilators may be administered to correct any bronchoconstriction that may occur.

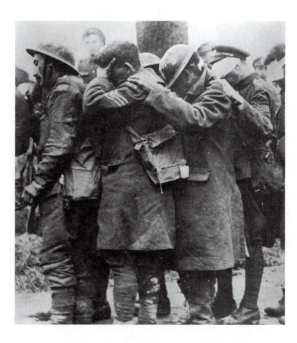

■ Figure 33-4 British casualties blinded by mustard gas in a German attack at Bethune, France. *(Getty Images, Inc.—Hulton Archive Photos)*

🗝⊸ ───────

Vesicants pose not only a potential military threat, but also may be a threat to civilian populations. Because they are relatively easy to synthesize and manufacture, they are a likely choice for groups that decide to develop a capacity for CWs.

LEWISITE

Lewisite exposure will result in many of the same clinical features as mustard exposure. The most important difference is that lewisite will produce immediate severe pain to exposed areas. In large doses, lewisite is also capable of causing an increase in the permeability of systemic capillary beds. This may result in significant intravascular fluid loss that may develop into hypovolemic shock. Lewisite exposure also may lead to hepatic or renal necrosis, and is typically characterized by more prominent GI effects than mustard exposure. However, unlike the mustard agents, lewisite does not cause immunosuppression.

A specific antidote for lewisite exposure exists. British anti-lewisite (Dimercaprol), also known as BAL, has demonstrated usefulness in treating lewisite exposure. For acute exposure, BAL is administered as an IM injection of 0.04 cc/kg (up to 4 cc) of a 10% solution in oil. This dose may be repeated up to three times in 4-hour intervals. BAL is, however, available in extremely limited quantities across the United States. Otherwise, treatment for lewisite exposure is supportive and aimed at patient comfort and maintenance of normal hemodynamic status.

PHOSGENE OXIME

The urticant phosgene oxime will also cause immediate signs and symptoms, because it is corrosive to the skin, eyes, and respiratory tract. The clinical signs and symptoms of phosgene oxime exposure will not differ greatly from that of mustard. The key difference is that, rather than blister formation, phosgene oxime casualties will report immediate pain on contact with spontaneous blanching of the skin. This is followed by the development of an erythematous ring within the first minute of exposure. Wheals commonly form within the first hour of exposure, and the associated extreme pain may persist for days after the exposure. No specific antidotes are known, and treatment is supportive.

INCAPACITATING AND IRRITANT AGENTS

incacitating and irritant agents *chemical agents that produce transient pain and involuntary eye closures, incapacitating the exposed patient for short periods of time.*

In some forms, **incapacitating and irritant agents** are commonly employed throughout society for both defensive and law enforcement purposes. Agents within this category include the tear gases known formally as chlorobenzylidenemalononitrile (CS) and chloroacetophenone (CN), and common pepper spray, which is oleoresin capsicum (OC). These substances produce transient local pain and involuntary eye closure that can render the exposed patient temporarily incapable of normal activity. Law enforcement agencies commonly use these agents for riot control, barricade situations, or to control violent subjects. These agents cause immediate pain and burning sensation of exposed mucous membranes and skin. Clinical effects occur almost immediately following exposure, but seldom persist longer than a few minutes after exposure has ended. Although unlikely, bronchospasm is a concern following exposure to these types of agents. Acute exacerbation of preexisting reactive airway disease may occur. In these cases, bronchoconstriction is usually transient when treated with bronchodilating agents. For these reasons, it is very unlikely that the critical care paramedic will encounter patients needing specific care related to exposure to an incapacitating agent.

BIOLOGICAL AGENTS

Biological agents include any living organism or toxin that can be developed for use to cause illness or death in a population.

Biological agents include any living organism or toxin that can be developed for use to cause illness or death in a population. Because many of the agents historically developed for use as biological weapons are also naturally occurring, it is important that the critical care paramedic be prepared to care for victims of these illnesses. Biological weapons (BWs) distinguish themselves as a lucrative tool in the arsenal of terror groups for several reasons. They can be utilized in a low-profile manner, some are communicable and therefore have the potential to cause a high yield of casualties, and some agents are relatively easy to obtain. Agents can be used alone, or several different agents can be used simultaneously to make a combined biological weapon. Important variables used to distinguish biological agents as potential weapons include communicability, survivability in the environment, the infectious dose, and the nature of the disease itself.

Biological weapons are relatively inexpensive and simple to produce. Although the most sophisticated and effective versions of these BW systems require highly developed expertise and expensive equipment, countless recipes and techniques are widely available that allow the general public enough information to potentially create crude, but operational, BW systems in a discrete location with nominal equipment and training. Although these groups may develop BW with varying levels of refinement and quality, even an ineffective distribution can potentially cause great stress on health care and public safety systems. An additional attractive feature of BW use is that smaller-scale BW events, perhaps using common naturally occurring disease organisms, may be overlooked as a natural epidemic. Often, the clinical effects of a BW attack are not realized for days, which affords terrorists time to distance themselves from the scene and any focal point of the initial investigation. This also provides a small group or individual with the opportunity to affect a large geographic area prior to detection.

The continuum of possible bioterrorism situations ranges from "white powder" hoaxes, to the use of small quantities of an agent by an individual or small group, to state-sponsored terrorism or military BW agent tactics aimed at producing mass casualties. Any successful use of BW agents against a population will present unique challenges to society and its health care systems.

There are widespread incidents of BW use throughout world history, including the intentional poisoning of food, water, and textiles with communicable diseases such as plague and smallpox. During the last century, the development of BWs has become a very sophisticated science, and BWs are a real threat to public health. Several countries are suspected of having technically proficient offensive BW programs. In 1994, a sect of the Aum Shinrikyo cult attempted, on several occasions, to release an aerosolized form of anthrax from rooftops in Tokyo, Japan. No casualties resulted from the Aum's attempts at bioterrorism, but the cult demonstrated that it is possible to release a biological agent in an urban environment with potentially disastrous consequences. One year later, two members of a militia group in Minnesota were convicted of possessing the toxin ricin, which they claimed to be producing for use against local government officials.

During the months of September through November 2001, there were 23 cases of terrorism-related anthrax releases in the United States, in an event that is now known as "Amerithrax." Postal workers in New Jersey and Washington, D.C., and members of the media in New York and Florida fell victim to inhalational anthrax when they came into contact with the contents of letters tainted with the deadly organism. Amerithrax incidents resulted in the potential exposure of more than 32,000 people, all of whom received antibiotic prophylaxis.

A significant number of biological agents have the potential for terrorist use. As stated previously, the Centers for Disease Control and Prevention (CDC) has placed many of the potential biological agents into categories based on their likelihood of usage and potential impact if effectively disseminated in a civilian population. This categorization allows us to focus on the more likely of the potential threat agents. As such, most of this section will focus on discussion of the CDC Category A agents. The critical care paramedic must always remember, however, that a number of agents exist that could be encountered which are not discussed within the limits of this section. Regardless of the specific disease process or agent used, the principles of patient care and personal protection are similar for nearly all of the known possible agents. We will begin with a review of the CDC Category A bacterial, viral, and toxin threats (which can be reviewed in Table 33–1).

There are widespread incidents of BW use throughout world history, including the intentional poisoning of food, water, and textiles with communicable diseases such as plague and smallpox.

BACTERIAL AGENTS

Bacteria are, by definition, microscopic free-living organisms that contain all of the requisite machinery to exist independently in the environment. They surround us everyday, and in fact are even present on the very pages that you hold in your hands as you are reading these words. As you are surely already aware, most bacteria pose little threat to humans; however, many common diseases and infections are caused by bacteria. Fortunately, most of the bacterially produced diseases respond to antibiotic therapy. Several bacterial agents have been specifically identified as potential biological weapon agents in the past, and many are still considered possible threats to this day.

Table 33–1	Critical Biological Agent Categories for Public Health Preparedness

Biological Agent(s)	Disease
Category A	
Variola major	Smallpox
Bacillus anthracis	Anthrax
Yersinia pestis	Plague
Clostridium botulinum (botulinum toxins)	Botulism
Francisella tularensis	Tularemia
Filoviruses and Arenaviruses (e.g., *Ebola virus, Lassa virus*)	Viral hemorrhagic fevers
Category B	
Coxiella burnetii	Q fever
Brucella spp.	Brucellosis
Burkholderia mallei	Glanders
Burkholderia pseudomallei	Melioidosis
Alphaviruses (VEE, EEE, WEE[a])	Encephalitis
Rickettsia prowazekii	Typhus fever
Toxins (e.g., Ricin, Staphylococcal enterotoxin B)	Toxic syndromes
Chlamydia psittaci	Psittacosis
Food safety threats (e.g., *Salmonella spp., Escherichia coli* O157:H7)	
Water safety threats (e.g., *Vibrio cholerae, Cryptosporidium parvum*)	
Category C	
Emerging threat agents (e.g., *Nipah virus*, hantavirus)	

[a]Venezuelan equine (VEE), eastern equine (EEE), and western equine encephalomyelitis (WEE) viruses

ANTHRAX

anthrax *caused by the* Bacillus anthracis *bacterium, anthrax manifests itself in three syndromes described as cutaneous, gastrointestinal, and inhalational, depending upon location or method of exposure.*

Anthrax is caused by a bacterium known as *Bacillus anthracis,* and can manifest itself in any of three different syndromes depending on where the exposure and subsequent infection has occurred in the body. These three potential presentations of anthrax infection are known as the cutaneous, gastrointestinal, and inhalational forms. As mentioned in the introduction, the Amerithrax incidents of 2001 were all manifestations of either the inhalational or cutaneous forms of the disease.

Cutaneous anthrax occurs when the bacteria breech the skin barrier. It is characterized by sores or blisters that form at the site of inoculation, typically on the hands or forearms, often associated with fever and malaise. Historically, this was caused by exposure to the contaminated wool, hides, or tissues of infected cattle, sheep, or goats. Although the cutaneous form of anthrax may progress to cause systemic septicemia, typically this form is successfully treated with antibiotics. Although unlikely, direct contact with the lesions may result in dermal contamination and subsequent secondary infection, making use of standard infection controls and precautions of paramount importance. Untreated cutaneous anthrax can have a mortality rate of up to 25%; however, aggressive antibiotic therapy will decrease this mortality rate to less than 1%.

Gastrointestinal anthrax is rare in humans, and is typically caused by the ingestion of meat from an infected animal. It presents with nausea, vomiting, and fever, which may be followed by severe abdominal pain with hematemesis, ascites, and diarrhea. Some cases may present with associated oropharyngeal lesions and sore throat. Systemic symptoms may include fever, chills, and malaise. Mortality is approximately 50% despite aggressive supportive care and antibiotic therapy. Gastrointestinal anthrax is not considered to be transmissible from person to person; however, strict use of Standard Precautions is still recommended. Critical care transport of gastrointestinal anthrax victims may include the need for fluid replacement therapy and vasopressors as well as management of various intravenous antibiotics as described at the end of this section.

Inhalational anthrax occurs when anthrax spores are inhaled. It is extremely uncommon, and is the form of anthrax that caused all of the deaths associated with the 2001 Amerithrax cases. This form is characterized by malaise, fatigue, myalgia, and fever, followed by nonproductive cough and mild chest discomfort persisting for 2 or 3 days. There may be a short phase of symptom improvement, a prodromal phase, before the patient experiences an acute onset of increasing respiratory distress with dyspnea, stridor, cyanosis, increased chest pain, and diaphoresis, sometimes associated with edema of the chest and neck. The disease can progress very rapidly, often resulting in the rapid onset of shock and death within 24 to 36 hours. Meningitis may be associated with up to 50% of the inhalational cases, causing an initial presentation of seizures. It was previously thought that mortality rates were likely to be as high as 100% despite appropriate treatment; however, early diagnosis followed by aggressive antibiotic therapy and supportive care has proven to be somewhat effective in lowering mortality to much lower rates. In fact, 6 of the 11 Amerithrax inhalational anthrax victims were successfully treated using this aggressive approach.

Like victims of the gastrointestinal form, these patients may require critical care transport. Multiple intravenous antibiotics, corticosteroids, chest tubes, and ventilators are likely to be encountered, as well as any of a number of other interventions and medications as described throughout this text. It is also important to note that, like the gastrointestinal form, inhalational anthrax is not considered to be communicable; however, Standard Precautions are certainly still strongly recommended.

Transport care is supportive in nature, and may include such things as intravenous hydration or vasopressors for shock, supplemental oxygen, invasive monitoring, and ventilator usage. Many different antibiotics have been used in the treatment of anthrax infections. The critical care paramedic may encounter ciprofloxacin, doxycycline, penicillin derivatives, rifampin, tetracycline, vancomycin, and clindamycin. Antibiotic treatment will be initiated on all patients considered to be infected. A decision regarding specific therapy is typically made after antibiotic susceptibility testing is performed. It will be the responsibility of the transport team to ensure familiarity with and understanding of the specific pharmacologic agents being used during transport.

PLAGUE

Plague is caused by the bacteria *Yersinia pestis,* and is probably best known as the causative agent of the "Black Death" of 14th-century Europe. The disease presents in two primary forms: bubonic and pneumonic plague. Plague is a naturally occurring disease, and is still endemic to certain portions of the United States to this day. In fact, in North America plague is found from the Pacific Coast eastward to the western Great Plains and from British Columbia and Alberta, Canada, southward to Mexico. Bubonic plague is the most common form of the disease, and is typically transmitted to humans from the bite of infected fleas. These fleas also feed from animal populations such as rats, mice, ground squirrels, prairie dogs, and even domestic cats. These animal populations serve as a reservoir for the disease.

plague *caused by the bacteria* Yersinia pestis. *The bubonic form presents as abrupt onset of high fever, headache, and painful, swollen regional lymph nodes. The pneumonic (and highly contagious) form presents with additional respiratory symptoms.*

Forms of Plague

Bubonic plague is characterized by the abrupt onset of high fever and headache, followed by the development of painful, swollen regional lymph nodes known as *buboes.* If untreated, the bubonic form can lead to bacteremia, which can eventually progress to the stage of full systemic septicemia. This septicemic form of the disease is sometimes known as *septicemic plague.* Although septicemic plague is not considered transmissible, patients with septicemic plague may develop a secondary pneumonic plague. Patients with pneumonic plague are considered communicable. Unfortunately, it may be difficult to know exactly when pneumonic plague has developed, so all patients with septicemic plague should be considered communicable and appropriate personal protective equipment should be used and respiratory isolation strictly followed.

Pneumonic plague typically presents with high fever, cough, chills, chest pain, and hemoptysis, and it appears clinically similar to a pneumonia or acute tuberculosis. Without treatment the disease may progress to complete respiratory failure and have a mortality near 100%. Even with treatment, pneumonic plague carries with it a mortality rate as high as 50%. When caring for a possible pneumonic plague victim, respiratory droplet precautions, including the use of a mask for patient care, are imperative. These patients may have coughs that can produce infectious particle droplets, allowing transmission of the disease in a manner similar to that of common influenza.

Transport care is supportive in nature, and may include such things as intravenous hydration, supplemental oxygen, invasive monitoring, and ventilator management. Because plague infection is bacterial in nature, antibiotic therapy is likely to be encountered by the critical care paramedic who may come in contact with these patients. Antibiotic choices to treat the infection may include gentamicin, streptomycin, tetracyclines, chloramphenicol, or doxycycline. Again, it is the responsibility of the transport team to ensure familiarity with and understanding of the specific pharmacologic agents being used during transport.

TULAREMIA

tularemia *a bacterial disease caused by* Francisella tularensis: *one of the most infective agents known on earth, it requires as few as ten organisms to cause disease.*

The last of the CDC Category A bacterial agents is **tularemia,** which is caused by the bacteria *Francisella tularensis.* Tularemia is endemic to the majority of the Northern Hemisphere, and within the United States has been reported in every state except Hawaii. It exists in a wide variety of animal and arthropod hosts, the most notable of which are ticks, rabbits, hares, mice, and squirrels. Tularemia is one of the most infective agents known, requiring as few as 10 organisms to cause disease. This is in sharp contrast with the 8,000 to 10,000 anthrax spores typically required to cause a case of inhalational anthrax. Like all of the other bacterial agents mentioned thus far, the clinical presentation of this disease varies depending on the portal of entry and specific organ system infected. Tularemia therefore may present in several different forms: ulceroglandular, oculoglandular, pneumonic, and typhoidal (septicemic). Regardless of form, typical symptoms of infection with tularemia include abrupt onset of fever, chills, rigors, myalgia, cough, and headache.

Forms of Tularemia

Tularemia is usually introduced through breaks in the skin, or through the mucous membranes of the eye or mouth. When this occurs, the accompanying disease process is referred to as ulceroglandular tularemia. This form of the disease is characterized by the formation of a lesion at the site of exposure, either on the skin or mucous membranes (including the conjunctiva; known as oculoglandular tularemia), associated with enlargement of associated regional lymph nodes.

Although less common, tularemia can also be contracted through primary inoculation of the respiratory tract. In these cases, the disease process is referred to as pneumonic tularemia. These patients typically present in a manner similar to pneumonia, with either a dry or mildly productive cough, and less commonly with pleuritic chest pain, shortness of breath, or hemoptysis.

All forms of tularemia infection can progress to the typhoidal (septicemic) tularemia. This systemic infection may also present without an ulcerative phase.

Tularemia is not considered contagious, so patients need not be isolated, although Universal Precautions are advised.

Primary treatment concerns for the critical care paramedic include supportive care and antibiotic therapy. Streptomycin is generally considered to be the drug of choice, although ciprofloxacin, gentamicin, chloramphenicol, or tetracycline may also be used. Other supportive care measures are likely to include ventilator support and hydration. With appropriate treatment, tularemia has an overall mortality rate of approximately 1% to 2.5%.

VIRAL AGENTS

Viruses are much smaller than bacteria and, due to the fact that they do not possess the cellular machinery necessary to live and reproduce independently, require a host in order to reproduce and cause infection. They function as intracellular parasites, using the cellular machinery of their target cells to reproduce. The stability of viruses in the ambient environment varies.

Diseases caused by viral agents do not respond to antibiotic therapy. Therefore, care is typically limited during transport to supportive measures. Like bacterial agents, several viral agents have been specifically identified as possible biological weapons.

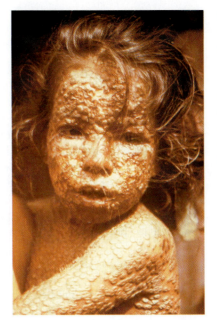

■ **Figure 33-5** A young girl in Bangladesh shows the typical raised bumps of the smallpox infection, which she contracted in 1973. In 1977, the World Health Organization announced that smallpox, a potentially fatal disease, had been eradicated from the country. *(CDC/Phil, CORBIS-NY)*

SMALLPOX

The first of the CDC Category A viral agents is **smallpox,** which is caused by the *variola* virus. Although the fully developed cutaneous eruption of smallpox is quite unique and identifiable, earlier stages of the rash could be mistaken for *varicella* (chickenpox). The incubation period for smallpox ranges from 7 to 17 days. Patients will initially present with malaise, fever, rigors, vomiting, headache, and backache. Two to 4 days later, a discrete rash will begin to appear about the face and extremities. The rash then spreads centrally to the trunk; however, lesions will still be found in higher concentrations on the extremities and face. This centrifugal distribution is an important diagnostic feature of smallpox. The lesions also develop synchronously, with all of the lesions appearing in the same stage of development at the same time. This is directly in contrast with *varicella* infection (chickenpox), where the lesions concentrate primarily on the trunk of the body (centripetally) and develop asynchronously, with some lesions healing as new ones are just developing. Figure 33-5 ■ illustrates what smallpox lesions typically look like.

Smallpox is considered to be highly contagious, and is spread primarily through direct contact with patient body fluids. Respiratory droplet transmission, however, has been known to occur. Therefore, strict contact and respiratory isolation practices should always be followed. Patients are considered contagious until all scabs separate. The mortality of smallpox in unvaccinated patients is approximately 30%.

Management of the smallpox victim during critical care transport primarily consists of supportive care measures. Antibiotic therapy may be instituted in an effort to combat secondary infections. In addition, the use of antiviral agents, such as Cidofovir, may be considered. The critical care team is responsible for ensuring familiarity with and understanding of any pharmacologic agents being used during transport.

smallpox *a manifestation of the usually lethal* variola *virus, this disease presents with malaise, fever, rigors, vomiting, headache, backache and a subsequent discrete rash that spreads from the face and extremities to the entire body.*

VIRAL HEMORRHAGIC FEVERS

The **viral hemorrhagic fevers** (**VHFs**) are a diverse group of illnesses caused by a multitude of different viruses. Specific diseases that fall under this general classification include:

★ Argentine hemorrhagic fever
★ Bolivian hemorrhagic fever
★ Venezuelan hemorrhagic fever
★ Lassa fever
★ Congo-Crimean hemorrhagic fever

viral hemorrhagic fevers (**VHFs**) *a diverse group of illnesses caused by a multitude of different viruses that attack the vascular bed causing hemorrhaging.*

- ★ Rift Valley fever
- ★ Ebola
- ★ Marburg
- ★ Dengue fever
- ★ Yellow fever

These diseases are categorized together primarily due to the similarity of their clinical presentation. All of these diseases target the vascular bed, causing changes in vascular permeability.

Initial presenting symptoms may include fatigue, fever, myalgias, and prostration. Physical examination may reveal conjunctival injection, periorbital edema, petechial rash, flushing, and mild hypotension. As the disease progresses, the patient may develop generalized mucous membrane hemorrhage, disseminated intravascular coagulation (DIC), shock, multiple organ system failure, or death. Often these patients will also display signs of pulmonary, hematopoietic, and neurologic involvement. The incubation period varies depending on the specific infective agent, and can range from days to months.

These viruses are all considered to be contagious, and may be spread through contact with body fluids, respiratory droplets, and secondarily contaminated surfaces. Special caution must be exercised in handling sharps, needles, and other potential sources of parenteral exposure. Strict adherence to Standard Precautions has been shown to be very effective in preventing nosocomial transmission of most VHF infections. As a general rule, all caregivers must wear gloves, gowns, and eye protection. Respiratory protection should consist of a mask or respiratory protection device capable of 100% high-efficiency particulate air (HEPA) filtration. Mortality rates for the viral hemorrhagic fevers are variable, dependent on the strain of virus, and range from less than 10% to as high as 90% (Ebola, Marburg). Figure 33-6 ■ shows a care provider who has donned the personal protective equipment (PPE) necessary for entering the scene for this kind of exposure.

Critical care transport of the VHF patient poses some unique challenges. Regardless of the specific etiologic agent, general principles of care are supportive. Fluid resuscitation, management of electrolyte balance, and maintenance of vasopressor agents may be required. Antibiotic therapy is often utilized to combat commonly occurring secondary infections. Patients may require treatment for shock, blood loss, renal failure, seizures, and coma. Treatment for severe bleeding may include fresh frozen plasma and other clotting factor concentrates. Patients administered too much IV fluid tend to develop pulmonary edema, so fluid balance should be monitored closely. In many cases, transportation of these patients, especially by air, is deemed contraindicated because of the effects of drastic changes in ambient pressure on pulmonary fluid balance. Intravenous lines, catheters, and invasive monitoring should be avoided unless clearly indicated for appropriate management of the patient.

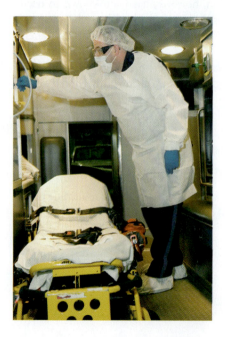

■ **Figure 33-6** First responder in highest level of personal protective equipment (PPE). *(Craig Jackson/In the Dark Photography)*

Pharmacologic agents used during transport are generally standard and supportive in nature. The antiviral drug ribavirin is sometimes considered for use in these patients, but would not normally pose any specific challenge during transport. As always, however, the transport team is responsible for ensuring familiarity with and understanding of any pharmacologic agents being used during transport.

BIOLOGICAL TOXINS

In the context of biological agents, toxins are defined as harmful substances, or poisons, which are produced by living organisms (animals, plants, microbes). They behave in a manner very similar to that of chemical agents, do not grow or reproduce, are nonvolatile, and do not pose a vapor hazard. Unlike many chemicals, toxins are generally not able to be absorbed through the skin. Toxins are, however, generally much more toxic per weight than chemical agents. Fortunately, due to their nonvolatile nature, they are unlikely in most circumstances to pose any threat to health care workers.

Because the effects of toxins on the body are direct, the symptoms of an exposure may appear very rapidly. The potency of many of these toxins is such that even very small doses may cause illness and/or death. The only toxin that appears in the listing of CDC Category A agents is botulinum toxin.

In the context of biological agents, toxins are defined as harmful substances, or poisons, which are produced by living organisms (animals, plants, microbes).

BOTULINUM TOXIN

Botulinum toxin is produced by the bacteria *Clostridium botulinum.* On a dose/weight basis, botulinum is the most toxic substance known. In fact, botulinum is up to 15,000 times more toxic by weight than VX nerve agent and 100,000 times more toxic than sarin. Paradoxically, it has been used therapeutically to treat certain spastic conditions (strabismus, blepharospasm, torticollis, and tetanus) and to cosmetically treat wrinkles.

Exposure to botulinum is most frequently caused by the ingestion of contaminated foods and is usually associated with improper canning. The possibility also exists, however, of direct respiratory exposure to the toxin following an intentional dissemination. The toxin produces similar effects regardless of exposure route, although the time course may vary depending on the route of exposure and the dose received. This toxin exerts its effect by inhibiting the release of acetycholine from cholinergic nerves that control both autonomic and skeletal muscle function. This interruption of neurotransmission causes cranial nerve and skeletal muscle paralysis.

The motor complications of botulism feature a descending bilateral paralysis, usually beginning with cranial nerve palsies leading to blurred vision, diplopia, dysphonia, and dysphagia. Flaccid skeletal muscle paralysis follows, in a symmetrical, descending, and progressive manner. Collapse of the upper airway may occur due to weakness of the oropharyngeal musculature. Because the descending motor weakness involves the diaphragm and accessory muscles of respiration, respiratory failure may occur. The initial presentation of botulism may be mistaken for a stroke, but unlike stroke, symptoms of botulism exposure will appear bilaterally. Symptoms usually begin 12 to 36 hours following intoxication, although this can vary depending on the dose and route of exposure. The untreated mortality rate is approximately 60%, however it drops to less than 5% with appropriate management. Recovery of neurologic function can take weeks to months.

Treatment during critical care transportation of the botulism patient is primarily supportive, and will most likely include respiratory support and hydration. Antibiotics may be used for secondary bacterial infections. Specific therapy consists of giving trivalent botulinum antitoxin, however this antitoxin will typically be administered prior to transport.

botulinum toxin *a neurotoxic bacteria,* Clostridium botulinum, *is the most toxic substance known to medicine on a dose/weight basis.*

OTHER POTENTIAL AGENTS

In addition to those described in the earlier section, the CDC has also identified several other potential agents that could be used as biological weapons. In general, these Category B agents have some potential for large-scale dissemination with resultant illness, but generally cause less morbidity and mortality and therefore would be expected to have lower medical and public health impact. Some of the Category B agents are briefly described here:

★ *Q fever:* A rickettsial disease found in sheep, cattle, and goats. Humans acquire the disease by inhalation of contaminated particles. Typically self-limiting, it causes a febrile illness with headache, general malaise, and myalgias. The illness typically lasts 2 days to 2 weeks. Complications of the disease are pneumonia and endocarditis.

★ *Brucellosis:* A systemic bacterial disease acquired through broken skin while handling infected animals or through the ingestion of nonpasteurized dairy products. The acute form typically presents with a sudden nonspecific febrile illness with chills, sweats, headache, fatigue, myalgia, arthralgia, and anorexia.

★ *Glanders and melioidosis:* Bacterial diseases that cause similar human disease complexes and are highly communicable. Infection produces fever, rigors, sweating, myalgia, headache, and pleuritic chest pain. Glanders sometimes presents with a generalized papular/pustular rash that may be mistaken for smallpox. These diseases are almost always fatal without treatment.

★ *Alphaviruses (VEE, EEE, WEEa)—encephalitics:* This subcategory includes Venezuelan, eastern, and western equine encephalitis. Carried by mosquitoes, these viral diseases cause generalized malaise, spiking fever, severe headache, photophobia, and myalgias. Nausea, vomiting, cough, sore throat, and diarrhea are typically also associated with illness. Severe cases progress to encephalitis.

★ *Typhus fever:* A rickettsial disease characterized by severe headaches, sustained high fever, generalized muscle aches, and skin rash.

★ *Ricin:* A toxin generated as a by-product of castor bean processing. Ingestion can cause nausea, vomiting, abdominal cramps, severe diarrhea, and vascular collapse. Inhalation may cause more nonspecific symptoms such as weakness, fever, cough, and hypothermia followed by hypotension and cardiovascular collapse.

★ *Staphylococcal enterotoxin B (SEB):* One of several exotoxins produced by *Staphylococcus aureus,* the causative agent in typical food poisoning. If inhaled, SEB may cause sudden onset of fever, chills, headache, myalgia, nonproductive cough, dyspnea, retrosternal chest pain, and pulmonary edema.

RADIOLOGICAL/NUCLEAR CONCERNS

Radiological and nuclear concerns are the most commonly misunderstood aspects of CBRNE preparedness.

Radiological and nuclear concerns are the most commonly misunderstood aspects of CBRNE preparedness. Although not considered to be the most likely of the threats, the possibility of an intentional use of radiological materials against a civilian population has been receiving increased attention during the past several years. The term *nuclear* refers to the use of a traditional or improvised nuclear weapon. With the end of the cold war, we have enjoyed a reduction in the likelihood of nuclear weapon use. The term *radiological* refers to the use of radioactive substances in a manner that may cause injury, other than associated with a nuclear detonation. In this age of potential terrorism, the possibility of the use of radiological weapons is considered more likely than an actual nuclear weapon detonation.

It is common knowledge that exposure to high levels of radiation may occur following a nuclear detonation. Another potential, and probably more likely scenario, involves the use of a radiological dispersal device (RDD). RDDs are defined as devices that cause the purposeful dissemination of radioactive material across an area, often by explosive means, but without a nuclear detonation. The material can originate from any location that uses radioactive sources, such as a nuclear waste processor, a nuclear power plant, a university research facility, a medical radiotherapy clinic, or an industrial complex. The radioactive material is disseminated by means of a conventional explosive, scattering radioactive debris throughout the area. This type of dissemination would likely cause conventional traumatic injuries as well as contamination with radioactive materials.

Several significant radiological accidents have occurred in the past, and can serve as a reference for us when considering the possible consequences of significant dissemination of radioactive materials. One such incident occurred in Goiania, Brazil, in September 1987, when a junkyard worker dismantled the containment vessel from an abandoned radiotherapy machine. A glowing blue dust, radioactive cesium-137, was found inside. Over the following days, scores of local citizens were exposed to the radioactive substance. In fact, many children and adults rubbed the powder on their bodies, leading to one of the largest accidental radioactive substance dispersions in history. In the end, 244 people were found to be contaminated, 54 seriously enough to be hospitalized for further tests or treatment. Of these, more than 20 patients were internally contaminated due to either inhalation or accidental ingestion of the dust. Tens of thousands of people had to be surveyed for radioactive contamination. Despite the magnitude of this event and the high doses of radiation received by many of the victims, only four victims had died within the first several months following exposure. It is important to note, when looking at Goiania, that even in this widespread dispersion of significantly radioactive material, the patient volumes and acute mortality were quite low. This is, in fact, a common trend related to radiological dispersion, and provides a framework with which to base care decisions.

TYPES OF IONIZING RADIATION

When radiation interacts with atoms, energy is deposited, resulting in a process called **ionization.** This ionization may damage certain critical molecules or structures in a cell. The damage from this is irreparable, causing the cell to either die or malfunction. There are several types of ionizing radiation, including alpha particles, beta particles, and gamma rays:

ionization when radiation interacts with atoms, energy is deposited, resulting in the process called ionization.

★ *Alpha particles* are massive, charged particles that travel only a few inches in air. Intact skin and clothing provide adequate shielding from alpha particles.

★ *Beta particles* are very small charged particles that can travel several feet in air. The energy released from beta particles is able to penetrate the first few layers of intact skin, causing "beta burns," a condition very similar to a thermal burn. Both alpha and beta particles pose their most significant hazard if inhaled or ingested.

★ *Gamma rays* are high-energy waves of ionizing radiation similar to X-rays. Gamma radiation is highly penetrating, and can cause whole-body exposure. Shielding from gamma radiation is accomplished through use of lead or other very dense substances.

Figure 33-7 ■ shows the penetrability of these various forms of ionizing radiation.

EXPOSURE AND CONTAMINATION

When radioactive materials are encountered, the result may be exposure, contamination, or both. *Exposure* is defined as irradiation from a radioactive source that comes into proximity with the body. In these cases, direct contact does not have to occur between the victim and the radiation source. Once the person has been removed from the source of radiation, the irradiation ceases. The victim is not a secondary source of radiation and individuals providing support and treatment are in no danger of receiving radiation from the victim. A person exposed to external irradiation does not become radioactive and poses no hazard to nearby individuals. *Contamination* has occurred when radioactive material is found either in or on the body. Caregivers and support personnel must be careful not to spread the contamination to uncontaminated parts of the victim's body, themselves, or the surrounding area. External contamination may result from direct contact with material. Internal contamination can result from inhalation, ingestion, or direct absorption of these materials through either the skin or open wounds.

RADIATION INJURY

In reality, the medical consequences of radiation injury are quite predictable, and treatment of radiation victims is typically straightforward. (See Table 33–2.) Depending on the particular means of agent delivery, such as in the case of explosive injuries following detonation of an RDD, secondary traumatic injuries may also exist. In these cases, initial care is directed specifically at treating these conventional injuries.

■ **Figure 33-7** Nuclear radiation.

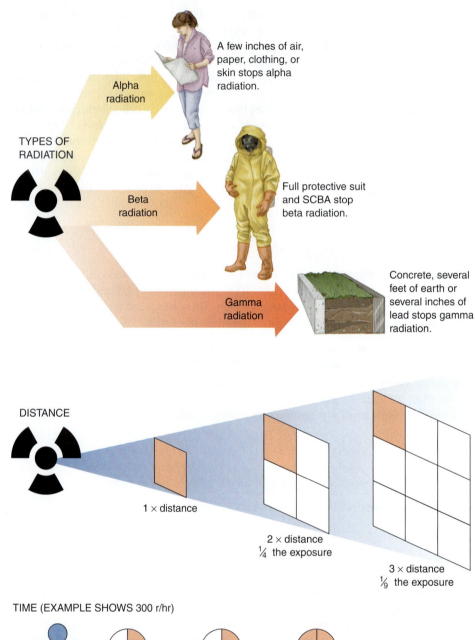

TYPES OF RADIATION

Alpha radiation

A few inches of air, paper, clothing, or skin stops alpha radiation.

Beta radiation

Full protective suit and SCBA stop beta radiation.

Gamma radiation

Concrete, several feet of earth or several inches of lead stops gamma radiation.

DISTANCE

1 × distance

2 × distance
¼ the exposure

3 × distance
⅑ the exposure

TIME (EXAMPLE SHOWS 300 r/hr)

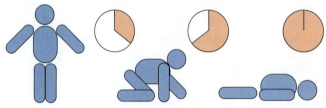

acute radiation syndrome (ARS) *a condition that develops following exposure to high doses of ionizing radiation, ARS presents as a sequence of phased and usually lethal symptoms that vary with onset and severity of exposure, including gastrointestinal, respiratory, and CNS deterioration.*

A condition known as **acute radiation syndrome (ARS)** can develop following exposure to high doses of ionizing radiation. ARS presents as a sequence of phased symptoms. The specific onset and severity of symptoms will vary and is dependent on the total radiation dose received. ARS starts with a *prodromal phase,* which may begin within hours of exposure. This phase is characterized by nausea, vomiting, diarrhea, fatigue, weakness, fever, and headache. A *latent period* typically follows in which the patient is relatively symptom free for a period of days to weeks. Following this, the patient enters the *manifest illness phase.* At this point, bone marrow function is often affected, causing decreased resistance to infection and anemia. At higher doses, gastrointestinal system

Table 33-2 — Dose-Effect Relationships to Ionizing Radiation

Whole Body Exposure

Dose (RAD)	Effect
5–25	Asymptomatic. Blood studies are normal.
50–75	Asymptomatic. Minor depressions of white blood cells and platelets in a few patients.
75–125	May produce anorexia, nausea, and vomiting, and fatigue in approximately 10–20 percent of patients within 2 days.
125–200	Possible nausea and vomiting. Diarrhea, anxiety, tachycardia. Fatal to less than 5 percent of patients.
200–600	Nausea and vomiting, diarrhea in the first several hours, weakness, fatigue. Fatal to approximately 50 percent of patients within 6 weeks without prompt medical attention.
600–1,000	Severe nausea and vomiting, diarrhea in the first several hours. Fatal to 100 percent of patients within 2 weeks without prompt medical attention.
1,000 or more	"Burning sensation" within minutes, nausea and vomiting within 10 minutes, confusion ataxia, and prostration within one hour, watery diarrhea within 1–2 hr. Fatal to 100 percent within short time without prompt medical attention.

Localized Exposure

Dose (RAD)	Effect
50	Asymptomatic.
500	Asymptomatic (usually). May have risk of altered function of exposed area.
2,500	Atrophy, vascular lesion, and altered pigmentation.
5,000	Chronic ulcer, risk of carcinogenesis.
50,000	Permanent destruction of exposed tissue.

degradation occurs, causing diarrhea, hemorrhage, and severe fluid loss. Neurovascular changes are associated with very high radiation doses and are characterized by a steadily deteriorating state of consciousness with eventual coma and death. Convulsions may or may not occur, and there may be little or no indication of increased intracranial pressure. Table 33–3 summarizes the phases of an acute radiation syndrome.

MANAGEMENT OF RADIATION ILLNESS

During critical care transport, care of the radiation illness patient is primarily supportive. Despite the minimal risk of provider contamination at this phase in the patient's care, it is better to err on the side of safety and ensure that adequate decontamination has occurred. In the majority of cases, standard BSI precautions will provide more than adequate protection.

The need for ventilatory support and intravenous fluid administration should be expected. Pharmacologic therapy may include standard antiemetics, antibiotics, and medications to assist with pain management. In addition, several pharmacologic agents are available that can be used to promote the dilution or blocking of internal contaminants. These agents may include ferric ferrocyanide (Prussian blue), stable iodine compounds (potassium iodide), diethylenetriamine-pentaacetic acid (DTPA), and calcium edetate (caEDTA). Colony-stimulating factors are also sometimes used in an attempt to combat hematopoietic deficiency. Several of these specific pharmacologic agents are investigational, and it is likely that they would not be continued during transport.

Table 33-3 | Acute Radiation Syndromes

Syndrome	Dose*	Prodromal Stage	Latent Stage	Manifest Illness Stage	Recovery
Hematopoietic (Bone marrow)	> 0.7 Gy (> 70 rads) (*mild symptoms may occur as low as 0.3 Gy or 30 rads*)	• Symptoms are anorexia, nausea, and vomiting. • Onset occurs 1 hour to 2 days after exposure. • Stage lasts for minutes to days.	• Stem cells in bone marrow are dying, although patient may appear and feel well. • Stage lasts 1 to 6 weeks.	• Symptoms are anorexia, fever, and malaise. • Drop in all blood cell counts occurs for several weeks. • Primary cause of death is infection and hemorrhage. • Survival decreases with increasing dose. • Most deaths occur within a few months after exposure.	• In most cases, bone marrow cells will begin to repopulate the marrow. • There should be full recovery for a large percentage of individuals from a few weeks up to two years after exposure. • Death may occur in some individuals at 1.2 Gy (120 rads). • The LD$_{50/60}$ [†] is about 2.5 to 5 Gy (250 to 500 rads).
Gastrointestinal (GI)	> 10 Gy (> 1,000 rads) (*some symptoms may occur as low as 6 Gy or 600 rads*)	• Symptoms are anorexia, severe nausea, vomiting, cramps, and diarrhea. • Onset occurs within a few hours after exposure. • Stage lasts about 2 days.	• Stem cells in bone marrow and cells lining GI tract are dying, although patient may appear and feel well. • Stage lasts less than 1 week.	• Symptoms are malaise, anorexia, severe diarrhea, fever, dehydration, and electrolyte imbalance. • Death is due to infection, dehydration, and electrolyte imbalance. • Death occurs within 2 weeks of exposure.	• The LD$_{100}$ [‡] is about 10 Gy (1,000 rads).
Cardiovascular (CV)/ Central Nervous System (CNS)	> 50 Gy (5,000 rads) (*some symptoms may occur as low as 20 Gy or 2,000 rads*)	• Symptoms are extreme nervousness and confusion; severe nausea, vomiting, and watery diarrhea; loss of consciousness; and burning sensations of the skin. • Onset occurs within minutes of exposure. • Stage lasts for minutes to hours.	• Patient may return to partial functionality. • Stage may last for hours but often is less.	• Symptoms are return of watery diarrhea, convulsions, and coma. • Onset occurs 5 to 6 hours after exposure. • Death occurs within 3 days of exposure.	• No recovery is expected.

* The absorbed doses quoted here are "gamma equivalent" values. Neutrons or protons generally produce the same effects as gamma, beta, or X-rays but at lower doses. If the patient has been exposed to neutrons or protons, consult radiation experts on how to interpret the dose.

† The LD$_{50/60}$ is the dose necessary to kill 50% of the exposed population in 60 days.

‡ The LD$_{100}$ is the dose necessary to kill 100% of the exposed population.

EXPLOSIVES

Of the various forms of terrorist activity that may be encountered by the critical care paramedic, the most widely used WMD remains explosive devices (bombs and incendiary devices). The critical care paramedic must be familiar with the effects of these types of devices along with the necessary treatment modalities for those who have fallen victim to them. However, fortunately for the critical care paramedic, the discussion of explosive agents will probably be familiar because they typically result in traumatic injury and burn patterns that the critical care paramedic is already well versed in from his or her initial EMS education.

Explosives work as a result of the ignition of special fuels that burn extremely rapidly, causing the hot gases created to displace air in a violent fashion from the resultant shock wave. The blast wave typically moves out in concentric circles from the blast at a sonic speed, as long as no structure or shielding device was present that channels the shock wave in a specific direction. Naturally, the greater the distance from the center of the explosion that a person is situated, the lesser the injuries sustained as a result. Additionally, the presence of barriers (protective clothing, walls, vehicles, and so on) may offer some protection from the shock wave or blast. Conversely, the absence of barriers or the presence of an explosive in a closed room or space results in an amplification of the shock wave with resultant increases in the number and severity of the injuries. It behooves the critical care paramedic to always gain a history surrounding any explosion regarding the patient's physical proximity to the explosion.

Of the various forms of terrorist activity that may be encountered by the critical care paramedic, the most widely used WMD remains explosive devices (bombs and incendiary devices).

EFFECTS OF EXPLOSIONS

Consistent with your initial education from earlier EMS courses regarding the phases of an explosion, explosions that are secondary to a WMD event share the same phases and create the same patterns of blast injuries.

The initial phase of the explosion is the actual detonation of material. This phase involves the sudden and violent release of energy in the form of rapidly moving molecules. During this phase the rapid expansion of hot gases causes a pressure wave to move outward in all directions. The initial movement of air from the epicenter is termed *overpressure*. The overpressure results in a drastic but brief increase, and then a decrease in the air pressure as it passes. Although the overpressure wave may be violent near the epicenter of the explosion, it rapidly loses its strength as it travels outward.

Following the initial pressure wave is the blast wind. This is a slower moving (less violent) wave of air traveling behind the pressure wave. The blast wind has less strength, but is of longer duration compared to the initial pressure wave. As such, it may result in the propelling of a victim or the showering of the victim with thrown debris.

Projectiles that may strike the patient could be from the casing that held the explosive, building components if the explosion happened in a structure, or nearby objects that were picked up and thrown by the blast. Since the projectiles may be large at times, they can potentially cause great bodily harm to the person they strike.

Personal displacement refers to the ability of the pressure wave and blast wind to physically propel the victim from his original location when the bomb detonated. This in essence makes the individual a projectile that can impact the ground or other nearby objects (walls, trees, vehicles, and so on) or strike other objects in flight. The resulting injuries from this phase can be extreme when the patient is near the epicenter of the explosion.

BLAST INJURY PHASES

The injuries sustained by the victim(s) subjected to a WMD event in which an explosion occurred can be classified into three types of injuries:

★ *Primary blast injuries* are those caused by the heat of the explosion and by the overpressure wave. This typically results in burn injuries as well as damage to tympanic membranes and hollow organs of the body (lungs, GI tract, and so on).

★ *Secondary blast injuries* are traumatic injuries that occur from projectiles striking the body. These projectiles may be large, causing extensive blunt trauma; they may be small and penetrate into the body; and they may be hot from the explosion and cause burns.

★ *Tertiary blast injuries* are those that result from the person being thrown away from the explosion and striking other objects, or may also occur if there is some type of structural collapse that pins or crushes the victim. The types of injury patterns from this phase may be blunt, penetrating, or a mix thereof (depending on the size of explosion and the patient's proximity to it).

INCENDIARY DEVICES

Incendiary devices are those that burn at extremely high temperatures. Incendiary devices include napalm, thermite, magnesium, and white phosphorus. Since the devices are made to burn at an extremely high temperature, patient burns from these devices are often severe.

A terrorist could easily obtain a number of readily available chemical structures and improvise a devastating incendiary device (recall the concept of "agents of opportunity" discussed earlier in the chapter). Gasoline, propane, or even natural gas is easily obtainable for these types of devices. A sabotaged natural gas line in a home, in a factory, or even a gas line serving a community could create escalating damage.

ASSESSMENT AND MANAGEMENT CONSIDERATIONS

As discussed in the opening of this section, the assessment and management of injuries found secondary to an explosive device follow the same assessment and management regime for traumatic injuries (blunt and penetrating) and burn injuries. As with any WMD scene, the personal safety of the critical care paramedic and other emergency personnel takes precedence. Beyond that, rely on your previous knowledge of trauma care to guide your actions. Also remain cognizant for any secondary explosive devices that may yet detonate, as well as the potential for structural collapse. Finally, remember that an explosive device may be the method by which other forms of CBRNE are released into a population.

ADDITIONAL INFORMATION RESOURCES

In the event that the transport of a CBRNE victim is required, a rapid review of the specific pathophysiology and treatment for the specific agent is strongly recommended. Because this information may be updated frequently, such as was the case with the Amerithrax incidents, reliable Internet-based resources often provide the best source for current information. Many such resources exist that can provide a quick reference to information regarding patient presentation, clinical interventions, and specific pharmacologic agents. Frequently updated Internet-based information sites are maintained by both the CDC (**http://www.cdc.gov**) and the World Health Organization (**http://www.who.int**). Additional information can be obtained through the U.S. Department of Homeland Security's Internet site. Several of the references mentioned in the chapter bibliography can also be accessed online through the Virtual Naval Hospital website found at **http://www.vnh.org**. Beware that some Internet sites that may provide inaccurate or incorrect information. To avoid this, use only sites operated by reputable organizations.

Summary

 Since the proliferation of terrorism, groups have been increasing their capacity to utilize weapons of mass destruction. The entire medical system continues to prepare for the worst scenarios, including the use of CBRNE agents against civilian populations. Most of the preparation has been directed at the response phase immediately following the event, and emergency responders have been dedicating vast resources to increasing their response capabilities for such an event. Critical care paramedics will play a significant role in the days and weeks following an event and must be prepared to understand and appropriately manage the clinical effects of these agents. These agents present unique challenges. For example, biological agents may be covertly deployed, leave no definitive crime scene, and remain undetected for several days, and thus many patients may be in varying stages of development of disease. Effective response to CBRNE deployment depends on cooperation and coordination between all levels of the health care system.

Although the likelihood of a mass casualty CBRNE agent terrorist attack may be relatively small, it is not negligible. The potential consequences are severe enough to justify continual clinical training and preparedness activities. By conducting continuing clinical education for the critical care paramedic, the health care system's domestic response capability will be strengthened.

The safety of the crew is of paramount importance, and all patients must be thoroughly and definitively decontaminated prior to critical care management. Nerve agent casualties may require prolonged treatment aimed at ventilatory maintenance and prevention of overstimulation of ACh receptors with the use of atropine, oximes, and anticonvulsants. Patients exposed to pulmonary agents may require aggressive ventilatory management with the use of PEEP, high concentrations of oxygen, and beta-agonists. Cyanide casualties will rarely require critical care for prolonged periods of time. However, critical care paramedics must be prepared to administer a cyanide antidote in cases of latent absorption of the poison, especially in cases of ingestion. The treatment of vesicant casualties will require supportive and symptomatic care, and frequently will require specific ophthalmologic care and antibiotic therapy to prevent systemic infection. Incapacitating agents represent an extremely low likelihood of a need for critical care.

BW events may be covert and unrecognized for several days. The most important concept for treating BW casualties is to employ strict personal protective measures and body substance isolation. Bacterial agents such as anthrax, plague, and tularemia may respond to aggressive antibiotic therapy, while viral agents such as viral hemorrhagic fevers and smallpox have very few treatment options outside of supportive critical care. Toxins represent a great threat to demand of critical care resources. Successful treatment of botulism casualties may result in the need for extended periods of ventilator support.

Management of ionizing radiation illness will be primarily supportive, however, several pharmacologic agents are available that can assist in diluting or blocking internal radioactive contaminate.

Review Questions

1. CBRNE agents include what types of substances?
2. What general personal protective measures should be taken during the transport of a victim exposed to a CBRNE agent?
3. What are the most likely chemical agents to be used as weapons?
4. What types of agent-specific antidotes exist for the standard chemical weapons agents?
5. What are the most likely biological agents to be used as weapons?
6. What is the general approach to care of the biological weapons victim?
7. What personal protective measures should be taken during the transport of a radiological agent victim?
8. What is an RDD, and what types of injuries could be expected following the use of one?
9. Where can up-to-date information regarding CBRNE agents be found?

See Answers to Review Questions at the back of this book.

Further Reading

De Lorenzo RA, Porter RS. *Weapons of Mass Destruction Emergency Care.* Upper Saddle River, NJ: Pearson Prentice Hall, 2000.

Gusev I, Guskova A, Mettler FA. *Medical Management of Radiation Accidents,* 2nd ed. Boca Raton, FL: CRC Press, 2001.

Khan AS, Levitt AM, Sage MJ. *Biological and Chemical Terrorism: Strategic Plan for Preparedness and Response Recommendations of the CDC Strategic Planning Workgroup.* Centers for Disease Control, April 2000.

LeBlanc FN, Benson BE, Gilg AD. "A Severe Organophosphate Poisoning Requiring the Use of an Atropine Drip." *Journal of Toxicology—Clinical Toxicology,* Vol. 24, No. 1 (1986): 69–76.

Maniscalco PM, Christen H. *Terrorism Response: Field Guide for Fire and EMS Organizations.* Upper Saddle River, NJ: Pearson Prentice Hall, 2002.

Medical Management of Biological Casualties, 4th ed. U.S. Army Medical Research Institute of Infectious Diseases, February 2001.

Medical Management of Chemical Casualties, 3rd ed. U.S. Army Medical Research Institute of Chemical Defense, July 2000.

Medical Management of Radiological Casualties, 2nd ed. Armed Forces Radiobiology Research Institute, April 2003.

The Medical NBC Battlebook. U.S. Army Center for Health Promotion and Preventive Medicine (USACHPPM) Tech Guide 244, August 2000.

Medical Treatment of Radiological Casualties. U.S. Department of Homeland Security Working Group on Radiological Dispersal Device (RDD) Preparedness Medical Preparedness and Response Sub-Group, May 2003.

Rotz LD, Khan AS, Lillibridge SR, Ostroff SM, Hughes JM. "Report Summary: Public Health Assessment of Potential Biological Terrorism Agents." *Emerging Infectious Diseases,* Vol. 8, No. 2 (February 2002).

Sidell FR, Patrick WC, Dashiell T. *Jane's Chem Bio Handbook.* Alexandria, VA: Jane's Information Group, 2000.

Textbook of Military Medicine: Medical Aspects of Chemical and Biological Warfare. Office of the Surgeon General, U.S. Department of the Army, May 1997.

Organ Donation and Retrieval

P.J. Geraghty, EMT-P, BS, CPTC, CTBS and Sean Conley, EMT-P, CTBS

Objectives

Upon the completion of this chapter, the student should be able to:

1. Describe indications for organ transplantation and the need for solid organ donors. (p. 990)
2. List the clinical indications to notify the organ procurement organization of a potential donor. (p. 991)
3. Define neurologic death and identify signs that neurologic death may be impending. (p. 991)
4. Identify the hallmarks of neurologic death testing. (p. 991)
5. Describe the systems in place for one to indicate one's wishes regarding donation prior to death. (p. 992)
6. Discuss the process of obtaining consent from the patient's legal next-of-kin. (p. 992)
7. Describe the system for matching donated organs with recipients. (p. 993)
8. Identify clinical management challenges encountered and the therapies indicated when managing the organ donor. (p. 994)
9. List the testing and evaluations performed to assess viability for each organ system. (p. 995)
10. Describe anesthesia requirements for the organ recovery procedure. (p. 996)
11. Discuss the organ recovery procedure and organ preservation. (p. 996)
12. Identify tissues that can be donated and differences between tissue and organ donation. (p. 997)

Key Terms

Case Study

EMS is activated to respond to a reported seizure. Upon arrival at the local mall, the paramedics find Bill Johnson, age 43, unconscious in the atrium of the food court. His wife, Laura, reports that he grabbed his head suddenly and fell out of his chair, and has been unresponsive since then. She reports some seizure-like activity immediately following his collapse, but states that he has been still ever since. The patient is incontinent of urine and stool, and a tray of fast food sits untouched at his table.

The paramedics do a rapid assessment and find the patient's airway to be patent, though his respirations are shallow. They quickly intubate him, checking tube placement using an $ETCO_2$ detector, and assist respirations at a rate of 12 per minute. He has no gag reflex when the tube is placed. His vital signs reveal a blood pressure of 190/106, heart rate of 56, and shallow respirations at 8. His lungs are clear bilaterally. His pupils are equal, round, and nonreactive. They cannot elicit any response to painful stimuli. His GCS is 3.

The paramedics transport the man to the local stroke center, establishing an IV en route and notifying the receiving facility via mobile phone. Upon arrival the emergency physician orders a stat CT of the brain. The radiologist reports a massive subarachnoid hemorrhage, with a marked left shift. Upon return to the ED, the patient's emergency nurse notes that he is no longer making any respiratory effort and that his blood pressure is dropping. She notifies the emergency physician of the change and quietly asks the unit clerk to notify the local organ procurement organization (OPO). Neurosurgery is consulted and performs a clinical exam. The resident cannot elicit any cranial nerve responses and, after consulting with her attending, reports to the emergency physician that the patient is not a surgical candidate.

The patient's wife has arrived and is met by members of the pastoral care team who take her to a small family consultation room. The emergency physician explains the findings of the CT and the examinations, and tells her that her husband has suffered a massive stroke. He explains that he will do one final test, but his suspicion is that the patient's brain has ceased to function. The patient's wife contacts their children and her husband's parents to meet her at the hospital, and asks if she can see her husband before the test is performed. The nurse and pastoral care staff escort her to her husband's bedside where she spends a few tearful minutes holding his hand.

The emergency physician ensures that the patient has been receiving 100% oxygen via the ventilator and that the patient's initial arterial blood gas measurement has normal values. He confirms that the patient has received no sedatives, is not hypothermic, and is not suffering from metabolic derangement. He then orders that the ventilator be disconnected and that the patient receive oxygen at 6 liters per minute through a cannula in his ET tube. He observes the patient for any signs of respiratory effort and orders a blood gas at 6 minutes. The results reveal a pCO_2 of 83 mmHg. The emergency physician orders that the ventilator be reconnected. He writes a note in the patient's medical record documenting his exam and certifying that brain death has occurred.

During this time, the organ procurement coordinator (OPC) has arrived and reviewed the patient's medical record. He meets with the nurse, physician, and pastoral care staff and together they come up with a plan for letting the patient's family know what has happened. The physician and nurse go with the pastoral care representative and tell the patient's wife (who has been joined by her children and in-laws) of the results of the exam. He is thorough but compassionate as he explains what has happened, answering all the family's questions. He explains that there will be some decisions for them to make and introduces the OPC as a member of the health care team who will assist with those decisions.

The OPC explains to the family that they have the opportunity to donate organs and tissues for transplantation. He explains how the procedure works, the amount of time it takes, and its lack of impact on funeral arrangements. Through all of this, he takes care to emphasize how this will help other people who will die without an organ transplant. The family agrees that this is something Bill would want to do, and agree to donate everything that can be used. The OPC reviews the authorization form and asks the family members some questions about Bill's medical and social history. He also invites them to spend some more time at Bill's bedside. They spend about 30 more minutes before leaving the hospital.

The OPC leaves the family at Bill's bedside and reviews the plan of care with the emergency nurse. Because the hospital is full, it may be some time before an ICU bed becomes available, and the OPC wants to begin the assessment of organ function as rapidly as possible. He writes orders transferring responsibility for the patient's care to the OPO as well as for laboratory tests to assess the function of Bill's organs. He requests the placement of a pulmonary artery (PA) catheter to monitor Bill's fluid status and asks the nurse to start a dopamine infusion to ensure adequate blood pressure and renal perfusion. He also sends blood specimens for infectious disease and human leukocyte antigen (HLA) testing.

While waiting for these and other studies to be completed, the OPC registers Bill with the United Network for Organ Sharing (UNOS) and obtains a list of potential recipients for Bill's organs. He documents Bill's history and current status on the OPO's donor information system and begins contacting the transplant centers. Within 3 hours he has placed Bill's heart, lungs, liver, and intestine with five different recipients. Shortly thereafter, the HLA typing results are completed revealing a perfect match for the pancreas and kidney with a patient three states away. The OPC contacts that transplant center and they accept the organs. A local kidney transplant center accepts the remaining kidney.

The OPC makes arrangements with the hospital OR for the organ recovery to take place, ensuring adequate instrumentation and staff support, including an anesthesiologist to monitor Bill's vital signs and administer medication as necessary. The OPC arranges the timing of the teams' arrival to the OR so that all the teams are ready at the same time. In the OR, each transplant team assesses the organ and performs the necessary dissection to allow the recovery of each organ. When all the teams are ready, the aorta is cross-clamped and the organs are recovered and packaged. The transplant teams return to the transplant centers and transplant the organs. Meanwhile, the ocular recovery technician recovers Bill's corneas for transplantation. Tissue recovery technicians come to the hospital and recover Bill's long bones and associated connective tissues from his arms and legs. These will be processed into usable grafts for surgeries. They close all the incisions and notify the funeral home that the body is ready to be picked up.

During the next few weeks, Bill's family has a memorial service and their pastor mentions that Bill gave the gift of life to seven different people. The OPC sends the family a letter detailing what organs and tissues were recovered as well as some information about the organ recipients. The OPC also follows up with the hospital staff to thank them for their efforts and to let them know the outcome.

Always consider your patient a possible organ donor. Many lives are lost because needed organs are not available.

When in doubt about whether a patient is a candidate for organ donation, contact your local organ procurement organization because organ transplantation is an evolving science.

organ procurement organizations (OPOs) *organizations designated by the federal government to recover organs for transplantation.*

INTRODUCTION

Critical care paramedics may find themselves more involved in the organ procurement and transplantation process than their non-critical care counterparts. Critical care paramedics can be involved in virtually any aspect of the transplant process and must be familiar with the issues and procedures involved. (See Figure 34-1 ■.) Organ transplantation can save many lives, although there remains more demand than supply.

Organ transplantation is the primary therapy for end-stage failure of the heart, lungs, liver, kidneys, pancreas, or small intestine. Patients suffering from organ failure due to any number of diseases can benefit from organ transplantation. Hundreds of thousands of people in the United States develop organ failure each year, but only a small percentage of these patients is suitable for organ transplantation, and due to the shortage of organ donors, even fewer will actually receive an organ. Since 1995 almost 400,000 people have been listed for transplantation in the United States, and only about 223,000 transplants have been performed. The primary reason for the disparity is a lack of donated organs. The estimated number of suitable organ donors in the United States is between 10,500 and 13,800 but each year only about 42% of these become organ donors. For this reason, **organ procurement organizations (OPOs)** and hospitals across the country continue to work on improving consent rates and removing barriers to organ donation.

■ **Figure 34-1** Transporting organs for transplantation. *(Courtesy of LifeGift Organ Donation Center, Houston)*

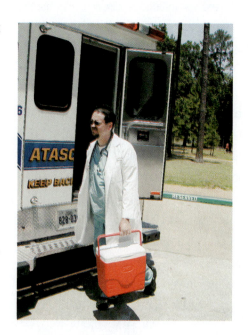

INDICATIONS FOR ORGAN DONATION

OPOs and hospitals are required by the Centers for Medicare and Medicaid Services (CMS) to identify and establish mutually agreed-on triggers for referral of potential organ donors. Many hospitals and OPOs have agreed that a ventilator-dependent, neurologically devastated patient with a Glasgow Coma Scale (GCS) of 5 or less is a patient who must be referred to the OPO. Because criteria for organ donation can vary so widely, OPOs discourage hospital staff from making further clinical judgments about a potential donor's suitability. OPOs receive calls about potential organ donors around the clock. While specific responses vary by agency, most OPOs will immediately send a staff member to the hospital to review the patient's medical record and work with the hospital staff to include assessment for brain death and organ donation in the patient's plan of care.

Historically, patients have been excluded from organ donation for a variety of clinical reasons. However, the critical need for organs has driven many transplant centers to expand their criteria for suitability and patients that once would have been refused as organ donors are now accepted routinely. Patients with histories of hepatitis, drug use, chronic disease, and other conditions can be suitable organ donors.

As a rule, physicians involved in death pronouncement should not be involved in the organ transplantation process or decisions.

NEUROLOGIC DEATH

Neurologic death, or **brain death,** is defined as the complete irreversible cessation of all brain and brainstem activity. The critical findings in a brain death examination are:

★ Explained loss of consciousness

★ No motor response to painful stimuli

★ No brainstem reflexes

★ Apnea

An explanation of the loss of consciousness is an important step in determining brain death. Most brain-dead patients have suffered some type of brain insult (severe head injury, subarachnoid hemorrhage, or intracerebral hemorrhage) that can be identified easily on computerized tomography (CT) scan. In some cases, brain insults such as anoxic brain injury may not be easily identifiable on CT, but can explain the presence of coma if the cause of the anoxic injury (e.g., cardiopulmonary arrest) is well documented.

Some factors or conditions can mimic brain death. It is important to exclude any condition that may cause the suppression of brainstem reflexes, including hypothermia, drug or alcohol intoxication, or metabolic derangement.

neurologic death *defined as the complete irreversible cessation of all brain and brain-stem activity.*

brain death *synonymous with neurological death; neurological death is the preferred term*

DETERMINING NEUROLOGIC DEATH

A brain death exam should demonstrate the following:

★ *Coma:* Lack of motor response to painful stimuli.

★ *Absence of pupillary reflexes:* Pupils should be dilated and unresponsive to light.

★ *Absence of ocular movement:* No eye movement occurs when the head is turned or when ice water is injected into the ear canal.

★ *Absence of response to corneal stimulation:* No blink or other response when a cotton swab touches the cornea.

★ *Absence of pharyngeal/tracheal reflex:* No gag reflex is noted when the posterior pharynx is stimulated, nor any couch reflex during bronchial suctioning.

An *apnea test* is performed to verify the complete cessation of brainstem function. The patient is preoxygenated with 100% FiO_2 and a baseline arterial blood gas (ABG) demonstrating normocarbia (pCO_2 >40 mmHg) is obtained. The ventilator is disconnected and 6 liters per minute (lpm) of O_2 is delivered via a cannula inserted into the endotracheal tube to the level of the carina. The patient is observed closely for respiratory movements or efforts; if any are observed, the test is terminated and the patient reconnected to the ventilator. If the patient does not breathe during the exam, an ABG sample is obtained and the patient reconnected to the ventilator. Arterial blood gases should be sampled at no later than 8 minutes; a pCO_2 of greater than 60 in the absence of respiratory effort is considered consistent with loss of brainstem function.

In cases where a clinical exam cannot be performed or when the patient's condition may confound the exam (e.g., drug intoxication, high cervical spine injury), other tests may be performed. These include tests to confirm the absence of blood flow to the brain (four-vessel angiography, isotope angiography, or portable cerebral blood flow study) or the absence of cortical brain activity (electroencephalography, somatosensory evoked potentials).

Any declaration of death by neurologic criteria should clearly document the injury that led to the death, the examinations performed and the results of those examinations, and the statement that the patient is declared dead, including the date and time of that declaration. This declaration of death is the legal declaration of death that will appear on the patient's death certificate.

Physicians who take part in determining neurologic death may not play a role in the subsequent procurement and transplantation of organs or tissues. This ethical (and in some instances legal) consideration helps to ensure that a totally unbiased assessment of the patient will be made. Likewise, in the United States and most Western nations, organs cannot be sold. This ensures that all people, regardless of their financial status, have access to organ transplantation and, more importantly, prevents black market exploitation.

ORGAN DONORS

All states have a version of the **Uniform Anatomical Gift Act (UAGA),** which describes the process by which consent is granted for organ and tissue donation, including donation by donor designation on a donor document (referred to in some areas as "first-person consent"). Historically, OPOs have been hesitant to act on donor cards without consent from the donor's legal next-of-kin (LNOK). In recent years, though, many OPOs have begun to embrace the concept of first-person consent, and to date no OPO has suffered any legal action when acting in good faith on such a document. Many different states have established online registries of donors so that OPOs can establish first-person consent without the need for an actual donor card at the time of the patient's death. Some states allow anyone to register; others require that registrants be residents of the state itself. Although no formal information-sharing agreements exist among registries, OPOs frequently will check a state donor registry at the request of another OPO handling a potential donor from that state.

Federal regulations require that an OPO staff member or someone trained by the OPO be the one to approach families about donation. OPOs and hospitals usually adopt a team effort to this discussion.

consent *consent for organ or tissue donation normally received from the donor's legal next-of-kin (LNOK) or donor document.*

Some states require physicians and other health care workers to initially approach families of recently deceased persons about possible organ donation.

Organ transplantation does not disfigure the body and is approved by most of the world's major religions.

CONSENT IN ORGAN DONATION

In the absence of a donor document or registration in a state donor registry, the OPO staff obtains **consent** for donation from the LNOK. Understandably, this is a process that requires a great deal of sensitivity and compassion, as the organ procurement coordinator (OPC) must guide the family through the acute stages of grief while helping them to understand what has happened and how organ and tissue donation can benefit them and others. (See Figure 34-2 ■.) Some OPOs have begun to employ staff solely for the task of working with families during this difficult time.

Frequently, families do not understand how their loved one can be dead. The body is still warm, the kidneys continue to produce urine, and the heart continues to beat. In many cases their loved one looks no different than shortly before, when he was alive. While it is the responsibility of the doctors to explain how the diagnosis of brain death was made, often the OPC must reiterate and reinforce this explanation. Using careful and compassionate language, the OPC can help the family understand that death has occurred, and help guide them toward the decision to donate organs and tissues. Often the OPC will talk about the potential recipients of the organs, and reiterate that the patient, through donation, can save many lives.

Some families are concerned about the patient's appearance after donation, and the OPC will explain that normal funeral arrangements are possible. Other families may worry that their religious leaders may object to donation, and the OPC can explain that no major religion opposes donation, and that many endorse it. Families will also struggle with the question of whether the

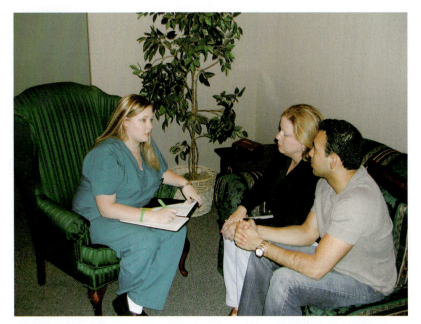

patient can feel or hear any part of what's going on. The OPC takes this opportunity to explain that all sensation is controlled and processed by the brain and, without the brain, no feeling or hearing is possible.

Families who agree to donate sign an authorization form detailing what organs and tissues will be donated. Most authorization forms describe the testing that is performed, the fact that the OPO is responsible for the costs associated with donation, how organs and tissues are allocated (including any other organizations that may be involved in the recovery of the gifts), and that the donor family will receive information from the OPO regarding the specifics about the donated organs.

The OPC will also complete a **medical/social/behavioral history** interview with the family or other appropriate historian. The interview is designed to identify donors who may be at high risk for hepatitis or HIV, as well as identify underlying medical conditions that may affect the safety and quality of the organs and tissues. In some cases, the legal next-of-kin may not be the best historian, especially if she or he has been living apart from the donor for a prolonged period of time. In these cases, the OPC will attempt to locate a close friend of the donor who may be able to provide more complete information about the donor's recent history and behavior.

medical/social/behavioral history *an interview conducted to identify donors who may be at high risk for hepatitis or HIV, and/or to identify underlying medical conditions that may affect the safety and quality of the organs and tissues.*

DONATED ORGAN/ORGAN RECIPIENT MATCHING

In the United States, the **United Network for Organ Sharing (UNOS)** oversees organ donation and transplantation. UNOS is the contractor operating the organ procurement and transplantation network (OPTN) on behalf of the federal government. All transplant candidates and recipients are listed with and matched by UNOS using matching criteria agreed on by the UNOS members, which include all transplant centers and OPOs in the United States.

While the exact criteria for matching varies slightly by organ, all donated organs are matched by blood type (ABO), donor/recipient size match, and donor/recipient distance. Organs must be from a donor who is ABO identical or ABO compatible with the recipient, or the recipient's body will quickly reject the organ. (See Table 34–1.) In addition, organs from donors who are substantially larger or smaller than the recipient's may not work well for the recipient. Finally, organs are usually allocated locally, then regionally, then nationally, with the sickest patients in each area being offered the organs first.

Candidates are listed for transplantation and their demographics and clinical data are entered in the UNOS computer system. Clinical data can be updated as often as is necessary to keep the candidate information current in the system.

United Network for Organ Sharing (UNOS) *the organizational contractor responsible for operation and oversight of the Organ Procurement and Transplantation Network (OPTN) on behalf of the U.S. government.*

Table 34–1	ABO-Identical or ABO-Compatible Organ Donations			
		Donor ABO		
		A	B	AB	O
Recipient ABO	A	Yes	No	No	Yes
	B	No	Yes	No	Yes
	AB	Yes	Yes	Yes	Yes
	O	No	No	No	Yes

When a donor is identified, the OPO lists the donor's demographic and clinical information in the UNOS computer system and requests a "match run" for the organs for which the donor or his or her next-of-kin has consented to donate. The computer assigns a unique identifier to the donor (commonly referred to as a UNOS ID), compares the donor demographics against all the candidates listed for each organ, and ranks the candidates according to the matching algorithm for each organ.

Once the match is complete, the organ procurement coordinator prints the list and contacts the transplant centers in order. The OPC shares the donor information with the transplant center so that the center can decide if the donor's clinical situation will provide a good outcome for their recipient. The transplant center may decline the organ for that particular candidate or for all candidates. The OPC notes the refusal reason and contacts the transplant center for the next candidate on the list.

CLINICAL MANAGEMENT OF THE ORGAN DONOR

Organ donors can present unique management challenges related to the original injury as well as to the complete cessation of function of the brain, brainstem, and central nervous system. The normal regulatory mechanisms performed by the brain must be supported or replaced by therapeutic interventions. **Organ donors** are critically ill patients who must be carefully monitored and managed in order to optimize organ function for the organ recipients.

organ donors
neurologically-dead patients who must be carefully monitored and managed in order to optimize organ function for the organ recipients.

The most common complication in the brain-dead organ donor is hypotension caused by hypovolemia related to the loss of vasomotor tone, which occurs as a result of the loss of the autonomic nervous system in brain death. This is commonly mistreated with vasopressors by well-meaning ICU staff but is best treated by infusion of IV fluids, including 0.45% saline, lactated Ringer's, albumin, or blood products if indicated. Organ donors should have central venous or pulmonary artery catheter monitoring and should be fluid resuscitated for a central venous pressure (CVP) of 6–9 or a pulmonary artery wedge pressure (PAWP) of 8–11. Once the donor has been adequately fluid resuscitated, IV vasopressors may be used to maintain a mean arterial pressure (MAP) of 60 or greater. Vasopressors of choice include dopamine, neosynephrine, or vasopressin. Norepinephrine and epinephrine should only be used as a last resort because they cause severe vasoconstriction and can lead to end-organ damage.

Hypovolemia can be complicated by diabetes insipidus (DI). DI is caused by the loss of antidiuretic hormone at the time of cerebral death. Without antidiuretic hormone, the body cannot regulate the retention of free water, and urine output increases to as much as 1,500–2,000 mL/hr. A vasopressin IV infusion can be titrated to maintain urine output between 7 and 10 mL/kg/hr. Vasopressin has the additional benefit of vasoconstriction, which can assist in maintaining blood pressure, but may be unwelcome in the face of a hypertensive donor. In this case, the OPC may consider the use of 1–2 mcg IV DDVAP (desmopressin) instead.

Some brain-dead patients may exhibit depressed cardiac function. Brain-dead patients lose all respiratory drive and function, and thus must be maintained on a ventilator. As with all ventilated patients, ventilator management is designed to maximize end-organ oxygenation and reduce the risk of infection. Donors with traumatic injuries may have additional pulmonary complications such as aspiration, pulmonary contusion, or pulmonary edema. While the lungs are constantly exposed to the environment, the donor has no protective mechanisms (coughing, sighing, and so on) to prevent infection in the lungs. The OPC must ensure good pulmonary toilet, including frequent turning and suctioning of the donor. As well, most organ donors receive broad-spectrum IV antibiotics such as cefazolin (Ancef) or piperacillin/tazobactam (Zosyn) to help fight infection. Donors suffering from pulmonary edema may be managed with increasing levels of oxygen, positive end-expiratory pressure, or other ventilator therapies in order to maintain proper oxygenation. In some cases, the OPC may elect to use furosemide (Lasix) to reduce the donor's preload and thus reduce the fluid collecting in the lungs.

ASSESSING ORGAN VIABILITY

Part of evaluating an organ donor is evaluating the status and function of transplantable organ systems. The OPC must order different studies to assess organ function before making organ offers to the transplant centers.

Hearts are evaluated by echocardiogram. A cardiologist or echocardiogram technologist will obtain cardiac images using ultrasonic waves. The heart and valves are assessed for size, structural abnormalities, and overall function. Ejection fraction (EF) is a measurement of how much blood the left ventricle pumps with each stroke and is measured as a percentage. A normal EF is 55% to 65%; an EF of less than 40% usually indicates a nontransplantable heart. The walls of the heart can be assessed for function and thickness. Akinetic or dyskinetic wall motion abnormalities can indicate ischemic damage to the cardiac tissue. Thickening (greater than 1 cm) of the septal or left ventricular walls may indicate hypertrophy (thickening of the cardiac muscle) and is frequently seen in patients with a history of poorly treated hypertension. Hypertrophic hearts frequently have bad outcomes after transplantation because the preservation solution cannot penetrate the thickened walls of the heart and the cells are not well preserved. Incompetent valves can also be identified via echocardiogram using Doppler mode to assess blood flow through the valves.

In some cases the transplant centers may request coronary angiography of the donor. This is usually requested in cases where the donor has increased risk of coronary artery disease, such as smoking, hypertension, or age greater than 40. When performing coronary angiography on a donor patient, the cardiologist should be reminded to minimize the amount of dye used to visualize the coronary arteries because the dye can have a nephrotoxic effect.

Pulmonary function is assessed via chest X-ray (CXR), bronchoscopy and ABGs. The transplant center will want measurements taken of both lungs from the CXR to determine the fit with the recipients. The center will also want to know about any abnormalities seen on CXR, including pulmonary contusions, infiltrates, reduced lung volumes, and airspace disease.

The OPC should perform an oxygen challenge to determine how well the donor lungs are processing oxygen. The ventilator FiO_2 is turned to 100% for 30 minutes, and an ABG is drawn. Thereafter, the FiO_2 is turned to 40% for 30 minutes and another ABG is drawn. At that point, the FiO_2 is returned to its original setting. A pO_2 greater than 300 mmHg on 100% FiO_2 is an indicator of transplantable lungs.

Some centers may request a bedside bronchoscopy. A pulmonologist should be consulted to perform this examination. Using a fiber-optic bronchoscope, the pulmonologist will examine the airways of both lungs, looking for evidence of trauma or infection. He will also take samples of secretions found in each lung and send these for culture and sensitivity. The OPC should request a STAT gram on all respiratory secretion samples to report organisms to the transplant center. The pulmonologist will note the nature of the secretions and whether they clear easily with suctioning. All of this information should be reported to the transplant center.

Liver function is assessed primarily via lab studies. The OPC will order studies of different hepatic enzymes to assess function of the liver. Especially after a hypotensive or anoxic event, or in the case of hepatic trauma, these enzymes may be elevated, but should return to near-normal levels after 24–48 hours. In some cases, if the donor is obese or has a history of heavy alcohol use, the liver transplant team may request a biopsy of the liver. A physician trained in such procedures, usually a hepatologist, can perform this in the ICU under ultrasound guidance. In some cases, it may be preferable to obtain a CT-guided biopsy by a radiologist. A pathologist will evaluate the biopsy frozen section for evidence of fatty infiltration (steatosis), inflammation, and other chronic changes. Pancreas function is assessed by studying the donor's serum glucose level as well as serum levels of amylase and lipase. Elevations of any of these may indicate pancreatic dysfunction, especially in the case of abdominal trauma. Facial injuries, however, can produce an elevated amylase level due to damage to the salivary glands in the mouth. Kidney function is assessed by monitoring urine output as well as BUN and serum creatinine levels. The OPC should ensure that the donor is properly hydrated before treating decreased urine output with a diuretic or other therapy. In a properly hydrated donor, urine output should average 7–10 cc/kg/hr.

Intestine function is difficult to assess directly, but can be determined by evaluating the liver and pancreas function. As well, the OPC should look for evidence of abdominal trauma and listen for bowel sounds.

ANESTHESIA REQUIREMENTS FOR ORGAN RECOVERY

Because organ donors have experienced neurologic death, they are incapable of feeling pain and thus do not require anesthesia for pain control. Most OPOs, however, use an anesthesiologist or nurse anesthetist to monitor the donor during the procurement surgery and titrate medications and IV fluids to optimize organ function throughout the surgical organ recovery process. In addition, toward the end of the case, prior to the placement of the cannulas, the anesthesiologist will give 300 units/kg of IV heparin to prevent blood clotting around the cannulas and in the organs after aortic cross-clamp.

ORGAN RECOVERY AND PRESERVATION

In preparation for surgical recovery of the organs, the OPC should establish contact with the hospital's operating room staff early in the process of donor evaluation. The OPC should explain the process to the OR staff and review with them which supplies the OPO will provide and which supplies should be provided by the hospital. The division of supplies varies by OPO, but in general the OPO will supply donor-specific items (like retractors, storage basins, and flush solutions) while the hospital will provide more standard surgical supplies (gloves, gowns, table drapes, suture, electrocautery equipment, and so on). The OPC and OR staff will agree on what OR staff members will be needed (usually a circulating nurse and a scrub nurse or scrub technician). The OPC will review with the circulating nurse the documentation of brain death, the authorization for donation, and the credentials of the surgical teams coming to recover the organs. The OPC will ensure that the team members behave appropriately and that contact is maintained as necessary between the donor site and the transplant center.

In general, the sooner an organ is retrieved and transplanted, the better the chances of success.

When the teams are ready, the donor is transported to the OR and moved to the operating table. The donor is prepped and draped in normal surgical fashion according to established hospital procedure. A midline incision is made from just above the pubic bone to the sternal notch. The organs are exposed and examined for any obvious anatomical abnormalities. The surgical teams isolate the vasculature of each organ in preparation for removal from the body. The teams place cannulas into the great vessels to allow preservation solution to be flushed into the organs. When everything is ready, the aorta is cross-clamped, the chest and abdominal cavities are cooled rapidly using sterile ice, and cold preservation solutions are flushed through the vessels into the organs. The organs are further examined to ensure that the preservation solution flows well and that there are no vascular abnormalities. The organs are removed from the body and taken to a back table for further inspection and packaging. Once packaged, they are transported back to the transplant center for implantation into the recipient. (See Table 34–2 and Figure 34-3 ■.)

Table 34–2	Preservation Times
Heart	4 hours
Lungs	4–6 hours
Liver	12–24 hours
Pancreas	16–24 hours
Intestine	8–12 hours
Kidney	24–72 hours
Corneas	5–7 days
Skin	Fresh: 10 days
	Frozen: 5 years
Dura	5 years

TISSUE DONATION

In 2004, the waiting list for an organ transplant in the United States grew to nearly 90,000 people. However, 625,000 people are waiting for a tissue graft. The demand for both organs and tissues is dramatically higher than the supply. Facilitating donation for thousands of people takes a special group of clinicians. They have to convince family members to put their grief on hold and take the time to help someone else in need of transplant; carefully screen the viability of an organ or tissue to ensure compatibility and prevent disease transmission; and coordinate numerous events to ensure that they all come together at the just right moment to prevent critical delays or even the death of another.

A variety of human tissue can be donated by anyone who has suffered a cardiac death and has a suitable medical and social history, unlike organ donation, which requires brain death and has strict legislative requirements to determine brain death. Organ donors can always be tissue donors following the organ recovery, unless something in the decedent's history excludes them as a donor. Medical and social history requirements also differ between organ and tissue donors. In the United States, the Food and Drug Administration strictly regulates the transplantation of tissues. Tissues are often considered life enhancing, rather than lifesaving. Very few tissues are transplanted quickly

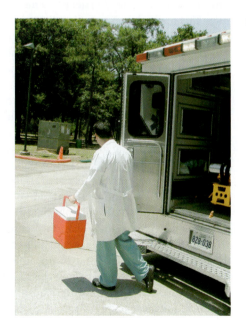

■ Figure 34-3   An organ, packaged for transport to the transplant center. *(Courtesy of LifeGift Organ Donation Center, Houston)*

and only under emergent situations. Organs have to be transplanted immediately and this is accomplished at a greater risk and expense. If waiting recipients do not receive the organ that they need, they will certainly die. Therefore, certain medical conditions are overlooked for organs, as long as the organ functions properly. Tissue donation does not overlook any disease. If there is a risk of transmission of communicable disease or a risk to the quality of the tissue, then the tissue is ruled unsuitable and is not recovered.

Tissue donation involves all areas of the human body. Similar to organ recovery, tissues are recovered in a sterile environment, usually in an operating room, and removed aseptically. This is done to reduce the risk of contamination and transmission of bacteria to a recipient. Tissues must be recovered within 24 hours of death if the decedent has been cooled, 15 hours if the decedent has not been cooled after death.

Starting from the head, the *dura mater* is a tough fibrous lining around the brain and can be used for transplantation. Dura mater is usually recovered during an autopsy and can only be used to replace the dura mater in patients who have undergone invasive brain surgery. Brain surgeries may include resection or removal of brain tumors, traumatic repair, and dura replacement following craniotomy. Dura mater must be recovered within 40 hours after death. After processing, dura mater can be kept for 5 years before being transplanted.

Whole eyes or *corneas* can be recovered and used to give sight to those with correctable diseases and disorders. Corneas are the hard glassy surfaces of the eyes that allow light to pass into the retina, which is then processed into an image by the brain. Corneas are usually sutured onto the recipient's eye after the diseased cornea is removed. The cornea has a very short shelf life and must be transplanted within 2 days after recovery. The whole eye can be recovered, with the cornea being removed and used as stated previously. The sclera or white portion of the whole eye can be used as a whole globe for eye prosthesis or the sclera can be cut into strips and used as straps for the eye in the treatment of glaucoma.

Though rare, the *mandible* can be used as a bone graft for patients suffering from bone cancer, traumatic injuries, or serious dental diseases. The mandible can be transplanted whole or cut into segments and used accordingly.

Skin grafts can be recovered using a device known as a dermatome. The dermatome is a surgical instrument and can be powered by electricity or compressed air. The dermatome removes a thin layer of the skin that includes both the epidermis and dermis. The skin is then processed in two different ways. The traditional method of skin processing is cryopreservation, which is a form of freezing. When a surgeon is ready for a skin graft, he will thaw the graft and then mesh the graft to two or thee times the graft's original size. The graft is used in conjunction with other dressings and burn care products to create a barrier and a media for the patient's own skin to grow back. Unfortunately, using this method does not allow for the graft to adhere to the patient and after about 7 days the graft will die and have to be removed.

A more advanced method of skin grafting is known as Alloderm. Alloderm is a proprietary method of removing the epidermal layer and de-cellularizing the graft. This process leaves behind a biomatrix of collagen. The graft can be sutured directly to a burn patient after traditional debridement. The Alloderm graft will grow with the patient and the patient's own cells will populate the graft. This creates an immediate barrier reducing infection, pain, and the need to debride the patient as often. Alloderm also reduces the number of skin grafts needed to treat a single patient and reduces the amount of scarring for the patient. In the traditional cryopreserved method, a single burn patient can use 80 to 100 square feet of skin every 7 to 10 days. Alloderm alleviates this 7- to 10-day process and reduces the number of grafts because the grafts will adhere and grow with the patient.

The whole *heart* can be removed in order to use the valves of the heart. The heart valves used are commonly the aortic and pulmonary valves and occasionally the mitral valve. The aortic valve is used along with a conduit of aorta to ensure the surgeon of a perfect fit inside the recipient. Likewise, the pulmonary valve is used with a conduit of pulmonary artery. Heart valves are commonly used in pediatric patients and young adults. Pediatric recipients may need as many as five to six heart valve transplants throughout their lives since the valves do not grow with the patient. The mitral valves are more commonly transplanted into older patients with mitral valve prolapse.

Bone and *tendons* are the most significant tissues recovered, because they provide the most usable grafts and help the most people. One bone donor can help up to 75 people, depending on the us-

tissue donation *involves all areas of the human body. Similar to organ recovery, tissues include heart valves, corneas, bone, skin, and other non-vascularized body parts.*

age and planning of the grafts. Bone is recovered from the arms, including the humerus, radius, and ulna, and from the lower body, including the pelvis, femurs, tibias, fibulas, calcaneus, and talus. Multiple tendons can be transplanted as well, including the patella, semitendinosus, and gracilis tendons.

Some specialty uses for bone are fresh frozen grafts known as *osteoarticular* (OA) grafts or *osteochondral* (OC) grafts. An OA graft is a complete joint that has been processed and frozen intact. This could be a complete knee, elbow, or shoulder joint. These grafts are used in an urgent situation, often to prevent amputation of limbs. The best example is with treatment of osteosarcomas. Osteosarcoma is a type of bone cancer that usually involves a tumor-like lesion in the growth plate of the humerus or tibia. This type of cancer is commonly seen in children and young adults and can be very aggressive. Therefore, immediate radical amputation of the limb can result, giving doctors the comfort that the cancer has been completely removed. However, with the use of an OA graft the limb can be spared. Doctors can surgically remove the diseased joint and all surrounding muscle tissue to be certain about the complete removal of the cancer lesion. Then the doctor will place the OA graft joint using various tools, rods, and other support prostheses. The OA graft will then grow with the patient.

Finally, *veins* from the legs can be recovered and used in patients requiring coronary bypass or bypass to save a limb. The *greater saphenous vein* and *femoral vein* are typically recovered after being flushed with an antispasmotic solution. The vein is recovered in its full length from the groin to the foot, usually yielding 70–80 cm of usable graft. The veins are processed and cryopreserved to await the high demand of cardiovascular surgeons. Recently, femoral veins have been used as shunts in patients requiring hemodialysis. Traditional synthetic grafts tend to clot easier and develop resistant infections. With the femoral vein these side effects are reduced dramatically and the dialysis process is less painful for the patient.

EMS SCENE DEATH REFERRAL PROGRAM

Currently in the United States a federal mandate is in place to ensure that a compliant relationship exists between organ procurement organizations and hospitals. Prior to 1998 it was the hospital's responsibility to recognize potential tissue donors, to determine if the decedent was suitable to donate tissues, and to offer the family the option of donation and perform the legal consent process. This process was found to be an extreme burden on the hospital staff and resulted in numerous inconsistencies and miscommunications regarding donation.

The federal mandates of 1998 instituted policies to have hospitals refer all deaths, regardless of age or disease, to an OPO. After the referral it is up to the OPO to determine suitability for donation and obtain consent. This revolutionized the tissue donation industry, resulting in numerous OPO call centers emerging and a dramatic increase in tissue donation nationwide.

Unfortunately, this mandate only covers hospital deaths; deaths that occur outside of a hospital are not covered or addressed, leaving a number of families without the option of donation. However, a new program involving EMS agencies is gradually being introduced. This program empowers EMS personnel to get involved in saving lives by a different means.

All over the country, tens of thousands of EMTs and paramedics respond to calls everyday. Some of these calls involve people who die at a scene for various reasons. Some EMS agencies have protocols to terminate nonviable cardiac arrest patients; others have patients who have injuries incompatible with life. Either way every scene death has the potential to yield a tissue donor and involving EMS personnel is critical.

EMS personnel respond quickly and can provide important clinical and scene survey information that can be important in determining suitability. Time is one of the most important factors in donation. Tissue donation has to occur within 24 hours of the death, and time becomes critical when the person has been down for a long or unknown amount of time. Time for donation can expire if an OPO has to wait on a medical examiner, coroner, or a justice of the peace to make a referral.

The procedure can be adapted to format any agency protocol and is very simple to follow. The referral process is usually a brief phone call from the EMT or paramedic at the scene. The step-by-step procedure is listed in Table 34–3.

Table 34–3	Donation Referral Process

Death on Scene Identified by EMS

1. Obvious trauma incompatible with life
2. Extended downtime with evidence of rigor mortis or dependent lividity
3. Field termination protocol implemented

Vital Information Obtained from Scene by Paramedic

1. Location of deceased
2. Next-of-kin or contact person
3. Next-of-kin or contact person phone number
4. Name, age, sex, and race of deceased
5. Mechanism of injury
6. Brief medical history (if available)

Call Initiated from Scene by Paramedic
Information Needed by OPO:

1. Name of referring EMS employee
2. Agency name and unit/medic number
3. Station or communication center phone number
4. Location of death and deceased
5. Vital information gathered at the scene (above)

OPO Provides Follow-Up

1. By phone within 24 hours (if applicable)
2. Referring medic will receive a letter

Summary

Organ and tissue donation represent a new chance at life for recipients as well as solace for the donor's family and friends. As health care professionals, it is incumbent on us to provide families with the opportunity to donate whenever that opportunity arises, and to preserve the option of donation in order to maximize the potential for the recipients of the donated organs and tissues. Through a complex medical and emotional process, one person can save and/or enhance the lives of many.

Review Questions

1. Discuss the role of the critical care paramedic in organ recovery and transplantation.
2. Detail the indications for organ procurement.
3. Define neurologic death.
4. Discuss the importance of consent with regard to organ and tissue procurement.
5. Briefly describe the organ recovery process.
6. Discuss the importance of tissue donation and describe the types of tissues usually harvested.
7. Discuss the role of EMS in death scene referral for organ donation.

See Answers to Review Questions at the back of this book.

Further Reading

Medicare and Medicaid Programs; Hospital Conditions of Participation; Identification of Potential Organ, Tissue, and Eye Donors and Transplant Hospitals' Provision of Transplant-Related Data, 42 CFR Part 482, (June 22, 1998).

Organ Donation: A Medical Dictionary, Bibliography, and Annotated Research Guide to Internet References. San Diego, CA: Icon Health Publications, 2004.

Organ Procurement and Transplantation Network. http://www.optn.org.

Rosendale JD, Kauffman HM, McBride MA, Chabalewski FL, Zaroff JG, Garrity ER, Delmonico FL, Rosengard BR. "Aggressive Pharmacologic Donor Management Results in More Transplanted Organs." *Transplantation,* Vol. 75, No. 4 (February 27, 2003): 482–487.

Sheehy E, Conrad SL, Brigham LE, Luskin R, Weber P, Eakin M, Schkade L, Hunsicker L. "Estimating the Number of Potential Organ Donors in the United States." *New England Journal of Medicine,* Vol. 349, No. 7 (2003): 667–674.

Wijdicks, EFM. "Determining Brain Death in Adults." *Neurology,* Vol. 45 (1995): 1003–1011.

Wood KE, Becker BN, McCartney JG, D'Alessandro AM, Coursin DB. "Care of the Potential Organ Donor." *New England Journal of Medicine,* Vol. 351 (2004): 2730–2739.

Quality Improvement in Critical Care Transport

Darryl A. Coontz, MBA, EMT-P and Bryan E. Bledsoe, DO, FACEP

Objectives

Upon completion of this chapter, the student should be able to:

1. Describe why quality improvement processes and practices are essential for any critical care transport operation. (p. 1004)
2. Describe the importance of ongoing monitoring of key performance indicators in critical care practice. (p. 1007)
3. Detail items and information than can be gleaned from environmental scanning. (p. 1007)
4. List and define some of the key performance areas in critical care transport medicine. (p. 1007)
5. Describe the QCDSM model of information analysis. (p. 1009)
6. Discuss the advantages and disadvantages of various schemes for reporting data and trends including:
   A. Flowcharts (p. 1011)
   B. Cause-and-effect (fishbone) diagrams (p. 1011)
   C. Run (trend) charts (p. 1011)
   D. Histograms (p. 1012)
   E. Scatter diagram (p. 1012)
   F. Pareto charts (p. 1013)
   G. Control charts (p. 1013)
7. Discuss the traits of an effective leader. (p. 1015)
8. Contrast the difference between common cause and special cause variations. (p. 1015)

Key Terms

Case Study

You are a shift supervisor for a busy critical care transport program that is a part of a large EMS operation. One day, while retrieving some supplies, the supply manager mentioned that they were out of intraosseous (IO) needles again. At that time, you did not give much thought to the statement. Later, while reviewing some QI data for the critical care department, you noticed that the IV success rate for the past 2 months had dropped from 92% to 71%. You rechecked the figures and the math to ensure this was correct. Then, you remembered what the supply clerk had said about the IO needles. You wondered whether there might be a relationship. You accessed the QI database and pulled all IV start success rates by paramedic. Much as you suspected, four critical care paramedics had IV success rates less than 80% with one at 44%. These four happened to be on another shift and were the graduates from the most recent critical care paramedic class. A quick query into the database revealed that these four critical care paramedics had used more IO needles than all of the other paramedics in the system combined.

Based on this, a remedy was in order. The problem, while limited to the four critical care paramedics in question, was still a system issue. Instead of punishing the four, you elect to have the current month's continuing education focus (CE) on "Improving IV Success Rates." You look and find four paramedics with the highest IV success rate (which also happen to be the four most experienced paramedics in your division) and ask them to conduct the in-service. After the in-service you found, through your ongoing QI program, that the IV success rate for these four paramedics (and the system in general) improved, while the IO usage rate for the system was reduced by 50%.

In this case, you used the QI program as it was designed: for system improvement and not individual employee punishment. All involved left the CE session with improved skills and were not threatened by the process. Most important though was the fact that patient care improved because a less invasive way of accessing the circulation was used in more patients.

INTRODUCTION

The term quality is difficult to define. When used as a noun, quality typically means a superiority of kind. When used as an adjective, it usually describes something with a high degree of excellence. From a business standpoint, quality can be defined as a dynamic state associated with products, services, people, processes, and environments that meets or exceeds expectations. A fundamental tenet of quality is customer satisfaction—the purpose of business is to satisfy the customer. People have come to expect quality in every product or service. Health care, including EMS and critical care transport providers, is certainly no different.

Throughout the history of business, there has been continued evolution in the notion of what quality is, in both theory and practice. In order for the critical care paramedic to better understand this concept of quality (or what is generically stated as "quality assurance or quality management") which attempts to improve a system's performance, this chapter will present an overview of the work by leaders in the field of quality assurance and discuss these theories as they pertain to critical care paramedic services.

In the 1980s, many businesses adopted an approach to quality that affected all aspects of the operation. This concept, called *total quality management*, varies based upon the service or product provided. However, it is a top-down, company-wide commitment to excellence in all aspects of operation. Today, businesses define quality using specific specifications, standards, and other measures. Thus, quality can be defined and measured. Health care and EMS are no different. We are there to serve the patients who are functionally our customers. Thus, one measure of EMS quality is customer satisfaction.

Dr. W. Edwards Deming detailed how a product must be developed in order to meet customer needs. This concept, usually referred to as the Deming Cycle, is as follows:

1. Consumer research is performed and used to plan the product (plan).
2. Product production (do).
3. Assure the product was produced in accordance with the plan (check).
4. Market the product (act).
5. Analyze the reception of the product by the consumers in terms of quality, cost, and other criteria (analyze).

A hospital or company might use this model to try and determine the feasibility of a helicopter operation. First, they would research the market and try and determine the need (demand) for the service. Second, they would establish the service which would include hiring personnel, acquiring assets, establishing policies and procedures, and performing other essential details. Third, and prior to beginning operation, management and employees will check the assembled program against the plan and correct any deficiencies. Fourth, the business is opened and operations begin. Finally, the company should evaluate customer feedback, outcomes, and other indicators. Any deficiencies identified should be corrected. Analysis is a continuous process in organizations committed to total quality management.

Another prominent leader in the quality management (or assurance) movement was Joseph M. Juran who enumerated 10 steps to quality improvement:

1. *Build awareness of both the need for improvement and opportunities for improvement.* An example of this in critical care transport would be a policy that any member of the operation, from the CEO on down, can point out problems or make recommendations without fear of retribution. For example, a critical care paramedic on several occasions sees a popular pilot fail to adhere to all routine safety measures. There must be an avenue to bring these concerns forward without fear of retribution.

2. *Set goals for improvement.* In order to set goals for improvement, performance must be measured. For example, certain procedures in emergency medicine have zero tolerance. Of these, unrecognized esophageal intubations can be a problem in EMS. The goal should be 0 percent unrecognized intubations. To achieve this, performance must be measured, deficiencies identified, a remedy proposed and initiated, and continuing follow-up used to assure that the remedy is working.

3. *Organize to meet the goals that have been set.* To meet established goals requires commitment from every employee. An organized system, often overseen by a committee or quality management person, is necessary in order to engage all personnel in quality improvement. Each deficiency must have a plan to remedy it. However, the plan must be dynamic to assure that it adapts to the problem identified.

4. *Provide training.* Training (or education) assures that everyone in the operation follows the same policies and procedures. For example, American Airlines has several thousand pilots. Despite their various degrees of experience on myriad aircraft types, they all operate American Airlines jets in exactly the same manner. Through initial and ongoing training, pilots are reminded of the standards, policies, and procedures the airline expects. Thus, you will see virtually identical takeoffs and landings despite personnel and equipment differences. In helicopter operations, the aviation policies and procedures are often company-wide to minimize deviations by individual pilots.

5. *Implement projects aimed at solving problems.* Problems should be identified and a system to remedy the problem established. For example, in one EMS system ongoing quality measures revealed that paramedics were only administering aspirin to 53% of eligible chest pain patients. Thus, an educational program was provided and the mnemonic "MONA" (morphine, oxygen, nitroglycerin, and aspirin) was taped on the wall above the stretcher. Compliance with aspirin administration increased appreciably.

6. *Report progress.* In order to make changes, quality must be measured and progress reported. People cannot be expected to make changes unless they are aware of the severity of the issue or where they personally stand in respect to others. For example, several critical care crews were submitting documentation that was substandard. In order to change the behavior, an education class was held and then a weekly graphic was posted with the acceptable percentage documents by crew. This allowed the crews with poor documentation to know where they stood and encouraged them to improve in a competitive environment.

7. *Give recognition.* Human nature demands that we be recognized for good performance. Recognition is a positive reinforcement for good behavior and good performance. This reinforcement may be simply recognition or it could be something more elaborate such as money, trips, products, or similar enticements. This promotes loyalty and can lead to beneficial competition.

8. *Communicate results.* People today need information. Feedback is important and results, either negative or positive, need to be reported. For example, a critical care transport system was having an increasing number of expired drugs go unreplaced. A program was developed to check the drugs (including those in backup vehicles) on a regular basis. After a predetermined interval, the results of the action should be reported. If the program is working and expired drugs are replaced, then the results are reported and the program continued. If the program is not working, the results are also reported except the program is changed in order to facilitate better quality control of expired drugs.

9. *Keep score.* The idea of keeping score in health care seems strange—something more expected from car dealers and aluminum siding salesmen. However, keeping score allows you to know how one employee is performing compared to another, how one team or shift is performing when compared to another, or how the whole company is performing compared to another. Medicare and the insurance companies keep score. They know which hospitals have the lowest costs, best outcomes, lowest mortalities, and fewest complications. They also know a great deal about EMS operations in terms of patient demographics, average charges, and so on. To be able to survive in such a highly measured and regulated environment, organizations must "keep score" at numerous levels.

10. *Maintain momentum by building improvement into the organizations regular system.* The commitment to quality must integrate into every aspect of the operation. In a critical care operation this should include such areas as supply, dispatch, operations, and management as failure in one area will adversely affect the other and can adversely impact patient care and thus customer satisfaction.

Juran was also responsible for espousing the *Pareto Principle* that is sometimes referred to as he "80/20 rule." This principle states that 80 percent of trouble in an organization comes from 20 percent of the problems. Juran encouraged management to concentrate on the few sources of problems and not be distracted by those of lesser importance.

Another leader in the quality management field was Phillip B. Crosby who advocated the idea of "zero defects" instead of statistically acceptable levels. The idea of "zero defects" has particular application to medicine and critical care transport systems as defects in a health care system can lead to patient injury or even death. Crosby described four absolutes of quality management:

1. Quality must be defined as conformance to requirements—not just as a good thing to do.

2. The best way to ensure quality is prevention and not inspection.

3. The standard for quality must be zero defects and not "close is good enough."

4. Quality is measured by nonconformance and not indexes.

RECENT TRENDS IN QUALITY MANAGEMENT

Several recent trends in quality management have begun to integrate into EMS and critical care quality management. Of these, the ISO 9000 and Six Sigma systems are encountered. ISO 9000 is a series of international quality standards developed in 1979 by a committee with participants from 20 countries. This served to provide a clear, international set of quality requirements. It is most commonly used in manufacturing operations although it is finding utility in other aspects of business. The Six Sigma concept was developed by Motorola in the mid-1980s. The term Six Sigma comes from the Greek letter sigma (σ) which, in statistics, is used to represent a standard deviation unit. (For additional information on standard deviation and Gaussian curves, see Chapter 12.) The *standard deviation* is a statistic that tells you how tightly all the various examples are clustered around the mean in a set of data. When the examples are tightly bunched together and the bell-shaped curve is steep, the standard deviation is small. When the examples are spread apart and the bell curve is relatively flat, that tells you that you have a relatively large standard deviation. With each increasing standard deviation, a greater percentage of the sample is included. For example:

σ = 68.26895 percent confidence level

2σ = 95.44997 percent confidence level

3σ = 99.73002 percent confidence level

4σ = 99.99366 percent confidence level

5σ = 99.99994 percent confidence level

6σ = 99.99999 percent confidence level

Thus, if a company strives for a 6-sigma quality plan, they will have 99.9999998 percent acceptable products or, stated another way, only 0.002 defective products per million. In summary, Six Sigma assures that all customer requirements are met. The Six Sigma system is detailed in the Six Sigma Road Map:

1. Appoint a champion.

2. Select a cross-functional team.

3. Develop quantifiable goals.

4. Develop an implementation plan that establishes training, addresses data collection, and includes a program maintenance plan.

5. Coordinate the road map.

In today's competitive and highly litigious society, the only acceptable product or service, is quality based upon customer satisfaction. EMS and critical care transport are no different. This is especially important given that flaws in a health care organization have the direct capability to harm the patient. Because of this, quality management must be a part of every aspect of the operation.

QUALITY ASSURANCE VERSUS QUALITY IMPROVEMENT

While both quality assurance (QA) and quality improvement (QI) fall under the realm of quality management, there are significant functional differences between quality assurance and quality improvement. In general, QA and QI are used in reference to clinical care but the processes may also be applied to administrative and educational review.

In quality assurance, the primary objective is to "assure" that quality care and service are being provided. In quality improvement, the aim is to develop strategies that will have a global impact on the efficiency and accuracy of patient care delivery. QA is accomplished through the review of patient records or documentation of clinical performance. QI is a dynamic process that is initiated following identification of trends in procedural failure or recurrent deficits in QA outcome data. QI is frequently driven by data obtained during the QA process and should be continuously reevaluated.

MEASURING PERFORMANCE AND QUALITY IN CRITICAL CARE TRANSPORT

There are numerous methods of measuring quality in EMS and critica care transport. Each has a specific feature for which it is best used. The following discussion will detail common measures used in EMS and critical care quality management. (See Figure 35-1 ■.)

CHART REVIEW AND FEEDBACK TO CLINICIANS

One component of your clinical quality improvement process can be a review of individual cases or groups of cases. This process can be a helpful learning tool, however, it's important to keep in mind that the big improvements usually come from looking at processes rather than individual paramedics. There are many different ways to coordinate this activity. Some of the most effective systems use peers to review the charts and provide feedback on patient management and documentation. Often the feedback is provided in a **morbidity and mortality (M&M) conference** that is modeled after how residents critique each other in their advanced medical training programs.

morbidity and mortality (M&M) conference *a meeting to audit and discuss cases that address or identify quality assurance issues raised by the resident medical staff in an effort to evaluate performance and patient care modality or outcomes.*

environmental scanning *operational scanning that looks for changes in clinical literature that might affect the protocols and clinical management of patients in your system.*

ENVIRONMENTAL SCANNING

The last part of an ongoing quality management process for a critical care program is **environmental scanning.** This scan should look for changes in the clinical literature that might affect the protocols

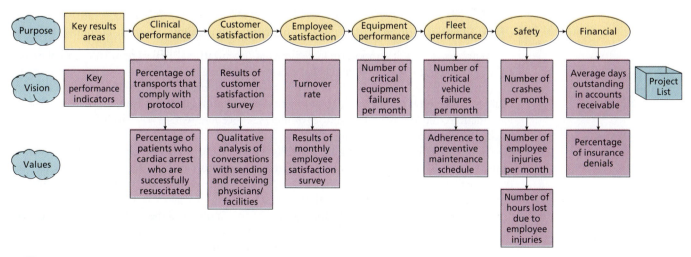

■ Figure 35-1   Critical care transport quality management system.

and clinical management of patients in your system. There are several options for making this process easy and low maintenance. If your system has access to a hospital or medical school library, the librarian can help set up a monthly photocopy of the table of contents of selected medical journals. These can be reviewed for relevant articles. There are also ways to set up regular Internet searches of current literature.

Your environmental scan should also pay attention to what is happening in your local health care arena. Which hospitals are opening day surgery centers? Which neurosurgical groups are moving to another hospital? Keeping a good handle on what is going on in your local environment allows you to stay ahead of the changes so your system can provide the best possible service.

It is best to employ a fourfold approach to environmental scanning:

1. Identify local clinical practices and quality issues including potential threats.
2. Use evidence-based medicine guidelines (Class I or II research) to identify KPIs and develop improvement plans.
3. Promote future orientation in the thinking of the management and staff.
4. Alert management and staff to trends that are converging, diverging, speeding up, slowing down, or interacting.

HOW IS THE ORGANIZATION PERFORMING?

Management educator Ken Blanchard says, "Feedback is the breakfast of champions." Feedback is essential to our ability to optimize performance in any endeavor. Can you imagine flying a helicopter with no gauges to tell you the fuel level, altitude, speed, and the like? In order for a critical care service to answer the "How are we doing?" question, it needs a set of gauges that provide feedback on performance. Typically organizations focus only on direct clinical performance, outcomes, and adherence to protocol. Although these areas are essential, they are incomplete. Organizations first need to define the **key results areas (KRAs)** of the organization necessary to provide their service. For example, a typical critical care organization might include the following as KRAs:

key results areas (KRAs)
areas of interest that may include clinical performance, customer satisfaction, employee satisfaction, equipment performance, fleet performance, safety, and financial operations.

★ Clinical performance (i.e., Is the prehospital practice state of the art?)
★ Customer satisfaction (i.e., Are customers satisfied and do they feel they received value?)
★ Employee satisfaction (i.e., Are employees happy and motivated?)
★ Equipment performance (i.e., Is equipment state of the art without incidence of critical failures?)
★ Fleet performance (i.e., Is the fleet well maintained and dependable?)
★ Safety (i.e., Is the work environment safe for customer and employee?)
★ Financial performance (i.e., Are billings correct? Is accounts receivable current?)

Within each KRA it's important to define a few organizational vital signs or KPIs. Just like a patient's vital signs, these should be regularly monitored to see how the organization is performing, to identify problems, and to assess the results of interventions. For example, in the safety area you could track the total number of hours of work each month that are lost from employees' primary job functions due to on-the-job injuries or illnesses. (See Figure 35-2 ■.) This information can be tracked on a run chart or control chart.

To be used effectively the quantitative KPIs should be tracked over time and plotted on a chart in their naturally occurring order. This will give you a picture of how the process performs over time. It will also help you get a handle on the process's natural variation, which can guide any actions that you might take to improve the process.

All processes have variation in their performance. Sometimes the variation is dramatic, like that seen in the stock market. At other times it is subtle, like differences in the angle of bevels on a set of 18-gauge IV needles. The variation that is inherent in a process is called *common cause variation*. If something special happens to the process it can cause variation that is outside the expected common cause. When that happens it is referred to as *special cause variation*. For example, one EMS

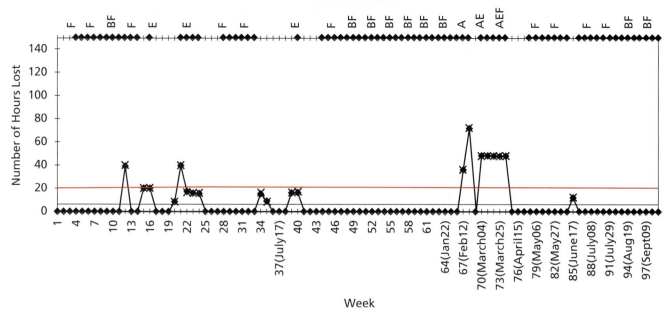

OK C Hours Lost

■ **Figure 35-2**   Hours lost due to work-related injuries.

system was averaging 95% compliance with their chest pain protocol. Some months it was 98%, others 92%, and over the course of several years it hovered around 95%. Then there was a sudden dramatic drop in performance to 70%, a special cause variation. Exploration of the shift revealed that the protocol had been modified to include the early administration of aspirin to patients with cardiac chest pain. Many paramedics were failing to administer aspirin and thus compliance fell.

Further investigation revealed that the noncompliance with protocol was almost all related to aspirin administration. An old-style manager would want the names of the paramedics who had failed to comply with the protocol. However, managers who practice quality improvement know that their biggest leverage for improvement is in the process, not the people. Further investigation revealed that paramedics who did not give aspirin felt that their patients were having severe myocardial infarctions accompanied by lots of pain that needed to be managed with morphine not aspirin. It became clear that the system had failed to properly educate paramedics that the reason patients with cardiogenic chest pain need aspirin was to decrease the agglutination of cells that contribute to the occlusion and to decrease the inflammation in the walls of the coronary arteries. The system provided redesigned education on the new chest pain protocol and the use of aspirin. The protocol compliance rose to an average of 98% and has stayed there ever since.

Most critical care transport programs will have both quantitative and qualitative measures in their KPI list. It's important that people with a scientific quantitative mind don't dismiss qualitative information from their span of consideration. For example, interviews with physicians who order critical care transport from your service can be a powerful and valid source of ideas for improvement even though the results can't be plotted on a chart.

Every critical care transport system, whether ground, fixed-wing, or rotor-wing, must have an ongoing quality management program.

INFORMATION AND ANALYSIS

As mentioned earlier, to better serve your customers, you must measure many aspects of your program to ensure that you are operating in a manner that takes into account all aspects of critical care transportation. An organization that blindly sends its people out in the world hoping they are doing what we expect will soon be out of business. For this reason information is required and we must learn how to manage and interpret the information. The first question that needs to be answered is "What should we measure?" You should measure things that are important to the delivery of your service. One model that is used is the **QCDSM model.** QCDSM stands for quality, cost,

QCDSM model *an information and analysis model that assesses* **quality,** **cost, delivery, safety,** *and* **morale.**

delivery, safety, and morale. Each component consists of a subset of KPIs that tell you how you are doing. Each one of the following indicators should be reviewed on a scheduled basis whereby management can determine where best to implement improvements.

★ *Quality*—can be described as a degree of excellence. Some examples of quality measurements for a critical care transport program:

  – Customer satisfaction

  – IV or intubation success rates

  – Medication or documentation errors

★ *Cost*—sustaining a critical care transport program requires managers to understand where the money is being spent. Some examples of cost measurements that may be helpful:

  – Fleet maintenance (tire wear, brake wear, fuel usage)

  – Payroll (unscheduled overtime)

  – Supplies (disposable medical, durable medical)

★ *Delivery*—usually refers to cycle times:

  – Time from call received until critical care team arrival (response time)

  – Time from arriving on scene to departure (bedside time)

  – Time from arrival at destination to available (turnaround time)

  – Miles between ambulance breakdowns (mission failures)

★ *Safety*—may describe incidents or accidents. May also be used as a subjective measurement to determine compliance with policies. Some examples of measurements of safety in critical care service:

  – Days between injury

  – Lost workdays due to injury

  – Cost per injury

  – Compliance with safety goggle use

  – Compliance with ear protection use (for helicopters)

★ *Morale*—a measurement of the employee's well-being:

  – Annual employee satisfaction surveys

  – Attendance and tardiness

DATA ANALYSIS: COMMON TOOLS OF QUALITY IMPROVEMENT

Because you will use data for your QI program, seven charts that can help you analyze the data are discussed next. The following charts will also help when you uncover problems in your program and you need to analyze them. These seven charts are relatively simple to use, yet extremely informative:

★ Flowchart

★ Cause-and-effect chart (fishbone diagram)

★ Run (trend) chart

★ Histogram

★ Scatter diagram

★ Pareto chart

★ Control chart

FLOWCHART

A **flowchart** is used to document a given process. Some processes are extremely complicated, like building a jet fighter, and some are extremely simple, like getting dressed in the morning. The goal when creating your flowchart is to understand what the current process looks like, then find inefficiencies and remove them. A flowchart allows everyone to view the system and understand their roles. A good method to try is to document how you think a process should work, then document how the process actually works today. Most often, you will find redundancies and inefficient practices when you finally see the system in a simplified flowchart. Figure 35-3 ■ shows a flowchart that demonstrates the process of ruling out spinal motion restriction.

flowchart *used to document a given process with the goal of understanding what the current process looks like, finding inefficiencies, and removing them.*

CAUSE-AND-EFFECT CHARTS

Cause-and-effect charts, otherwise known as Ishikawa or **fishbone diagrams,** are often used during brainstorming sessions when a group is trying to understand all of the variables that cause a problem. Some groupings that are common in the service industry are policies, procedures, equipment, and personnel, but you can use as many others as you need. Each bone can have as many "bones" as needed to document the variables. (See Figure 35-4 ■.)

cause-and-effect charts (fishbone diagrams) *useful during brainstorming sessions when a group is trying to understand all the variables that cause a problem.*

RUN (TREND) CHART

Run or trend charts are perhaps the simplest of all the charts to understand. A run chart simply charts data points over a given period of time to see if there is any detectable trend. For example, an EMS agency found that there were not enough ambulances on duty during the midday hours. After creating a run chart they were able to determine the cycles of higher volume and staff accordingly. (See Figure 35-5 ■.)

run or trend charts *charts that diagram data points over a given period of time to see if there is any detectable trend.*

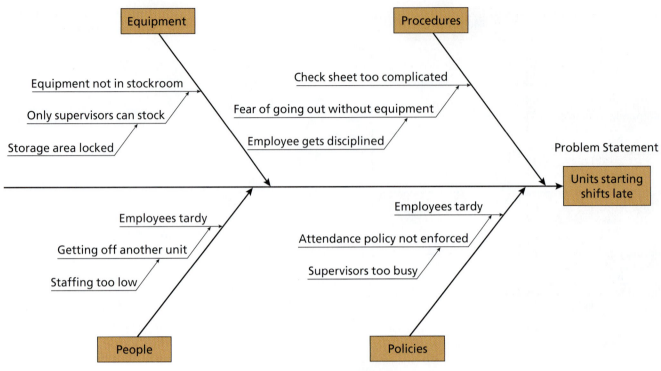

■ **Figure 35-4** Cause and effect diagram: units starting shifts late.

HISTOGRAM

histogram data chart used to demonstrate how frequently something occurs.

A **histogram** is used to see how frequently something occurs. For example, your local mayor wants to know your response time to a specific area of town. A histogram is a good chart to display the information. (See Figure 35-6 ■.)

SCATTER DIAGRAM

scatter diagram a visual representation of the relationship between two variables.

A **scatter diagram** is used to show the relationship between two variables. Suppose your system's intubation success rate is not very good and you wonder if it is due to the experience level of

■ **Figure 35-5** A trend chart: run volume.

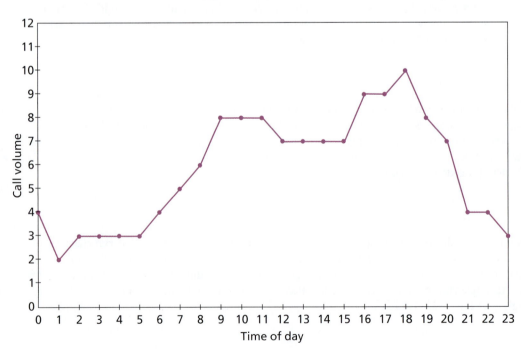

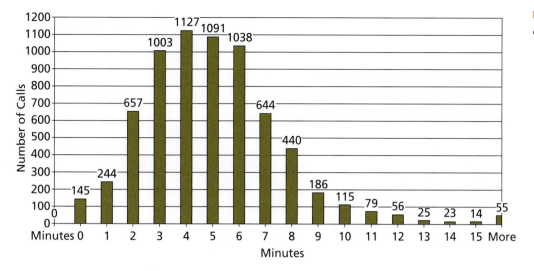

your paramedics. A scatter diagram would be a good tool to determine that information. (See Figure 35-7 ■.)

PARETO CHART

In a given process you may want to investigate problems that keep occurring. A **Pareto chart** is a vertical bar-based chart that visually demonstrates which problem is the most frequent. Understanding the true root cause of the problem will allow you to focus on the larger problem and thus you will have a greater potential for system improvement. The proven Pareto principle states that 20% of the sources cause 80% of the problem. (See Figure 35-8 ■.)

Pareto chart *a vertical bar-based chart that visually demonstrates which problem is the most frequent.*

CONTROL CHART

A process **control chart** is simply a graph that plots data points in a timeline. All process control charts have the same basic structure; they have a centerline (the mean), an upper control limit (UCL), and a lower control limit (LCL). A control chart is used to improve process performance by

control chart *a graph that plots data points in a timeline.*

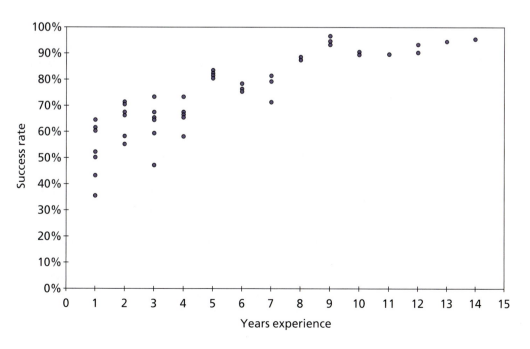

■ Figure 35-7 A scatter diagram: IV first attempt percent.

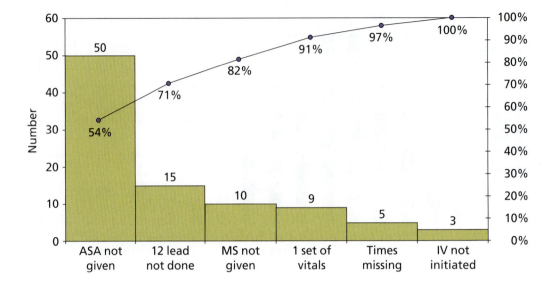

Figure 35-8 A Pareto chart: acute coronary syndrome outliers.

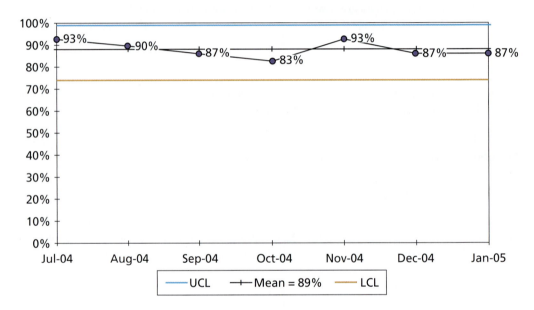

Figure 35-9 A control chart: system intubation success rate.

viewing it over a period of time and studying its variation. Control charts are very powerful and they tell you if a process is in statistical control or out of statistical control. (See Figure 35-9 ■.)

QUALITY IMPROVEMENT SOP

Every critical care service should specify all aspects of the quality improvement program. This is generally done by creating a quality improvement standard operating procedure (SOP) manual. The manual, at a minimum should include the following:

★ *Continuous Quality Improvement (CQI) program description.* The description outlines the intent behind the CQI program for the evaluation and continued improvement of the critical care service. The outline may describe activities such as how evaluations will take place, how QI initiatives will be handled, and responsibility to applicable laws and ordinances.

★ *Template for fixing problems.* Problems will arise in your agency and they will need to be addressed in a consistent manner. The template describes target selection, current situation, root cause analysis, countermeasures, results, and recommendations.

- ★ *Quality improvement forms.* Every employee has an idea about how to improve the operations. Management should include a method for receiving these ideas. A QI request form may be created and a process should be followed for handling these suggestions.

- ★ *CME training requirements.* All critical care providers have specific education and training requirements to maintain. A policy should include the specific license or certification and the methods by which the agency intends to maintain each provider's CME. The policy should also include local, state, and federal requirements for that certification level.

- ★ *Concurrent and retrospective initiatives.* A good QI program develops a process by which all aspects of clinical care and operational processes are evaluated and measured. These processes serve to provide key performance indicators for your agency. Examples of retrospective analysis may include the critical care team patient care report and documentation, treatment evaluations, or hospital pickup times. Concurrent initiatives may be compiled by direct supervision of tasks or skills. Concurrent evaluations should also be included in the KPI report. These KPIs should also be very descriptive and tell the reader all of the details about the measurement. The policy may include who is responsible for the measuring, why it is being measured, how to gather data, how to document the data, and who receives the report.

- ★ *Prospective initiatives.* This describes methods by which your agency improves through good hiring practices and a solid orientation and evaluation processes. These processes should be well documented and consistently followed. Only then can you measure if they are having the beneficial effect you desire.

- ★ *Reporting.* Collecting all of the above information does little good if the results are not summarized in a report. Management makes decisions based on the outcomes of these data and a reporting process should be documented and followed. This process may include items such as which reports are reviewed, who reviews them, and when they are due. Agencies may wish to publicize these reports to customers. A process should be defined as to which reports are for public consumption and how they will be distributed.

- ★ *Meeting attendance.* A critical care service does not generally operate in a vacuum. There are entities or bodies that require progress reports in order to make decisions regarding the direction of the program. Bodies such as advisory boards, steering committees, and the medical director may have set meeting dates and times to review the data. The dates, times, locations, personnel required, and reports required should be well documented.

This chapter's appendix includes a sample QI SOP that can be adapted by your agency. As you become more familiar with your own processes you may add or subtract from the SOP.

LEADERSHIP AND QUALITY IMPROVEMENT

You may be surprised to learn that **leadership** is not necessarily supervision. A good leader does not follow his or her employees around and point out every failure or weakness in an effort to get them to improve. When a leader notices something is not working correctly he or she does not automatically look for who is to blame. According to Deming, 94% of the problems in any organization are due to the system and thus management's responsibility and not the individual's. So why do we always look for someone to blame when a problem arises? When you start blaming the workers for problems they have no control over, it breeds resentment and poor morale, and robs the worker of pride. A leader instead focuses on the system as a whole to determine what is wrong. A leader understands that all processes, whether they be intubating a crashing patient or training an employee, contain variables called **common cause variation.** For example, if you were to track a group of

QI programs must be constructed and operated so that they are constructive and not punitive.

leadership *the ability to focus on the system as a whole and understand all applicable processes in an effort to determine what is wrong and effect positive change.*

common cause variation *variations that can be explained by the numerous causes that affect a process.*

employees for multiple months to assess their IV success rates, you would find that the success rate varies from month to month. One month the group may have been successful 90% of the time, while the next month only 85%. This variation can be explained by the numerous causes that conspire to make you miss such as the size of the patient, employee skill level, nature of illness, lighting, and a myriad of other factors.

There is a significant difference between common cause variation and special cause variation. **Special cause variation** can be simply described as a result so unusual and out of the ordinary for the given system that it cannot possibly be due to common cause variation. Example, if the critical care service received an influx of brand new nurses and paramedics who are now starting IVs, the overall success rate may fall to 50% in 1 month. Something is definitely different about the success rate this month compared to last month. The goal is to uncover the root cause and eliminate it from occurring again.

A leader also recognizes that employees have strengths and weaknesses. One employee may produce quick hospital turnaround times, yet need improvement in intubation skills. Another employee may be an expert at intubation, yet is rude to patients. The leader recognizes when an employee is in need of help and ensures that the employee who is falling behind receives the proper instruction to perform well in the job. A leader is also very patient and educates the employee to ensure that not only does the employee know what the task is, but how that task is important to the goals and mission of the organization.

A leader excels at making sure that all parts of the system work seamlessly together. One should not improve one process only to destroy the success of another process. For example, mandating that all critical care paramedics reduce their pickup time to within 20 minutes may improve your pickup times, but the cost may be missed information in pass-on.

Another function of the leader is to remove obstacles that prevent employees from being proud of their work. When a critical care team runs a call in a poorly maintained unit with frequent breakdowns it is hard for them to be supportive of the goals and missions of the organization. Sometimes the leader's job is to simply ensure that the policies, procedures, equipment, and training are adequate to ensure that quality care can be delivered by the team.

While there are some good examples of agencies that have made attempts at introducing these philosophies, there are also good examples of agencies that have misapplied or ignored the principles. QI is often viewed as a purely clinical subject and therefore relegated to a "QI manager" for implementation. Some in upper management believe that to bring quality to an organization all that needs to be done is hire a QI manager. They believe that "quality" has nothing to do with how to run the operations, communications center, or fleet maintenance, for example.

To fully appreciate the benefits of a quality improvement program the philosophies of Deming, Juran, Crosby, and others should be implemented system-wide, not just clinically. The most important predictor of a successful quality improvement program depends on the involvement of senior management. A great example of how important senior management is to an agency's quality mind set is found throughout the pages of "The Quality Journey: How Winning the Baldrige Sparked the Remaking of IBM" by Joseph H. Boyett Quality improvement theory and methods can be taught to all supervisors, critical care paramedic teams, communications personnel, and so on, but the real success of the quality philosophies will never be realized until senior management buys into the program.

Quality improvement in its simplest form can be described as improving on a process to ensure a better outcome. Here are a few examples of quality improvement in EMS:

★ Too many needle sticks prompted IV catheter manufacturers to develop "self-sheathing" needles and "needle-less" systems.

★ For years EMTs had to tape the nasal cannula to the C-collar in order to keep it in place. Manufacturers have since developed a small hook on either side of the C-collar where the cannula tubing can simply be looped to be held in place.

★ Cot manufacturers used to build cots that required a crew to lower the patient to the ground and then pick up the whole cot to load in the back of an ambulance. Cots nowadays come with roll-in features and power-assist lifts that eliminate this back-breaking chore.

special cause variation
results so unusual and out of the ordinary for the given system that the variation(s) cannot possibly be due to a common cause variation.

Quality in critical care transport is a top-down commitment—from management to the lowest-ranking employee.

quality improvement
improving a process to ensure a better outcome.

These types of improvements also occur in critical care services everyday. Hard-working people gather to determine a better way to provide care or a better way to improve the lives of the employees with better equipment and better processes.

DRIVE OUT FEAR

There is a strong desire on the part of managers to set arbitrary goals or targets for performance. Some managers may insist on 20-minute hospital turnaround times or have a zero-tolerance policy on vehicle collisions. These targets and others like them may be unrealistic and employees may not be able to perform to that level 100% of the time. When you fail to meet these targets you feel as if you have somehow failed and you lose the pride of a job well done. When employees are pressured into meeting unobtainable targets like those listed above they can only do three things:

1. *Work to improve the system.* This is the most desirable, but most difficult for frontline employees. After all, the only people authorized to change policies, procedures, and equipment are management.
2. *Distort the data.* An employee may neglect to document multiple intubation attempts or the administration of an incorrect dose of a medication.
3. *Distort the system.* In the case of an unrealistic turnaround time, an employee may neglect to contact dispatch when he actually arrives at the hospital. He may wait until the patient is dropped off and he is back at the unit before he informs dispatch.

These behaviors do occur and it is not necessarily because the employees are dishonest; rather they are given a choice of reporting what management wants or being disciplined for poor performance. Instead of managing through fear, management must understand that most of the problems in an organization are due to the *system* and not the individual. When managers notice an increase in vehicle collisions they must set about trying to understand the system in place that allows collisions to happen. Their job is to look at the root causes of collisions, then make changes in education/training, hiring practices, policies, and perhaps introduce performance-enhancing technology that results in safer driving all around. This is true quality improvement.

Summary

A viable QI program cannot simply happen on its own. The program requires thoughtful intent and strong leadership. The leader sets the tone for the operation of the agency and oversees all aspects of the operation. The leader requires a full understanding of the concepts of quality improvement and an appreciation for the system. The leader is also responsible for driving out fear in the organization through commonsense practices and through having the discipline not to react to every blip in the system. The leader must understand the difference between common cause and special cause variations. Data are the most important tools for the leader so that informed decisions can be made in a timely fashion. Key performance indicators should be developed and monitored to detect any unusual variations in the processes. All of the quality improvement initiatives, policies, and procedures should be meticulously documented to ensure a consistent application of the management practices. Consistency in your critical care service will provide you with the best chance of operational viability.

Review Questions

1. Discuss the importance of ongoing QI in critical care transport.
2. Describe how the QI system can be used for monitoring the system performance.
3. Discuss the importance of system and individual skills and protocol performance.

See Answers to Review Questions at the back of this book.

Further Reading

Boyett JH. *The Quality Journey: How Winning the Baldrige Sparked the Remaking of IBM.* New York, NY: Dutton, 1993.

Collins J, Porras J. *Built to Last: Successful Habits of Visionary Companies.* Harper Business Essentials, 2002.

Deming WE. *Out of the Crisis.* Cambridge, MA: Massachusetts Institute of Technology, 1995.

Memory Jogger. Methuen, MA: Goal/QPC, 1994.

Wheeler D. *Understanding Variation: The Key to Managing Chaos.* Knoxville, TN: SPC, 1993.

Sample QI Programs and Forms

QI Standard Operating Procedures

The sections in the SOP book will be given the following letter notations. This letter notation will precede any numeric notation given in order to group the contents of the book. The letter notations will be as follows:

CQI =   Quality Improvement Tools
E =   Education
M =   Metrics (concurrent and retrospective initiatives)
P =   Prospective Initiatives
R =   Reporting
Appendix   Resource Materials

As new sections are identified in the future, this will allow the creation of these sections without disrupting the other sections.

Within each section, the policy, protocol, and so on, will be given a number that will usually coincide with the current numbering sequence for existing contents. For example, the current policy 1 will become P 1. New policies, protocols, and so on, will be given the next open number in the ascending sequence. For example, the current policies ascend from 1 to 12. The next number assigned would be 13. If a policy, protocol, and so on, has been deleted, that number will remain open without assigning new policies, protocols, and so on, to it. For example, if policy 12 were deleted at a future date, no other policy would be assigned that number.

Every policy, protocol, and so on, will have the .00 suffix designation. Any revisions to that policy, protocol, and so on, will be given the .01 assignment for the first revision, .02 for the second revision, and so forth. Any *new* policies, protocols, and so on, will be given the .00 suffix designation for the original version and future revisions will have the suffix increments as discussed above.

When all parts of the new system are combined, each policy, protocol, and so on, will have a section letter, designated permanent number, and revision suffix. An example would appear as P 1.01 meaning this is policy 1, first revision.

Finally, a date for each version will be listed. The effective date is that date on which the procedure or policy actually goes into effect. These dates will be listed as footnotes on the last page of the documents.

Table of Contents

Last Update xx/xx/xx

Continuous Quality Improvement

Continuous Quality Improvement Program

GENERAL GUIDELINES

1. **CCT, Inc.,** shall maintain a system-wide continuous quality improvement (CQI) program to monitor, review, evaluate, and improve the delivery of medical transportation services. The program shall involve all system participants and shall include, but not be limited to, the following activities:

   A. Prospective—designed to prevent potential problems.
   B. Concurrent—designed to identify problems or potential problems during patient care.
   C. Retrospective—designed to identify potential or known problems and prevent their recurrence.
   D. Reporting/feedback—all CQI activities will be reported to management in report format and oral presentations at specified intervals described herein. As a result of CQI activities, changes in system design may be made.

2. **CCT, Inc.,** shall maintain a CQI Steering Committee. Membership of the CQI committee is limited to the medical director, and **CCT, Inc.,** senior management. The CQI committee shall meet at regular intervals to coincide with senior management meetings.

   A. The CQI databases used to enter clinical and operational data are tools of the CQI committee.
   B. The CQI committee may assign task forces to deal with recurring issues.
   C. All proceedings of the CQI committee, its subcommittees, and the contents of the CQI databases are confidential and protected under **Section XXXXX of your state's QI protection code.**
   D. No copies of EMS patient/system data records shall leave **CCT Inc.**'s custody, and all unessential copies shall be destroyed by paper shredder.
   E. All correspondence addressed to the CQI committee will be stamped "Confidential," remain unopened, and personally handed to the addressee.
   F. Any outgoing CQI correspondence will be stamped "Confidential."
   G. All CQI records shall be stored in a locked cabinet at the **CCT, Inc.,** offices, and dedicated for CQI Committee use.

3. Appropriate revisions shall be made as requested by CQI Committee.

1. Prospective

    A. Comply with federal, state, and county rules, regulations, laws, and codes applicable to EMS.
    B. Plan, implement, and evaluate the EMS system.
    C. Approve and monitor all EMS training programs.
    D. Certify/accredit prehospital personnel where applicable.
    E. Establish policies and procedures to ensure medical direction, which may include, but not be limited to, dispatch, basic life support, patient destination, patient care guidelines, and CQI requirements.
    F. Facilitate implementation by system participants of required CQI programs.
    G. Design system-wide reports for monitoring identified problems and/or trends analysis.
    H. Approve standardized corrective action plan for isolated and trend deficiencies with prehospital and base hospital personnel.

2. Concurrent

    A. Site visits to monitor and evaluate EMS system components to include CCT unit inspections.

3. Retrospective

    A. Evaluate system providers for retrospective analysis of prehospital care.
    B. Evaluate identified trends in the quality of care delivered in the system.
    C. Monitor and evaluate the Crew Event Resolution Process.
    D. Conduct MCI critiques.

4. Reporting/feedback

    A. Evaluate data submitted from system participants and make changes in system design as necessary.
    B. Provide feedback to system participants when applicable or when requested on CQI issues.

Medical Director Approval __/__/__   **Effective Date __/__/__**

_____

Your Medical Director   **Last Update xx/xx/xx**

Quality Management Template for Fixing Problems

Philosophy—Remember that most problems in any company are most likely a cause of the system and not individuals. Lean toward examining the system before blaming any person.

Target Selection—Will be provided by either the QI manager or the individual department or person wishing to solve a problem.

CURRENT SITUATION

1. You will need to gather data in order to determine your course of action.

    A. Plot the dots—To determine if this is a common or special cause situation you will need to evaluate the system using control charts.
    B. Process maps—To determine the true work flow.
    C. Surveys—To determine subjective or difficult to track information.

ANALYSIS OF ROOT CAUSE

–Depends on whether this is a special cause or common cause problem.

1. *Special Cause*—Determine what is different this time as compared to last time. Once you have discovered this, eliminate the possibility of it reoccurring by engineering the problem out.
2. Common Cause
   A. Stratification—Generally a process of segregating different layers of people and how they fit into the process. Example: If the system is having long pickup times look at new crew members, old crew members, crew members who work part-time, crew members who work full-time, and so on.
   B. Desegregation—Take the component parts and see if there is a problem at different stages of the process. Example: If the system is having long pickup times look at all of the components that go into pickup times like the run reports, individual hospitals, the training, and so on.
   C. Experimentation—Just as it sounds. If something sounds, in theory, like it should work, go ahead and try it and track the results.

COUNTERMEASURES

1. After you have analyzed the data, brainstorm some solutions that you believe will have an effect on the system. Remember to have all stakeholders present at this time so another process or system is not adversely affected.
2. Put the countermeasures into effect and track the results with control charts.

RESULTS

1. Continue to track the results of your fixes to determine if you made a positive change in the system.
2. A positive change will cause the UCL and LCL to narrow, or the dots may go out of control, but in the right direction. Going out of control on a chart is not necessarily a bad thing.

RECOMMENDATIONS

1. After all of this, you are able to decide if the changes you made were good or bad. If they were good, make sure that the system is permanently changed to reflect the new process.
2. Update the process map of how the procedure or policy should be done. This ensures continuous learning down the road for newcomers.

Quality Improvement Request Form

INSTRUCTIONS

1. This form may be used by any employee of *CCT, Inc.,* for process improvements.
2. The purpose of this form is to address process or system deficiencies in a standardized format and to ensure that all improvements are adequately addressed by the management staff.
3. Complete this form in as much detail as possible and submit to the QI manager.

SUBMISSION INFORMATION

1. In your own words, what is the problem?
2. How long has problem been around?
3. Who are the individuals that this problem affects?
4. What changes do you suggest to solve this problem?
5. Your name (not required) _____

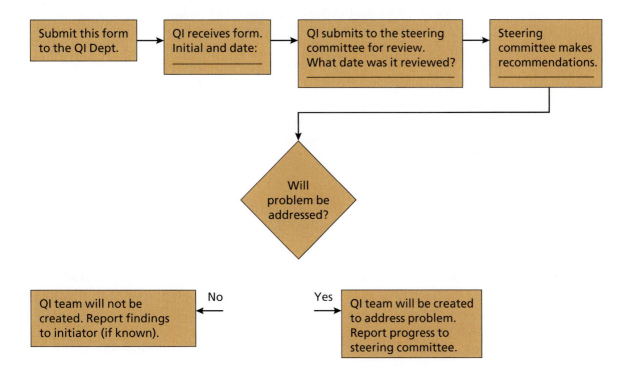

Last Update xx/xx/xx

Education

CME Training Requirements

1. It is the policy of **CCT, Inc.,** to offer continuing medical education to our employees that meets all county and state guidelines for CCT certified providers.

2. It is the policy of **CCT, Inc.,** that all employees must meet the county and state requirements to operate emergency vehicles and practice as attendants. **CCT, Inc.,** requires all certified employees to maintain their certification at the appropriate level.

Description—**CCT, Inc.** offers continuing medical education to all full- and part-time certified employees as follows:

Program	CME Hours	Frequency
CPR	4	Monthly
CEVO II (driving)	20	W/new employee orientation
OSHA Bloodborne pathogens	2–4	W/new employee orientation (4 hours) and monthly (2 hours)
New employee orientation	40	PRN
Pediatric assessment	5	Two classes bimonthly
Online continuing education program	24	Annually

1. *CPR*—Depends on the institution that issued your CPR card.
   A. AHA—every two years
   B. American Red Cross—annually
2. *CEVO II*—All employees are given a 20-hour course upon employment. Employee driving is to be monitored and refreshers are targeted to poor drivers.
3. *OSHA*—All employees will be given a 4-hour course upon employment. Employees thereafter are required to take a refresher class each year.
4. *Online CEU*—All employees are required to attain 10 hours of online continuing education annually.

PREHOSPITAL CME PROVIDER APPROVAL

1. ***CCT, Inc.,*** has applied for, and been approved by ***Your Jurisdiction*** to provide CE for a(n) ***X***-year certification period beginning ***Insert date.***
2. A copy of the approval letter with attachments is provided in the following pages.

I am familiar with the educational offerings and I submit my approval of the CME program.

_____

Your Medical Director

Last Update xx/xx/xx   **Date**

Concurrent and Retrospective Initiatives

CCT Run Report Documentation

[The following are three examples to use]

RN DOCUMENTATION COMPLETENESS

1. **Nature of the measurement.** Successful completion of a CCT run report is defined as a report that contains all relevant information pertaining to the quality of patient care; the correct billing and demographic information as well as patient or guarantor signatures; and run data such as times and caregiver names with signatures; all documentation should be neat and legible.
2. **Responsible parties for measurement.** The ***CCT, Inc.,*** CCT program director in coordination with the quality improvement office measures this key performance indicator.
3. **Gathering of the measurement.** The run reports are collected by the CCT program director.
4. **Documentation of the measure.** The measurements are documented first by the RN completing the report.
5. **Frequency and count of the measure.** Randomly sampled run reports will be reviewed on a monthly basis and will include not less than 30 reports per month.
6. **Specified tolerances.** These should be based on historical data and the reliability verified. Tolerances will be set through the use of statistical process controls (SPC).

7. **Items to be tracked.** Current process will track the following KPIs *(**You may insert your own here**):*

    A. Chief complaint
    B. On scene times documented
    C. En route times documented
    D. At least two sets of vital signs
    E. Appropriate documentation of the initial assessment
    F. Appropriate documentation of a reassessment

8. **Performance correction**

    A. ***CCT, Inc.,*** will track both individual performance and system performance.
    B. Individuals will be compared to the rest of the system and, using SPC, we will determine if the individual is operating within the norms of the system.
    C. Should the individual be operating below the specified limit, the management team will attempt to ascertain the reasons for the deficiency and use reeducation as necessary to effect a positive change.

9. **Process map.** See the process map section to view how this process should look.

Last Update xx/xx/xx

CCT Care and Treatment

RN TREATMENT

1. **Nature of the measurement.** Appropriate treatment of a patient is defined as care that is rendered in a timely manner, is appropriate for the patient's condition, and the care does not exceed the provider's skill level as set forth by the jurisdiction of the treatment.

2. **Responsible parties for measurement.** This key performance indicator is measured by the ***CCT, Inc.,*** quality improvement office through peer review.

3. **Gathering of the measurement.** The run reports are collected by the CCT program director and copies are forwarded to a designated RN for review.

4. **Documentation of the measure.** The measurements are documented first by the RN completing the report.

5. **Frequency and count of the measure.** Randomly sampled run reports will be reviewed on a monthly basis and will include not less than 30 reports per month.

6. **Specified tolerances.** These should be based on historical data and the reliability verified. Tolerances will be set through the use of statistical process controls (SPC).

7. **Items to be tracked.** Our current process will track the following KPIs *(**You may insert your own here**):*

    A. Was the treatment rendered required?
    B. Was the treatment rendered in a timely fashion?
    C. Was the treatment within the RN's scope of practice?
    D. Was appropriate care withheld?
    E. Was the treatment appropriate?

8. **Performance correction**

    A. ***CCT, Inc.,*** will track both individual performance and system performance.
    B. Individuals will be compared to the rest of the system and, using SPC, we will determine if the individual is operating within the norms of the system.

C. Should the individual be operating negatively outside the specified limit, the management team will attempt to ascertain the reasons for the deficiency and use reeducation or reengineering as necessary to effect a positive change.

9. **Process map.** See the process map section to view how this process should look.

Last Update xx/xx/xx

Hospital Pickup Times

PICKUP TIMES GENERAL

1. **Nature of the measurement.** The efficiency and effectiveness of an EMS system are largely dependant on critical time factors. Quick response times, scene times, and transport times are all important in ensuring the availability of ambulances when they are needed. This KPI will establish the system norms for hospital pickup times.

2. **Responsible parties for measurement.** This key performance indicator is measured by the *CCT, Inc.,* quality improvement office through the dispatch center.

3. **Gathering of the measurement.** The key data points are exported from the CAD.

4. **Frequency of the measure.** Since the data are generated by the CAD, a 100% sample will be the goal, but not less than 30 per month.

5. **Specified tolerances.** These should be based on historical data and the reliability verified. Tolerances will be set through the use of statistical process controls (SPC).

6. **Items to be tracked.** Our current process will track the following KPIs:

   A. Pickup times by individual
   B. Pickup time as a system

7. **Performance correction**

   A. Individuals will be compared to the rest of the system and, using SPC, we will determine if the individual is operating within the norms of the system.
   B. Should the individual be operating negatively outside the specified limit, the management team will attempt to ascertain the reasons for the deficiency and use reeducation or reengineering as necessary to effect a positive change.

Last Update xx/xx/xx

Prospective Initiatives

Hiring Process

INTRODUCTION

1. *CCT, Inc.,* believes that hiring the right individual is paramount to a smooth-running organization. *CCT, Inc.,* is committed to searching for applicants who possess the specific personality profile and temperament characteristics of an EMS worker.

2. *CCT, Inc.,* utilizes a behavior-based interview process to screen prospective employees for the above-mentioned attributes. The attributes were determined using intensive job analysis studies.

3. The prospective employees are asked a series of questions about how they handled situations in their past. *CCT, Inc.,* is looking for individuals who have an ability to match our expectations as close as possible.

1. The prospective employees are invited to attend an interview process with *CCT, Inc.,* management. They are then asked a series of questions designed to assess their ability to handle problems, communicate, lead people, handle stress, and various other components.

2. See the following pages for samples of the interview questions, the scoring sheet, and the final report. *[Insert your own description].*

Last Update xx/xx/xx

Orientation Process

INTRODUCTION

1. The *CCT, Inc.,* orientation process is geared toward providing new hires with the knowledge, skills, and attitudes it will take to become a successful employee.

2. The orientation program is divided into two components, classroom and lab work (see following pages for course description) *[Insert your own course description].*

Last Update xx/xx/xx

CCT Training

PROCEDURE

1. The training of an employee is performed by a field training officer (FTO).

2. An FTO has at least 1 year of experience in the system and has demonstrated proficiency in performing his tasks.

3. Evaluation measurements (see following pages) *[Insert your own description].*

Last Update xx/xx/xx

Reporting

Meeting Attendance

GENERAL

1. Medical Director Advisory Meeting

   A. When
   B. Duration
   C. Where
   D. Miscellaneous

2. *Your Jurisdiction* Fire Response Meeting

   A. When
   B. Duration
   C. Where
   D. Miscellaneous

3. *Your Jurisdiction* Physicians Advisory Board Meeting
   A. When
   B. Duration
   C. Where
   D. Miscellaneous

Last Update xx/xx/xx

Reports

GENERAL

These reports are to be created and reported at the following intervals and to the following individuals:

1. CCT Run Report Evaluations
   A. When due: on the 10th day of each month
   B. Reported to: senior management staff, medical director, and posted for all crews
2. Ambulance Pickup Times
   A. When due: on the 10th day of each month
   B. Reported to: senior management staff, medical director, and posted for all crews
3. Hiring Process and Interview Report
   A. When due: on the 10th day of each month
   B. Reported to: senior management staff and medical director
4. Annual CQI Report
   A. When due: on the second week of January each year
   B. Reported to list may include, but not limited to: all employees of *CCT, Inc.,* the medical director, and local hospitals in our service area

Last Update xx/xx/xx

Communications and Documentation

Randall W. Benner, M.Ed., MICP, NREMT-P

Objectives

Upon completion of this chapter, the student should be able to:

1. Understand the importance of verbal, written, and electronic communication to the success of any critical care mission. (p. 1031)
2. Identify current technology used to collect and exchange information in the critical care environment. (p. 1036)
3. Explain the responsibility of the FCC in the licensing and use of communication equipment and radio frequencies. (p. 1037)
4. Understand dispatch center considerations and the dynamics of verbal communication as they pertain to the:
   A. Communication specialist (p. 1032)
   B. Aeromedical pilot (p. 1039)
   C. Critical care team members (p. 1041)
   D. Sending and receiving health care facilities (p. 1043)
5. Identify and differentiate between the following communication system components:
   A. Simplex (p. 1037)
   B. Half-duplex and full duplex (p. 1037)
   C. Multiplex (p. 1037)
   D. Trunking systems (p. 1037)
   E. Digital systems (p. 1037)

F. Logging recorders (p. 1038)

G. Computer terminals (p. 1038)

H. Camera monitors (p. 1038)

I. Weather radar (p. 1038)

J. Mapping systems (p. 1039)

K. Facsimile (p. 1039)

6. Properly use the phonetic alphabet and numbering system for verbal communication. (p. 1041)

7. Discuss additional documentation needs and strategies as they pertain to the critical care paramedic. (p. 1041)

8. Identify and properly use medical terminology, medical abbreviations, and acronyms. (p. 1042)

9. Describe the desired characteristics of a properly completed patient care report. (p. 1045)

10. Describe at least one effective system for providing thorough documentation on a patient care report. (p. 1047)

11. Describe the potential complications of illegible, incomplete, or inaccurate documentation in the critical care transport realm. (p. 1048)

Key Terms

air traffic controllers, p. 1041
communications specialist,
  p. 1032
digital systems, p. 1039
Federal Communications
  Commission (FCC),
  p. 1037
full duplex system, p. 1038

half-duplex system, p. 1038
multiplex systems, p. 1039
patient care report (PCR),
  p. 1045
phonetic alphabet and
  numeric system, p. 1041
simplex system, p. 1038
trunking systems, p. 1039

ultra high frequency (UHF),
  p. 1038
very high frequency (VHF),
  p. 1037
VHF AM, p. 1037
VHF high-band, p. 1037
VHF low-band, p. 1037

Case Study

It's a warm summer Saturday, a beautiful day for flying and your service has been busy all morning. You are currently at a local airport refueling your EC 130 when the pager tones you to go on "standby." Once everyone is aboard and the engines are running, the pilot gets the "go ahead" from dispatch. You are dispatched for a three-car MVC with entrapment, and the pager includes the following coordinates, which are dialed into the autopilot: 41.43.35 longitude, 83.51.21 latitude. The coordinates take you to a remote stretch of road on the border of your state and a neighboring state.

The pilot calls the local scene command and finds out that the accident is right on the border, and involves three different fire jurisdictions. Apparently there has been some confusion about which fire department called which flight service because as the pilot is speaking with the ground command, your partner catches a glimpse of an aircraft at her eleven o'clock position. She relays this information to the pilot who switches to the air traffic frequency and speaks with the other aircraft. Apparently this second aircraft is from a competing flight service that was also called by one of the ground units.

You can tell that there is a little bit of a heated discussion about who was on final and who was landing where. Cooler heads prevail, however, and both helicopters land safely at the landing zone. After hot off-loading and approaching the scene, you are advised by the fire department scene commander that you will need all the help you can get. Your crew is directed to a car where two kids are trapped, and the fire department is working on extricating them. While you partner works with local EMS to stabilize the patients, you walk across the road where you find the second aeromedical flight crew working on immobilizing another critically injured patient who has already been extricated from the car the children are in. You quickly confirm with the crew that the patient is the father of your two patients. Conferring with the flight crew you find that they intend to transport the father to their trauma center in the neighboring state, about 30 miles away.

After a clinically fruitful discussion, consensus is reached to keep the family together by transporting them to the same Level I trauma center. The fire chief calls over the radio and says that it will be another 30 minutes at least before they can get the kids out. After receiving this information you give your pilot the shutdown signal, and confirm with him to set up for two patients. After 35 minutes you are able to extricate the children, who are fairly stable, and load them into the helicopter.

After taking off, the pilot heads west toward the trauma center. As you begin your journey home, you notice that the clouds are beginning to turn a dark gray. The pilot seems busier than usual, and you listen in on the air traffic control (ATC) traffic. Apparently the approaching storm has forced more air traffic into your airspace in order to land at a local airport. ATC tells your pilot that he will have to travel around the traffic, adding another 15–20 minutes to your total travel time. Realizing that this time could adversely affect your patients' outcome, you have the pilot declare "lifeguard status" with ATC and you are directed straight through to the hospital helipad.

After off-loading the patients and giving your report, you confirm the status of the parent and relay the information to both children. Following this you debrief with your crew and pilot and, on returning to base, complete an incident report so that the administrative teams from all services can work out a more fluid mutual aid plan for next time.

INTRODUCTION

Communication and documentation for the critical care paramedic hold the same degree of importance as they do for those working as prehospital care providers. In either realm of patient care, the practitioner must interact and communicate with a wide variety of individuals, including fellow care providers (crew members, hospital staff, physicians), noncare providers (the patient and patient's family), and other emergency service providers (such as law enforcement, fire department, hospital security personnel, and possibly air traffic controllers). In all of these situations, the communication that occurs must be concise, timely, objective, and provided (encoded) in such a way that the person receiving the verbal communication can properly understand (or decode) the message for accurate interpretation.

Documentation is also an integral component for an effective critical care organization. Your patient care report is the sole factual document that commits to paper what occurred during the critical care mission. The need for it to be factual, comprehensive, well written, and appropriately

Communication and documentation for the critical care paramedic hold the same degree of importance as they do for those working as prehospital care providers.

Your patient care report is the sole factual document that commits to paper what occurred during the critical care mission.

completed cannot be overstated—especially in the litigious society that we live in today. Even though partial elements of a mission may be documented elsewhere (for example, hospital transfer papers or the audio tapes in the communications center), these records are often incomplete and do not hold the same credibility as a well-written patient care report. In any instance, the axiom "If it wasn't written, it wasn't done" holds just as true for the critical care paramedic as it does for all other prehospital care providers.

The purpose of this chapter, then, is to instill on the critical care paramedic the importance of communication and documentation in the overall success of any ground or aeromedical critical care program. Communication and documentation are not just begrudged "aspects" of a critical care program; rather they are the common link that will bind all other aspects of the program together. Effective communication optimizes patient care and transport, and documentation provides the needed information to ensure that quality care progresses at the receiving facility, and allows the transport service to know that patient care decisions and interventions meet the expected standard of care.

COMMUNICATIONS

The role communication plays in the critical care paramedic's world cannot be overemphasized. It is impossible for any health care system to properly care for patients without some way of relaying information among those individuals working in the system.

Loosely defined as it pertains to the critical care environment, communications refers to the open transference of patient information by verbal, written, or electronic means. This is necessary so that patients can receive the very best care possible regardless of what phase or realm of health care they are currently in. Understanding the importance of communication starts first by understanding the myriad of components that make up the system. This understanding not only makes the critical care paramedic a more effective communicator, but it also allows him to better interact with other players in the health care continuum by anticipating what their communication needs will be also.

Some general terms the critical care paramedic should ensure familiarity with regarding this aspect of an organization include communications center and communications specialist. The communications center (sometimes referred to also as the communications department) typically refers to the department of an agency that handles all communication needs for the organization. The communications center typically regulates the flow of information to and from the critical care transport units, as well as intradepartmental communication. Within the communications center you typically have the dispatch center, where transport missions are received and transport requests are sent out to the critical care units. The term *dispatch center* is often used synonymously with communications center by the field providers, even though the communications center typically envelops tasks beyond the taking and dispatching of calls.

The **communications specialist** is the individual who answers the phone and dispatches missions to the critical care transport units. Similar to prehospital agencies, this person is known more informally as the *dispatcher*, even though his role within a communications center has grown considerably during the past several years. (See Figure 36-1 ■.)

DISPATCH CENTER CONSIDERATIONS

PLANNING

Although critical care paramedics may not be directly involved with the planning elements of a communications center, they may be involved in committee work designed to improve the efficiency of communication and information flow within an organization. This often includes the dispatch center because all forms of communication will inevitably pass through this department. It is also important from an organizational standpoint that the communications center *not* be viewed as a "nonrevenue" earning component of a critical care transport agency that doesn't warrant full

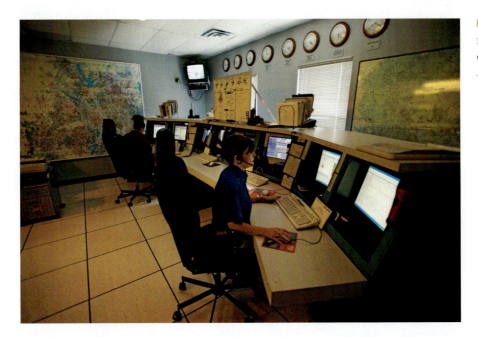

consideration by administration. The communications center is often the first contact potential patients and hospitals have with the critical care agency, so the organization must be sure that the communication specialists answering the phone do so in a courteous and professional manner. Beyond interfacing with the public, the communication specialists and the dispatch center are also integral links to other departments within the organization. As will be discussed later in the chapter, everyone from the flight crews to the billing department must rely on information gained initially by the communications specialist in dispatch. So the way in which the administration views the communications center—as an integral component of the organization by providing strategic planning initiatives, equipping the communication specialist, and investing in the technology for a state-of-the-art communications center—will contribute significantly to the overall success of the organization.

Everyone from the flight crews to the billing department must rely on information gained initially by the communications specialist in dispatch.

LOCATION

Important to the functioning of a communications center is its physical location in relation to other system components. The ideal arrangement would find the communications center housed within the same physical structure as the billing, marketing, and administrative offices of the organization. The only off-site buildings would be the hangers and bases that house the aircraft and/or ground units. This arrangement would allow those individuals responsible for the day-to-day operations (management, billing, communications, marketing, and so on) of the organization to be located within the same physical environment. The bases, naturally, would be distributed throughout the geographic or geopolitical boundaries served by the organization. The location must also be one in which there is very little influence from atmospheric, industrial, or seismic disturbances. While these influences are usually beyond the control of the organization, they should not be taken for granted and ignored during the planning stages of a communications center.

PERSONNEL

The communications center can be characterized as the nerve center for the critical care transport service. And despite the heavy reliance on technology, the human component can be either the strongest or weakest addition to this nerve center. Unlike early EMS systems that would sometimes employ injured or off-duty care providers as dispatchers, the dispatch centers of modern-day services must employ those individuals with the critical thinking skills, computer skills, and even temperament needed to survive the demands placed on the communications specialist. This can only

The communications center can be characterized as the nerve center for the critical care transport service.

Table 36–1	Common Requirements or Tasks Routinely Assigned to Communications Specialists

- Using computer terminals and software programs
- Answering phone calls and routing them internally as needed
- Receiving appropriate information regarding program missions or calls by phone, fax, or electronic means
- Interfacing (verbally) with care providers both inside and outside the organization
- Coordinating the movements of air and/or ground units within the system
- Interfacing with other emergency services on an as needed basis
- Monitoring video cameras that may be installed in ground unit garages or helipads
- Utilizing the mission or tracking board
- Help coordinate the flow of patient care information for internal uses such as quality assurance, billing, or administration

be ensured through the proper screening of applicants to ensure they have the required basic computer skills, the ability to speak clearly and concisely, and the ability to multitask across several different missions that may be progressing simultaneously. Almost invariably, the number of ground units and aeromedical units in the system exceeds the number of communications specialists sitting in the dispatch center.

The successful applicant may also receive training in emergency medical dispatching (EMD) and should complete periodic evaluations or testing of abilities inherent to the position. An educational curriculum has been developed by the Association of Air Medical Services (AAMS) for the training of communication specialists, and can be accessed by critical care services (The AAMS Manual for Air Medical Communications Operations). Table 36–1 lists common requirements or tasks that are routinely assigned to communications specialists.

CONSOLE DESIGN

The console is the large structure within the dispatch center that houses the various computers, keyboards, microphone jacks, telephones, and monitors that are needed in order to carry out the duties of dispatching. (See Figure 36-2 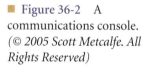.) These consoles are often specially designed to fit

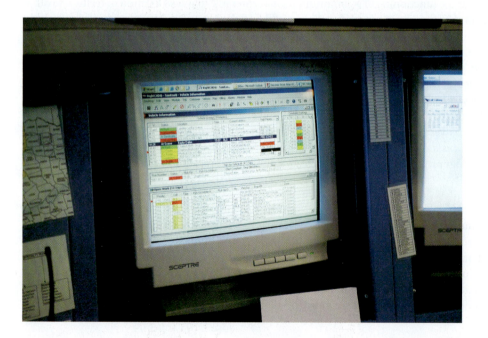

■ Figure 36-2   A communications console. (© 2005 Scott Metcalfe. All Rights Reserved)

the physical structure and needs of the communications specialist, and are costly and difficult to alter once built and installed. This underscores the need for those employed within a critical care transport service to maintain an active voice in the design or refurbishing of the communications center. The fundamental goal of any console is to allow easy access to the computer system, paging system, phone terminals, and computer screens without undue reaching, twisting, or stretching.

ERGONOMICS

Because the communications specialist is seated in front of the console for up to 12 hours at a time (or even longer in some organizations), it is important for the console and dispatch center to be designed in such a way as to minimize fatigue to communications specialists and help them stay effective in their duties. At the top of the list for these ergonomic designs is the appropriate use of lighting. It has been well documented that extremes in lighting can have a fatiguing effect on persons working within that environment. The architectural design of soft but sufficient lighting will help avoid this complication. The lighting should also not be positioned in such a way that it creates a glare on the computer screen. Generally speaking, lighting within any office space or dispatch center should not be so harsh that it is "noticeable." Finally, there should be provisions for emergency backup lighting in case of an electrical power failure to the organization.

Secondly, the dispatch center should have separate controls to the heating and cooling systems of the building. Because dispatch centers rarely have windows that can be opened, it is difficult to regulate the internal environment by other means. And because communications specialists must work overnight, when many of the other office personnel are at home, they should be able to alter their own internal ambient temperature for comfort.

Another consideration within this same vein of ensuring comfort in the work environment for communication specialists includes restroom, lounging, and kitchen facilities. Since access to a rest room is necessary for everyone, the layout of the dispatch center should place one nearby, especially for those smaller critical care services that may only utilize one communications specialist during the overnight or off-peak hours. Access to a properly appointed break room or lounge is also important so that the communications specialist may have a space away from the radios in which to relax, eat lunch, or simply take a break if the dispatch traffic has been extremely heavy or light (for example, in inclement weather). Finally, for the comfort of communications specialists a kitchenette should be available for the simple preparation of food or drink.

The acoustic design is also another consideration for any dispatch center. One general guide is that there should be sufficient acoustic insulation to isolate the communications specialist from ambient environmental noise outside the dispatch center. Since many dispatch centers are located at airports, the acoustic insulation should be sufficient enough to deaden the noise created by an aircraft engine located outside the building in which the dispatch center is housed.

EMERGENCY ELECTRICAL POWER

Every dispatch center should have a provision plan should there be a sudden or unexpected loss of electrical power. Although a dispatch center should have its own individual power supply from a different source than the building within which it is housed, there should also be allowance for emergency electrical power. Given the technology as it exists today, it is not problematic to design a system that allows for a seamless transition from the primary electrical source to a battery backup/generator system should a power failure occur. The transfer from the normal power source to the battery backup system should be seamless for the radio and telephone systems, and should have no longer than a 5-second delay for the transfer of the lighting system. In fact, with the exception of a "power supply status" light that may illuminate on the dispatch console, the transition from main power to the backup batteries (or generator) should be fluid and not encumber normal dispatch activity. Since many critical care programs employ the use of remote antennae towers and repeaters, they too should have an alternative electrical source should a power failure occur.

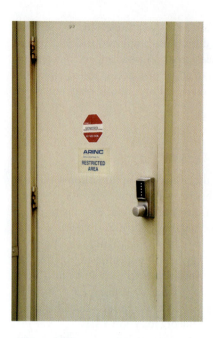

SECURITY

Security as it pertains to a dispatch or communications center is actually twofold. First is the consideration of physical security for the dispatch center, as defined by limited access by nonauthorized personnel. Second is the limitation of access to private information, as determined by the Health Insurance Portability and Accountability Act (HIPAA) of 1996, by communications specialists not directly involved with a particular mission.

The location of the dispatch center relative to other departments within a critical care organization will affect the level of needed security. This is especially true if the dispatch center is housed in a building that is either not attached to the main office building or is located in a remote building. (See Figure 36-3 ■.)

The first component of physical security is the limitation of access into the dispatch center by individuals not directly involved with normal dispatch activities. The use of a reinforced steel door with a numeric combination lock or a keyless entry card system is the industry standard, although a traditional lock-and-key mechanism will accomplish the same thing. Dispatch entry doors should also be lockable with a dead bolt from the inside should a situation occur where there may be some type of terrorist or criminal attempt at forced entry into the dispatch center. Also included with security is allowance for fire protection by the presence of fire/smoke alarms and a fire suppression system. Some dispatch centers also employ the use of video (or video and voice) monitoring to add another level of security.

As mentioned, not only is physical security a need, but information security for sensitive documents and information must also be ensured. With the current status of HIPAA law in the United States, a system must be in place that excludes unauthorized access to patient information via the communications specialist terminals. Although HIPAA law does allow for the intraorganizational sharing of personal information that is gathered for billing or administrative purposes, routine access to mission data should not be readily available to unauthorized personnel using the same mainframe computer programs that store these types of data. The establishment of encrypted passwords will ensure that unauthorized individuals (both inside and outside the company) cannot gain access to sensitive information and ensures HIPAA regulations are met.

⚷—◦

Although HIPAA law does allow for the intraorganizational sharing of personal information that is gathered for billing or administrative purposes, routine access to mission data should not be readily available to unauthorized personnel using the same mainframe computer programs that store these types of data.

EQUIPMENT

The use of technology in dispatch centers will vary significantly from service to service although some basic commonalities will be seen in all critical care organizations. The type of equipment chosen should ensure that communications (both digital and voice) are smoothly relayed within the organization and with the many outside entities that critical care services are often engaged with (such as fire departments, police departments, hospitals, air traffic controllers, and other critical care transport services). Most critical care transport organizations have a policy in which newly hired employees must complete an orientation within the communications center so they become more familiar with the equipment and procedures followed. The following is a brief overview of the components a critical care paramedic may see utilized within their organization:

Telephones

This is probably the most basic type of equipment found in a dispatch center. This is the primary means by which potential missions are received by communications specialists. All incoming lines into a dispatch center are commonly recorded, as are outgoing lines that are dedicated to alerting other agencies for assistance. It is not uncommon, given the diverse size of critical care organizations, to have multiple incoming and outgoing lines. The telephone technology used with these systems usually includes speed-dialing, hands free headsets, automatic redialing, and last number call-back features.

Radios

Radio systems are the other key piece of equipment at the disposal of the communications specialist. Radio frequencies utilized by the critical care organization are assigned by the **Federal Communications Commission (FCC)** in conjunction with the state's chapter of Associated Public Safety Communications Officers. The FCC is an independent U.S. government agency, directly responsible to Congress. The FCC was established by the Communications Act of 1934 and is charged with regulating interstate and international communications by radio, television, wire, satellite, and cable. The FCC also issues frequency licenses and assigns call letters to be utilized on one of several radio bands. The basic characteristics of these radio bands, which are labeled **very high frequency (VHF)** follow:

- ★ VHF high-band (148 to 174 MHz)
- ★ VHF low-band (30 to 50 MHz)
- ★ VHF AM (118 to 136 MHz)
- ★ Ultra high frequency (UHF) (403 to 941 MHz)

Found within the UHF frequency range are the channels that have been set aside by the FCC for the exclusive use of emergency medical services.

For completeness of the discussion, the critical care paramedic should be reminded of the various types of radio systems employed in emergency services. These include:

- ★ **Simplex system** is one that can only send and receive on the same frequency; it cannot simultaneously transmit in both directions.
- ★ **Full duplex system** is one that can transmit and receive simultaneously by employing one frequency for transmitting and a different one for receiving (usually use UHF). These systems also allow the transmission of voice or data.
- ★ **Half-duplex system** is one that uses two different frequencies for transmitting and receiving, but the hardware only allows for one direction of communication flow at a time (typically use UHF high-bands).
- ★ **Multiplex systems** have the ability to transmit data and voice simultaneously. This allows ongoing conversation between individuals while sending data information concurrently.
- ★ **Trunking systems** use a computer to pool all available frequencies. When a transmission arrives, the system assigns it to an open frequency. When that transmission ends, the frequency is then available and is added back into the pool.
- ★ **Digital systems** are an increasingly popular mode for emergency service and aeromedical service systems. This technology translates voice (analog) into digital code for broadcast. This type of radio equipment is much faster and accurate than the

Federal Communications Commission (FCC) *an independent United States government agency for regulating interstate and international communications, as well as issuing frequency licenses and assigning call letters utilized on assigned radio bands.*

very high frequency (VHF) *radio communications bands designated 30 MHz through 174 MHz.*

VHF high-band *FM radio bands used for business, new unlicensed Multi-Use Radio Service (MURS), and two-way land mobile radio technologies.*

VHF low-band *FM radio bands used by the U.S. military (including SINCGARS—Single Channel Ground and Airborne Radio System), cordless telephones, walkie-talkies, and mixed two-way mobile communication systems, in the 30–50 MHz range.*

VHF AM *Amplitude Modulation bands used for general and commercial aviation, Air Traffic Control Centers, AM radio, auxiliary civil service, space research, and other miscellaneous services. (121.5 MHz is the designated aviation emergency frequency.)*

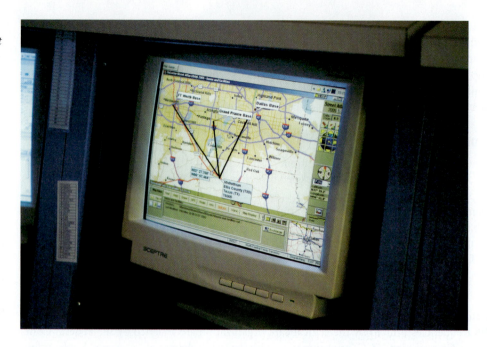

aforementioned systems. Plus they are not detectable by scanners, which allows the transmitted data to be more secure.

Logging Recorders

Emergency services and critical care agencies routinely utilize some type of recording technology for archiving incoming and outgoing transmissions. This capability is usually done through redundant mechanisms that allow continuous recording of dispatch activity (should one of the mechanisms fail). The method(s) by which this may be done can utilize a reel-to-reel recorder (referred to as a Dictaphone) that records all activity constantly for up to 24 hours on a single reel. The recorded reels can then either be stored or re-recorded after a given number of days. A second recording device is called the DAT recorder, which records transmissions on the recorded lines only when there is activity, and then saves the information to a cassette. A type of short-term recording device made by Eventide provides recordings of transmission activity for about 4 hours of recent time. This last recording method, generically known as the "callbox," is used primarily for immediate retrieval of names or information that is tied to a recent call or event.

Computer Terminals

Most (if not all) critical care services utilize computer terminals within their dispatch centers. The ability of computers and software programs to make the work of communications specialists more effective is well understood. Computer terminals often have common software applications preloaded (such as word processing, spreadsheet, Internet software), as well as computer-aided dispatch (CAD) software that is capable of integrating patient information, mapping of directions, coordinates of latitude and longitude, trip times, and paging into one seamless program (other features may be available as well).

Camera Monitors

Many communication centers have mounted remote cameras that monitor the various helipads and hangers employed by the service. This allows the communications specialist to have visual contact with the crew during downtimes, loading, lift-off, or landing procedures.

Weather Radar

Most communications centers as well as off-site bases and hangers have weather radar display monitors available for the pilot to consult prior to the acceptance of any aeromedical mission. While the

ultra high frequency (UHF) *radio bands assigned for restricted government use, Amatuer ("HAM") Radio, GPS (Global Positioning Services), GMRS (General Mobile Radio Service), FRS (Family Radio Service) television, cell phone short wave service, and cordless or mobile telephones.*

simplex system *system that sends and receives on the same frequency, but cannot transmit simultaneously in both directions.*

full duplex system *system that can transmit and receive voice or data simultaneously that employs one frequency for transmitting and a different one for receiving (usually found in the UHF bands).*

half-duplex system *system that uses two different frequencies for transmitting and receiving, but only allows for unidirectional communication flow (typically found in the UHF "high-bands").*

decision to fly or not ultimately rests with the pilot, the advantage of having a weather monitor in the communications center is to allow the communications specialist the ability to monitor the meteorological conditions that the aircraft may be flying into (or away from). This is especially beneficial for programs that do not have aircraft equipped with weather radar. If the conditions suddenly deteriorate, or if the pilot needs an update while in flight, the communications specialist can provide this important information.

Mapping System

The mapping system employed in the communications center could be as elaborate as a large flat-screen monitor that shows the terrain covered by each unit, to a simplistic system that uses a large geographical map with the radius of each base drawn on it. This allows the communications specialist to quickly determine the headings for any aeromedical missions that originate in the base's service area. Street maps should be available (either paper copy or software driven) that show the street index of localities in that service area. All of these will help increase the efficiency and functionality of the communications specialist in providing the pilot and crews with terrain-specific or location-specific information.

Facsimile Machine

A facsimile (Fax) machine allows for rapid transmission of printed material across phone lines. The machine "reads" the printed material and digitizes it for transmission across the phone line to the receiving fax machine, which decodes and prints the material. Some dispatch centers use this mode of communication to receive scheduled trips from hospitals or to send information regarding the trip to off-site bases.

multiplex systems *system that combines two or more information channels into a common transmission medium using a multiplexer (MUX); capable of concurrent voice and data communications.*

trunking systems *system controlled by a computer (called a "Site Controller" or "Master Control Center") linked to repeater sites by microwave or dedicated telephone circuits. This system pools all available frequencies, assigning incoming transmissions to an open frequency as needed.*

digital systems *systems capable of translating analog voice transmission into digital code for fast, accurate, and secured broadcast.*

BACKUP AND ALTERNATIVE SITES

A final component of communications centers includes a contingency plan should there be some malfunction or failure of the computer-aided dispatch system. This usually employs a pen-and-paper system for tracking the units and their assigned missions until the regular system is again functional. Additionally, some services have an alternative site where communications could be resumed should the primary center fail. The alternative site may also be incorporated into a vehicle with the capability of making the alternative dispatch location "mobile."

MISSION STATUS OR TRACKING BOARD

Most critical care communication centers employ a large tracking board, or a large computer screen, that allows anyone in the dispatch center to quickly review where each ground and airborne unit is at any given point in time. (See Figure 36-4 ■.) In larger systems the tracking board may incorporate a GPS system that will show the actual location of the critical care air or ground units as they proceed toward their next destination. Also commonly shown on the tracking boards are the call letters of the aircraft and the pilot/crew configuration (along with personnel names). One commercially available program called Garlin® allows the communications specialist to enter in the city and two crossroads relative to the scene, and the program produces the latitude and longitude coordinates, which can then be relayed to the pilot. The program also is integrated with the tracking board so information relative to the trip appears there also.

Other material that should be available within the dispatch center to aid in the tracking of units includes a full complement of paper maps, phone books, and topographical maps.

AEROMEDICAL PILOT CONSIDERATIONS

While the tasks for the pilot are drastically different than those for the critical care flight team, it behooves the flight team to be cognizant of the basic roles, responsibilities, and special communication needs of the pilot. Obviously the primary task of the pilot is the safe navigation of the aircraft, in fact, a common saying among flight program pilots about there position is that their job "is not to complete every mission, only to complete those missions you accept safely . . . . " This simple statement clearly specifies their purity of purpose in flight medicine. And just as communication is integral to the critical care team, communication is also critical to the pilot's job as well.

All pilots who fly for a critical care service must be "rated" for the type of aircraft to which they are assigned. This involves completing a set of prescribed guidelines for the type of aircraft flown as found in the Federal Aviation Regulations (FAR), as well as maintenance of either visual flight regulations (VFR) or instrument flight regulations (IFR) ratings as appropriate. Communication needs regarding this aspect of piloting the aircraft usually involve a dialogue between the communications specialist and the lead pilot. After being alerted by digital pager or voice that a mission is pending, the pilot will communicate (by radio or phone) with the communications center regarding the pilot's unilateral decision to either accept or decline the mission. The pilot will access the weather radar display at his disposal and make a determination about whether the weather conditions are favorable for completing the mission. This decision is influenced not only by the weather, but by the pilot's ability to fly under VFR or IFR status, the distance of the mission, the time of day, the terrain of the destination, and the type of aircraft the pilot is using. Almost everything influences the pilot's decision to accept the mission *except* for the knowledge about the specific mission or, in other words, the type of patient that the crew is summoned for. This information is purposely not communicated to the pilot to remove any influence on the pilot's part about the nature of the mission. After the pilot has objectively evaluated the mission dynamics, he communicates his decision to the communications specialist and the flight crew so that appropriate actions can proceed from there (either preparing for flight, or arranging ground transportation).

INTERACTION WITH THE COMMUNICATIONS CENTER

Once the decision to accept the mission is made, the pilot then communicates this to the dispatch center and the crew who prepare for flight. The communications specialist then normally pages the destination heading and coordinates to the pilot and crew so that the onboard autopilot and GPS unit can be programmed with this information. The pilot will, prior to actual liftoff, typically communicate with the crew via the internal headset communications of the aircraft to ensure that all personnel and equipment have been readied for liftoff. (Refer to Chapter 5, "Flight Safety and Survival," for more information.) Once this is ensured, the pilot will notify the communications specialist that he is now lifting off and give the direction of travel. Immediately after liftoff, the pilot will select the "ship to air" frequency and announce the aircraft departure location and general heading. This is to alert any aircraft in the immediate vicinity that your ship is entering the airspace. The next step for the pilot is to contact the local air traffic control (using yet another frequency) and advise them of your travel. The air traffic controller will then assign a specific frequency for the aircraft to use should it need to contact the air traffic tower with other information.

During flight, normally at 10-minute intervals the pilot (or occasionally a flight member), will communicate with the dispatch center via radio to give his current location using latitude and longitude coordinates as displayed by the onboard GPS unit. Simultaneously, the communications specialist should be able to track the flight via the mission tracking board, which is tied into the computer and GPS system as described earlier. Finally, should there be any sudden change in weather conditions as seen on the weather monitor in the dispatch center, the communications specialist can relay that information to the pilot so corrective actions, if required, can be taken.

The pilot may also need to communicate with alternative aeromedical services that they may be flying over while en route to their destination. It is not uncommon during longer distance flights for the communications centers of other services to "track" the aircraft traveling in their area. This would include noting the coordinates every 10 minutes or so, and then relaying that information back to the pilot's communications center by telephone. Although this is not an FAA requirement, it is a common courtesy among aeromedical services.

INTERACTION WITH AIR TRAFFIC CONTROLLERS

Air traffic controllers are those individuals who work at the various airports across the United States and abroad. Air traffic controllers (ATCs) are responsible for the safe and efficient flow of air traffic throughout the nation's airspace. Their primary role is to monitor the airways, help pilots pass other planes safely, navigate pilots through fog and rough weather, and allow safe landing at busy airports.

Most civilian ATCs work for the FAA or the Department of Defense (DOD). Air traffic controllers regulate a specific airport's traffic by using direct radio communication with the aircraft's pilot, giving permission to take off and land and recommending altitudes of travel. They also direct the ground traffic, which includes taxiing aircraft, vehicles, and airport workers. Tower controllers normally direct air traffic within 3 to 30 miles of an airport.

When the aeromedical flight leaves the airspace of the current ATC through which it is traveling, the monitoring and communication of the flight is then passed on to an en route center. En route controllers regulate flights between airports. They contact pilots by radio and control their positions in the airways between tower jurisdictions. Using sophisticated radar and computer equipment, they maintain a progressive check on aircraft and issue instructions, clearance, and advice. When an aircraft leaves the airspace assigned to an en route center, control passes on to the next center or to a tower controller. Within this elaborate system of monitoring and controlling air traffic, if a pilot is lost or having trouble, he is provided orientation instructions and directions to the nearest emergency landing field.

Another consideration for pilots of aeromedical aircraft as it pertains to communicating with air traffic controllers is the declaration of "lifeguard status." This declaration to the ATC identifies that your aircraft's mission is one of patient care, and gives priority status to your flight plans over all other flights (even the presidential Air Force One). Although this status could be given as the pilot passes through various tower airspaces, it is typically reserved for extreme situations in which the pilot must rapidly enter into the tower's airspace and arrive at the desired destination.

The single most important thought with pilot-controller communications is mutual understanding. To help achieve this, pilots and air traffic controllers use a unified vocabulary for certain words or numbers. The International Civil Aviation Organization (ICAO) has created a **phonetic alphabet and numeric system** to be used by air traffic controllers and aircraft pilots for consistency and accuracy in radio communications. Table 36–2 lists the alphanumeric table along with the related phonetic pronunciation of the words.

INTERACTION WITH EMERGENCY SERVICE AGENCIES

Because aeromedical flight programs also provide transport *from* emergency scenes, the pilot must be able to communicate directly with the landing zone (LZ) coordinator. As a reminder, the LZ coordinator must prepare a spot (identified by lights or other visible markers) that provides a safe landing surface for the aircraft. The LZ coordinator (if equipped with a portable GPS) can also relay the LZ coordinates to the communications specialist who then relays them to the pilot. As the aircraft nears the scene coordinates, the pilot will attempt to contact the LZ coordinator via the appropriate radio frequency used by the requesting agency (this frequency is usually in the 800-MHz range of the UHF band). The purpose of this communication is to identify any potential hazards as the pilot approaches. When there is visual identification of the landing zone, the pilot will perform one recon orbit around the landing zone to visualize the LZ from all directions and then communicate with the flight crew about the final descent. The critical care paramedic should be reminded at this point about the maintenance of a "sterile cockpit" during this final descent. Upon safe touchdown, the pilot will communicate to the dispatch center that the aircraft has landed.

CRITICAL CARE PROVIDER CONSIDERATIONS

At this point in time, there is minimal new information regarding the critical care paramedic and the use of communication skills or communication equipment while providing care in this environment. The principles discussed earlier about proper communication skills of dispatchers and pilots apply equally to the paramedic. There are, however, a few items worth mentioning.

air traffic controllers
professionals responsible for the safety and efficiency of aviation traffic flow.

phonetic alphabet and numeric system   *a set of radio protocols created by The International Civil Aviation Organization (ICAO); used by air traffic controllers and aircraft pilots for consistency and accurate communications.*

Table 36–2	Phonetic Alphabet for Use in Aircraft Communications

Letters:

Alpha	November
Bravo	Oscar
Charlie	Papa
Delta	Quebec
Echo	Romeo
Foxtrot	Sierra
Golf	Tango
Hotel	Uniform
India	Victor
Juliet	Whiskey
Kilo	Xray
Lima	Yankee
Mike	Zulu

Numbers:

0	Zero	6	Six
1	Wun	7	Seven
2	Too	8	Ait
3	Tree	9	Niner
4	Fower	.	(decimal) Point
5	Fife		

FAMILIARITY WITH COMMUNICATIONS HARDWARE AND FREQUENCY

Along with the task of knowing how to use all of the specialized medical equipment found aboard the aircraft, the critical care paramedic should also be efficient at using the onboard radio systems employed by the flight program.

Along with the task of knowing how to use all of the specialized medical equipment found aboard the aircraft, the critical care paramedic should also be efficient at using the onboard radio systems employed by the flight program. Like many prehospital services, the aircraft may be equipped with both a UHF and VHF radio as well as the radio the pilot uses for speaking with the control tower. The critical care paramedic should be familiar with the programming of the radios so that he can select the appropriate frequency for communicating with the dispatch center, fire departments, EMS agencies in the service area, and HEAR frequencies of receiving hospitals. The critical care paramedic is also encouraged to "think before speaking" so that the use of the frequency is specific yet short.

FAMILIARITY WITH PILOT AND COMMUNICATIONS CENTER PROCEDURES

The critical care paramedic is not responsible for communicating with air traffic controllers. The critical care team should, however, know about the phases of the transport in which the pilot will be communicating with the traffic control tower. This is usually after liftoff when the pilot advises the tower of their direction of travel (heading) and altitude, when the aircraft is passing from one tower airspace into another, and when landing at the airport following a mission (returning to base) or for refueling, which is commonly done at a local airport. To help isolate the critical care provider's communication from the pilot's communication with the air traffic control or dispatch center, the pilot can "isolate" his communication procedures from the crew with the flip of a switch.

The critical care paramedic should also be intimately familiar with the flight program's requirements of when to contact the dispatch center during the various phases of a mission. This allows the communications specialist to time-stamp these phases of the mission to ensure accurate documentation. The communications center should be contacted during a mission at these points:

★ When the mission is accepted by the pilot
★ When the aircraft lifts off
★ Every 10 minutes or so during flight (to give coordinates)
★ On final descent for landing
★ On aircraft landing
★ At patient contact (on scene or in hospital)
★ When lifting off with the patient loaded
★ During final descent at destination
★ On landing at final destination
★ When patient transfer of care has occurred and the aircraft is back in service

Other times when the dispatch center should be contacted include:

★ When the aircraft is in need of refueling
★ If a warning light illuminates or a sensor alarms
★ If the aircraft suddenly encounters significant weather turbulence
★ If the mission needs to be abandoned due to inclement weather conditions
★ When the flight heading is changed by the air traffic control tower
★ When unable to land at a designated LZ or hospital helipad
★ When any other unique or uncharacteristic incident occurs during a flight

COMMUNICATION WITH OTHER CARE PROVIDERS

Of particular significance regarding the success of any aeromedical transport system is the face-to-face communication between health care providers. While completing interhospital transport missions, the critical care paramedic will very often interface with a much wider array of health care providers than when working as a prehospital provider. Due to the nature of critical care transport environments, the critical care team will find itself in many hospital departments that a prehospital provider would not commonly access. To this end, there are two considerations of which the team should remain aware. First, any communication with other health care providers should incorporate appropriate medical terminology so that clarity in the message is maintained. Second, due to the specialization of departments within a hospital, the staff there usually have a specific way of assessing and treating the patient. This may translate in the department being unfamiliar with what procedures the critical care crew considers "routine" (for example, performing a thorough patient assessment when transporting a burn patient to a larger burn hospital). The perception may be that the crew is "wasting time" by performing an unnecessary assessment. Although this is a misunderstanding, it can be cleared up easily by taking a moment to communicate verbally with the hospital staff about the importance of obtaining a baseline assessment evaluation prior to flying. This could be explained to the staff as "necessary" so that crew has a baseline clinical impression of the patient. If the patient's stability changes en route, the critical care paramedic will be better prepared to recognize the abnormality rather than attributing it to the patient's general condition.

While completing interhospital transport missions, the critical care paramedic will very often interface with a much wider array of health care providers than when working as a prehospital provider.

COMMUNICATION WITH RECEIVING FACILITIES

The critical care team will often give patient information via the aircraft radio while en route to the receiving facility. Akin to the "call-in" performed by EMS providers to the receiving emergency department, the critical care team routinely calls ahead to the receiving facility to provide a patient update and allow the receiving facility time to make preparations to receive the patient. The critical care team should have the following information ready prior to establishing radio contact with the facility (although most systems or receiving facilities may request just portions or specifics of this information):

- ★ Age, gender, ethnicity
- ★ Chief complaint, purpose of transport
- ★ Significant medical history and history of the chief complaint
- ★ Current mental status
- ★ Airway and breathing status
- ★ Invasive/noninvasive assessment of hemodynamics
- ★ Care being provided currently (meds, fluids, vent settings, and so on)
- ★ Response of patient to current therapy
- ★ Confirmation of medical records/documentation
- ★ Estimated arrival at the department
- ★ Requests for additional personnel or equipment on arrival

RECEIVING AND PROVIDING BEDSIDE REPORTS

Another component regarding the communication needs of the critical care paramedic would include the oral transmission of patient information when either receiving or providing a bedside update about the patient. Usually the critical care team will be advised of the nature of transport by the communications center either on receiving the initial alert tones or while traveling en route to the patient's location. This communication is generally limited and includes only the age, gender, and the major disturbance the patient is experiencing. Here is an example of the information the crew may initially receive from the dispatch center:

> "Medevac 8, you will be transporting a 3-year-old male patient with 60% BSA burns back to Children's Hospital. Patient is sedated, intubated, and mechanically ventilated."

Obviously the initial dispatch information is very limited, and there is still a significant amount of information the critical care team will need in order to complete this transport. On arrival at the patient's bedside at the originating hospital, the balance of the information will be communicated to the team in an oral format. Given the diversity of the hospitals and departments that the critical care team will be transporting from, it is almost impossible to predict the exact format in which this information will be relayed. The best advice to the critical care team regarding this instance of communication is to listen keenly for pertinent bits of information during the oral report. The same also applies when the critical care team is receiving an oral report from an on-scene EMS provider. (In these latter situations, the tension is usually high and the report from the EMS provider may come in broken bits and pieces.) The components of patient information that the critical care team should keenly listen for include the following (and if any is missing, the critical care paramedic needs to ask for it):

- ★ MOI/NOI (mechanism of injury/nature of illness)
- ★ Current vitals
- ★ Specific airway, breathing, and circulatory parameters
- ★ Significant medical history, allergies, medications
- ★ Current therapies (medications, IV fluids)
- ★ Important physiological or hemodynamic findings relative to the medical/traumatic condition the patient is experiencing
- ★ Any uncommon medical technology being used on the patient (IABP, VAD, and so on)

When arriving at the destination facility with the patient, it is the responsibility of the critical care team to communicate patient information to the receiving staff so that appropriate medical care can be continued. Since you are providing this information, you can control the structure and flow of information. Organizing the patient data prior to communicating it will enhance this verbal exchange of information. One way of organizing it follows:

- ★ Age, gender
- ★ Primary medical/traumatic condition
- ★ Significant physical findings
  - – Head
  - – Neck
  - – Thorax
  - – Abdomen
  - – Pelvis
  - – Extremities
- ★ Last set of vitals
- ★ Current interventions
- ★ Response to therapy
- ★ Significant treatment limitations (e.g., important allergies, max dose of medications reached)

The critical care crew should *always* end this verbal exchange of information with the following question: "Is there anything else you need or questions I can answer?" This allows staff at the receiving facility the specific opportunity to obtain any other information they feel relevant to their acceptance of patient responsibility.

DOCUMENTATION

Documentation of every mission and each patient contact is another expectation of the critical care provider team. In many instances, the documentation needs of the critical care paramedic mirror the documentation procedures seen prehospitally by EMS providers. As such, the upcoming section should not present any new or unusual uses of documentation practices.

Documentation of every mission and each patient contact is another expectation of the critical care provider team.

SIMILARITIES WITH PREHOSPITAL EMS DOCUMENTATION PRACTICES

The **patient care report (PCR),** or simply the written documentation that is prepared following completion of a patient transport, will be utilized by numerous individuals within the health care continuum. These include medical professionals, program administrators, researchers, billing department personnel, and occasionally lawyers. Fortunately, the documentation requirements of critical care providers are very similar to those of prehospital providers. As such, becoming acclimated to this process should not be exceedingly difficult.

The first and foremost reason for providing documentation is to ensure that a written document exists for the health care providers who are responsible for carrying on patient care after your departure. The written documentation left with the receiving facility is often more thorough than the bedside oral report you gave when you delivered the patient to the receiving facility. The staff at the hospital may need to review the patient's original physiological status, establish what medications or interventions have already been provided, ascertain any pertinent medical history or known allergies, determine if there is any relevant information available from the people originally on scene with the patient, or find out how the patient has been responding to various treatment

patient care report (PCR)
the written documentation that is prepared following completion of a patient contact or transport.

The first and foremost reason for providing documentation is to ensure that a written document exists for the health care providers who are responsible for carrying on patient care after your departure.

modalities to date. In any instance, the PCR that you leave at the hospital becomes an important document that helps ensure the patient receives appropriate and continuous care.

Administrative needs also exist for the PCR. The patient care report is the one sole source of all information regarding the completed mission, and it is often accessed by administration for quality assurance needs. From the PCR, the administrative team can ensure that thorough documentation practices are being maintained, that the time from dispatch to liftoff of the aircraft is acceptable, and that appropriate protocols are being followed during patient management en route to the receiving facility, as well as other quality assurance needs. Administratively, the PCR may also be accessed by the billing department to ensure that a proper bill is created based on the care provided to the patient.

In support of the billing purpose, the written documentation obtained/created by the critical care team may also include additional needs. The critical care team may be responsible for ensuring that the physician certification statement (PCS) is included within the written records provided by the hospital requesting the transport of the patient. The PCS is a legal document that bears the patient's name and demographic information, and documents why the transport by the critical care team is warranted (versus transport by a traditional EMS ground unit). The PCS must be signed by the physician requesting transport. Another written document that the critical care team may be responsible for obtaining prior to departing with the patient is the advanced beneficiary notice (ABN). This document applies to patients who receive Medicare, and provides the legal documents needed by the billing department to ensure that the service is reimbursed by Medicare for the transport services provided.

Research is another use for the PCR. Critical care paramedicine is one area of health care that has not received much attention as far as research, in defining the role it occupies in health care. Without adequate research, decisions that need to be made regarding staffing, equipping, educational preparation, quality assurance needs, and reimbursement rates will be made by administrative or state officials without any real evidence on which to base these important decisions. This in turn may not prove beneficial to those involved in critical care transport medicine. Research is the only way that any health care entity can justify its existence; hence, adequate written documents that allow for the collection of research data are important. To illustrate the positive effects of research, one need only look at the nursing profession. About 15 to 20 years ago, there was a large expansion in the body of knowledge about nursing professionals. The information gained allowed nursing professionals to objectively establish themselves and their roles as professional care providers. In addition, enhancements were realized in both the working environment and pay as the scope of practice provided by nursing was confirmed. These advancements came through completed research that demonstrated the benefits provided by nurses. Critical care paramedicine needs to follow this lead.

One other use of written documentation is for legal concerns. In this sense, the PCR you complete and leave with the receiving facility becomes a permanent part of the patient's medical records. Because of the litigious society we live in today, critical care providers may find themselves one day defending their actions in a court of law. In this situation, the legal teams on both side of the lawsuit will use the PCR report you submitted as evidence to either support your care, or demonstrate that inadequate or inappropriate care was rendered. Please note: You may provide the best care possible, but if your PCR does not objectively demonstrate this, then the prosecution will have little trouble convincing the judge and jury that you were negligent in your actions.

Always prepare your PCR as if you knew for certain that it would be referred to in a court of law. Although general PCR documentation practices are discussed in the next section, the critical care provider must ensure that all necessary elements are present on the PCR. These elements include how the patient was found, what interventions were already being provided, the patient's response to these interventions, the clinical findings (and pertinent negatives) of your complete physical exam, medical therapies you rendered on behalf of the patient, the patient's response to your treatment, and any extraneous situations that had a bearing on the patient transport (for example, a long on-scene time due to patient extrication by the fire department or rescue squad during an MVC scene flight).

The patient care report is the one sole source of all information regarding the completed mission.

Always prepare your PCR as if you knew for certain that it would be referred to in a court of law.

GENERAL CONSIDERATIONS FOR COMPLETING A PATIENT CARE REPORT

The first consideration you will encounter with completing patient care reports in the critical care transport realm is the fashion in which you will do it. This varies from system to system, but may include both handwritten documentation as well as using a computer software program or electronic clipboard for documenting the mission. Some organizations submit a complete handwritten document to the receiving facility on arrival or prior to departure from the facility. Other organizations may submit a short (one-page) form that documents only pertinent information regarding the transport, but then complete a thorough PCR with a computer software program back at base, which is then faxed to the receiving facility. The critical care paramedic has the responsibility of following whatever procedure has been established within his respective system.

The next component of completing the PCR follows the same medicolegal documentation practices consistent with prehospital report completion. This refers specifically to how the report should be completed, and includes the following characteristics:

★ Use of appropriate medical terminology. The use of medical terms transforms your report into a universally accepted medical document. Ensure that your spelling and use of medical terms is accurate.

★ Use of medical abbreviations and acronyms. The use of abbreviations and acronyms allows the critical care paramedic to increase the amount of information contained in the PCR. Be certain, however, to only use abbreviations or acronyms that have a specific meaning. Never be creative and attempt to use ones that you have "thought up."

★ Ensure that your report is objective. Similar to completing a prehospital PCR, the document should not be used as a venue for the critical care paramedic to write what he "believes" happened or occurred.

★ Every PCR has spots designed to enter incident times. The standard for medical documentation is to use military times, which are based on the 24-hour clock. Not only are the incident times necessary, but also the documentation of times when vitals were obtained, medications administered, communications held with other medical professionals, and significant changes occurred in the patient's physiological status.

★ Finally, the PCR should have the following elements of proper documentation: It should be completed in its entirety, be highly accurate, be legible (especially when not using an electronic clipboard or computer software program), be submitted in a timely fashion, be devoid of excessive mistakes, and be submitted with the intent of not needing additional addendums or alterations.

Another component in the completion of a PCR by the critical care paramedic is the documentation of information that is characteristically not done in the prehospital environment. This includes the documentation of electrolytes, certain laboratory values, and oftentimes ventilator settings. Although the documentation of this information is not inherently difficult, it is usually done in a conventional manner with which the critical care paramedic should be familiar.

One such method for documenting patient variables uses a "fishbone" diagram. This diagram allows the rapid documentation of the following variables: sodium, chloride, blood urea nitrogen (BUN), glucose, creatinine, bicarbonate, and potassium. The "fishbone" is completed as follows:

$$\frac{Na^+ \mid Cl^-}{K^+ \mid HCO_3} \begin{array}{l} \diagup BUN \\ \!\!\!\!\!\!\!\!\!\!\!\!\! < \!-Glucose \\ \diagdown Creatinine \end{array}$$

Other electrolytes may be documented as well (calcium, magnesium, phosphate, and so on) in the appropriate space on the report. Other values, however, are documented in a specific fashion and include the following:

★ White blood cell count
★ Hemoglobin level

* ★ Hematocrit
* ★ Platelets

The format for these values is as follows:

$$WBC \diagdown \frac{Hgb}{Hct} \diagup Platelets$$

The critical care paramedic is referred to Chapter 12 for a full explanation of what these various lab and diagnostic values mean.

MODES OF DOCUMENTATION

It has been alluded to numerous times that PCRs take a multitude of forms. The first and most traditional is the narrative report. With a narrative report, the call is depicted at length and there is less structure with this type of written documentation due to the absence of check boxes. The narrative format provides the critical care team the freedom to describe the mission events and patient's condition as they deem necessary. The narrative reporting style is favored by many practitioners due to the freedom in documentation; this freedom though comes with a trade-off of time. This type of reporting typically takes a great deal longer to complete, and is more prone to "missing" information that the provider forgot to include.

Patient care reports can also be prepared with a series of check-off boxes or fill-in-the-bubble spaces, also called "bubble sheets," to denote the patient's care. The great advantage of this type of format is that it consumes very little time, and often the PCR can be scanned by an organization's computer system to allow the generation of research data. Where this mode of documentation fails is that it is less specific in nature. The use of bubble sheets inherently reduces the depth and breadth of information gathered.

The final type of PCR to mention is the style that uses technology to its advantage. The availability of electronic clipboards for documenting allows for a PCR to be designed to meet an organization's specific needs. It could be a combination of fill-in boxes and narrative sections that can be uploaded immediately to the organization's mainframe computer system by way of a wireless link. The use of PDA (personal digital assistant) technology is also gaining favor in EMS and critical care realms due to the size, cost effectiveness, and availability of software programs.

Also gaining increased popularity is the use of computer software for generating patient care reports. Like electronic clipboards and PDAs, the availability of software programs that can be modified to meet program needs makes this option extremely attractive. Many times this software can also be dovetailed into the agency's mainframe computer system so that the information entered by the critical care paramedic can also be used for quality assurance, administrative, and billing purposes automatically.

CONSEQUENCES OF POOR DOCUMENTATION PRACTICES

Inappropriate documentation carries with it both medical and legal consequences. Of these two, the medical consequences are naturally most severe since care decisions may be made based on your submitted patient care report, and if there are errors or omissions, the consequence can be poor subsequent patient care. From a legal standpoint, there are significant ramifications of poor documentation as well. In a court of law, what you documented is many times what is debated, not what you actually did. Even though your patient care may have been exemplary on a particular mission, if the documentation does not bear this out, you may be found libel or negligent for the damages the plaintiff is claiming. Additionally, poor documentation practices will lead your program's administration, quality assurance committees, and billing departments to become more aware of your practices. These aforementioned intraorganizational departments rely heavily on the quality of the documentation provided by the critical care teams, and progressive correctional action (up to and including dismissal) may be taken against the critical care provider who continually fails to document appropriately.

Summary

As a critical care paramedic you will be assuming a large responsibility in not only caring for seriously ill or injured patients, but in being able to competently and accurately relay information in verbal and written form to other practitioners. The number of health care providers you will encounter is innumerable, and the reliance of these individuals on your written documentation cannot be overemphasized. The best practice for the critical care paramedic is to become familiar with common medical terminology and documentation practices, and make them your habit with each patient, practitioner, and written documentation encounter.

Review Questions

1. Discuss the differences between the various modes of radio communication (simplex, duplex, multiplex, and so on).
2. What is the role of the FCC in critical care paramedic radio communications?
3. Other than fellow care providers, name other individuals the critical care paramedic must interact with on a daily basis using good communication skills.
4. What role does the air traffic controller have in determining the flight of an aeromedical aircraft?
5. What information is usually included in the radio report given to the receiving facility during a critical care interhospital transport?
6. Name three types of PCR documenting systems used in critical care transport.
7. List five elements of an appropriately completed PCR.
8. What are the medical and legal consequences of a poorly written PCR?

See Answers to Review Questions at the back of this book.

Further Reading

Association of Air Medical Services. http://www.aams.org (last updated November 23, 2004).

Bledsoe BE, Porter RS, Cherry RA. *Essentials of Paramedic Care*, 2nd ed. Upper Saddle River NJ: Pearson Prentice Hall, 2007.

Federal Aviation Adminstration. http://www.faa.gov/ (last updated March 4, 2005).

Holleran, RS. *Flight Nursing: Principles and Practice*, 2nd ed. St Louis, Mo: Mosby, 1996.

International Civil Aviation Administration. http://www.icao.org/ (copyright 1995–2005).

Sole ML, Lamborn ML, Hartshorn JC. *Introduction to Critical Care Nursing*, 3rd ed. Philadelphia: W. B. Saunders, 2001.

The Critical Care Paramedic in the Hospital Environment

Randall W. Benner, M.Ed., MICP, NREMT-P

Objectives

Upon completion of this chapter, the student should be able to:

1. Understand the evolution of the paramedic in both the prehospital and hospital environment. (p. 1052)
2. Value the importance of skills and knowledge that the critical care paramedic brings into the hospital environment. (p. 1053)
3. Discuss how state law and medical direction can influence the critical care paramedic's role in the hospital. (p. 1053)
4. Understand and be able to discuss the common pros and cons of paramedics working in the hospital as maintained by political entities involved with this ongoing debate. (p. 1054)
5. Name common hospital departments where the critical care paramedic may work alongside other health care providers. (p. 1056)
6. Name the most common skills the critical care paramedic is already familiar with that may be employed in the hospital setting. (p. 1058)
7. Discuss additional skills beyond those of the critical care paramedic that may be used within the hospital. (p. 1058)

8. Discuss common techniques aimed at smoothing the transition of patient care from prehospital to emergency department care, as well as between hospital departments. (p. 1056)

Key Terms

American Nurses Association (ANA), p. 1055

cardiac catheterization and electrophysiology lab, p. 1060

cardiovascular intensive care unit (CVICU), p. 1059

certification and licensure, p. 1053

diagnostic noninvasive cardiology laboratory, p. 1060

interventional radiology laboratory, p. 1060

medical intensive care unit (MICU), p. 1059

medical practice act, p. 1053

neonatal intensive care unit (NICU), p. 1059

patient care associate, p. 1059

pediatric intensive care unit (PICU), p. 1059

scope of practice, p. 1053

surgical intensive care unit (SICU), p. 1059

Case Study

You have been employed full-time as a critical care paramedic for a hospital-based mobile and air critical care service for several years. Recently your hospital opened an off-site urgent care facility in your rural community about 70 miles south of the original hospital. Since the opening of the urgent care facility, you have picked up some weekend shifts for the overtime pay.

The urgent care facility is a six-bed "clinic" staffed by a paramedic, an RN, and a physician assistant (PA), and is open from 0800 to 2330 seven days a week. In general its easy overtime pay and you enjoy the laid-back atmosphere. Around 2315 on a Saturday evening, a heavy set gentlemen walks in the clinic. You notice that he is not moving too quickly; in fact, he is kind of "shuffling" his way to the triage desk. You offer him a seat and begin to ascertain his name and chief complaint. "Charte" is a 48-year-old male with a long-standing history of hypertension, and is currently complaining of a "gnawing pain" in his stomach and an inability to move his bowels—even though he feels like he needs to.

You triage Charte and take him back to medical examination room 1. His vital signs are all within normal limits; however, he is slightly diaphoretic. You let the nurse know that he is ready to be assessed. While giving the RN his chart you take one more glance in the room and notice Charte leaning forward on the hospital bed while rubbing his lower lumbar region.

You hurry off to close the front window so nobody else can come in after hours, and after doing so the RN finds you and asks you to help take a second look at Charte. The PA is conducting her physician examination and all three of you agree something just isn't right with him. Charte only speaks broken English, enough to tell you that he has a "gnawing" pain in his epigastric region and an inability to evacuate his bowels even though he says "they feel full." The PA motions for everyone to step out, so that the three of you can discuss the patient's condition.

Agreeing the something doesn't look right, the RN decides to obtain orthostatic vital signs, the PA wants to look at the CXR, and you decide to run a quick 12-lead ECG. The patient nearly passes out as he stands for his orthostatic vital signs, and the 12-lead ECG shows ST elevation in leads II,

III, and AVF. You begin to run through your protocol for MONA and beta-blockers, when the PA asks if you performed a right-sided ECG. You place electrodes for V4R and V5R on the right chest wall, identifying a proximal right coronary artery occlusion. By this time the RN is on the phone with your ED approximately 90 minutes away by ground travel. Although commonplace treatment for a left ventricular infarction (LVI) would call for MONA therapy, the three of you discuss the pathophysiology of a right ventricular infarction (RVI,) and agree that an initial 0.9% saline bolus would increase preload to the ventricles and increase CO and perfusion pressures prior to administration of nitrates or opioids. The PA goes to review the case with the ED attending, and consensus is reached between the care providers noting that the patient meets the STEMI inclusion criteria and needs an emergent cardiac catheterization. Given the drive time by ground transport, the flight crew from the hospital is dispatched to your facility.

You explain to the RN and PA how the patient needs to be packaged for flight, after which you gather all the car keys to clear the surface parking lot so the helicopter can land. After completing this task and walking back inside the facility, the RN tells you the patient lapsed into an episode of pulseless V-fib which converted with one countershock at 200 joules. Currently the patient displays a perfusing idioventricular rhythm.

By the time the BK-117 lands with the flight crew, the patient's rhythm has increased to 82 beats per minute, creating a systolic blood pressure of 98 mmHg. The patient is quickly transferred to the flight crew's cot and portable equipment, records are gathered, and they load "hot" and lift for the hospital.

When you return for your next shift a week later, you learn that the patient survived his trip to the catheterization table and was discharged home with an automatic implanted cardiac defibrillator (AICD) and coronary artery stents 5 days later.

INTRODUCTION

There is no other profession that endures such rigorous and continuous change as that of medicine. Take, for instance, physicians. The processes by which these health care providers are educated and practice medicine is starkly different now than how it was done 50 or even 100 years ago. And due to the rapidity of change, there continues to be a rippling effect within all other health care professions. This is no less true for critical care paramedics as it is for physicians. At one time, ambulances were staffed by untrained people who simply picked up the ill or injured person and provided transport to a hospital. However, in a scant 40 years or so, these early ambulances have grown into a well-organized and sophisticated system of certified practitioners who provide care in emergencies with the assets of enhanced education, improved clinical competence, sophisticated medical technology, and liberal protocols that will allow them to intervene on many situations where the patient's condition itself is in jeopardy. Likewise, all signs indicate that there is no slowing down in the future trends for the critical care paramedic.

In fact, both the paramedic and the critical care paramedic are finding additional employment opportunities with differing responsibilities within the hospital environment. Hospital departments that have employed critical care paramedics include the emergency department (ED), critical care units (CCU), and special procedure units such as the cardiac catheterization lab, stress lab, and radiologic suite. Although the idea of using paramedics in the hospital environment is not a new idea (some hospital systems have been using paramedics for more than 10 years now), the idea is not widespread. As will be discussed in this chapter, not only have political barriers kept the idea from spreading, but also differences in the focus of medical care, delivery of medical care, and the utilization of techniques and procedures that may be unfamiliar to the street-level paramedic. The intent of this

Both the paramedic and the critical care paramedic are finding additional employment opportunities with differing responsibilities within the hospital environment.

chapter is to provide an overview of the differing roles the critical care paramedic may fill with their expanded scope of practice. It is important to remember, however, that even within the walls of a hospital the critical care paramedic must still function under the auspices of a medical physician.

As a final note, the critical care paramedic must remember that practicing in a hospital can be starkly different from practicing in the prehospital environment. The paramedic may have *more* or *less* autonomy than in the prehospital or critical care transport environments. The extent to which a paramedic is utilized in the hospital is extremely diverse across the United States. This is because of a lack in the standardization of in-hospital practice. Many political boundaries still exist for health care providers, and these boundaries are being challenged both by organizations that utilize paramedics and those that do not. The only thing consistent with the paramedic in the hospital is that the scope of allowed practice is highly diverse and highly specific to the hospital's needs. As such, this chapter will provide an overview of areas where critical care paramedics have been utilized in some hospitals, or may be utilized in the future. At the time of this writing, it is difficult to go into any greater specifics because there are no uniform specifics to discuss.

The extent to which a paramedic is utilized in the hospital is extremely diverse across the United States.

DEFINING THE ROLE OF THE CRITICAL CARE PARAMEDIC IN THE HOSPITAL

STATE LAW

As with all levels of prehospital care, the EMS regulations for each state clearly define what a prehospital care provider can and cannot do. This **scope of practice** is usually defined in what is known as a **medical practice act.** There is for each level of care provider (both prehospital and allied health specialties) a specific medical practice act that governs their practice of medicine. The medical practice act may also define how and to what extent a physician may delegate additional authority to a paramedic. Also included in the language of state regulations are the specifics regarding state certification and/or licensure as they pertain to the paramedic. Although the line between what a certification and licensure is (or is not) for the paramedic is sometimes blurred, they both govern paramedic practice. For legal as well as practical purposes, a state-issued "certification" for the paramedic is the same thing as a state-issued "license" for the nurse. A certification in this regard does not require (nor provide) any more or less responsibility, or legal liability, than does a licensure. **Certification and licensure** are mechanisms by which the state regulates health care providers practicing within the state's boundaries. It is ultimately the responsibility of the individual critical care paramedic to stay abreast of his state's scope of practice.

Since critical care paramedicine is a new and rapidly expanding subspecialty for the paramedic, many states are currently enacting regulations intended to define how this new breed of paramedic is expected to operate within their respective state. This was an ongoing process at the time this chapter was written; however, until a national standard emerges and states have adopted uniform terminology for this level of care provider, it is the responsibility of the critical care paramedic to know exactly his limitations when working in a hospital environment. One consistency, however, that is certain to be present in all state regulations is that the practice of medicine by the critical care paramedic will only occur with appropriate physician medical direction and oversight.

Other legal requirements will also impact the critical care paramedic who is now operating within a hospital. These are the same ones that you are familiar with regarding your role as a prehospital care provider and include regulations such as mandatory reporting requirements, negligence and medical liability, confidentiality, Health Insurance Portability and Accountability Act (HIPAA) requirements, defamation of character, obtaining patient consent, patient withdrawal of consent (refusal of care), advanced directives, and potential crime and/or accident scenes.

scope of practice *a state law that defines and regulates the practice of medicine in a state. In some states, EMS is regulated under a general medical practice act.*

medical practice act *state-level legislation that includes language clearly defining what a prehospital care provider can and cannot do, as well as where and when they can do it.*

certification and licensure *the mechanism by which a state regulates health care providers practicing within the state's boundaries.*

There is for each level of care provider (both prehospital and allied health specialties) a specific medical practice act that governs their practice of medicine.

Since critical care paramedicine is a new and rapidly expanding subspecialty for the paramedic, many states are currently enacting regulations intending to define how this new breed of paramedic is expected to operate within their respective state.

MEDICAL DIRECTOR

As mentioned, the critical care paramedic will only be legally permitted to provide care when doing so under the auspices of a medical director. While in the hospital environment, the critical care paramedic (CCP) will be less likely to have a set of standing orders or protocols to follow; rather CCPs are typically provided a set of job functions they are allowed to perform. Depending upon the state in which critical care paramedics may function, their direct oversight may be from a physician or from a nurse who has the legal permission to delegate responsibility to the critical care paramedic. Again, it is the responsibility of the critical care paramedic to be intimately familiar with the hierarchy of supervision and medical oversight prior to engaging in any type of patient care in the hospital, regardless of the department in which they function.

STATE LAWS GOVERNING MEDICATIONS AND PROCEDURES

As the scope and role of critical care paramedics becomes more standardized nationally, so will the state medical practice act governing them. In the absence of this direction, critical care paramedics are left in the dark regarding what patient skills or medications they are allowed to administer in this new environment. As mentioned previously, the critical care paramedic's medical oversight will provide some direction regarding procedures they can perform. And since the critical care paramedic is *still* a paramedic (i.e., licensed or certified), often the medical direction will review what the scope of practice is for the paramedic in that state, and then determine what they are permitted to do within the hospital setting based on that. If a skill is not permitted to be performed in the prehospital environment by paramedics due to a limited scope of practice, it is rare that they will be allowed to engage in that skill while in the hospital. Generally speaking though, the paramedic may have the latitude to perform skills common to the prehospital environment including, but not limited to:

★ Patient assessment and reassessment

★ Advanced airway skills

★ ECG monitoring

★ Patient movement and handling

★ Charting and documentation tasks

★ Medication administration (IVP, IM/SQ, IO, infusions)

★ IV initiation

★ Immobilization

★ Equipment preparation (for central lines, suturing, ECG, EEG, IABP, casting and splinting, wound dressings, and so on)

★ Arterial and venous blood sampling

★ Capnography, bedside BGL determination, and pulse oximetry

POLITICAL ENTITIES INFLUENCING PARAMEDIC PRACTICE IN THE HOSPITAL

Given the dynamic and sometimes volatile nature of lobbying entities that view the presence of paramedics in the hospital as hostile, it behooves the critical care paramedic to have an appreciation as to what their agenda may be. Understanding what motivates other health care lobbyists and what beliefs these care providers have may better prepare the critical care paramedic to interface with them in the hospital. It would not be prudent for the paramedic to take the stance of "we are better" or "you just don't want us here because you fear for your jobs" because this is really not the case. The only thing that sowing this attitude will reap is a greater divide between the paramedic and other hospital care providers.

Within any hospital are a number of health care specialties that provide very specific care to patients based on their need. The use of the critical care paramedic in the hospital is not to eliminate any of these positions (although that is often what is thought), but rather to use the critical care paramedic to support these other health care professionals. The operating paradigm is not replacement; it is integration and enhancement. Consensus on the role of the paramedic will only occur after all of the hospital administration, physicians, nurses, ancillary allied health professions, and paramedics learn to agree on what is best for the patient, rather than on what is best for their respective profession. To this end, rarely will a patient in need of airway management or acute bleeding control, or one simply needing someone to talk to, ever ask what the credentials are of the person standing in front of him. If the provider's intent is to offer care and provide hope, the patient will not mind.

One health care profession that has been challenging the use of paramedics in the hospital is the nursing profession. From the paramedic's viewpoint, the notion is generally that the paramedic's thought processes and assessment style are most akin to those of a physician. Hence, CCPs should flourish well in the emergency department or other critical care units because of their proven assessment and intervention skills for airway, breathing, and circulatory compromises. The paramedic's ability to interpret 3-lead and 12-lead ECGs, utilize various pharmacologic regimens, and think independently should make them useful additions in the critical care units. Additionally, the orientation of paramedics to be skill driven makes them eager to learn and accept more patient care responsibilities.

From the nursing perspective, however, a slightly different picture emerges. The primary nursing arguments *against* the use of paramedics in the hospital are (1) paramedics are unlicensed providers (in some states they are "certified," not "licensed"), (2) they lack the breadth of general pathophysiology that nursing students typically receive (remember that nursing programs are hour-for-hour longer than paramedic programs), and (3) they are often attuned more to skill provision than "holistic patient management" as nursing is.

The treatment pathways and priorities established by emergency nursing vary drastically from similar EMS pathways. Whereas the paramedic is usually concerned with "keeping the patient alive for 20 minutes," the emergency nurse is concerned with identifying the problem and instituting a treatment pathway that involves a holistic assessment and management of the patient.

In further illustration of the nursing profession's perspective on the use of paramedics in the ED, consider the following 1992 position statement from the **American Nurses Association (ANA)**, a professional organization that serves the nursing profession. This statement was released at a time when nursing shortages and forced lowering of nurse staffing spawned considerations for the use of paramedics in the emergency department:

> Other regulatory entities have been pressured to lower agency staffing standards, for instance by allowing emergency medical technicians to function in the emergency room without registered nurse supervision or by substituting unlicensed personnel for licensed nurses. These unlicensed persons have not completed nursing education programs or met other licensing requirements. In many instances, substitution of unlicensed personnel for licensed nurses clearly violates state nurse practice acts. At the very least, it is not in the interest of the health, safety and welfare of the public.

American Nurses Association (ANA) *a professional organization that serves the nursing profession in the United States, the ANA "advances the nursing profession by fostering high standards of nursing practice, promoting the economic and general welfare of nurses in the workplace, projecting a positive and realistic view of nursing."*

Here, the assumed belief by nursing organizations is that the best way to solve understaffing is by hiring more nurses or by rehiring nurses released during downsizing of departments due to budgetary constraints. The use of paramedics to augment the emergency department staff in order to meet budgetary confinements and patient needs is viewed as detrimental due to the belief that paramedics are, in nurses' views, less skilled care providers. Despite the fact that the ANA has updated this position statement in later documents, the thrust of their message remains the same over a decade later: If paramedics are to be used at all in the ED, they should simply serve as assistants to the RN.

There are also those EMS providers who are vocally against the use of paramedics in the emergency department due to the notion that they often are nothing more than "glorified orderlies." This perception has persisted from the initial paramedics who worked in the emergency department but were only allowed to provide routine bathing, cleaning, feeding, and transporting of patients between departments. Initially, paramedics were not hired for their expanded knowledge base and ability to provide critical skills; they were hired because they were an extra set of hands. Fortunately, however, this notion is starting to wane; some hospitals now allow paramedics to function in almost the same capacity as they do in the prehospital environment.

In any instance, both arguments are flawed, and the "turf" war continues regarding the optimal staffing of hospital departments and the role the paramedic provider has in resolving these issues. The best advice for all engaged in the decision-making process is to be respectful of each other's professions and understand that each has benefits and limitations. Fostering the preconceived notions that the battle will never end, and contributing to that battle will only widen the

Multiskill tasking of health care providers has become commonplace in medicine.

chasm that already separates the professions. Multiskill tasking of health care providers has become commonplace in medicine, and the integration of various certified/licensed professionals will be the only solution to this problem. It is best that all parties involved embrace this opportunity to change rather than stoically defending a "turf" that no longer exists.

HOSPITAL WORK ENVIRONMENTS FOR THE CRITICAL CARE PARAMEDIC

EMERGENCY DEPARTMENT

Years of cost cutting in medicine as a result of changing reimbursement patterns from the government and insurance companies, coupled with the yearly growth of patient visits to the emergency department by individuals without health care insurance, have led to an unprecedented crisis in health care. Hospitals have been forced to close, emergency departments are becoming overcrowded causing undue wait times, and some hospitals that are victims of downsizing do not have beds available for those patients who need admitting. All of this places the patient in need of medical attention at risk.

This problem, which has been steadily worsening during the past 10 years, is finally getting much needed attention. A report in the January 2000 issue of the *Annals of Emergency Medicine* warned, "Unless the problem is solved, the general public may no longer be able to rely on emergency departments for quality and timely emergency care, placing the people of this country at risk." Note that this report did not cite the root of the problem, just that the external influences that a hospital must deal with are resulting in overtaxing of the system.

One technique used to lessen the load on the ED staff is to employ one or more physicians so that more patients may be seen simultaneously. While good in theory, what it plays out to is needing almost a duplicate number of ancillary health care providers (nurses, clerks, technicians) to support the second physician's needs. Without this, the staff is usually committed to the first physician and the second physician cannot perform to her full potential. While it is easy to assume that employing more nurses may solve the dilemma, that is not an option due to the financial constraints imposed by government, insurance companies, and health maintenance organizations that dictate reimbursement rates. Hospitals nowadays are running as lean as possible in order to stretch the health care dollar. Paramedics offer a cost-effective way of ensuring patient care when appropriately incorporated into the ED staff, but despite this only 20% of hospitals employ paramedics according to a 1999 survey by the American College of Emergency Physicians (ACEP). This may change because ACEP has formed a task force to examine alternative scenarios for ED staffing using nurses, nurse practitioners, physician assistants, EMTs, and paramedics. Hence, the role of the paramedic in the emergency department is destined to increase. (See Figure 37-1 ■.)

When functioning in the emergency department, the critical care paramedic will be able to draw from his knowledge of the many tasks necessary in the critical care environment. To avoid unnecessary duplication of material presented in other chapters, those skills that the critical care paramedic will be performing under most situations are mentioned, but not described a second time (i.e., how to initiate an IV or insert a Foley catheter).

First and probably most common are patient assessment skills. Whenever the paramedic enters a patient's room in order to perform some task, an assessment of some extent will naturally occur. You may be providing a nebulizer treatment, but you will listen to breath sounds before and after the therapy. You may be applying a 12-lead ECG, but you will assess the thorax for surgical scars and implanted pacer/defibrillators. You may note abnormalities to the 12-lead, and then listen to heart tones because you suspect an underlying cardiac pathology. In these situations your knowledge and experience as a critical care paramedic will dictate what assessment techniques to use, and your understanding of pathology and symptomatology will alert you to abnormal findings.

One area that needs special attention is that of triaging patients into the emergency department. Given the current regulations in many states, if a paramedic triages patients, he may actually be violating the Emergency Medical Treatment and Active Labor Act (EMTALA), which is a subset of regulations within a larger legal body of laws known as COBRA or the Patient Anti-Dumping

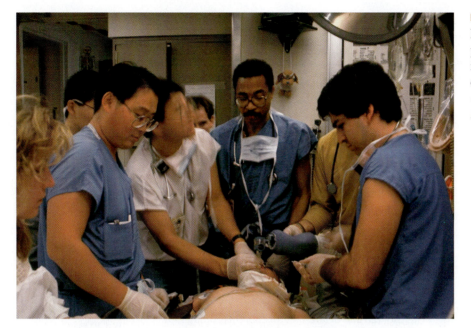

■ Figure 37-1 The hospital-based critical care paramedic is playing an increasingly important role in emergency medical care. *(Hank Morgan/Photo Researchers, Inc.)*

Law (COBRA stands for the Consolidated Omnibus Budget Reconciliation Act of 1986). Current EMTALA regulations are often interpreted to mean that patients entering the ED for treatment must first be triaged by an RN. A paramedic can assist with this triage process but a nurse must be present simultaneously. Any physical assessments performed by the paramedic subsequent to this as the patient is seen and treated in the emergency department are usually cosigned by the RN delegating that responsibility to the paramedic.

The critical care paramedic working in the ED is also commonly called on to be part of "special teams" such as trauma alerts or cardiac arrests. In either scenario, the critical care paramedic has a wealth of knowledge and experience to draw from while care is being provided simultaneously by a number of care providers. The paramedic can also serve as a "go-between" between EMS crews and the trauma staff, because paramedics understand the situational dynamics and the equipment common to prehospital care. Although rare, a transporting EMS crew may arrive with some type of immobilization device or automatic CPR compression device that may be unfamiliar to the ED providers. In this situation the critical care paramedic can help make the transition from the EMS cot to the hospital bed more fluid while facilitating a seamless transition from care being rendered by the prehospital crew to the ED staff. Likewise, if a patient is being transported from the ED to another facility by an EMS crew, and the EMS crew is unfamiliar with the type of medication infusion pump being used, the critical care paramedic can ease this transition by assisting with the transfer of care to the EMS equipment.

Depending on the procedures that the critical care paramedic is permitted to use in the emergency department, additional training may be required. As mentioned previously the breadth of practice varies greatly from hospital to hospital, so it is the responsibility of the critical care paramedic to become familiar with procedures he is responsible for administering under medical direction. Although not an exhaustive list, Table 37–1 outlines most of the skills that the paramedic may utilize in the ED.

Researchers of the ACEP investigated the skills performed by paramedics and EMTs in the emergency department and found the following breakdown of skills reported:

★ Performing basic skills (94%)

★ Intermediate skills (89%)

★ Advanced level skills (50%)

★ Administering ACLS drugs (51%)

★ Administering non-ACLS drugs (38%)

★ Administering medications via IM/SQ (48%)

Depending on the procedures that the critical care paramedic is permitted to use in the emergency department, additional training may be required.

Table 37–1	Most Commonly Used Paramedic Skills in the Emergency Department Setting

- Patient assessment and reassessment
- Airway skills (suctioning, OPA/NPA, BVM, ETT, ETC, LMA)
- ECG monitoring (3-lead and 12-lead)
- Patient movement and handling
- Charting and documentation tasks (Some hospitals utilize a fully computerized system that is integrated with the hospital's mainframe system.)
- Medication administration (IVP, IM/SQ, IO, infusions)
- IV initiation
- Immobilization
- Equipment preparation (central lines, suturing, ECG, EEG, IABP, casting and splinting, and wound dressing)
- Venous blood sampling
- Bedside cardiac enzyme testing
- Capnography, bedside BGL determination, and pulse oximetry
- Aerosolized and nebulized bronchodilitation therapy

★ Administering medications IV (46%)
★ Administering medications oral (45%)

The study went on to describe the types and variety of patient problems encountered, including:

★ Wound care (86%)
★ Medical emergencies (79%)
★ Suturing (23%)
★ Rape intervention (17%)

About two-thirds (67%) of EMTs indicated that they performed triage; however, in a national survey of 1,380 emergency departments, only 6% of emergency departments reported that paramedics/EMTs performed triage.

There may also be skills that the critical care paramedic is relatively unfamiliar with (or uses infrequently in critical care transport) that may be a common aspect of your job delineation. These are listed in Table 37–2.

Table 37–2	Less-Frequently Used Paramedic Skills in the Emergency Department Setting

- Foley catheter insertion
- NG/OG tube insertion
- Tracheal airway replacement
- Sterile techniques (tracheal suctioning, surgical procedures)
- ABG blood draw
- Conscious sedation monitoring
- Billing procedures if task done by critical care paramedic

It has been noted anecdotally by many experienced ED paramedics that it takes a certain personality to flourish in this environment. Generally speaking, the degree of autonomy is significantly less than when working prehospitally or in a critical care transport setting. The paramedic must also interface with a much larger number of care providers, which means you must have good interpersonal communication skills and be able to speak as an advocate for the patient. The environment is more controlled than the prehospital environment, and on any given shift, you will be much busier when working in an ED. A medium-size emergency department (of 25 to 30 beds) may see more than 45,000 patients per year (this equals roughly 65 patients per 12-hour shift). Compare that to a 12-hour shift on an ambulance where the paramedic in an average size EMS system may have six to eight trips.

The benefits usually include a higher pay scale than prehospital providers, as well as better benefits and a more reliable schedule. Additional benefits include the ability to practice skills that are rare to the prehospital environment and uncommon to the critical care environment, and the ability to gain a tremendous amount of clinical experience. Additionally, the critical care paramedic will interface with many departments within the hospital (radiology, lab, surgery, physical therapy, and so on), and this allows CCPs to become more familiar with other practitioners in an environment that is more conducive to learning.

In summary, regarding the tasks that may be performed by the critical care paramedic in the emergency department, it must always be remembered that patient care only happens in accordance with the physician's approval. Like the RN or respiratory therapist in the ED, the paramedic functions with a limited amount of autonomy and all patient care decisions are made by the physician responsible for that patient. The role of the paramedic is to be supportive of the physician's requests and to integrate well with the other care providers (regardless of certification/licensure level) who also have responsibility to caring for that patient.

CRITICAL CARE UNITS

Critical care units that the paramedic may find themselves working within include a **surgical intensive care unit (SICU), medical intensive care unit (MICU), cardiovascular intensive care unit (CVICU)**, and, to a lesser extent, the **pediatric intensive care unit (PICU)** and **neonatal intensive care unit (NICU)**. These critical care units will be discussed simultaneously since they share many of the same characteristics as they pertain to the critical care paramedic.

The role of the paramedic in these environments is much more limited in nature as compared to working in the emergency department, but that does not mean that it is any less challenging, because in these critical care units you will find the "sickest of the sick" patients. These patients are placed in these units because of the need for highly intensive care, which is often dependent on numerous medications and sophisticated medical equipment. (See Figure 37-2 ■.)

In this role the paramedic may be referred to as a **patient care associate** a person who works in conjunction with other heath care providers in caring for patients and who has the primary responsibility of monitoring the cardiac rhythms of those patients admitted to that unit. They also have additional duties, including documentation and charting of the patient's status; ordering therapies or diagnostics such as X-rays, lab values, or arterial gases according the physician's standing orders for that patient; and ensuring that the morning weaning parameters are set on ventilator-dependent patients (when working in an SICU).

Clinically the critical care paramedic will assist the RN staff with routine procedures such as endotracheal suctioning, dressing changes, emptying of drainage bags or devices, bathing and repositioning of the patient, and changing bed linens. As opportunity presents, the critical care paramedic may also assist the physician with skills such as spinal taps and central line insertion. Here the paramedic's role is primarily supportive in nature by way of holding the patient getting a spinal tap in a knee-chest position or limiting the motion of the body or extremities in a patient receiving central line insertion. The paramedic may also help set up equipment and hand various medical implements to the physician as he completes these skills.

Along with benefits similar to those received when working in the ED regarding pay, scheduling, and health care benefits, the critical care paramedic will also enjoy the ability to interact with various other health care practitioners. And, as in the ED, oftentimes these individuals are very

surgical intensive care unit (SICU) *a specialized unit dedicated to the intensive care of critical postsurgical patients.*

medical intensive care unit (MICU) *a specialized unit dedicated to the intensive care of critically ill patients.*

cardiovascular intensive care unit (CVICU) *a specialized unit dedicated to the care of patients with critical cardiovascular insults.*

pediatric intensive care unit (PICU) *a specialized unit dedicated to the care of critically ill or injured pediatric patients.*

neonatal intensive care unit (NICU) *a specialized unit dedicated to the care of critically ill or injured neonatal patients.*

patient care associate *a person who works in conjunction with other health care providers in caring for patients.*

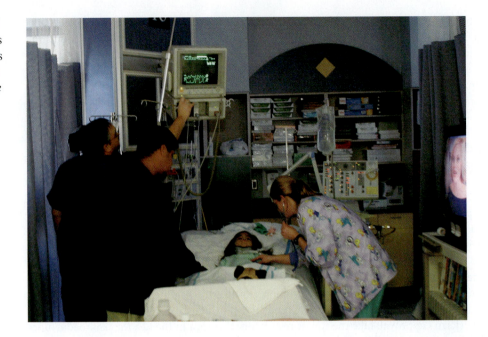

■ **Figure 37-2** The role of the critical care paramedic is expanding to meet the needs of both out-of-hospital and in-hospital patients. *(George Dodson)*

eager to teach and explain the interventions they are providing. This also greatly enhances the clinical knowledge of the critical care paramedic. The paramedic can also become very adept at 12-lead interpretation, X-ray interpretation, blood gas analysis, ventilatory assist devices, and cardiopulmonary bypass machines and can gain an understanding of advanced pharmacology. ARDS patients may be found on extracorpreal membrane oxygneator (ECMO) machines, and patients who are intolerable of normal renal hemodialysis may be receiving central veno-venous hemofiltration (CVVH). Also seen in this arena are those patients receiving hemodynamic support via left ventricular assist devices (LVADs).

Disadvantages to working in this environment may be construed by the paramedic as doing those skills that are considered "less glamorous," but still equally important to the patient's overall condition. These tasks include changing bed linen, bathing patients, and emptying bed pans. In summary of this intrahospital critical care department, the paramedic is even further removed from his traditional role in emergency medicine, and will acquire knowledge and skills integral to patient management in these critical care units.

SPECIAL PROCEDURE UNITS

As the name implies, special procedure units are components of hospital systems where specific diagnostic tests are performed in order to help diagnose or manage conditions. These units include the **cardiac catheterization and electrophysiology lab**, the **diagnostic noninvasive cardiology lab,** and the **interventional radiology lab**.

Fundamentally, the role of the critical care paramedic in these units is supportive in nature, assisting the team that is administering these interventions with the tasks inherent to each. Medical direction is provided to the critical care paramedic by the physician who is overseeing the procedure, and the critical care paramedic usually receives "on-the-job training" during initial employment.

CARDIAC CATHETERIZATION AND ELECTROPHYSIOLOGY LABORATORY

In the cardiac catheterization lab, the paramedic may help in setting up the sterile field for the procedure, assisting with transfer of the patient to the table, and assisting the physician with the machines (under direct supervision). On-the-job training is usually required to familiarize the medic with sterile procedures and the equipment.

cardiac catheterization and electrophysiology lab *a specialized unit where specific diagnostic tests and procedures are performed in order to help diagnose or manage cardiac conditions.*

diagnostic noninvasive cardiology lab *a specialized unit where specific diagnostic tests and procedures are performed in order to help diagnose or manage cardiac conditions.*

interventional radiology lab *a specialized unit where specific radiological tests are performed in order to help diagnose or manage a variety of conditions, either medical or trauma related.*

DIAGNOSTIC NONINVASIVE CARDIOLOGY LABORATORY

There is an increasing need for paramedics in this arena. Many physicians perform noninvasive cardiology procedures in their offices or at off-hospital locations where they can be billed under a separate DRG (diagnosis-related group). The critical care paramedic is usually required to assist with obtaining IV access, drawing baseline labs, prepping the patient's chest (shaving and applying EKG pads), and monitoring the patient's vital signs during the test. Cardiologists may be benefited by having critical care paramedics in this environment because of their familiarity with cardiac arrest management and the use of the monitor/defibrillator. They may also be called on as a backup if a patient arrests and the intubation is difficult (especially if they are off the hospital main campus where there is no anesthesia available).

INTERVENTIONAL RADIOLOGY

This is yet another area where critical care paramedics are seeing increased utilization. Many magnetic resonance imaging (MRI) and computed tomography (CT) suites are located off the hospital campus. While this may allow billing under a new DRG, its remoteness from the hospital increases the possibility of adverse outcomes if the patient suddenly deteriorates. The MD (radiologist) and critical care paramedic are commonly the only ACLS-certified health care practitioners at such a facility. The paramedic is usually responsible for starting the IV and then administering IV contrast under the physician's supervision. Should a complication occur such as a patient becomes dyspneic suffering an anaphylactic reaction or even cardiac arrest, it is usually the paramedic who can initiate and run the arrest team if required until additional help arrives. Even though the radiologist may have completed an ACLS class, he may not be as intimately familiar with the arrest management.

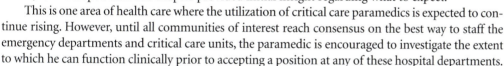

Summary

The intent of this chapter was to provide an overview of the differing roles and tasks the critical care paramedic may provide when employed in a hospital environment. Currently, there is no national standard as to what the scope of practice is for the paramedic working in these hospital departments, so it is hoped that this chapter provided initial insight regarding what to expect.

This is one area of health care where the utilization of critical care paramedics is expected to continue rising. However, until all communities of interest reach consensus on the best way to staff the emergency departments and critical care units, the paramedic is encouraged to investigate the extent to which he can function clinically prior to accepting a position at any of these hospital departments.

Overall the job market for the critical care paramedic is very good. With the RN shortage, most institutions are utilizing "patient care associates" in a number of different roles, and physicians usually enjoy having paramedics available because of the ability to manage critical situations (IV access, airway management, cardiac rhythm interpretation, ALCS, and so on).

Many aspiring flight paramedics have found that by taking jobs in the ED or ICU they get to know the flight crews/physicians very well, which usually translates into a much broader knowledge base because they tend to share information with them. The job is also well suited for the critical care paramedic who is tired of completing 24-hour shifts in an unstable and dynamic environment, and instead wants a more stable and potentially better paying position.

Review Questions

1. Why must a critical care paramedic still function under medical direction in the hospital?
2. Name some hospital departments that have employed paramedics historically.

3. What are some competing external influences that impact the paramedic's function inside the hospital?

4. Discuss common advantages to hospitals employing paramedics.

5. Describe the most commonly sited disadvantages made by those opposing the use of paramedics in the hospital.

6. List patient care skills the critical care paramedic will have to become more familiar with while working in the emergency department.

7. What would be a disadvantage to the paramedic working in the emergency department between missions?

8. How can a paramedic who is working in the emergency department ease the transition of patients from prehospital care providers to the emergency department staff?

See Answers to Review Questions at the back of this book.

Further Reading

American College of Emergency Physicians. *A Report of the EMT/Paramedic Working in the Emergency Department Survey.* Dallas, TX: Author, 1999.

American Nurses Association. "Joint Statement on Maintaining Professional and Legal Standards During a Shortage of Nursing Personnel." *NursingWorld.* http://www.nursingworld.org/readroom/position/joint/jtshort.htm.(1992).

Bledsoe BE, Porter RS, Cherry RA. *Essentials of Paramedic Care,* 2nd ed. Upper Saddle River NJ: Pearson Prentice Hall, 2007.

Derlet RW, Richards JR(2000). "Overcrowding in the Nation's Emergency Departments: Complex Causes and Disturbing Effects." *Annals of Emergency Medicine;* 35: 63–68.

Emergency Nurses Association. *ENA 2001 National Benchmark Guide: Emergency Departments.* Des Plaines, IL: Author, 2002.

National Council of State Boards of Nursing. *Delegation: Concepts and Decision-Making Process. National Council Position Paper.* http://www.ncsbn.org/public/regulation/delegation_documents_delegati.htm (1995).

Precautions on Bloodborne Pathogens and Infectious Diseases

Critical care transport providers, like all health care workers, are at risk for exposure to bloodborne pathogens and infectious diseases. In emergency situations it is often difficult to take or enforce proper infection control measures. However, as a paramedic, you must recognize your high-risk status. Study the following information on infection control carefully.

Infection control is designed to protect emergency personnel, their families, and their patients from unnecessary exposure to communicable diseases. Laws, regulations, and standards regarding infection control include:

★ *Centers for Disease Control and Prevention (CDC) Guidelines.* The CDC has published extensive guidelines on infection control. Proper equipment and techniques that should be used by emergency response personnel to prevent or minimize risk of exposure are defined.

★ *The Ryan White Act.* The Ryan White Act of 1990 allows emergency personnel to find out if they were exposed to an infectious disease while rendering patient care. Employers are required to name a "designated officer" to coordinate communications with the treating hospital.

★ *Americans with Disabilities Act.* This act prohibits discrimination against individuals with disabilities including those with contagious diseases. It guarantees equal employment opportunities and job protection if the infected individual can perform essential job functions and does not pose a threat to the safety and health of patients and coworkers.

★ *Occupational Safety and Health Administration (OSHA) Regulations.* OSHA has enacted a regulation entitled Occupational Exposure to Bloodborne Pathogens that classifies emergency response personnel as being at the greatest risk of occupational exposure to communicable diseases. This regulation requires employers to provide hepatitis B (HBV) vaccinations free of charge, maintain a written exposure control plan, and provide personal protective equipment. These requirements primarily apply to private employers. Applicability to local and state governmental employees varies by locality. Many states have developed their own OSHA plans.

★ *National Fire Protection Association (NFPA) Guidelines.* This is a national organization that has established specific guidelines and requirements regarding infection control for emergency response agencies, particularly fire departments and EMS services.

BODY SUBSTANCE ISOLATION PRECAUTIONS AND PERSONAL PROTECTIVE EQUIPMENT

Critical care personnel should practice body substance isolation (BSI), a strategy that considers ALL body substances potentially infectious. To achieve this, all emergency personnel should utilize personal protective equipment (PPE). Appropriate PPE should be available on every type of vehicle used for critical care transport. The minimum recommended PPE includes the following:

★ *Gloves.* Disposable gloves should be donned by all emergency response personnel BEFORE initiating any care. When a mission involves more than one patient, you should attempt to change gloves between patients. When gloves have been contaminated, they should be removed as soon as possible. To properly remove contaminated gloves, grasp one glove approximately 1 inch from the wrist. Without touching the inside of the glove, pull the glove halfway off and stop. With that half-gloved hand, pull the glove on the opposite hand completely off. Place the removed glove in the palm of the other glove, with the inside of the removed glove exposed. Pull the second glove completely off with the ungloved hand, only touching the inside of the glove. Always wash hands after gloves are removed, even when the gloves appear intact.

★ *Masks and Protective Eyewear.* Masks and protective equipment should be present on all critical care transport vehicles and used in accordance with the level of exposure encountered. Masks and protective eyewear should be worn together whenever blood spatter is likely to occur, such as during arterial bleeding, childbirth, endotracheal intubation, invasive procedures, oral suctioning, and cleanup of equipment that requires heavy scrubbing or brushing. Both you and the patient should wear masks whenever the potential for airborne transmission of disease exists.

★ *HEPA and N-95 Respirators.* Due to the resurgence of tuberculosis (TB), critical care providers should protect themselves from TB infection through use of an N-95 or a high-efficiency particulate air (HEPA) respirator, as approved by the National Institute of Occupational Safety and Health (NIOSH). It should fit snugly and be capable of filtering out the tuberculosis bacillus. An N-95 or HEPA respirator should be worn when caring for patients with confirmed or suspected TB. This is especially true when performing "high-hazard" procedures such as administration of nebulized medications, endotracheal intubation, or suctioning on such a patient.

★ *Gowns.* Gowns protect clothing from blood splashes. If large splashes of blood are expected, such as with childbirth, wear impervious gowns.

★ *Resuscitation Equipment.* Disposable resuscitation equipment should be the primary means of artificial ventilation in emergency care. Such items should be used once, then disposed of.

Remember, the proper use of personal protective equipment ensures effective infection control and minimizes risk. Use ALL protective equipment recommended for any particular situation to ensure maximum protection.

Consider ALL body substances potentially infectious and ALWAYS practice BSI.

Chapter 1

1. Transport of patients essentially had its beginnings during wartime. Soldiers from the battlefield were transported to hospitals where they could be cared for by surgeons. The first use of an ambulance in the United States occurred during the Civil War around 1865. In the latter half of the 19th century, civilian ambulances began to appear in various states such as Ohio, New York, and Illinois. Advanced life support was introduced to the prehospital setting in Belfast, Northern Ireland, in the late 1950s. In 1970, advanced life support was first introduced in the United States by Dr. Eugene Nagel in Miami, Florida. Today, EMS is a sophisticated part of the health care system. Paramedics are filling more roles in both hospital and prehospital settings. The development of the *EMS Agenda for the Future* will guide EMS programs well into the 21st century.

2. Although the first use of aircraft for the transport of patients is lost in history, there are records of hot air balloons being used to transport wounded during the Prussian siege of Paris in 1870. During World War I and wars thereafter, selected patients were transported by airplane. Helicopters were first used for medical transport during the Korean War in the early 1950s, and were relied on heavily during the Vietnam conflict. Injured soldiers were provided first aid at the scene and transported rapidly by helicopter to medical facilities such as a Mobile Army Surgical Hospital (MASH) or battalion aid station. Although some sporadic use was made of aircraft for civilian medical transport, the first aircraft dedicated primarily used for ambulance work operated out of Samaritan Air Evac in Phoenix in 1969. The Maryland State Police began providing a combination of police/ambulance helicopter service in 1970. In 1972, Saint Anthony's Hospital in Denver established the first helicopter service dedicated exclusively to patient care. Today, air transport is a common part of EMS.

3. Critical care medicine evolved with the recognition that better care was needed for patients who had a life-threatening illness or injury beyond routine nursing floor care. Specialized areas of the hospital were subsequently devoted to care of these very ill patients. Intensive care in the United States began early in the 20th century when a noted neurosurgeon established a three-bed intensive care unit (ICU) for neurosurgical patients at the Johns Hopkins Hospital in Baltimore, Maryland. By 1958, approximately 25% of community hospitals with more than 300 beds had an ICU. By the late 1960s, virtually every hospital had at least one ICU bed. In 1970, the Society of Critical Care Medicine (SCCM) was formed, and in 1973, the American Association of Critical-Care Nurses (AACN) developed achievement examinations for the purpose of recognizing the expertise of registered nurses who were practicing in the specialty of critical care. In 1986, the American Board of Medical Specialties recognized the specialty of critical care medicine by approving a certificate of special competence for physicians certified by one of four primary boards (anesthesiology, internal medicine, pediatrics, and surgery). By 1997, more than 5,000 ICUs were operational in the United States. The development of the critical care paramedic happened somewhat by happenstance. Essentially the increased specialty of hospitals required the transport of patients from facility to facility to take advantage of special needs care available at certain facilities. Although a nurse would initially accompany the patient, the trend moved toward educating an EMT paramedic in many advanced skills and knowledge, who, when equipped with the appropriate medical equipment, can provide a high level of care to these critical patients during transport between facilities.

4. The role of the critical care paramedic varies significantly. Critical care paramedics may be assigned to dedicated ground critical care transport vehicles or they may be assigned to standard EMS units and summoned when a critical care transport call is received. Many hospitals operate critical care transport services as part of their emergency department or ICU. In these cases, critical care paramedics will often work in the emergency department or ICU when not involved in a critical care transport. Critical care paramedics also work as flight paramedics for aeromedical operations. In critical care transport, paramedics are often called on to use advanced skills much more frequently than they would in the standard prehospital environment. In addition, critical care paramedics will usually acquire skills in procedures that are not commonly used in routine prehospital care. Like all aspects of EMS, critical care paramedics must function under the authority of a licensed physician. Likewise, care must be guided by medical protocols and standing orders that provide guidelines and direction for care of individual patients. Critical care protocols must be customized for the specific operation (adult medicine, pediatrics, neonatal, cardiac).

Chapter 2

1. As discussed in Chapter 1, the present-day paramedic evolved from the ranks of initial care providers who were active during wartime. As time passed and EMS system designs grew more comprehensive, a need arose to staff ambulances with highly skilled providers for the management of acutely ill or injured patients being transported to specialty hospitals. Although in a state of flux, the role of the critical care paramedic is becoming more solidified within the domain of prehospital and interhospital medicine. Critical care paramedics can be found in both ground transport and aeromedical systems.

2. Specialty care transport (SCT) pertains to the interfacility critical care transports of patients, and is defined by Medicare as "hospital-to-hospital" transportation of a critically injured or ill beneficiary by a ground ambulance vehicle, including the provision of medically necessary supplies and services, at a level of service beyond the scope of the EMT-Paramedic. SCT is necessary when a beneficiary's condition requires ongoing care that must be furnished by one or more health professionals in a specialty area, for example, emergency or critical care nursing, emergency medicine, respiratory care, cardiovascular care, or a paramedic with additional training."

3. Three instances when the critical care transport of a patient by ground may be preferable to air include when inclement weather or challenging geographic influences exist, when a considerable amount of medical equipment is needed for transport (such as an intra-aortic balloon pump or a pediatric isolate) and additional room is needed, or when the health care system needs to remain cognizant of the expenditure of health care dollars because, generally, ground systems are more cost effective to operate than aeromedical systems. Finally, other considerations may include environmental factors that can affect both the patient and care providers in air medical operations that might not be experienced in ground transportation. Although more prevalent to fixed-wing operations, some of these factors may include oxygen levels, acceleration/deceleration forces, gas volume changes at altitude, cabin pressurization, humidity, noise, and vibration.

4. Medical direction for the critical care paramedic is typically provided through off-line standing orders via medical protocols. On-line medical direction is also utilized, but because of the advanced skill training and education, as well as the rigorous QA/QI programs of critical care transport systems, it is relied on with less frequency than off-line control. Contributing to this, especially in the case of ground transport units that operate in geographic locations where transport distances to remote locations are great, the use of on-line control may be inhibited. In the absence of on-line medical control, critical care paramedics must rely on standing orders and their clinical expertise to provide appropriate patient care. The critical care practitioner usually possesses a great deal of autonomy for this reason.

Chapter 3

1. The program director is responsible for coordinating all of the daily operations of the flight program, including the direction of the program in terms of strategy and growth. The main responsibilities of the program director include creating administrative policy, establishing a continuous quality improvement program, ensuring the fleet of aircraft is maintained (although some air medical systems use external vendors to purchase or lease aircraft), maintaining the communications center, preparing and planning the operating budget, directing the marketing and growth strategies, and serving as a figurehead of the organization to hospital and nonhospital health care organizations.

2. The medical director is responsible for creating medical protocols, ensuring proper training of the flight crews, and providing on-line medical direction in the event that a patient case falls outside of the existing written protocol. Many states have specific laws and guidelines on who can perform the duties of the medical director, and in many cases these physicians have backgrounds in emergency or critical care medicine.

3. Air medical transport offers a number of advantages and disadvantages. The advantages include much more rapid transport speed; access to remote locations; access to specialty teams (e.g., neonate, transplant, burn centers); access to personnel with specialized skills such as surgical airway, thoracotomy, RSI, hemodynamic; and critical care experience.

4. Clinical situations for air transport and interfacility transfers are best summarized as being present when patients have diagnostic and/or therapeutic needs that cannot be met at the referring hospital, and when factors such as time, distance, and/or intratransport level of care requirements render ground transport unfeasible. A more expansive and clinically based description of recommendations has been developed by the National Association of EMS Physicians that is available for use by critical care transporting systems.

5. Using basic mechanism of injury criteria, another list of indications for utilizing aeromedical critical care services would include:
   a. Trauma score < 12
   b. Unstable vital signs (e.g., hypotension or tachypnea)
   c. Significant trauma in patients < 12 years old, > 55 years old, or pregnant patients
   d. Multisystem injuries (e.g., long-bone fractures in different extremities, injury to more than two body regions)
   e. Ejection from vehicle
   f. Pedestrian or cyclist struck by motor vehicle
   g. Death in same passenger compartment as patient
   h. Ground provider perception of significant damage to patient's passenger compartment
   i. Penetrating trauma to the abdomen, pelvis, chest, neck, or head
   j. Crush injury to the abdomen, chest, or head
   k. Fall from significant height

6. Visual Flight Rules (VFR) and Instrument Flight Rules (IFR) are two modes of flight navigation available for aircraft. All helicopters and certified pilots have the ability to fly VFR, while only specially equipped helicopters can fly IFR. VFR applies when the pilot can clearly see outside the aircraft, uses visual landmarks and cues as to the safe operation of the aircraft, and requires the weather to meet minimum standards as outlined and mandated by the FAA.

7. Fixed-wing transport of the critical care patient is predominantly considered when transport of the patient will exceed 100 miles, and for some international and intercontinental flight missions.

8. The communications center is responsible for all incoming requests for air medical transports, as well as the gathering of specific required information such as coordinates,

ground contact frequencies, destinations, and patient information. Beyond these initial duties, the communications specialists must perform multiple follow-up duties such as flight following of the aircraft, communications with the accepting hospital, and call-back to the requesting agency to get any additional medical or logistical data. The communications center and the communications specialists are very important members of the air medical team and are often not recognized for their importance in the program.

9. The indications for patient transport by helicopter include medical emergencies, trauma emergencies, and search-and-rescue missions. Determining whether or not the patient needs air medical transport depends on two factors. The first is the clinical status and/or the mechanism of injury, and the second is the transport time by ground vs. the arrival time and transport time of the aircraft.

Chapter 4

1. Boyle's law is the most important gas law to critical care flight medicine. Boyle's law states that the volume of a gas is inversely proportional to its pressure (assuming temperature remains constant). As such, whenever a patient is flown, the care provider must remain cognizant of potential pressure changes that may occur during flight. The PASG, the delivered tidal volume for patients who are ventilator dependent, any inflated cuff of a medical device (for example, an endotracheal tube), and even intravenous flow rates at altitude can vary (which is why mechanical infusion pumps are commonly used). Due to gas expansion at altitude, patients may experience nausea, vomiting, or a need to urinate.

2. It is important for the critical care paramedic to closely monitor all air-filled cuffs that are employed for patient management during flight (endotracheal tubes, central lines, PASG, and so on). The best way to do this is to either remove pressure from the cuff as needed as you ascend to altitude, use water or saline instead of air in the cuff to minimize this effect, or employ a commercial device to regulate cuff pressure.

3. Stresses of altitude and flight can affect the critical care paramedic as much as the patient. Stresses of altitude include hypoxia, barometric pressure changes, fatigue, and thermal dehydration. Stresses of flight include noise, vibration, gravitational forces, third spacing, spatial disorientation, and flicker vertigo. These effects can be individually or collectively detrimental to the flight crew because they may precipitate confused thought, visual disturbances, extreme fatigue, motion sickness, dizziness, and an inability to concentrate or think clearly. The best way for critical care transport team paramedics to avoid these stresses of flight and altitude is by simply maintaining good health, obtaining adequate rest between shifts and missions, eating properly, avoiding smoking, avoiding flying with ear infections or head colds, learning to recognize disturbances in other crew members, and finally realizing when these stressors of flight and altitude are starting to affect themselves.

4. Hypoxia is the most significant problem following decompression. The rapid reduction of ambient pressure produces a corresponding drop in the partial pressure of oxygen and reduces the alveolar oxygen tension. A twofold to threefold performance decrement occurs regardless of altitude. The reduced tolerance to hypoxia after decompression is due to a reversal in the direction of oxygen flow in the lung, and also diminished respiratory activity at the time of decompression, and decreased cardiac activity. Fortunately, pressurized aircraft have supplemental oxygen delivery systems that deploy in the event of a depressurization.

5. G-forces may be relevant to the patient's position in some types of aircraft. Their effect on the patient is influenced by weight and distribution, gravitational pull and centrifugal force, which collectively affect blood pooling. Centrifugal force tends to alter the blood flow in the body in proportion to the amount of force imposed. When positive

($+G_z$) forces are applied to the body, blood tends to pool in the lower portions of the body; the opposite occurs during negative ($-G_z$) application. Patient positioning in some aircraft may minimize or enhance the effects of G-forces.

Chapter 5

1. Maintaining "safety consciousness" refers simply to the ability of flight crew members to actively look for risks, rather than simply noticing them. To operate with a safety consciousness, the provider must understand his job as well as those external influences that impact it. The critical care paramedic need not be a pilot, but he does need to understand the dynamics of how helicopters fly. He need not be a meteorologist, but the critical care paramedic needs to understand how the weather impacts aircraft operations. The critical care paramedic need not be an aviation mechanic, but he needs to be aware of how he can assist the mechanic in identifying and isolating mechanical problems. And finally, the critical care paramedic need not be an engineer, but he needs to realize how workplace controls and the mounting of medical equipment can impact safe movement around the patient compartment of the aircraft.

2. The pilot safety brief is the process of the pilot discussing with the medical crew issues such as weights and balances of the aircraft, fuel capacity, weather conditions and forecast, and any operational issues existing with the aircraft. The pilot safety brief not only serves the purpose of maintaining a safe working environment, but also facilitates an understanding of normal flight operations and reinforces the constant need for communication between pilot and crew members.

3. Preflight responsibilities include those procedures that should be completed prior to each mission. These help ensure that the highest degree of safety for flight is being maintained and include looking for foreign material on the ground that may be picked up or thrown by the turning rotors; inspecting for "cords, covers, and cowlings"; and finally ensuring that all safety harnesses and helmets are donned and portable equipment secured prior to liftoff.

4. The sterile cockpit is an FAA regulation that requires all nonessential communication to cease during critical phases of flight. Critical phases include lifting off, taxiing, and landing. The sterile cockpit serves numerous purposes. First, it eliminates any distraction of the pilot from nonessential or casual conversation by the crew. Second, if any noise is heard on the headset, it is probably either the airport or your communications center relaying important information that the pilot may need to immediately receive. Third, it allows the pilot to carefully listen to the sounds of the engines during these critical power phases (landing, lifting, and taxiing are three instances when the aircraft's engines are typically run at maximum power). The only time the medical crew can violate the sterile cockpit is when they identify some type of safety concern to themselves or the aircraft.

5. An in-flight emergency is one that influences the flight of the helicopter (or airplane) itself. And since many of these in-flight emergencies that lead to an accident occur due to pilot error (64%) or mechanical failure (22%), they are caused by something that the medical flight crew cannot necessarily prevent—but must deal with nonetheless. In-flight emergencies can generally be broken into two categories: controlled flight into terrain (CFIT) and mechanical failure.

6. If an in-flight emergency is called by the pilot, the critical care paramedic should first obey any specific pilot directions, and secondly (or simultaneously if possible) tend to the following tasks should a forced landing be inevitable: Relay as much information as possible to your communications center about your current coordinates and a brief description of emergency, disable the power inverter and shut off the main oxygen supply,

prepare the patient for an emergency landing, and then prepare the crew for an emergency landing.

7. Following a forced landing, the critical care paramedic should ensure that certain aircraft components are shut down. This is normally a task for the pilot; however, if the pilot is incapacitated, the critical care paramedic should know how to shut off the engines, the fuel supply, and the main batteries (all of these reduce the chance for fires following impact).

8. Following a forced landing, the critical care paramedic needs to inventory usable aircraft material and establish priorities pertaining to survival. One way of doing this is by understanding the "rule of threes" when in outdoor survival situations. The rule states that a person can survive 3 minutes without oxygen, 3 hours in extreme weather without shelter, 3 days without water, and 3 weeks without food.

9. In situations where rescue may be several days away, the critical care paramedic can use the "rule of threes" as a guide to establish priorities given the estimated likelihood and time frame for rescue personnel to reach the crash site. After tending to immediate medical needs of those injured, the first priority would be creating shelter, the second priority is fire to create heat and allow the boiling of water, and the last priority is food. Unless rescue is 4 to 5 days off, rationing of the emergency food supply on board should suffice.

10. Although not expressly listed within the "rule of threes," the flight crew should be prepared to signal rescuers and implement the plan at first notice of rescuer arrival. The critical care paramedic should ready the flare gun (be cautious, however, when discharging the flare gun in extremely dry wooded areas), have items near the fire that will easily produce smoke (leaves, upholstery, or tires), and attempt communication via the radios on the aircraft (if still operable) or via the use of satellite or cellular/digital phones that may be carried by flight personnel.

Chapter 6

1. Each phase of assessment has a "purpose," or a reason why the steps of that phase are completed. And for the scene size-up phase of assessment, the purpose is to *control the scene*. Controlling the scene means employing those techniques that will best ensure your safety and that of your crew and patient immediately on arrival at the patient's side. It also includes considering additional resources to better enable you to control the ongoing assessment and management of the patient.

2. The six individual steps of the initial assessment that should be completed by the critical care paramedic with each patient contact include (in order of normal occurrence) forming a general impression; assessing mental status, airway assessment, determination of breathing adequacy, completing the circulatory assessment, and determination or classification of the patient's priority status.

3. The overall goal for the initial assessment is to identify and support any lost vital bodily function. Although you may be assessing clinical parameters not directly related to vital bodily functions, everything that the critical care paramedic does in this phase should be performed with the express purpose of determining if a life-threatening injury or illness is present that must be expediently treated.

4. The rapid physical exam is a head-to-toe assessment geared toward rapid assessment of key findings in order to provide specific interventions. The overall goal is to assess the patient rapidly from head to toe, looking for those critical injuries or clinical findings that contributed to the loss of function identified earlier in the initial assessment phase. Whereas the initial assessment includes treatment interventions geared to support lost

function, treatment interventions in this phase are geared to correct the physiological disturbance that caused the lost function that you are already supporting.

5. Concurrently with the critical care team's assessment of the patient, the other team members can begin the preparation of the patient and necessary documents for transport. Several important documents need to be gathered prior to the initiation of the transport. These documents are outlined in the COBRA/EMTALA legislation, and typically include the following paperwork: physician certification for flight; written request for the transfer by the patient; advanced acceptance by the destination hospital, which is documented in the record; signed consent to transfer the patient; medical orders for the ongoing treatment of the patient by the transporting critical care team; and copies of the medical records, tests, and X-rays unless delays for these might jeopardize the patient. The majority of this information is usually found on a special consent to transfer form provided by the sending facility.

6. Three non-patient care centered tasks that should be completed by the critical care transport team prior to departure with the patient (especially with interfacility transfers) include procurement and documentation of medical records and EMTALA/COBRA considerations, proper securing of the patient and all portable medical equipment, and briefly discussing the patient's condition and care plan with the patient's family so they can remain abreast of the patient's condition.

7. The critical care paramedic should still complete a thorough patient assessment rather than simply reviewing and documenting the patient's status according to any medical records already available. This is to ensure that the provider is intimately familiar with the patient's condition, as well as to determine any changes in the patient's clinical status given the treatment rendered thus far by other care providers. Remember, the medical records document the patient's status historically (i.e., after the assessment and management have been ongoing). If the critical care paramedic needs to know how the patient is doing *now*, she must perform a physical exam *now* to find out.

8. Although the specific reasons for transport missions are varied, the request for critical care transport usually falls into one of the following categories: The patient is still in the prehospital environment due to entrapment or isolation issues (remote locations) and flying him to a medical facility is a viable option due to distance and time concerns; the patient needs to be transported for medical treatment not available at current facility; the patient is being admitted to another facility due to economic or insurance reasons; and finally the patient or their family has requested the transport.

9. During interfacility transports, the critical care paramedic should review with the providers already caring for the patient any of the pertinent diagnostic studies. Several of the things that should be reviewed are lab results, X-rays, 12-leads, capnograms, hemodynamic waveforms, and any other diagnostic studies that may have been performed prior to the critical care team's arrival. In the event that the patient's clinical condition appears to differ from the diagnostic findings or current diagnosis, err on the side of concern for the patient and be more diligent in your assessment and thorough in your management. If necessary, ask for a chance to converse with the physician responsible for the patient regarding your concerns.

10. Generally speaking, the critical care staff completes interfacility and prehospital missions for patients who are in real or potentially dangerous degrees of hemodynamic compromise. Despite this, there are those situations when the critical care crew should not depart the scene with a patient. These include (but are not limited to) current or incoming inclement weather, inadequate preparation of accompanying medical records, if the patient has a high likelihood of arresting while transport is occurring, if there is disagreement between what the critical care team believes is warranted care versus what the sending physician believes

to be appropriate (until the crew's medical director makes the final decision), or if the patient's body habitus precludes transport safely (i.e., obesity, aggression, danger to self or crew, combative). Almost all the aforementioned problems can be resolved adequately, but may require more forethought and planning by the care providers.

Chapter 7

1. Numerous devices and techniques are available to assist in airway management. Normal EMS operations will usually carry a basic airway kit that includes an assortment of laryngoscope blades (Miller and MacIntosh), tubes of various sizes, McGill forceps, stylets, a rescue airway, and equipment for creating a surgical airway. In the critical care setting, airway problems should be anticipated and additional equipment and supplies should be readily available. This includes the ability to identify the following equipment as well as perform the related skills: rapid-sequence induction; use of *Grandview* and *Viewmax* blades, the Burden nasoscope, the BAAM device, and the gum elastic bougie; digital, lighted stylet, and retrograde intubation; use of the "sky-hook" technique; and use of the LMA, the intubating LMA, the cobra perilaryngeal airway, and the King LT airway. Finally, if the paramedic is unfamiliar or unexperienced with needle and surgical cricothyrotomy techniques, they should be reviewed as well.

2. If a patient clearly is precipitously failing maximal aggressive medical management, or if the history of his problem clearly indicates that he will not be able to or already cannot protect his airway, then active intervention is appropriate to control the airway and provide adequate ventilation. The safest way to do this is by means of an advanced airway procedure called rapid-sequence induction or rapid-sequence intubation (RSI). Because of the risk of disastrous outcomes should the procedure be inappropriately administered, it should be performed by only the most skilled and confident care providers available.

3. From a process point of view, the critical care paramedic should follow a prescribed method of achieving intubation when performing the RSI technique. The steps for this include (in relative order that they should be completed) preoxygenation and preparation of airway equipment and medications, induction with a sedative (using analgesic for traumatic pain as warranted), application of the *Sellick* maneuver after adequate induction has occurred, consideration of premedication (defasciculating agent, atropine, lidocaine, and so on), administration of a paralytic, performance of intubation, confirmation of intubation, securing of the endotracheal tube, and provision of long-term sedation and paralysis.

4. Confirming intubation placement for the critical care paramedic is done in essentially the same way as in the prehospital environment. The critical care paramedic should ensure proper placement of the ETT by visualizing the tube passing into the trachea, auscultate with each ventilation for bilateral breath sounds over the chest after ensuring gastric sounds are absent over the stomach, employ a secondary confirmation device such as a self-inflating bulb syringe and/or use of a colorimetric end-tidal CO_2 detector, and watching for the chest to rise and fall with ventilations and for condensation in the ETT.

5. The use of analgesics and hypnotics in the RSI procedure is to allow for patient induction. Induction refers to the sedation provided to the patient prior to paralysis. Since neuromuscular blockers (paralytics) do not affect mental status, all patients (except those already unconscious) must receive sedation with a blocking agent prior to administration of neuromuscular blockade. Drugs from the barbiturate, opiate, neuroleptic, and benzodiazepine families are commonly used in EMS, critical care, and emergency medicine.

6. Perhaps no other part of medical documentation is more important than the documentation of airway management. A significant percentage of claims and lawsuits that are filed against critical care providers involve inadequate patient ventilation. Therefore, it is crucial that the provider learn to document in medically correct and legally sufficient

terms exactly what was done in managing the airway. Since airway management literally determines whether the patient lives or dies, it stands to reason that the greatest emphasis should be placed on detailed documentation. Such documentation can save you from a claim or lawsuit being filed or, in the unfortunate event that one is filed, can help the critical care provider prevail.

7. There will be multiple instances when the critical care provider must utilize mechanical ventilation while transporting a patient by either air or ground. In any situation, the provider must remain cognizant that the mechanical ventilations provided, although they result in air flow in and out of the lungs, DO NOT mimic normal spontaneous ventilations. By this it is meant that with mechanical ventilation in a ventilator-dependent patient, there is no opportunity for negative intrathoracic pressure created by spontaneous inhalation efforts. As such, this may result in diminished cardiac preload with subsequent drop in left ventricular ejection. In addition, there may be retention of carbon dioxide if the minute ventilation is not meeting the patient's needs. As such, it is imperative that the critical care provider closely monitor ventilatory volumes and other clinical indicators that illustrate desired ventilator function.

Chapter 8

1. Oxygen cannot be stored in the peripheral tissues. Thus, the amount of oxygen delivered to the tissues must meet the oxygen requirements of the tissues. The oxygen delivered to the tissues is commonly referred to as the rate of oxygen uptake (VO_2). The metabolic demand for oxygen at the tissue level (MRO_2) is the rate at which oxygen is utilized in the conversion of glucose to energy and water through glycolysis and the tricarboxylic acid (TCA) cycle. When the rate of oxygen uptake fails to meet the metabolic demand for oxygen, shock occurs.

2. Normally, one molecule of glucose will yield 36 molecules of energy in the form of adenosine triphosphate (ATP) and water as an end product. If oxygen is not present, the glucose will be metabolized through glycolysis only. In this case, 1 molecule of glucose will result in only 2 moles of ATP and the production of pyruvic acid as an end product. Pyruvic acid is converted to lactic acid (a toxic metabolic acid). In summary, when the oxygen supply to the tissues falls, the energy yield from glucose then drops dramatically, resulting in a phenomenon known as dysoxia. When cellular dysoxia causes a change in organ function, the condition is referred to as shock.

3. For the critical care paramedic, the common denominator of shock is the amount of oxygen consumed by the cells. When the body is under normal conditions, the oxygen uptake (VO_2) is independent of oxygen delivery (DaO_2), which means if the cells need to consume additional oxygen to produce energy, they can extract the necessary amount of oxygen required to produce energy in the form of ATP. Thus the equation:

$$VO_2 = \text{Cardiac output (CO)} \times 13.4 \times Hb \times (SaO_2 - SvO_2)$$

From this equation it is apparent that a problem with cardiac output, available hemoglobin, or arterial oxygen saturation can result in shock. It is the critical care paramedic's role to recognize disturbances to these parameters and provide corrective measures in an attempt to prevent shock.

4. In compensated shock the body is still able to compensate for the fall in cardiac output. When baroreceptors in the body detect a fall in cardiac output, it immediately begins to compensate for the decrease via release of various neurotransmitters. Primarily vasoconstriction of nonvital organs causes an increase in peripheral vascular resistance, which increases preload, stroke volume, and ultimately cardiac output. Vasoconstriction also causes several clinical signs common to this stage of shock, including pallor, which is most noticeable around the skin under the eyes, around the mouth and nose, and in

the extremities. The critical care paramedic may also note a normal blood pressure, increases in the heart and respiratory rates, and normalcy to the level of consciousness. At this stage, with appropriate assessment and treatments, the shock can still be reversed.

5. Numerous neurohumoral agents work together to produce a stress response while the body is in a shock state. The overall effects of the neurohumoral response are to support cardiac output by increasing heart rate and contractility, produce vasoconstriction to distribute the cardiac output to vital organs, retain salt and water to maintain circulating plasma, and assemble metabolic fuels for use. Activation of these responses can only be tolerated for a short period of time (during compensation).

6. Shock is ultimately an event that takes place at the cellular level and progresses in stages ranging from mild to lethal—from compensated, to decompensated, to irreversible. In compensated shock, the body is able to compensate for the fall in cardiac output. At this stage, with appropriate assessment and treatments, the shock can be reversed. If the cause of the shock is not found and treated, the compensatory mechanism will eventually collapse, leading to the next stage, which is called decompensated (or progressive) shock. In the decompensated stage, further compensatory mechanisms are engaged. Additional neurotransmitters are secreted into the circulation, which promotes even more vasoconstriction and reabsorption of sodium which acts to conserve water. With shock yet unabated there will be eventual hypoxemia, tissue hypoxia, and diminished cardiac output. Eventually, in the irreversible stage of shock, permanent cellular damage will occur. At this stage, patients typically present unresponsive and have decreasing pulse rates, dysrhythmias, nondetectable blood pressure, and agonal respirations. ARDS is commonly seen as a result at this stage, and the patient will likely suffer multiple system organ failure (kidney failure, heart failure, and hypoxic brain syndrome). Even if the patient is successfully resuscitated at this phase, her prognosis is poor.

7. Shock is classified into four categories: hypovolemic, obstructive, distributive, and cardiogenic. Hypovolemic shock results from a reduction in circulating intravascular volume. Obstructive shock is a result of impedance of the circulatory flow. Distributive shock occurs from a decrease in vascular resistance or increased venous capacity from a vasomotor dysfunction. Distributive shock can further be classified into septic shock, neurogenic shock, and anaphylactic shock. Finally, cardiogenic shock occurs when the heart is unable to maintain a sufficient cardiac output. Damage to either the right or left ventricle can cause a decrease in the amount of blood pumped to the cells to maintain normal activity.

8. Proper fluid management is critical to the survival of patients with fluid loss because it is sometimes needed to maintain homeostasis. The initial step to fluid resuscitation is with two large-bore peripheral IVs. In hypovolemia from trauma it is now common practice to not elevate a patient's blood pressure to more than 75% of the patient's preinjury blood pressure. Several of the body's compensatory mechanisms operate best at a systolic blood pressure between 70 and 85 mmHg. Increasing the blood pressure to normal levels in patients where the bleeding has not been controlled (i.e., blunt abdominal trauma) can actually worsen bleeding, resulting in a fall in circulating hemoglobin and coagulation factors. If IV access cannot be obtained, consider the placement of a central line early if peripheral access is difficult to obtain, or when large volumes of fluid are anticipated (such as a severe burn injury). In these cases, these lines can be used to facilitate further hemodynamic monitoring if needed. A fluid bolus can be tried to improve the patient's blood pressure if no signs of pulmonary edema are present. A bolus of 100–200 mL of a crystalloid solution may be instituted.

Chapter 9

1. Ways to invasively determine the patient's hemodynamic status that may be utilized during critical care transport include (but are not limited to) the assessment of central venous pressure, arterial pressure, cardiac output, pulmonary capillary wedge pres-

sure, stroke volume, and oxygen delivery. Assessment of these parameters as well as noninvasive indicators (such as skin characteristics, heart rate, and mental status) will provide the critical care paramedic with a solid interpretation of the patient's physiological status.

2. The critical care paramedic will commonly be responsible for the care of unstable patients during transport, and will frequently transport patients with various hemodynamic monitors in place. In these critical patients, subtle changes in a hemodynamic parameter may be the earliest indicator of deterioration in the patient's condition. Because of this, it is important to understand the common monitoring devices used in modern critical care. It is also important to interpret what changes in the patient's various physiological parameters may indicate.

3. Starting with the most distal aspect of the pulmonary artery catheter, the distal port is where the monitoring of the wedge pressure is done. The distal tip has a small balloon that, when inflated, allows the tip of the device to occlude a small pulmonary artery vessel, and the pressure sensor in the tip of the PA catheter can then calculate the pressure between the catheter's tip and the left side of the heart. The balloon inflation port is equipped with a special 3-cc syringe that will only inject 1.5 cc into the distal balloon. The next port moving proximally opens into the right ventricle. This port, when present, allows for medication administration, and on some types of PA lines it also allows the insertion of a ventricular pacing wire should the patient be in need of intracardiac pacing. The most proximal port on the PA line is the CVP port, which opens into the right atrium and is used for determining central venous pressure.

4. To get the most accurate pressures within the waveform of any invasive line, the transducer of the flush system must be in a fixed position that is relative to the system being monitored (the cardiovascular system). The transducer must be placed at a level corresponding to the right atrium in order to provide the most accurate measures. The *phlebostatic axis,* located at the fourth intercostal space, midaxillary line, is the approximate level of the right atrium. Placement of the transducer at the phlebostatic axis is best accomplished initially while the patient is supine. Once this is established, the transducer is ready to be zeroed to atmospheric pressure. Having the transducer placed at a level either higher or lower than the phlebostatic axis will result in dangerously erroneous hemodynamic readings.

5. Low central venous pressure, diminished cardiac output, and elevations in the patient's systemic vascular resistance would be consistent with intravascular volume deficit. Etiologies underlying this arrangement of hemodynamic parameters may include traumatic blood loss, severe dehydration, excessive fluid loss from uncontrolled or prolonged diarrhea, or blood loss from a medical cause such as GI bleeding.

6. A continuous wedged waveform on the monitor of a PA line may be caused by accidental migration of the PA tip into a pulmonary artery branch. In this situation (assuming the cuff is deflated), the critical care paramedic should attempt repositioning maneuvers (left side lying) while flushing catheters; if still unsuccessful in correcting the situation, contact medical direction.

7. A loss of waveform with hemodynamic monitoring may be from numerous causes. These causes can include disconnection of the communicating cable, disconnection of the flush system, kinking of the catheter, improper stopcock positioning on lines, improperly scaled waveform, and a clotted catheter.

8. A superwedge occurs when the balloon of a PA catheter is overinflated beyond the distal tip. It is avoided by using the correct amount of volume in inflating the balloon (0.8–1.2 mL). Should this occur, however, the critical care paramedic should first remove the balloon syringe from the port to ensure the balloon port is open and allowed to passively deflate. Then reinflate the balloon with 0.8–1.2 cc air and observe for PCWP waveform.

9. The cardiac index is derived by taking the cardiac output and dividing it by the BSA of the patient. This derived value may be more reflective of left ventricular function because it does in fact take into consideration the actual cardiac output *and* the size of the patient (rather than *just* the amount of cardiac output). This may be necessary, for example, when infusing vasoactive drugs or when the patient is receiving IABP therapy.

10. This should occur when there is identification of significant ventricular irritability, and the observance of a right ventricular waveform is noted. This means the distal tip of the PA catheter has migrated back into the right ventricle (contributing to the ventricular irritability). Should this occur, observe for a change in PA catheter reference point (point where PA catheter enters introducer). If the patient is hemodynamically stable, contact medical direction. If the patient is hemodynamically unstable, pull the PA catheter back until RA waveform is observed or until ventricular irritability ceases and still contact medical direction.

Chapter 10

1. Critical care patients can easily display any one of a number of dysrhythmias. Some dysrhythmias are benign, and a number of them are lethal. Some dysrhythmias are easy to see (ventricular fibrillation and asystole), whereas others are complex and deceiving for a single lead analysis. As such, the critical care provider should be adept at monitoring and interpreting multiple-lead ECGs, which view the electrical activity of the heart from multiple views, in order to best interpret the true underlying rhythm.

2. It has been consistently shown that leads V1 and V6 (or their bipolar equivalents MCL-1 and MCL-6) are the best leads for differentiating wide QRS rhythms. The morphology of the QRS complexes as displayed in these leads has been shown to be invaluable in differentiating ventricular tachycardia from supraventricular tachycardia with aberrant conduction. However, recent studies have shown that lead V1 may be even better than MCL-1 in that QRS morphology differed between V1 and MCL-1 in 40% of patients with ventricular tachycardia. Because of this, the American Heart Association does not recommend MCL-1 for diagnosing wide QRS complex tachycardia. However, if you do not have a 12-lead monitor, the MCL-1 lead is better than anything else available. In addition, other findings such as the presence of AV dissociation, QRS width, QRS axis, and the presence of fusion or capture beats can often be better observed in these leads as well.

3. The critical care paramedic should remain keenly aware of the patient's current ECG findings in order to manage significant dysrhythmias as well as predict if a life-threatening dysrhythmia may develop. One such example of identifying risk factors is for a third-degree block. If the provider should observe fascicular blocks, bundle branch blocks, or a combination of two or more blocks in the patient's ECG, a third-degree block may be imminent.

4. Two ways to determine axis exist. The first uses the Rapid Axis and Hemiblock Chart and is used by looking at leads I, II, and III on the ECG. Determine whether the QRS complex is more positively or negatively deflected in each lead. Compare your findings to the Rapid Axis and Hemiblock Chart. If a 12-lead machine is being used and if it provides a calculated axis angle (the number to look for is the R axis or QRS axis), simply use this information. This number represents the exact geometrical axis angle, based on the hexaxial system.

5. A *left-anterior hemiblock* occurs when the anterior hemifascicle of the left bundle branch system becomes blocked, thereby causing (in effect), a pathological left-axis deviation. Other clues to a left-anterior hemiblock are a small Q wave in lead I and a small R wave in lead III. A *left-posterior hemiblock* occurs when the posterior fascicle of the left bundle

branch system is blocked. For practical purposes, in a patient with cardiovascular symptomatology, a right axis deviation is indicative of a left-posterior hemiblock. Other clues include small R waves in lead I and small Q waves in lead III. A *left* or *right bundle branch block* is initially suspected when the QRS is greater than 120 milliseconds and there is evidence of atrial activity (a P wave) preceding the wide QRS. If the terminal force of the QRS is negative in V1 (or a QS complex), then a left bundle branch is interpreted. If the terminal force of the QRS is positive (or a RSR' complex), then a right bundle branch block is interpreted.

6. The clinical significance of a bundle branch block is that it represents an increased risk for developing complete heart block, hemodynamic compromise, and sudden cardiac death when associated with an MI due to the proximal occlusion of the LAD coronary artery. As the ischemic conduction cells within the bundle branches start to fail from LAD occlusion, a bundle branch block develops. Left untreated, the ischemic cells will eventually die and a complete block will occur. New onset of a bundle branch block in a patient suffering a myocardial infarction is correlated with both a higher morbidity rate and mortality rate.

7. A wide complex tachydysrhythmia results essentially from one of two etiologies. Obviously, if a true ectopic site in the ventricles is discharging faster than the normal conduction system (in this sense, a true ventricular tachycardia), the ECG will appear rapid with a wide QRS complex. The other etiology of a wide complex tachycardia is from a supraventricular pacemaker that is discharging at a rate faster than the bundle branches can handle. The atrial tachydysrhythmia accounts for the rapid rate, while the conduction defect in the bundle branches (which may be new or chronic) accounts for the wide and aberrant-looking QRS complex.

8. Specialized ECG leads can be used to more effectively evaluate the right ventricle. Lead V4R looks at the right ventricle. The 15-lead ECG, lead V4R in particular, can be helpful in discovering the presence of RVI. In addition to 15-lead ECG evidence, the following clinical triad of signs and symptoms provides further clues for the condition:
   - Jugular vein distention (JVD)
   - Hypotension, either presenting or following nitroglycerin administration
   - Clear lung sounds

   A right ventricular infarction presents with ST segment elevation in lead V4R. Reciprocal changes are uncommon, owing to the small size of the ventricle and the fact that it is across the septum from a reciprocal lead.

9. Most standard 12-lead machines do not have the extra leads to run the posterior and right ventricular leads. To acquire the 15-lead ECG, follow these steps:
   a. Run the initial 12-lead ECG as usual.
   b. Place an electrode pad on the midclavicular line at the fifth intercostal space on the right side of the patient—the same as V4 on the left side.
   c. On the back, place an electrode pad in the fifth intercostal space, midscapular line—the lead V8 (posterior) position.
   d. Place another electrode between V8 and the spine in the same intercostal space—the lead V9 (posterior) position.
   e. Remove the electrode wires for leads V4, V5, and V6.
   f. Attach the V4 wire to the V4R lead placement.
   g. Attach the V5 wire to the lead V8 placement and the V6 wire to the lead V9 placement.
   h. Run a second 12-lead ECG with the new lead placements.
   i. Label the second 12-lead ECG to reflect the new leads: V4 as V4R, V5 as V8, and V6 as V9.

Chapter 11

Initial Case Study

- *Best initial agent for the induction needed to facilitate intubation.*
  - With rapid-sequence induction (RSI) intubation, the critical care paramedic must consider the possibility of difficult airway management. The administration of etomidate (Amidate) provides sedation without hemodynamic compromise. An acceptable initial dose would be 0.3 mg/kg IVP.
- *Best agent to maintain proper sedation and paralysis for the long transport.*
  - The administration of midazolam (Versed) and vecuronium (Norcuron) would provide the necessary chemical paralysis and sedation for transport. Additional doses of midazolam may be required if the patient becomes hypertensive, tachycardic, or has other hemodynamic changes from agitation and anxiety. An appropriate dose for midazolam could be 0.5 mg/kg IVP, and for vecuronium a dose of 0.1 mg/kg IVP could be used.
- *Best agent to consider for the bilateral wheezing, and if the patient is refractory to this, what else could be considered given the patient's age, history, and physical condition.*
  - The administration of albuterol (Proventil) provides direct beta-2 stimulation to promote bronchiole relaxation. Furthermore, the administration of ipatropium (Atrovent), a parasympatholytic drug that promotes indirect sympathomimetic effects, will enhance the actions of albuterol to promote and prolong bronchodilation without the adverse reactions of providing additional beta agonist stimulation.

Case 1

- *Given the above information, your diagnostic impression is:*
  - With an acute anteroseptal wall MI, hyperacute ST elevation is seen in leads V1–V4 on the 12-lead ECG. The depression found in the inferior leads (II, III and AVF) represents reciprocal changes that sometimes accompanies MIs viewed on the frontal plane (i.e., the "V" leads).
- *The critical care paramedic's next pharmacological intervention would be to administer what agent?*
  - The development of reperfusion ventricular rhythms is common after the administration of fibrinolytics such as reteplase. These events are transient in nature, and normally subside spontaneously as oxygen is restored to ischemic myocardial cells. As such, the administration of any antidysrhythmics may not yet be warranted. If the resulting rhythm remains, consideration of a worsening MI could be assumed.
- *Emergent treatment would include what?*
  - The administration of morphine and furosemide at traditional doses will rapidly decrease preload pressures through vasodilation and diuresis, while intravenous nitro will decrease both preload and afterload. Nesiritide may then be indicated for the acute congestive heart failure unresponsive to normal front-line therapy. Emergent intubation utilizing etomidate and vecuronium is an intervention that may be required if symptoms persist or worsen, but is not an immediate need.

Case 2

- *Based on the above information, which intervention would the critical care paramedic complete first?*
  - Intravenous nitroprusside (Nipride), a fast-acting and potent vasodilator, will allow the critical care paramedic to rapidly control this episode of hypertension. A titrated dose starting at 0.5 mcg/kg/min can be considered.
- *After establishing airway control, the critical care paramedic would administer what hyperosmolar medication?*

- The symptoms are indicative of Cushing's reflex, a sign of increased intracranial pressure. The drastic changes in the physical assessment finding in addition to vitals would lead the critical care paramedic to the belief that the patient may be herniating. The administration of mannitol (Osmitrol) at a dose of 1.5–2 g/kg over 30 minutes may be considered for this emergent treatment of herniation syndrome.
- *The critical care paramedic must then consider the administration of what?*
  - After the administration of vecuronium for long-term paralysis during transport, the critical care paramedic must also administer an analgesic or benzodiazepine to the patient because neuromuscular blockades do not have sedating or analgesic effects.

Chapter 12

1. Usually prior to transport on most interhospital missions, certain diagnostic and laboratory tests will have been conducted by the transferring facility prior to transport. These tests provide valuable information about the patient. Because of this, the critical care paramedic must have a basic understanding of common lab tests routinely encountered during interfacility transfer.

2. After undergoing a certain test or diagnostic procedure, people who are found to have the disease and test positive are called true-positives. People who do not have the disease and test negative are called true-negatives. People who test positive, yet do not have the disease are called false-positives. People test negative, yet have the disease are called false-negatives.

3. The terms *specificity* and *sensitivity* are often used in relation to laboratory testing. The *specificity* of a test is a measure of how well it detects a disease. If a test is 100% specific, it will identify the disease in question in 100% of patients who have the disease. A test with a high specificity has few false-positives. The sensitivity of a test is the degree to which a test detects disease without yielding a false-negative result. No test is 100% sensitive. A test with high sensitivity has few false-negatives.

4. Hemoglobin is the amount of hemoglobin present in blood. Hematocrit is the percentage of RBCs in the plasma. The WBC count represents the number of white blood cells per cubic millimeter of blood. The RBC count is the number of red blood cells per cubic millimeter of blood. MCV is the mean corpuscular volume (size of RBC). MCH represents the mean corpuscular hemoglobin (amount of hemoglobin present in one cell). MCHC is the mean corpuscular hemoglobin concentration (the proportion of each cell occupied by hemoglobin). RDW is the red blood cell distribution width (calculated from the MCV and RBC).

5. The basic metabolic panel (BMP) is an assessment of various electrolytes and various kidney indicators. The substances commonly assayed in the basic metabolic panel are sodium, potassium, chloride, bicarbonate, glucose, blood urea nitrogen, and creatinine.

6. The measurement of enzymes and markers associated with cardiac disease is an important aspect of medical practice—especially emergency medicine and critical care transport. Numerous tests and findings can be used to help diagnose and classify cardiac disease. The enzymatic and cardiac markers assessed include *creatine kinase (CK or CPK)*, *lactic dehydrogenase (LD or LDH), myoglobin, troponin I, T, and C,* and *B-natriuretic peptide (BNP).*

Chapter 13

1. The American College of Surgeons' Committee on Trauma publishes guidelines and provides accreditation of regional trauma centers, as do most states. Numerous components

must be considered when developing a regional trauma system, one of the central ideas being that enough serious trauma cases must be available to as to maintain a high level of expertise among the specialists at the receiving trauma centers. These components include (and are required of designated Level I trauma centers) the ability to offer comprehensive trauma care (from initial evaluation to rehabilitation), to manage any type of trauma patient, to offer many specialized services such as burn, neurologic, and cardiovascular surgical subspecialties, and to maintain a predetermined number of available operating rooms, resuscitation areas, and ICU beds. They should also remain active in planning and research.

2. In the United States, trauma is the leading cause of death for all persons under the age of 44, and is the fifth leading cause of death in all ages. Each year trauma kills more people than AIDS, cancer, or heart disease. Trauma is the leading cause of death in children in the United States. In a typical year, approximately 150,000 Americans die from trauma. In the United States, more than 400 people—50 of whom are children—die of an injury every day. Approximately 90,000 of these deaths annually are due to unintentional injury, with the rest resulting from violence.

3. Organized trauma systems can contribute to a reduction in trauma-related mortality and morbidity along a number of lines. First and foremost is participation in trauma reduction strategies, commonly referred to as prevention methods (for example, participating in educational programs designed to improve seat belt usage, or safety device utilization with dangerous jobs or sports). Beyond the prevention strategies, the trauma system can be optimally prepared for the traumatic event by having well-integrated trauma identification, organized EMS providers, carefully defined trauma treatment protocols, and transport destination criteria.

4. The original Trauma Score (TS) included four physiological parameters and ranged from 1 to 16 points. Patients with a score of 12 or less were deemed to be seriously injured and required specialized trauma care. The TS was revised in 1989 and became the Revised Trauma Score (RTS). The range of the RTS is 0 to 12. Patients with a score of 11 or less are deemed to require specialized trauma care. For pediatrics, the Pediatric Trauma Score (PTS) is a version of the trauma score that is extensively modified to take into account the different physiological considerations that pediatrics possess as compared to adults. The Abbreviated Injury Scale (AIS) is a severity scale that was developed jointly by the American Medical Association, the American Association for Automotive Medicine, and the Society of Automotive Engineers in order to collect detailed data on the types and severity of injuries suffered by victims of motor vehicle crashes. The Trauma Score, Injury Severity Score, Age Combination Index (TRISS) method combines the physiological measurements of the RTS with the anatomical components of the ISS, along with the patient's age, to attempt to provide a comprehensive and accurate indication of the overall severity and survivability of a given patient's injuries. The TRISS score is used primarily by trauma registries and is impractical for clinical use.

5. A Level I trauma center offers comprehensive trauma care, from initial evaluation (and often transport) to rehabilitation. Such a center can manage any type of patient and offers many specialized services, such as burn, neurological, and cardiovascular surgical subspecialists. A Level II trauma center can appropriately manage most seriously injured patients, but lacks some surgical subspecialties. They also may not focus as much on research and education as a Level I, but still must adhere to rigorous staff educational and credentialing requirements.

6. Courses such as prehospital trauma life support and basic trauma life support teach a systematic framework for the approach and management of the trauma patient in the prehospital setting. Regardless of the course or reference, the priorities for management of the trauma patient in the critical care setting are universal and clear. They include:

a. Safety of the rescuer(s)
b. Safety of the victim(s)
c. Management of airway and/or respiratory system compromise
d. Management of life-threatening hemorrhage
e. Protection/prevention of actual or potential spinal cord injury
f. Rapid transport to an appropriate facility
g. Maintenance of body temperature
h. Consideration for pain control

7. The primary difference between the critical care paramedic and the "street" paramedic is that the critical care paramedic specializes in the interfacility transport of critical patients who require therapies or interventions not usually implemented or performed in the field. The management priorities when transporting a trauma patient from a referring facility are identical to those when transporting from a prehospital scene, however, in most cases immediately life-threatening injuries have been managed or controlled by the time the critical care paramedic has arrived to transport the patient to the next level of care.

8. First, the critical care paramedic must report on the patient; the transporting crew must understand the mechanism of injury, what the suspected or known injuries are, and what has been done to manage the patient thus far. The next task is to perform a patient assessment that focuses on ensuring that all critical elements of patient management and preparation have been performed (such as appropriate ETT placement and appropriate intravenous access), that appropriate medications or blood products are available during transport, that the patient is properly immobilized if indicated, and so on. Just as in the prehospital setting, a judgment must be made as to whether to perform interventions before or during transport. After the critical interventions have been confirmed, the patient is placed on the transport equipment and medications are switched to the transport IV. Finally, the patient is moved to the transport stretcher and then to the transport vehicle. The patient is, of course, closely monitored throughout the transport, and managed per the designated plan of care.

Chapter 14

1. The clinical signs of brain death include the absence of corneal, cough, gag, oculocephalic, and oculovestibular reflexes. There must be no purposeful motor response to pain anywhere on the body, and no reflexive motor response in the facial muscles. The pupils will be nonreactive to light. Patients must also be apneic. Brain death testing can be supported by other diagnostic tools; however, clinical declaration should only be done when pharmacologic and metabolic causes of brain death signs can be absolutely ruled out.

2. Cerebral perfusion pressure (CPP) is a measure of the efficacy of cellular perfusion within the brain. It is determined by subtracting the intracranial pressure from the mean arterial pressure: $CPP = MAP - ICP$. If there is a drop in the mean arterial pressure, or an excessive increase in the pressure within the cranial vault, cerebral perfusion pressure will suffer and brain injury may occur (or worsen).

3. Autoregulation refers to the ability of cerebral vasculature to control its own vascular tone to maintain a normal perfusion status in the brain given changes in MAP or ICP. Cerebral autoregulation is most effective in the presence of CPP values ranging from 60 to 160 mmHg.

4. Increases in the partial pressure of serum carbon dioxide ($PaCO_2$) will cause the vasodilation of cerebral vasculature. This causes increased cerebral blood flow and therefore increased intracranial pressure. Hypocapnia results in vasoconstriction, which causes a

decrease in ICP, but creates the potential for ischemia. The ideal $PaCO_2$ for patients with significantly elevated ICP and poor compliance is 30 to 35 mmHg.

5. Cytoxic cerebral edema occurs when histopathologic changes result in the accumulation of edema within the cells of the brain. This pattern is generally seen as the result of global injury, such as from hypoxia and anoxic injury, or metabolic injury. The end result is diminishment in cerebral perfusion pressure as intracranial pressure rises.

6. Vasogenic cerebral edema is interstitial edema that forms subsequent to changes in vascular wall permeability, such as in the presence of tumors or similar localized lesions. In essence, the cause of vasogenic edema is direct tissue damage. Like cytotoxic edema, however, the end result is cellular dysfunction from ICP changes and direct nerve damage.

7. The Monroe-Kellie hypothesis (or doctrine) states that, because the cranium is a nondistensible fixed space, an increase in the volume of any of the three substances that occupy it (blood, brain tissue, and CSF), will cause an increase in ICP if a compensatory reduction of one or both of the other substances does not also occur.

8. Normal ICP ranges from 0 to 10 mmHg. ICP levels from 10 to 20 are considered elevated, and ICP > 20 mmHg is dangerously elevated. ICP that is sustained > 40 mmHg for any significant length of time is associated with a tremendous increase in mortality and morbidity.

9. The external auditory meatus (EAM) landmarks the level of the lateral ventricles within the brain, and is used as the leveling point for extraventricular drains. This is necessary information while preparing your head-injured patient for transport, should he have a drain placed.

10. In the normal brain, P1 should be the tallest component of the ICP waveform. Elevations of P2 and other components above P1 are reflective of poor cerebral compliance. Additional clinical symptomatology will help identify the significance of pressure changes as the neurologic status of the patient deteriorates.

11. The stopcock connecting the catheter from an EVD to its collection system must be turned off to the collection system in order to accurately measure an ICP.

12. The stopcock must always be turned off to the collection system to prevent excessive drainage of CSF when moving a patient. Always ensure that the EVD is returned to its prescribed level before reopening the stopcock to allow drainage.

13. Hypotonic IV fluids and admixture diluents such as D_5W and D_5W with 0.45% NS are readily absorbed as free water by edematous brain tissue, and can thus cause worsening of cerebral edema and worsen the perfusion of blood through the edematous brain.

14. Neurogenic shock typically occurs in the presence of spinal cord injury at the level of the sixth thoracic vertebra (T-6) or higher. At this level, a significant amount of sympathetic nerve tone will be lost.

15. The most common cause of autonomic dysreflexia in patients with spinal cord injury is a noxious stimulant such as a distended bladder or fecal impaction. Cutaneous stimuli may also cause autonomic dysreflexia. The result is a dramatic increase in sympathetic tone to still functioning sympathetic innervated tissue, which then causes a severe hypertensive crisis. Bradycardia, as well as peripheral vasodilation and diaphoresis above the level of the lesion, may also occur.

Chapter 15

1. The most common types of thoracic trauma that will likely be seen by the critical care paramedic include motor vehicle crashes (MVCs), falls, sports injuries, crush injuries,

stab wounds, and gunshot wounds. By understanding the severity of the injury, the MOI, management concerns of specific thoracic injuries, and the unique challenges associated with transporting these patients (especially in the air), the critical care paramedic can anticipate potential complications and be ready to manage them promptly.

2. Multiple processes are involved in the act of breathing, all of which can be altered by thoracic trauma. These processes include the mechanics of ventilation and the neurochemical control of respiration. With chest trauma, any structure or organ within the thoracic cavity may be injured. Tissue hypoxia results from inadequate delivery of oxygenated blood to the tissue cells. This can result from hypoperfusion (typically hypovolemia) or decreased oxygenation of the red blood cells (RBCs) (such as occurs with ventilation/perfusion mismatch caused by pulmonary contusions, hematomas, or alveolar collapse). Hypercarbia results from decreased ventilation, which is typically a result of changes in intrathoracic pressure relationships and/or depressed levels of consciousness. Acidosis (typically metabolic) is secondary to the anaerobic metabolism created by the inadequately oxygenated cells (hypoperfusion).

3. This condition is characterized by progressive air accumulation under pressure, within the pleural space of the injured lung. As the injury progresses in severity, ventilation is severely compromised due to the increases in intrapleural pressure with each breath, causing ipsilateral lung collapse and a mediastinal shift to the opposite side, leading to compression of the contralateral lung. Perfusion becomes inadequate because of decreased venous return to the heart as a result of the increased pressure and mediastinal shifting of the thoracic structures. Emergent treatment for this condition is thoracic decompression, which is accomplished by inserting a large-bore catheter into the thoracic wall on the side of initial lung injury, to relieve the air pressure and allow the lung to reinflate.

4. Injuries to intrathoracic organs or lacerations to major vessels will cause rapid accumulation of blood and fluid in the pleural cavity, which can result in severe respiratory and hemodynamic compromise. Hypovolemic shock may also be present because the uninjured lung can offer little or no resistance to a large amount of blood accumulating in the pleural space. Emergency treatment by the critical care paramedic includes the administration of high-flow oxygen, possible endotracheal intubation, and tube thoracotomy. Additional treatment commonly consists of administering fluids to maintain adequate perfusion until the source of bleeding can be controlled.

5. By definition a flail chest is three or more ribs broken in two or more places. A flail chest is usually a result of blunt trauma, such as MVCs or falls, and typically involves either anterior or lateral ribs. (Posterior ribs have more protection from muscles and the scapula.) The resulting hypoventilation, hypoxemia, and respiratory acidosis is best treated by immediately stabilizing the flailed segment, administering high-flow oxygen, supporting inadequate breathing with positive-pressure ventilation if present, and ensuring peripheral perfusion is maintained. CPAP may be considered for the spontaneously breathing patient with a flail segment as well.

6. Beck's triad is a collection of three clinical findings that, when present with a suggestive MOI, indicate the patient may be suffering from pericardial tamponade. The symptoms include jugular venous distention (JVD), diminished or muffled heart sounds, and a decreased blood pressure.

7. Pericardial tamponade is a condition caused by the accumulation of blood in the pericardial space between the pericardial sac and the heart itself. While a rapid accumulation of 150–200 mL may be fatal, the slow accumulation of up to 2 liters of blood or fluid may occur without significant hemodynamic compromise. Management for this emergency includes ensuring the patient's airway and providing for oxygenation and ventilation. The next most important intervention is the rapid administration of volume to improve filling pressures. This will in turn improve, although temporarily, cardiac output until a

more definitive intervention can be made (i.e., pericardiocentesis). A pericardiocentesis is a procedure in which a needle is placed into the pericardial sac and blood or fluid is withdrawn. A significant improvement in the patient's condition may be seen with removal of as little as 20 mL of blood.

8. While the following injuries may not be initially life threatening to the patient, they may progress in severity and contribute to continuous deterioration in the patient's overall condition. Some of the common, yet less severe, injuries in this class include myocardial contusion, pulmonary contusion, tracheobronchial disruption, and esophageal perforation.

9. In your work as a critical care paramedic you will commonly encounter chest tubes in your postsurgical and chest trauma patients. Management of the chest tube includes ensuring that it is not displaced from the thoracic insertion point, that suction and the drainage system remain intact, and that the chest tube itself remains free from obstructions. The critical care paramedic should be aware that the amount of suction applied to the chest tube is determined by the water level in the suction chamber and not the amount of suction applied by the suction unit. The goal is to maintain a minimal amount of bubbling.

Chapter 16

1. If the critical care provider's patient has a liver injury that is described as a laceration that extends 3 cm into the renal parenchyma, is 6 cm in length, and is bleeding actively, it would be categorized as a Grade I or II injury. These injuries account for 70% to 80% of all liver injuries, and carry with them roughly a 10% mortality rate.

2. A urinalysis would be warranted after identifying that the serum urea is disproportionately higher than the creatinine level. The injury suspected with the lower abdominal pain and lab values as described are consistent with traumatic rupture of the urinary bladder. The urinalysis will determine if there is blood in the urine, which is suggestive of GU insult.

3. Injury to the lower right rib cage should raise the index of suspicion for hepatic injury. Given the proximity of the liver to the inferior aspect of the right costal margin, blunt and penetrating trauma to this region can easily cause additional trauma to the liver.

4. During a FAST exam, placement of the transducer to allow a sagittal view of the abdomen from the right midaxillary line between the 11th and 12th rib is needed to evaluate the hepatorenal space, or Morrison's pouch, for blood.

5. The recent trend in volume resuscitation suggests that critical care providers should avoid the blind administration of crystalloid solutions in large volumes (that was the old standard of care for hypotensive trauma patients). Instead, the critical care paramedic should endeavor to achieve a blood pressure of about three-quarters the patient's normal blood pressure. This can be achieved by calculating a 20 mL/kg bolus amount, and then infusing 250 mL of fluid rapidly followed by hemodynamic reassessment. The goal is to achieve a blood pressure of 75–80 mmHg systolic. It has been fairly well established that this practice of "permissive hypotension" results in less bleeding in patients with uncontrolled hemorrhage, while still maintaining an acceptable perfusion pressure to the heart, lungs, brain, and kidneys.

6. A retrograde cystogram can be useful in the diagnosis of urethral or bladder injury. In this study approximately 300–500 mL of contrast media is infused into the urethra and serial radiographs performed. Any extravasation of contrast from the urethra or bladder indicates perforation. Evaluation of the urine for blood is required in trauma patients to assess for hematuria secondary to GU insult. Determination of gross blood can be made clinically by direct observation of the urine after catheterization. Urine reagent strips are useful for a rapid assessment of the urine.

1. The first statement is true. Injuries to Zone I are associated with high mortality because they can involve the great vascular structures of the chest, the inferior larynx, and trachea, as well as intrathoracic structures such as the lungs. The second statement is also true because Zone II injuries commonly involve the carotid arteries and airway structures and are readily identifiable (owing to the exposed nature of this area of the neck). The third statement is false and the fourth statement is true based on the fact that Zone III injuries often involve the internal and external carotid arteries, the vertebral artery, and the cranial nerves.

2. The concern with neck and facial trauma is the associated loss of function that can cause rapid deterioration and death of the patient. Airway trauma may result in either an occluded airway or impaired ventilations, and neck injuries can bleed heavily or impinge on the airway. Proper care of the patient with blunt or penetrating face or neck trauma can prove to be extremely challenging for the critical care paramedic. Seemingly benign injuries can quickly turn life threatening, and delayed or inappropriate treatment can easily result in disability or death.

3. Avulsed but intact teeth can be reinserted within 20 minutes of removal into their sockets as long as there are no serious injuries that would demand the critical care paramedic's attention. Care should be taken to handle the tooth by the crown and avoid injuring the root or periodontal fibers. The tooth and socket should both be rinsed clean with Hank's solution if available. If rinsing the avulsed tooth is warranted, rinsing of the socket to remove dirt and clots should be performed gently, with as little manipulation as possible. The tooth should be properly aligned after reinsertion, comparing it to the surrounding dentition. If able, the patient should be instructed to bite down on a roll of gauze for a minimum of 20 minutes.

4. The first statement is false because a Le Forte I maxillary fracture is a transverse fracture just superior to the apices of the teeth, through the maxillary sinus and across the nasal septum. The second statement is false because a Le Forte III maxillary fracture includes the zygomatic arches, frontozygomatic suture, sphenoid bone, and nasal bone. This would allow for movement of the facial structures, including the eyes, when manipulated. The third statement is also false since a Le Forte II fracture does not involve the full facial skeleton, hence no movement of the eyes with manipulation. Finally, the final statement is also false because the description of the fracture is more in line with a La Forte III, rather than a La Forte II, injury.

5. With penetrating neck trauma, injury to the paired phrenic nerves will cause some degree of disturbance to the diaphragm since this is the nerve that carries efferent messages from the brain. While isolated injury to one of the paired phrenic nerves can cause a marked insult to normal respiration, insult to both phrenic nerves (however unlikely) would result in paralysis of the diaphragm.

6. Unless it interferes with airway control, any object impaled in the neck should be immobilized in place. If it is impossible to either obtain or maintain an open airway due to the penetration of a foreign object into the neck, the only option is to remove it in order to secure the airway, and then provide appropriate soft-tissue and hemorrhage control techniques.

7. An occlusive dressing would be used in the neck-injured patient if the mechanism of injury caused an open soft-tissue wound to a major blood vessel. The concern with a laceration to one of the large jugular veins is the possible entrainment of air that could result in embolization once the air reaches the myocardium. If it is difficult to ascertain whether an artery or large vein was injured, the application of an occlusive dressing to the injury is a good precautionary idea.

8. Direct injury to nerves located outside of the spinal cord is the most common etiology of neurologic deficits secondary to neck trauma. Of particular concern are injuries to the

recurrent laryngeal nerves. The paired recurrent laryngeal nerves provide innervation, allowing for opening of the vocal cords. Insult results in vocal cord paralysis and airway obstruction secondary to a closed glottic opening.

9. With severe facial trauma, the critical care paramedic must maintain a high degree of suspicion that the basilar skull may also be fractured. In that case, the insertion of either an NPA or NG tube may result in additional injury should the tube advance through the basilar fracture and into the base of the brain. Although an extremely rare occurrence, cases of this happening have been documented, and should serve as a warning to other critical care providers.

Chapter 18

1. Burn injuries in the United States and other developed countries have been steadily declining for several decades, but burns still rank as the fourth leading cause of trauma deaths of all age groups, and is the second leading cause of death in children under the age of 12 years. Each year, in the United States, an estimated 1.25 to 2 million Americans are treated for burns and 50,000 are hospitalized. Approximately 3% to 5% of these burns are considered life threatening. Persons at greatest risk for serious burns include the very young, the elderly, and the infirm. This group makes up the majority of the injured and its members are approximately five times more likely to die from burns than members of other groups.

2. Thermal burns cause a number of effects that are collectively referred to as Jackson's theory of thermal wounds. When a burn occurs, the central area of the burn wound, that is, the skin nearest the heat source, typically suffers the most profound effect or changes. This most damaged area is called the *zone of coagulation*. Extending peripherally from the zone of coagulation is a labile area of injured cells with decreased blood flow, which under ideal circumstances may survive, but which more often than not undergo necrosis in the ensuing 24–48 hours post-burn. This zone is called the *zone of stasis*. Lying farther peripherally is an area where inflammation and changes in blood flow are limited. This area will typically recover in 7–10 days post-burn. This area is called the *zone of hyperemia*.

3. The most critical component of the initial assessment regarding burn patients is the airway assessment. Given the mechanism of the burn, the patient may inhale superheated gases or steam or be subjected to direct burning to the face and airway. The resulting injury can cause rapidly developing laryngeal edema with complete airway obstruction if management is not efficient nor appropriate.

4. When determining total body surface area affected by a burn, the critical care paramedic can use one of several measures. The first is called the "rule of nines" and is based on the fact that in the adult body each anatomical region represents approximately 9%, or a multiple thereof, of the total body surface area (TBSA). Another method that works particularly well with scattered burns is called the "rule of palms" or "walking out the burn." This method is based on the fact that the size of the patient's palm represents approximately 1% of the patient's TBSA. The last method, which is the "Lund and Browder method," is more commonly used in the hospital. This method is difficult to use in the critical care environment because it takes more time to calculate, but this method is the most accurate, especially in infants and children, because it allows for developmental changes in percentage of TBSA.

5. The Parkland formula calculation for a 101-kg burn patient with 65% TBSA burned is as follows: *Parkland formula = 4 milliliters × kg weight × TBSA*. Half of the volume is to be given during the first 8 hours post-burn, with the remaining half of the volume to be given during the next 16 hours.

i. 4 mL × 101 kg × 65% = 26,260 mL of fluid

ii. 13,130 mL to be given during first 8 hours

iii. 13,130 mL to be given during next 16 hours

6. The critical care paramedic must be aware that typical signs/symptoms such as severe bronchospasms may occur in the first minutes to hours post-burn, and the severity of the overall inhalation injury and the amount of damage done to the underlying respiratory structures are clinically unpredictable in the first few hours post-burn. Thus, the patient who presents with possible inhalation injury should be closely observed for signs/symptoms of complications for at least 24 hours. Routine treatment during this time includes high-flow oxygen, pulse oximetry, capnography, cardiac monitoring, intravenous therapy, and elective intubation should the glottis become edematous and occlude the airway.

7. The effects of carbon monoxide inhalation to the burn patient may be subtle, but can still be deadly. It is not uncommon to find carboxyhemoglobin levels of 50% to 70% or more. Carboxyhemoglobin levels should be checked, whenever possible, especially in those patients who present with respiratory complaints and those with altered mental status. Since carbon monoxide will displace oxygen off of hemoglobin, dysfunction of hypoxia-sensitive organs (such as the brain) may cause coma, seizures, and death.

8. The care for electrical burn injuries includes the potential management of cardiac arrest, muscle compartment syndrome, and hemochromogens in the urine. Treatment guidelines according to the type of injury include:

- *Cardiac arrest.* Treatment should follow the standard guidelines outlined in the advanced cardiac life support course.
- *Muscle compartment syndrome.* If signs of muscle compartment syndrome are present, consider performing either an escharotomy or fasciotomy.
- *Hemochromogens.* This is the presence of rhabdomyolsis in the urine and serves as an indication of significant damage to underlying muscles. In these cases the urine output must be maintained between 75 and 100 mL/hr to ensure clearing of the kidneys. Fluid resuscitation should be titrated to facilitate this amount of urine output. Also, sodium bicarbonate (44 mEq in each liter of RL) should be administered until the pH of the urine is >6.0. Finally, mannitol may be given if hemochromogens are seen in the urine.

9. Treatment for chemical burn injuries differs somewhat from other burns because you must take extra precautions to protect yourself and others from chemical exposure. Although this may prolong the time interval to start patient treatment, you cannot help anyone if you become a victim. Prior to initiating treatment, care must be taken to remove as much of the chemical as possible. This means brushing off any powder agents, removing all contaminated clothing, and then beginning copious irrigation.

10. The injury or damage caused by exposure to nuclear radiation is called *ionization*. Injury is caused when radioactive energy particles travel into a substance and change an internal atom. In the body, for instance, one of three things happens in the cell: It either repairs the damage, dies, or produces damaged cells (cancer). There are cells within the human body that are more susceptible to radiation than others. Typically these are the cells that reproduce quickly, such as those responsible for red blood cells (erythrocyte) and white blood cells (leukocyte and platelet production). Also susceptible are cells that line the intestinal tract and those involved in reproduction.

11. According to the American Burn Association the following burn injuries should be referred to a burn center:

- Partial-thickness burns greater than 10% TBSA
- Any burns involving the face, hands, feet, genitalia, perineum, or major joints

- Full-thickness burns in any age group
- Any electrical burns, including lightning injuries
- Any chemical or inhalation burns
- Any burn patient who has some preexisting condition that may complicate management, prolong recovery, or affect mortality
- Any patient who has sustained concomitant significant trauma
- Burned pediatric patients in hospitals without qualified personnel or equipment to care for the child
- Burn injury in patients who will require special social, emotional, and/or long-term rehabilitative intervention

Chapter 19

1. In 2000, 1.6 million geriatrics were treated in emergency departments for fall-related injuries and 353,000 were hospitalized. Of those who fall, 20% to 30% suffer moderate to severe injuries such as hip fractures or head traumas that reduce mobility and independence, and increase the risk of premature death. Approximately 3% to 5% of older adult falls cause fractures. Based on the 2000 census, this translates to 360,000 to 480,000 fall-related fractures each year. The most common fractures are of the vertebrae, hip, forearm, leg, ankle, pelvis, upper arm, and hand. The total cost of all fall injuries for people age 65 or older in 1994 was $20.2 billion. By 2020, the cost of fall injuries is expected to reach $32.4 billion. Each year in the United States, emergency departments treat more than 200,000 children ages 14 and younger for playground-related injuries. About 45% of playground-related injuries are severe—fractures, internal injuries, concussions, dislocations, and amputations.

2. There are numerous descriptions for fractures. These include the open fracture in which the fractured bone is protruding through the skin, the closed fracture in which the fractured bone does not break the skin, the complete fracture in which the bone is broken completely through all layers, an incomplete fracture in which the fracture line does not extend through the entire bone, a displaced fracture in which the broken ends of the bone are no longer aligned, a greenstick fracture in which part of the bone is broken along the length of one side, a comminuted fracture in which the bone is fragmented into several small parts, a segmental fracture in which two complete fractures of the same bone cause a segment to be free floating, a butterfly fracture in which a small portion of the bone breaks free (but there is no complete fracture), and a spiral fracture in which the fracture line extends circumferentially around the bone. A hairline fracture is a minute fracture that is often difficult to see on a radiograph.

3. Further descriptive grading systems can be applied to open and closed fractures. Closed fractures are typically graded using the Tscherne method:

Grade 0	Negligible soft-tissue injury
Grade 1	Abrasions or contusions (superficial) over the site of the fracture
Grade 2	Significant muscle contusion, contaminated abrasions
Grade 3	Severe soft-tissue injury, including degloving, crush injury, or vascular damage

Open fractures are classified using the Gustilo grading system:

Type I	Small and clean wound (<1 cm), minimal muscle injury, no stripping of periosteum
Type II	Larger open wound (> 1 cm), no significant soft-tissue damage; minimal, if any, periosteum damage
Type III	Larger open wounds; extensive muscle and soft-tissue damage; subdivided into three types (a, b, and c)
Type IIIa	Extensive contamination of underlying soft tissue; still enough soft tissue to cover bone and vasculature
Type IIIb	Extensive muscle and soft-tissue damage; will require muscle transfer; major contamination
Type IIIc	Open injury with vascular damage that requires surgical repair

4. In children, the bone growth plate is still active. Fractures involving the growth plate can result in various growth abnormalities. The cartilaginous epiphyseal plate, also called the physis, is readily injured in that it is weaker than ossified bone or ligaments. Damage to the epiphyscal plate during a child's growth may destroy all or part of the bone's ability to produce new bone. The potential for a growth disturbance from a growth-plate injury is related to the number of years the child has to grow. Thus, the older the child, the less time remaining for a deformity to develop.

5. The *Salter-Harris* system is often used to classify growth-plate injuries. The potential for growth disturbances increases as the classification number increases. The prognosis is best for Type 1 fractures and worst for Type 5 fractures.

6. The general treatment modalities of orthopedic injuries is, at the fundamental level, very straightforward. The goal is simply to place the bone into proper alignment, keep it in place, and let it heal. The manner in which the orthopedic surgeon elects to accomplish this goal will vary greatly, depending on the nature of the injury and the capability of the hospital. With the exception of pelvic fractures, most orthopedic injuries can be stabilized with one of several methods: splinting, casting, external fixation, internal fixation, or amputation.

7. Most fractures are not a major concern for a critical patient. While they do need to be addressed in the course of the treatment plan, definitive care can be delayed, often for 24 hours or more. A few fractures, however, require immediate management to prevent hemodynamic instability, specifically, pelvic fractures, femur fractures, spinal fractures, humerus fractures, and certain rib fractures. These bones can be the source of life-threatening hemorrhage, permanent neurologic damage, or pulmonary injury.

8. During the course of treating an orthopedic injury or disease, various pharmacological agents are used for the treatment of pain, inflammation, infection, and thrombus. The

critical care paramedic should have a working knowledge of the properties of these medications, including indications, contraindications, pharmacokinetics, pharmacodynamics, side effects, and dosing. Generally, the medications used will fall into one of several categories: nonsteroidal anti-inflammatory drugs (NSAIDs), opiate analgesics, antibiotics, muscle relaxants, or anticoagulants.

Chapter 20

1. Injuries are the leading cause of death and disabilities in children and adolescents older than 1 year. According to the National Pediatric Trauma Registry (NPTR), trauma kills more children than all other diseases combined. Annually in children and adolescents, trauma is responsible for approximately 25,000 deaths, more than 500,000 hospitalizations, and 16 million emergency department visits, at a cost of more than $7.5 billion. More than 30,000 children will have permanent disabilities because of injuries to the brain. Blunt trauma accounts for approximately 85% of all injuries.

2. The approach to the pediatric patient varies with the age of the patient and with the problem being treated. Foremost in approaching any pediatric emergency is consideration of the patient's emotional and physiological development. Care also involves the family members or caregivers responsible for the child. They will demand information, express fears, and, ultimately, give or refuse consent for treatment and/or transport.

3. Children progress through developmental stages on their way to adulthood. The critical care paramedic should tailor her approach to the developmental level of the pediatric patient, as briefly discussed:

   - *Neonates (ages birth to 1 month):* The child should always be kept warm. Observe skin color, tone, and respiratory activity. The lungs should be auscultated early during the exam, while the infant is quiet. You might find it helpful to have the child suck on a pacifier during the examination. Allowing the infant to remain in a parent's or caregiver's lap may help keep the child calm.
   - *Infants (ages 1 to 5 months):* The infant's personality at this stage still centers closely on the parents or caregivers. The history must be obtained from these individuals, with close attention to possible illnesses and accidents, including SIDS, vomiting, dehydration, meningitis, child abuse, and household accidents. Concentrate on keeping these patients warm and comfortable. Allow the infant to remain in the parent's or caregiver's lap. A pacifier or bottle can be used to help keep the baby quiet during the examination.
   - *Infants (ages 6 to 12 months):* These children should be examined while sitting in the lap of the parent or caregiver. The exam should progress in a toe-to-head order, since starting at the face may upset the child. If time and conditions permit, allow the child to become familiar with you before beginning the examination.
   - *Toddlers (ages 1 to 3 years):* Be cautious when treating toddlers. Approach toddlers slowly and try to gain their confidence. Conduct the exam in a toe-to-head order. The child may be difficult to examine and may resist being touched. Speak quietly and use only simple words. Avoid asking questions that allow the child to say "no." If the situation permits, allow toddlers to hold transitional objects such as a favorite blanket or toy. Be sure to tell the child if something will hurt. If possible, avoid procedures on the dominant arm and hand, which the child will try to pull away.
   - *Preschoolers (ages 3 to 5 years):* when evaluating children in this age group, question the child first, keeping in mind that imagination may interfere with the facts. The child often has a distorted sense of time, and thus you must rely on the parents or caregivers to fill in the gaps. If time and situation permit, give the child health care choices. Often the use of a doll or stuffed animal will assist in the examination. Allow the child to hold a piece of equipment, such as a stethoscope, and to use it. Let the child sit on your lap.

Start the examination with the chest and evaluate the head last. Avoid misleading comments. Do not trick or lie to the child, and always explain what you are going to do.

- *School-age children (ages 6–12 years):* When examining school-age children, give them the responsibility of providing the history, if possible. However, remember that children may be reluctant to provide information if they sustained an injury while doing something forbidden. The parents or caregivers can fill in the pertinent details. When assessing children in this age group, it is important to respect their modesty. Be honest and tell the child what is wrong. A small toy may help to calm the child.

- *Adolescents (ages 13–18 years):* Adolescents vary significantly in their development. Regardless of physical maturity, remember that teenagers as a group are "body conscious." You should tactfully address their stated concerns about body integrity or disfigurement. They may take offense at the use of the word "child." They have a strong desire to be liked by their peers and to be included. Relationships with parents and caregivers may at times be strained as the adolescent demands greater independence. They value the opinions of other adolescents, especially members of the opposite sex. Generally, these patients make good historians. Do not be surprised, however, if their perception of events differs from that of their parents or caregivers. In gathering a history, be factual and address the patient's questions. It may be wise to interview the patient away from the parents or caregivers. Listen to what the teenager is saying, as well as what he or she is not saying. If you must perform a detailed physical exam, respect the teenager's sense of privacy. If the patient exhibits modesty or bodily shame, try to have a paramedic of the same sex as the teenager conduct the examination. Regardless of the situation, provide psychological support and reassurance.

4. There has been a significant change in the way pediatric trauma is definitively managed. Formerly, most children who sustained serious trauma received an exploratory operation. Today, however, with the significant advances in diagnostic imaging (CT scanning, ultrasound, magnetic resonance imaging), it is easy to detect internal injuries without an exploratory operation. In addition, we have found that children are amazingly resilient and most injuries will heal without operative intervention. The changes in pediatric trauma care during the last decade have been remarkable and pediatric trauma mortality rates continue to improve.

5. In using the Glasgow Coma Scale with pediatric patients, you will have to make certain modifications. Verbal responses, for example, will not be possible for neonates and infants. However, motor function may be assessed in very young children by observing voluntary movement. Infants under 4 months of age should have a grasp reflex when an object is placed on the palmar surface of their hand. The grasp should be immediate. Children older than 3 years of age will follow directions, when encouraged. Sensory function can be observed by the withdrawal reaction from "tickling" the patient. After you score the GCS for the patient, prioritize the patient according to severity:

- *Mild*—GCS 13 to 15
- *Moderate*—GCS 9 to 12
- *Severe*—GCS less than or equal to 8

6. When possible, use an objective measure, such as the Pediatric Trauma Score, to evaluate the patient objectively when traumatized. The scoring system uses several determinates to assess the status of the patient. The scores that can be applied range from +2 to −1 (as the given parameter worsens). The trauma score assesses the patient's weight, airway status, blood pressure, level of consciousness, open wound findings, and presence of fractures to compute the overall score.

7. Many times, geriatric patients may display a decrease in mental status. This makes assessment and management more difficult. Senility and organic brain syndrome may manifest themselves similarly. The priorities of care, however, for the elderly trauma

patient are similar to those for any trauma patient. While keeping in mind age-related systemic changes and the presence of chronic diseases, treat any alteration in mental status as an acute change if evidence to the contrary is not present. As such, ensure patency of the airway, provide for adequate ventilations, and support the hemodynamic status of the patient.

8. First and foremost the traumatized female needs airway, breathing, and circulatory support if any of these functions are lost. She is equally in need of appropriate spinal immobilization and rapid transport to a trauma center. During this transport, the pregnant patient should be placed in a supine position unless she is hypotensive. If so, tilt or rotate the patient 20–30 degrees to the left. Manually displace the uterus to the left side during transport, especially in the 7-month or later gestation. Venous return to the maternal heart may be decreased up to 30% because of uterine compression by the fetus.

Chapter 21

1. Acute respiratory failure (ARF) can be defined as a state of inadequate gas exchange, and it occurs when the respiratory system is unable to absorb oxygen and/or excrete carbon dioxide. While ARF can be suspected based on purely clinical findings, the best method of diagnosing ARF is arterial blood gas (ABG) analysis. While no rigid criteria exist, it is generally accepted that ARF exists when the arterial oxygenation level (PaO_2) is less than 60 mmHg and the level of arterial carbon dioxide ($PaCO_2$) is greater than 50 mmHg, with an arterial pH of less than 7.30 on room air.

2. ARF can be categorized as a failure of oxygenation resulting in hypoxemia, a failure of ventilation resulting in high levels of arterial carbon dioxide (hypercapnia), or a combination of both. Oxygenation failure resulting in hypoxemia has six generally accepted mechanisms: hypoventilation, ventilation perfusion mismatch, intrapulmonary shunting, cardiogenic shock, diffusion defects, and low FiO_2. Common mechanisms for ventilatory failure inducing ARF include CNS depression, brainstem injury, depressant drug overdose, and neuromuscular disorders.

3. Oxygenation failure occurs when the inspired or delivered oxygen makes it to the alveoli, but is unable to cross the alveolar-capillary membrane to oxygenate the blood. As such, with this type of etiology for acute respiratory failure, the critical care paramedic needs to consider whether the patient is receiving (or is displaying) an adequate tidal volume with alveolar aeration but has a low pulse oximetry finding and indications of hypoxemia. In such a case, oxygen failure should be suspected.

4. Ventilatory failure (hypoventilation) will allow the development of hypercapnia and CO_2 accumulation in the alveoli, thereby eliminating the concentration gradient necessary for CO_2 to diffuse from the blood into the alveoli. Ventilation failure resulting in hypercapnia is measured by evaluating the $PaCO_2$ via ABG analysis.

5. The basic goals of management in acute respiratory failure are to ensure adequate ventilation, oxygenation, and CO_2 elimination. All patients in respiratory distress should receive high-flow oxygen, and ventilations can be assisted or provided to those patients who have a labored or absent respiratory drive. The decision to intubate, when possible, should be made prior to the initiation of transport, in the transporting facility or on scene. Airway and ventilation control aside (needed to ensure adequate ventilations), the pharmacologic management for ARF is aimed at the underlying cause (asthma, ARDS, and so on), and commonly includes the use of oxygen, bronchodilators, diuretics, and steroids in the acute phase.

6. ARDS should be ventilated at low tidal volumes to prevent overpressure injuries to the lung. The damage to the lung in ARDS is not equally distributed, with some areas expe-

riencing significant insult and others seemingly none. These unaffected regions receive the majority of delivered tidal volume and experience high peak inspiratory pressures (PIP), resulting in hyperinflation and barotrauma including disruption of the alveolar-capillary membrane and surfactant depletion. To prevent overinflation injury, an effort should be made to limit PIP to 35 cm H_2O by utilizing tidal volumes of 7–10 mL/kg.

7. The provision of RSI to a spontaneously breathing patient is done to ensure that the patient is well oxygenated and ventilated despite the pulmonary disturbance he is experiencing. While no set criteria exist for the indication of intubation, it is generally accepted that intubation is warranted when the PaO_2 is less than 60 mmHg, the $PaCO_2$ is greater than 50 mmHg, and the arterial pH is less than 7.30 on room air.

8. ARDS is considered when bilateral infiltrates on chest radiograph are present. Also, ABG analysis is usually significant for hypoxia, and respiratory alkalosis may be present early in the disease from the initial tachypnea. In addition to the bilateral diffuse infiltrates evident in the early stage of ARDS, chest radiograph findings will progress to complete bilateral whiteout of the lung fields late in the disease state.

9. The decision to decompress a tension pneumothorax is made from clinical assessment findings, not diagnostic interpretations. As such, if the patient is displaying consistently worsening dyspnea, diminishment of or absence of breathsounds on the affected side, a decrease in lung compliance, or hyperresonance, the critical care provider should evaluate the need to provide emergency thoracic decompression.

Chapter 22

1. The heart has three intrinsic pacemaker sites to ensure depolarization of the ventricles. The primary site, the sinoatrial node, has an intrinsic discharge rate of 60–100 impulses per minute. The sinoatrial (SA) node is influenced by both the sympathetic and parasympathetic nervous systems. The second pacemaker site is the atrioventricular (AV) node, which discharges spontaneously at a rate of 40–60 impulses per minute should the SA node fail. This node is also influenced by the sympathetic and parasympathetic nervous systems. The third impulse site is the Purkinje network, which can discharge spontaneously at 20–40 impulses per minute with failure or blockage of the higher pacer sites. The Purkinje network is primarily influenced by the sympathetic nervous system.

2. The primary difference between myocardial angina and myocardial infarction is the amount of tissue destruction present. Myocardial angina occurs when the heart cells start to starve for oxygen because the supply to the heart muscle is insufficient to meet the demand. In this scenario muscle cells are being injured, but they have not become necrotic yet. In myocardial infarction, permanent cellular muscle death occurs from a lack of oxygen to the heart. While ischemia can be reversed, infarction is permanent. Myocardial ischemia is commonly caused from partially blocked coronary blood vessels, whereas infarction occurs commonly when a vessel becomes totally occluded.

3. A patent with occlusion to the left anterior descending artery could affect the septal wall, anterior wall, and perhaps a small portion of the lateral wall of the left ventricle. As such, the findings of infarction would be present primarily in leads V1, V2, V3, and V4.

4. The goal of treating an evolving MI include reversing hypercapnia and hypoxia if present, minimizing the extent of the infarction, and making the patient feel more comfortable. To do this, the pharmacologic categories of drugs used include oxygen, nitrates, narcotics, beta-blockers, fibrinolytics, and antihypertensives. The patient may also receive antidysrhythmics should the electrical system of the heart start to fail.

5. Aortic aneurysms are commonly confused with aortic dissections. In aortic dissections, blood enters the media of the aorta and splits (dissects) the aortic wall. Unlike aneurysms

they seldom originate in the abdominal aorta. They commonly originate in the thoracic aorta but they may extend throughout the entire aorta. An aneurysm, conversely, is more typical to the abdominal vascular and is a disorder that involves a weakening of all vascular layers that results in a "bleb"-like structure that may burst and result in significant hemorrhage into the abdominal cavity.

6. All patients suspected of having an aortic dissection should have ongoing monitoring of cardiac rhythm, blood pressure, and urine output. Therapy is geared at decreasing the forces that favor progression of the dissection. This is accomplished by maintaining systolic blood pressure between 100 and 120 mmHg and by reduction of cardiac contractility. These goals are most commonly accomplished by the use of beta-adrenergic blockers and vasodilators.

7. The cardiomyopathies are a group of cardiac disorders in which the dominant feature is involvement of the heart muscle itself. Cardiomyopathies are characterized as primary or secondary. Primary cardiomyopathies are those in which no cause can be identified. Secondary cardiomyopathies are those in which there is a demonstrable underlying cause. The cardiomyopathies are also classified into three major categories: dilated cardiomyopathies, hypertrophic cardiomyopathies, and restrictive cardiomyopathies.

8. If the cardiogenic shock is due to a right ventricular infarct, the patient will need volume resuscitation. Avoid diuretics and nitroglycerin, which reduce preload and can worsen the hypotension. Dobutamine can be considered if fluids do not lead to improvement, or if an inotropic and vasopressor agent is needed that does not simultaneously vasoconstrict pulmonary vasculature. Dopamine should also be avoided in right ventricular infarct since it increases pulmonary vascular resistance and can worsen hypotension.

9. A faulty aortic valve may present in one of several ways, depending on the type of problem the valve is experiencing. For example, if the valve is stenosed, then the clinician may auscultate an S_4 sound or a high-pitched ejection snap. If during ventricular systole (between S_1 and S_2) a sound is heard and can be described as crescendo–decrescendo, a systolic murmer may be suspected. If the sound is heard after S_2 but prior to the next S_1, then a diastolic murmer may be suspected. In both the latter examples, the sound is created by blood passing through or regurgitating backward across an incompetent aortic valve.

10. Balloon-pump counterpulsation can augment cardiac output by as much as 10% to 20%. Raising the intra-aortic pressure during diastole and lowering the intra-aortic pressure during systole accomplish this augmentation in cardiac output. The balloon, after placement into the thoracic aorta, is inflated and deflated synchronously with the cardiac cycle. During diastole, the balloon is inflated, thereby displacing blood both proximally and distally to the balloon. Proximal displacement of blood enhances both coronary artery and cerebral perfusion; distal displacement of blood enhances systemic perfusion. The deflation of the cuff at the onset of ventricular systole causes a rapid drop in afterload pressure in the aorta, and the ejection fraction of the patient improves.

Chapter 23

1. The circle of Willis is a vascular structure that completely encircles itself around the base of the brain. The internal carotid and vertebral arteries form the foundation of the circle of Willis.

2. The left hemisphere is dominant in all right-handed persons, as well as roughly 75% to 85% of left-handed persons. Dominance is determined by the presence of the speech centers, known as Wernicke's and Broca's areas, in one hemisphere or the other.

3. The ACCP recommends that fibrinolysis be given to otherwise eligible patients whose symptoms began less than 3 hours prior. Patients in some areas may be eligible for intra-arterial intervention up to 6 hours after the onset of symptoms.

4. Myocardial stunning causing dysrhythmias, myocardial infarction, and left ventricular wall dysfunction after atraumatic subarachnoid hemorrhage (SAH) is believed to be the result of a sudden surge in endogenous catecholamines.

5. Cerebral vasospasm is most likely to occur between days 3 and 21 after a traumatic sub-arachnoid hemorrhage. Some cases may persist for up to a month, with persistent signs and symptoms.

6. *HHH* stands for "hypertense, hypervolumize, and hemodilute" and can be considered for the treatment of cerebral vasospasms that are inhibiting normal cerebral blood flow. Central venous pressure is maintained abnormally high with isotonic crystalloids and colloids, and vasopressor agents are used to elevate the blood pressure.

7. The most common cause for atraumatic intracerebral hemorrhage in deep white matter structures is from chronic hypertension or hypertensive crises.

8. Todd's paralysis is a phenomenon of transient hemiplegia that occurs as the result of a seizure. The hemiplegia occurs on the side of the body contralateral to the seizure focus, and may cause ipsilateral deviation of the gaze.

9. Any patient complaining of a fever and headache should be regarded as having the potential for meningitis. As such, respiratory precautions should be observed in addition to standard Body Substance Isolation Precautions.

10. The most sensitive and noninvasive tool for brain tumor diagnosis is the MRI with gadolinium dye administration. It has been found to be the most sensitive tool for neoplastic CNS lesions without performing a tissue biopsy.

Chapter 24

1. Due to the lack of a specific, identifiable clinical syndrome, a diagnosis of pancreatitis cannot be obtained by clinical evaluation alone. Laboratory and imaging studies are helpful in the ruling out of alternative diagnoses of abdominal pain, and to an extent can be helpful in determining the severity of pancreatitis. While serum amylase and lipase are the two most commonly utilized serum markers for pancreatitis, both lack the sensitivity and specificity to be used as the sole indicators of disease and should be used in conjunction with the entire clinical picture.

2. Of those listed, the use of a broad-spectrum antibiotic in the management of hemorrhage associated with esophageal varicies is not warranted. In fact, the IV antibiotic will not contribute at all to cessation of blood flow. The use of the Sengstaken-Blakemore tube and IV octreotide will help to slow the bleed, and the use of whole blood will replace lost volume and clotting factors from the ongoing hemorrhage.

3. Imaging studies are helpful in the ruling out of alternative diagnoses of abdominal pain, but abdominal radiographs are of little use in the diagnosis of acute pancreatitis because of the relative inability to visualize the pancreas itself.

4. Fulminant hepatic failure (FHF) is a medical emergency that is described as acute liver failure associated with hepatic encephalopathy. No cure for liver failure exists, and the definitive treatment is liver transplant. Thus, its management is mostly supportive, with particular attention to the airway, breathing, and circulation deserving obvious attention from the critical care transport team.

5. Potential complications from liver failure can be initially subtle, but ultimately widespread and fatal. Among other things, the patient may display third spacing of fluids, especially into the abdomen if portal congestion coexists with the liver failure. Additionally, coagulation abnormalities may occur due to a disturbance in clotting factor synthesis, and alterations in mental status may be present from hepatic encephalopathy. However, perforation or rupture of any hepatic vascular structure will most likely be the result of blunt or penetrating trauma, rather than a disease process.

6. Lower GI bleeds (LGIBs) occur in about 20 individuals per 100,000 population per year, and also occur more often in the elderly and males. Mortality rates are between 10% and 20%. The most common cause of LGIBs is diverticular disease (43% of cases), with angiodysplasia (20%), undetermined etiologies (12%), neoplasia (9%), and colitis (9%) accounting for the majority of remaining cases.

7. Priority is placed on ensuring that your patient has an adequate airway, is breathing appropriately, and has a pulse. Patients with UGIBs and hematemesis may require aggressive suctioning and an advanced airway to prevent the aspiration of blood. Oxygen should be administered to all patients suffering from GI bleeding. In addition, significant blood loss may lead to shock and inadequate breathing, necessitating artificial ventilation. Signs and symptoms consistent with shock require the aggressive administration of volume expanding agents. Initial volume replacement can be accomplished with crystalloid solutions; blood products should be administered based on clinical findings suggestive of severe volume depletion (greater than 2 L of crystalloid used). Despite concerns to the contrary, NG tube placement will not result in bleeding in patients with varicies, and all patients with significant GI bleeding should have an NG tube placed.

8. CT scanning may be helpful in assessing various gastrointestinal disorders due to its unsurpassed anatomical detailing. One disorder that is commonly evaluated by CT is pancreatitis due to the ability to visualize the size of the pancreas and to identify the presence of pancreatic fluid, pseudocysts, and abcesses.

9. The decision to minimize the amount of gastric acid in the stomach of a patient with a UGIB should be a conscious one. This is accomplished immediately by allowing stomach evacuation of acid via an NG tube attached to suction, and administration of pharmacologic agents that minimize the production of gastric acid.

Chapter 25

Additional Case Study 1

1. The correct answer is **C** for the first question of Case Study 1. As with most poisonings causing metabolic acidosis, hemodialysis is the definitive treatment for salicylate poisoning. For the critical care paramedic, the treatment priorities include fluid resuscitation, urine alkalization, and GI decontamination after airway management and ventilatory maintenance have been ensured. There is conflicting research regarding the efficacy of gastric decontamination, so the critical care paramedic should consult on-line medical direction before attempting this intervention. Also, the administration of bicarbonate is usually done by adding it to the intravenous solution, rather than direct IVP.

2. The correct answer is **A** for the second question of Case Study 1. The critical care paramedic is met in this case with many pieces of lab data information in the patient suffering from acute salicylate poisoning. Arterial blood gases reveal metabolic acidosis, coagulation studies reveal a prolonged prothrombin time (normal range being 7–10 seconds), and the salicylate level is fatally high. In this situation the critical care paramedic needs to avoid unnecessary cannulations, especially arterial, because significant bleeding may occur due to a deranged clotting mechanism from the overdose.

3. The correct answer is **B** for the third question of Case Study 1. In this situation, the only correct answer (at the correct dose and administration rate) is bicarbonate and IV fluids. The use of potassium and continued activated charcoal administration may be warranted, but the doses as listed are incorrect. Hemodialysis is not a treatment modality carried out in the back of a critical care transport vehicle (air or ground).

Additional Case Study 2

1. The correct answer is **D** for the first question of Case Study 2. The purpose of this question was simply to underscore the importance of your initial assessment and critical interventions for an unstable pediatric patient (regardless of cause). While it seems evident from the history that this pediatric patient is probably suffering from a methanol overdose, the critical care paramedic must first ensure adequate support of the airway and breathing functions. And for a decompensating pediatric patient who is intubated, endotracheal tube displacement, obstruction, or development of a tension pneumothorax could all be explanatory for the bradycardia, hypotension, and drop in pulse oximetry reading.

Chapter 26

1. All health care workers, including critical care paramedics have a professional responsibility to prevent the spread of infectious and communicable diseases. This includes stopping (or minimizing) the spread of infection to and from patients, coworkers, themselves, and their families and friends. To fulfill this obligation it is incumbent on every health care professional to be knowledgeable in the principles of infection control and the recognition and treatment of those infectious diseases that they may reasonably expect to encounter in their work.

2. Preventing the transmission of infectious agents requires practicing good infection control measures including general precautions and transmission-specific isolation precautions. Critical care paramedics are recommend to adopt the Standard Precautions as their primary strategy for preventing the transmission of diseases regardless of a patient's diagnosis or presumed infection status. A second strategy is Transmission-Based Precautions intended for patients known or suspected to be infected by epidemiologically important pathogens spread by airborne or droplet transmission or by contact with dry skin or contaminated surfaces.

3. Some of the currently epidemiologically important infectious diseases include human immunodeficiency virus (HIV) and acquired immunodeficiency syndrome (AIDS), hepatitis, epiglottitis, influenza, tuberculosis, SARS, meningitis, meningococcal infections, the childhood diseases, gastroenteritis, tetanus, and septicemia.

4. The CDC not only recommends that all children be immunized against highly infectious diseases, they further recommend that health care workers without documentation of immunity from acquired disease, serological evidence, or effective vaccination be immunized per guidelines published by the CDC as well.

5. Agents that are now important because of their potential use in bioterrorism include anthrax, botulism, tularemia, filoviruses, arenaviruses, cholera, brucellosis, ricin, saxitoxin, and mycotoxins. Although many countries have signed treaties resulting in the destruction of all biochemical warfare agents, some counties continue to manufacture and stockpile these agents.

Chapter 27

1. Infants and small children are at a greater risk for the development of acute hypoglycemia because of decreased glycogen stores, inability to stimulate the release of stored glycogen from an immature liver, and an increased metabolic rate that demands a higher utilization of serum glucose stores to maintain normalicy.

2. Anatomical differences that cause pediatric intubation to be more challenging than adult intubation include the tongue of the pediatric being proportionally larger in the oral cavity, the relative flaccidity of the epiglottis due to immature cartilagenous development, a prominent occipital region that results in neck flexion when placed supine, increased flexibility of the trachea, and the relative location of the glottic opening being more cephalad and anterior than in the adult patient.

3. It is important to remember at all times with neonatal, infant, and pediatric patients that the leading cause of cardiopulmonary arrest is airway and breathing insufficiency. If the airway and ventilatory systems are not carefully monitored and managed appropriately when compromises arise, the pediatric patient will degrade rapidly into cardiopulmonary failure and arrest, which carries with it even more abysmal rates for successful resuscitation than seen in the adult population.

4. The findings of respiratory distress, when the pediatric patient is still achieving adequate alveolar ventilation at the expense of a heightened work of breathing, include:
   - Tachypnea (to include "quiet" tachypnea)
   - Use of accessory respiratory muscles
   - Nasal flaring
   - Diaphoresis
   - Tachycardia (as defined by patient's age)
   - Irritation
   - Inspiratory retractions
   - Excessive abdominal motion
   - Grunting (physiological PEEP)
   - Pulse oximetry and end-tidal capnography changes

   The patient is said to be in respiratory failure when the following clinical findings are present:
   - Altered mental status (as appropriate for age)
   - Muscular hypotonia
   - Tachycardia giving way to bradycardia
   - Diminishment in systolic perfusion pressure
   - Pallor and eventual cyanosis
   - Loss of vesicular breath sounds
   - Irregular respirations
   - Alterations to normal breath sounds

5. Croup is a viral infection primarily found in children and is most common in children with a recent history of upper respiratory infections (URIs). The typical presentation of croup includes respiratory distress findings along with croup's hallmark "barking cough," which may be accompanied by stridor and a low-grade fever. Epiglottitis is an acute, severe, life-threatening disease of the upper airway. The epiglottis and the structures connected to or immediately surrounding it become inflamed and edematous, leading to a compromised airway at the level of the epiglottis and resultant respiratory compromise. The typical presentation for epiglottitis is rapid onset of a fever that may or may not be accompanied by a sore throat. The child will likely refuse to eat or drink because of the irritation this may cause, and will eventually be unable to tolerate his own secretions, which leads to the characteristic drooling seen in these patients. The child may also develop signs of upper airway obstruction with inspiratory stridor and some degree of respiratory compromise.

6. Asthma is a respiratory disease that is associated more with older children, and is characterized by general respiratory distress findings, wheezing on auscultation, and a history

consistent with allergenic respiratory exposure. Bronchiolitis typically occurs in children between 2 and 24 months of age and is most commonly caused by a virus. Symptoms of bronchiolitis include a fever, tachycardia and/or tachypnea, shortness of breath, chest tightness, wheezing, and coughing.

7. Treatment of asthma is focused on reversing bronchospasm, correcting hypoxia, and treating airway inflammation. The following agents help to reverse these pathological changes to return normal ventilations and oxygenation:
   - Oxygen
   - Intravenous fluids
   - Beta-specific agonists
   - Corticosteroids
   - Methylxanthines
   - Anticholinergics

8. The four etiologies for hypoperfusion (shock) discussed in the chapter include distributive shock (e.g., fluid loss), nondistributive shock (e.g., systemic vasodilation), cardiogenic shock (e.g., poor contractility), and obstructive shock (e.g., cardiac tamponade).

9. While in a water submersion/drowning episode, if a significant amount of fluid enters the child's lungs, the resulting death is referred to as a wet drowning (which accounts for the majority of all pediatric drownings). A dry drowning occurs when laryngospasm occurs as a protective reflex and prevents fluids from entering the lungs. Although this laryngospasm may prevent fluids from entering the lungs, cellular hypoxia is sustained. If this spasm persists throughout the event, the resulting death is referred to as a dry drowning.

Chapter 28

1. The HELLP syndrome is an acronym for **H**emolysis, **E**levated **L**iver function tests, and **L**ow **P**latelets, and is thought to be a subcategory of severe preeclampsia.

2. Beta-adrenergic agonists, magnesium sulfate, calcium channel blockers, and prostaglandin synthetase inhibitors are the agents most commonly used for tocolysis, with IV terbutaline or magnesium sulfate commonly utilized by critical care transport teams.

3. They can worsen the vasoconstriction and vascular depletion characteristic of preeclampsia.

4. Oxytocin 20–40 units (mixed in 1000 mL) at 100 mL/hr.

5. Once shoulder dystocia has been recognized, the immediate draining of the urinary bladder and a generous mediolateral episiotomy may facilitate delivery.

6. Late deceleration begins at the peak of a uterine contraction, and then returns to the FHR baseline after the contraction is finished. Late decelerations can be a serious sign of fetal distress, indicating hypoxia and acidosis secondary to uteroplacental insufficiency (i.e., inadequate oxygen exchange is taking place across the placenta during uterine contractions).

7. Early decelerations are generally considered normal, in that they represent an event that can be expected to occur with each uterine contraction. It is very important, however, for the critical care paramedic to be able to differentiate an early deceleration from a late deceleration, because late decelerations are an indicator of fetal distress, as are variable decelerations.

8. A low platelet count ($<100,000/mm^3$) is one indicator of preeclampsia. Others include SBP > 160 mmHg or DBP > 110 mmHg two times at least 6 hours apart. Others include proteinuria > 5 g in 24 hours, cerebral or visual symptoms, oliguria, pulmonary edema, right upper quadrant pain, elevated liver enzymes, and restricted fetal growth.

9. Ultrasound cannot diagnose the presence or absence of abruptio placenta itself, although it can demonstrate a placental hematoma that is consistent with abruption. Retroplacental hematomas may be recognized in 2% to 25% of all abruptions, but recognition of a retroplacental hematoma depends on the severity of hematoma and on the operator's skill level. Ultrasound can, however, rule out placenta previa as a cause of vaginal bleeding by determining the location of the placenta. As such, ultrasound does have a place, albeit limited, in the assessment of the high-risk OB-GYN patient.

10. Digital or speculum examination is to be avoided in all cases of suspected placenta previa because this may cause hemorrhage. Diagnosis of previa is confirmed with transabdominal ultrasound, which has an accuracy of 93% to 98% and a false-negative rate of only 7%.

Chapter 29

1. Anatomical differences that cause neonatal intubation to be more challenging than adult intubation include the tongue of the pediatric being proportionally larger in the oral cavity, the relative flaccidity of the epiglottis due to immature cartilagenous development, a prominent occipital region that results in neck flexion when placed supine, increased flexibility of the trachea, and the relative location of the glottic opening being more cephalad and anterior than in the adult patient.

2. At birth, the neonatal body surface area-to-volume ratio is four times that of an adult, while their heat production (thermogenesis) is only one and a half as high. This leaves the neonate at significant risk for hypothermia with resultant physiological compromise. Despite the larger surface area, the neonate has little adipose tissue and, as a result, a limited ability to maintain core body temperature. Additionally, neonatal muscle tone is immature and cannot effectively induce shivering to promote heat generation.

3. Respiratory distress indicates that the patient is still compensating and maintaining adequate minute ventilation. However, the signs and symptoms seen indicate that the neonate is struggling harder to breathe, and further pulmonary deterioration will probably occur if left untreated. Respiratory failure is considered to be present when the patient has exhausted all of her compensatory mechanisms, and the respiratory effort present is now insufficient in meeting the metabolic demands being made by the body. The neonate may still be breathing spontaneously, however, the ventilatory effort is insufficient for the body's needs. A patient in respiratory distress can progress to respiratory failure rapidly, and a patient in respiratory failure will progress to respiratory arrest (apnea) if management is not rapid and aggressive.

4. Neonatal respiratory distress syndrome is also known as hyaline membrane disease and primarily affects the lungs of premature infants. This disease is caused by a lack of pulmonary surfactant in the alveoli. During transport by the critical care team, the focus is not on providing curative treatment to the patient, but on suporting ventilations until the patient can be delivered to the receiving hospital for definitive care. Long-term management for IRDS includes surfactant replacement therapy.

5. In left-to-right shunt defects, oxygenated blood is shifted from the left side of the heart to the right side. This type of defect is considered to be acyanotic because the oxygenated blood received by the left side of the heart remains in the left side and there is no right-sided (venous) blood mixture. Types of acyanotic defects include atrial septal defect, ventricular septal defect, and patent ductus arteriosus.

6. In these types of defects, the offending problem is somehow related to a diminishment of pulmonary blood flow. The result is cyanosis due to poor pulmonary perfusion and inadequate oxygenation. Two conditions placed in this category of heart defects are complete transposition of the great vessels and tetralogy of Fallot.

7. A preterm infant is one who is less than 37 weeks gestational age.

8. PPHN can occur from multiple etiologies but is most commonly associated with severe hypoxia, meconium aspiration syndrome, or congenital diaphragmatic hernia. It is not related however, to hypoglycemia (nor even diabetes mellitus).

9. Treatment of sepsis is generally centered on antibiotic therapy and blood pressure support. Neonates have immature renal and hepatic systems and, as a result, the administration of antibiotics should be done judiciously and with regard for potential complications related to drug clearance. Sepsis that is refractory to antibiotic therapy may be caused by a virus rather than bacteria. If the sepsis is related to a virus, central nervous system and hepatic function will most likely be compromised.

Chapter 30

1. The thermostatic control is in the preoptic region of the hypothalamus, and serves as the principal center for thermoregulation. To aid in themoregulation, several thermoreceptor sites monitor information about the current temperature of the body. These sites are located in the skin (peripheral thermoreceptors), the core of the body, interior vessel walls (central thermoreceptors), and in the hypothalamus itself. Information from each of these locations is integrated and analyzed in the preoptic region. Based on the thermostatic "set point" that the hypothalamus has established for the body, versus the relative temperature of the body, certain compensatory mechanisms are set in motion.

2. Heat production arises primarily as a result of many of the biochemical processes that normally occur within the body. Most of the body's heat production occurs within the deep organs of the body, especially the liver, brain, and heart. During physical activity, the skeletal muscles produce heat that is subsequently transferred to the deep organs and tissues via the circulatory system. To retain heat, the body can utilize the vascular system in transporting heat to the core or limiting heat loss in the periphery by vasoconstricting. Additionally, adipose layers of the body can allow preservation of heat as well.

3. When the body needs to be cooled, heat is transferred from the deeper structures to the periphery. Blood vessels within the skin are dilated, allowing heat to be transferred to the skin. Once there, it is lost to the air and other surroundings. The rate of heat loss is determined by how rapidly heat can be conducted from the deep tissues to the skin and how rapidly heat can be transferred from the skin to the environment. Heat is also eliminated through the pulmonary system with exhalation.

4. Heat is a common by-product of many biochemical processes. The rate of heat production is referred to as the metabolic rate of the body. The rate of heat production while the body is at rest is a function of the *basal metabolic rate (BMR)*. The BMR refers specifically to the amount of energy needed to maintain homeostasis when the individual is at digestive, physical, and emotional rest.

5. Heat exhaustion is the result of cardiovascular strain as the body strives to maintain a normal temperature. Although heat exhaustion is an ill-defined syndrome, the body dysfunctions start to occur at temperatures between 102.9° and 104° F (39.4° and 40° C). The symptoms of heat exhaustion include dizziness, headache, fatigue, irritability, anxiety, chills, nausea, vomiting, and heat cramps. On physical examination the skin is commonly found to be diaphoretic; there will also be tachycardia, hyperventilation, hypotension, and, in some cases, syncope. Heat exhaustion is treated by removing the patient from the warm environment, providing rest, and replacing fluids and electrolytes.

6. Hypothermia is defined as a core temperature of less than 95° F (35° C) and occurs because the body can no longer generate sufficient heat to maintain body functions. The emergencies that can occur secondary to hypothermia are based on core temperature of the body, and the resulting altered physiology and symptomatology. The three categories of hypothermia are mild hypothermia (34°–35° C), moderate hypothermia (29°–32° C), and severe hypothermia (<29° C).

7. The assessment of the hypothermic emergency starts first with ensuring your safety as a care provider. After ensuring this, your assessment should follow the same initial assessment format as described for any other clinical situation. Attention should be paid to the patient's airway, ventilatory status, circulatory function, and mental status. At all times the hypothermic patient should be handled very carefully, and interventions employed only when necessary. Treatment of hypothermia is dependent on the severity. Generally speaking, all wet garments should be removed and the patient protected from additional heat loss. The patient should be maintained in a horizontal position. Particular care should be taken to avoid handling the patient in a rough manner because this may trigger a dysrhythmia. If possible, measure and monitor the core temperature as well as the ECG and vital signs.

8. The three categories of hypothermia are mild hypothermia (34°–35° C), moderate hypothermia (29°–32° C), and severe hypothermia (<29° C).

9. Patients with mild hypothermia should receive rewarming with active external methods (blankets, heat packs, and occasionally warm water immersion). With the advent of portable prehospital IV fluid warmers, active internal rewarming with heated IV fluids may also be initiated. If available, warmed humidified oxygen can be administered. Patients with severe hypothermia tend to develop numerous complications during the rewarming process. Most patients who die during active rewarming hypothermia do so from ventricular fibrillation. Because of this, rewarming of severe hypothermia patients is best deferred to a hospital setting using a predefined protocol. However, if transport times exceed 15 minutes, rewarming may need to be started in the field.

10. The principal insult in drowning is hypoxia. Once immersion occurs there is a natural tendency to hold one's breath. At some point, however, the victim will succumb to the situation and gasp for air; this will occur when the stimulus to breath overrides the voluntary effort of breath holding. This gasping and the sudden influx of fluid will cause either laryngospasm or inhalation of fluid. Special attention must be given to the maintenance of a patent airway for these patients. Vigilant monitoring of breath sounds and a review of blood gas values should be obtained. Decompression of the stomach can be accomplished via NG/OG tube, and remember to provide spinal immobilization should there be a history of trauma or if the exact mechanism underlying the episode is unknown.

Chapter 31

1. As a diver descends below the surface, pressure changes occur almost immediately. The ear is most often affected, but problems with the sinuses and blood vessels of the eye are also possible. The tympanic membrane experiences the pressure changes when the eustachian tube is compressed and no longer allows equalization of the pressure in the middle ear. When air in the sinus becomes trapped during the diver's descent, the shrinking volume is replaced by fluids or blood from the sinus linings. Known as a sinus squeeze, the diver will experience pressure or pain in the areas above the eye, over the upper teeth, or from deep in the skull.

2. Decompression sickness is also known as *caisson disease,* the *bends, diver's paralysis,* and *dysbarism.* This condition is caused by the expansion of nitrogen in the tissues following

a dive of significant depth and duration. The signs and symptoms of decompression sickness start small and worsen as small bubbles expand and combine to form larger bubbles. This causes occlusions of larger blood vessels, affecting greater tissue fields. Tissue ischemia and occasionally infarction can occur. The definitive treatment of decompression sickness is recompression in a hyperbaric chamber so that the nitrogen in the body can safely exit over time.

3. In the commercial diving industry, deep dives are performed utilizing mixed gases in place of compressed air. When oxygen and helium are used at depths exceeding 400 feet, a condition known as high-pressure neurologic syndrome (HPNS) can develop. Also known as helium tremors, HPNS is the result of breathing helium and may be more related to the effects of helium on nervous tissues than the pressurization of helium itself. HPNS starts with a tremor in the hands and arms similar to shivering, and difficulty in general muscle coordination. As the diver continues to descend, alterations in level of consciousness may occur. Confusion, unconsciousness, and seizures are possible. Difficulty breathing develops as the degree of muscle incoordination worsens.

4. During a diver's rapid or uncontrolled ascent, nitrogen gases that have dissolved into the tissues and bloodstream at depth will begin to expand as the pressure exerted on the body lessens. As the gas expands, the result is nitrogen bubbles emerging into the bloodstream, joint capsules, and tissues, which can result in pain, vascular occlusion, and tissue damage. As well, the amount of air in the lungs will expand if the diver fails to exhale during ascent and can potentially result in significant barotraumas (pneumothorax, bronchiole rupture, and so on).

5. *Ciguatera* is an accumulated toxin encountered in reef-dwelling fish. It is found in small planktonic organisms that serve as food for small fish. As larger fish eat the small fish, the toxin is concentrated in the tissues, growing stronger with each contaminated fish eaten. Signs and symptoms of ciguatera poisoning develop within 15 minutes to 3 hours from ingestion, with symptoms worsening within 12–24 hours. Initially, nausea, abdominal pain, vomiting, and diarrhea will occur. A tingling sensation to the lips and mouth and running down the extremities is followed in a few days with itching to the soles and palms. Other signs include fatigue, blisters, skin rash, difficulty walking, leg and arm pain, headache, vision disturbances, sweating, insomnia, hypotension, irregular cardiac rhythms, dyspnea, seizures, and coma. The treatment of ciguatera in the prehospital setting is supportive. IV fluids can be helpful in preventing dehydration associated with vomiting and diarrhea. Diphenhydramine may help to relieve the itching sensation.

6. The majority of factors related to diving deaths can be separated into three groups (listed in order of most common causes): human error, environmental causes, and equipment failure. Human error includes diving with a disqualifying medical condition, panic, fatigue, buoyancy problems, low-on-air or out-of-air situations, failure to ditch the weight belt in difficult situations, ignoring the buddy system, and improper use of equipment. Adverse sea conditions, water movement, and extreme temperatures make up the list of environmental factors. Finally, failure of the equipment itself may be the cause of death, but has been a factor in amazingly few cases.

7. The definitive treatment of decompression sickness is recompression in a hyperbaric chamber so that the nitrogen in the body can safely exit over time. When the body is subjected to increased atmospheric pressure in a recompression chamber, the gas that is dissolved in the tissues cannot rapidly form bubbles. The pressure is slowly decreased in the chamber (this process may take several hours), and the dissolved gases will reemerge slowly into the vascular system and be eliminated harmlessly by the pulmonary system.

8. The Divers Alert Network (DAN) is a nonprofit medical and research organization dedicated to the safety and health of scuba divers and associated with Duke University Medical Center. Founded in 1980, DAN has served as a lifeline for the scuba industry by

operating diving's only 24-hour emergency hotline, which is an emergency service for injured divers. Additionally, DAN operates a diving medical information line, conducts vital diving medical research, and develops and provides a number of educational programs for everyone from beginning divers to medical professionals. What DAN can do in support of the critical care paramedic's role is provide emergency medical advice and assistance for underwater diving injuries. The Divers Alert Network should be contacted for referral to hyperbaric chambers worldwide, and can be of great benefit in arranging transportation and technical assistance.

Chapter 32

1. Because every patient is unique, a discussion with your regional poison center, medical direction, or a medical toxicologist may help to establish the best treatment approach. During the interfacility transport of these patients by the critical care team, management is still largely supportive of lost function due to the toxic exposure. These interventions include airway skills (to included medication-assisted intubation), ventilatory support, circulatory management by way of IV fluids and vasopressor, and the continued management of lethal dysrhythmias.

2. The ways in which a toxin may gain entry into the body include inhalation (across the pulmonary vasculature), absorption (across the skin), injection (toxin is allowed to penetrate the skin to the tissues beneath), and ingestion (toxin is absorbed across the GI tract). Limiting continued exposure by any of the routes is largely done by simply removing the exposure to the toxin. This means either removing the patient from the toxic environment, or removing the toxin from the patient.

3. Arriving at a clinical decision that your patient has been exposed to a toxic substance relies both on the history and clinical signs present. In concert with each other, the patient may display what is referred to as a *toxidrome*, which is a constellation of clinical signs and symptoms that, taken together, reliably suggest an exposure to a specific drug class. Many patients, when exposed to an adequate dose of a drug, display the specific clinical effects of that drug class.

4. Scene characteristics suggestive of a toxicologic exposure would include the assessment of the mechanism of injury and/or nature of illness. The critical care provider would want to remain aware of possible environmental exposure (for example, smoke from a factory fire) and potential contamination from an industrial accident. If multiple people are affected simultaneously, the toxic emergency could be from an inhalation or ingestion mechanism. Finally, if the patient was bitten or stung it could suggest that the patient is experiencing an emergency from a toxic injection.

5. The availability of herbal medications has rapidly increased since the passage of the Dietary Supplement Health and Education Act in 1994. Since then, dietary supplements (including herbal medications) have not been stringently regulated by the FDA or other government agency. Therefore, these "natural" products do not undergo any scientific testing and are potentially dangerous for several reasons: first, no verification of ingredients; second, no testing for biological effects; and third, no knowledge of drug interactions. These potential dangers increase for those patients with significant underlying disease and those taking prescription medications. Common prescription drugs with herbal interactions include warfarins, digoxin, and several anticonvulsants. Furthermore, the manufacturing of herbal medications is not regulated and there have been numerous reports in the literature about herbal medications being contaminated with other compounds, microbes, medications, or heavy metals.

6. Beta-blocker (BB) overdose typically manifests with bradycardia, hypotension, or dysrhythmias (often associated with ECG changes such as a prolonged PR interval). Severe

toxicity can cause hypoglycemia (particularly in children), pulmonary edema, or coma. Propranolol toxicity can lead to QRS widening and seizures, due to sodium channel blockade. For BB toxicity, hypotension and bradycardia may respond to IV calcium chloride (one ampule) or glucagon (up to 10 mg). Often, the hypotension present in these patients will only respond to the use of vasoactive pressors, such as norepinephrine, and should be used if available. Dysrhythmias and hypotension associated with QRS widening, and propranolol-induced seizures respond well to IV boluses of sodium bicarbonate.

7. After cyanide exposure, the patient rapidly develops severe hypoxia and metabolic acidosis, leading to abrupt coma, cardiovascular collapse, and death. The management of cyanide toxicity includes aggressive control of the airway, supporting circulation, treatment of seizures, and the immediate administration of a cyanide antidote kit.

8. One of the many roles of U.S. Poison Control Centers (PCCs) is to assist with the triage and management of patients with (potentially) toxic exposures. Critical care paramedics should take full advantage of the knowledge and resources available through consultation of a poison control center. They can be reached by phone at 1-800-222-1222, when caring for a poisoned patient. Information that may be requested by the PPC specialist includes the type of exposure, the amount of exposure, the route of entry, the presenting signs and symptoms, the presence of concurrent trauma or significant medical history, and the transport time to the receiving facility.

Chapter 33

1. CBRNE are agents that fit into the categories of chemical, biological, radiological, nuclear, and explosive weapons. These are often referred to as *weapons of mass destruction* (WMD) and have received extensive public media and emergency service attention in recent years as potential agents of terrorist use.

2. The first priority for the critical care paramedic is the safety of the crew and the patient. An important component of this is the separation of what can be considered operational and clinical issues. The critical care paramedic will not (if ever) be involved in the rescue of a patient subjected to a CBRNE event (this is operations). Once the individual has been safely extricated from the situation by experts, and has received appropriate decontamination, then the issue now becomes a clinical one that the critical care paramedic becomes involved in during the assessment and management phases. During this time specifically, the provider should employ those personal protective measures commonly used to limit exposure to bloodborne pathogens.

3. Industrial chemicals that affect the ability of the nervous system to function properly by inhibiting acetylcholinesterase (AChE) are referred to as *nerve agents,* which are extremely potent compounds that are lethal in very small doses. Additionally, pulmonary agents, such as chlorine and phosgene, are easy to acquire and transport. Due to the fact that large quantities of these chemicals may be so easily found in our society, their potential for accidental release or intentional use as a weapon is very high.

4. The treatment of patients with significant exposure to organophosphorous compounds includes the use of atropine sulfate, pralidoxime chloride (2-PamCl), and diazepam. For exposure to pulmonary agents, the treatment of resultant bronchospasm may include administration of beta-2-specific bronchodilators such as albuterol or metaproterenol. Cyanide exposure should be treated with cyanide antidote kits. A specific antidote for lewisite exposure exists, British Anti-Lewisite (Dimercaprol), also known as BAL, has demonstrated usefulness in treating this type of exposure.

5. Biological agents include any living organism or toxin that can be developed for use to cause illness or death in a population. From a categorical standpoint, the types of agents

that could be used include bacterial agents (anthrax, plague, tularemia), viral agents (such as smallpox), and biological toxins (such as botulinum).

6. Regardless of the specific disease process or agent used, the principles of patient care and personal protection are similar for nearly all of the known possible agents. Beyond ensuring that the patient's airway, breathing, and circulatory systems are intact (and supporting them if they are not), most of the bacterially produced diseases respond favorably to antibiotic therapy.

7. A person exposed to external irradiation does not become radioactive and poses no hazard to nearby individuals. If, however, contamination has occurred when radioactive material is found either in or on the body, care providers must be careful not to spread the contamination to uncontaminated parts of the victim's body, to themselves, or to the surrounding area. Despite the minimal risk of provider contamination at this phase in the patient's care, it is better to err on the side of safety and ensure that adequate decontamination has occurred. Afterwhich, in the majority of cases, standard Body Substance Isolation Precautions will provide more than adequate protection.

8. RDD stands for radiological dispersal device and is defined as a device that causes the purposeful dissemination of radioactive material across an area, often by explosive means, but without a nuclear detonation. The material can originate from any location that uses radioactive sources, such as a nuclear waste processor, a nuclear power plant, a university research facility, a medical radiotherapy clinic, or an industrial complex. The radioactive material is disseminated by means of a conventional explosive, scattering radioactive debris throughout the area. This type of dissemination would likely cause conventional traumatic injuries as well as contamination with radioactive materials.

9. When looking for updated information on CBRNE, reliable Internet-based resources often provide the best source for current information. Many resources exist that can provide a quick reference to information regarding patient presentation, clinical interventions, and specific pharmacologic agents. Frequently updated Internet-based information sites are maintained by both the Centers for Disease Control and Prevention (CDC), www.cdc.gov, and the World Health Organization (WHO), www.who.int. Additional information can also be obtained through the U.S. Department of Homeland Security's Internet site.

Chapter 34

1. Critical care paramedics may find themselves more involved in the organ procurement and transplantation process than their non-critical care counterparts. Critical care paramedics can be involved in virtually any aspect of the transplant process and must be familiar with the issues and procedures involved, but primarily the critical care transport team is responsible for the rapid transport of harvested organs, or physiological maintenance of the "brain dead" patient until such time that the organs are harvested.

2. Organ Procurement Organizations (OPOs) and hospitals are required by the Centers for Medicare and Medical Services (CMS) to identify and establish mutually agreed-on triggers for referral of potential organ donors. Many hospitals and OPOs have agreed that a ventilator-dependent, neurologically devastated patient with a Glasgow Coma Scale (GCS) of 5 or less is a patient who must be referred to the OPO. Because criteria for organ donation can vary so widely, OPOs discourage hospital staff from making further clinical judgments about a potential donor's suitability.

3. Neurologic death, or brain death, is defined as the complete irreversible cessation of all brain and brainstem activity. The critical findings in a brain death examination include explained loss of consciousness, no motor response to painful stimuli, no brainstem reflexes, and apnea. Any declaration of death by neurologic criteria should clearly docu-

ment the injury that led to the death, the examinations performed (and the results of those examinations), and the statement that the patient is declared dead, including the date and time of that declaration. This declaration of death is the legal declaration of death and will appear on the patient's death certificate.

4. In the absence of a donor document or registration in a state donor registry, the OPO staff obtains consent for donation from the legal next-of-kin (LNOK). Understandably, this is a process that requires a great deal of sensitivity and compassion, as the organ procurement coordinator must guide the family through the acute stages of grief while helping them to understand what has happened and how organ and tissue donation can benefit them and others. Some OPOs have begun to employ staff solely for the task of working with families in this difficult time.

5. The OPC and OR staff initially determine necessary surgical supplies and agree on what OR staff members will be needed. The OPC will review with the circulating nurse the documentation of brain death, the authorization for donation, and the credentials of the surgical teams coming to recover the organs. When the teams are ready, the donor is transported to the OR and the organs are exposed and examined for any obvious anatomical abnormalities. The chest and abdominal cavities are cooled rapidly using sterile ice, and cold preservation solutions are flushed through the vessels into the organs. The organs are further examined to ensure that the preservation solution flows well and that there are no vascular abnormalities. The organs are removed from the body and taken to a back table for further inspection and packaging. Once packaged, they are transported back to the transplant center for implantation into the recipient.

6. In 2004, the waiting list for an organ transplant in the United States grew to nearly 90,000 people. However, 625,000 people are waiting for a tissue graft. Tissues typically harvested include the dura mater, eyes or corneas, skin, heart valves, bones, tendons, and veins.

7. Because of the likelihood of EMS providers to have patients who are dead on arrival due to some traumatic incident, see patients with injuries that are incompatible with ultimate survival, or be permitted to terminate resuscitative efforts on an arrested patient, they too may be an important component to the organ donation program. In these instances, there should be a step-wise procedure the EMS provider can utilize to identify the potential donor and initiate the procurement procedure.

Chapter 35

1. Given that critical care paramedics often see the most significantly injured or critically ill patients, the care rendered by these providers is often very intensive and complicated. The quality assurance program within that critical care transport organization can help monitor and improve the care provided by identifying those components or individuals who are not meeting the expectations of the patient, the medical community, and the service. The QI process will become an intertwined and ongoing process of improvement in all aspects of the program.

2. When properly designed and implemented, the quality improvement program of a service can allow continuous monitoring of critical care provider performance. This can be done by establishing program or service goals, determining how to monitor and measure the goals, employing the monitoring process, reviewing data gained through monitoring, arriving at informed decisions regarding what to do with the level of compliancy attained versus goal establishment, and finally employing strategies designed to enhance the outcomes desired.

3. The skill and system performance is unequivocally tied to ultimate program success and, as such, is extremely important to monitor. If the skill of the providers is not meeting the needs of the patient or system, the patient will suffer and the system will eventually fail.

If the program system conversely is not meeting the needs of the provider, then the provider will be unable to perform at his/her ultimate capacity and again, the patient will suffer and the system will eventually fail.

Chapter 36

1. The various types of radio systems employed in emergency services include the simplex system, which can only send and receive on the same frequency, and cannot simultaneously transmit in both directions. The full-duplex system can transmit and receive simultaneously. The half-duplex system is one that uses two different frequencies for transmitting and receiving, but the hardware only allows for one direction of communication flow at a time. The multiplex system provides the capability of transmitting data and voice simultaneously. Trunking systems use a computer to pool all available frequencies and then assign communication to an open frequency. Digital systems are those that translate voice (analog) into digital code for broadcast.

2. Radio frequencies utilized by the critical care organization are assigned by the Federal Communications Commission (FCC) in conjunction with the state's chapter of Associated Public Safety Communications Officers. The FCC is an independent U.S. government agency, directly responsible to Congress. The FCC was established by the Communications Act of 1934 and is charged with regulating interstate and international communications by radio, television, wire, satellite, and cable.

3. The critical care provider must interact with a multitude of individuals on a daily basis as well as a mission-to-mission basis. These individuals include the communication specialist (dispatcher), physicians and nurses involved in the patient's care, the operator of the vehicle (ground or air transport), family members, other prehospital providers (fire, police, and EMS), and finally the patients themselves.

4. Air traffic controllers are those individuals who work at the various airports across the United States and abroad. Air traffic controllers are responsible for the safe and efficient flow of air traffic throughout the nation's airspace. Their primary role is to monitor the airways, help pilots pass other planes safely, navigate pilots through fog and rough weather, and allow safe landing at busy airports. As such, it is the air traffic controller who will determine if the pilot can fly in the direction and altitude that they desire to.

5. The critical care paramedic should have the following information ready prior to establishing radio contact with the receiving facility (although most systems or receiving facilities may request just portions or specifics of the following information):
   - Age, gender, ethnicity
   - Chief complaint, purpose of transport
   - Significant medical history and history of the chief complaint
   - Current mental status
   - Airway and breathing status
   - Invasive/noninvasive assessment of hemodynamics
   - Care being provided currently (meds, fluids, vent settings, and so on)
   - Response of patient to current therapy
   - Confirmation of medical records/documentation
   - Estimated arrival at the department
   - Requests for additional personnel or equipment upon arrival

6. The patient care report (PCR) should be filled out by the critical care provider following each mission. Depending on the system, the PCR type employed may be one of three types. The first type is narrative, where the provider has the freedom to describe the mis-

sion events and patient's condition as he deems necessary. Patient care reports can also be prepared with a series of check-off boxes or bubble-in spaces to denote the patient's care. Finally, the system may use technology to its advantage and utilize a software program on a PDA or a laptop computer in which the patient data can be uploaded immediately to the organization's mainframe computer system by way of a wireless link.

7. The PCR should have the following elements of proper documentation: It should be completed in its entirety, it should be highly accurate, it must be legible (especially when not using an electronic clipboard or computer software program), it must be submitted in a timely fashion, it must be devoid of excessive mistakes, and it should be submitted with the intent of not needing additional addendums or alterations.

8. Inappropriate documentation carries with it both medical and legal consequences. Of these two, the medical consequences are naturally most severe since care decisions may be made based on your submitted patient care report, and if there are errors or omissions, the consequence can be poor subsequent patient care. From a legal standpoint, there are significant ramifications of poor documentation as well. In a court of law, what you documented is many times what is debated, not what you actually did. Even though your patient care may have been exemplary on a particular mission, if the documentation does not bear this out, you may be found libel or negligent for the damages the plaintiff is claiming.

Chapter 37

1. The critical care paramedic will only be legally permitted to provide care in any environment (prehospital, critical care transport, or in-hospital) when doing so under the auspices of a medical director. While in the hospital environment, the critical care paramedic will be less likely to have a set of standing orders or protocols to follow; rather she is typically provided a set of job functions that she is allowed to perform. Depending on the state in which the critical care paramedic may function, her direct oversight may be from a physician or a nurse who has the legal permission to delegate responsibility to the critical care paramedic.

2. The critical care paramedic has historically found employment in the emergency departments of hospitals since this domain would be most functional to the paramedic's skills. Other departments of employment include critical care units and some specialty procedure units.

3. Influences that impact the role of critical care paramedics in the hospital include other health care providers (for example, nurses), insurance agencies, quality assurance programs, physician medical direction, and state medical practice acts.

4. For the critical care provider advantages include the opportunity to interface with numerous health care providers, clinical experience, the chance to utilize many skills, a more stable (typically) work schedule, and commonly the pay is higher. For the hospital, the employment of paramedics allows them to utilize a care provider who is extremely well educated and skilled for an hourly wage that is less than most other providers in the hospital.

5. Disadvantages to the paramedic in the hospital as cited by opponents include the perception that the paramedic is not educated nor trained high enough to competently care for patients, the fact that many paramedics are "certified" rather than "licensed," the fact that there is a lack of research "justifying" the advantage of paramedics in the hospital, and finally that the paramedic is not adequately oriented to the in-hospital environment.

6. Skills that may be required by critical care paramedics in the hospital that they may be less familiar with include Foley catheter insertion, NG/OG tube insertion, tracheal airway

replacement, sterile techniques (tracheal suctioning, surgical procedures), ABG blood draw, setting up equipment (central lines, chest tubes, and so on), conscious sedation monitoring, monitoring critical patients during transport to other departments, and billing procedures.

7. The primary disadvantage of the critical care paramedic taking care of patients between missions is that there could be a potential break in the continuity of care. Important information such as drug dose, patient response, and current vital signs may not yet be documented in the patient chart when the paramedic must suddenly leave on another mission.

8. Since the critical care paramedic in the hospital environment is familiar with both pre-hospital and in-hospital nuances, he can ease the transition of the patient from EMS providers to the nursing and physician staff by seeking out needed information from the EMS providers and relaying it to the ED staff. As well, he can help the EMS crew replace equipment, get patient demographic information if needed for the PCR, and serve as a feedback loop for patient disposition should it be required later.

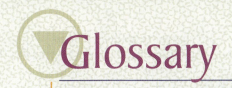

Glossary

Abbreviated Injury Scale (AIS)   developed to collect detailed data on the types and severity of injuries suffered by victims of motor vehicle crashes.

ABO typing   the ABO typing determines which of the four blood groups a sample belongs to.

abruptio placentae   the premature separation of a normally implanted placenta from the uterine wall.

absolute zero   the temperature at which molecular motion stops, described as "−460°F" or "−273°C."

acceleration   during uterine contraction, an abrupt increase in FHR of 15 bpm (or more) above baseline, lasting from 15 seconds to 2 minutes.

accidental hypothermia   a spontaneous decrease in core temperature that falls below 35°C (95°F); usually a direct result of exposure to a colder environment.

acclimatization   a gradual physiologic process where the body learns to adjust its retention or release of heat according to environmental conditions.

acquired immunodeficiency syndrome (AIDS)   a severe life-threatening disease caused by the Human Immunodeficiency Virus (HIV); the terminal clinical manifestation of HIV infection.

actual acidosis   overproduction of hydrogen ions.

actual alkalosis   overproduction of bicarbonate ions.

acute coronary syndrome (ACS)   a spectrum of coronary artery disease (CAD) processes including myocardial ischemia, myocardial injury, and myocardial infarction.

acute radiation syndrome (ARS)   a condition that develops following exposure to high doses of ionizing radiation, ARS presents as a sequence of phased and usually lethal symptoms that vary with onset and severity of exposure, including gastrointestinal, respiratory, and CNS deterioration.

acute respiratory failure (ARF)   defined as a state of inadequate gas exchange resulting from the inability of the respiratory system to absorb O_2 and/or excrete CO_2.

addiction   characterized by one or more behaviors that may include impaired control over drug use, compulsive use, continued use despite harm, and cravings.

agents of opportunity   describes both common and unusual industrial agents, along with a myriad of other potential toxic chemicals, readily available in our society.

agonists   drugs that stimulate receptor sites inhibit in order to cause an effect.

air traffic controllers   professionals responsible for the safety and efficiency of aviation traffic flow.

air transport systems   specialized medical transport of critically ill or injured patients via helicopter or fixed-wing aircraft.

airborne   diseases transmitted by microorganisms capable of being transmitted as droplet nuclei or on dust particles through the atmosphere.

airframe   generally refers to the "type" of aircraft, main structure that all other components are attached to.

Ambu Laryngeal Mask (ALM)   a supraglottic, single-use, disposable airway designed for insertion when maintaining neutral position is desired.

ambulance chassis   type of vehicle/cab frame, such as a van or truck, upon which the patient care compartment is mounted.

ambulance configuration   vehicle type, physical layout, electrical, and mechanical design of an ambulance. (Example: USDOT KKK-1822 specifications.)

ambulances   vehicles designed for the safe transport of injured or ill patients.

American Nurses Association (ANA)   a professional organization that serves the nursing profession in the United States, the ANA "advances the nursing profession by fostering high standards of nursing practice, promoting the economic and general welfare of nurses in the workplace, projecting a positive and realistic view of nursing."

amphiarthrosis   joints, or the connection between two bones, classified as slightly movable.

anaphylactic shock   shock caused by exaggerated systemic response to an allergen.

Anderson, Miller-Abbott, and Cantor tubes   long (up to 10 feet), wide-diameter tubes used to clear obstructions of the small bowel in patients considered high-risk surgical candidates.

angiography   diagnostic study of the inside of vasculature by injection of radio-opaque dye, then inspection under a fluoroscope.

anion gap   an indirect measurement of negatively charged ions including phosphates, sulfates, and organic acids.

antagonists   drugs that block receptor sites in order to inhibit a certain cellular function.

anterior cavity   the anterior cornea, separated from the posterior lens by the pupil.

anthrax   an acute bacterial infection caused by *Bacillus anthracis*, a gram-positive, encapsulated, spore-forming rod.

antibiotic-resistant organisms (AROs)   multi-drug resistant pathogenic microorganisms, including methicillin-resistant *Staphylococcus aureus* and vancomycin-resistant enterococcus (VRE).

aortic aneurysm   a localized dilatation of the aorta caused by weakening of the aortic wall; can involve all three layers of the aorta (intima, media, and adventitia).

aortic dissection   a potentially lethal dissection of the intimal layers of the aorta. Blood, under the force of arterial pressure, goes through an intimal tear and enters the media of the aorta and splits (dissects) the aortic wall.

aortic rupture   lethal injury with high potential for immediate exsanguination; associated with blunt and/or penetrating chest trauma.

aqueous humor   a clear fluid in the anterior cavity that circulates freely between the anterior and posterior chambers through the pupil.

arenavirus   class of viruses, such as Lassa fever; another hemorrhagic fever with symptoms similar to Ebola and Marburg.

arterial blood gas   dissolved gases in the arterial circulation. Generally consists of: pH, pCO_2, pO_2, oxygen saturation, and hemoglobin.

arterial gas embolism (AGE)   a serious over-expansion syndrome, secondary to air being forced into the capillary system of the alveoli. Gases combine in the circulatory system to form larger "bubbles" that block arterial vasculature of the heart.

arteriovenous malformation (AVM)   a vascular abnormality caused by the abnormal anastomosis of veins and arteries; a tortuous collection of structurally weak veins and arteries that are vulnerable to rupture.

arthrodia   gliding movable joints.

Asherman chest seal   commercial device commonly used to mitigate effects of sucking chest wounds.

Association of Air Medical Services (AAMS)   an international association, serving the air and surface medical transportation industries.

atmosphere (earth)   the gas cloud surrounding earth.

atmospheres of absolute pressure (ATA)   describes underwater pressure; includes the weight of the water *plus* the atmospheric pressure at the surface. Every 33 feet of depth is equal to 1 atmosphere (or 14.7 psi in pressure); surface pressure is also equal to 1 atmosphere. (A diver at a depth of 33 feet is at an ATA of 2 atmospheres.)

atmospheric pressure   pressure on the earth and its inhabitants, caused by the weight of atmospheric gases in conjunction with gravity.

atria   thin-walled, upper chambers of the heart that receive venous blood from the pulmonary or systemic circulation.

atrial septal defect (ASD)   a hole in the atrial septum thought to be from incomplete closure of the foramen ovale.

atrioventricular (AV) blocks   conduction blocks that occur in the AV node and include 1st degree and both 2nd degree blocks.

atrioventricular (AV) node   secondary "pacemaker" of the heart, comprised of nodal cells embedded in the floor of the right atria near the opening of the coronary sinus.

auditory ossicles   three bones in the middle ear that transmit vibrations of the tympanic membrane to the vestibulocochlear complex in the inner ear.

automatic transport ventilators   compact mechanical ventilators that can be used in out-of-hospital transport.

autoregulation   inherent ability of the arterial system within the brain to adjust in attempts to maintain adequate cerebral perfusion, despite changes in systemic pressure.

autorotation   a sequence of collective pitch and foot pedal controls that allow a pilot to harness air flowing through the main rotor to control the aircraft's descent and landing.

Avogadro's law   equal volume of all gases under identical conditions of pressure and temperature contain the same number of molecules.

B-natriuretic peptide (BNP)   peptide found in the ventricles of the heart, increases when ventricular filling pressures are high; can be used to detect CHF.

bacteria   unicellular microorganisms that are round, spiral, or rod-shaped; capable of being pathogenic.

barodontalgia   toothache reported by individuals at actual or simulated altitudes, varying from 5,000 to 15,000 feet. Relieved by descent.

basal metabolic rate (BMR)   the amount of energy needed to maintain homeostasis at rest.

basic mechanical airways   nasopharyngeal airway; oropharyngeal airway.

Beck airway airflow monitor (BAAM)   a device used to facilitate blind nasotracheal intubation in patients who are breathing.

Beck's triad   the clinical presentation of cardiac tamponade, first described by Dr. Claude Beck in the early 1930s, it includes hypotension (often with narrowing pulse pressures), jugular venous distension, and muffled heart tones.

"bends"   also known as decompression sickness, "caisson disease," "diver's paralysis," and "dysbarism."

bilirubin   by-product of red cell destruction, the liver processes and removes the bilirubin from the blood, excreting it in the stool.

bioavailability   free, unbound state of a drug molecule, making it capable of exerting an action.

biotransformation   method by which a drug changes into inactive metabolites for elimination from the body.

blood banking   routine tests that include ABO typing, Rh factor and direct Coombs test (RBC antibody screening).

blood urea nitrogen (BUN)   a diagnostic test for the determination of renal function that measures the amount of urea nitrogen present in the bloodstream.

Body Substance Isolation (BSI) Precautions   protective gear designed to reduce the risk of transmission of diseases via moist body substances.

Boerhaave syndrome   an esophageal perforation that can lead to leakage of gastric contents into the mediastinal space. It can have a high mortality rate.

botulinum toxin   a neurotoxic bacteria, *Clostridium botulinum,* is the most toxic substance known to medicine on a dose/weight basis.

botulism   a spore-forming anaerobic bacillus caused by *Clostridium botulinum.*

Boyle's law   The volume of a gas is inversely proportional to its pressure, assuming temperature remains constant.

brain death   synonymous with neurological death; neurological death is the preferred term.

bronchiolitis   an acute infectious process of the lower respiratory tract common in children under 24 months of age; most often attributed to respiratory syncytial virus or *Mycoplasma pneumoniae.*

brucellosis   debilitating illness caused by the gram-negative, rod-shaped, non-spore-forming bacilli, *Brucella (suis, melitensis, abortus).*

bundle branch block (BBB)   block of either the right or left bundle branch system, associated with an MI, congenital defects, ischemic tissue, or RF ablation.

buoyancy   determined by the density of an object and the specific gravity of the liquid in which it is suspended.

Burden nasoscope   a type of nasotracheal tube auscultation device.

BURP (Backward, Upward, Rightward Pressure) maneuver   technique for facilitating visualization of the vocal cords during endotracheal intubation.

caisson disease   also known as "decompression sickness," the "bends," "diver's paralysis," and "dysbarism."

capnogram   the visual representation of the expired CO_2 waveform.

capnography   a monitoring device that samples and reports the concentration of carbon dioxide (CO_2) in exhaled gases.

cardiac catheterization and electrophysiology lab   a specialized unit where specific diagnostic tests and procedures are performed in order to help diagnose or manage cardiac conditions.

cardiac index (CI)   compares O_2 consumption and CO of different people.

cardiac output   the amount of blood pumped by the heart in one minute.

cardiogenic shock   shock caused by failure or inability of the heart to maintain a level of cardiac output sufficient to perfuse tissues with oxygenated blood.

cardiomyopathies   a group of cardiac disorders in which the dominant feature is dysfunctional involvement of the heart muscle itself.

cardiopulmonary arrest   the absence of organized ventricular contractions, resulting in the cessation of effective blood flow and systemic circulatory failure.

cardiovascular intensive care unit (CVICU)   a specialized unit dedicated to the care of patients with critical cardiovascular insults.

cause-and-effect charts (fishbone diagrams)   useful during brainstorming sessions when a group is trying to understand all the variables that cause a problem.

CBRNE agents   defined as chemical, biological, radiological, nuclear, and/or explosive agents or substances that can cause illness or injury to exposed victims.

central venous pressure (CVP)   the pressure of blood within the vena cava or right atrium.

cerebellum   area of the brain responsible for coordination and stabilization of fine and complex movements; helps determine body's external spatial relationships.

cerebral perfusion pressure (CPP)   measures efficacy of brain perfusion, determined by subtracting the intracranial pressure from the mean arterial pressure. Represented in formula as: MAP − ICP = CPP.

certification and licensure   the mechanism by which a state regulates health care providers practicing within the state's boundaries.

Charles' law   The volume of a quantity of gas, held at constant pressure, varies directly with the temperature of said gas.

chemical thermogenesis   the principal effect of the futile cycle—heat generation.

chickenpox varicella   a rapidly developing, highly infectious disease caused by the human herpesvirus. Presents with slight fever, general malaise, and maculopapular rash that becomes vesicular, then pustular, before crusting over (sometimes called chickenpox, herpes zoster or shingles depending upon the location on/in the body).

"chokes"   a potentially lethal condition hallmarked by chest pain, dyspnea, and pulmonary edema, secondary to pulmonary capillary occlusions.

cholera   debilitating syndrome attributed to enterotoxins produced by the bacteria *Vibrio cholerae;* transmitted through infected food or water.

cholesterol   an important lipid for digestion; required for production of bile slats.

chronic renal failure (CRF)   disruption of normal kidney function that results in patient use of artificial means to filter blood and maintain electrolyte and fluid balance.

chronotrope an agent that causes an increase in heart rate (positive effect).

ciguatera an accumulated toxin encountered in large, reef-dwelling fish that feed on small planktonic organisms and other smaller fish, thus concentrating the toxin.

ciliary body muscle group that connects to the lens via the suspensory ligaments; holds the lens in place and divides the eye into the anterior and posterior chambers.

circle of Willis a series of constituent cerebral arteries located at the midline, anterior portion of the brain that form a circle around the brainstem; the foundation of the arterial system that perfuses the brain, and other collateral areas.

Cnidaria stinging marine animals belonging to the phylum *coelenterates*. Includes jellyfish, Portugese man-of-war, hydroids, fire coral, and sea anemones.

Cobra Perilaryngeal Airway (PLA) a single lumen airway device designed to occlude the supraglottic area and facilitate ventilation.

collective pitch control changes the pitch angle of the main rotor blades to control altitude.

colonoscopy diagnostic examination of the insides of the colon by use of a remote camera on the end of a scope; can be utilized to treat LGIBs.

coma state in which a patient has had no meaningful response to external stimuli for a significant period of time.

common cause variation variations that can be explained by the numerous causes that affect a process.

communication center receives, gathers, disseminates, and coordinates operational and logistical information for each mission.

communication specialist the individual who answers the phone, and/or dispatches missions out to the critical care transport units.

computed tomography (CT) a process by which transverse planes of tissues are swept by a pinpoint radiographic beam allowing the construction of a computerized image.

conduction heat loss due to direct contact with another cooler solid object.

condyloid pivot movable joints.

congenital heart defects congenital abnormalities of the heart, often classified by increased pulmonary blood flow (PDA, ASD), decreased pulmonary blood flow (tetralogy of Fallot), or obstructed blood flow (coarctation of the aorta, aortic, or mitral (tricuspid) or pulmonary stenosis/atresia, and hypoplastic left heart syndrome).

congestive heart failure (CHF) a pathophysiologic state in which the heart is unable to maintain sufficient cardiac output to meet the metabolic needs of the body, leading to increased dyspnea and pulmonary or systemic edema.

consent consent for organ or tissue donation normally received from the donor's legal next-of-kin (LNOK) or donor document.

continuous ambulatory peritoneal dialysis (CAPD) also known as hemodialysis.

continuous intracranial pressure monitoring (ICP) a continuous, direct intracranial pressure measurement technique using an intracranial sensor, transducer, and recording device.

control chart a graph that plots data points in a timeline.

controlled flight into terrain (CFIT) refers to any aircraft flying into the ground, into water, or in/on some other stationary object without adequate awareness or warning by the pilot.

convection heat loss from air currents passing over a surface.

Coombs' test crossmatching blood to check for hemolytic transfusion reactions, and/or to assess for hemolytic disease of the newborn.

Cormack and Lehane classification system four "grade" level airway assessment for use in unconscious patients, defined by the ability to visualize all, part, or none of the glottic opening and/or the vocal cords.

coronary artery bypass graft (CABG) surgical reperfusion technique used to improve the myocardial blood supply for patients with significant coronary artery occlusion, complications of PTCA (such as coronary artery dissection), or AMI.

corrected QT interval (QTc) QT interval adjusted for current heart rate.

cortex a thin layer in the brain comprised of neuronal cell bodies and supporting structures; the epicenter of higher forms of consciousness, thought, and control.

creatine kinase (CK or CPK) isoenzymes important in energy utilization.

creatinine a waste product derived from skeletal muscle, associated with renal function.

crew resource management (CRM) operational implementation of pilot safety briefings, flight crew "comfort levels," education, and a safety conscious culture.

critical care medicine (CCM) medical specialty dedicated to the care and transport of critically ill or injured patients.

critical care paramedics EMT-paramedics who have completed additional formal education in the care and transport of critically ill or injured patients.

critical thermal maximum a core temperature equal to or greater than 43°C (109.4°F).

critical values life-threatening values or "panic" values.

croup (laryngotracheobronchitis) a viral pulmonary infection most common in children with a recent history of upper respiratory infections (URIs).

CT (CAT) scanning use of focused X-ray beams to examine various body areas.

Cullen's sign   blood in the abdomen that has tracked to the umbilicus through the ligamentum teres, resulting in periumbilical bruising.

cyanotic heart defects   systemic cyanosis due to poor pulmonary perfusion, shunting of deoxygenated blood from right to left, or structural deformity of the heart.

cyclic pitch control   controls the direction and airspeed of the helicopter, and is commonly referred to as the "stick."

cystogram   X-ray study used in the diagnosis of urethral or bladder injury; contrast media is placed into the urethra. Any extravasation of contrast from the urethra or bladder seen on serial radiograph indicates injury.

D-dimer   the degradation products of cross-linked fibrin.

Dalton's law   the total pressure in a container is the sum of the partial pressures of all the gases in the container.

deceleration   during uterine contraction, a normal, gradual decrease in FHR below baseline of greater than 30 seconds duration, then gradual return to baseline.

decompression sickness   a condition caused by the expansion of nitrogen in the tissues following a dive of significant depth and duration. Also known as; "caisson disease," the "bends," "diver's paralysis," and "dysbarism."

deep peroneal reflex   reflex arc involving L_4, L_5, and S_1 spinal segments mediated through deep peroneal nerve.

Denis system   method most commonly used to describe lumbar vertebral fractures.

depolarizing blocking agent   short acting medications that depolarize the synaptic membrane of the muscle, causing total paralysis from 3 to 5 minutes.

detailed physical exam   methodical assessment designed to identify non-life-threatening conditions, general abnormalities, and adequacy of interventions.

devascularization   loss of blood supply to an organ or a part of the body.

diagnostic noninvasive cardiology lab   a specialized unit where specific diagnostic tests and procedures are performed in order to help diagnose or manage cardiac conditions.

diagnostic peritoneal lavage (DPL)   technique for ascertaining the presence of blood in the abdomen via insertion of a catheter into the peritoneal cavity, then aspirating fluids for examination.

diaphragmatic rupture   a defect in the diaphragm that occurs as a result of severe blunt or penetrating injury to the abdomen or lower thorax.

diarthrosis   joints, or the connection between two bones, classified as movable.

difficult airway   a clinical situation in which a conventionally trained paramedic experiences difficulty with mask ventilation and/or endotracheal intubation.

digital systems   systems capable of translating analog voice transmission into digital code for fast, accurate, and secured broadcast.

dilation and curettage (D&C)   a surgical procedure used to diagnose or treat abnormal bleeding from the uterus; involves *dilation* of the cervix and *curettage* of endometrial tissue for later examination.

diplopia   double vision.

distributive shock   shock caused by decreased vascular resistance, or increased venous capacity, resulting from vasomotor dysfunction.

Divers Alert Network (DAN)   a nonprofit medical and research organization dedicated to the safety and health of scuba divers.

diverticula   a defect in the wall of the colon; an "outpouching" of the colonic mucosa.

drowning   death from suffocation due to submersion in a liquid within 24 hours of insult.

drug abuse   the intentional abuse of medication or illicit drugs; includes addiction, physical dependence, and tolerance.

drug toxicity   harmful levels of a drug in the blood stream.

ductus arteriosus (DA)   during fetal development, a vascular connection that joins the right ventricle and pulmonary artery directly to the descending aorta, bypassing the immature lungs.

ductus venosus   vessel that leads directly into the vena cava that allows some oxygenated blood and nutrients to be pumped directly out of the body, bypassing the kidneys.

dysoxia   falling energy yield from glucose when oxygen supply to tissue fails or is reduced dramatically.

eclamptic   broadly defined as seizure activity or coma unrelated to other cerebral conditions in an obstetrical patient; usually associated with preeclampsia.

egophony   describes the distortion of voice transmission, as heard through the stethoscope, when a patient is instructed to speak during auscultation of the lungs.

electrolytes   chemical substances that take on an electrical charge when dissolved in water.

electronic fetal monitoring (EFM)   the electronic evaluation and/or monitoring of uterine contractions and fetal heart rate by *Doppler wave* or other methods.

emergency locator transmitter (ELT)   device mounted to the aircraft designed to emit a distress radio signal upon impact of the aircraft.

emergent phase   the initial phase immediately following the burn; includes pain response and the systemic effects of massive catecholamine release, as well as the physical and emotional stresses associated with being burned.

empty weight   weight of the helicopter (includes structure, fixed equipment, fuel/hydraulic liquids) minus passengers and portable equipment.

EMTALA and COBRA legislation   federal legislation addressing appropriate licensure and skills of medical personnel involved with patient care and transport, as well as stabilization of patients prior to transport.

enarthrosis   ball and socket movable joints.

endoscopy   diagnostic examination of the insides of organs or body cavities by use of a remote camera on the end of a scope; can be utilized to identify and treat UGIBs.

engines   affixed directly to the airframe and supply power to both rotor systems.

enophthalmos   a posterior displacement of the eye.

enucleation   traumatic removal of the globe from the orbit.

environmental scanning   operational scanning that looks for changes in clinical literature that might affect the protocols and clinical management of patients in your system.

epiglottitis   an acute, severe, life-threatening disease characterized by inflammation and edema of the epiglottis and surrounding connected tissues.

epiphysis   the cartilaginous bone growth plate, also called the physis.

erythrocyte sedimentation rate (sed rate)   a nonspecific hematologic test that can point to various problems. An elevated sed rate is associated with pregnancy, autoimmune disease, and inflammation, as well as diagnostic for temporal arteritis.

esophageal perforation   tear or rupture of the esophagus.

Esophageal Tracheal CombiTube® (ETC)   a dual-lumen airway device with a ventilation port for each lumen, designed for blind insertion that permits ventilation with BVM via either tube, as required.

ethics   self-imposed standards or rules governing conduct by members of a group, profession, or society.

eustachian tube   the auditory tube; found between the middle ear and the nasopharynx.

evaporation   heat loss that occurs as water changes from a liquid to a vapor.

external auditory meatus (EAM)   external landmark, a.k.a. the "ear canal." Visually correlates with the level of the lateral ventricles within the brain.

external fixation   application of external metal or composite framework applied with pins, screws, and rods to the bone, keeping proper alignment, while fracture is visualized under fluoroscopy.

extrauterine   life and growth outside the uterus.

Federal Aviation Administration (FAA)   federal agency whose mission is to regulate, control, and provide for a safe and efficient aerospace system.

Federal Communications Commission (FCC)   an independent United States government agency for regulating interstate and international communications, as well as issuing frequency licenses and assigning call letters utilized on assigned radio bands.

fibrinolytics   chemicals/drugs used to lyse coronary thrombi, thus improving oxygen supply to the myocardium. Also known as thrombolytics.

Fick method   standard technique for measuring CO in pulmonary blood flow.

Fick's law   the net diffusion rate of a gas across a fluid membrane is proportional to the difference in partial pressure, proportional to the area of the membrane, and inversely proportional to the thickness of the membrane.

filoviruses   class of viruses, such as the Ebola and Marburg fevers, that cause systemic hemorrhage and are often fatal.

filtration   filtration of blood through a complex arrangement of capillaries that maintain pressure through the glomerulus during transient fluctuations in systemic blood pressure.

fixed-wing transport   the transport of a patient by fixed-wing aircraft.

flail chest   defined as 3 or more ribs broken in 2 or more places.

flicker vertigo   an imbalance in brain cell activity created by light sources that emit a flickering (rather than steady) light.

flight paramedics   paramedics with specialized skills and education in the care of critically injured or ill patients transported via helicopter or fixed-wing aircraft.

flowchart   used to document a given process with the goal of understanding what the current process looks like, finding inefficiencies, and removing them.

fluid shift phase   phase in which fluid movement occurs; begins shortly after the burn, reaches a peak in 6–8 hours, and can last for up to 18–24 hours.

focused assessment with sonography for trauma (FAST)   ultrasound assessment designed to detect blood in the pericardium or abdomen, secondary to traumatic injury.

Foley catheter   A large diameter tube attached to a metered drainage bag; inserted into the urethral meatus for bladder drainage and to measure urine output.

foot pedals   allows the pilot to control the pitch angle of the tail rotor.

foramen ovale   during fetal development, an opening between the left and right atria that allows blood to enter the left atrium of the heart from the right atrium.

full duplex system   system that can transmit and receive voice or data simultaneously that employs one frequency for transmitting and a different one for receiving (usually found in the UHF bands).

fulminant hepatic failure (FHF)   described as acute liver failure associated with hepatic encephalopathy; presents a life-threatening medical emergency.

fungus   a saprophytic and parasitic spore-producing organism that lacks chlorophyll; includes mold, rust, mildew, smut, mushroom, and yeast.

fuselage   external body of the aircraft surrounding the airframe and all of its components.

futile cycles a metabolic process, most often occurring in muscles, when the body activates specialized biochemical pathways in order to generate heat.

gastritis a superficial erosion and chronic inflammation of the gastric mucosa; can be a precursor to peptic ulcers.

gastroenteritis an inflammation and infection within the GI tract.

Gay-Lussac's law the pressure of a fixed amount of gas (fixed number of moles) at a fixed volume, proportional to the temperature.

gestation the time between fertilization of an oocyte until birth; in humans the average is 266 days.

gestational diabetes mellitus (GDM) diabetes, regardless of type, that initially presents during pregnancy, and usually resolves postdelivery.

ginglymus hinge movable joints.

glossoptosis a downward or posterior displacement of the tongue.

glycohemoglobin the amount of glucose bound to hemoglobin; indicates recent regulation of glucose levels in diabetic patients.

Graham's law the rate at which gasses diffuse, inversely proportional to the square root of their densities.

Gram stains bacteria identified with various stains and then classified as gram positive or gram negative (whether they take the stain(s) or not).

Grandview™ blade laryngoscope blade with an 80% wider blade surface and anatomically appropriate curve for improved visualization.

gravitational forces the forces of attraction between all masses in the universe; more commonly the attraction of the Earth's mass for bodies near its surface.

Grey Turner's sign retroperitoneal bleeding that causes bruising to the flank.

gross weight total of empty weight plus useful payload.

ground transport systems medical transport of ill or injured patients via ground ambulance.

gum elastic bougie a straight, semirigid stylette-like device with a tip bent at about 30 degrees to facilitate difficult intubations. (Also called Eschmann tracheal tube.)

Gustilo grading system method of grading open fractures.

Haddon matrix applied theory about injury prevention. The core concept is that the energy transfer that causes trauma is predictable, and can be prevented in many cases by manipulating the environment, agent, the host's behavior, or a combination of these.

half-duplex system system that uses two different frequencies for transmitting and receiving, but only allows for unidirectional communication flow (typically found in the UHF "high-bands").

half-life the time in which it takes one-half of a particular drug to be eliminated from the blood/body.

hangman's fracture injury and fracture of the C2 vertebral body; usually without obvious neurological deficit, unless a C2–C3 facet dislocation is present.

hantavirus group of viruses that cause potentially lethal respiratory syndromes in humans; transmitted by respiratory exposure to the aerosolized feces of infected mice.

hazardous materials describes the significant danger from chemicals and/or biological agents, with regard to type, volume, and concentrations of such agents.

HDL high-density lipoproteins, a component of cholesterol.

heat cramps painful muscle cramps that are a frequent complication of heat exhaustion, secondary to salt depletion, and other electrolyte and fluid abnormalities.

heat exhaustion heat emergency resulting from cardiovascular strain as the body struggles against derangements in bodily functions occurring at temperatures between 39.4°–40°C (102.9°–104°F).

heat index system based on the Fahrenheit scale; allows an accurate measure of how it really feels when relative humidity is added to actual air temperature.

heat syncope postural hypotension, secondary to massive peripheral vasodilation and dehydration, that occurs when the body attempts to rapidly cool itself.

heat tetany hyperventilation syndrome in conjunction with respiratory alkalosis and carpopedal spasms.

heat the kinetic energy of molecules in motion.

heatstroke a life-threatening emergency described by a triad of signs and symptoms that include a core temperature greater that 104.9°F (40.5°C), anhidrosis, and CNS dysfunction.

HELLP an acronym for *H*emolysis, *E*levated *L*iver function tests, and *L*ow *P*latelets that describes a subcategory of severe preeclampsia.

hematology the testing and study of blood and its various elements.

hemiblock a block of one of the two fascicles of the left-bundle-branch system.

hemochromogens oxygen-carrying compounds (hemoglobin and myoglobin) found in the body; they are released through the process of rhabdomyolysis.

hemodialysis external process for filtering waste products from the blood stream by means of scheduled and continuous ambulatory peritoneal dialysis (CAPD).

hemodynamic parameters may include ECG, ABP, CVP, CO, PCWP, SV, and DO_2 saturation. These (and others) can assist the practitioner in trending and diagnosis.

hemothorax rapid accumulation of blood and fluid in the pleural cavity which can result in severe respiratory and hemodynamic compromise.

Hemovac drainage system rigid plastic housing with internal springs that is compressed and attached to the proximal end of a drainage tube, thereby plugging a vent hole and creating a closed, low-pressure system.

Henry's law at equilibrium, the amount of gas dissolved in a given volume of liquid, directly proportional to the partial pressure of that gas in the gas phase.

hepatitis an inflammation of the liver that can lead to organ failure and death.

herbal medications "natural" products that may not have been subjected to the rigors of scientific testing, as are prescription or other over-the-counter (OTC) drugs.

high-altitude cerebral edema (HACE) considered to be end-stage, severe, acute mountain sickness (AMS). Classic initial symptoms include headache, insomnia, anorexia, nausea, and dizziness.

high-altitude pulmonary edema (HAPE) a potentially lethal condition caused by accumulation of fluid in the lungs following rapid ascent to high altitude.

high-pressure neurologic syndrome (HPNS) also known as "helium tremors," HPNS is the result of breathing pressurized helium and oxygen at depths exceeding 400 feet.

histogram data chart used to demonstrate how frequently something occurs.

horizontal and vertical stabilizers provide stabilization of flight altitude while airborne.

Horner's syndrome caused by injury to the sympathetic nerves of the face, it causes a triad of constricted pupil, ptosis, and facial dryness (anhidrosis).

hospice medical institutions designed to care for and relieve the physical and emotional suffering of the dying.

hosts persons or animals who may become (or are) infected with pathogenic microorganisms.

human immunodeficiency virus (HIV) a retrovirus that attacks the immune system, consisting of two identified types similar in epidemiologic characteristics; HIV-1 appears more pathogenic than HIV-2.

hydrocephalus describes the abnormal accumulation of cerebrospinal fluid in the brain.

hyperbaric chamber a medical device used to recompress internal gases in patients suffering from decompression sickness or *AGE*, as well as injuries related to necropsy in diabetes, and so on.

hypercapnia high levels of carbon dioxide in arterial blood.

hyperkalemia abnormally elevated potassium.

hypermetabolic phase the healing phase of a burn; may last from days to weeks depending on the severity of the injury.

hypertensive emergency severe, accelerated hypertension, with a diastolic blood pressure greater than 140 mmHg, leading to a constellation of systemic findings that can include end-organ damage or "shut down."

hyphema a collection of blood in the anterior chamber of the eye.

hypokalemia abnormally low potassium.

hypoperfusion lack of adequately oxygenated blood to effectively sustain tissue at the cellular, organ, or system level.

hypothalamus a portion of the diencephalon, located immediately superior to the brainstem and inferior to the thalamus. Primarily responsible for regulation of body temperature, water balance, and thirst.

hypothermia defined as a body core temperature of less than 95°F (35°C).

hypovolemic shock shock caused by reduced intravascular circulating volume, resulting from hemorrhage, third-space fluid shifts, and/or systemic fluid loss (dehydration).

ICP waveform representation of the pulsations created by the cardiovascular system, translated through CSF into the brain parenchyma via the choroid plexus.

ideal gas law an ideal gas (perfect gas) is one that obeys Boyle's law, Charles' law, and Avogadro's law exactly.

in-flight emergency situation affecting flight stability or safety of the aircraft itself.

in-flight procedures safety tasks designed to assure the highest degree of safety is maintained during flight operations.

incapacitating and irritant agents chemical agents that produce transient pain and involuntary eye closures, incapacitating the exposed patient for short periods of time.

induction agents medications used for sedation, prior to paralysis, during RSI.

infectious disease a condition caused by the invasion and multiplication of pathogenic microorganisms within the body.

influenza (the flu) dangerous respiratory infection caused by a virus that may lead to complications of pneumonia and death.

initial assessment immediate assessment of life threats and transport priority.

Injury Severity Score (ISS) scoring system calculated retrospectively by adding the squares of the highest of the seven Abbreviated Injury Scale (AIS) scores (score of 1 to 75).

inotropic an agent that causes the myocardium to contract more forcefully.

Instrument Flight Rules (IFR) FAA regulations setting minimum standards for use of VFR in conjunction with specialized flight instruments during times of low visibility and/or poor weather.

instrument landing system (ILS) system that provides information to the pilot about vertical movement (that is, gaining or losing of altitude) of the aircraft via the instruments.

internal fixation the internal placement of rods, plates, screws, and nails is performed through a surgical opening in the skin to stabilize a fractured bone.

International Normalized Ratio (INR) the INR reports PT in a more standardized form, comparing it to a preestablished control.

interventional radiology lab a specialized unit where specific radiological tests are performed in order to help diagnose or manage a variety of conditions, either medical or trauma related.

interventricular (IV) blocks conduction blocks that occur in the interventricular pathways and include fascicular and bundle branch blocks.

intra-aortic balloon pump (IABP) a balloon inserted into the aortic arch controlled by an external pulsating pump; used to augment cardiac output when other therapies available for cardiogenic shock have failed or cannot be used.

intracranial pressure (ICP) the pressure within the cranial vault.

intrarenal failure trauma, infection, or disease that causes direct damage to kidney parenchyma; causes disruption of normal kidney function and can result in total organ failure.

intrauterine growth and development within the uterus.

intubating laryngeal mask airway (LMA Fastrach®) a single lumen airway device designed to facilitate endotracheal intubation and ventilation.

ionization when radiation interacts with atoms, energy is deposited, resulting in the process called ionization.

ischemia injury to an area of myocardial cells that may be followed by cellular death (infarction) if perfusion of oxygenated blood is not restored.

J (or Osborne) wave thought to represent a distortion of the earliest stage of repolarization; causes a "hitched up" appearance at the beginning of the ST segment.

Jackson-Pratt drainage system tubing placed at or near a surgical incision site with the proximal end attached to a "hand-grenade"-sized compressed bulb creating a closed, low-pressure drainage system.

Jackson's theory of thermal wounds a zone theory that reflects the effects of high heat on human tissue (zone of coagulation, stasis, and hyperemia).

jaundice results from high serum bilirubin levels (due to immature liver function) in neonates; presents as a yellowish discoloration of the skin and the sclera of the eyes.

Jefferson (burst) fracture vertebral fractures normally associated with spinal compression injury, as in anterior arch, posterior arch, and lateral mass fractures.

Kehr's sign blood in the peritoneum that irritates the diaphragm and causes referred pain in the shoulder as nerve impulses travel to nerve roots in the lower cervical spine.

key results areas (KRAs) areas of interest that may include clinical performance, customer satisfaction, employee satisfaction, equipment performance, fleet performance, safety, and financial operations.

King LT airway a supraglottic, reuseable, airway that stabilizes the airway at the base of the tongue, via the inflation of a large silicone cuff.

laboratory tests specific studies or assays performed on various body tissues.

laboratory values analysis of a specimen in comparison with a set of controls and known parameters.

lacrimal glands glands that secrete lacrimal fluid, which moistens and lubricates the surface of the eye.

lacrimators irritant gases and solutions (i.e., tear gas and capsaicin spray); induce temporary debilitation by means of irritation to the mucous membranes and respiratory tree, as well as uncontrolled watering of the affected eyes(s) and the nose.

lactic acid toxic metabolic by-product of pyruvic acid, as a result of anaerobic metabolism.

lactic acidosis a common cause of metabolic acidosis; a result of abnormal conversion of pyruvate (pyruvic acid) into lactate during hypoxic or anaerobic states.

lactic dehydrogenase (LD or LDH) enzyme found in heart muscle, skeletal muscle, liver, erythrocytes, kidney, and some types of tumors.

laparotomy a surgical incision into a cavity of the abdomen.

Laryngeal Mask Airway (LMA) a noninvasive, single lumen airway device designed to occlude the supraglottic area and facilitate ventilation.

LDL low-density lipoproteins, transport cholesterol in the plasma.

Le Fort system classification system for defining maxillary fractures according to structure(s) involved and seriousness.

Le Système International d'Unités a comprehensive form of the metric system that deals in more precise measurements (abbreviated SI units) than standard metric.

leadership the ability to focus on the system as a whole and understand all applicable processes in an effort to determine what is wrong and effect positive change.

left-anterior hemiblock anterior hemi-fascicular block of the left bundle branch, effectively causes a pathological left-axis deviation.

left-posterior hemiblock posterior fascicular block of the left-bundle branch, effectively causes a pathological right-axis deviation.

lipoproteins specialized proteins that transport the lipids in the blood serum.

Lown-Ganong-Levine syndrome (LGL) pre-excitation syndrome characterized by possible existence of intra- and/or para-nodal fibers that bypass all or part of the (AV) node.

Lund and Browder method accurate method of determining the area of a burn; calculates TBSA while accounting for developmental (age) changes in percentage.

magnetic resonance imaging (MRI) high-quality magnetic images of body areas without the use of ionizing radiation.

main rotor system horizontal blade above the fuselage that produces lift and thrust for the aircraft as it spins.

malignant hypertension persistent state resulting from end-organ damage, secondary to both acute and chronic episodes of hypertension, clinical signs and symptoms vary depending upon the organs involved.

Mallampati classification system four "class" level airway assessment for use in conscious patients, defined by the ability to visualize all, part, or none of the tonsillar pillars and/or the uvula.

Mallory-Weiss syndrome upper GI bleed secondary to a longitudinal tear in the cardio-esophageal region: can be caused by retching, vomiting, forceful coughing, long-term use of NSAIDs, salicylates, and/or alcohol use.

malocclusion a misfit of the occlusal surfaces of the teeth upon mouth closure.

manual airway maneuvers manual manipulations of the airway, including head-tilt/chin-lift, jaw-thrust maneuver, and modified jaw-thrust.

Marfan's disease a genetic connective tissue disorder that causes a weakening of vascular tissue, among other problems.

Marriott lead same as MCL-1, also know as the "Gold Mine Lead."

Material Safety Data Sheet (MSDS) federally mandated product descriptions that contain specific information about an individual product, including the chemical name, brand name, health effects, and the Chemical Abstracts Service number (CAS#).

maximum gross weight certified maximum weight for safe flight operations.

mean arterial pressure (MAP) true systemic "driving" pressure for peripheral blood flow.

measles rubeola a highly contagious viral infection characterized by prodromal symptoms of cough, fever, conjunctivitis, coryza, malaise, and anorexia (sometimes called hard measles and/or red measles).

mediastinal emphysema described as a tear in pulmonary tissues along the central area of the mediastinum. Symptoms can include dysphasia and tracheal pressure; extreme cases may present as *cardiac tamponade*.

medical crew configurations the crew mix for any particular mission, as determined jointly by the program director and the medical director.

medical director physician who creates and implements medical protocols, ensures proper crew training, conducts quality assurance program, and provides on-line medical direction.

medical imaging use of technology to electronically visualize the body.

medical intensive care unit (MICU) a specialized unit dedicated to the intensive care of critically ill patients.

medical practice act state-level legislation that includes language clearly defining what a prehospital care provider can and cannot do, as well as where and when they can do it.

medical/social/behavioral history an interview conducted to identify donors who may be at high risk for hepatitis or HIV, and/or to identify underlying medical conditions that may affect the safety and quality of the organs and tissues.

meningitis potentially life-threatening inflammation of the meningeal layers; can be either bacterial or viral.

meningococcal infections caused by a gram-negative diplococcus bacteria called *Neisseria meningitidis;* responsible for several serious infections including meningococcal meningitis and meningococcemia.

metabolic requirement for oxygen (MRO$_2$) the rate at which oxygen is utilized in the conversion of glucose to energy and water, via the glycolysis/tricarboxylic acid (TCA) cycle.

metazoa/helminths parasitic segmented worms; includes tapeworms, liver flukes, roundworms, and pinworms.

microwave landing system (MLS) system that provides information to the pilot about vertical movement (that is, gaining or losing of altitude) of the aircraft via the instruments.

Minnesota tube similar to the Sengstaken-Blakemore, but also has an esophageal aspiration lumen that allows for suctioning of collected esophageal secretions.

modified central lead 1 (MCL-1) a bipolar version of lead V$_1$. With ECG monitor set to Lead III or V$_1$, electrode placement is RA (white), LA (black), and LL (red), at the right side, 4th intercostal space.

modified chest lead 6 (MCL-6) same as V6 on 12-lead. Set monitor to Lead III, rotate LL (red) electrode wire (LL) to the 5th IC space, mid-axillary, left side.

MODS multiple organ dysfunction syndrome a sequential or concomitant occurrence of a significant derangement of function in two or more organ systems of the body, against a background of a critical illness.

Monroe-Kellie hypothesis the intracranial vault is a fixed space that contains brain tissue, blood, and cerebrospinal fluid. Volume expansion of any (or all) of these components will increase ICP unless the volume of one of the other components is reduced.

morbidity and mortality (M&M) conference a meeting to audit and discuss cases that address or identify quality assurance issues raised by the resident medical staff in an effort to evaluate performance and patient care modality or outcomes.

Morrison's pouch the hepatorenal space, a recess of the peritoneal cavity that lies between the liver in front and the kidney and adrenal behind.

mucosa a layer of simple or stratified epithelium (depending upon the location), moistened by the secretions of mucous glands.

MUDPILES mnemonic used to identify the most common causes of metabolic acidosis, as in–*M*ethanol; *U*remia; *D*iabetic ketoacidosis; *P*araldehyde; *I*nfection; *L*actic acidosis; *E*thylene *g*lycol; *S*alicylates.

multiplex systems system that combines two or more information channels into a common transmission medium using a multiplexer (MUX); capable of concurrent voice and data communications.

mumps a virus that causes an acute infection of one or both parotid glands (sometimes involves salivary glands), characterized by fever and swollen, tender glands.

muscularis externa smooth muscle layers arranged in an inner, circular layer covered by an outer, longitudinal layer, as in the muscularis mucosae.

mycotoxins agents, Trichothecene mycotoxins, produced by filamentous fungae; may be inhaled, ingested, or absorbed through the skin and mucous membranes.

myocardial contusions a result of severe blunt force trauma, the heart is compressed between the sternum and the spinal column, resulting in a "bruised heart."

myocardial rupture the most lethal of all thoracic injuries, occurs as a result of major blunt force trauma.

myoglobin hemeprotein found in striated muscle; contains iron, stores oxygen, gives muscle its red color.

nasointestinal tubes small-bore (8- to 10-French) tubes inserted via a nare into the small intestine to support nutrition: commonly referred to as feeding tubes.

National Fire Protection Association (NFPA) "Risk Watch" program injury prevention and public education campaigns aimed primarily at school aged children.

National Pediatric Trauma Registry (NPTR) organization that monitors and tracks annual statistical figures related to injuries and deaths in children and adolescents.

National Transportation Safety Board (NTSB) federal agency charged with investigating civil aviation accidents and other transportation accidents in the United States.

near-drowning survival of suffocation due to submersion in a liquid past the 24-hour point of insult.

necrotizing enterocolitis (NEC) ischemic damage to the lining of the stomach and/or intestines and bacterial growth that results in acute inflammation of the large intestine with subsequent necrosis of the intestinal mucosa.

necrotizing fasciitis (NF) an insidious soft tissue infection characterized by widespread fascial necrosis.

negative feedback loop a response that continually reacts in a negative manner to a particular stimulus.

neonatal intensive care unit (NICU) a specialized unit dedicated to the care of critically ill or injured neonatal patients.

neonatal respiratory distress syndrome a lack of pulmonary surfactant causes significant difficulty in breathing; also known as hyaline membrane disease.

nerve agents chemicals developed for war (CWs) or industrial chemicals that inhibit the uptake of acetylcholinesterase (AChE), and affect the function of the CNS.

neurogenic shock shock caused by damage to the sympathetic nervous system causing reduction in PVR secondary to widespread vasodilation.

neuroglia various cells within the brain that comprise the supportive structures surrounding neurons.

neurohumoral response stress mechanism that increases cardiac output through increased heart rate contractility, vasoconstriction, fluid retention, and supports other metabolic functions in response to shock states.

neurologic death defined as the complete irreversible cessation of all brain and brainstem activity.

neuromuscular-blocking agents medications used to induce muscle relaxation, thus facilitating endotracheal intubation.

nitrogen narcosis an intoxicating effect of unclear etiology that appears to affect the brain in a manner similar to alcohol or narcotics, and affects diver judgment.

nondepolarizing blocking agents medications that block acetylcholine's neurotransmitter action, rendering muscles flaccid without depolarizing the synaptic membrane.

nondistributive shock also known as hypovolemic or hemorrhagic shock, the circulating volume is diminished or lost from within the vascular space.

noninvasive monitoring devices devices used to assist in patient trending and care; they include pulse oximeters, continuous waveform capnography units, automated blood pressure devices, self-registering or digital thermometers, and ECG machines.

noninvasive positive-pressure ventilation (NPPV) ventilatory therapy that provides constant positive gas pressure via mask. Also known as CPAP (continuous positive airway pressure) and BiPaP (bilevel positive airway pressure).

normal reference values nationally established parameters based upon a large number of lab tests conducted over several years, affected by gender and age.

obstructive shock shock caused by impedance of the circulatory flow, resulting from blockage, compression, embolic, dissecting, and/or tamponade type insults.

optic canal the passageway for the optic nerve (CN II), from the optic disc to the sphenoid bone.

orbit the bony recess that contains the eye, comprised of the frontal, zygomatic, and temporal bones.

organ donors neurologically dead patients who must be carefully monitored and managed in order to optimize organ function for the organ recipients.

organ procurement organizations (OPOs) organizations designated by the federal government to recover organs for transplantation.

organophosphate (OP) compounds potent warfare agents that may be lethal to humans; includes nerve agents (such as tabun, sarin, soman, and VX).

osteoarthritis inflammation of a joint resulting from wearing of the articular cartilage.

ostomy removal of the diseased bowel, and surgical attachment of the proximal bowel to the surface of the abdomen with a portal that facilitates defecation.

oxygen delivery (DO_2) the amount of measurable oxygen delivered to the tissues.

oxygen uptake (VO_2) the actual amount of oxygen withdrawn from the circulation at the capillary level.

$PaCO_2$ carbon dioxide level in arterial blood.

pancreatitis inflammation of the pancreas caused by disruption of the pancreatic ducts; interferes with the normal release of digestive enzymes.

PaO_2 oxygen level in arterial blood.

Pareto chart a vertical bar-based chart that visually demonstrates which problem is the most frequent.

Parkland formula widely used standard for fluid resuscitation (partial- and full-thickness burns); utilizes patient's weight, and percentage of TBSA involved. Represented in formula as: 4 mL × kg of body wt × TBSA%.

partial thromboplastin time (PTT) the PTT, also called the activated partial thromboplastin time. Used to detect coagulation disorders and monitor heparin therapy.

patient care associate a person who works in conjunction with other health care providers in caring for patients.

patient care report (PCR) the written documentation that is prepared following completion of a patient contact or transport.

pediatric assessment triangle (PAT) method assessment that uses appearance, breathing, and circulation status to determine a child's overall condition.

pediatric Glasgow Coma Scale a method of assessing and monitoring neurological status; assigns a numerical value to different levels of verbal response, motor function, and eye movement.

pediatric intensive care unit (PICU) a specialized unit dedicated to the care of critically ill or injured pediatric patients.

Pediatric Trauma Score (PTS) modified version of the trauma score accounting for pediatric differences in normal vital sign ranges, developmental levels, and increased physiological reserve, as compared to adults.

Penrose drain a flat, 0.5–1.0 inch diameter, single-lumen tube inserted into a surgical site to promote drainage of large amounts of fluid.

penumbra describes a region of tissue that will become necrotic after an infarct occurs if perfusion is not restored.

peptic ulcer disease (PUD) mucosal defect in a portion of the stomach or duodenum exposed to acid or peptic secretions.

percutaneous transluminal coronary angioplasty (PTCA) mechanical method used to restore perfusion in coronary arteries blocked or constricted by atherosclerotic disease.

perialveolar capillary bed the network of capillaries surrounding the alveoli.

pericardial tamponade hemodynamic compromise resulting in decreased cardiac output, as a result of blood accumulation in the pericardial space between the pericardial sac and the heart itself.

pericardiocentesis insertion of a specialized needle into the pericardial sac as a means of aspirating blood or other fluids.

perimeter guards ground personnel who secure the landing zone, normally stationed at least 50 feet from the aircraft, and remain in direct visualization of the pilot.

peritoneal dialysis catheter a flexible, siliconized rubber catheter surgically placed into the abdominal cavity to facilitate the administration and removal of dialysate solutions.

permissive hypotension purposeful maintenance of a lower systolic pressure that will maintain perfusion to the heart, brain, lungs, and kidneys during the initial phases of trauma resuscitation, without "popping the clot."

persistent pulmonary hypertension of the newborn (PPHN) a clinical syndrome in which the ductus arteriosus and foramen ovale remain open after birth, increasing pulmonary vascular resistance and causing cardio-respiratory distress.

pharmacodynamics the study of what a drug does to the body as it alters cellular and tissue activity in order to achieve a clinical response.

pharmacokinetics the study of how the body absorbs, distributes, transports, inactivates, and eliminates a drug.

pharmacology the study of drugs, and how they relate to altering the body's activities.

pharyngotracheal lumen (PtL) airway a dual-lumen airway device designed for blind insertion that permits ventilation with BVM via either tube, as required.

phonetic alphabet and numeric system a set of radio protocols created by The International Civil Aviation Organization (ICAO); used by air traffic controllers and aircraft pilots for consistency and accurate communications.

physical dependence a syndrome wherein withdrawal syndromes can be produced by abrupt cessation, rapid dose reduction, decreasing blood level of drug, or administration of an antagonist.

physiologic shunt introduction of deoxygenated blood into the pulmonary vein from drainage of the coronary and bronchial veins, combined with the normal variances of alveolar perfusion and ventilation secondary to gravity.

physiologic zone the atmospheric zone in which oxygen levels are sufficient to sustain a normal, healthy individual—up to 10,000 feet above sea level.

physiologically deficient zone the atmospheric zone in which barometric pressure is decreased, trapping evolved gases potentially harmful to humans, and causing hypoxia—10,000 to 15,000 feet above sea level.

piloerection physiological response that causes the hairs in the skin to stand erect; commonly referred to as "goose bumps" or "goose flesh."

pilot safety brief a mission specific operational discussion led by the pilot that includes aircraft and weather information, as well as landing zone and other safety issues.

pinna the portion of the ear (auricle) that is visually exposed.

placenta previa occurs when the placenta implants and develops in the lower third of the uterus, totally or partially covering the cervical os.

placenta the blood-rich structure that facilitates the exchange of nutrients and wastes between the mother and fetus; also produces hormones necessary for the maintenance of pregnancy and fetal development.

plague caused by the bacteria *Yersinia pestis*. The bubonic form presents as abrupt onset of high fever, headache, and painful, swollen regional lymph nodes. The pneumonic (and highly contagious) form presents with additional respiratory symptoms.

platysma a thin, superficial muscle covering mostly the neck; located just below the subcutaneous tissue and surrounded by the superficial fascial layer.

pneumonia swelling and obstruction of the lungs by fiberlike fluids and/or mucus; commonly contracted by inhalation of the *Diplococcus pneumoniae* bacteria, rickettsiae, a virus, or a fungi.

POGO classification system airway assessment used by some EMS personnel to rate the percentage of glottic opening (POGO) one can visualize from "0" to "100" percent (all).

poison control center (PCC) information banks that assist with the triage and management of patients with (potentially) toxic exposures.

positron emission tomography (PET) imaging modalities capable of observing organ function, especially in the brain.

post-accident duties hazard mitigation, rescue operations, and location and/or activation of emergency locator transmitter (ELT) immediately following an unplanned landing (regardless of significance of impact).

post-flight safety procedures tasks designed for safe landing and exiting of the aircraft upon arrival.

post-renal failure result of clinical conditions that cause obstruction to urine flow.

posterior cavity the larger of the two cavities, encompassing all of the area behind the lens.

preeclampsia potentially life-threatening (both mother and fetus) syndrome of combined hypertension and proteinuria in the third trimester of pregnancy.

preflight procedures tasks completed prior to each mission designed to ensure the highest degree of flight safety for each flight is maintained.

premature rupture of membranes (PROM) a significant risk factor associated with premature labor and can lead to endometritis, septicemia and septic shock, chorioamnionitis, premature delivery, and fetal or neonatal death.

premedications medications used to blunt or attenuate various adverse side effects of neuromuscular blockers.

preoptic region located in the hypothalamus, this area is the principal center for thermoregulation.

prerenal failure a decrease or loss of perfusion to the kidney, causing ischemic changes that are reflected in the subsequent loss of renal function.

prions protein particles that lack nucleic acid; cause of various infectious diseases of the nervous system (formerly referred to as "slow viruses").

professionalism the conduct or qualities that characterize the standard of excellence in a particular field or occupation.

program director person who coordinates daily operations and directs flight program strategy and growth.

prothrombin time (PT) prothrombin is factor II in the coagulation cascade, produced by the liver and essential to normal blood coagulation.

protozoa unicellular organisms, including some pathogenic parasites that can infect humans.

ptosis drooping of the eyelid.

pulmonary agents chemicals that can be readily absorbed across pulmonary tissue; commonly released as a vapor and may be lethal in relatively low concentrations.

pulmonary artery pressure (PAP) pressure within the pulmonary artery throughout the cardiac cycle.

pulmonary artery wedge pressure (PAWP) measures left atrial and left ventricular end-diastolic pressure, normal range is 8 to 12 mmHg.

pulmonary contusions an area of "bruised lung" resulting from blunt force trauma to the thoracic wall, most commonly seen in conjunction with flail segments.

pulmonary surfactant a combination of phospholipids that serve to decrease the surface tension of water in the alveoli, preventing alveolar collapse and atelectasis.

pulse oximetry use of an electronic device to measure hemoglobin-oxygen saturation in peripheral tissues.

pulsus paradoxus a physical manifestation felt on palpation of arterial pulses; may reveal either a decreased or absent arterial pulse wave during inspiratory phase.

Purkinje fibers   conductive fibers that carry impulses to the contractile cells of the ventricular myocardium to promote uniform contraction of the ventricles.

Q fever   an acute illness caused by the rickettsia *Coxiella burnetii*, a spore-forming, gram-negative coccobacillus.

QCDSM model   an information and analysis model that assesses *q*uality, *c*ost, *d*elivery, *s*afety, and *m*orale.

QT interval   an indirect measure of ventricular repolarization.

quality improvement   improving a process to ensure a better outcome.

radiation   heat loss in the form of infrared rays (electromagnetic waves).

rapid decompressions   at altitude, perforations of the cockpit or cabin wall, or unintentional loss of the canopy or a hatch, causing rapid decrease in pressure (also known as "explosive decompressions").

rapid physical exam   a head-to-toe assessment designed to identify critical injuries or findings that may contribute to the loss of function or life.

rapid-sequence induction (RSI)   advanced airway technique; includes the use of sedation, anesthesia, neuromuscular blockade, oxygen therapy, and endotracheal intubation.

rectal tubes   tubes, 25–35 cm long and 18–30 French, that may have a distal balloon to keep them in place; used for temporary measure and collection of liquid stool.

relative acidosis   overelimination of bicarbonate ions.

relative alkalosis   overelimination of hydrogen ions.

rescue airways   alternative airway management tools and techniques used when endotracheal intubation (including RSI) fails.

resolution phase   scar tissue is laid down and remodeled, allowing rehabilitation to begin.

respiratory distress   breathing difficulty hallmarked by inadequate alveolar gas exchange.

respiratory failure   progressive decompensation of the respiratory system ultimately resulting in respiratory arrest.

respiratory syncytial virus (RSV)   a highly contagious subgroup of myxoviruses that are the predominant causative agent for bronchial infections in children.

reticulocyte count   measures less mature types of RBCs in the bloodstream; a function of bone marrow production.

retrograde intubation   intubation technique involving placing a needle into the patient's cricothyroid membrane through which a flexible wire is "snaked" upwards into the oropharynx, facilitating orotracheal intubation.

Revised Trauma Score (RTS)   triage tool that requires evaluation of respiratory rate, systolic blood pressure, and the result of the Glasgow Coma Score.

ricin   an extremely lethal cytotoxin derived from a component of the castor bean. It is transmitted by ingestion, injection or inhalation, and kills cells upon contact.

rickettsia   rod-shaped, coccoid, or diplococcus-shaped bacteria transmitted to humans by the bite of infected lice or ticks.

right atrial pressure (RAP)   the pressure in the right atrium, normally less than 8 mmHg.

right ventricular infarction (RVI)   tissue damage to the right ventricle that can affect systemic preload, causing decreased cardiac output and cardiogenic shock.

right ventricular pressure (RVP)   pressure within the right ventricle; required to open pulmonic valve and release blood into pulmonary arteries.

roentgenogram   X-ray; the primary imaging method for orthopedic injuries.

rotor wash   the airflow (wind currents) produced around a helicopter while the rotor systems are spinning.

rotor-wing transport   the transport of a patient by rotor-wing (helicopter) transport.

rotorcraft (helicopter) airframes   aircraft that is kept airborne by air foils rotation, around a vertical axis.

rubella   a highly contagious viral infection characterized by mild fever and a diffuse maculopapular rash (sometimes called German or 3-day measles).

rule of nines   anatomic regions of the body are assigned percentage designations that represent approximately 9 percent (or multiples thereof); the sum is TBSA.

rule of palms (palmar method)   method of measuring the area of a burn based upon the size of a patient's own palm (approximately 1 percent of TBSA).

run or trend charts   charts that diagram data points over a given period of time to see if there is any detectable trend.

Salter-Harris system   method of classifying growth plate injuries.

saltwater aspiration syndrome   faulty regulators or leaking seals allow small amounts of water to enter the diver's lungs, producing dyspnea, a labored cough, and hemoptysis.

saxitoxin   a neurotoxin produced by marine dinoflagellates, blue-green algae, crabs, and blue-ringed octopus; transmitted by ingestion, can cause respiratory paralysis.

scatter diagram   a visual representation of the relationship between two variables.

scene size-up   assessment of scene safety and the resources needed to control a scene, effect appropriate rescue or extrication, and initiate transport of patients.

scintigraphy   diagnostic test to detect bleeding in the GI tract.

scombroid   toxin created by improper preservation of tuna and related species. Bacterial growth causes decomposition of the muscle in the fish and triggers a chemical reaction that releases histamines. Ingestion of affected fish will cause allergic reactions.

scope of practice   a state law that defines and regulates the practice of medicine in a state. In some states, EMS is regulated under a general medical practice act.

SCUBA or scuba   self-contained underwater breathing apparatus.

secondary (intentional) hypothermia   characterized by a compromised thermoregulatory mechanism, a side effect of medications or induced by medical procedures.

Sengstaken-Blakemore tube   a triple-lumen tube with ports for the inflation of an esophageal balloon, inflation of a gastric balloon, and gastric aspiration.

sensitivity   the degree to which a test detects disease without yielding a false-negative result (high sensitivity = low false-negatives).

septic shock   shock caused by toxins in the blood, as a result of disease or infection, that can cause potentially lethal systemic vasodilation.

septicemia   a potentially lethal condition in which bacteria are spread from an infected part of the body via the bloodstream causing an overwhelming infection.

serosa   serous membrane that is continuous with the mesentery, and covers the muscularis externa of all parts of the intestinal tract located in the peritoneal cavity.

set point   the internal temperature that the body "wants" to maintain and controlled in the hypothalamus.

severe acute respiratory syndrome (SARS)   a potentially deadly coronavirus spread by close personal exposure or person-to-contaminated surface contact, via droplet method.

shock   a state of inadequate tissue perfusion associated with anaerobic cellular metabolism.

simplex system   system that sends and receives on the same frequency, but cannot transmit simultaneously in both directions.

sinoatrial (SA) blocks   conduction blocks occurring in the SA node and include sinus arrest, sinus pause, and sinus block.

sinoatrial (SA) node   primary "pacemaker" of the heart; comprised of nodal cells embedded in the posterior wall of the right atria near the superior vena cava.

sinus squeeze   pressure or pain in the areas above the eye, over the upper teeth, or from deep in the skull, while diving at depth.

sky hook technique   a two-person technique facilitating visualization of the glottis in a seated or upright patient.

smallpox   a manifestation of the usually lethal *variola* virus, this disease presents with malaise, fever, rigors, vomiting, headache, backache and a subsequent discrete rash that spreads from the face and extremities to the entire body.

sodium/potassium pump   maintains the ionic gradient across cell walls; driven by energy produced in the cells.

sonography   inaudible sounds (ultrasonic echoes) that are recorded as they strike the tissues of various densities in order to produce an image of an organ or tissue.

sources   host or vector of infection; includes persons with acute illnesses, asymptomatic carriers of pathogenic microorganisms or diseases during incubation periods, endogenous flora and/or contaminated inanimate objects.

space-equivalent zone   the atmospheric zone, sometimes referred to as "space," beginning at 50,000 feet above sea level. Human survival requires the use of pressure suits, self-contained oxygen systems, sealed cabins, and a heat source.

spatial disorientation   an inability to determine position, attitude, and motion relative to the surface of the earth or significant fixed objects.

special cause variation   results so unusual and out of the ordinary for the given system that the variation(s) cannot possibly be due to a common cause variation.

specialty care transport (SCT)   interfacility critical care ground transport of patients by specially trained and educated medical personnel.

specific gravity   determined by the density of an object compared to the density of freshwater (which has a specific gravity of 1.0).

specificity   the measure of how well a test detects a disease without yielding a false-positive result (high specificity = low false-positives).

staphylococcus enterotoxin (B) (SEB)   an agent responsible for food poisoning; transmitted by ingestion or inhalation, causes severe, debilitating syndromes.

stenosis   abnormal narrowing of a structure, inhibiting normal blood flow.

stress-related erosive syndrome (SRES)   stress ulcers in the stomach and duodenum of critically ill patients; secondary to stress from trauma, burns, sepsis, hypotension, cranial or CNS disease, or exposure to long-term ventilatory support.

stroke volume index (SVI)   the amount of blood ejected by the ventricles during one contraction.

sublingual capnometry   an electrode is placed under the tongue to evaluate the sublingual PCO_2, (essentially the visceral PCO_2); an early diagnostic marker for shock.

subluxation   orthopedic injury classified as partial dislocation.

submucosa   a layer of dense connective tissue surrounding the mucosal and muscularis layers; contains exocrine glands, larger blood vessels, lymphatic tissue, and collections of nerve fibers called *Meissner's plexus*.

sucking chest wound   external penetration of the chest wall allowing air to enter the pleural cavity.

supine hypotensive syndrome   a transient decrease in venous return to the heart when the gravid uterus compresses the inferior vena cava (IVC); occurs most often when the pregnant female is supine.

surfactant   a mixture of phospholipids and proteins with a primary function of reducing surface tension within the alveoli and increasing lung compliance.

surgical intensive care unit (SICU) a specialized unit dedicated to the intensive care of critical postsurgical patients.

survival techniques the gathering of resources—shelter, fire, water, food, and signaling devices—and methods for use of these resources during survival operations.

synarthrosis joints, or the connection between two bones, classified as nonmovable.

systemic vascular resistance (SVR) refers to the resistance to blood flow offered by all of the systemic vasculature excluding the pulmonary vasculature.

T-tube a tube used to collect bile from the gallbladder after liver transplant, cholecystectomy, or other surgery of the common bile duct.

tail boom aft of the airframe, it houses the tail rotor and serves as point of fixation for the stabilizers.

tail rotor system vertical rotor blade at the end of the tail boom that compensates for torque induced by the main rotor system.

teardrop fracture displaced fracture of the antero-inferior corner of the superior vertebral body, with segmental disc disruption, posterior ligament injury, and retropulsion of the proximal body into the neural canal.

temporomandibular joint (TMJ) the hinge joint for the mandible; articulation point of the condylar process and the mandibular fossae of the temporal bone.

tension pneumothorax increased pressure within the pleural space of the hemithorax from accumulation of air resulting in collapse of the ipsilateral lung, mediastinal shift to the opposite side, compression of the contralateral lung and decreased venous return to the heart.

tentorium cerebelli section of dura mater invaginated into the cranial vault, forming a barrier between the cerebrum and the cerebellum, and defined by the posterior fossa.

tetanus infectious process resulting from exposure to exotoxins produced by the gram-negative, spore-forming, anaerobic bacilli, *Clostridium tetani.*

thermal equilibrium a warmer object will transfer heat to a cooler object until a steady state is reached.

thermal gradient the difference in temperature between two objects.

thermoreceptor temperature sensors located in the skin (peripheral thermoreceptors), the body core, interior vessel walls (central thermoreceptors), and in the hypothalamus itself.

third spacing the loss of fluids from the intravascular space into the tissues, caused by increased intravascular pressures and/or an increased permeability of the cell membranes.

throttle control valve assembly that controls air and fuel flow into an engine, controls desired thrust to the rotor systems.

time of useful consciousness the time from initial exposure to an oxygen-deficient environment until useful consciousness is lost.

tissue donation involves all areas of the human body. Similar to organ recovery, tissues include heart valves, corneas, bone, skin, and other non-vascularized body parts.

tocodynamometer an intrauterine pressure-monitoring catheter utilized to detect and record uterine contractions.

tocolytic agents medications used to help limit or stop contractions in patients who present in preterm labor between 24 and 36 weeks' gestation.

tolerance a state of adaptation in which exposure to a drug induces changes that result in a diminution of one or more of the drug's effects over time.

total body surface area (TBSA) the total extent of body surface area by the burn. TBSA, specific locations, and depth combine to determine severity of the injury.

toxic alcohols methanol, ethylene glycol, and isopropanol; ingestion of these is associated with significant mortality.

toxic industrial chemicals (TICs) chemicals used in the industrial setting with less potential for severe toxicity in small amounts, however accessibility of large volumes may render them an effective potential weapon.

toxic shock syndrome (TSS) potentially lethal systemic infection resulting from toxins produced by *Staphylococcus aureas.*

toxidrome clinical syndromes essential for the successful recognition of poisoning patterns; a constellation of clinical signs and symptoms that together, reliably suggest an exposure to a specific drug class.

tracheobronchial disruption thoracic injury, most commonly from blunt force trauma; allows air to pass from the trachea and/or bronchi into the pleural or mediastinal space.

transabdominal feeding tube tube used to support nutrition, and placed via open surgical technique, under endoscopy, or percutaneously. The three types often utilized are gastrostomy, jejunostomy, and gastrojejunostomy.

transient tachypnea of the newborn (TTN) a normally self-limiting syndrome of neonatal acute respiratory distress caused by delayed clearing of excess fluid in the lungs; also called "wet lung," or "Type II Respiratory Distress Syndrome" (RDS).

transjugular intrahepatic portosystemic shunt (TIPS) a radiologic procedure that creates an intrahepatic shunt in an attempt to decrease portal pressure and slow the hemorrhage of esophageal varices when other methods have failed.

transmission converts power from the engines into rotational power that is then transferred to both rotors via drive shafts.

trauma system combined triage and transport protocols, referral guidelines, transfer agreements, education, consultation, research and injury prevention programs; designed to assist EMS, hospitals, physicians, and tertiary centers in providing patient access to appropriate care.

triglycerides the most abundant of the lipids; derived from both plant and animal fats and oils.

trochoid pivot movable joints.

troponins contractile proteins of the myofibril.

trunking systems system controlled by a computer (called a "Site Controller" or "Master Control Center") linked to repeater sites by microwave or dedicated telephone circuits. This system pools all available frequencies, assigning incoming transmissions to an open frequency as needed.

Tscherne method method of grading closed fractures.

tuberculosis (TB) a potentially deadly pulmonary disease caused primarily by infection with the bacillus *Mycobacterium tuberculosis.*

tularemia febrile syndrome caused by the bacterium, *Francisella tularensis* (formerly *Pasturella tularensis*) a gram-negative coccobacillus (also known as "Rabbit fever" and "deer-fly fever").

ultra high frequency (UHF) radio bands assigned for restricted government use, Amatuer ("HAM") Radio, GPS (Global Positioning Services), GMRS (General Mobile Radio Service), FRS (Family Radio Service), television, cell phone short wave service, and cordless or mobile telephones.

ultrasound diagnostic sound waves transmitted into an area of specific interest.

Uniform Anatomical Gift Act (UAGA) in the U. S., a state specific legal act that describes the process by which consent is granted for organ and tissue donation.

United Network for Organ Sharing (UNOS) the organizational contractor responsible for operation and oversight of the Organ Procurement and Transplantation Network (OPTN) on behalf of the U.S. government.

Universal Precautions work practice controls designed to reduce the risk of transmission of bloodborne pathogens.

uremia the accumulation of urea and other nitrogen-containing waste products in the blood.

urinalysis urine test designed to detect medication/drug use, blood, infection, pH, density, protein, glucose, ketones, bilirubin, nitrites, and other formed elements.

useful load (payload) total weight of pilot, passengers, and portable medical equipment.

variability variability of FHR (Fetal Heart Rate) occurs as the sympathetic and parasympathetic nervous systems alternate short- or long-term influence on the fetus; abnormalities can indicate differing levels of fetal distress.

vector-borne diseases that are transmitted through an intermediate host such as a fly, mosquito, or tick.

ventilation/perfusion (V/Q) mismatch phenomenon where either perfusion or ventilation to an area of lung decreases; results in diminished gas exchange, hypoxemia, and hypercapnia.

ventricles thick-walled, lower chambers of the heart that discharge blood into the pulmonary or systemic circulation.

ventricular septal defect (VSD) a hole in the ventricular septum between the left and right ventricles.

vertigo disturbance of the inner ear characterized by a "spinning" sensation.

very high frequency (VHF) radio communications bands designated 30 MHz through 174 MHz.

vesicants potentially lethal chemical agents that cause severe blistering of human and animal tissue, both internally and externally (i.e., "sulfur mustard").

vestibulocochlear complex inner ear structure comprised of the vestibular complex (semicircular canals and the vestibule) and the cochlea.

VHF AM Amplitude Modulation bands used for general and commercial aviation, Air Traffic Control Centers, AM radio, auxiliary civil service, space research, and other miscellaneous services. (121.5 MHz is the designated aviation emergency frequency.)

VHF high-band FM radio bands used for business, new unlicensed Multi-Use Radio Service (MURS), and two-way land mobile radio technologies.

VHF low-band FM radio bands used by the U.S. military (including SINCGARS—*S*ingle *C*hannel *G*round and *A*irborne *R*adio *S*ystem), cordless telephones, walkie-talkies, and mixed two-way mobile communication systems, in the 30–50 MHz range.

Viewmax™ blade laryngoscope blade with built-in viewing tube and lens system that refracts images approximately 20 degrees from horizontal useful for intubation of very anterior airways.

viral hemorrhagic fevers (VHFs) a diverse group of illnesses caused by a multitude of different viruses that attack the vascular bed causing hemorrhaging.

virus one of the smallest microorganisms; can only replicate and grow in the cell of another host or animal.

Visual Flight Rules (VFR) FAA regulations mandating minimum visual flight standards for landmark recognition, altitude variables, and weather conditions.

vitreous humor a clear, gelatinous fluid that fills the posterior cavity.

VLDL very-low-density lipoproteins; transports triglycerides and cholesterol.

whispered pectoriloquy assessment tool used to determine areas of consolidation in the lung tissues.

wide-area augmentation system with global positioning satellites (WAAS/GPS) system that provides information to the pilot about vertical movement (that is, gaining or losing of altitude) of the aircraft via the instruments.

wind chill factor   refers to the increased body heat lost from convection on windy days, especially in the cold.

withdrawal syndrome   requires both a preexisting physical adaptation (i.e., tolerance) to a specific and decreasing concentration or availability of that drug.

Wolff-Parkinson-White syndrome (WPW)   pre-excitation syndrome characterized by errant excitation of the bundle of Kent, causing early depolarization.

X-rays   electromagnetic radiation with a very short wavelength, capable of penetrating most body tissues.

zone of coagulation   area of burn where cell membranes rupture and are destroyed, blood coagulates, and structural proteins denature (coagulation necrosis).

zone of hyperemia   area of burn where inflammation and changes in blood flow are limited.

zone of infarction   a component of ischemic stroke, describes the area of brain tissue distal to an occluded vessel, and without collateral circulation.

zone of stasis   labile area of injured cells with decreased blood flow where tissue can undergo necrosis in the 24–48 hours post-burn.

zygomatic bone   facial bone that articulates with the frontal bone and maxilla to complete the lateral wall of the orbit.

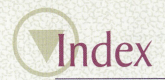

Index